Solved Papers
Medicine
for PG Students

A must for MD and DNB Medicine
Past 10 years exams across various universities

Solved Papers
Medicine
for PG Students

A must for MD and DNB Medicine
Past 10 years exams across various universities

SECOND EDITION

Volume 1

Ashis Kumar Saha
MD(Cal) DTM & H(Cal) FRCP(Edin, Glasgow, UK) FACP(USA) FICP(India) MNAMS(India)
PhD(Honoris Causa) DSc(Honoris Causa) Fellow of Royal Asiatic Society of Great Britain and Ireland
MBA(Hospital Administration)
Professor and Head
Department of Medicine, Deputy Medical Superintendent
Jagannath Gupta Institute of Medical Sciences and Hospital, Budge, Budge, Kolkata
Ex-Professor, College of Medicine and JNM Hospital, Kalyani, West Bengal, India
Ex-Professor and Head in MGM Medical College and LSK Hospital, Kishanganj, Bihar, India
Ex-Professor and Head in KPC Medical College and Hospital, Jadavpur, Kolkata, West Bengal, India

Foreword
Gurpreet S Wander

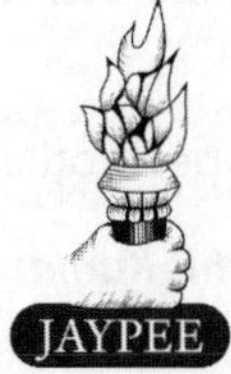

JAYPEE BROTHERS MEDICAL PUBLISHERS
The Health Sciences Publisher
New Delhi | London

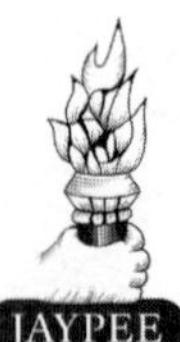

JAYPEE **Jaypee Brothers Medical Publishers (P) Ltd**

Headquarters
EMCA House, 23/23-B
Ansari Road, Daryaganj
New Delhi 110 002, India
Landline: +91-11-23272143, +91-11-23272703
+91-11-23282021, +91-11-23245672
e-mail: jaypee@jaypeebrothers.com

Corporate Office
4838/24, Ansari Road, Daryaganj
New Delhi 110 002, India
Phone: +91-11-43574357
Fax: +91-11-43574314
e-mail: jaypee@jaypeebrothers.com

Overseas Office
JP Medical Ltd.
83, Victoria Street, London
SW1H 0HW (UK)
Phone: +44-20 3170 8910
e-mail: info@jpmedpub.com

EU GPSR Authorised Representative
Logos Europe, 9 rue Nicolas Poussin
17000, La Rochelle, France
Phone: +33 (0) 6 67 93 73 78
e-mail: contact@logoseurope.eu

Website: www.jaypeebrothers.com
Website: www.jaypeedigital.com

Inquiries for bulk sales may be solicited at: jaypee@jaypeebrothers.com

Solved Papers Medicine for PG Students (Volume 1) / Ashis Kumar Saha

First Edition: 2022

Second Edition: **2026**

ISBN: 978-93-7202-416-6

Printed in India by K.K. Printers, Kundli, Haryana-131 028.

Dedication

This marathon and thoroughly updated book is dedicated with deepest respect and gratitude to all my teachers and patients. Without their guidance, trust, and invaluable lessons, this long and difficult journey toward success would never have been possible.

I remain forever indebted for the wisdom imparted by my teachers and the knowledge gained through the experiences of my patients. Their contributions have shaped not only this book but also my growth as a physician and lifelong learner.

Foreword

"He who studies medicine without books sails an uncharted sea, but he who studies medicine without patients does not go to sea at all".

—**William Osler**

It is a pleasure and an honor to write a foreword for the book *"Solved Papers Medicine for PG Students"*. It is going to be of great use for postgraduate students for the theory examination since it provides answers to questions from various universities for the MD/DNB medicine exit examination. This is the first book of its kind for the MD Medicine students. The book has been written in a format in which one is expected to answer the theory questions. It gives an insight into the kind of questions that are asked in the examination. Clinical medicine is learned and practiced in the bedside of the patients. However, unless we have a strong understanding of the theoretical aspects of the subject, we will not be able to manage patients well.

The text of the book is simple, easy to understand, and evidence based. The answers are backed with appropriate tables and algorithms. This makes the answers easy to understand. The examiner can scan through your paper in case you attempt in the format in which it has been done in the book. Dr Ashis Kumar Saha, the author of the book, is a brilliant academician. He himself has been a very bright student and is now a very popular Professor of medicine. No foreign book can provide you answers in the manner in which this book is written. He has used the latest textbooks for preparing the answers. We today live in the era of instant and comprehensive solutions to the problems. This book serves this purpose completely and perfectly. The print of the book is easy to read and Jaypee Brothers Medical publishers (P) Ltd needs to be complimented for coming out with excellent editing and presentation. I strongly recommend this book for postgraduate students in medicine. In fact, this book will be useful for practicing physicians also.

Gurpreet S Wander DM FACC FAMS
Professor and Head of Cardiology
Hero DMC Heart Institute
Chairman, Research and Development Centre
Dayanand Medical College and Hospital, Ludhiana
Past President Association of Physicians of India
Past President Hypertension Society of India
Director Physicians Research Foundation (of API) India

Preface to the Second Edition

Medicine and medical education is an ever-evolving science, with a strong emphasis on clinical presentation, recent advances in pathophysiology and immunology, and continuously updated diagnostic and treatment protocols.

During my years as a postgraduate teacher, I observed a persistent gap—students often struggled due to the lack of concise, updated, and lucid answer books for postgraduate examinations. While multiple publications exist for undergraduate students, there has been a scarcity of equivalent resources tailored to the needs of postgraduates. This realization inspired me to prepare a book that would fill this void by compiling authentic questions from different universities across the country.

After collecting these questions, I undertook the task of carefully consulting standard monographs and textbooks to provide structured, reliable, and exam-oriented answers. This process was both rigorous and time-consuming but essential to ensure that the answers remained clinically relevant and academically sound.

In this new edition, a major addition is the inclusion of the last 10 years' MD (Medicine) and DNB (Medicine) examination questions. This expansion not only provides a comprehensive repository of authentic material but also highlights current trends in postgraduate assessments. By practicing with these questions, students will gain the ability to approach exams with clarity and confidence.

Ultimately, the aim of this book is to serve as both a preparatory tool and a clinical guide, enabling postgraduate students to strengthen their conceptual knowledge while also excelling in examinations. I sincerely hope that this effort will support aspiring physicians in their academic journey and professional growth.

Every postgraduate student must face examinations as an inevitable milestone in their academic journey. While students may go through numerous textbooks and monographs, many often find it difficult to prepare effectively for the final examination. Despite investing substantial effort, success may elude them if their preparation is not systematic and exam-oriented. No single book can comprehensively cover every theoretical aspect of medicine; rather, the key lies in adopting the right approach to answering questions.

Examiners usually test not only the breadth but also the depth of a candidate's knowledge, and the manner in which answers are structured often reflects this understanding. A well-organized approach to answering can demonstrate clarity of thought, precision, and command over the subject. Thus, instead of being anxious about the questions, students should focus on practicing how to present concise yet meaningful answers under examination conditions.

It is also important to note that marks allocated for similar questions may vary widely across different universities in India. To address this variation, this book has been designed to provide model answers that can be adapted flexibly. The content is structured in such a way that students can either write a detailed response for long-answer questions or extract succinct bullet points for short-answer formats. This adaptability allows learners to refine their examination technique while simultaneously strengthening their conceptual grasp of medicine.

Jai Hind!

Ashis Kumar Saha

Preface to the Second Edition

Medicine and medical education have [illegible] with emphasis on clinical presentation, recent advances in pathophysiology and [illegible], and continuously updated diagnostic and treatment protocols.

During my years as a postgraduate teacher, I observed a persistent gap—students often struggle due to the lack of concise, updated, and [illegible] answer books for postgraduate examinations. While multiple publications exist for undergraduate students, there has been a scarcity of equivalent resources geared to the needs of postgraduates. This realization inspired me to prepare a book that would fill this void by compiling authentic questions from different universities across the country.

After collecting these questions, I undertook the task of carefully consulting standard monographs and textbooks to provide structured, readable, and exam-oriented answers. This process was both rigorous and time-consuming but essential to ensure that the answers remained clinically relevant and academically sound.

In this new edition, a major addition is the inclusion of the last 10 years' MD (Medicine) and DNB (Medicine) examination questions. This expansion not only provides a comprehensive repository of authentic material but also highlights current trends in postgraduate assessment. By practicing with these questions, students will gain the ability to tackle challenges with clarity and confidence.

Ultimately, the aim of this book is to serve as a [illegible] guide, enabling postgraduate students to strengthen their conceptual knowledge while also excelling in examinations. I sincerely hope that this effort will support aspiring physicians in their academic journey and professional growth.

Every postgraduate student [illegible] examinations as an inevitable milestone in their academic journey. While students may go through numerous textbooks and monographs, many often find it difficult to [illegible] comprehensively cover every theoretical aspect of medicine, rather the key lies in adopting the right approach to answering questions.

Examiners usually test not only the depth of a candidate's knowledge but the manner in which answers are structured [illegible] approach to answering [illegible]. Thus, instead of being anxious about the questions, students should focus on practicing how to present concise yet meaningful answers under examination conditions.

It is also important to note that the pattern of questions may vary widely across different universities. To address this variation, this book has been designed to provide model answers that can be adapted flexibly. The content is structured in such a way that students can either write a detailed answer for long-answer questions or extract relevant bullet points for short-answer formats. This adaptability allows learners to refine their examination technique while simultaneously strengthening their conceptual grasp of medicine.

Jai Hind

Ashis Kumar Saha

Preface to the First Edition

Medicine and medical education is a continuously evolving science with a sharp focus on clinical presentation of recent pathophysiology, immunology, and recent updated information in the diagnosis and treatment protocols.

After being a postgraduate teacher for years the thing that struck with me was that there is currently a dearth of books for a concise updated lucid answers in different textbooks. It took a long time for the students to prepare notes. At the same time the fact that there are many answer books for undergraduates in different publishing house, but no such books for postgraduates made me determined to write a book for them by collecting questions from various universities of our country. After collection of the questions, I started reading different monograms as well as textbooks to make a sketch of answers. Ultimately I decided to write the huge tasks to help the students appearing in MD final or DNB Final Examinations.

This book contains a large number of questions collected from different universities such as All India Institute of Medical Sciences (AIIMS), New Delhi, Armed Forces Medical College, Pune, Aligarh Mullana University (Aligarh), SN Medical College (Agra), Allahabad University (Prayagraj), Baba Farid University (Faridkot), Era Lucknow Medical College (Lucknow), Government Medical College (Haldwani), Mahatma Jyotiba Phule Rohilkhand University (Bareilly), Maharashtra University of Higher Studies (Maharashtra), Muzaffarnagar Medical College (Muzaffarnagar), Post Graduate Institute of Medical Education and Research (Chandigarh), Maharani Laxmi Bai Medical College (Jhansi), West Bengal University of Health Sciences (West Bengal), and Diplomate National Board by National Board of Examinations (Delhi).

All the students have to face the examinations in their lives, so this must be taken as natural incidence in their lives. Students may read a large number of books, different monograms, but cannot prepare themselves either mentally or physically prior to final examination, so all the hard work that they put may ultimately go in vain if they do not prepare smartly. In any book, it is not possible to cover all the theoretical questions. All depend upon the approach of the candidate to answer the questions asked by the examiners. Approach of answering the question can indicate the quantity as well as quality of knowledge gathered by the students on those topics. One should not panic after listening to the questions, rather answer that after taking a little pause.

In these books same question has large variation of marks allotted by different universities in India. Here my aim is to write the answer in such a way that one can write as either long question form or can take salient points with slight elaboration of those points in case short question.

Shri Jitendar P Vij (Group Chairman), always searching for a novelty in the field of Medicine accepted my brain-storming idea and asked me to materialize this huge tasks, I took the challenge and ultimately finished the job. I think, this book will throw a light and enlighten the students with recent knowledge written in this book. But, ultimately success depends upon the students who will read, produce it in the theory paper, remember it, and apply it in their practical life.

Jai Hind!

Ashis Kumar Saha

Acknowledgments

I extend my heartfelt gratitude to Mr Krishna Kumar Gupta, Chairman of JIMSH, Budge Budge, Kolkata, West Bengal, India. His unwavering support, visionary leadership, and encouragement have been instrumental in shaping this work. His constant motivation and keen interest in academic excellence have provided me with the strength to continue writing with dedication.

I am deeply thankful to Dr Balaram Gupta, Vice Chairman of JIMSH, Budge Budge, Kolkata, West Bengal, whose invaluable guidance and continuous encouragement have always inspired me to pursue greater goals. His academic vision and personal support have been a beacon of light in my journey.

My wife, Mrs Kalyani Saha, deserves special recognition for her exuberant inspiration. Her constant enthusiasm, patience, and unconditional support have been the greatest source of motivation in my life, and without her encouragement, this book would not have been possible.

I am blessed with my sons, Mr Subhra Kanti Saha and Mr Abhrokanti Saha. Their constant smiling faces and cheerful encouragement have provided me with enthusiasm for further writing. Their presence fills my life with positivity and energy, pushing me forward even during the most challenging times.

I extend my heartfelt appreciation to my daughters-in-law, Mrs Shilpi Saha and Mrs Tania Saha. Their warmth, kindness, and continuous support have brought immense joy and comfort to my life. They have made this journey lighter and more fulfilling with their constant care and encouragement.

I acknowledge with deep gratitude my nephew, Mr Soumya Kanti Saha, and his wife, Mrs Trisha Saha, for their dedicated help in providing the updated printing chapters. Their timely assistance and enthusiasm have significantly contributed to the successful completion of this work.

I express my heartfelt thanks to my brother, Mr Kaushik Saha, and his wife, Mrs Rinku Saha. Their words of encouragement and constant inspiration have motivated me at every step, reminding me of the importance of family support in all endeavors.

My youngest grandson, Rudranksh, though only 2 years old, has been a constant source of happiness and inspiration. His cheerful smiling face and innocent laughter have cheered me up countless times and given me fresh energy to continue my work with renewed enthusiasm.

I am extremely grateful to Shri Jitendar P Vij for his valuable guidance in writing this book. His thoughtful suggestions, intellectual input, and constructive feedback have helped me refine and polish my ideas. His mentorship has been a cornerstone in the shaping of this manuscript.

I also acknowledge with appreciation Mr Sabyasachi Hazra for his continuous inspiration. His encouragement has been vital in keeping me motivated throughout this project, providing me with the confidence to move ahead.

Last but not the least, I dedicate my sincere thanks to my students from my institution and from all over India. Their constant writing inspiration, thoughtful questions, and active participation have encouraged me to keep striving for excellence.

Even some depressive words from certain individuals have paradoxically given me strength, as they became a source of renewed determination and inspired me to write further with greater passion and commitment.

Solving Papers for MD and DNB Medicine

Purpose and Scope

This compendium curates 10 years of MD/DNB Medicine question papers from nearly 25 Indian universities/teaching hospitals, mapped across all major chapters/systems. It is designed to sharpen examination technique, update core concepts, and align preparation with current patterns.

Coverage (Chapter-wise)

- *General principles*: Ethics, EBM, biostatistics, and research methods
- *Systems*: Cardiology, Pulmonology, Gastro-Hepatology, Nephrology, Endocrinology, Hematology, Neurology, Rheumatology, Infectious Diseases, Dermatology, Psychiatry in Medicine, Toxicology, Oncology, Geriatrics, Critical Care, and Emergency Medicine
- *Cross-cutting*: Imaging, genomics, therapeutics, vaccines, and antimicrobial stewardship

What's New (Last 10 Years)

Integration of national guidelines, outbreak learning (COVID-19 and Nipah updates), novel therapies (DOACs, SGLT-2/GLP-1, and biologics), point-of-care ultrasound, AI/decision support, and ethics/medicolegal scenarios. "Recent advances" tags are appended to relevant questions.

Format and Features

- Year–University index, Chapter-wise sorting, Short/Long/Case-based segregation
- Model answer frames: Key headings, flowcharts, scoring rubrics, and common pitfalls
- 30-, 60-, 120-minute drill sets with difficulty gradation
- Recall→Reason→Revise boxes: One-page last-minute notes

How to Use

1. Start with diagnostic drill (2–3 papers).
2. Build a chapter loop: Read core, solve 5–7 past questions, then revise.
3. Weekly grand test + error log; convert errors into flashcards.
4. Practice case-based writing: Differential, investigations with justification, management + guideline citation.
5. Simulate timing; aim ≥10% buffer.

Ethics and Academic Integrity

Use past papers for learning and practice only; cite guidelines and avoid rote replication.

Message to Postgraduate Students Across India

Dear Colleagues,

Medicine rewards clarity, compassion, and consistency. Solve widely, read deeply, and reflect after every test. Anchor answers in first principles, guidelines, and patient safety. Learn from mentors, discuss with peers, and keep an error log—it becomes your finest teacher. Guard your wellbeing: Sleep, exercise, and humility sustain excellence. You are preparing not just for an examination, but for a lifetime of service. Study hard, stay kind, and trust your training. All the best!

Solving Papers for MD and DNB Medicine

Purpose and Scope

This compendium curates 10 years of MD/DNB Medicine [illegible] papers from nearly 25 [illegible], including [illegible] repeated across all major [illegible]. It is designed to sharpen [illegible] technique, update core concepts, and align preparation with current patterns.

Coverage (Chapter-wise)

- General: [illegible], ethics, EBM, biostatistics and research methods
- Systems: Cardiology, Pulmonology, [illegible], Gastroenterology, Nephrology, Endocrinology, Hematology, Neurology, Rheumatology, Infectious Diseases, [illegible], Psychiatry, [illegible] Medicine, Toxicology, Geriatrics, Critical Care and Emergency Medicine
- Cross-cutting: [illegible] therapeutics, [illegible], and antimicrobial stewardship

What's New (Last 10 Years)

Integration of [illegible] guidelines [illegible] COVID-19 and Nipah [illegible], novel therapies [illegible] [illegible], and ethics/medicolegal scenarios, [illegible] advances [illegible] relevant [illegible]

Format and Features

- Year/University-wise [illegible] Chapter-wise [illegible] case-based segregation
- Model [illegible] headings, flowcharts, tables, [illegible] and common pitfalls
- [illegible]

How to Use

1. Start with diagnostic [illegible]
2. [illegible] past questions [illegible]
3. Weekly [illegible] convert [illegible] into [illegible]
4. Practice case-based writing: differential, investigations with interpretation, management + guideline citation
5. Simulate timing [illegible]

Ethics and Academic Integrity

Use past papers for learning and practice only; cite guidelines and avoid [illegible].

Message to Postgraduate Students Across India

Dear Colleagues,

Medicine rewards clarity, compassion, and consistency. [illegible] widely, read deeply, and reflect after every test. Anchor your answers in first principles, guidelines, and patient safety. [illegible] with peers, and keep an error log. [illegible] becomes your [illegible]. [illegible] your wellbeing [illegible] and humility sustain excellence. You are preparing not just for an examination, but for a lifetime of service. [illegible] and trust your training. All the best.

Review

As this book is student-centered because they are the pillar and backbone of the future DOCTOR community, I am adding the following four reviews of already passed postgraduate students and one dedicated professor.

Recently finishing my own postgraduate journey, I can attest—on behalf of the present batch—that this book is a remarkable guide. Concise solutions, evidence-based explanations, and a focus on practical reasoning make it indispensable for every resident preparing for exams. It not only streamlines revision but also reinforces sound clinical thinking, helping students translate textbook knowledge into bedside decision-making. The structured approach saves precious time in a busy residency schedule and offers the confidence that comes from truly understanding core concepts. For the current generation of postgraduate trainees, it stands as both a reliable exam companion and a lasting reference in everyday practice.

Dr Ankan Pathak
MD(Medicine) DNB(Cardiology)

Most intimidating aspect of PG examination is answering the theory questions. Esoteric questions are frequently asked in the final examination making it the most daunting task for the students. Professor Ashis Kumar Saha has come up with a wonderful solution to this problem in the form of his current book. Not only does it provide single-stop solution but also goes a long way in building concepts. I really wish that I had such a book when I was a student.

Dr Nirmalya Roy
MD
Professor
Department of Medicine
KPC Medical College, Kolkata, West Bengal
Consultant Physician and Diabetologist
BM Birla Heart Research Centre
Kolkata, West Bengal, India

Solved Papers Medicine for PG students by Dr Ashis Kumar Saha is an ultimate help book for every postgraduate student. This resource brings together years of real exam questions with simple, clear explanations coupled with latest guidelines that make preparation both focused and effective. Dr Saha has designed the content keeping students' struggles in mind, making this book a true companion during the most crucial phase of exam readiness. With its exam-oriented solutions and high-yield coverage, it saves time while boosting confidence. This book is the go-to guide for students aiming to crack the DNB exams with success.

Dr Oendri Bhattacharyya
MBBS DNB(General Medicine) PDT DrNB(Nephrology)

This comprehensive guide is designed to support postgraduate students in medicine by presenting key concepts in a clear, question-and-answer format. It effectively bridges theoretical knowledge with clinical application, making it an invaluable resource for examination preparation and clinical practice. By strengthening clinical reasoning and decision-making skills, this book aims to empower postgraduate learners on their journey toward academic and professional excellence.

Dr Mukesh Kumar
MD(Medicine)
MGM Medical College
Kishanganj, Bihar, India

It is my immense pleasure to write for Solved Papers Medicine for PG Students and my heartfelt gratitude to Professor Dr Ashis Kumar Saha.

I have been immensely helped from this book and it is a must read for every postgraduate trainee in General Medicine.

Enriched in information and updated regarding recent advancements, the overall coverage of topics has been exceptional.

I wish all the very best to Professor Dr Ashis Kumar Saha for his tremendous hard work and sharing his vast knowledge with us through this book.

Dr Arnab Kumar Gayen
Senior Resident
Department of General Medicine
KPC Medical College and Hospital
Kolkata, West Bengal, India

Contents

VOLUME 1

Section 1: Hepatology

Section 2: Hematology

Section 3: Pancreatology

Section 4: Gastroenterology

Section 5: Nephrology

Section 6: Cardiovascular Systems

Section 7: Pulmonology

Section 8: Rheumatology

COLLAGEN VASCULAR DISEASE

VOLUME 2

Section 9: Diabetes and Endocrinology

DIABETES

Section 12: Infectious Disease

Miscellaneous

Section 13: General Metabolism, Poisoning in the Body, General Topic, and Geriatrics

Section 14: Miscellaneous

Section 1 Hepatology

Q1. Pathogenesis and complications of Wilson's disease.

PGI/NOV2012 (10)

Discuss biochemical defect and management of a child with Wilson's disease.

BF/JUNE2016/MDI (10)

Wilson's disease.

MGR/MAR2006/MDIV (5)

MGR/MAR2008/MDIV (6)

Diagnosis and management of Wilson's disease.

DNB (DEC2022) (10)

Diagnosis of Wilson's disease

DNB (DEC2020) (4)

Bilirubin synthesis and metabolism. Diagnosis and treatment of Wilson's disease.

DNB (DEC2019) (10)

Wilson disease clinical manifestations and diagnosis.

DELHI UNI, 2024 (10)

Management of Wilson's disease.

KERALA UNIVERSITY, 2019 (10)

Write the diagnosis and management of Wilson's disease.

MANIPUR UNIVERSITY, 2019 (10)

ANSWER

Wilson's disease is a rare inherited familial disorder characterized by progressive neurological features with evidence of cirrhosis and Kayser–Fleischer (K–F) ring in the cornea.

Pathogenesis

There are two genes responsible for metal-transporting enzyme P-type ATPase (adenosine triphosphatase):

- **A.** One is ATP7A; it is abnormal in Menkes disease.
- **B.** The other is ATP7B found in chromosome 13; ATP7B is present in liver, kidney, and in small amount in brain, placenta, and lung. This gene product is Wilson-ATPase in intracellular.

Transport of copper and its defect in homeostasis:

Copper is present in plasma in cupric form bounded with albumin and histidine. Cupric form must be transformed to cuprous form prior to intake by hepatocytes. It is transported into hepatocytes in cuprous form via the copper-binding N-terminal domain of transmembrane transporter (CTR1). But in presence of high concentration of copper CTR1 will be degraded leading high rise of nonceruloplasmin-bounded copper—it is responsible for neurological manifestation of Wilson's disease prior to hepatocellular necrosis.

Now within the hepatocytes coppers bound to low-molecular protein metallochaperones, it will ultimately directs the copper molecules to the following molecules:

- **A.** Some coppers metallothioneins store copper as non-toxic form.
- **B.** Some coppers form complexes with glutathione.
- **C.** Intracellular ceruloplasmin such as ferroxidase oxidizes iron from iron to transferrin. When ceruloplasmin is devoid of copper it is called apoceruloplasmin. When intracellular copper combines with apoceruloplasmin, holoceruloplasmin is formed, it is enzymatically active.
- **D.** CCS1 protein delivers the copper to Cu/Zn superoxide dismutase.
- **E.** COX17 delivers copper to subunit II cytochrome c oxidase within the mitochondria mediated by SCO1 and SCO2.
- **F.** ATOX1 by virtue of its copper-binding domain CXXC will transport copper Wilson ATPase present in the trans-Golgi network region. Now Wilson-ATPase has two-fold of actions:

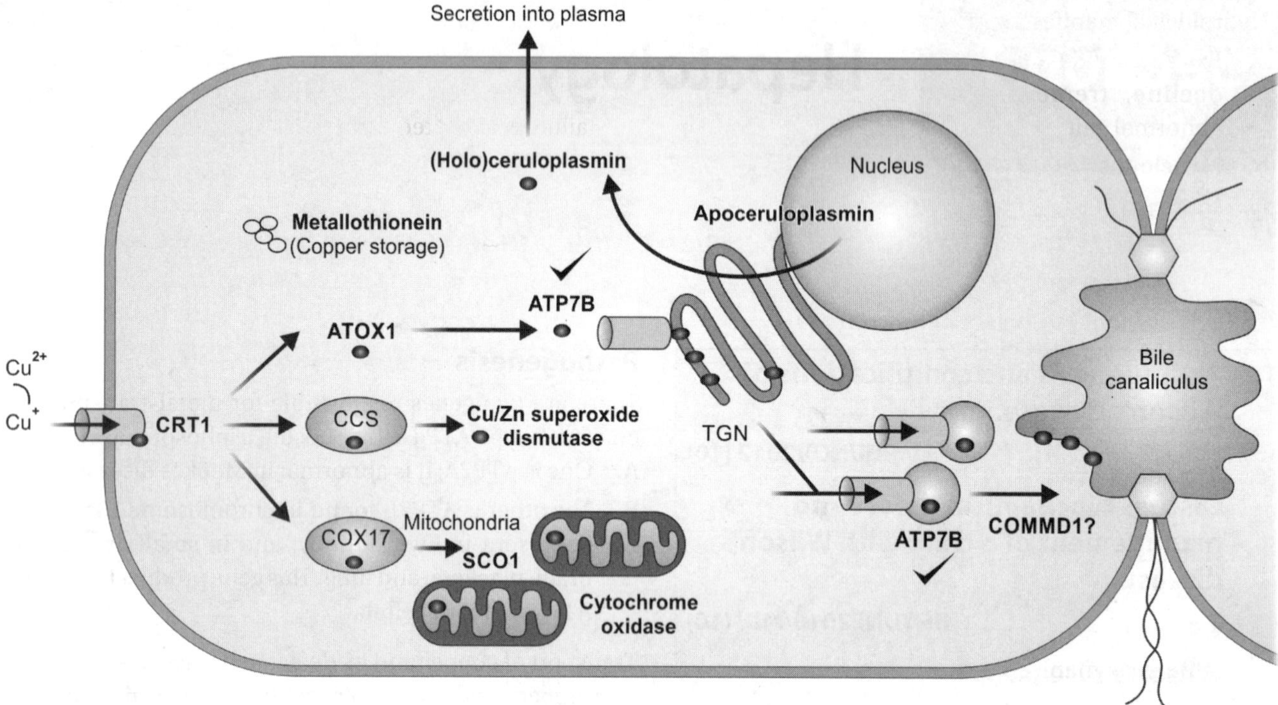

a. It will incorporate copper into apoceruloplasmin.

b. It will help in excretion of copper into biliary canaliculi.

If the intracellular concentration of copper will be elevated Wilson ATPase redistributes to the apical region of hepatocytes near the area of biliary canalicular membrane.

When the concentration of copper is elevated Wilson ATPase moves to lysozyme and imports copper into the lumen where it interacts with p62 subunit dynactin and translocate lysozyme toward canalicular pole and release copper into the bile. This exocytosis is governed by a gene *COMMDI*. Protein encoded by *COMMDI* will interact with copper-binding domain of Wilson's ATPase, ATP7B. It inhibits transcription factor κβ and thus affects immune response as well as cell cycle regulation.

So defect in ATP7B for the copper-related damage of hepatocytes is in the following ways:

Being prooxidant accumulated copper produces liver damage by oxidative stress through "Fenton-type" reaction. Generated peroxides and hydroxyl radicals in this reaction produce damage of deoxyribonucleic acid (DNA) in hepatocytes.

In the brain action of copper is regulated by amyloid protein. If the concentration of copper in brain will be increased or the activities of key copper-containing enzymes are altered, both will lead to neuronal damage in brain.

Other mechanisms in case of Wilson's disease are:

A. Focal deletion of DNA in mitochondria found usually in aging.

B. Antioxidant vitamin E is found in untreated Wilson's disease.

C. There is evidence of increased mutation of tumor suppressor gene *TP53*.

D. Nitric oxide synthase (NOS) will be increased.

So natural history of Wilson's disease is divided into four stages:

A. Stage 1: In this initial period accumulation of copper present within hepatic binding sites.

B. Stage 2: Acute redistribution of copper in the liver and its release into the circulation.

C. Stage 3: In this stage, there is chronic accumulation of copper within the brain along with other extrahepatic tissues and eventually fatal disease.

D. Stage 4: Long-term chelation therapy will restore the copper balance.

Clinical Features in Wilson's Disease

A. Different spectrum of liver diseases:

- **a.** Acute hepatitis
- **b.** Chronic hepatitis
- **c.** Decompensated or compensated cirrhosis
- **d.** Acute fulminant hepatic failure
- **e.** Persistent transaminases elevation

B. Neurological manifestation:

- **a.** Extrapyramidal manifestations, such as cognitive decline, tremor, dysarthria, seizures, and abnormal gait
- **b.** Myoclonus
- **c.** Chorea
- **d.** Insomnia
- **e.** Metabolic myopathy

C. Psychiatric manifestations:

- **a.** Depression
- **b.** Personality changes
- **c.** Bipolar disorders
- **d.** Schizophrenia
- **e.** Mental retardation

D. Eye changes:

- **a.** Sunflower cataract
- **b.** K–F ring

E. Hematological manifestations:

- **a.** Anemia
- **b.** Bleeding gum
- **c.** Hematemesis

F. Genitourinary abnormalities:

- **a.** Menstrual irregularities
- **b.** Acute tubular necrosis

Most important complication is Wilsonian fulminant hepatic failure. It occurs mainly in 10–30 years females. This complication can be differentiated from liver failure of other etiologies by combining the clinical and biochemical features together.

Biochemical features are:

A. Disproportionate low level of aminotransferases to <2,000 U/L from the onset of this disease.

B. Serum alkaline phosphatase (ALP) level is normal or mildly reduced.

C. Bilirubin level is highly increased where there is associated hemolysis.

D. Following biochemical index is suggestive of this failure (calculated in American unit):

- **a.** Ratio of ALP to serum bilirubin is <4
- **b.** Ratio of aspartate aminotransferase (AST) to alanine aminotransferase (ALT) is <2.2
- **c.** In case of children ratio of ALP to bilirubin level is <1
- **d.** NAZZER index: It is based on serum AST, bilirubin concentration, and prolongation of prothrombin time (PT); it identifies Wilsonian failure but cannot detect the prognosis of the failure.

E. Associated intercurrent viral illness or hepatitis C may precipitate liver failure in case of Wilson's disease.

Management

Drugs recommended for treating the Wilson's disease:

Disease state	First choice	Second choice
Hepatitis or compensated cirrhosis	Zinc	Trientine
Decompensated cirrhosis		
Mild	Trientine and zinc	Penicillamine and zinc
Moderate	Trientine and zinc	Liver transplantation
Severe	Liver transplantation	Trientine and zinc
Initial neurologic or psychiatric features	Tetrathiomolybdate and zinc	Zinc
Maintenance	Zinc	Trientine
Presymptomatic	Zinc	Trientine
Pediatric	Zinc	Trientine
Pregnant	Zinc	Trientine

Drugs with dosages and side-effects:

Drugs	Dose	Efficacy assessment	Monitoring of side effects
D-penicillamine	• Initially 1–1.5 g/day in twice or thrice equally divided doses • Maintenance dose is 0.75–1 g/day in thrice equally divided doses	Target is 24 h urinary copper excretion 200–500 µg/day	• Complete blood count • Dermatological examination • Urinalysis
Trientine	• Initially 1–1.5 g/day in twice or thrice equally divided doses • Maintenance dose is 1–1.5 g/day in thrice equally divided doses	Target is 24 h urinary copper excretion 200–500 µg/day	• Complete blood count • Serum iron and iron-binding capacity • Urinalysis
Zinc	• Initially 50 mg elemental zinc orally thrice daily ≥1 h meals • Maintenance dose is titration of the dose as required to achieve the efficacy	Target is 24 h urinary copper excretion <0.75 µg/day	• Serum creatinine, zinc (to monitor adherence) • Urinalysis • Serum AST and ALT

In case of decompensation of liver following score as suggested by Nazer has to be followed:

Laboratory test	Normal value	Score				
		0	1	2	3	4
Bilirubin	0.2–1.2 mg/dL	<5.8	5.8–8.8	8.8–11.7	11.7–17.5	>17.5
AST	10–35 IU/L	<100	100–150	151–200	201–300	>300
Prolongation of prothrombin time	→	<4	4–8	9–12	13–20	>20

Note: If the score is <7—oral therapy will be recommended.

If the score is >9—liver transplantation is recommended.

If the score is between 7 and 9, then clinical judgment is required whether oral therapy or transplantation is best for that patient.

If the score is >9 bridge should be combination of zinc and trientine prior to transplantation.

Q2. Discuss etiology, clinical features, investigations and management of acute liver failure.

MUHS/NOV2010/MDIII (25)

Describe pathophysiology, clinical features, complications, and management of acute hepatic failure.

MUHS/MAY2010/MDIII (25)

Management of acute hepatic failure.

BF/MAY2010/MDIII (10)

Discuss etiology, clinical features and management of acute liver failure.

ERA/MAY2012/MDII (15)

Discuss etiology, clinical features, prognostic markers and management of acute liver failure.

DNB/JUNE2012 (10)

Clinical manifestations of liver dysfunction.

SCB MED COL, 2017 (20)

Define fulminant hepatic failure. Describe its clinical features, investigations and management.

MAHARASHTRA UNI OF HEALTH SC. 2022 (25)

Acute liver failure.

TEERTHANKER MAHAVEER UNIVERSITY, 2018 (10)

ANSWER

Definition

Acute liver failure is a devastating syndrome characterized by impairment of liver function test, such as hemodynamic instability, coagulopathy, cerebral edema, renal failure, severe metabolic disturbances, and propensity to develop bacterial or fungal infections.

Acute liver failure is divided into three subtype depending upon the appearance of jaundice and development of hepatic encephalopathy:

A. Hyperacute or fulminant liver failure, the interval is <2 weeks.

B. Acute or subfulminant liver failure where the interval is >2 weeks but <8 weeks.

C. Subacute liver failure where the interval is >8 weeks but <24 weeks.

Etiology

A. Infections:
- **a.** Hepatitis A, B, C, D, and E
- **b.** Epstein–Barr virus
- **c.** Dengue fever
- **d.** Herpes simplex virus

B. Drugs and toxins:
- **a.** Acetaminophen
- **b.** Carbon tetrachloride
- **c.** Idiosyncratic drug reactions
- **d.** Mushroom poisoning

C. Ischemic:
- **a.** Hypotension
- **b.** Heat stroke
- **c.** Cardiogenic stroke

D. Vascular causes:

   a. Acute Budd–Chiari syndrome

   b. Sinusoidal obstruction syndrome

E. Acute liver failure of pregnancy

F. Wilson's disease

G. Malignancy

Spectrum of liver damage histologically according to etiologies of hepatic failure:

A. Confluent necrosis (+ activation of nonparenchymal cells, Kupffer cells, stellate cells, endothelial cells)—drugs such as acetaminophen, toxins, viruses, and ischemia

B. Microvascular steatosis—drugs such as tetracycline, valproic acid, mitochondrial toxins, and fatty liver of pregnancy

C. Malignant infiltration—metastatic deposits, leukemia, and lymphoma

Molecular mechanism of cell injury and death:
Death of hepatocytes is of two types:

A. Apoptosis: Here there is shrinkage of cytoplasm and cell nucleus without disruption of the cell membrane integrity and release of liberation of intracellular content. So, there is no secondary inflammation. It occurs following sequential activation of cysteine proteases called Caspases. There are two mechanisms by which apoptosis can occur:

   a. Extrinsic mechanism: Here death receptor is present on the cell membrane

   b. Intrinsic mechanism: Here oxidative stress of mitochondria and endoplasmic reticulum are responsible.

   Caspase-8 and 9 mediate signals for extrinsic and intrinsic mechanisms, respectively.

B. Necrosis: Here as a consequence of depletion of adenosine triphosphate cell will swell followed by disruption of membrane and release of cell content associated with secondary inflammation.

Pathophysiology

A. Hemodynamic changes:

   a. Marked splanchnic vasodilatation

   b. Marked systemic arteriolar vasodilatation

   c. Hyperdynamic vasodilatation

   d. Low arteriovenous oxygen difference. It may be due to endothelial damage, generation of oxygen-free radicals, production of vasoactive cytokines and microcirculatory plugging by platelet-rich thrombi, and increased adhesion to endothelium by leukocytes.

B. Hepatic encephalopathy: It occurs due to cerebral edema as a result of following mechanisms:

   a. Accumulation of ammonia

   b. Disturbances in different pathways, such as glutamatergic, noradrenergic, and serotonergic pathways

   c. Accumulation of false neurotransmitters

   d. Activation of γ-aminobutyric acid receptors

   e. Altered metabolism of cerebral energy

   f. Failure of autoregulation with cerebral perfusion due to cerebral vasodilatation and impaired cerebral resistance vessel constriction in response to systemic arterial pressure

C. Renal impairment: It may occur through following mechanisms:

   a. Relative hypovolemia due to:

      1. Vasodilatation

      2. Microcirculatory disturbances

      3. Vasodilatation

      4. Acute tubular necrosis due to sepsis

      5. Direct nephrotoxic injury by acetaminophen

D. Susceptibility to infection: Patients are susceptible to infection due to following mechanisms:

   a. Impaired phagocytic function of neutrophils

   b. Impaired phagocytic function of Kupffer cells

   c. Reduced complement function by hepatocytes

   d. Different types of invasive procedures

   e. Increased translocation of bacteria from the gut

   Infective organisms are bacteria and fungi. Sometime these patients may be afebrile with normal white blood cell count.

E. Nutritional disturbances:

   a. Energy requirement in these patients is nearly increased up to 60% with mean energy expenditure is 4.05 kJ/kg/h in spite of reduction of liver cell mass.

   b. Glycogen storage capacity and gluconeogenesis will be reduced

   c. Increased breakdown of skeletal muscles

   d. Impaired whole body protein degradation due to:

      1. Reduced synthesis of insulin-like growth factor-1

   e. Electrolyte disturbances, such as hyponatremia, hypokalemia, hypophosphatemia, and hypomagnesemia

   f. Hypoglycemia

F. Coagulation disorders may develop due to following:

   a. Reduced synthesis of clotting factors leading to impaired coagulation and anticlotting factors, like protein S and C and antithrombin III leading to microvascular thrombosis and thus producing clogging of dialysis circuit.

b. Consumption of clotting factors and platelets due to disseminated intravascular coagulation.

G. Platelet abnormality due to following:

a. Thrombocytopenia

b. Increased adhesion and impaired aggregation of platelets

Clinical Manifestations

A. Symptoms such as malaise, nausea, vomiting, progressively increasing yellow discoloration of eyes and dark urine, fever, progressively increasing alteration in consciousness, bleeding abnormalities, gastrointestinal bleeding, and wasting

B. Signs include:

a. General signs such as anemia, jaundice, tachycardia, hypotension, and tachypnea in case of respiratory infections

b. Loss of hepatic mass leading to shrunken liver which can be palpable in midclavicular line

c. Features of hypoglycemia

d. Features of electrolyte disturbances

C. In case of subacute and chronic liver failure ascites, edema, cerebral edema, renal failure, features of chronic liver disease, and hypotension.

Investigations

A. Hematology:

a. Complete blood count to detect anemia due to disease and bleeding

b. WBC—it is increased in case of infection.

c. Hematocrit

d. Hemoglobin

e. Blood group

B. Biochemical tests:

a. Liver function test: Bilirubin level >10 mg/dL and aminotransferase level >3,500 IU/L are suggestive of paracetamol toxicity.

b. Serum electrolytes

c. Urea and creatinine

d. Fasting serum glucose

e. Serum ceruloplasmin, copper, and cortisol level at 8 AM

f. Cosyntropin test to detect Addison's disease

C. Virology:

a. Viral profile of hepatitis B, C, D. D virus should be sought if the patient is hepatitis B virus (HBV) positive.

b. If the patient is HBV or HCV positive, HBV DNA or HCV RNA (ribonucleic acid) has to be done.

c. In case of endemic areas immunoglobulin M (IgM) HAV and IgM HEV are indicated.

d. Polymerase chain reaction (PCR) for cytomegalovirus or herpes simplex virus and Epstein–Barr virus in immunosuppressed patients

e. HIV screening

D. Toxicology screening:

a. Drug

b. Toxin

c. Alcohol

d. Urine drug screening

E. Autoimmune disorders:

a. Antinuclear antibody (ANA)

b. Antismooth muscle cell antibody

c. Anti-liver-kidney microsomal (LKM) antibody

F. Microbiology:

a. Culture of aerobic and anaerobic blood culture

b. Urine microscopy and culture

c. Sputum microscopy and culture

G. Radiological investigations:

a. Ultrasound of abdomen to detect liver condition, spleen, pregnancy or not.

b. Electroencephalogram (EEG)—slowing of cortical activity in 50% patients with liver disease with epileptiform activity. There are five grades found in EEG in this disease.

1. Grade A to D—wave of decreasing frequency but increasing amplitude—it suggests increasing drowsiness.
2. At D—triphasic wave appears.
3. There is an interrupted line at D—on the right of that line recovery is unlikely.
4. From E to F grade—amplitude decreases but frequency changes little—it suggests patient is going to deep unconsciousness.
5. At F grade—there is no cerebral activity.

c. CT scan of brain—it can rule out cerebral hemorrhage in case of unconscious patients.

d. Chest X-ray to detect hepatic hydrothorax, or infective features

e. Doppler ultrasound of portal vein to see any obstruction, reversal of flow

H. Invasive studies:
   a. Liver biopsy to detect status of liver architecture, vascular pattern, reduction in liver size, viral inclusions, and copper estimation
   b. Drainage of ascetic fluid to detect character of the fluid, culture
I. Miscellaneous studies:
   a. 24-hour urinary copper
   b. Pregnancy test

Treatment

Treatment of liver failure mainly consists of treatment of complications and treatment of the etiologies.

Treatment of Hepatic Encephalopathy

Neurological support is aimed at:
A. Optimizing cerebral blood flow
B. Optimizing cerebral perfusion pressure
C. Oxygen administration
D. Treatment of cerebral edema

So, management is:
A. Head end should be elevated by 30°
B. Elective mechanical ventilation with muscle paralysis with propofol, minimal endotracheal suctioning, and tactile stimulation to prevent surge of intracranial pressure (ICP)
C. Infusion of prostacyclin can be given
D. International normalized ratio (INR) and platelet count should be 2 or less and 50,000/cc, respectively prior to introduction of transducer which can guide the therapy in patient with grade III or IV encephalopathy. But it should be removed within 5 days as there is chance of infection and bleeding.
E. Cerebral perfusion pressure = Mean arterial pressure - Intracranial pressure
   a. If it is <50 mm Hg due to hypotension, it has to be corrected by vasopressor agents but intravascular volume is normal.
   b. If cerebral perfusion pressure is low due to increased ICP or if later is increased >25 mm Hg, intravenous 20% mannitol has to be administered at a rate of 0.25–1 g/kg and it can be repeated if the serum osmolarity is <320 mOsm/L
   c. If there is volume overload and the patient is oliguric renal replacement therapy should be given.
F. To induce cerebral vasoconstriction to reduce cerebral flow hyperventilation can be tried or in some cases intravenous indomethacin to treat refractory intracranial hypertension.
G. In case of impending herniation:
   a. Thiopentone has to be given in bolus dose of 5–10 mg/kg intravenously followed by 3–5 mg/kg/h; or
   b. Phenobarbital at a dose of 3–5 mg/kg bolus intravenously followed by 1–3 mg/kg slow infusion
H. Induction of hypothermia to core body temperature to 32–33°C with cooler blankets for period of 10–118 hours may reduce ICP by reduction of cerebral blood flow, glutathione synthesis, and decreasing the arterial ammonia.
I. Correction of acidosis and electrolytes:
   a. Administration of hypertonic saline to raise the serum sodium 145–155 mmol prophylactically in case of severe encephalopathy.

   Lactulose: But it has been shown having no benefit because of following reasons:
   a. There is chance of aspiration
   b. Bowel distension which complicates transplantation.

Treatment of Coagulopathy

A. If platelet is <10,000/cc—platelet transfusion should be given.
B. In case of any active procedure required or there is active bleeding—fresh frozen plasma (FFP) has to be given.
C. If the coagulopathy is refractory to FFP then 40 μg/kg recombinant factor VII has to be given 30 minutes before the procedure.
D. In case of severe bleeding with fibrinogen level of <100 mg/dL cryoprecipitate should be administered.
E. If INR is >1.5, injection of vitamin K has to be given through intravenous or intramuscular route required.
F. In case of requirement of large amount of FFP, plasmapheresis is of choice.
G. Prophylactically for stress ulceration proton-pump inhibitor is required.

Treatment of Renal Failure

Renal complication in case of acute liver failure may occur due to the following:
A. Hepatorenal syndrome (HRS) due to lowering of renal perfusion pressure, sympathetic nervous system activation, decreased filtration through glomerulus, and increased vasoactive mediator synthesis
B. Direct nephrotoxicity to drugs

Secondary complications due to bleeding, sepsis, and hypotension.

Treatment should be:

A. Administration of 1–1.5 L intravenous fluid to treat prerenal azotemia.

B. To increase renal perfusion pressure low-dose dopamine is to be given. Continuous renal replacement therapy with bicarbonate buffer is given in case of hemodynamically stable patients to prevent ICP fluctuation.

Treatment of Hemodynamic Changes

Hemodynamic changes are characterized by increased cardiac output in the face decreased peripheral vascular resistance.

Treatment:

A. Intravenous administration of crystalloid or albumin

B. Administration of vasopressors to maintain the mean arterial pressure of >60 mm Hg or cerebral perfusion of <50 mm Hg.

C. Administration of vasopressin to cause cerebral vasodilatation

D. If serum cortisol level is low intravenous hydrocortisone 200–30 mg/day may be beneficial.

Treatment of Infection

A. Prophylactic antibiotic treatment with surveillance for prompt antibiotic treatment

B. If the patient is not responding to antibiotic treatment, antifungal treatment should be given.

C. Invasive procedure should be done under strict aseptic control.

Treatment of Pulmonary Complication

A. To prevent increased intracranial hypertension sedation should be given in case of endotracheal intubation and suction.

B. If the patient is under ventilation following parameter should be followed:

- **a.** Tidal volume 6 mL/kg
- **b.** Low positive end-expiratory pressure
- **c.** $PaCO_2$ of 30–40 mm Hg

Treatment of Metabolic Causes

A. Treatment of electrolyte imbalance

B. In acute liver failure it is persistent and intractable. It produces neurological deterioration and death. If blood glucose is <60 mg/dL continuous infusion of 5–10% dextrose should be administered.

Treatment of Specific Causes

Paracetamol overdose:

A. N-acetyl cysteine can be given orally 140 mg/kg bolus followed by 70 mg/kg every 4 hourly for total 17 doses. It can be given intravenously at 150 mg/kg in 5% dextrose over 15 minutes followed by 50 mg/kg over 4 hours then 100 mg/kg over 16 hours.

Mushroom poisoning:

A. Gastric lavage with activated charcoal in case of acute ingestion with nausea and vomiting.

B. Most common antidote penicillin G at a dose of 300,000–1 million units/kg.

C. Silibinin at 30–40 mg/kg/day orally or intravenously along with or without N-acetyl cysteine is more effective.

Hepatitis B or C treatment: Effective antiviral treatment has to be given.

Herpes simplex treatment: It occurs mainly in immunosuppressed or pregnant patient. Diagnosis is suspected by vesicular rash with high aminotransferase level. Prognosis is poor in spite of acyclovir treatment.

Autoimmune hepatitis (AIH):

A. This patient has to be treated by prednisolone 60 mg/day.

B. If there is multilobar collapse, persistent elevated bilirubin, and the patient fails to respond to steroid within 2 weeks, transplantation is the treatment of choice.

Wilson's disease:

A. Penicillamine or trientine is the drug of choice.

B. Albumin dialysis

C. Plasmapheresis to remove copper

D. Continuous renal replacement therapy

Liver transplantation: It should be done in patient with grade III to IV hepatic encephalopathy due to hepatic failure. It is used on following validated criteria, such as age, pH, interval between onset of jaundice and encephalopathy, etiology, PT, raised bilirubin level, and <20% of normal factor V.

Contraindications

A. Malignancy

B. Infection

C. Brain death

D. Cardiac disease

E. Pulmonary disease

F. Multiorgan failure
G. Fixed dilated pupil for prolonged periods
H. Cerebral perfusion pressure <40 mm Hg
I. Intracranial pressure >35 mm Hg. For than 1–2 hours

Relative Contraindications

A. More than 70 years
B. Infections under treatment
C. History of psychiatric problem
D. Rapidly increasing requirement for vasopressor support

Outcomes

A. Control of cachexia, portal venous collateral
B. Correction of coagulant defects by plasma derivatives and platelets
C. Within 3 months of surgery death is due to sepsis and neurological complications.
D. Survival rate is better in acute liver failure as compared to cirrhosis.

Q3. Pathophysiology, diagnostic approach, and management of Budd–Chiari syndrome.

PGI/NOV2013/MDIII (10)

Budd–Chiari syndrome.

KHUS/MAY2014/MDIII (10)

Anatomy of vascular system of liver. Management of Budd–Chiari syndrome.

ODISHA UNI, 2020 (10)

Vascular supply will be described in question number 28.

ANSWER

Budd first described this disease as triad of hepatomegaly, abdominal pain, and ascites and Chiari provided the pathological description of it. So, it can be defined as a potentially life-threatening disorder characterized by hepatic venous outflow obstruction manifested by abdominal pain, hepatomegaly, and ascites. Obstruction can arise from the site of efferent vein of the acinus to inferior vena cava prior to its drainage into right atrium.

Etiopathogenesis

A. Myeloproliferative disorders:
   a. Polycythemia rubra vera
   b. Essential thrombocytosis
   c. Idiopathic myelofibrosis
   d. Occult myeloproliferative disorders

   First three are called Philadelphia-negative myeloproliferative neoplasia. Last one can be diagnosed by erythroid bone marrow colony test. All are JAK2 positive.
B. Collagen vascular disease:
   a. Systemic lupus erythematosus
   b. Antiphospholipid syndrome
   c. Idiopathic granulomatous venulitis
C. Paroxysmal nocturnal hemoglobinuria
D. Other hypercoagulable state:
   a. Mutation of factor V Leiden
   b. Deficiency of antithrombin III
   c. Deficiency of protein S and C due to poor liver synthesis
   d. Oral contraceptive pregnancy
E. Trauma produces membrane obstruction to inferior vena cava.
F. Mechanical obstruction:
   a. Polycystic liver disease
G. Metastasis from tumor produces obstruction to inferior vena cava:
   a. Hepatocellular cancer
   b. Renal carcinoma
   c. Angiosarcoma
   d. Leiomyosarcoma
   e. Wilm's tumor
H. Systemic diseases:
   a. Sarcoidosis
   b. Inflammatory bowel disease (IBD)

Pathological changes include the following:

A. In acute case occlusion of inferior vena cava by thrombus—it may be purulent or fibrous strand. Site of block starts from hepatic venule to end of inferior vena cava prior to its entry to right atrium.
B. In acute stage:
   a. Liver is enlarged, smooth with venous congestion, cut surface shows "nutmeg," and in acute stage subcapsular lymphatics are prominent and dilated.
C. In chronic case:
   a. Enlarged caudate lobe compresses the inferior vena cava.
   b. Regenerative nodules after first hepatic vein thrombosis progress to involve portal venous system.

c. Spleen is enlarged.
d. Mesenteric vessels will thrombose.

D. Histology demonstrated:
a. Zone 3 venous dilatation associated with hemorrhage and necrosis.
b. Hepatic venule obstruction leads to venocentric cirrhosis whereas, portal vein obstruction leads to venoportal cirrhosis.

Diagnosis

The diagnosis is composed of clinical features and different investigations.

Clinical Features

Clinical features depend upon:

A. Speed of occlusion
B. Site of obstruction
C. Severity of liver dysfunction

Spectrum of disease varies from severe fulminant form to chronic slow growing form or even asymptomatic.

In acute form:

A. Precipitating causes will continue and present according to the nature of the diseases, such as:
a. Polycythemia
b. Hepatocellular or renal carcinoma
c. Diarrhea
d. Liver enlargement
e. Watery diarrhea

B. In case total obstruction of hepatic vein:
a. Different grades of unconsciousness
b. Hepatocellular failure
c. Death

In chronic form:

A. Jaundice
B. Abdominal pain
C. Hepatomegaly mainly caudate lobe of liver in the epigastrium
D. Ascites
E. Splenomegaly
F. In case of inferior venacaval obstruction:
a. Edema
b. Venous distension over the flanks and back

Asymptomatic form: It occurs in 15% of patients. These patients demonstrate no ascites, hepatomegaly or splenomegaly or abdominal pain. These patient are usually diagnosed by accidental detection of abnormal liver function test.

Investigations

A. Liver function test:
a. Bilirubin rarely increases >2 mg/mL.
b. Alkaline phosphatase is reduced.
c. Albumin will be reduced due to liver failure of protein-losing enteropathy.
d. Transaminases level >1,000 IU/L suggests acute outflow obstruction or hepatocellular failure.

B. Prothrombin time is normal
C. Ascitic fluid protein is high 25 g/L
D. Radiology:
a. Ultrasound:
1. Shrunken liver with caudate lobe hypertrophy
2. Abnormalities of hepatic vein
3. In acute stage hyperechogenic but in later stage hyperechogenic with fibrosis
4. Presence of ascites

E. Doppler ultrasound:
a. Abnormalities of direction of flow of blood in hepatic vein and retrohepatic inferior vena cava.
b. Blood flow in inferior vena cava and hepatic vein will be absent, reversed or turbulent or continuous.

F. Color Doppler studies: It will detect abnormalities in hepatic veins, inferior vena cava, and portal vein.
G. CT scan of abdomen: It demonstrates:
a. Enlargement of liver with:
1. Diffuse hypodensity prior the contrast
2. Patchy enhancement but completely hypodense in case of complete obstruction of hepatic vein after contrast.
3. Caudate lobe is dense with surrounding under perfused parenchyma.

H. Magnetic resonance imaging (MRI):
a. Absence of normal hepatic venous drainage
b. Absence of normal inferior venacaval drainage
c. Alteration of signal intensity
d. Deformity of inferior vena cava by enlarged caudate lobe

I. Hepatic venography:
a. Narrowed hepatic veins
b. Tortuous, lace-like adjacent veins, pattern spiderweb like signifying patent collaterals

J. Inferior venography:
a. In the hepatic segment, there is side-to-side narrowing of inferior vena cava.

b. Pressure measurement of throughout the inferior vena cava to the uniform patency and any membranous obstruction or caudate lobe obstruction

K. Celiac angiography:
   a. Branches of hepatic artery are stretched and displaced.
   b. Multiplying space-occupying lesions in the liver looking like metastases

L. Liver biopsy:
   a. Speckled zone 3 congestion

Treatment

A. Drug treatment:
   a. In case of hypercoagulability—anticoagulation
   b. In case of polycythemia and thrombocytosis—venesection or cytotoxic therapies
   c. In case of PNH—molecular therapies, such as eculizumab.
   d. Ascites—low sodium in the diet, diuretics

B. Percutaneous transluminal angioplasty:
   a. After liver transplantation to dilate the web and narrowing of inferior vena cava this procedure is of choice in case of suprahepatic portion of inferior vena cava.
   b. In case of hepatic vein multiple dilatation followed by administration of metallic stent. This should be tried in case of failed angioplasty.

C. Transjugular intrahepatic stent shunt: It should be done in case of failed anticoagulation and percutaneous angioplasty.

   Aim is:
   a. Decompression of liver
   b. There is reversal of portal venous flow.
   c. In case of acute state it will rescue the patients where emergency transplantation cannot be done.

   It will avoid:
   a. Open surgery
   b. Mortality

   In case where hepatic vein cannot be entered the approach should be transcaval.

D. Surgical portosystemic shunt:
   Indications:
   a. Liver transplantation is not feasible
   b. TIPS are not available

   Contraindications:
   a. Acute Budd-Chiari syndrome as here salvage transplantation is required in case of liver failure.
   b. In case of portal venous obstruction

   Prognosis: 5-year survival rate is 87% but it will be reduced to 38% in case of shunt thrombosis.

   Anticoagulation is required throughout the life.

   If the pressure in the infrahepatic portion of inferior vena cava exceeds 20 mm Hg due to pressure of enlarged caudate lobe, venacaval stenting has to be done first followed by shunting.

   Type of shunt: Interposition mesocaval graft as it will not affect the subsequent hepatic transplantation. If inferior vena cava is obstructed Mesoatrial shunt is used.

E. Liver transplantation:
   Indications:
   a. In case of progression to cirrhosis with hepatocellular failure
   b. In case of deterioration in spite of medical and radiological treatment

   But TIPS should be done as a stop-gap step so that more time will be present for procuring the donor-liver.

   If the underlying is hypercoagulability then life-long anticoagulation has to be given.

   One year and 5-year survival rates are 85% and 80%, respectively.

Q4. Discuss the management of hepatic encephalopathy.

BF/NOV2013/MDIII (10)

Hepatic encephalopathy.

MGR/MA2006/MDI (5)

Precipitating factors and management of hepatic encephalopathy.

MGR/FEB2005/MDI (5)

Clinical features and management of hepatic encephalopathy.

RGUHS/SEP2002/MDII (10)

West Haven classification of hepatic encephalopathy.

DNB (2020) (4)

Hepatic encephalopathy.

KERALA UNI, 2021 (10)

BHARATI VIDYAPEETH DEEMED UNI, JHELUM (10)

Acute hepatic encephalopathy.

MAHARASHTRA UNI OF HEALTH SC, VIJAYAWADA, 2020 (10)

Hepatic encephalopathy.

MGU, 2024 (5)

Hepatic encephalopathy and its management.

RAJASTHAN UNIVERSITY, 2023, (8)

ANSWER

Hepatic encephalopathy is a reversible metabolic encephalopathy occurred as a consequence of advanced hepatic failure due to various etiologies. If the inciting events are not treated successfully the survival of the patients will be shortened.

Though ammonia level in the blood is high in patient with hepatic encephalopathy but there is lack of correlation between the two which means that factors other than ammonia may come into play in the development of hepatic encephalopathy.

Precipitating Factors

Ammonia:

A. In the gastrointestinal tract:

  a. In the small intestine ammonia is produced through the deamination of glutamine via deaminase.

  b. In the large intestine through the bacterial degradation of urea and proteins.

B. Kidney produces small amount of ammonia which is aggravated by treatment with diuretics and in hypokalemia.

C. In liver disease in the state of sarcopenia glutamine is also released from the muscles.

Normally, ammonia enters into the liver and is converted to urea through urea cycle which will be ultimately cleared by kidney. But in case of cirrhosis with portosystemic shunting ammonia will bypass the liver thus increasing its concentration in the blood and it crosses the blood–brain barrier into brain where astrocytes will convert ammonia and glutamate into glutamine by glutamine synthetase. Glutamine will be accumulated in the astrocytes and it will draw water as it is osmotically active leading the swelling of these cells. Glutamine also enters mitochondria and is cleaved into ammonia and glutamate by glutaminase leading to increased concentration of ammonia in the cells which is responsible for "Feed forward loop"—according to it increased intracellular ammonia concentration leads to production of reactive oxygen and also nitrogen species perpetuating further edema.

In case of long-standing exposure of brain to ammonia myo-inositol and taurine will be released from the brain cells leading to lowering of myo-inositol in the cells producing decompensated hepatic encephalopathy.

Cerebral perfusion will be altered in hyperammonemia leading to redistribution of cerebral blood flow to subcortical areas from cerebral cortex which produces impaired neuropsychiatric performances.

Effect of inflammation:

Inflammation occurs in following conditions: (1) Sepsis, (2) Acute liver failure, (3) Cirrhosis, (4) Obesity, (5) Gastrointestinal bleeding, and (6) Alteration of gastrointestinal microbiota. As a result proinflammatory cytokines, tumor necrosis factor-alpha (TNF-α), interleukin-1 (IL-1), and IL-6 are released which alter the morphology of astrocytes leading to increased permeability of blood–brain barrier.

Effect of microbiota:

A. There is release of ammonia, indoles, oxindoles, and endotoxins leading to cognitive impairment.

B. In case of cirrhosis, in case dysbiosis, there is reduced level of members of autochthonous taxa, such as Clostridiales, Ruminococcaceae, and Lachnospiraceae and increased level of Streptococcaceae and Enterobacteriaceae. In hepatic encephalopathy, there is endotoxemia and lower dysbiosis rate and this endotoxemia activates immune response and inflammatory cascade leading to liver damage as well as augmentation of cerebral edema.

Neuromodulators:

A. Gamma-aminobutyric acid (GABA): Increase sensitivity of benzodiazepine receptors on astrocytes will activate GABA system increasing the tone of GABAergic tone in the brain

B. Excess benzodiazepine like compounds derived from vegetable diet, intestinal flora, and medications contribute to hepatic encephalopathy.

C. Ammonia binds to GAB receptor presents on the astrocytes triggering neurosteroid synthesis

D. Serotonin

E. Acetylcholine

F. Monoamines

G. Glutamate

Manganese deposition: Usually manganese is excreted in bile from the liver. But in case of cirrhosis with portosystemic shunting manganese leading to increased blood level and deposition of manganese in the brain augmenting hepatic encephalopathy.

Clinical Features of Hepatic Encephalopathy

There is wide spectrum of mental changes from near normal which can be diagnosed by specialized testing to extremes of mental changes. This hepatic encephalopathy is of following types:

Type	Definitions	Grade	Term	Course	Spontaneous or not
A	Hepatic encephalopathy associated with acute liver failure	Minimal change	Covert hepatic encephalopathy	Episodic	Spontaneous
B	Hepatic encephalopathy associated with portosystemic bypass and no acute liver failure	2	Overt hepatic encephalopathy	Recurrent	Precipitated
		3			
C	Hepatic encephalopathy associated with cirrhosis or portal hypertension/portosystemic shunt	4		Persistent	

In case of minimal changes: Encephalopathic changes are always below clinical detection level, hence this type of covert in hepatic encephalopathy can be diagnosed by specialized testing.

Overt encephalopathy may be of two types:

A. Persistent encephalopathy: In it mental changes are always above the clinical detection level with minimal fluctuation.

B. Episodic encephalopathy: In this condition neurological changes are episodic with upper limit and are always above the clinical detection level but in between the episode the patient will be completely normal.

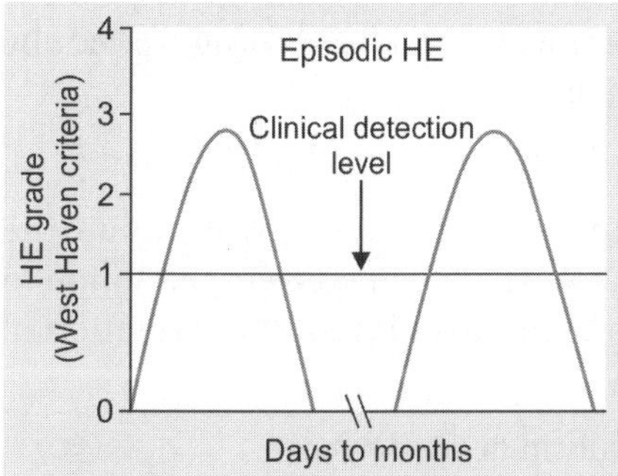

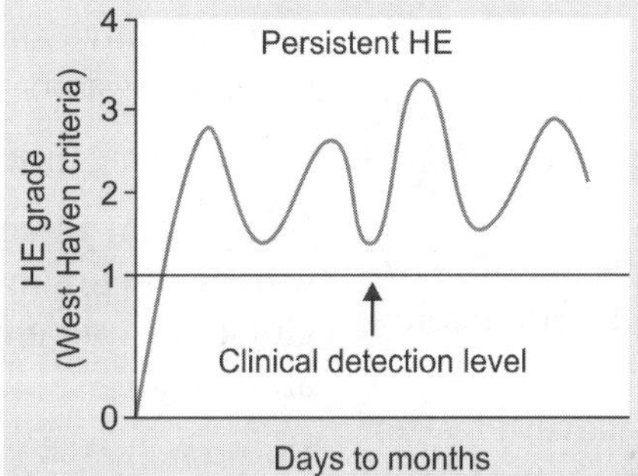

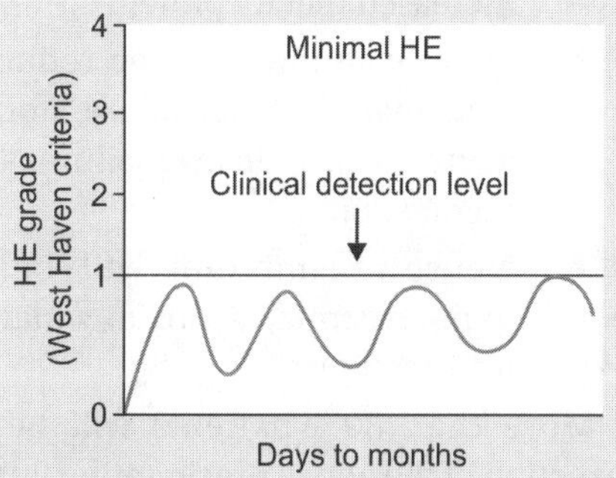

(HE: hepatic encephalopathy)

Different modalities of sensations in patients with different types of encephalopathies:

Tests	Functions	CHE	OHE	Late OHE
Psychomotor	Normal	Abnormal	Abnormal	Not done
Neurophysiologic	Normal	Abnormal	Abnormal	Not done
Clinical	Normal	Normal	Abnormal	Abnormal

(CHE: covert hepatic encephalopathy; OHE: overt hepatic encephalopathy)

Clinical classifications of hepatic encephalopathy are based on West Haven criteria:

Grade	Features
0	No abnormality detected
1	Euphoria, anxiety, trivial loss of awareness, impairment of addition or subtraction, and attention span is shortened
2	Lethargy, disorientation of time, apathy, personality changes, and inappropriate behavior
3	Somnolence to stupor, confused, response to stimuli will be lowered, gross disorientation, confused, and bizarre behavior
4	Coma

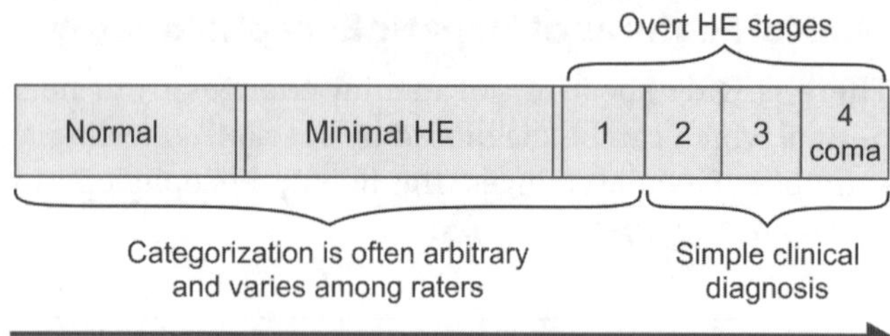

(HE: hepatic encephalopathy)

Physical signs:
In case of overt hepatic encephalopathy:

- **a.** Hyperreflexia
- **b.** Positive Babinski sign
- **c.** Asterixis: It occurs due to disturbance in oscillatory network of the brain. It is shown in upper and lower extremities and tongue.

Management of Hepatic Encephalopathy

A. Correction of precipitating factors:

- **a.** Increased load of nitrogen occurred from gastrointestinal bleeding, infections, and increased dietary protein
- **b.** Toxin clearance will be reduced as a result of constipation, renal failure, portosystemic shunt, acute on chronic liver failure, and noncompliant medication
- **c.** Neurotransmission will be altered due to hypoglycemia, hypoxia, sedation, and alcohol intoxication.

More than 80% patients will be recovered after correction of the above precipitating factors. Patients with grade III encephalopathy will be treated in intensive care unit as there is facility of mechanical ventilation.

Medical Therapy in Case of Overt and Persistent Hepatic Encephalopathy

It includes the management of episodic hepatic encephalopathy and persistent hepatic encephalopathy and this should be followed by prevention of secondary hepatic encephalopathy. With the first line of therapy if the patient responds within 24–48 hours it will support the diagnosis, but if the patient will not respond for >72 hours then other cause of altered mentation has to be sought.

Nonabsorbable disaccharides: These are lactulose and lactitol.

Mechanism of actions: In the colon lactulose will be converted to acetic acid and lactic acid and colonic pH will be reduced. In low pH survival of urease-producing bacteria will be decreased thereby facilitating the conversion of ammonia to less readily absorbable ammonium. It will act as cathartic to increase excretion of the nitrogenous waste.

Adverse effect: Cramping abdominal pain, diarrhea which may be so severe that patient develop hypovolemia and dehydration and electrolyte imbalance.

Dose:

A. Initial dose is 20–30 mL twice daily to maintain two semisolid stool per day, this followed by dose should be adjusted according to the patients. This drug has to be continued indefinitely in patient with persistent hepatic encephalopathy.

B. In case of comatose patients this drug has to be administered as 300 mL in 1 L of water every 6–8 hours till the patient will initiate oral intake.

Antibiotics: The drug is rifaximin, neomycin, and metronidazole.

Mechanism of action of rifaximin: It will change the microbiota in the gut and create more favorable microbiome so that endogenous ammonia production by bacteria will be reduced. It is active against gram-positive, gram-negative anaerobic bacteria. This drug will not be absorbed systematically.

Dose: 550 mg thrice daily

Mechanism of action of neomycin: It will inhibit the activity of glutaminase which will convert glutamine to glutamate and ammonia thus prevent the formation of ammonia.

Dose: Orally 1–4 g daily in divided doses

Adverse effects: Nephrotoxicity and ototoxicity—for these complications this drug is not used now.

Mechanism of actions of metronidazole: It acts against gram-negative anaerobic bacteria in the gut which will hydrolyze urea to ammonia leading to decreased formation of ammonia.

Dose: 400 mg twice daily orally

Toxicity: Abdominal cramps, metallic taste. Long-term use may lead to potential toxicity.

Nutrition: Most of these patients may suffer from severe protein energy malnutrition. The patient with overt encephalopathy usually requires 35–40 kcal/kg in addition to small nutritional supplements throughout the day.

Protein intake: In this patient no restriction of protein intake should be advised because skeletal muscles metabolize ammonia. Daily requirement is 1.2–1.5 g/kg/day.

Nonabsorbable vegetable fiber: It should be taken in large amount to increase clearance of nitrogenous waste via stool.

Branched chain amino acid (BCAA): Cirrhotic patients have altered ratio of amino acids with increase in aromatic amino acid (AAA) as compared to BCAA leading to development of encephalopathy by changing the cerebral neurotransmitter balance. Orally BCAA alters the ratio and is effective in patients with hepatic encephalopathy who are not responding to oral lactulose and rifaximin.

Leucine stimulates the production of hepatocyte growth factor with the help of stellate cells leading to regeneration of hepatocytes and thus compensate death of liver cells.

L-ornithine L-aspartate (LOLA): It improves the patient with encephalopathy and LOLA will reverse the ratio of AAA to BCAA and thus lowering the amount of ammonia.

Dose: 6 g thrice daily orally in grade II encephalopathy. Since aspartate moiety will undergo transamination in the gut mucosa hence, the efficacy of this drug depends upon the ornithine moiety alone.

Zinc: It is a cofactor for urea cycle enzyme and ammonia detoxification by reducing the activity of glutathione synthetase. Its level is commonly low in patients with cirrhosis. So, zinc supplementation commonly helps the patient from intoxication of ammonia.

Bromocriptine: These patients have deficit in dopaminergic neurotransmission. So, chronic stable persistent hepatic encephalopathy having extrapyramidal features which are resistant to previous agent can respond to this dopamine agonist bromocriptine.

Dose: 2.5 mg daily to maximum 5 mg twice daily.

Complication: Ototoxicity. So, every 6 month audiogram should be done in this patient.

Flumazenil: In patient with hepatic encephalopathy has

A. Deficit in GABAergic neurotransmission.

B. Increased level of circulating benzodiazepine like ligands.

This drug is benzodiazepine receptor antagonist, thus when given intravenously it will improve the encephalopathy for a short time.

Surgical Therapy

Shunt Occlusion

Spontaneous or artificial shunt, like TIPS, may be responsible for persistent hepatic encephalopathy which may be difficult to treat. So these shunt should be occluded to prevent or worsen the encephalopathy. The methods included are:

A. Vascular embolization

B. Vascular plugging with Amplatzer device

C. Balloon occlusion

D. Laparoscopic disconnection of periumbilical vein shunt.

Liver Transplantation

Model for End-stage Liver Disease (MELD) is used to prioritize the patient for liver transplant. This scoring system does not include neuropsychiatric status. Now selection of the patients is based on presence of hepatic encephalopathy with preservation of liver function test with exclusion of other types of neuropsychiatric manifestation.

Postliver transplant patient shows following improvement:

A. Parkinsonian features resistant to treatment

B. Resolution of electroencephalography, cerebral MRI, cerebral positron emission tomography (PET)

C. Improvement of cognitive functions

These patients may also unmask following effects:

A. Preexisting unrecognized abnormalities

B. Effects of immunosuppressive therapy

C. Effect of comorbidities, like systemic hypertension

D. Development of neurological complications.

Artificial liver support system: Patients with severe encephalopathy having decompensated cirrhosis who do not respond to conventional therapy may require support.

A. To provide time during which the inciting event may be corrected

B. It acts as a bridge for future liver transplantation.

Most extensively studied liver support is Molecular Adsorption Recirculating System (MARS). It removes both lipophilic albumin-bound as well as water-soluble molecules and thus purifies blood. Thus it will improve cerebral hemodynamics by removing:

A. Circulating ammonia

B. Endotoxin

C. Inflammatory mediators

Colectomy/Colonic exclusion: It will reduce intestinal production of ammonia. But operative morbidity and mortality is very high.

Future Therapies

Hepatic encephalopathy is mainly based on increased production and decreased excretion of ammonia. So, treatment should be based on:

A. Prevention of ammonia production in the intestine: Enterocytes breakdown glutamine after its uptake from the intestine. Phosphate activated glutaminase (PAG) is responsible for catabolizing the glutamine to produce ammonia. Concentration of PAG is about four times higher in duodenum in cirrhotic patients. So, inhibitors of this PAG may reduce the blood ammonia level and provide therapeutic benefit.

B. Kidney is the organ where ammonia is produced and excreted. In cirrhotic patient expansion of plasma leads to excretion of ammonia.

C. Skeletal muscle cells detoxify ammonia by converting it to glutamine by glutamine synthetase which is promoted by ornithine and phenylacetate promotes excretion of this glutamine through kidney.

Recently newer pathogenic and potentially harmful agents are recognized and possible potentially alternative treatments are:

A. *L-carnitine:*

It is used:

a. In children having urea-cycle deficiency with hyperammonemia

b. Valproic acid-induced hyperammonemia

Mechanism of actions:

a. It acts on metabotropic glutamate receptors at the level of brain in ammonia uptake.

b. It acts on mitochondrial metabolism.

B. *Rivastigmine*:

Mechanism of action: In cirrhotic patient with hepatic encephalopathy acetylcholine is considerably low. This drug inhibits reversibly cholinesterase and thus improves the psychomotor performance in this patient.

C. *Endocannabinoids*:

Mechanism of action: In patient with hepatic encephalopathy neural intoxication disrupts cerebral energy flux. This drug augments the adenosine monophosphate (AMP)-activated protein kinase and thus improves the cellular energy store in response to metabolic injury.

D. *Sildenafil*:

Mechanism of action: In hepatic encephalopathy altered function of glutamate-nitric oxide-cyclic guanosine monophosphate (cGMP) pathway and decrease in extracellular cGMP in the brain lead to cognitive function decline. This drug modulates cGMP concentration thus restoring the learning episode. This is under phase III trial.

E. *Metabotropic glutamate receptors 1 (mGluR1)*:

Mechanism of action: In the pars reticulata of the substantia nigra of this patient there is alteration of glutamatergic neurotransmission leading to psychomotor slowing. This drug blocks the mGluR1 receptor and thus normalizes the brain activity. This is in phase III trial.

Q5. Bilirubin metabolism and outline of diagnostic approach to a patient with hyperbilirubinemia.

PGI/APR2013/MDI (10)

Bilirubin metabolism, classify hyperbilirubinemia syndrome, outline approach to diagnosis.

DNBIV/JUN2011 (10)

Bile pigment metabolism.

MGR/OCT2012/MDI (5)

Congenital hyperbilirubinemia.

MGR/OCT2003/MDIII (10)

Jaundice.

MGR/MAR2008/MDI (5)

Write bilirubin metabolism and causes of portal hypertension.

ODISHA UNI, 2021 (10)

Briefly describe bilirubin metabolism. How do you classify jaundice? Outline the clinicopathological approach to a case of jaundice.

BHARATI VIDYAPEETH DEEMED UNIVERSITY, 2019 (15)

Outline the bilirubin metabolism and describe the histopathology of chronic viral hepatitis.

AIIMS (BHU), 2024 (10)

Bilirubin metabolism.

MANIPUR UNIVERSITY, 2018 (10)

Histological changes in chronic viral hepatitis has been described in question number 35.

ANSWER

Bilirubin Metabolism

Bilirubin is derived mainly from hemoglobin but small fractions also derived from myoglobin, cytochrome 450, and immature bone marrow cells. Nearly daily 300 mg of bilirubin is formed. In the reticuloendothelial system the enzyme hem oxygenase breaks hemoglobin at α-methane bridge porphyrin ring to globin, hem, biliverdin, and carbon monoxide. This biliverdin will be at once converted into bilirubin by biliverdin reductase, a cytosolic enzyme. This bilirubin due to its water insolubility is bound to albumin and transported into plasma. Bilirubin is transported from the blood into bile through four distinct steps:

A. Hepatocellular uptake: This albumin bound bilirubin in the sinusoidal blood reaches the surface of hepatocytes through the endothelial cell fenestrae. Then bilirubin is removed from albumin and enters into the hepatocytes by two processes, one is facilitated diffusion and second is by simple diffusion.

B. Intracellular binding: Within the hepatocyte bilirubin binds to cytosolic carrier protein glutathione-S-transferase, called ligandin.

C. Conjugation of bilirubin: Bilirubin will be conjugated with one and two glucuronic acids to monoglucuronide and diglucuronide, respectively with the help of UDP-glucuronosyltransferase thus by disrupting the internal hydrogen bonding making it highly soluble in water. Major bilirubin conjugate is diglucuronide but sulfate, xylose glucose conjugation may occur.

D. Biliary excretion: Conjugated bile is excreted across the canalicular membrane into bile by ATP-dependent multidrug resistance-associated protein 2 (MRP2). Some amount of conjugated bilirubin is secreted into portal circulation with the help of MRP3 which will be taken back into hepatocyte by sinusoidal uptake transporter, organ anion transport protein 1B1 (OATP 1B1).

Extrahepatic Aspect of Bilirubin Metabolism

After the secretion of bile into bile it will reach into duodenum and from there it will pass down the gastrointestinal tract without its reabsorption through the mucosa.

In the gut through bacterial β-glucuronidase and other enzymes large fraction will be converted into water-soluble colorless compound urobilinogen. Most of the urobilinogen will be converted into stercobilinogen and excreted in stool.

Rest of urobilinogen undergoes enterohepatic cycling. Urobilinogen that enters into the hepatocytes will reach systemic circulation and will be excreted through kidney. If urobilinogen excretion in urine is increased it indicates high plasma level—it may be due to overproduction of urobilinogen or decreased hepatic clearance of it.

Classification of Hyperbilirubinemia

A. Disorders associated with unconjugated hyperbilirubinemia (>85% of total):
   - **a.** Physiological jaundice of newborn
   - **b.** Hemolysis
   - **c.** Resorption of hematoma
   - **d.** Ineffective erythropoiesis:
     - Thalassemia
     - Megaloblastic anemia
   - **e.** Maternal milk jaundice
   - **f.** Congenital diseases:
     - Gilbert's syndrome
     - Crigler–Najjar syndrome I and II

B. Predominantly conjugated hyperbilirubinemia:
   - **a.** Hepatitis
   - **b.** Cirrhosis
   - **c.** Cholelithiasis
   - **d.** Toxins
   - **e.** Drugs:
     - Anabolic steroid
     - Oral contraceptive pills
   - **f.** Congenital:
     - Dubin–Johnson syndrome
     - Rotor syndrome
     - Benign intrahepatic cholestasis
     - Progressive familial intrahepatic cholestasis (PFIC)

C. Mixed (unconjugated and unconjugated) hyperbilirubinemia (conjugated 20–25% of total):
   - **a.** Viral hepatitis
   - **b.** Alcoholic hepatitis

Congenital Hyperbilirubinemia

Gilbert Syndrome

A. It is autosomal recessive disease; it occurs in 5% of the population.

B. Bilirubin level is never above 5–8 mg/dL.

C. Routine liver function test is normal.

D. Serum bile acid is normal.

E. Liver histology is normal.

F. Oral cholecystography is normal.

G. Increased proportion of bilirubin monoglucuronide
H. Uridine-diphosphoglucuronate glucuronosyltransferase family 1 memberA1 (UDT1A1) is 25–40% normal.
I. Serum bilirubin will be reduced due to its effect of phenobarbitone administration.
J. Few drugs, such as rifampin, flavaspidic acid, and novobiocin, inhibit the uptake of bilirubin which can be reversed by cessation of these drugs.
K. Prognosis is benign.

Crigler–Najjar Type 1 Syndrome

A. It is autosomal recessive. It occurs due to 30 different lesions in *UDT1* gene having common features of absent or trace amount of UDT attached to genetic proteins. There is history of consanguinity in family.
B. There is defect in conjugation of bilirubin as well as other xenobiotics.
C. Nearly virtual absence of bilirubin from the bile so bile will be colorless.
D. Unconjugated bilirubin will be accumulated in the plasma and it will be slowly eliminated through alternate pathway, like directly through bile and small intestine possibly via bilirubin photoisomers but no bilirubin is found in urine and small amount of urobilinogen in feces.
E. Bilirubin level is 18–45 mg/dL. With normal transaminases and ALP level.
F. Unconjugated bilirubin will appear stating from birth to last day of life.
G. Trace amount of UDP-transferase present in the liver.
H. Treatment is liver transplantation. Patient may die of bilirubin encephalopathy in infancy or childhood. In absence of liver transplantation patient may die from bilirubin encephalopathy.

Crigler–Najjar Type 2 Syndrome

A. It occurs due to missense mutation of *UGT1* gene. According to molecular analysis most patients are homozygotes or compound heterozygotes.
B. Presence of unconjugated hyperbilirubinemia of 6–25 mg/dL with normal transaminases and ALP and liver histology.
C. Incidence of kernicterus is low but may occur in infancy to adulthood in case of intercurrent infection or fasting which is responsible for temporary rise in serum bilirubin of reduction of albumin level.
D. Hyperbilirubinemia is not recognized in some cases until adulthood.
E. Administration of phenobarbital reduces the bilirubin level to >25% but never to <3-5 g/dL.
F. These patients can be treated by phenobarbitone.

Dubin–Johnson Syndrome

A. It is autosomal recessive. There is defective expression of ATP-dependent canalicular membrane transporter, MRP2 which prevents transport of conjugated bilirubin across the canalicular membrane and other compounds except bile acids. But in absence of MRP2, bile pigment is still excreted into the bile suggesting that other transport protein may be responsible secondarily in this transport process.
B. Total bilirubin level may be normal, typically within 2–5 mg/dL but may increase up to 20–25 mg/dL. But other liver biochemical tests are normal. Since it is conjugated bilirubin predominantly hence bilirubinuria occurs.
C. Hyperbilirubinemia may be increased in case of pregnancy, oral contraceptives, or intercurrent illness.
D. On physical examination, except jaundice, occasionally there may be hepatosplenomegaly and other constitutional symptoms.
E. There is nonvisualization of gallbladder in oral cholecystography.
F. Due to accumulation of black pigments in the lysosomes of centrilobular hepatocytes liver becomes grossly black color. These black pigments are thought to be generated from epinephrine metabolites but it will disappear if the patient develops viral hepatitis but reappears after recovery.
G. Bromsulphalein (BSP) excretion test demonstrates rise in BSP at 90 minutes after its injection.
H. Among the coproporphyrin I and III normally 75% type III is excreted through urine but in this patient more than excreted coproporphyrin is type I though total coproporphyrin is normal.

Rotor Syndrome

A. This disorder is autosomal recessive.
B. There is no black pigment in the liver and liver appears normal.
C. Total bilirubin is increased in the blood with increased fraction of direct part but with other hepatic biochemical tests is normal.
D. Gallbladder is normally visualized in oral cholecystography.
E. Major coproporphyrin is type I isomer present in the bile and it will be refluxed into the circulation followed by excretion in urine.

F. BSP excretion is delayed but there is no evidence of second rise in blood.

G. There is reduced reuptake of conjugated bilirubin due to deficiency of hepatocyte plasma membrane transporters OATP1B1 and OATP1B3. So, this conjugated bilirubin will be pumped out to portal circulation.

Benign Recurrent Intrahepatic Cholestasis

A. This disease started in childhood or occasionally adulthood with malaise followed by jaundice and severe pruritus. This disorder is familial.

B. Mutation of the gene *FIC1* is responsible for this disorder. In case of a second type of BRIC called type 2, mutation of another type of protein—bile salt excretory protein—which is also defective in case of PFIC type 2.

C. Duration of this episode may be weeks to months followed by complete resolution of symptoms. In between the episodes of months to years the patient is completely normal.

D. Biochemically, there are elevation of bilirubin with increased fraction of conjugated bilirubin, transaminases, bile acids, and ALP.

E. It will never end in cirrhosis or end-stage liver disease.

Progressive Familial Intrahepatic Cholestasis

A. Three types of PFIC:
   - a. Type 1 PFIC (Byler's disease):
     - It occurs in infancy, episodic
     - It will progress to growth retardation, malnutrition, and ultimately to end-stage liver disease in childhood.
     - Gamma-glutamyl transferase (GGT) will be normal.
     - It occurs as a consequence of mutation of *FIC1*.
   - b. Type 2 PFIC:
     - It is associated with mutation of bile salt excretory protein, a major exporter of bile acid in the biliary canaliculi, similar mutation is also demonstrated in BRIC type 2. But recently, it has been demonstrated that mutation of the gene NR1H4 encodes farnesoid X receptor—nuclear hormone receptor which is activated by bile acids, it is absent in BRIC type 2.
     - Increased conjugated fraction of bilirubin but GGT will be normal.
     - There is severe cholestasis started in the childhood.
   - c. Type 3 PFIC:
     - It is associated with the mutation of *MDR3* gene, responsible for normal phospholipid secretion across the biliary canaliculi.
     - There is severe cholestasis in childhood.
     - GGT will be raised in blood.
     - There is decreased level of phospholipid in the bile.

Approach to a Patient with Hyperbilirubinemia

To diagnose causes of hyperbilirubinemia firstly we have to classify the causes according to result of liver function test, such as serum aminotransferases, ALP, serum albumin, and PT.

Jaundice may be of three types:

A. Hemolytic jaundice

B. Hepatic jaundice

C. Posthepatic jaundice

Causes of hemolytic jaundice:

A. Congenital: Different types of congenital hemolytic anemia, such as thalassemia, sickle cell crisis, congenital red blood cell (RBC) enzyme deficiency, abnormal shape of RBC, etc.

B. Acquired hemolytic jaundice:
   - a. Mismatched blood transfusion
   - b. Trauma
   - c. Infections
   - d. Thrombotic thrombocytopenic purpura
   - e. March disorder
   - f. Disseminated intravascular coagulation (DIC)
   - g. Hemolytic uremic syndrome (HUS)

In this type of jaundice history or presentations are:

a. History of long march, snake bite, fever suggestive of infection, blood transfusion, diarrhea (HUS), and anemia from birth

b. Anemia

c. Jaundice

d. Purpuric spot in the limbs

e. Dark yellow brown color urine

f. Investigation shows:
   1. Low hemoglobin
   2. Different shapes of RBC, such as tear drop cells, elliptical cells, small round RBC, sickle cells, and spherocytes

3. Peripheral blood smear may show malarial parasite
4. White blood cell count may be high in DIC or malarial infection
5. High bilirubin, mainly unconjugated variety
6. Normal liver enzymes and ALP
7. Serum phosphate level will be low—hypophosphatemia
8. Serum vitamin B12 and folic acid level will be low in vitamin B12 and folic acid deficiency anemia
9. Osmotic fragility test positive in case of spherocytosis.
10. Urinary urobilirubin will be low
11. Liver biopsy is normal
12. All radiological investigation will be normal.

Hepatic jaundice: In this jaundice the basic defect lies in the hepatocytes. These hepatocytes are responsible for capturing, conjugating, and excreting the bilirubin in the bile. So, defect in any of the three above processes may produce hepatic jaundice. If there is any defect in the UDP-glucuronosyltransferase, there will be defect in conjugation due to abnormal mutation of the gene present in the chromosome number 2, and there will be jaundice. Similarly any defect in the bile acid dependent and bile acid-independent secretion lead to defective secretion into biliary canaliculi. So, causes are:

A. Congenital causes:
- **a.** Wilson's disease
- **b.** Rotor syndrome
- **c.** Crigler-Najjar syndrome
- **d.** Dubin-Johnson syndrome
- **e.** Gilbert syndrome
- **f.** Hemochromatosis

B. Acquired causes:
- **a.** Hepatitis—viral, alcoholic, autoimmune, and drug-related
- **b.** Sepsis
- **c.** Pregnancy
- **d.** Malnutrition
- **e.** Systemic disease—celiac disease
- **f.** Hepatic adenoma

In above cases the clinical presentations are the following:

A. Sex predilection—mainly in males—hemochromatosis because it does not occur in female usually because of menstruation

B. Jaundice from birth in all congenital diseases, except Wilson's disease and hemochromatosis

C. Abdominal pain, nausea, and vomiting—viral hepatitis, alcoholic hepatitis, hemochromatosis, and pregnancy

D. Severe infection in any organ with septicemia—sepsis

E. Malabsorption, chronic diarrhea with progressive weight loss, and steatorrhea—celiac disease

F. History of exposure, such as blood transfusion, hair cutting in salon, tattooing, needle prick—viral hepatitis

G. History intake of alcohol for long duration—alcoholic hepatitis

H. History of jaundice developed during pregnancy—pregnancy-induced hepatitis

I. Blackening of the skin—hemochromatosis

J. History of abnormal tremor, neuropsychiatric manifestation—Wilson's disease

K. History of intolerance to rye, wheat, and cereals—celiac disease.

L. Physical examination:
1. Anemia—alcoholic hepatitis and celiac disease
2. High temperature—sepsis
3. Wasting—celiac disease
4. Lymphadenopathy—viral hepatitis and sepsis
5. Slate-gray pigmentation mainly in groins, axilla, genitalia, and already present scar due to deposition of excess melanin in the basal layer—hemochromatosis
6. Eye findings:
   - Greenish brown corneal KF ring present in the periphery of the iris
   - Sun flower cataract in the posterior of lens capsule—Wilson's disease

M. Liver:
- **a.** Enlarged tender soft to firm smooth liver—viral and alcoholic hepatitis
- **b.** Liver shrunken—Wilson's disease
- **c.** Enlarged firm tender liver—hemochromatosis
- **d.** Splenomegaly—hemochromatosis and viral hepatitis

N. Ascites—hemochromatosis, any causes of fulminant hepatic failure

O. Hematological investigations:
- **a.** Low hemoglobin—celiac disease and alcoholism
- **b.** WBC count—raised or <3,000/cc with polymorphonuclear leukocytosis—sepsis

P. Biochemical investigations:
- **a.** Increased conjugate bilirubin in presence of other features of liver function test normal—congenital liver disease

b. High bilirubin with more conjugate function, with high liver enzymes and ALP level—viral hepatitis and alcoholic hepatitis
c. High serum bilirubin with moderately high serum enzymes—hemochromatosis
d. Serum iron increased, transferrin concentration/ total iron-binding capacity, and high serum ferritin—hemochromatosis
e. Normal transferrin saturation with high serum ferritin—inflammation, hepatic steatosis, and alcohol excess
f. Low serum ceruloplasmin and high 24 hours urinary copper—Wilson's disease

Q. Other tests:
a. Serum anti-tissue transglutaminase (tTG) antibody IgA and compare with serum IgA—Celiac disease
b. Serum antiendomysial antibody—high in celiac disease
c. Hepatitis B surface antigen (HBsAg)—high titer, HBeAg—HBV
d. HCV antibody—HCV-related hepatitis

R. Ultrasonography:
a. Increased size of liver with increased splenic size—viral hepatitis and alcoholic hepatitis

S. Biopsy:
a. Liver biopsy:
1. Completely normal—congenital disease
2. Panlobular infiltration of mononuclear cells, Kupffer cell hyperplasia, necrosis of hepatic cells, variable degree of cholestasis—viral hepatitis
3. Increased fat globules in perivenular hepatocytes, distortion of hepatocytes by perivenular cells, giant mitochondria, perivenular fibrosis—alcoholic hepatitis
4. Accumulation of iron in liver cells as diagnosed by visual scoring system when it is stained by Perl's reagent.

b. Intestinal biopsy in celiac disease:
1. Increased number of intraepithelial lymphocytes
2. Flattening of the villi with increased cryptic cell proliferation
3. Nuclei are cuboidal in appearance
4. Increased number of lymphocytes and plasma cells in lamina propria.

Posthepatic Disease

Causes of Posthepatic Jaundice

A. Congenital disease:
a. Biliary atresia
b. Cystic fibrosis
c. Pancreatic biliary malfunction

B. Acquired causes:
a. Cholecystitis with or without choledocholithiasis
b. Pancreatitis
c. Trauma
d. Strictures
e. Tumor
f. Common bile duct (CBD) obstruction
g. Primary biliary cirrhosis

Clinical Presentation

Main presentations are:

A. Female sex—primary biliary cirrhosis
B. Clay-colored stool
C. Progressively increasing jaundice
D. Dark urine
E. Generalized pruritus
F. Fever, biliary colic, and abdominal pain—suggest cholecystitis with or without cholangitis along with cholangitis
G. Painless jaundice, abdominal mass—pancreatic carcinoma.

Physical Signs

A. Anemia—malignancy
B. Whole body will be yellow colored with scratch marks all over the body but mainly on limbs.
C. Clubbing—sclerosing cholangitis
D. Grey Turner sign and Cullen sign positive—acute pancreatitis
E. Shining nails—in all obstructive jaundice
F. Right upper quadrant area—tender
G. Whole abdomen tender—acute pancreatitis

Investigations

A. Hematological features:
a. Anemia—malignancy
b. Raised WBC with polymorphonuclear leukocytosis—acute pancreatitis and acute cholecystitis

B. Biochemistry:
  a. Liver function test:
    1. Raised bilirubin with highly increased conjugate fraction with mildly elevated liver enzymes but highly raised ALP—obstructive jaundice of any etiology
    2. Highly increased serum amylase and lipase—acute pancreatitis

C. Others:
  a. Cancer biomarkers like CA 19.9—high in pancreatic and biliary cancer

D. Radiology:
  a. Radiopaque round material in CBD—choledocholithiasis
  b. Increased echogenic pancreas with dilatation of lower end of CBD—acute pancreatitis, pancreatic carcinoma, and stone in lower end of CBD
  c. Magnetic resonance cholangiopancreatography (MRCP) of hepato-pancreatico-biliary region—acute pancreatitis, pancreatic carcinoma, and stone in lower end of CBD

Q6. Biosynthetic function of liver.

BF/MAY/2011/MDI (9)

ANSWER

Liver is the main source of synthesis of albumin, fibrinogen, and other coagulation factors and α and β globulins. But commonly measured synthetic functions of liver are albumin and PT.

Albumin: It is exclusively synthesized by liver. Normal value in the serum is 3.5–4.5 g/dL. Liver synthesizes 15 g/day or 200 mg/kg/day. Approximately 300–500 g of albumin has distributed in the body fluids. Its half-life of albumin is approximately 20 days. Its synthesis is regulated by following factors:

A. Inflammation
B. Osmotic pressure
C. Nutritional status
D. Hormone level

Mechanism of albumin synthesis is unknown. But synthesis of albumin is related to formation of albumin messenger RNA called polysomes.

The factors that stimulate each ribosome to bind with albumin mRNA to form polysomes increase albumin synthesis. These are:

A. Amino acids, such as tryptophan, phenylalanine, glutamine and lysine, and arginine
B. Ornithine will be converted to polyamine spermine thus increases polysomes formations
C. Corticosteroid
D. Thyroid hormone

Last two hormones increase the formation of polysomes transferring the increased concentration of albumin mRNA into hepatocytes by decreasing their degradation or increasing their synthesis.

Factors decrease the synthesis of albumin:

A. Heavy alcohol ingestion
B. Chronic inflammation

Serum albumin level is normal in:

A. Viral hepatitis
B. Drugs-related hepatotoxicity
C. Obstructive jaundice

Serum albumin level of <3 g/dL is found in:

A. Chronic liver disease
B. Cirrhosis

Ascites is the one condition where albumin synthesis is normal but serum level will be low due to its increased volume of distribution.

Prothrombin Time

Clotting is the complex interaction of 13 clotting factors through intrinsic and extrinsic pathways, amongst 13 factors, 11 factors are synthesized by liver. These are:

A. Factor I—Fibrinogen
B. Factor II—Prothrombin
C. Factor V—Labile factor
D. Factor VII—Stable factor
E. Factor IX—Plasma thromboplastin component, Christmas factor
F. Factor X—Stuart factor
G. Factor XII—Prekallikrein
H. Factor XIII—High-molecular-weight kininogen

Prothrombin time is the measuring method of choice where action of number of factors, such as factor I, II, V, VII, and X, is measured. It will measure the rate of conversion time of prothrombin to thrombin in presence of the above activated factors in presence of tissue extract, calcium ions. Result is declared in seconds as compared to control. Normal control is usually 9–11 seconds. If the PT is >2 seconds, it is considered as abnormal and if it is >4 seconds, it may be considered as severe liver disease.

Vitamin K helps addition of carboxylic acid in the gamma position of glutamic acid residues of factor II, V, VII, and X. Again these proteins bind to calcium ion avidly in the gamma-carboxylation step of post-translational process. Vitamin K antagonist, absence of vitamin K, and hepatocellular carcinoma (HCC) inhibit vitamin K-dependent carboxylation and release of des-γ-carboxy prothrombin, an abnormal prothrombin in the serum. Serum concentration of des-γ-carboxy prothrombin is very useful in case of HCC but it do not correlate with alpha-fetoprotein (AFP) in HCC. The level of des-γ-carboxy prothrombin will be decreased with the excision of tumor and increased with the recurrence of tumor.

Following factors decrease the vitamin K level which can be restored within 24 hours by single injection of vitamin K:

A. Inadequate dietary intake

B. Obstructive jaundice

C. Steatorrhea

D. Malabsorption

E. Administration of antibiotics altering the gut flora

Following factors decrease the vitamin K level which cannot be restored by injection of vitamin K:

A. Severe chronic liver disease

Prognosis of the condition of patient can be correlated with the magnitude of elevation of vitamin K:

A. Elevation of PT of >5 seconds above control suggests fulminant hepatic failure in patient suffering from acute viral or alcoholic or toxic hepatitis.

B. If PT is >100 seconds above normal, it suggests urgent liver transplantation.

C. If the patient suffers from acetaminophen overdose he can recover from it in spite of raise PT.

International Normalized Ratio

International normalized ratio standardizes PT based on characteristic of thromboplastin reagent that is used in different laboratory. It is used to express the level of anticoagulation who has been receiving warfarin. But INR is not the best expression of irregularity of coagulation in patients with liver failure where the same thromboplastin is not consistently used for the measurement.

Q7. Portal vein anatomy and classification of portal hypertension.

MUHS/MAY2009/MDI (10)

SNMC/MAY2013/MDIII (10)

Classify portal hypertension. Enumerate the causes of extrahepatic portal hypertension.

MGR/APR2012/MDIV (10)

Applied anatomy of portal vein, definition, causes and complications of portal hypertension.

MANIPUR UNIVERSITY, 2024 (10)

Complications of portal hypertension has been described in the question number 37.

ANSWER

Anatomy of Portal Vein

Embryologically, portal venous system develops in 4th to 12th gestational week from vitelline venous system which is in close relation with umbilical venous system. Over time there selective involution of venous network, as a result dorsal and cranial-ventral vitelline system anastomoses leading to rise of main and left portal veins.

Anatomically

Splenic vein arises as five to six tributaries taking the blood from spleen unite and form single tortuous vessel which runs in the posterior abdominal wall along the groove in the upper part of pancreas. During its course it collects small branches from the pancreas. In the groove splenic vein combines with superior mesenteric vein at right angle to form portal vein anterior to inferior vena cava and posterior to pancreatic neck, ascends upward and to the right within hepatoduodenal ligament posterior to hepatic artery and CBD to reach hilum where it will be divided into right and left portal vein before entering the portal fissure.

A. Longer and smaller left branch of portal vein joins with umbilical vein and paraumbilical vein runs horizontally for some distance then turns upward to supply Couinaud segments of the liver (I, II, III, and IV).

B. Right branch of portal vein is short and thick receives cystic vein, divides into two branches:

- **a.** Anterior branch supplies hepatic segments V and VIII
- **b.** Posterior branch supplies hepatic segment VI and VII

Other branches of portal vein are left and right gastric vein, cystic vein, and Sappey vein.

Inferior vena cava joins splenic and superior mesenteric vein or at the joining area in 40%, 40% and 20% cases, respectively.

Within the liver portal vein will be divided into smallest tributaries which are present in the portal triad with hepatic artery and bile duct in the periportal zone.

Ultimately, all the portal venules join to form hepatic vein which will drain to inferior vena cava.

Superior mesenteric vein receives blood from following organs:

A. Small intestine
B. Cecum
C. Right colon
D. Right two-thirds of transverse colon
E. Head of the pancreas
F. Stomach via right gastroepiploic vein

Splenic vein receives tributaries from following organs:

A. Head of the pancreas
B. Left gastroepiploic vein

Inferior mesenteric vein receives blood from following organs:

A. Left one-third of transverse colon
B. Descending colon
C. Sigmoid colon
D. Rectum

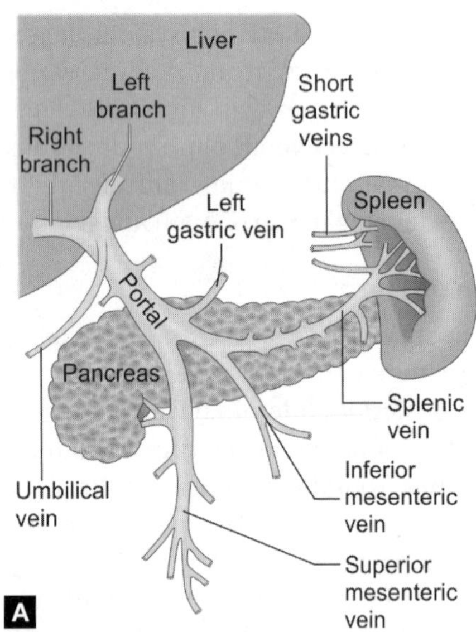

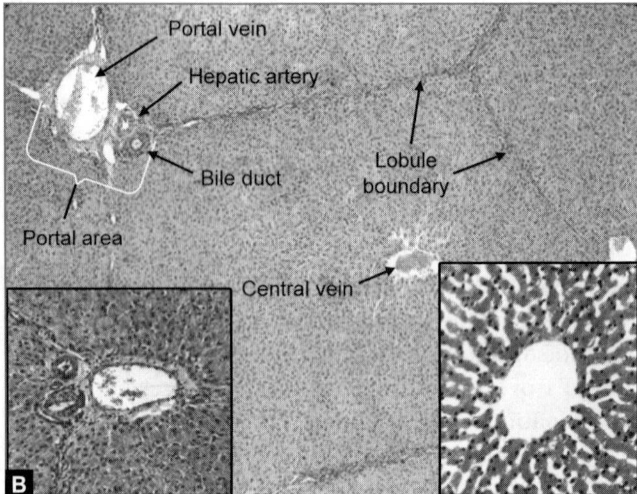

Anatomical Variation and Congenital Variation of Portal Vein

Common anatomical variants include:

A. Trifurcation of main portal vein—left portal vein, right anterior portal vein, and right posterior portal vein.
B. Main portal vein divides into right posterior portal vein and common trunk which is divided into left portal vein and right anterior portal vein.

The above anomalies may be associated with duplication of portal vein, annular pancreas which can produce duodenal obstruction.

Classification of Portal Hypertension

Portal hypertension can be defined as constellation of features due to increased pressure in portal vein above 10–12 mm Hg.

Portal hypertension can be divided in to following:

A. Presinusoidal hypertension:
   a. Presinusoidal extrahepatic causes:

1. Infections: It will spread from umbilical vein to left portal vein then to main portal vein. Infections come from:
   - Acute appendicitis
   - Ulcerative colitis
   - Crohn's disease
   - Biliary obstruction
2. Postoperative thrombosis:
   - It occurs mainly after splenectomy. It spreads to main portal vein.
   - Occlusion of portosystemic shunt
   - Difficult biliary surgery
3. Trauma: It occurs following accident and stabbing.
4. Hypercoagulable state: It is responsible for portal venous thrombosis as a consequence of following factors:
   - Myeloproliferative disorders
   - Presence of G20210A prothrombin gene mutation
   - Deficiency of protein C, S, and antithrombin III

5. Invasion and compression:
   - Carcinoma from the body of pancreas and adjacent organ
   - Chronic pancreatitis: It produces splenic vein obstruction.
6. Cirrhosis:
   - Invasion from HCC
   - Postsplenectomy thrombocytosis
7. Congenital:
   - Obstruction present along the line of right and left vitelline veins.
   - In absence of portal vein, visceral venous blood will return to systemic veins directly.
8. Miscellaneous:
   - Pregnancy
   - Long use of oral contraceptives in case of old women
   - Thrombophlebitis migrans

b. *Pre-sinusoidal intrahepatic portal hypertension*:
   1. Schistosomiasis: It occurs due to reaction of ova in the minute portal venous system.
   2. Congenital hepatic fibrosis: It occurs due to deficiency of terminal branches of portal vein in the area of fibrotic portal zones.
   3. Myeloproliferative disorders: These occur due to hematopoietic tissue infiltration of the portal zones.
      - Myeloid leukemia
      - Hodgkin's disease
   4. Systemic mastocytosis:
      - Due to mast cell infiltration there is increased intrahepatic resistance.
      - Due to histamine release there is increased splenic blood flow.
   5. Primary biliary cirrhosis is due to portal zone lesion with narrowing of sinusoid.
   6. Toxic causes: The agents are vinyl chloride, copper, and inorganic arsenic. These fibrogenic toxic substances are taken up by hepatic stellate cells and Disse's space.
   7. Cytotoxic drugs, such as methotrexate, 6-mercaptopurine, and azathioprine

c. *Intrahepatic sinusoidal hypertension*: Cirrhosis

d. *Postsinusoidal intrahepatic hypertension*:
   1. Veno-occlusive disease
   2. Thrombosis
   3. Congenital web
   4. Invasion by the tumor

e. Post-sinusoidal extrahepatic hypertension:
   1. Inferior venacaval occlusion:
      - Web
      - Tumor
      - Budd–Chiari syndrome
      - Invasion by tumor
   2. Heart causes:
      - Constrictive pericarditis
      - Right heart failure

Complications of Portal Hypertension

A. Gastroesophageal varices leading to bleeding
B. Hypersplenism
C. Ascites
D. Spontaneous bacterial peritonitis
E. Hepatic encephalopathy
F. Hepatorenal syndrome
G. Hepatopulmonary syndrome

Q8. HBsAg positive mother during pregnancy.

MJPRU/2015/MDIII (15)

ANSWER

Effect of Pregnancy on Natural Course of HBV Infection

If the pregnant mother is HBsAg positive, she is susceptible to be attacked by delta group of virus and this virus can be transmitted to the fetus from mother leading to development of severe hepatitis. The course of HBV infection may be present in any of the four phases:

A. Immune tolerant (HBeAg positive, HBV DNA > 200,000 IU/mL)
B. Immune active phase (HBeAg positive, HBV DNA ≥ 20,000 IU/mL)
C. Inactive chronic hepatitis (HBeAg negative, HBV DNA low or undetectable)
D. Reactivation phase (HBeAg negative, HBV DNA ≥ 2,000 IU/mL)

Physiological changes in pregnancy as a result of altered immune activity can also affect the natural history of HBV infection. There may be increase in flare of HBV infection in postpartum period rather than pregnancy. This flare may be mild but in case of preexisting liver disease or liver fibrosis flare may be so severe that she may enter into the stage of decompensated hepatic failure.

Impact of HBV Infection in Pregnancy

A. In case of chronic HBV infection in pregnancy there is increased risk of:

- **a.** Miscarriage
- **b.** Gestational diabetes
- **c.** Preterm labor
- **d.** Maternal and fetal morbidity and mortality in advanced liver disease in the form of:
  - **1.** Decreased fertility due to frequent occurrence of anovulatory cycles
  - **2.** Amenorrhea
  - **3.** Spontaneous abortion
- **e.** Increased level of cytokines IL-2, IL-6, IL-10, TNF-α, and macrophage migration inhibitory factor produce adverse event in these patients.

B. In case of patient with cirrhosis there is risk of:

- **a.** Perinatal complications
- **b.** Poor pregnancy outcomes:
  - Intrauterine infection
  - Uterine growth retardation
  - Premature delivery
  - Intrauterine fetal death

Investigations in HBV-related Chronic Liver Disease Affected Pregnant Patients

Some symptoms such as fatigue and abdominal pain are present and isolated during pregnancy. Again clinical signs such as palmar erythema, spider angioma, and edema are present also in third trimester of pregnancy, few laboratory parameters such as protein, albumin, and ALP also physiologically altered in pregnancy.

Like other immune-mediated diseases during pregnancy there is less activity of hepatitis virus but after delivery there will be significant flare up of chronic hepatitis B. So, presumptive diagnoses during pregnancy can be diagnosed and are based on following information, such as:

A. Duration of the disease

B. Past history of disease

C. Blood tests like, platelets and ALT

D. Status of HBeAg

E. Viral load

F. Noninvasive imaging

G. In case of advanced liver disease upper gastrointestinal endoscopy to diagnose portal hypertension

H. Noninvasive liver fibrosis tests like fibroscan and AST-to-platelet ratio index can be done but cannot be validated.

Mother to Child Transmission

There are three modes of transmission:

A. Prenatal or transplacental transmission:

- **a.** Leakage of maternal blood due to disruption of placental barrier by uterine contraction
- **b.** As a result of presence of HBV DNA in the sperm or oocyte there may be infection at the time of conception.
- **c.** Ascent of intrauterine transmission of vaginal secretion from HBV-infected mother.

In this type of transmission the child can born with HBV markers in spite of getting immunoglobulin and vaccination with HBV.

B. Natal infection is due to exposure of maternal blood, vaginal, or cervical secretions at the time of child birth. So, elective cesarean section prior to membrane rupture or before labor is performed.

C. Postnatal transmission: It may occur in case of postnatal care and breastfeeding. But this is negligible if the child receives immunoprophylaxis already.

In case of pregnant women:

A. If mother is HBeAg negative with hepatitis B infection + low viral load—transmission rate is 10% to child without immunoprophylaxis at birth.

B. If mother is HBeAg positive with hepatitis B infection + high viral load—transmission rate in child is 90% without immunoprophylaxis at birth.

C. Mother with high viral load—transmission rate to child is very high even after immunoprophylaxis.

Mother to child transmission can be prevented by following methods:

A. HBsAg screening in all pregnant women in first trimester:

- **a.** If it is negative—they should be vaccinated at once.
- **b.** If it is positive—HBeAg, HBV DNA, and liver function tests should be done.

B. Immunization in infants born to HBsAg positive mother:

- **a.** About 0.5 mL/kg hepatitis B immunoglobulin (HBIg) should be given to all the children within 12 hours of birth in different sites followed by two doses at 1 and 6 months.
- **b.** In case of preterm infants (<2 kg) first dose of vaccine usually is not included in the vaccine schedule due to its low immunogenicity of that dose. So in this case total 4 doses have to be administered.

At the age of 9–18 months HBsAg and anti-HBs tests have to be done:

a. If anti-HBs is >10 mIU/mL, these children are considered as protected from HBV.

b. If anti-HBs is <10 mIU/mL, they have to be vaccinated again after 1–2 months of final dose.

C. In case of infants born to female with unknown HBsAg status: Blood of the mother has to be sent for HBsAg and in the meantime children have to be vaccinated without HVIg within 12 hours of birth.

a. If the mother is HBsAg positive, HBIg and HBV vaccine according to schedule should be administered to new born child within 7 days after birth.

b. If the mother is HBsAg negative, HBV vaccine has to be completed according to schedule.

Management of HBV Infection in Pregnancy

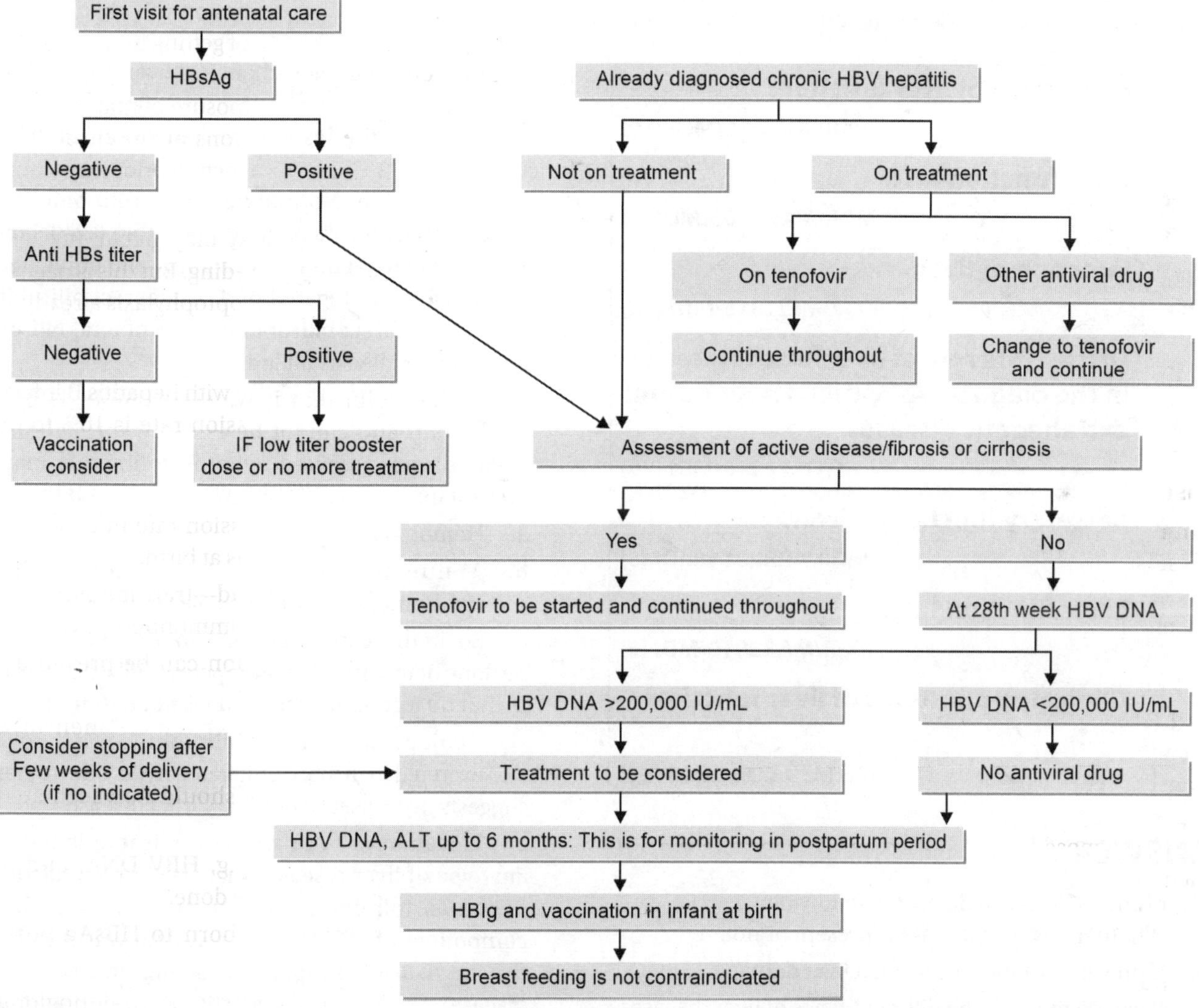

Treatment options during pregnancy:

Drug and dose	Indication	Pregnancy category	Side effects	Risk of resistance
Pegylated interferon-α	HBeAg positive or negative but HBV positive, compensated disease	No data	Flu-like syndrome, cytopenias, autoimmune disorders	Low
Lamivudine 100 mg/day	Chronic HBV but active viral replication, liver inflammation	No data	Pancreatitis, lactic acidosis	High

Continued

Continued

Drug and dose	Indication	Pregnancy category	Side effects	Risk of resistance
Telbivudine 600 mg/day	Chronic HBV but active viral replication	No data but can be used for its potential benefit	Myopathy, CPK elevation, lactic acidosis	Moderate
Entecavir 0.5 mg/day	Chronic HBV but active viral replication	No data	Lactic acidosis	Low in HBV native
Adefovir 10 mg/day	Chronic HBV hepatitis	No data	Nephropathy, Fanconi syndrome, lactic acidosis	Moderate
Tenofovir 300 mg/day	Chronic HBV hepatitis	No data but can be used for its potential benefit	Nephropathy, Fanconi syndrome, lactic acidosis	Low

(CPK: creatine phosphokinase; HBeAg: hepatitis B e antigen; HBV: hepatitis B virus)

Q9. Evaluation of liver function.

MJPRU/2015/MDI (10)

Liver function test.

MGR/MAR2009/MDI (5)

Function of liver.

GMC/2015/MDI (10)

Discuss the role of liver function tests in the diagnosis of various hepatic and extrahepatic diseases.

BF/OCT2010/MDI (25)

Secretary function of liver.

MGR/APR2016/MDI (5)

Liver function test.

MGR/MAR2010/MDI (5)

Clinical applications of liver function test.

SCB MED COL, 2018 (10)

ANSWER

Liver function test can detect the following:

A. Whether any liver disease is present or not.

B. If present, what is the extent if liver damage.

C. It can distinguish the different types of liver diseases.

D. It can also demonstrate the follow-up of the treatment of the liver disease by serial estimation.

Liver function test is neither specific nor sensitive, because in case serious liver disease this test may be normal, again abnormal test may not reflect the presence of liver disease. It can specify whether this disease is hepatocellular or obstructive. To evaluate liver function a battery of tests has to be done. If more than one tests are persistently abnormal then chance of liver disease is very high.

Following are the tests to be done to evaluate liver function:

A. Serum bilirubin: Normal level of serum bilirubin is 1–1.5 mg% with 95% patients fall within 0.2–0.9 mg%. There are two fractions of bilirubin—unconjugated or indirect and conjugated of direct. Direct bilirubin is 0.3 mg%. If direct bilirubin is <15% of total bilirubin, bilirubin is called as all indirect.

Indirect bilirubin is water insoluble, is bound to albumin and cannot be excreted through urine. Isolated unconjugated hyperbilirubinemia may be present in:

a. Hemolysis

b. A number of genetic conditions, Gilbert syndrome, and Crigler–Najjar disease

So, in this case total work-up of hemolysis has to be done before it will be stamped as Gilbert syndrome, in that no further investigation is not required.

Conjugated or direct bilirubin is water soluble and excreted in urine. Conjugated hyperbilirubinemia suggests liver disease or biliary tract disease.

Elevation of both types of bilirubin is found in any type of liver disease, such as viral and alcoholic hepatitis, fulminant hepatic failure. Again it is a component of MELD scoring system which estimate the survival of the patient having end-stage liver disease.

Again, bilirubin in urine is found in case of liver disease. Urine dip-stick can detect it and it is 100% accurate. It can also estimate the recovery of patient as urine bilirubin clears prior to clearing of serum bilirubin.

B. Serum enzymes: There are thousands of enzymes secreted by liver and they are present in the serum in low concentration but their process of catabolism is not known. These enzymes are divided into two categories:

a. Enzymes secreted by the hepatocytes: These are ALT and AST. AST is found in following organ in decreasing order of concentration:
  1. Liver
  2. Cardiac muscle
  3. Skeletal muscle
  4. Kidneys
  5. Brain
  6. Pancreas
  7. Lung
  8. Leukocytes
  9. Erythrocytes

  Alanine aminotransferase is primarily found in liver. It is released in large concentration in case of liver cell injury due to increased permeability but not due to liver cell necrosis, but there is no positive correlation between the level of aminotransferase and extent of liver disease and hence its absolute elevation is of no prognostic significance in hepatocellular damage.

  Normal range of these enzymes is 10–40 IU/L, but there is interlaboratory variation due to technical reasons.

  Elevation of aminotransferases to 300 IU/L is nonspecifically in any type of liver disorders. If these are >1,000 IU/L, it suggests following causes producing extensive hepatocellular injury:

  1. Viral hepatitis
  2. Ischemic liver damage due to prolonged hypotension or acute right heart failure
  3. Drug- or toxin-induced liver injury

  In case of alcoholic liver disease AST level rarely >300 IU/L but ALT level is low due to alcohol-induced deficiency of pyridoxal phosphate.

  Again, pattern of rise in aminotransferases are diagnostic type of liver damage:

  1. AST:ALT <1—
     - Chronic viral hepatitis
     - Nonalcoholic fatty liver disease (NAFLD)
  2. If AST:ALT >1—suggests cirrhosis
  3. If AST:ALT 2:1 to 3:1—It suggests alcoholic liver disease.

  In acute phase of biliary obstruction due to passage of gallstone in the CBD these enzymes rise up to 2,000 IU/L transiently but it will decrease quickly.

b. Enzymes which reflect cholestasis: Three enzymes are elevated in cholestasis, these are:
  1. Alkaline phosphatase
  2. 5′-nucleotidase
  3. Gamma-glutamyl transferase

  First two are secreted from near the canalicular membrane and last one is secreted from bile duct epithelial cells and is located in endoplasmic reticulum thus less specific for cholestasis.

Alkaline phosphatase has many isoenzymes that are found in:

  1. Liver
  2. Bone
  3. Placenta
  4. Small intestine

In case of healthy individual:

  1. Patient over the age of 60 years
  2. Patient with blood group O and B: In these patients there is secretion of ALP from the intestine after intake of fatty meal.
  3. Adolescent during rapid bone growth
  4. In case late phase of pregnancy due to increased secretion from the placenta.

In case of isolated elevation of ALP in apparently healthy patient two following methods has to be undertaken:

  1. Fractionation of ALP by electrophoresis
  2. Measurement of GGT and 5′-nucleotidase—because elevation of these enzymes is found in liver disease.

Following diseases are responsible for elevation of ALP:

  1. Early cholestasis
  2. Hepatic infiltration by tumors or granuloma
  3. Hodgkin's disease
  4. Diabetes
  5. Hyperthyroidism
  6. Congestive heart failure
  7. Inflammatory bowel disease
  8. Sarcoidosis
  9. AIDS: In this disease it is greatly elevated due to:
     - *Cryptosporidium* infection
     - Cytomegalovirus infection

  Alkaline phosphatase elevation cannot differentiate between intrahepatic and extrahepatic cholestasis.

Tests measuring the synthetic function of liver:

A. Albumin: It is exclusively synthesized by hepatocytes, half-life is 18–20 days.

- **a.** It is not a good indicator of mild hepatocyte injury.
- **b.** It is minimally decreased in acute viral hepatitis, drug-induced hepatic injury, and obstructive jaundice.
- **c.** If it is <3 g/dL, it indicates chronic liver disease reflecting severe liver damage.

Other causes of hypoalbuminemia are the following:

- **a.** Nephrotic syndrome
- **b.** Protein-losing enteropathy
- **c.** Protein energy malnutrition
- **d.** Chronic infection with:
  1. Increased level of serum IL-1
  2. Increased TNF
  3. Cytokines those inhibit albumin synthesis
- **e.** Ascites: Here though albumin synthesis is normal or increased but serum level will be decreased due to increased volume of distribution.

B. Globulins: Globulins are composed of:

- **a.** γ-globulin (immunoglobulin): It is formed from B lymphocytes. It is increased in cirrhosis and chronic hepatitis due to increased synthesis of antibodies directing toward intestinal bacteria. It happens because bacterial antigen is failed to be cleared by cirrhotic liver when it reaches liver through hepatic circulation.
- **b.** β-globulin: It is produced by hepatocytes.

Isotypes of γ-globulins are increased in different conditions:

- **a.** Polyclonal IgG is increased in AIH
- **b.** IgM is increased in primary biliary cirrhosis
- **c.** IgA is increased in alcoholic liver disease.

Coagulation Factors

All the coagulation factors except factor V (which is synthesized by vascular endothelial cells) are synthesized in liver. Due to their short half-life, their measurement is single best indicator of:

- **a.** Measurement of hepatic synthetic function
- **b.** Diagnosis and assessment of prognosis of acute parenchymal liver disease

The test that measures the factor is PT. In this test factor II, V, VII, and X can be assessed. PT is elevated in:

- **a.** Viral hepatitis
- **b.** Cirrhosis
- **c.** Obstructive jaundice
- **d.** Fat malabsorption

In case of fulminant hepatic failure PT of >5 seconds above control cannot be corrected by injection of vitamin K. It is also component of MELD score to assess the level of hepatic decompensation.

International normalized ratio is used to measure the degree of anticoagulation after therapy with warfarin.

Other Diagnostic Tests

Ammonia

It is produced by protein metabolism by the intestinal bacteria. Ammonia then will be detoxified in the liver to form urea and in the skeletal muscles by combining it with the glutamic acid to glutamine. In case of cirrhosis with severe wasting ammonia level will be increased. There is poor correlation between presence and severity of liver disease and hepatic function and blood level of ammonia. In some cases of portal hypertension with portal shunting ammonia level will be elevated in presence of normal or near normal liver function.

Liver Biopsy

Percutaneous liver biopsy is the safe procedures in the following cases:

- **A.** Unexplained hepatomegaly
- **B.** Unexplained splenomegaly
- **C.** Prolonged hepatitis may be of autoimmune origin
- **D.** Hepatocellular carcinoma
- **E.** Hepatocellular disease of uncertain origin
- **F.** Fever of unknown etiology
- **G.** Staging of malignant lymphoma
- **H.** Radiologic imaging failed to characterize the hepatic lesion

Contraindications

- **a.** Significant ascites
- **b.** Prolonged INR

It should not be the first procedure in case of cholestasis.

Noninvasive Tests for Detecting Fibrosis

A. Fibrotest: It is a multiparameter test requiring haptoglobin, bilirubin, apolipoprotein A-1, GGT, and α_2-microglobulin. It can diagnose with high positive and negative predictive value in following cases:

- **a.** Chronic hepatitis C
- **b.** Chronic hepatitis B

c. Alcoholic liver disease
d. Patient taking methotrexate

B. Elastography: It measures the hepatic stiffness and advanced fibrosis in following cases:
   a. Chronic hepatitis C
   b. Nonalcoholic fatty liver disease
   c. Alcoholic liver disease
   d. Primary biliary cirrhosis
   e. Hemochromatosis
   f. Post-transplant recurrent chronic hepatitis

   There are three types of elastography:
   a. Vibration-controlled transient elastography (VCTE):
      1. It provides stiffness of the liver measured in kilopascals. Its detection in cirrhosis is both specific and sensitive. But its sensitivity is limited by thick chest wall, ascites.
      2. It provides two-dimensional view.
      3. It employs Young's elastic modulus.
   b. Magnetic resonance elastography:
      1. It provides three-dimensional views
      2. It uses shear elastic modulus.
      3. It is not confounded by body mass index (BMI).
   c. Acoustic radiation force impulse elastography:
      1. Here standard ultrasonography (USG) machine is retrofitted so that it will emit acoustic pulse to generate shear waves.
      2. It will provide two-dimensional image.
      3. Area coverage is smaller than that associated with VCTE.
      4. Inflammation is the main confounder but regarding BMI is not clear.

C. MRI: It can detect different stages of chronic active hepatitis.

D. Ultrasonography: This noninvasive procedure can identify the following cases:
   a. Presence of dilated intrahepatic or extrahepatic causes of biliary obstruction
   b. Identification of gallstones
   c. Identification of space-occupying lesions

E. Doppler ultrasound can identify:
   a. Patency of portal vein, hepatic vein, and artery
   b. Determination of direction of portal blood flow

F. Administration of 1–1.5 L intravenous fluid to treat prerenal azotemia.

G. To increase renal perfusion pressure low-dose dopamine is to be given. Continuous renal replacement therapy with bicarbonate buffer is given in case of hemodynamically stable patients to prevent ICP fluctuation.

Q10. Management of hepatitis B.

BF/MAY2013/MDII (10)

Immunopathogenesis of hepatitis B infection and management of chronic hepatitis B.

DNBII/JUN2010 (10)

Discuss the diagnosis and management of chronic hepatitis B infection.

DNBII/DEC2012 (10)

Antiviral therapy in hepatitis B.

MGR/APR2014/MDIII (7)

Classify hepatitis. Discuss in detail hepatitis B virus infection and add a note on hepatitis B vaccine.

MGR/SEP2010/MDII (20)

Bilirubin metabolism and a note on management of hepatitis B.

MGR/SEP2008/MDII (20)

Describe the structure of hepatitis B virus and the natural history of HBV infection. Describe the diagnosis, treatment and prevention of the infection.

MGR/APR2003/MDIII (25)

Australia antigen positive patient.

SNMC/MAY2005/MDIV (10)

Hepatitis B vaccination.

BF/MAY2011/MDII (13)

Hepatitis B—diagnosis and management.

BF/OCT2010/MDIII (10)

Discuss the serological markers in hepatitis B and their clinical significance.

BF/JUNE2016/MDIII (10)

Postexposure prophylaxis of Hepatitis B.
GMC/2016/MDI (5)

Plan for HBsAg positive patient.
MUZ/MAY2016/MDIV (10)

Hepatitis vaccination.
MGR/MAR2006/MDIII (5)

Extrahepatic complication of hepatitis B.
MGR/OCT2003/MDIII (5)

Acute hepatitis B infection: Virology and etiology, laboratory features and complications.
DNBIIIB/JUN2015 (10)

Describe pathophysiology, evaluation and management of hepatitis B induced chronic active hepatitis.
MUHS/NOV2014/MDII (25)

Clinical course of hepatitis B infection.
SNMC/MAY/2001/MDII (10)

Discuss the emerging trends in the drug treatment of chronic hepatitis B.
BF/MAY2011/MDIV (20)

Describe the pathogenesis of hepatitis B infection. List the various serological markers and their significance in clinical practice.
DNB (DEC 2020)(10)

Etiopathogenesis and management of hepatitis B infection.
DNB (DEC2018) (8)

Discuss the current concept of management of hepatitis B and C.
AIIMS, BBS, 2023 (10)

Investigations and treatment and complications of chronic hepatitis B infection.
SAURASHTRA UNI, 2022 (20)

Serological diagnosis and management of hepatitis B infection.
NTR UNI OF HEALTH SC, ANDHRA, 2022 (10)

Discuss the pathophysiology, clinical features, diagnosis and management of chronic hepatitis B.
KERALA UNI, 2021 (20)

Diagnosis and treatment of chronic hepatitis B infection.
BABA FARID UNI OF HEALTH SC, 2019 (10)

Discuss the approach to a patient with chronic hepatitis B infection including investigation and treatment.
BHARATI VIDYAPEETH DEEMED UNI, LHELAM, 2018 (15)

Describe genetic structure of hepatitis B virus. Write the causes of isolated hyperbilirubinemia.
MANIPUR UNIVERSITY, 2019 (10)

Describe the structure of hepatitis B virus. Write down the current treatment models of chronic hepatitis B infection.
MANIPUR UNIVERSITY, 2021 (10)

Discuss the serological markers in chronic hepatitis B. Outline the updated management.
WBUHS, 2020 (10)

Classification of hyperbilirubinemia has been described in question number 5.

Hepatitis C treatment has been discussed in question number 18.

ANSWER

Classification of Hepatitis

Acute Hepatitis

A. Viral hepatitis:
- **a.** Hepatitis A
- **b.** Hepatitis B
- **c.** Hepatitis C
- **d.** Hepatitis D

   e. Hepatitis E
   f. Hepatitis G
B. Nonviral hepatitis:
   a. Toxin-induced
   b. Drug-induced
   c. Alcoholic
   d. Nonalcoholic fatty liver disease
   e. Autoimmune diseases

Chronic Hepatitis

A. Chronic nonbiliary hepatitis:
   a. Autoimmune hepatitis
   b. Chronic B hepatitis
   c. Chronic B and D hepatitis
   d. Chronic C hepatitis
   e. Chronic drug hepatitis
   f. Wilson's disease
   g. Alpha-1 antitrypsin deficiency of liver
   h. Cryptogenic chronic hepatitis
B. Chronic biliary hepatitis:
   a. Primary biliary cirrhosis
   b. Primary sclerosing cholangitis
   c. Autoimmune cholangitis

Structure of Hepatitis B Virus

Complete virus particle is called Dane particle and is spherical lipid-containing double-shelled structure having diameter of 42 nm. Inner cell of this virus consists of icosahedral nucleocapsid assembled to form 120 dimers of core protein. This nucleocapsid is covered by three types of envelope proteins, namely, large (L), middle (M), and small (S), there are acquired together while it buds into endoplasmic reticulum. There are three surface proteins called HBsAg. They will translate from their own start codons but containing same C terminal amino acids known as S domain. M protein contains one extra domain, called "pre-S2" domain. On the other hand, S and L proteins contain two extra domain, known as pre-S1 and pre-S2.

Nucleocapsid contains one copy of HBV genome containing double-stranded relaxed circular DNA, it is linked with viral polymerase at the 5' end of complete strand, it is called viral minus strand DNA. During infection with HBV there is secretion of subviral particles containing empty viral envelope and empty virions consisting of outer envelope as well as inner capsid shell but devoid of viral genome. These subviral particles freely circulate in the blood and spread of virus by adsorbing viral neutralizing antibodies.

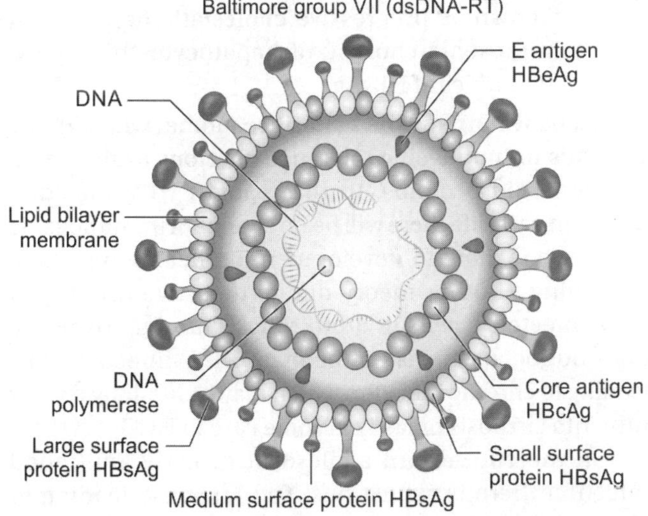

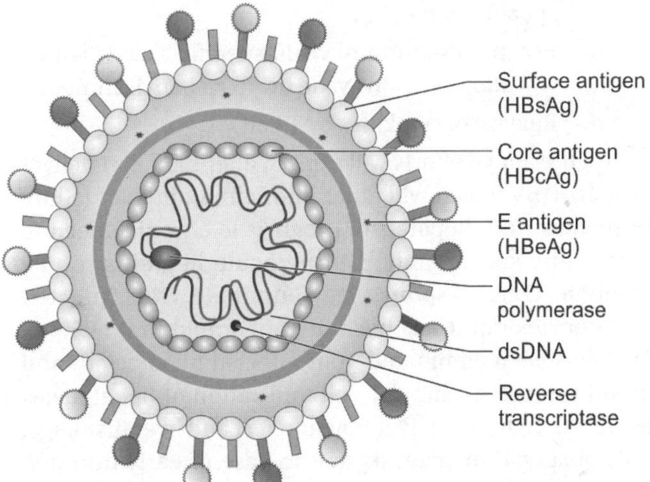

Viral polymerase is the main anchor during viral replication and it is divided into four main domains:

   a. TP (terminal protein) domain: It primes the reverse transcription and is very essential.
   b. RT (reverse transcriptase) domain: It contains the active site for polymerase and essential for viral polymerization.

c. RNase H domain: During minus strand DNA synthesis it is responsible for degradation of pregenomic RNA.
d. Spacer region: It is dispensable for all the required function of the enzyme.

Hepatitis B virus genome is also responsible encoding three nonstructural (NS) proteins:

a. HBeAg: It has immunoregulatory function.
b. X protein: It will initiate and maintain HBV transcription.
c. Hepatitis B spliced protein: It results from HBV messenger and RNA splicing. Its role in the pathogenesis of hepatitis is not exactly known.

Immunopathogenesis of Hepatitis B Virus

Hepatitis B virus is not directly cytopathic as evidenced by presence of normal liver histology, liver function in case of carriers. Cellular immune response is mainly responsible for chronic liver cell injury rather than clearing the HBV from the liver. Main target antigens, hepatitis B core antigen (HBcAg) and HBeAg, though present in minute quantities on the liver cell surface membrane along with host cell antigen will invite cytolytic T cells to destroy the infected liver cells. But the different responsiveness of CD8+ cytolytic cells in the form of polyclonality depends upon the following:

a. At the level of CD4+ T cells
b. Deletion, exhaustion, or attenuation of virus-specific liver cells
c. Escape mutation of virus-specific T cells which will allow virus to evade the T-cell environment
d. Release of cytokines by T cells

All the above efforts will explain after infection of liver cells by HBV which will enter into fulminant liver failure or recover from hepatitis or progress to chronic infection or chronic carrier state. During acute hepatitis robust cytolytic T-cell response may eliminate virus-infected hepatocytes but it has been demonstrated that >95% of HBV has been eliminated from infected hepatocytes and blood prior to maximal T-cell infiltration of hepatocytes as well as changes in liver function test and liver histology. This observation suggests that in case of early immune response to HBV infection both inflammatory cytokines and innate immunity will come into play independently without any relation with cytopathic antiviral mechanism, as result, HBV circular DNA from hepatocyte nucleus, and HBV intermediates from hepatocyte cytoplasm. Innate immune response works through natural killer (NK) cells being activated by following mechanism:

a. Immunosuppressive cytokines, such as IL-10 and transforming growth factor-β
b. Reduced or excitatory signals from inhibitory receptor expression on hepatocytes.

Natural killer cells:

a. Reduce helper CD4+ T cells leading to reduction of CD8+ cells
b. Exhaust virus-specific T-cell response in HBV infection.

Ultimately recovery from HBV infection results due to response of HBV-HLA (human leukocyte antigen)-specific cytolytic T cell of adaptive immune system.

Liver cell injury also depends upon viral factor as evidenced from following incidence:

a. Precore mutant of HBV may produce direct cytopathic effect on infected hepatocytes leading to development of fulminant hepatic failure or chronic hepatitis due to its relatively increased pathogenicity as compared to host.
b. If the hepatocytes are concomitantly infected with HDV and HBV, HDV damage infected hepatocytes by its direct cytopathic effect in absence of any host-specific immunogenic response.
c. If the liver is transplanted in case of end-stage chronic liver disease due to HBV and the patient is under immunosuppressive drugs to prevent allograft rejection, in the newly transplanted liver rapidly progressive injury appears leading to development of unusual histologic pattern, known as progressive cholestatic hepatitis—it represents choking of hepatocytes by a huge quantities of HBsAg.

If a baby born to HBeAg positive mother with chronic hepatitis immunogenic tolerance develops against both nucleocapsid proteins. In that baby if HBV infection occurs in early life there will be no chance of immunogenic clearance leading to development of lifelong infection. According to other theory due to defective priming of HBV-infected T cells in utero robust immune response does not occur in case of neonatal HBV infection thus leading to chronic infection which may be life-long or may turn into cirrhosis or lastly in some case to HCC.

On the contrary in adolescent or early adulthood infection there is robust host cell response leading to clearance of HBV-infected hepatocytes, so chronicity and incidence of HCC is low. Based on these above observations HBV infection can be divided into four phases:

a. Immunotolerant phase: In this phase:
    1. Presence of HBeAg in the blood
    2. High level of HBV DNA in the blood
    3. Normal ALT level

4. It typically occurs during perinatal and early childhood.
5. Absence of weak or no immune response.
6. Period last for 10–30 years—during this time there is very low rate of HBeAg seroconversion.
7. Very little hepatic injury
8. Prognosis is favorable in patients with spontaneous HBeAg seroconversion.

b. Immunoreactive phase (HBeAg positive chronic hepatitis): In this phase:
   1. It occurs during second to fourth decade of life and duration is few months to decades.
   2. Presence of HBeAg in the blood
   3. High of fluctuating level of HBV DNA in the blood.
   4. Occasionally high level of anti-HBc IgM.
   5. Presence of fluctuating or persistently high level of ALT due to:
      - Immune-mediated lysis of infected hepatocytes or
      - Distribution of HBcAg from nucleus to cytoplasm
   6. Liver histology shows active inflammation.

c. Inactive carrier phase: In this phase:
   1. There is seroconversion of HBeAg
   2. Very low (10^3 IU/mL) or undetectable level of HBV DNA
   3. Limited infectivity
   4. Normalization of serum ALT
   5. Reduction of microinflammation with regression of fibrosis in the liver histology.

Conversion from indolent phase to inactive carrier state occurs in 10% patients per year.

This phase can be diagnosed based on the presence of at least three normalization of serum ALT level and three HBV DNA level of <2,000 IU/mL during period of 12 months period. But if HBsAg level is <1,000 IU/mL during this period this phase can be declared as true inactive carrier phase.

d. Reactivation phase (HBeAg negative chronic hepatitis): In this phase:
   1. Absence of HBeAg in the serum
   2. Level of HBV DNA is 10^8–10^9 IU/mL
   3. Intermittently high level of ALT
   4. Inflammation in liver biopsy
   5. Hallmark of this phase is, it is fluctuating phase.
   6. In this phase patient develops more and more complications.
   7. This HBeAg negative chronic hepatitis is more common in people of genotype except Asia, Europe, and Mediterranean area. Histologic and biochemical activity in this case correlates with HBV DNA replication. This level of replication correlates with ultimate development of cirrhosis or HCC in both HBeAg positive or negative patients.

Antiviral therapy reduces the HBV DNA level to undetectable value in HBeAg negative patients and the patient will enter into inactive carrier state.

Natural History of HBV Infection

In Acute Infection

Incubation period is 30–180 days.

Prodromal period: Arthralgia-like syndrome manifested by fever and skin rash. But quite variable.

Constitutional symptoms: Anorexia, nausea, vomiting, arthralgia, fatigue, malaise, headache, myalgia, cough, pharyngitis, photophobia, and alteration of olfaction and taste.

Specific symptoms: Dark urine and clay stools and appearance of jaundice by 1–2 weeks, right upper quadrant pain. 70% patients present with anicteric hepatitis and 30% from icteric hepatitis only 1% develop fulminant hepatic failure.

In the icteric phase constitutional symptoms diminish but develop mild weight loss, right upper quadrant pain. On examination, there is jaundice, hepatomegaly, in some cases splenomegaly, in 10–20% patients cervical lymphadenopathy, and rarely few spider nevi. In early cholestatic phase, there is itching.

In the recovery phase of 2–12 weeks Constitutional symptoms disappear but some degree of hepatomegaly along with liver function test abnormalities.

Complete recovery occurs 3 to months after the onset of jaundice in 95–99% of cases and in the rest recovery will be delayed.

Laboratory Features

Liver function test:

a. In the prodromal phase: There is variable rise in transaminases within 400–4,000 IU/mL or more not correlating with liver damage but will decrease progressively during recovery.
b. Bilirubin will be raised to 5–20 mg/dL and it will continue to rise in spite of decrease in serum

transaminases. In the early phase, the conjugated fraction of bilirubin will be increased as it is the congestive phase, but in case of superimposed hemolysis, such as hemolytic anemia, total bilirubin will rise and in this case prognosis will be poor.

c. Alkaline phosphatase: It is raised in case of early congestive phase but later on it will decrease.
d. Serum albumin is normal.

Prothrombin time will be prolonged reflecting synthetic defect in liver from extensive hepatocellular necrosis.

Other biochemical test: Low blood sugar may occur from vomiting, inadequate intake of food along with poor glycogen reserve.

Hematological tests: There is neutropenia, lymphopenia with atypical lymphocyte in early phase, and transient lymphocytosis in late phase.

Urine microscopy may demonstrate hematuria and proteinuria.

Serological markers of HBV hepatitis: Diffuse mild elevation of γ-globulin with IgM and IgG occurs in acute viral hepatitis.

HBsAg is detected in the serum in early phase but in some cases it may be too low to be detected in the acute phase. But there is inverse relationship between serum concentration of HBsAg and the severity of hepatic damage, i.e., high level is found in immunosuppressive patients and low in case of chronic liver disease.

HBeAg is invariably present in early phase of acute hepatitis and it indicates relative infectivity. But it is usually done in chronic HBV infection. IgM anti-HBc is the only serological marker when HBsAg is not present and anti-HBs does not appear in the blood. This can reappear during the acute reactivation of chronic hepatitis B. It can be falsely positive in case of high titer of rheumatoid factor.

IgM anti-HBc can diagnose acute or recent infection but it is not present in chronic infection where *IgG anti-HBc* will be evident.

Anti-HBs is rarely present in presence of HBsAg but may be present in low titer in case of chronic infection. This antibody is detected against heterotypic subtype determinant, such as HBsAg of subtype ad with anti-HBs of subtype y.

HBV DNA: Its determination is quantitative and sensitive. It is detected by RT-PCR. In this method range of detection is between 5 and 10 IU/mL to largest dynamic range of 10^8—10^9 IU/mL. There is correlation between rise in HBV DNA and extent of hepatocyte damage. So, in case of immunocompetent patient increased expression of viral antigens, high level of HBV DNA, and necroinflammatory activity of hepatocytes because of cytolytic T-cell response to infected hepatocytes.

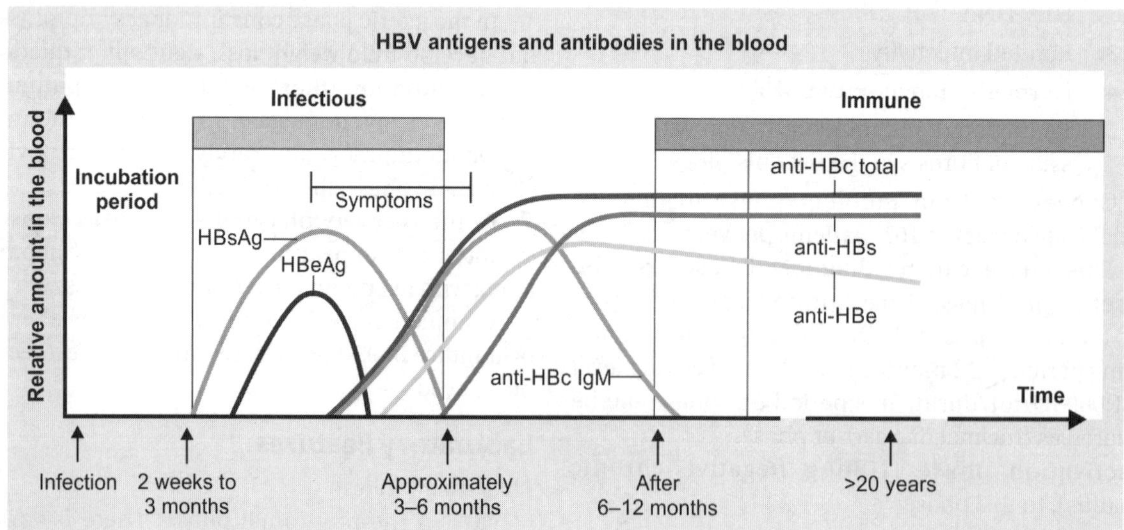

In Chronic Infection

Symptoms: In case of acute silent infection started at birth there is >90% chance of development of chronicity but in case of immunocompetent adolescent only <1% of acute hepatitis will enter into the chronicity. Most of the patients with chronic HBV hepatitis will never experience symptoms. Liver damage may be variable from none in case of inactive carrier to mild to moderate to severe. Most important is the degree of HBV replication.

Symptoms are intermittent deepening of jaundice, worsening of fatigue, anorexia, and recurrent malaise; these symptoms may coincide with viral replication.

Laboratory Features

Liver function test:

Bilirubin level is elevated to 3–10 mg/dL. Elevation of aminotransferases may range from 100–1,000 IU/mL. In case of acute viral hepatitis, ALT is greater than AST but it will be reverse in case of chronic hepatitis. ALP level is marginally elevated.

In case of late stage of chronic hepatitis, there will be hypoalbuminemia, and PT will be elevated. Hyperglobulinemia along with detectable autoantibodies are absent in chronic HBV hepatitis.

In the presence of HBeAg positive or HBeAg negative, chronic HBV hepatitis patient level of HBV DNA correlates with liver cell injury.

Treatment of Acute Hepatitis B

Ninety-nine percent patients suffering from acute hepatitis B infection will recover spontaneously, so there will be no requirement of antiviral therapy. But some authorities recommend most potent least resistant antiviral drug, tenofovir or entecavir for moderate or severe hepatitis. In these case treatment should be continued until:

A. 3 months after HBsAg seroconversion; or
B. 6 months after HBeAg seroconversion

Goal of Therapy for Chronic HBV Infection

A. To improve the disease-free survival
B. To improve the quality of life
C. To prevent progression of disease
D. To prevent the development of HCC
E. To prevent mother-to-child progression
F. To prevent hepatitis B reactivation
G. HBV-associated extrahepatic manifestation
H. To aggravate the regression of fibrosis and cirrhosis in patients with advanced fibrosis and cirrhosis.
I. In patient with HBV-induced HCC goal of nucleoside therapy to:
- **a.** To reduce viral replication
- **b.** To induce stabilization of HBV-induced liver disease
- **c.** To prevent the progression of the disease
- **d.** After curative therapy to reduce the recurrence of the disease.

Indications of Antiviral Therapy

A. Patients with chronic hepatitis B having HBeAg positive or HBeAg negative as defined by HBV DNA of >2,000 IU/mL and ALT level more than upper limit of normal and/or at least moderate liver microinflammation or fibrosis.

B. Decompensated or compensated cirrhosis with any level of DNA and regardless of ALT level.

C. Patient with HBV DNA level of >20,000 IU/mL and ALT level twice of upper limit if normal regardless of degree of fibrosis.

D. The patient of >30 years with HBe positive chronic HBV infection as defined by high HBV DNA level and normal ALT level regardless of the severity of histological lesion in the liver.

E. HBeAg positive or negative chronic hepatitis patient having family history of cirrhosis or HCC and extrahepatic manifestation even if nonfulfillment of typical treatment indication.

End-points of Therapy

A. Induction of long-term suppression of HBV DNA level

B. Induction of loss of HBeAg with or without seroconversion of anti-HBe in HBeAg positive chronic hepatitis B patient as it represents partial immune control of chronic hepatitis B infection.

C. Normalization of ALT level which is achieved in most of the patients with long-term suppression of replication of HBV.

D. Loss of HBsAg with or without seroconversion to anti-HBs is an end point as it indicates profound suppression of HBV DNA replication.

Following patients who are not getting treatment should be monitored:

A. Patients who are younger than 30 years, HBeAg positive, and has been suffering from chronic hepatitis B infection and do not fulfill above indications for treatment should be followed every 3–6 months at least.

B. Patients with chronic hepatitis B infection but HBeAg negative and serum HBV DNA level <2,000 IU/L and do not fulfill any above treatment indications should be followed every 6–12 months.

C. HBeAg negative chronic hepatitis B infected patients with HBV DNA ≥2,000 IU/mL who do not fulfill any above indication of treatment should be followed every 3 months for first year thereafter every 6 months.

Treatment Strategies

There are two main treatment options:

A. Interferon-α (IFN-α) currently known as pegylated interferon-α.

B. Nucleoside analogs: These drugs are further classified into two groups:

  a. Low barrier against HBV resistance—lamivudine, adefovir dipivoxil, and telbivudine

  b. High barrier against HBV resistance—tenofovir disoproxil, entecavir, and tenofovir alafenamide.

Features	Pegylated interferon	Nucleoside analog
Route	Subcutaneous	Orally
Duration of treatment	48 weeks	Till the loss of HBsAg
Tolerability	Low	High
Contraindications	Comorbidities, decompensated disease	Dose should be adjusted according to estimated glomerular filtration rate (eGFR)
Level of viral suppression	Moderate	Universally high
Effect on HBeAg loss	Moderate but it depends upon baseline	In first year low but it increases gradually with long-term treatment
Effect on HBsAg level	Moderate but it depends upon baseline	Low in the first year but gradually increases in HBeAg patient, but very low in case of HBeAg negative patients
Risk of relapse after completion of treatment	Low in case of sustained response for 6–12 months after cessation of treatment	Moderate if consolidation treatment is given after HBeAg seroconversion
Early stopping	Yes	No
Viral resistance	No	Minimal

Response can be divided into four types:

A. Virological response:

  a. In case of nucleoside therapy it can be defined as no detection of DNA with sensitive PCR having detection limit of 10 IU/mL.

    1. Primary response can be defined as less than one $\log_{10}$ IU/mL decrease in DNA in serum after 3 months of treatment

    2. Partial response can be defined as more than 1 $\log_{10}$ IU/mL decrease in DNA in serum but detectable DNA after 12 months of therapy.

    3. Virological breakthrough can be defined as confirmed increase in viral DNA level more than 1 $\log_{10}$ as compared to viral DNA level when the patient was on therapy.

    4. In case of discontinuation of this drug the response can be defined as serum viral DNA level <2,000 IU/mL for at least 12 months after the cessation of therapy.

  b. In case of pegylated IFN-α:

    1. Virological response can be defined as serum HBV DNA level <2,000 IU/mL evaluated at 6th month and at the completion of therapy.

    2. Sustained response can be defined as serum HBV DNA level <2,000 IU/mL for at least 12 months after the completion of therapy.

B. Serological response:

  a. For HBeAg—loss of HBeAg and development of HBeAb.

  b. For HBsAg—loss of HBsAg and development of anti HBs.

C. Biochemical response: It can be defined as normalization of ALT level. As it fluctuates over time hence every 3 months follow-up for about 1 year is required.

D. Histological response: It can be defined as decrease in necroinflammatory activity by ≥2 in histology activity index without worsening of fibrosis as compared to previous histology.

Management of Pre-exposure Prophylaxis

Following persons have to take prophylaxis:

A. Laboratory staff, hemodialysis and endoscopy staff

B. Patient under hemodialysis

C. Homosexuals

D. Persons with multiple sexual partners or with partners suffering from chronic HBV infection

E. Intravenous drug users

F. Persons having sexually transmitted disease

G. Persons living or traveling in endemic areas

H. Persons born in countries with high prevalence of HBV infection

I. Persons with end-stage renal failure

J. Diabetic patient having >60 years of age

K. Pregnant patient

Following are the types of vaccines:

A. Recombivax—HB containing 10 μg of HBsAg/mL

B. Engerix—B containing 20 μg of HBsAg/mL

C. Twinrix containing recombinant HBV vaccine plus inactivated hepatitis A vaccine

Site of injection is deltoid region not in gluteal region

Vaccine	Number of doses	Dose	Schedules in months
Recombivax—HB			
Infants and children of <1–10 years	3	5 µg	0, 1–2, 4–6
11–19 years	3 or 4	5 µg	0, 1–2, 4–6, 12
≥20 years	2	10 µg	0, 1, 4–6
Hemodialysis patients of <20 years	3	10 µg (double dose may be given)	0, 1, 2, 6
Hemodialysis patients of >20 years	3	40 µg	0, 1, 6
Engerix—B			
Infants and children of <1–10 years	3 or 4	10 µg	0, 1–2, 4–6
11–19 years	3 or 4	10 µg	0, 1–2, 4–6, 12
≥20 years	3 or 4	20 µg	0, 1, 4–6
Hemodialysis patients of <20 years	4	10 µg (double dose may be given)	0, 1, 2, 6
Hemodialysis patients of >20 years	4	40 µg	0, 1, 2, 6

Post exposure Prophylaxis

A. For perinatal prophylaxis in case of children born to HBsAg positive mother: Single dose of 0.5 mL HBIg intramuscularly in thigh immediately after birth, this is followed by complete course of hepatitis vaccine starting within 12 hours after birth.

B. For persons having direct percutaneous inoculation and direct transmucosal exposure to body fluids and blood of HBsAg patients, such as needle stick, ingestion: Single dose of 0.6 mL/kg HBIg as soon as after exposure followed by complete course of hepatitis vaccine starting within first week of exposure.

C. In case of pregnant female with HBV DNA level of >2,000 IU/mL: Antiviral therapy (most potent and least resistance) to be started in third trimester to reduce the risk of perinatal transmission.

D. In case of persons with sexual contact with HBV positive patients: Single dose of 0.6 mL/kg HBIg has to be given within 14 days after exposure and complete course of vaccine thereafter.

Duration of protection (maintenance of protective level of anti-HBs:

A. About 80–90% for 5 years and 60–80% for 10 years. After that in spite of undetectable level of anti-HBs protection persists against HBsAg antigenemia, chronic hepatitis B infection.

B. Booster dose is not recommended except in case of immunosuppressed patients or person sustaining percutaneous inoculation from HBsAg positive patients.

Following are the complications of hepatitis B infection:

Hepatic complications of hepatitis B infection:

A. Fulminant hepatic failure

B. Ascites

C. Edema

D. Bleeding from gastroesophageal varices

E. Hepatic encephalopathy

F. Coagulopathy

G. Pancytopenia due to hypersplenism

H. Hepatorenal syndrome

I. Hepatopulmonary syndrome (HPS)

Extrahepatic complications of hepatitis B infection:

A. Serum sickness-like syndrome: It occurs in 10% patient in the prodromal phase of acute hepatitis B infection. It is characterized by arthralgia, rash, arthritis, angioedema, and occasionally proteinuria and hematuria. The diagnosis is established by raised aminotransferases level and detection of HBsAg in the blood.

B. Polyarteritis nodosa: 10–30% patient with polyarteritis nodosa has been found to be HBsAg positive. This antigen combines with antibody to form immune complexes which lead to injury to small, medium, and large blood vessels producing vasculitis; it affects:

- **a.** Musculoskeletal system
- **b.** Gastrointestinal system
- **c.** Cardiovascular system
- **d.** Dermatological system
- **e.** Neurological system—peripheral neuropathy, Guillain-Barré syndrome

It may be fatal.

C. Glomerulonephritis: It is rare and mainly found in children. Different types of glomerulonephritis, such as:

- **a.** Membranous glomerulonephritis: It is present in Asiatic population. Diagnosis is based on presence of HBsAg in the renal tissue.

b. Membranoproliferative glomerulonephritis
c. Focal proliferative glomerulonephritis
d. Mesangiocapillary glomerulonephritis: Histologically, it is associated with mesangium and capillary deposits of HBsAg. In presence of persistent infection heightened immune response will lead to formation of immune complexes in the circulation and its deposition in the capillary membrane and ultimately dense deposit disease will be developed.
e. IgA nephropathy: In this case, there is subepithelial deposits of IgA

There is no correlation between HBV replication or severity of hepatic disease and severity of glomerulonephritis but it has been shown that treatment with antiviral therapy is associated with remission of this kidney disease.

D. Papular acrodermatitis (Gianotti-Crosti syndrome): It is strongly associated with hepatitis B antigenemia mainly in young children. This disease is characterized by nonitchy maculopapular rashes over the buttock, face, limbs, and trunk occasionally.
E. Oral lichen planus: Incidences of oral lichen planus and pitted keratolysis are found in HBsAg carriers
F. Bullous pemphigoid: It is autoimmune bullous disorder in elderly and may be triggered by:
  a. Hepatitis B surface antigen producing nonspecific immune reactivation.
  b. Production of specific antibody which cross-reacts with antigen of bullous pemphigoid.
G. Polymyalgia rheumatica: Serious dermatologic, neurological, arthritic, gastrointestinal, and immunologic reactions following adult vaccination with hepatitis B vaccine.
H. Rare complications:
  a. Aplastic anemia
  b. Acute pancreatitis
  c. Transverse myelitis

Q11. Relevance of genotypes in hepatitis B infection.

BF/NOV2012/MDII (12)

ANSWER

Hepatitis B virus is circular double-stranded DNA which encodes four overlapping open reading frames (ORFs):

A. *S* gene and pre-*S* genes. These encode following pre-*S* gene products:
  a. HBV surface receptor for polymerase human serum albumin
  b. HBV surface receptor for hepatocyte membrane

Pre S region is divided into two parts:
  a. Pre-S1
  b. Pre-S2

Depending upon the initiation of translation three types of *HBsAg* gene products are synthesized:
  a. *S* gene product is HBsAg (major protein)
  b. *S* gene product + product of adjacent pre-S2 region (middle protein)
  c. Product of pre-S1 region + product of pre-S2 region (large protein)

In case HBV infection both pre-S antigen and respective antibodies can be detected in the blood and coincides with other pre-S antigenemia of B virus replication. But the relevance of this pre-S antigen is of little value in routine testing.

B. This virion contains 27 nm nucleocapsid protein which is coded by *C* gene. The antigen present of the surface of nucleocapsid is called HBcAg and its corresponding antibody is anti-HBc.

There is another antigen known as HBeAg, a nucleocapsid protein. It is antigenically distinct from HBcAg but it is the product of same gene *C*. This *C* gene has two initiation codon—one is precore and the other one is core region.
  a. If translation starts at precore region, the protein product is HBeAg. It is a single peptide, bind to smooth endoplasmic reticulum leading to its release into circulation. So, it can be detected in the serum and indicates the infectivity and viral replicability.
  b. If translation starts at core region, the protein product is HBcAg. It is not single peptide, so it not secreted and it will assemble into nucleocapsid particles which bind to RNA and incorporate into it, ultimately it contains HBV DNA and DNA polymerase which are responsible for repair and replication of DNA. Hence, HBcAg will remain in the hepatocyte hence it cannot be detectable by immunohistochemistry but is exported after it is being encapsidated by envelope of HBsAg.

C. Third *HBV* gene called *P* gene. It is the largest of all. It encodes DNA polymerase has two activities:
  a. DNA-dependent DNA polymerase
  b. RNA-dependent reverse transcriptase

D. Fourth gene is *X* gene. It is small nonparticulate protein known as hepatitis X antigen. It transactivates the transcription of cellular and viral genes. It activates calcium channels in the mitochondria thus activating signal-transduction pathways which in turn stimulates HBV reverse transcriptase leading to HBV DNA replication. This shows the association between expression of HBxAg and anti-HBx and development of chronic hepatitis and HCC. This transcription activity can enhance replication of HIV. Cellular processes that are transactivated by *X* gene include:

a. Interferon γ-gene

b. Class I major histocompatibility gene

The overall effect is enhanced susceptibility of hepatocytes infected by HBV to cytotoxic T cells.

Hepatitis B virus has been classified into 8–10 main genotypes and four major serotypes. There is a common antigenic determinant "a" in all serotypes and other subtypic antigenic determinants are "d", "y", "r," and "w".

So, four major serotypes are "adr", "ayr", "adw," and "ayw". So, antibody developed against "a" will confer immunity to all the serotypes. Anti-HBs developed after recovery from HBV infection or after hepatitis B vaccination will be directed against "a" which ultimately cross-protects against other serotypes.

The 8–10 genotypes are A to J. There is geographical variation of genotypes and subtypes.

A. Genotype A (adw) and D (ayw) predominate in United States and Europe

B. Genotype B (adw) and C (adr) predominate in Asia

C. Genotype B is related to less rapid progression in liver disease and toward cirrhosis as well as delayed occurrence of HCC than genotype C and D

D. Genotype A responsible for rapid clearing of antigenemia and seroconversion of HBsAg and HBeAg

Q12. Hepatorenal syndrome.

ERA/NOV2012(S)/MDII (15)

Pathogenesis of hepatorenal syndrome. Discuss in brief its management and prognosis.

DNBIIIA/DEC2014 (10)

Describe a systemic evaluation and current management of renal dysfunction in cirrhosis of liver cases.

MUZ/MAY2016/MDIII (15)

Define hepatorenal syndrome. Describe its pathogenesis, diagnostic criteria, and treatment modalities.

DNBI/DEC2011 (10)

What are the diagnostic criteria for diagnosing hepatorenal syndrome?

DNB (DEC2020) (4)

Define hepatorenal syndrome. Write down the recent treatment guidelines of HRS.

AIIMS, BBS, 2023 (10)

Hepatorenal syndrome etiopathogenesis, laboratory findings and therapy.

SCB MED COL, 2015 (10)

Discuss the pathophysiology of ascites, spontaneous bacterial peritonitis and hepatorenal syndrome. Describe clinical features, investigations and treatment of spontaneous bacterial peritonitis and hepatorenal syndrome.

SARDAR PATEL UNIVERSITY, 2019 (25)

Hepatorenal syndrome.

TEERTHANKER MAHAVEER UNIVERSITY, 2018 (10)

Hepatorenal syndrome.

MANIPAL UNIVERSITY, 2018 (10)

What is hepatorenal syndrome? Classify and briefly outline the management strategies of each of them.

WBUHS, 2023 (10)

Write hepatorenal syndrome.

WBUHS, 2020 (10)

Spontaneous bacterial peritonitis has been described in the question 23.

ANSWER

Hepatorenal syndrome is characterized by circulatory and functional changes leading to reduction of glomerular functional rate which can be reverted back by vasoconstrictor drugs and liver transplantation. Serum creatinine cannot estimate accurately the renal function in cirrhosis due to following factors:

A. Impairment in production of creatinine, precursor of creatinine

B. Reduced muscle mass

C. Tubular secretion of creatinine

D. In presence of high bilirubin inaccurate measurement of creatinine by calorimetric methods

So, to get better diagnostic performance incorporation of newer biomarkers, cystatin C, cysteine proteinase inhibitor into conventional creatinine-based glomerular functional rate can accurately estimate the kidney function in cirrhosis.

Definition of HRS has been changed according to International Club of Ascites in 2015. Stages of acute kidney injury (AKI) according to this club are:

Stage 1: Increase in serum creatinine of ≥3 mg/dL or increase in serum creatinine ≥1.5-fold or 2-fold from baseline:

a. Stage 1a: Creatinine <1.5 mg/dL

b. Stage 1b: Creatinine ≥1.5 mg/dL

Stage 2: Serum creatinine will be increased at least two- to threefolds from the baseline.

Stage 3: Serum creatinine will be increased at least three-folds from the baseline or serum creatinine of ≥4 mg/dL with an acute increase of ≥3 mg/dL or initiation of renal replacement therapy.

Types of hepatorenal syndrome:

(Old name) Type 1 hepatorenal syndrome (HRS)	(New name) HRS-AKI
Doubling of serum creatinine to ≥2.5 mg/dL within 2 weeks	Increase in serum creatinine to ≥3 mg/dL within 48 h Or Increase in serum creatinine ≥1.5 mg/dL from the baseline (creatinine value within previous 3 months, when available, may be used as baseline. Value closest to baseline should be taken)
No response to diuretic withdrawal and 2 day after fluid challenge with 1 g/kg/day of 20–25% albumin	No response to diuretic withdrawal and 2 day after fluid challenge with 1 g/kg/day of 20–25% albumin
Cirrhosis with ascites	Cirrhosis with ascites
Absence of shock	Absence of shock
No current use of nephrotoxic drugs [nonsteroidal anti-inflammatory drugs (NSAIDs) and contrast media]	No current use of nephrotoxic drugs (NSAIDs and contrast media)
• Absence of signs relating to any structural kidney injury • Absence of proteinuria (>500 mg/day) • Absence of hematuria [50 RBCs/HPF (high-power field)] • Normal findings in ultrasonography	• Absence of signs relating to any structural kidney injury • Absence of proteinuria (>500 mg/day) • Absence of hematuria (50 RBCs/HPF) • Normal findings in ultrasonography
(Old name) Type II HRS	**(New name) HRS-non-AKI (NAKI)**
	HRS-AKD
Gradual increasing in creatinine not meeting the criteria above	eGFR <60 mL/min/1.73 m² for <3 months in absence of other potential causes of kidney disease
	Percentage increase in serum creatinine <50% using last available value of outpatient serum creatinine within 3 months as baseline value
	HRS-chronic kidney disease (CKD)
	eGFR <60 mL/min/1.73 m² for <3 months in absence of other potential causes of kidney disease

Pathophysiology of Hepatorenal Syndrome

A. Circulatory dysfunction:

a. Cirrhosis increases intrahepatic vascular resistance

b. Splanchnic vessels are dilated due to presence of vasodilators, such as nitric oxide, prostacyclins, carbon-monoxide as well as endocannabinoids.

It results in decrease in arterial pressure and effective circulating blood volume. As the liver disease progresses cardiac function will decline due to cirrhotic cardiomyopathy leading to HRS.

c. Renin–angiotensin–aldosterone system and arginine vasopressor are the vasoconstrictors that increase the effective circulating blood volume leading to constriction of renal blood vessels with reduction of renal blood flow and retention of sodium and water. In the early phase due to vasodilatory effect of prostaglandin I_2 and E_2 glomerular filtration will be maintained in spite of reduction of renal blood flow. But in the late stage of liver disease NSAIDs inhibit synthesis of prostaglandin as well as effective filtration fraction leading to development of AKI.

B. Systemic inflammation: Systemic inflammatory response in presence or absence of infection. Various proinflammatory cytokines, such as IL-6 and 8, TNF-α, vascular cell adhesion protein-1 as well as urinary concentration chemoattractant protein-1, are increased in patient with AKI with cirrhosis as compared to cirrhosis without AKI. Inflammation may develop from two group of molecules:

- **a.** Pathogens-associated molecular patterns (PAMPS): These are bacterial products translocated from the intestinal gut bacterial, such as flagellin, lipopolysaccharide (LPS), and nigericin
- **b.** Damage-associated molecular patterns (DAMPs): These are intracellular components released from damaged liver cells, such as high mobility group protein B1, heart block protein, double-stranded genomic DNA, and ATP.
  1. In absence of inflammation or infection both the above activate pattern recognition receptors, like toll-like receptors and release proinflammatory cytokines which in turn release vasodilators leading to reduction of decrease in vascular resistance and effective circulating blood volume.
  2. PAMPs and DAMPs directly affect the renal tubular cells by increasing the expression of toll-like receptor 4 and Caspase-3 as a result of renal ischemia.
  3. There is also impairment of hypothalamic pituitary axis and exhaustion of cortisol by proinflammatory cytokine and PAMPs.
- **c.** Cholemic nephropathy: In case of high bilirubin level bile acid cast is formed directly, obstructs the renal tubules, and develops direct toxicity to the tubular cells in patient with AKI-HRS. It also affects the outcome of treatment.
- **d.** Intra-abdominal hypertension: Increase in abdominal pressure of >12 mm Hg is an important cause of HRS in patient with refractory ascites. It can be best estimated by measuring the diameter of inferior vena cava and its collapsibility, this can also estimates which patient gets benefit from large volume paracentesis.
- **e.** Hepatorenal reflex hypothesis: Osmoreceptors, chemoreceptors, and baroreceptors in the hepatocytes through complex neurocircuits directly affect the kidney cells.

Risk Factors

A. Hyponatremia

B. High plasma rennin activity

C. Liver size

D. Severity of ascites

E. Large volume paracentesis without albumin administration produces hypotension, hyponatremia leading to AKI.

F. Spontaneous bacterial peritonitis (SBP) with bacterial infections: Infusion of albumin along with antibiotic treatment will improve circulatory dysfunction and renal function.

G. In patient at risk of SBP determined by ascitic protein of <1.5 mg/dL, dysfunction of liver/kidney as estimated by bilirubin of >3 mg/dL, serum sodium of <130 mEq/L, Child–Turcotte–Pugh score of >10, and/or serum creatinine level of >1.2 mg/dL antibiotic prophylaxis will prevent SBP as well as HRS.

Management of HRS

A. Stage 1A HRS due to hypovolemia can be corrected by volume depletion.

B. Stage 1B should be corrected by vasoconstrictor agents according to European Association of Study of Liver. After proper diagnosis of AKI following treatment has to be provided:

- **a.** Withdrawal of diuretics
- **b.** Administration of fluid
- **c.** Intravenous albumin infusion at a rate of 1 g/kg/day
- **d.** Withdrawal of nonselective beta blockers to abate negative inotropic effect
- **e.** Culture of ascitic fluid in case SBP, urine and blood
- **f.** Chest radiography to exclude any infection

C. Administration of vasoconstrictors: Constriction of splanchnic vessels reduces the portal pressure leading to increase in effective arterial blood volume and thus renal blood flow. Increased renal perfusion increases the mean arterial pressure resulting reversal of HRS.

Drugs available are: Terlipressin, noradrenaline, or combination of midodrine and octreotide.

- **a.** Terlipressin:
  1. It acts on vasopressin 1A and acts as primary vasoconstrictor.

2. It acts on vasopressin 1B and stimulates adrenocorticotropic and cortisol hormone counteracting adrenal insufficiency in case of decompensated cirrhosis. By activating this receptor it acutely reduces serum sodium mainly in cirrhotic patient without ascites treated for variceal bleeding.
3. Indirect vasopressin-mediated anti-inflammatory effect
4. Side effects are diarrhea and abdominal pain rarely intestinal and myocardial ischemia, so patient should be monitored twice daily.
5. In HRS fluid monitoring is needed when it is being used with albumin infusion.

b. Novel analog of vasopressin 1A agonist selepressin is used in the management of septic shock but without any hyponatremia or volume overload producing pulmonary edema in animal model.

c. Norepinephrine is intravenous drug used as vasoconstrictor through activation of α-1 receptor on the vascular smooth muscle cells. Complications are tachyarrhythmias.

d. Midodrine is an oral drug used as vasoconstrictor through activation of α-1 receptor on the vascular smooth muscle cells.

e. Octreotide being somatostatin analog:
1. Inhibits glucagon secretion
2. Splanchnic vasodilator
3. Direct mesenteric vasoconstrictor

D. Albumin infusion

E. Albumin administration reduces the incidence HRS by stabilizing the endothelial function due to following factors:
a. Volume expansion
b. Anti-inflammatory properties
c. Antioxidant properties
d. It will bind with bile acids, hormones, cytokines, nitric oxide, long-chain fatty acids, endotoxin, and bacterial products thus clearing of substances from the blood.

F. Transjugular intrahepatic portosystemic shunt: Its use is in investigational stage.

G. Renal replacement therapy: It is done in case of AKI-HRS who is unresponsive to drugs with uremia, volume overload, and dyselectrolytemia. But I cannot improve the survival of the patients.

H. Liver transplantation: It is the optimal treatment but recovery rates depend upon the duration of injury. In some centers combined liver–kidney transplantation is going on.

I. Emerging treatment:
a. Serelaxin: Recombinant human relaxin-2 acts on renal vessels thus reducing renal vascular resistance and increases renal blood flow.
b. Pentoxifylline, phosphodiesterase inhibitor, has anti-inflammatory activity and anti-TNF-α activity.

Predictor of Response

A. Serum creatinine concentration—low creatinine at the start of treatment will be associated with good HRS reversal but high creatinine >7 mg/dL there will be negligible response.

B. Pretreatment sepsis, other organ failure

Q13. Hepatocellular carcinoma.

MGR/APR2015/MDIII (7)

ANSWER

Introduction

Hepatocellular carcinoma arises from hepatocytes, it is the second leading cause of death, 6th most common cancer in the world, in USA 13th most common cancer but 4th leading cause of death. 5-year overall survival rate is only 17%. Highest incidence is found in Asia and Africa due to increased incidence of HBsAg infection.

Etiology

A. Relative risk of HCC is 100% in the HBsAg carriers. Risk increases with increased incidence of cirrhosis and presence of large plasma burden of HBV DNA through integration into host DNA.

B. There is increased incidence of HCC with HCV RNA due to its chronicity in USA (50%).

C. Alcoholic cirrhosis may be a factor when it is associated with HCV infection.

D. Other risk factors are:
a. Nonalcoholic steatotic hepatitis
b. Alpha-1 antitrypsin deficiency
c. Hemochromatosis
d. Increasing age mostly between 55–65 years
e. Male sex
f. Exposure to aflatoxin

Pathology

Development of HCC usually takes many years starting at genetic level.

A. Dysplasia: It is characterized by a recognizable cluster of hepatocytes differing from normal adjacent hepatocytes in the liver tissue—if it is <1 mm in diameter it is called foci but if it is 1 mm in diameter it is nodule. It is detected in USG as it is larger than cirrhotic nodule.

- **a.** Nodule may be of low grade if it is composed of minimally abnormal hepatocytes surrounded by fibrous scar.
- **b.** Nodule may be high grade contains more atypical cells which may be difficult to distinguish from carcinoma and having no capsule.
- **c.** Small cell dysplasia more characteristically is precursor of HCC because:
  - They have expression of proliferating cell nuclear antigen marker
  - There is transition between small cell dysplasia and HCC.

B. Very early dysplasia: Following are the characteristics—

- **a.** Varying grade of dysplasia
- **b.** >40% lesions contain fat
- **c.** Hepatocytes invade portal spaces
- **d.** Absence of vascular invasion

C. Progressed HCC: It can be categorized according to absence or presence of cord-like structure, pseudoacinar formation, and cellular morphology into:

- **a.** Well-differentiated HCC: Plate of cords of cells lined by endothelium.
- **b.** Moderately differentiated HCC: Presence of glandular structures called bile-stained pseudoacini.
- **c.** Poorly differentiated HCC: Cells are very large containing multiple bizarre nuclei, structure plates are absent.
- **d.** Other rare malignancies are fibrolamellar carcinoma, angiosarcoma, hepatoblastoma, and hemangiosarcoma.

D. Clinical presentation:

- **a.** It may be asymptomatic or accidentally found during routine screening of cirrhosis.
- **b.** Symptoms of advanced liver disease, such as abdominal pain, weight loss, palpable mass in the abdomen. May be jaundice of obstructive variety due to invasion or obstruction of intrahepatic duct.
- **c.** Acute pain indicates large superficial tumor indicating rupture.
- **d.** It is localized tumor but can metastasize if the tumor is very large; sites are bone, lung, adrenal gland, and lymph node.
- **e.** Paraneoplastic syndrome may develop; these are erythrocytosis, hypoglycemia, diarrhea, and hypercalcemia, dermatologic manifestations, such as pemphigus foliaceus, seborrheic keratosis, and pityriasis rotunda.

E. Diagnosis:

- **a.** Screening:
  - Population at risk should be screened at every 6 months
  - Abnormal USG finding should be followed by CT or MRI screening
  - Screening by AFP
- **b.** Screening of liver: Triphasic CT or MRI (arterial, venous and delayed phase): Characteristic features are: arterial phase enhancement and venous or delayed phase washout in patient with lesion of >2 mm. Less than 1 cm tumor should be screened every 3–6 months.
- **c.** Liver biopsy: In case of radiologically suspicious lesion biopsy should be performed, but percutaneous biopsy should not be performed in case of orthotropic transplantation of lever and there is chance of needle track seedling.
- **d.** Alpha-fetoprotein: It is most common marker. Presence of cirrhosis with a liver mass and >400 ng/mL AFP indicates HCC. It can be normal in 40% cases.

F. Staging: There are different types of staging found in HCC. But Barcelona clinic liver cancer (BCLC) is most common as it incorporates following parameters:

- **a.** Size of cancer
- **b.** Number of lesion
- **c.** Child–Pugh score (CP)
- **d.** Performance status (PS)
- **e.** Implications in regard to treatment option.

  Score 0: PS = 0, CP = A

  Score A–C: PS-0–1, CP = A/B

  Score D: PS = 2, CP = C

New extremely validated score is albumin-bilirubin score based on serum bilirubin and albumin alone providing simple assessment of liver function.

G. Treatment: Not candidates of surgical intervention—(1) Extent of tumor, (2) Underlying liver function

Surgical interventions include the following:

A. Surgery: Indications—

a. Presence of liver function

b. Tumor burden

c. Presence of portal hypertension

d. Macrovascular invasion

e. Regional lymph node involvement

Types of surgery:

a. Hepatic resection: Type of resection depends upon:

- Severity of cirrhosis
- Location of the lesion

Survival: 5-year survival rate is 50–70%. But adjuvant antiviral therapy increases the survival. It depends upon:

- Site of the lesion
- Number of the lesion

Complications include:

- Bile leak
- Pleural effusion
- Cirrhotic patient may develop postoperative liver failure.

b. Liver transplantation: Candidates must meet Milan criteria. These are the following:

- Single lesion of ≤5 cm or up to three lesions each ≤3 cm.
- Absence of macrovascular invasion or presence of portal vein thrombosis
- No metastasis or regional lymph node involvement

Transplant organ may be from cadaveric or living donor.

But locoregional control and chemoembolization act as bridge for liver transplantation.

B. Locoregional treatment:

a. Ablation therapy: Three methods are available. These are:

- Radiofrequency ablation and microwave ablation are percutaneously or laparoscopically and are very effective if the tumor size <4 cm.
- Following factors influencing the recurrences:
  - Larger size of tumor
  - Proximity to major vessels
  - Subcapsular lesions
  - Percutaneous approach
  - Ablation <1 cm

Choice of ablation depends upon local expense and institutional preference.

Contraindications of thermal ablation include: Lesion adjacent to diaphragm or intestine or major blood vessels.

b. Hepatic artery embolization: Methods are transarterial chemoembolization (TACE) and bland embolization. Tumor receives blood supply from hepatic artery but normal liver parenchyma receives blood from portal vein.

TACE is commonly done with drug-eluting beads laden with doxorubicin. It is done in:

- Patients with preserved liver function (CP A-B)
- Unrespectable disease
- Bridging therapy prior to liver transplantation.

Contraindications to TACE:

- Severely reduced portal venous flow
- Decompensated cirrhosis

Common side effects: Postembolization syndrome:

- Nausea, right upper abdominal pain, fever, and transient elevation of liver function test.

c. Radioembolization: Liver tolerates radiation dose up to 20 Gy. This method utilizes Yttrium-90, red and glass microspheres. Radioembolization produces radiation segmentectomy by providing high-radiation dose and better tumor necrosis.

Indications:

- Larger lesion
- Significant lobar involvement
- Diffuse disease

Contraindications:

- Decompensated liver function
- Bilirubin level > 2 mg/dL

Complications:

- Postembolization fatigue, abdominal pain
- Radiation-induced hepatic dysfunction
- Radiation-induced liver disease
- Radiation-induced pneumonitis

C. Radiation: It will deliver high dose to a specific area by external beam radiation. Total dose 20–60 Gy in 3–6 dose-fractional schedule should be given. Tumor thrombus can be treated with other locoregional treatment.

D. Systemic therapy: It is given in patients with advanced disease, metastatic disease. The drugs are sorafenib, sunitinib, brivanib, erlotinib, everolimus, linifanib, and ramucirumab. Sorafenib is multikinase inhibitor having antiangiogenic properties, its target is RAF-1, BRAF, VGEFR1, 2 and 3, and PDGFR-β. Dose is 400 mg twice daily with response rate 2–3%. Side effects are: diarrhea, hypotension, fatigue, mouth sore, depression of bone marrow, and hepatotoxicity. In 45% of case there will be palmar plantar erythema.

Q14. Amebic liver abscess.
MGR/MAR2010/MD (6)

Management of amebic liver abscess.
MGR/APR2013/MDIII (7)

Enumerate the various parasites that affect the liver and describe the life cycle and management of any one in detail.
MGR/MAY/2011/MDIII (15)

Amebic liver abscess.
BHARATI VIDYAPEETH DEEMED UNI, JHELUM, 2019 (10)
NTR UNI OF HEALTH SC, VIJAYAWADA, 2018 (10)

ANSWER

Introduction

Entamoeba histolytica is distributed throughout the world but mainly in low-income group families. *Entamoeba* species are composed of mainly two types: *E. histolytica* and *E. dispar*. Other types are *E. moshkovskii* and *E. bangladeshi*. Microscopy cannot differentiate between *E. histolytica* and *E. dispar*, only serology can differentiate them.

Transmission

There are two forms of *E. histolytica*: Tissue noninvasive form—cyst and tissue invasive form—trophozoite. Cyst is hardy, survives for 1 month at 4°C in sewage water and at room temperature in different vegetables for 48 hours, and dies immediately in boiling water.

Transmission occurs through:

a. Fecal-oral route from fecally contaminated food or water
b. Oral-anal route
c. In homosexual men

Risk factors:

a. It is disease of young of any sex.
b. Between the age of 20 and 40 years, male to female ratio is 10:1. Females at their menstruating age are less common to suffer because iron deficiency acts as natural immunity for them.
c. Alcoholic males
d. Iron content in liquor in males.
e. Breast-fed children are less likely to develop because IgA will be transmitted to the children through breast milk and this milk also contains low iron.

After ingestion of *Entamoeba* cyst along with food excystation occurs in the small intestine with release of large number of trophozoites; they will proliferate with bacterial flora, first adhere to colonic epithelium through the galactose/N-acetylgalactosamine-specific lectin then invade the mucosa and submucosa to form flask-shaped ulcers mainly in the cecum, ascending colon, sigmoid colon, and rectum.

Trophozoites reach the liver through:

a. Portal vein
b. Lymphatics
c. Intraperitoneal spread

Trophozoites portal vessels run through this vein and reach and are trapped in the interlobular vein. In the portal triad they multiply and block it producing infarction of the surrounding hepatocytes and proteolytic enzymes produced by the trophozoites lyse the hepatocytes leading to liquefaction necrosis. All the necrotic material coalesces to produce large hepatic abscess. The material of the abscess is composed of necrotic liver tissue and 20% blood called "Anchovy sauce". Trophozoites are found in the wall not in the pus. Glisson's capsule cannot be invaded by this abscess cavity until late stage. Abscess cavity is surrounded by a rim of connective tissue, large numbers of inflammatory cells, and trophozoite form of *E. histolytica*.

Clinical Features

Symptom may occur in absence/presence of intestinal symptoms, or there may be short course of diarrheal illness followed by symptoms of liver abscess. 80% patients develop within 2–4 weeks of exposure. Adult males between 20 and 40 years are affected. Onset may be acute, subacute, or insidious. In case of insidious onset the patients present with fever, dull aching right upper abdominal pain or in epigastrium, unproductive cough, and pleuritic chest pain in right lower quadrant. In subacute cases presentation may be with gradual weight loss, anorexia, mild right upper abdominal pain, and low-grade fever. In acute case fever is spiky with severe prostration. History of travel to endemic country must be taken.

On clinical examination, raised temperature, tachycardia, tachypnea, enlarge tender liver, intercostal tenderness in the right lower costal region, and atypical of liver abscess are found.

About 10–30% of patients may show gastrointestinal features, such as nausea, vomiting, diarrhea, and abdominal cramps.

Investigations

A. Hematological features demonstrate: Normochromic normocytic anemia, leukocytosis, and raised ESR

B. Biochemical features demonstrate in case of acute amebic abscess raised transaminases with normal ALP which is opposite in case of chronic form.

C. Culture of blood can differentiate the pyemic liver abscess.

D. Stool examination may demonstrate Charcot–Leyden crystals

E. Radiological investigations:

- **a.** Ultrasonography: Round hypoechoic lesion
- **b.** Contrast-enhanced CT scan shows single nonenhancing abscess center surrounded by irregular rim-like area of inflammation as highly enhanced area.

  Pyemic liver abscess can be differentiated by multiple cavities occasionally overlapping cavities.
- **c.** Chest X-ray demonstrates elevation of right dome diaphragm, right basal collapse, and may be right-sided pleural effusion.

F. Aspiration of amebic liver abscess demonstrates odorless anchovy sauce-like material and there may be presence of trophozoite form of *E. histolytica,* if scrapping from the wall of the cavity will be taken, Gram stain will be negative. Trophozoite with presence of RBC with in it may be found. If it is found in stool also it can only the differentiating point by which you can discard the other *Entamoeba*.

G. Serology:

- **a.** Cellabs kit demonstrates *E. histolytica*-derived Gal/GalNAc-specific lectin; it can differentiate other *Entamoeba*.
- **b.** PCR of stool or pus can confirm *E. histolytica*.
- **c.** Antibody to amebic antigen can be detected on 90% of cases of liver abscess and it will be positive for next 5 years. So, it is of only historical interest.

Differential Diagnosis

Amebic liver abscess	Pyemic liver abscess
Age <50 years	Age >50 years
Male to female ratio is 10:1	Male to female ratio is 1:1
Recent travel to endemic area	Risk factors, such as diabetes mellitus, malignancy, and immunocompromised
Diarrhea present	High spiky fever
Pulmonary complaint, like cough	Sepsis
Severe right upper abdominal pain	Jaundice
Fever	Pruritus
Enlarged tender liver	Palpable liver
Amebic serology positive	Pus/Blood culture positive for bacteria
Chest X-ray elevated diaphragm, pleural effusion	Chest may show secondary infection

Treatment

A. Medical treatment:

- **a.** Metronidazole—400–800 mg thrice daily orally or intravenously × 10 days.
- **b.** Ciprofloxacin orally 500 mg twice daily or 200 mg intravenously × 10 days.

- **c.** Chloroquine base 600 mg orally × 2 days followed by 300 mg/day × 2–3 weeks.

- **d.** Diloxanide furoate in case of chronic cyst passers 500 mg orally thrice daily × 10 days.

B. Surgical treatment:

Aspiration and percutaneous drainage:

- **a.** Large abscess containing 10 cm of pus at risk of rupture
- **b.** Left lobe abscess as there is chance of intrapericardial rupture
- **c.** Secondary infected abscess with highly elevated diaphragm.
- **d.** Complicated liver abscess, such as:
  - Impending rupture
  - Presence of jaundice
  - Rupture into pericardial cavity
  - Rupture into peritoneal cavity
  - Presence of inferior venacaval obstruction
  - Abscess resistant to recent medical therapy
  - In case of pregnancy where drug administration is contraindicated.

Open surgical drainage:

- Life-threatening hemorrhage
- Fistulization to hollow viscus
- Ruptured abscess into peritoneal cavity

Complications

A. Rupture:

  a. Thoracic rupture:
    - Pleural cavity
    - Lung
    - Bronchus

  b. Peritoneal cavity

  c. Intrapericardial rupture: In case of left lobe abscess, it will occur.

  d. Stomach

  e. Duodenum

  f. Biliary tree

B. Secondary infection: It occurs due to obstructive effect abscess of intrahepatic biliary radicles

C. Vascular obstruction: There is involvement of inferior vena cava and hepatic vein.

D. Rare complications:

  a. Hemobilia

  b. Hepatic vein thrombosis

  c. Fulminant hepatic failure

Q15. Serological markers of hepatitis B infection.

RGUHS/MDI (10)

ANSWER

Following are the serological markers along with the relevance in infection in hepatitis B:

A. HBsAg and anti-HBs:

  a. It will appear in the serum within 1–12 weeks after exposure to HBV and 2–6 weeks before the onset of hepatitis or increase in ALT.

  b. It will disappear after 4–6 months if the patient recovers. Few weeks to few months after its disappearance anti-HBs appears and persists throughout the life conferring life-long immunity.

  c. If it persists after 6 months it indicates chronic infection.

  d. HBV DNA is divided into eight genotypes and four serotypes. All genotypes have common antigenic determinant, i.e., "a," other two pairs are "w" or "y" and "d" or "y" making four following serotypes—"adr," "adw," "ayr," "ayw". So if antibody develops against "a" determinant it will confer protection against all four serotypes. Based on this theory hepatitis vaccine has been developed containing antibody against "a" determinant. If antibody will be developed against other antigenic determinant it will not be able to neutralize all the circulating virion hence these patients will be the carriers of hepatitis B.

  e. There are other two antigens, pre-S1 and pre-S2; these correlate with the detection of GBV DNA in the serum and indicate active viral replication. If the patient will recover from infection antibody will develop against these two antigens prior to appearance of anti-HBs.

B. Hepatitis core antigen (HBcAg) and anti-hepatitis core antibody (anti-HBc):

  a. HBcAg being an intracellular antigen is not circulating in the serum, only expressed in hepatocytes. Only anti-HBc will be present in the serum. In case of acute hepatitis B infection first antibody HBc IgM is found 1 month after the appearance of HBsAg but 1–2 weeks before the increase of ALT.

  b. But during convalescence IgM HBc disappears and titer of IgG HBc starts appearing. But in case of chronic infection low titer of IgM HBc will be present in low titer up to 2 years.

  c. Detection of anti-HBc in the serum depends upon the cutoff level of anti-HBc assay. In case high cutoff level also it can be detected in case of exacerbation of chronic HBC infection.

  d. Importance of anti-HBc in the serum:
    1. It can monitor the response to antiviral therapy
    2. It will correlate with ALT and HBV DNA level in case of exacerbation of hepatitis B infection.
    3. It will present with anti-HBs in patient recovering from HBV infection.
    4. It is only marker detected during window period.
    5. It can be detected in 10–20% blood donor in low endemic areas and nearly 40% in high endemic areas. So, there is chance of transmission from blood donation in 0.4% of cases.

C. HBeAg and anti-HBe:

  a. HBeAg is a secretary protein processed from precore protein indicates infectivity and replicability of the virus in the body. Its presence is associated with detection of HBV DNA.

b. It appears shortly after the appearance of HBsAg and in the recovering patient its seroconversion precedes the HBsAg seroconversion. After seroconversion, anti-HBe will persist for many years, but in case of chronic infection HBeAg will persist for many years to decades.

c. In case of seroconversion, it will correlate with decline of HBV DNA as well as remission of liver disease. But in some seroconverted patient HBV DNA and active liver disease will persist which may be due to wild type HBV infection or presence of precore mutant.

D. HBV DNA level: It can be estimated either by molecular hybridization having sensitivity of 100,000–1,000,000 copies/mL or by PCR with sensitivity of much more high sensitivity and very low detection limit up to 100 copies/mL. To diagnose chronic hepatitis B infection an arbitrary value of 100,000 copies/mL has been set.

a. Molecular hybridization assay detect HBV DNA 1 week after the appearance of HBsAg whereas PCR can detect it 2–3 weeks before the HBsAg appearance.

b. Recovery from hepatitis is associated with complete disappearance of HBV DNA by molecular assay but it will remain detectable for years.

c. Incaseofchronic HBVinfectionantiviraltreatment molecular assay cannot detect HBV DNA further in the serum but PCR frequently detect it except in case of complete seroconversion.

d. Patient with very high pretreatment HBV DNA level will less likely to respond to IFN therapy but in case of treatment with nucleosides HBV DNA level is less important.

Type of infection	HBsAg	Anti-HBs	Anti-HBc IgM	Anti-HBc IgG	HBeAg	Anti-HBe	HBV DNA	Interpretation
Acute infection	+	–	+	–	+	–	++++	Early phase
	–	–	+	–	–	+	++	Window period
	–	+	–	+	–	+	±	Recovery period
	+	–	–	+	+	–	+++	HBeAg positive chronic hepatitis
Chronic infection	+	–	–	+	–	+	±	Inactive carrier state
	+	–	–	+	+	–	++	HBeAg negative chronic hepatitis
	+	–	±	+	±	±	+++	Exacerbation of chronic hepatitis

Q16. Autoimmune hepatitis.

MJPRU/2015(S)/MDIII (10)

MGR/OCT2011/MDIII (7)

Define autoimmune hepatitis. Describe its immunopathogenesis and management.

DNBII/DEC2010 (10)

Autoimmune hepatitis.

DNB (DEC2019) (5)

Autoimmune hepatitis.

SCB MED COL, (10)

Autoimmune hepatitis.

MGR UNI, TAMIL NADU, 2022 (10)

ANSWER

Introduction

It is a chronic hepatitis with female preponderance, characterized by interface hepatitis with lymphoplasmacytic infiltration on histology, presence of circulating antibodies, hypergammaglobulinemia, and good response to immunosuppressives. This disease has been classified into three types: Type 1, type 2, and type 3.

Epidemiology

In spite of its occurrence in all age groups and in all ethnicities female sexes are predominantly involved. Type 1 is most common. Type 2 demonstrates regional prevalence. African-Americans mainly present with cirrhosis.

Pathogenesis

A. This disease is thought to arise from triggering of environmental factors, such as drugs, toxins, and infectious agents which stimulate a subsets of T cells leading to development of cell-mediated response against liver-specific antigen producing inflammatory reaction followed by scarring.

B. This autoimmune response can also be triggered by HLA class III; it presents specific antigenic peptide through antigen-presenting cells to T cells, as a result T cells will be activated to differentiate into T_h 1 and T_h 2 cells which ultimately release proinflammatory cytokines producing periportal inflammation; it is usually observed in viral or bacterial infections.

   a. HLA DR3is strongly associated with AIH in Caucasian population.

   b. HLA DRB1*0301 is associated with the younger age of onset of AIH and disease will be very severe.

C. Molecular mimicry: In this method in type 2 hepatitis LKM-autoimmune antibodies react with B cell epitope cytochrome-450 sharing homologous sequence with the antigen of virus herpes simplex.

   Normally through the removal of autoreactive cells by apoptosis as well as T- and B-cells homeostasis is tightly regulated. So failure of any of the mechanisms leads to initiation of autoimmunity.

D. Following genetic factors may also contribute to development of AIH:

   a. TNF-α

   b. Complement factor *C4* gene

   c. Cytotoxic T lymphocyte antigen-4

E. 10–18% of chronic hepatitis is associated with type 1 polyendocrine syndrome; it is autosomal recessive disorder.

Clinical Presentation

Spectrum of presentation may be from asymptomatic to acute severe hepatitis or smoldering cirrhosis. Following are the different types of presentations:

A. Like acute hepatitis patient may present with nausea, vomiting, abdominal pain, anorexia, and arthralgia. On physical examination, jaundice, hepatomegaly, and splenomegaly.

B. In case of severe disease along with above features, progressively increasing jaundice, raised AST and ALT levels, increased PT, alteration of consciousness—this is more common in children but rare after 30 years.

C. Many patients present with transient illness with spontaneous recovery but later on cirrhosis may develop in one-third adult patients. So these patients may present with decompensated cirrhosis, variceal bleeding, hepatic encephalopathy, or ascites.

D. In rare cases patient may be diagnosed during pregnancy while doing routine investigations or during flare up during postpartum period probably due to immune reconstitution.

E. Sometimes type 2 AIH may be diagnosed concomitantly in patients with autoimmune thyroiditis, ulcerative colitis, type 1 diabetes mellitus, rheumatoid arthritis, and celiac disease.

Investigations

A. Serum biochemistry demonstrates elevation of transaminases of any magnitude with very high in case of fulminant hepatic failure, mild elevation of ALP.

B. Generalized elevation of gamma globulin mainly IgG fraction.

C. Serology:

   a. To diagnose type 1 AIH:
      - Antinuclear antibody in HEP-2 method
      - Antismooth muscle cell antibody

   b. To diagnose type 2 AIH:
      - Anti-liver-kidney mitochondrial antibody-1 directed against P450 CYP 2D6 and uridine-5'-diphosphate-glucuronosyltransferase

   c. To diagnose type 3 AIH:
      - Antibodies against soluble liver antigen
      - Antibodies against liver-pancreas antigen

      These are directed toward UGA-suppressor transfer ribonucleic acid (RNA)-associated protein.

   d. Other antibodies:
      - Antibodies against asialoglycoprotein receptor:
         - It is closely associated with histologic activity of the liver.
         - It can define treatment end point.

D. Liver histology: Interface hepatitis is characterized by the following:

   a. Periportal inflammation is the main hallmark of this disease

   b. Hepatocyte rosette formation

   c. Dense plasma cell infiltrate

   d. Active penetration of lymphocytes into hepatocytes—emperipolesis.

Diagnosis

Prior to diagnose AIH following causes of hepatitis have to be excluded, such as alcoholic, viral causes, Wilson's disease, hemochromatosis, and alpha-1 antitrypsin deficiency. In 2008, a simplified scoring system for diagnosing AIH is proposed by International Autoimmune Hepatitis Group.

Parameter	Discriminator	Score
ANA or ASMA	≥1:40	+1
	≥1:80	+2
Anti-LKM antibody	≥1:40	+2
Anti-SLA/LP	Any titer	+2
Total IgG	Upper limit of normal (ULN)	+1
	1.1 × ULN	+2
Liver histology	Compatible with AIH	+1
	Typical of AIH	+2
Absence of viral hepatitis	No	0
	Yes	+2

(ASMA: antismooth muscle antibody; SLA/LP: soluble liver antigen/liver-pancreas)

Definite AIH: ≥7; probable AIH: ≥6. Typical histology of AIH as described above all should be present. Compatible liver histology with AIH will be chronic hepatitis with plasma cell infiltration without above typical features.

Natural Progression and Prognosis without Treatment

Following parameters are associated with very poor prognosis:

A. Presence of inflammatory activity at the onset of the disease

B. Presence of development of cirrhosis of liver

C. 5–10-fold increase in aminotransferases

D. 2-fold increase in gamma globulin level

Course of AIH is also influenced by:

A. HLA antigen profile of the affected individual

B. Presence of HLA B8-associated severe inflammation at presentation

C. In case of HLA DR3-associated AIH lower probability of treatment remission

D. More benign outcome and higher age of onset in HLA DR4 subgroup of patients

Treatment

Absolute treatment indications are:

A. Sustained elevation of AST more than 10-fold normal

B. Serum AST elevation of more than 5-fold normal along with 2-fold increase in gamma globulin level

C. Hepatic histologic evidence of bridging necrosis, multilobular necrosis

D. Severe hepatic and extrahepatic symptoms

Relative indication are:

A. Mild clinical symptoms

B. Less severe laboratory and histologic abnormalities

No treatment is required for:

A. Inactive cirrhosis

B. Complication of portal hypertension in absence of hepatitis

C. Mild interface hepatitis in absence of symptoms

Induction of remission:

Remission can be defined as:

A. Complete biochemical and histological resolution of inflammation, but histological remission lagging 6–12 behind the biochemical markers.

B. Disappearances of clinical symptoms

Drugs used are:

A. Prednisolone 40–60 mg/day in tapering dose. Isolated use of this drug is required in:
   - **a.** Severe cytopenias
   - **b.** Active malignancy
   - **c.** Pregnant woman
   - **d.** Woman who is planning for pregnancy
   - **e.** Absence of thiopurine methyltransferase activity

B. Or, Prednisolone 20–30 mg/day in tapering dose + azathioprine 1–2 mg/kg/day. This is preferred because dose of prednisolone can be tapered to 10 mg/day to minimize the toxicity of prednisolone.

Maintenance of remission:

In this stage oral prednisolone dose will gradually be reduced to 10 mg daily within 2–3 months along with 50 mg azathioprine.

Treatment endpoints are:

A. Normalization of laboratory test

B. Normalization histology of liver tissue

C. Failure of normalization of liver test even after 36 months of therapy

D. Despite with treatment regimen worsening of laboratory tests

E. Drug intolerance in the form of metabolic changes, cosmetic changes, severe cytopenia, or compression of vertebrae.

Addition of 6–9 mg daily budesonide in place of prednisolone in noncirrhotic patients with mild inflammatory activity or premorbid conditions can be done with 1–2 mg/kg of body weight azathioprine. But this is not effective salvage regimen in case of steroid dependent or refractory patients.

Outcome of these patients: Patients may progress into:

A. Cirrhosis
B. Hepatic failure
C. Hepatocellular carcinoma
D. Relapse after withdrawal of the drugs
E. Other extrahepatic malignancies, such as blood cancer, breast, bladder, cervix, skin, stomach cancers, and lymphoma

Outcomes of the patients under treatment:

A. Resolution:
   a. Liver function tests will improve within 2 weeks of therapy returns to near normal 3 ± 3 months.
   b. Histologic pictures resolute within 3–8 months.

   Average duration of treatment until normalization of liver function tests and liver histology is 22 months.
B. Incomplete response: These patients fail to achieve histologic and biochemical response even after 36 months of treatment, so in these cases aims are to suppress as well as stabilize the inflammatory activity at the same time avoiding the drug-induced complications. In this case low dose of steroid should be continued for 7–43 years. Complications are cryptococcal meningitis and aseptic necrosis of hip.
C. Treatment failure: In spite of compliance with drug regimens the patients will progress to hepatocellular failure or cirrhosis or association with other diseases, such as drug-induced liver injury, hepatic steatosis, and overlap syndrome has to be searched for. In this case following treatment is given:
   a. Daily 60 mg prednisolone in case of azathioprine intolerant patients or daily 30 mg prednisolone with 150 mg azathioprine for 1 month followed by gradual reduction of prednisolone 10 mg and azathioprine 50 mg monthly till the maintenance dose of 10 mg prednisolone and 50 mg azathioprine daily or 20 mg prednisolone only in azathioprine refractory cases, but monthly liver test has to be done.
   b. Cyclosporine: Dose is 2–5 mg orally with trough level 100–300 ng/mL.
   c. Tacrolimus: Initial dose is 0.5–1 mg daily, maintenance dose in ≤3 mg twice daily. No response in 2% of cases.
   d. Mycophenolate mofetil: To start with 1 g daily followed by 1.5–2 g daily, but should be avoided in case of pregnancy as there is chance of miscarriage, congenital defect of face and heart. Side effects are cytopenia and nausea.
D. Relapse after withdrawal of drugs: It occurs usually within 3 months of drug withdrawal.
   a. Elevation of aminotransferases ≥3 times of upper limit of normal
   b. Recurrence of interface hepatitis
   c. Incomplete histological resolution mainly plasma cell infiltration
   d. Progression to cirrhosis
   e. Genetic predisposition

   In this case steroid has to be continued until normalization of liver function test then steroid dose should be reduced with increase in up to azathioprine to 2 mg/kg, then steroid is withdrawn but azathioprine should be continued indefinitely.

Liver transplantation: It should be performed in following conditions:

a. In MELD score of more than 16 points
b. Fulminant hepatic failure
c. Poorly tolerated drug treatment
d. Intractable symptoms
e. Suspected liver cancer

Q17. Describe the guidelines for assessment and management of NAFLD.

BF/MAY2013/MDIV (10)

Diagnosis and management of nonalcoholic fatty liver disease.

BF/NOV2013/MDII (10)

Nonalcoholic steatohepatitis.

RGUHS/MDIII (10); KHUS/NOV2013(S)/MDIII (10)

NASH.

SNMC/MAY2005/MDIV (10)

Nonalcoholic fatty liver disease.

GMC/2016/MDI (5)

Nonalcoholic fatty liver disease: pathogenesis, pathology and consequences.

PGI/APR2013/MDIV (10)

Nonalcoholic fatty liver causes, clinical features and management.

DNBIII/JUN2011 (10)

Nonalcoholic steatohepatitis.

MGR/MAR2009/MDII (6)

Enumerate the causes of hepatic steatosis. Discuss clinical features, diagnosis and management of non-alcoholic fatty liver disease.

DNBIII/DEC2012 (10)

Define nonalcoholic fatty liver disease. Discuss its pathogenesis, diagnosis and management.

DNBIVA/DEC2013 (10)

Fatty liver.

MGR/SEP2007/MHI (5)

Differentiate between nonalcoholic fatty liver disease and nonalcoholic steatohepatitis. How will you diagnose and treat nonalcoholic fatty liver disease.

DNB (DEC2021)(10)

Define NASH. Describe its clinical features and management. Advantages and disadvantages of fibroscan in the hepatic pathology evaluation.

DNB (DEC2018) (10)

Management of NASH.

SCB MED COL, 2022 (20)

Complications of NAFLD.

VEER NARMAD SOUTH GUJARAT UNI, 2022 (12)

Describe etiology, clinical features, investigations and treatment of NAFLD.

VEER NARMAD SOUTH GUJARAT UNI, 2022 (10)

Nonalcoholic fatty liver disease.

MAHARASHTRA UNI OF HEALTH SC, VIJAYAWADA, 2022 (10)

Nonalcoholic steatohepatitis.

NTR UNI OF HEALTH SC, VIJAYAWADA, 2020 (10)

Nonalcoholic steatohepatitis.

NTR UN OF HEALTH SC, VIJAYAWADA, 2019 (10)

Nonalcoholic fatty liver disease.

BHARATI VIDYAPEETH DEEMED UNI, 2018 (10)

What is the new terminology used and discuss about the clinical features, diagnosis and recent treatment updates in the management of nonalcoholic fatty liver disease in adults.

WBUHS, 2024 (10)

Newer therapy in NAFLD.

MANIPUR UNIVERSITY, 2021 (5)

NASH RAJASTHAN UNIVERSITY, 2022 (8)

Discuss nonpharmacological management of NAFLD.

MAHATMA UNIVERSITY, 2022 (10)

Nonalcoholic steatohepatitis.

MAHATMA UNIVERSITY, 2019 (10)

Outline the guidelines on the management of metabolic dysfunction-associated steatotic liver disease.

WBUHS, 2024 (10)

New terminology of NAFLD is metabolic dysfunction associated fatty liver disease (MASLD).

ANSWER

Nonalcoholic fatty liver disease is a spectrum of diseases and can be defined as microvascular steatosis involving ≥5% of hepatocytes in absence of other etiologies, such as alcohol and drugs. Spectrums involved are steatosis, steatohepatitis, fibrosis, cirrhosis, and HCC; hence it can be called as a silent killer of human being and leading cause of chronic liver disease worldwide.

Pathophysiology

A. Role of hormones:

   a. In obese patients with NAFLD, there is imbalance between energy expenditure and energy gain in the form of large amount of food intake which occurs due to stimulation of opioid and dopamine receptors in the nucleus ambiens of brain which is an area for craving of foods. Again increased fructose intake increases blood flow to these centers and thus fails to reduce the satiety.

   b. Gut-derived hormones: Decreased concentration of glucagon-like peptide-1 decreases satiety and increased concentration of ghrelin overstimulates hunger.

   Above hormonal changes increase the triglyceride levels in the blood.

   c. Leptin and adiponectin: Leptin acts centrally to reduce intake of food and at the same time increases energy expenditure. Adiponectin increases the sensitivity of hepatic insulin and decreases the body fat. In patients with NAFLD leptin level will be elevated suggesting resistance to action of leptin, but adiponectin level will be low indicating decrease in sensitivity of hepatic insulin.

B. Role of nutrition and intestinal dysbiosis: Due to inherent challenges of human nutrition studies influences of specific nutrients on increased susceptibility to NAFLD are not known. Carbohydrate-rich diet and high-fat but low-fiber content of the food are responsible for development of NAFLD. High fructose and sucrose content of the diet increases the susceptibility of NAFLD by:

   a. Promotion of intestinal dysbiosis

   b. Dysregulation of key to lipid metabolic pathways

   Gut microbiota are censored by diet as macronutrients control the microflora composition in the gut. It has been shown that gut bacteria invade the tight junction of the gut by unknown mechanism to gain access of the circulation and inflammatory cytokines leading to promotion of hepatic steatosis and inflammation.

C. Insulin resistance, lipotoxicity, and liver inflammation in the liver: Normally insulin is secreted in response to high circulating glucose level from pancreatic beta cells.

   a. Insulin promotes esterification of fatty acids by acting on adipose tissue and store it in lipid droplets.

   b. It inhibits lipolysis.

   In the liver insulin has following actions:

   a. It promotes glycogen storage.

   b. It inhibits gluconeogenesis.

   c. It activates key regulators of lipogenesis de novo.

   But in case of NAFLD there is insulin resistance which leads to:

   a. Increased lipolysis in adipose tissue leading to increased circulating level of free fatty acids which ultimately will be taken by liver.

   b. Reduced storage of glycogen in liver

   c. Increased gluconeogenesis

   d. Due to hyperinsulinemia there is augmentation of hepatic lipogenesis de novo.

   Net result is:

   a. Increased lipid accumulation in the liver tissue leading to hepatic steatosis

   b. Increased secretion of triglycerides in the form of very low-density lipoprotein (VLDL)

   c. Increased lipid will reach the adipose tissue through circulation which will be compounded by the already reduced ability of this adipocyte cells in adipose tissue for storing this lipid within lipid droplets.

   Since lipid droplets cannot accommodate neutral lipid it will be exposed to lipotoxic bioactive lipid. This lipotoxicity will perform following downstream actions leading to progressing from isolated steatosis to fibrosis, cirrhosis, and HCC:

   a. It will impair insulin signaling further.

   b. It will produce further oxidative damage.

   c. It will promote inflammation further leading to fibrosis.

D. Proprotein convertase subtilisin/kexin type 9 secreted from hepatocytes acts on receptor for degradation of fat and inhibits the uptake of LDL and thus augments lipogenesis. This enzyme will be elevated in patient with NAFLD.

E. Influence of genes: There is association between patatin-like phospholipase domain-containing protein 3 (PNPLA3) with triacylglycerol lipase and acylglycerol transacylase activity. But single amino acid substitution of methionine to isoleucine at 148th position of PNPLA3 will lead to increased risk and severity of NAFLD in both adults and children. This "G" allele is most common with highest risk in Hispanic population and lowest risk and least common in African-Americans. On the other hand, replacement of serine to isoleucine in 453th position in PNPLA3 may be protective from hepatic steatosis and is more common in African-Americans.

Several additional loci are associated with NAFLD, these are:

- **a.** Neurocan
- **b.** Glucokinase regulator
- **c.** Lysophospholipase-like 1
- **d.** Protein phosphatase 1 regulatory subunit 3B

Risk Factors Associated NAFLD

- **a.** Obesity
- **b.** Type 2 diabetes mellitus
- **c.** Dyslipidemia
- **d.** Polycystic ovarian syndrome
- **e.** Hypothyroidism
- **f.** Obstructive sleep apnea
- **g.** Hypopituitarism
- **h.** Hypogonadism
- **i.** Pancreaticoduodenal secretion
- **j.** Psoriasis

Symptoms of NAFLD

- **a.** May be asymptomatic, only incidental radiological finding or biochemical derangement.
- **b.** Symptoms are in case of symptomatic patients:
    - Malaise
    - Fatigue
    - Right upper quadrant pain due to distended Glisson's capsule

Signs in NAFLD

- **a.** There is no specific sign which may not clench the diagnosis of NAFLD.
- **b.** Central obesity—it is most common finding
- **c.** Hepatomegaly
- **d.** Signs of hepatocellular failure may be found in case of steatohepatitis or cirrhosis
- **e.** Stigmata of cirrhosis

Biochemical Abnormalities

- **A.** Liver enzymes such as ALT or AST less than twice of upper limit of normal. In some cases these may be within normal limits. Characteristically, AST/ALT ratio is <1 in NAFLD but as the disease progresses toward hepatic fibrosis the ration will be reversed to >1.
- **B.** Elevation of GGT with mildly elevated ALP level
- **C.** Blood glucose level will be high with presence of hyperinsulinemia.
- **D.** Hypertriglyceridemia, low high-density lipoprotein (HDL), or cholesterol levels
- **E.** Elevated ferritin level with normal transferrin saturation indicates acute phase response.

Histological Features in NAFLD

- **A.** Steatosis—More than 5% hepatocytes are affected, centrilobular (zone 3) in distribution, macrovesicular or microvesicular or mixed disposition. Morphologically, fat distribution can be classified into three types:
    - **a.** Macrovascular distribution: Larger lipid droplets occupy the center displacing the nucleus and other organelles toward periphery.
    - **b.** Microvascular distribution: Here multiple small fat droplets occupy cell without displacing the nucleus but the cell appears foamy. It is not seen in metabolic syndrome but present in alcoholic liver disease.
    - **c.** Mixed variety: It is present as combination of above.

    As the disease progresses toward fibrosis steatosis level will fall.
- **B.** Steatohepatitis: Here steatosis is accompanied by infiltration of chronic mononuclear cells, monocytes, and plasma cells associated with mild or mixed portal inflammation and most important is hepatocyte ballooning.
- **C.** Fibrosis: Initially, perivenular to start with followed by pericellular in chicken-wire pattern, may be associated with portal or periportal fibrosis, bridging fibrosis between portal to portal, central to central, or central to portal septa ultimately leading to micronodular cirrhosis.

Different scores of NAFLD:

NASH Clinical Research Network NAFLD activity score		Steatosis activity fibrosis score	
Histologic features	Category definition	Histologic features	Category definition
Steatosis	0—<5%	Steatosis	0—<5%
	1—5–33%		1—5–33%
	2—34–66%		2—34–66%
	3—>66%		3—>66%
Hepatocyte ballooning	0—None	Hepatocyte ballooning	0—None
	1—Few		1—Clusters of round hepatocytes with pale cytoplasm
	2—Many		2—Same as grade 1q with enlarged hepatocytes
Inflammation	0—None	Inflammation	0—None
	1—1-2 foci/20 times field		2—<2 foci/20 times field
	2—2-4 foci/20 times field		2—>2 foci/20 times field
	3—>4 foci/20 times field		
Fibrosis	0—No fibrosis	Fibrosis	0—No fibrosis
	1a—Zone 3 mild perisinusoidal fibrosis		1a—Zone 3 mild perisinusoidal fibrosis
	1b—Zone 3 moderate perisinusoidal fibrosis		1b—Zone 3 moderate perisinusoidal fibrosis
	1c—Periportal/portal fibrosis		1c—Periportal/portal fibrosis
	2—Zone 3 plus portal/periportal fibrosis		2—Zone 3 plus portal/periportal fibrosis
	3—Bridging fibrosis		3—Bridging fibrosis
	4—Cirrhosis		4—Cirrhosis

(NASH: nonalcoholic steatohepatitis)

Following noninvasive tests and scores for predicting fibrosis severity in NAFLD:

Test type	Test	Formula	Risk
Simple panel	Aspartate transaminase to platelet ratio index (APRI)	AST/platelet count (10^9/L) × 100	High risk >1
	Predicted advanced fibrosis [NAFLD fibrosis score (NFS)]	NFS = 1.675 + 0.037 × age (year) + 0.094 × BMI (kg/m^2) + 1.13 × IFG or diabetes (yes = 1, no = 0) + 0.99 × AST/ALT ration – 0.013 × platelet count (10^9/L) – 0.66 × albumin (g/dL)	• High risk—>0.676 • Intermediate risk—1.455–0.676 • Low risk—<1.455
	Fibrosis-4 index (FIB-4 score)	FIB-4 score = age (year) × AST (IU/L)/platelet count (10^9/L) × √ALT (IU/L)	• High risk—score >2.67 • Intermediate risk—score 1.30–2.67 • Low risk—score <1.30
Radiologic technique	Fibroscan		• High risk—>9.6 kPa • Intermediate risk—7.9–9.6 kPa • Low risk—<7.9 kPa

Treatment

In each and every patient in the plan of treatment of nonalcoholic fatty liver disease following three components should be incorporated:

- **a.** Mediterranean diet to reduce the daily intake of calorie of at least 500 to 1000 Kcal.
- **b.** By diet and daily physical activity, weight loss should be 3–5% of body weight.
- **c.** Moderate physical activity should be 150–200 minute/week including the patient suffering from advanced chronic liver disease.

A. Lifestyle modification:

- **a.** Calorie restriction with increased physical activity improves biochemical and histological parameters in NAFLD. Combination of hypocaloric diet with moderately intense exercise will reduce 500–1,000 kcal per day. 3–5% weight loss is necessary to improve steatosis and 7–10% loss will improve steatohepatitis and fibrosis.
- **b.** Low fructose or sucrose-containing diet improves the metabolic syndrome.

B. Insulin sensitizers: Since this disease is associated with insulin resistance and metabolic syndrome, these therapies will obviously improve the condition.

- **a.** Metformin improves biochemical parameters but fails to improve histological improvement. But it should be given to improve diabetes; it is safe in cirrhosis and protects against the development of HCC.
- **b.** Thiazolidinediones: It will act through peroxisome proliferator-activated receptor (PPAR)-γ signaling and increases the tissue insulin sensitivity thus improving blood sugar. Drugs are pioglitazone and rosiglitazone. Pioglitazone improves both hepatic insulin sensitivity and fatty acid oxidation, and inhibits hepatic lipogenesis.

C. Antioxidants: Vitamin E administration at a dose of 800 mg/day especially nondiabetics helps in improving histological parameters, such as steatosis, hepatocyte ballooning, fibrosis, and lobular inflammation.

D. Incretin-based therapy: Both GLP-1 and DPP-4 inhibitors induce meal-induced pancreatic insulin secretion associated with extrapancreatic effects on multiple organs. Former drugs are associated with weight loss also; it will improve liver histology and biochemical tests in type 2 diabetes with NAFLD.

E. Lipid-lowering agents: Statin improves NAFLD associated with diabetes mellitus and metabolic syndrome associated with hyperlipidemia. Proprotein convertase subtilisin/kexin type 9 inhibitor has been highly effective in improving hypercholesterolemia in patients with NAFLD.

F. Drugs responsible for weight loss:

- **a.** Orlistat: It prevents fat absorption by inhibiting pancreatic lipase leading to weight loss.
- **b.** Lorcaserin: This suppresses the appetite and decreases weight by 4% associated with lifestyle modification within 12 months of therapy.
- **c.** Naltrexone/Bupropion: These drugs in combination are associated with weight loss of 5% along with improvement of liver biochemistry.
- **d.** Phentermine/Topiramate: This combination reduces body weight along with improvement of NAFLD.
- **e.** Liraglutide: 3 mg/day liraglutide is used for reducing body weight in nondiabetic patients.

G. Other novel agents:

- **a.** Pentoxifylline: This nonselective phosphodiesterase inhibitor increases cyclic AMP and decreases TNF-α and prevents inflammation in liver.
- **b.** Prebiotic and probiotic drugs: These prevent abnormal multiplication of microbiota and prevent hepatic steatohepatitis.
- **c.** Obeticholic acid: This synthetic bile acid is farnesoid X receptor agonist and can be used in case of NAFLD.
- **d.** Elafibranor: This PPAR-α/delta agonist is shown to improve moderate to severe NASH.

H. Bariatric surgery: It has been shown to improve the histological and biochemical parameters in patients with NAFLD.

I. Liver transplantation: One important and third most important indication is NASH-related end-stage hepatic failure in US in obesity pandemic. Survival rate in this case is as same as hepatic failure due to other liver diseases.

Current treatment guidelines of nonalcoholic fatty liver disease:

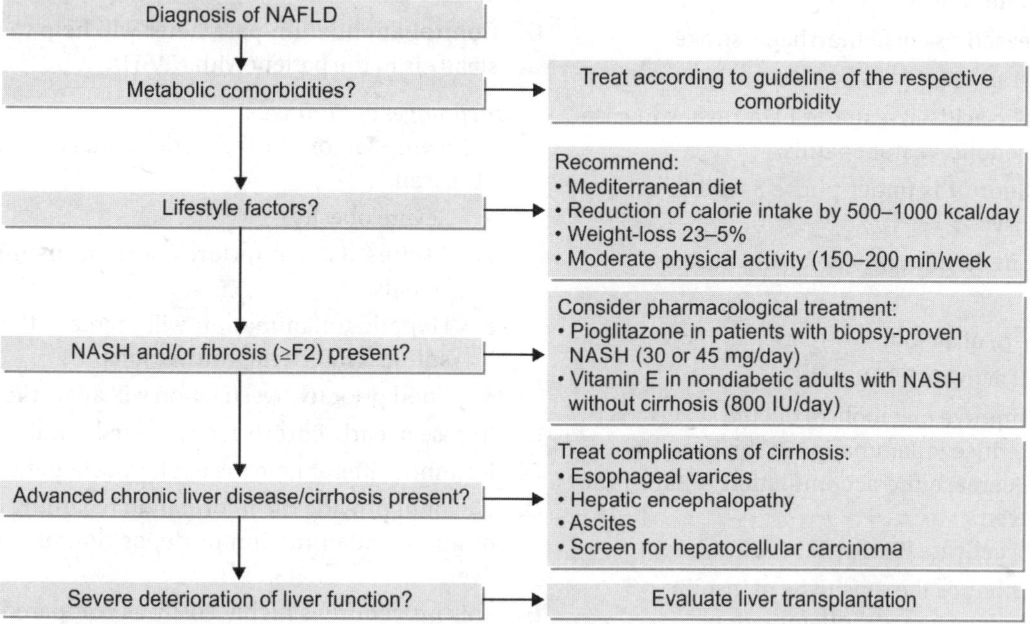

Drug treatment in case of nonalcoholic fatty liver disease:

A. Insulin sensitizer: Pioglitazone:

- **a.** Mechanisms:
  - **1.** Improves sensitivity to insulin
  - **2.** It reduces the fat content in the liver
  - **3.** It will decrease the inflammation in the liver.
- **b.** Clinical evidence:
  - **1.** There is histological improvement
  - **2.** Reduces fibrosis
- **c.** Side effects:
  - **1.** Weight gain
  - **2.** Increased risk of fracture
  - **3.** Retention of fluid

B. GLP-1 receptor antagonist: Semaglutide and liraglutide:

- **a.** Mechanism of action:
  - **1.** Increases secretion of insulin
  - **2.** Appetite will be reduced
  - **3.** Prolongs weight loss
- **b.** Clinical implications:
  - **1.** Reduction of fibrosis
  - **2.** Reduction of fat
- **c.** Side effects:
  - **1.** Nausea and vomiting
  - **2.** Chance of gallbladder disease

C. Fibroblast growth factor 21 and 19 (resmetirom):

- **a.** Mechanism of action is: The target receptor is β.
- **b.** Clinical implication:
  - **1.** Improves liver histology
  - **2.** Improves metabolism of lipid.
- **c.** Side effects:
  - **1.** Transaminitis
  - **2.** Possible cardiovascular effects

D. SGLT-2 inhibitor (dapagliflozin):

- **a.** Mechanism of actions:
  - **1.** Increases excretion of glucose
  - **2.** It improves resistance to insulin
  - **3.** It reduces liver fat
- **b.** Clinical implications:
  - **1.** It reduces hepatic steatosis along with inflammation.
- **c.** Side effects:
  - **1.** Dehydration
  - **2.** Urinary tract infection

E. Vitamin E:

- **a.** Mechanism of actions:
  - **1.** It reduces oxidative stress
  - **2.** It reduces inflammation in the hepatocytes.
- **b.** Clinical implications:
  - **1.** There is histological improvement.

c. Side effects:
   1. Prostate cancer
   2. Increased risk of hemorrhagic stroke

F. Other drugs are:
   a. Obeticholic acid—it is under FDA review in case of nonalcoholic steatohepatitis.
   b. Lanifibranor: It is under phase 3 trial in case of liver fibrosis.
   c. Aldafermin: It reduces liver fat and fibrosis.

G. Saroglitazar:
   a. Mechanism of action:
      1. It will activate PPAR-α to
         - Improve metabolism of lipid
         - Reduce inflammation in the liver
         - Decrease the accumulation of fat in the liver.
      2. It will activate PPAR-γ TO:
         - Enhance the sensitivity of insulin
         - Reduce hepatic inflammation
         - Slow the progression of fibrosis.
   b. Clinical implications:
      1. It improves the NAFLD activity score and decreases the liver enzymes.
      2. It reduces the accumulation of fat in the liver
      3. It improves the sensitivity of insulin thereby reduces the fasting plasma glucose.
      4. It lowers the LDL and triglyceride and increases the HDL.
      5. It will reduce the hepatic inflammation and fibrosis.

Fibroscan of Liver

Hepatic fibroscan is a noninvasive procedure to detect any steatosis, fibrosis in the liver and measures the stiffness in the liver.

Advantages of fibroscan:

A. It is noninvasive and painless, hence it does not require ant sedation. So it is comfortable to the patient.

B. It takes nearly 10 minutes to perform, so it is quick procedure.

C. Its data shows minimal observer variability as compared to ultrasound.

D. It can detect steatosis, different grades of fibrosis and cirrhosis.

E. It is devoid of any risk of bleeding, infection or pain during and after the procedure.

F. It can measure the improvement and monitor the disease after treatment.

G. Control attenuation parameter will help to grade of steatosis in the patient with NASH.

Disadvantages of fibroscan:

A. Following factors in the patient affect the result of fibroscan:
   a. Severe obesity
   b. Ascites as it interferes with transmission of signals.
   c. Hepatic inflammation will increase the hepatic stiffness interfering with results.
   d. Food prior to investigation will affect the results.

B. In case of early fibrosis it has limited value.

C. It cannot differentiate the etiology of hepatic stiffness.

D. It cannot provide the information regarding the types of micro-inflammation or deposition of iron in the liver.

E. This procedure is highly costly as compared to other investigation.

Nonpharmacological management in nonalcoholic fatty liver disease:

A. Weight loss with target of ≥7% to 10% weight to improve fibrosis, hepatic steatosis and inflammation.

B. Modification of diet:
   a. Caloric restriction to 500–1,000 kcal/day.
   b. Diet preferred is Mediterranean diet which is monosaturated fat, refined curb and red meat.
   c. Sugar, beverages and fructose containing fruit should be avoided.

C. Physical activity:
   a. 150–300 minute/week aerobic exercise of moderate intensity and 75–100 minutes vigorous exercise to reduce hepatic steatosis.
   b. Resistance exercise is better.

D. Control of blood pressure, diabetes and obesity and alcohol to reduce the weight loss.

E. Evaluate and treatment of obstructive sleep apnea.

Q18. Describe the etiopathogenesis, clinical presentation and management of hepatitis C infection.

DNBIII/DEC2011/(10)

Describe the clinical manifestation, diagnosis and management of chronic hepatitis C infection.

DNBIII/JUN2013(10)

Drugs used for the treatment of hepatitis C virus infection.

DNBII/APR2016 (4)

Management protocol of a patient with HCV genotype 3 infection.

DNBII/APR2016 (6)

Management of chronic hepatitis C infection.

DNBIIIB/JUN2016 (7)

Hepatitis C virus.

MGR/OCT2011/MDI (5)/MGR/SEP2010/MDI (5)/ MGR/SEP2009/MDIII (6)

Describe current management and newer drugs in hepatitis C infection.

MJPRU/2015(S)/MDIII (20)

Give a brief account of investigational approach and newer trends in the management of chronic hepatitis C.

MJPRU/2016/MDIV (20)

Describe the recent advances in the management of chronic hepatitis C.

BF/NOV2013/MDIV (10)

Discuss the current management of chronic hepatitis C.

BF/MAY2009/MDIV (20)

Treatment of hepatitis C.

BF/JUN2016/MDII (10)

How will you manage a case of hepatitis C?

MUZ/MAY2016/MGII (20)

PGI/APR2013/MDII (10)

Management of chronic hepatitis C infection.

DNBIIIB/JUNE2016 (7)

Discuss etiology, pathophysiology, clinical features and management of chronic hepatitis.

MGR/OCT2015/MDII (15)

Treatment of chronic hepatitis C infection.

AMU/2011/MDII (10)

What are the various viruses causing jaundice? Write down the clinical picture and management of hepatitis C.

MJPRU/2016/MDI (25)

Guidelines and management of hepatitis C infection.

PGI/APR2014/MDIII (10)

Diagnosis and management of hepatitis C infection.

DNB (DEC2022) (5)

Genotype based treatment of HCV infection.

DNB (DEC 2020) (5)

Treatment of hepatitis C infection.

DNB (DEC 2019) (5)

Recent advances in management of hepatitis C infection.

KERALA UNI, 2022 (10)

Clinical features, diagnosis and treatment of hepatitis C virus infection.

NTR UNI OF HEALTH SCIENCES, ANDHRA, 2022 (10)

Association of CD4/CD8 ratio with viral load, genotypes and cirrhosis with chronic hepatitis and management of chronic hepatitis C infection.

SAURASHTRA UNI, RAJKOT 2021 (20)

Treatment of hepatitis C.

NTR UNI OF HEALTH SC, VIJAYAWADA, 20121 (10)

Discuss the management of chronic hepatitis C.

TEERTHANKER MAHAVEER UNI, 2020 (10)

Hepatitis C infection.

SAURASHTRA UNIVERSITY, 2020 (20)

Outline the updated management of a case of HCV.

BWBUHS, 2020 (10)

Management of hepatitis C.

BABA FARID UNI OF HEALTH SC, 2019 (10)

Management of a case of hepatitis C infection.

BABA FARID UNI OF HEALTH SC, 2018 (10)

Management of hepatitis C syndrome.

BABA FARID UNI OF HEALTH SC, 2019 (10)

Management of hepatitis C infection.

TEERTHANKER MAHAVEER UNIVERSITY, 2018 (10)

Describe etiopathogenesis and management of hepatitis C infection.

GURU GOVIND SINGH NEW DELHI, 2018 (15)

Discuss the management of chronic hepatitis C infection.

WBUHS, 2024 (10)

Guidelines for management of hepatitis C infection.

MANIPUR UNIVERSITY, 2018 (10)

Discuss newer therapies in the management of chronic HCV infection.

MANIPUR UNIVERSITY, 2019 (10)

Discuss extra-hepatic features of HCV infection.

MANIPUR UNIVERSITY, 2024 (10)

Treatment of chronic hepatitis C infection.

RAJASTHAN UNIVERSITY, 2019 (8)

Diagnosis and treatment of hepatitis C virus infection.

MAHATMA UNIVERSITY, 2018 (10)

Discuss extrahepatic manifestations of hepatitis C. How can you manage a patient with hepatitis C infection?

WBUHS, 2024 (10)

ANSWER

Introduction

Structure

Hepatitis C virus identified in the year of 1989 is the most important cause of post-transfusion hepatitis. It is in the genus *Hepacivirus* in the family of Flaviviridae. This viral protein has been cleaved by host and viral protease into 10 viral proteins. 5' end of the genome consists of untranslated region adjacent to genes for structural proteins, such as core, envelope protein (E1 and E2) and 3' end contains nonstructural proteins, such as p7 viroporin, NS2-3, and NS3 NS4A proteases, NSE RNA helicase, NS4B and NS5A proteins, and NS5B RNA-dependent RNA polymerase. Envelope proteins are encoded by hypervariable region varying from isolate to isolate and this region helps to evade host immune response. High replicative activity as well as lack of proofreading function of RNA-dependent RNA polymerase is the main cause of genomic variability of HCV.

- **a.** P7 is membrane ion channel responsible for efficient assembly and HCV release.
- **b.** NS2, a cysteine protease responsible cleavage between NS3 from NS2.
- **c.** NS3-4A, serine protease is responsible for breakage of all downstream protein from polyprotein.

Life Cycle of Hepatitis C

Hepatitis C virus having highly restricted tropism invades human hepatocytes as main target in following steps:

Step 1: Hepatitis C virus enters into the hepatocytes through the attachment of the cell surface receptors, such as CD81, scavenger receptor class B type 1, tight junction protein claudin 1 as well as occluding along with LDL receptor and glycosaminoglycans as attachment factors. Virus can transmit from cell to cell.

Step 2: After its entry through receptor-mediated endocytosis it will release its RNA genome into the host cytoplasm after pH-dependent membrane fusion within acidic compartment.

Step 3: In a membrane web made of HCV NS protein and host cell protein called replication complex located near perinuclear membrane replication and post-translation of virus occurs. So replication complex is composed of (1) viral protein, (2) replicating RNA, (3) altered cellular membranes—these are the characteristics of positive-strand RNA.

Step 4: Now virus replicates in those webs where negative-strand RNA is synthesized by NS5B RNA-dependent RNA polymerase; this negative strand RNA is the future template for positive-strand RNA which ultimately leads to production of new viral protein; it acts as template for further viral replication.

Step 5: Packaging and assembly: After replication they are assembled in virion following incorporation of viral RNA—which will be facilitated by HCV core on lipid droplets.

Step 6: After the maturation of virion it will be leased from hepatocytes and it will be facilitated by lipid droplets and VLDL pathway.

Virus replication

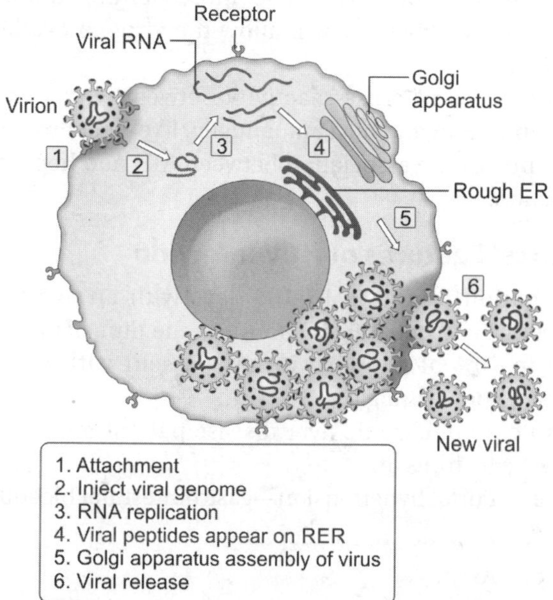

(RER: rough endoplasmic reticulum)

Each step of HCV life cycle is the target of antiviral drugs.

Mechanism of Hepatic Injury in HCV Infection

In case of acute hepatitis C: Virus control is mediated by CD8 T cells and NK cells through cytopathic and noncytopathic mechanisms.

In case of chronic hepatitis C: In this case balance between the virus and immune response is mainly responsible for future course of disease as this balance is very much complex. HCV will be adapted in the hepatic environment by following mechanisms:

- **a.** Increased number of infected cells
- **b.** Inhibition of cellular antiviral pathways
- **c.** Immune escape mutation
- **d.** Potential extrahepatic reservoir

Immune mechanisms prevent excessive damage of liver cells at the same time control replication of virus.

Virus-mediated Injury

In a viable or in immunosuppressed host virus will survive as noncytopathic host; HCV expresses in the liver in the form hepatic steatosis, hepatic injury, and liver cancer. Liver damage will be accelerated in case of HIV coinfection as well as HCV-infected liver transplant.

Immune-mediated Liver Cell Injury

- **A.** T cell-mediated injury: There is correlation between hepatocellular damage and CD8 activity as evidenced by correlation between T cells infiltration of hepatocytes by CD8 cells and induction of anti-HCV T-cell response and multi-month delay in rise of AST and ALT leading to release of chemokines, neutrophil, and platelets and recruitment of NK, NK T and macrophages, monocytes, and dendritic cells in the liver. There is also elaboration of IFN-γ which will clear the virus-infected hepatocytes which lead to viral clearance without producing fulminant hepatic failure.
- **B.** Involvement of chemokines in immune cells recruitment in the liver: Viral gene products and antiviral cytokines, like IFN-γ, increase the production of chemokines which are responsible for migration and inflammation. T-cells recruited HCV-infected hepatocytes express chemokine receptors CXCR3 and CCR5, again CXCL10 receptors expression is associated with liver cell inflammation and hepatic fibrosis. CXCL8 expression is associated with persistence of HCV as well as resistance to IFN-α.
- **C.** Influence of NK cells in liver cell injury: There is correlation between hepatitis flares and increased NK cell activation and TNF-related apoptosis-induced ligands. NK cells are involved in liver disease activity and control of viruses in case of HCV infection.
- **D.** Progression to fibrosis: Progression to fibrosis varies person to person and cannot be predicted but there are several factors that may increase the progression to fibrosis; these are alcohol abuse, diabetes mellitus, and obesity. So few patients will progress faster to cirrhosis but some cases are modifiable.

Genotypes and Serotypes of HCV

Nucleotide sequencing isolates 6 distinct genotypes and more than 50 subtypes within genotypes. By sequence homology genotypes differ from each other by 30% and subtypes differ by 20%. In the same host and in the same genotype there may be divergence—this is intragenomic differences called quasispecies. This intragenomic diversity is responsible for high mutation rate and it interferes with effective humoral immunity.

Neutralizing antibody against HCV is short-lasting and it will not produce long-lasting immunity, so it will not protect against reinfection with different or same isolates of viruses. So, homologous or heterologous immunity will not develop after acute HCV infection.

Few genotypes are distributed worldwide and some genotypes are more confined to specific geographical areas. Genotype 3 is responsible for hepatic steatosis along with clinical progression but other genotypes will respond to antiviral therapy.

Third-generation immunoassays can detect anti-HCV antibodies during acute infection by incorporating proteins from core, NS3 and NS5 regions. HCV RNA can be detected by PCR, it is expressed in IU/L. It can detect HCV RNA to as low as 5 IU/L and within few days of exposure and before the appearance of anti-HCV and will persist through the period of infection.

Most sensitive molecular assay detects presence of replicative HCV in peripheral lymphocytes in patient infected with HCV.

Pathogenesis of Hepatitis C

In case of HCV infection there will be T cell-mediated immune response in which elaborated cytokines produce both multicellular innate and adaptive immune response which are responsible for containment of infection and pathogenesis in liver. HCV is very efficient in evading the host immune response. Immediately after exposure to HCV host cells can identify viral product motif and distinguish from self-antigen and liberates cytokines and IFN leading to development of adaptive and innate immune response. In HCV-infected patients, viral NS protein, nucleocapsid, and envelope-specific intrahepatic HLA class I-restricted cytotoxic T cells do not correlate with degree of injury in hepatocytes or its recovery. But in case of HCV-associated liver injury CD4+ helper cells after being activated by virus stimulate HCV-specific CD8+ cytotoxic cells via release of cytokines. This response is more robust in patients recovered from HCV infections because in case of chronic infection there is defect in proliferation of CD8+ cells due to mutation of CD8+ cells resulting contraction of CD4+ cells, as a result HCV virus will escape the immune clearance and upregulation of inhibitory receptors. HCV proteins interfere with innate immunity by blocking type 1 IFN response and inhibit IFN signaling cascade. In case of underexpression of HLA class I molecule responsible for developing adaptive immunity NK cells of innate immunity system come into play to limit HCV infection, but in case of persistent viral infection both intrahepatic NK cell cytotoxicity and peripheral cytotoxicity are dysfunctional. In case of complex immune response core, NS4B and NS5B protein will reduce antiapoptotic proteins by suppressing the immunoregulatory nuclear factor-κβ pathway, as a result there is TNF-α-mediated cell death.

There is definite link between HLA allele and self-limited hepatitis C. CC haplotype of *IL2B* gene coded for IFN λ3, a component of antiviral innate immune response, has been seen and it is stronger when it is combined with HLA class II DQB1*03:01. In case of polymorphism of IL2B the hepatocyte fails to clear the virus from within. This unfavorable *IL2B* allele will depress the NK cells and innate immune response. Moreover appearance of quasispecies diversity will allow the virus to evade the hepatocyte.

Presence of cross-reactivity between viral antigen NS3 and NS5A and host autoantigen, like cytochrome 450 2D6, proves the association between AIH and hepatitis C infection.

Clinical Features of HCV Infection

Incubation period is 15–160 days with an average of 7 weeks. HCV hepatitis is chronic at the time of presentation in 70% of patients; it may present with malaise, fatigue, and arthralgia.

In case of chronic liver disease patient may present with the features of:

- **a.** Portal hypertension—gastrointestinal bleeding
- **b.** Hepatic encephalopathy
- **c.** Ascites
- **d.** Extrahepatic manifestations:
  - **1.** Arthralgia
  - **2.** Myalgia
  - **3.** Pruritus
  - **4.** Sicca syndrome

Physical Examinations

- **a.** Signs in hand: Palmar erythema, asterixis, leukonychia, clubbing, and Dupuytren's contracture
- **b.** Signs in head: Jaundice, temporal hollow, parotid enlargement, and cyanosis
- **c.** Fetor hepaticus
- **d.** Gynecomastia and small testes
- **e.** Edema feet
- **f.** Body hair scanty
- **g.** Skin signs: Spider nevi, petechiae, and excoriations

h. Extrahepatic manifestations:
   1. Mixed cryoglobulinemia
   2. Non-Hodgkin's lymphoma
   3. Monoclonal gammopathy of undetermined significance
   4. Thrombocytopenia
   5. Lichen planus
   6. Porphyria cutanea tarda
   7. Necrolytic acral erythema
   8. Leukocytoclastic vasculitis
   9. Membranoproliferative glomerulonephritis
   10. Membranous nephropathy
   11. Keratoconjunctivitis Sicca
   12. Sjögren's syndrome
   13. Porphyria cutanea tarda
   14. Raynaud syndrome
   15. Necrotizing cutaneous vasculitis
   16. Type 1 diabetes mellitus
   17. Autoimmune thyroid diseases:
       - Hashimoto thyroiditis
       - Grave's disease
   18. Peripheral neuropathy
   19. Mononeuritis multiplex
   20. Cognitive decline

Diagnosis of HCV Infection

After discovery of HCV in 1990s first-generation HCV screening test was based on yeast-expressed recombinant protein having epitope of NS4 region of HCV genome. Now third-generation anti-HCV assay with automated PCR testing reduces the risk to 1 in 2.3 million transfusions. Following are the laboratory features of HCV infection:

a. There is episodic pattern of elevation of aminotransferases.

b. Detection of anti-HCV in the serum.
   1. In case of acute hepatitis C infection during early phase when aminotransferases are raised.
   2. It will be detectable after recovery—which is rare.
   3. It is common to be present in case of chronic infection.

      In some cases of rheumatoid arthritis rheumatoid factor nonspecifically will bind to assay agents leading to false negative results.
   4. Gold standard estimation is detection of HCV RNA by RT-PCR. It can be detected:
      - Before the acute elevation of aminotransferases in the serum.
      - Before the detection of anti-HCV in the serum in acute HCV infection.
   5. It can be detected in most cases of chronic infection continuously or intermittently.
   6. It can be detected in case of chronic carrier.
   7. It can also be detected in anti-HCV negative patients.

      In recent process of measurement by RT-PCR lower limit of detection is 10–25 IU/mL and highest limit is 10^7 IU/mL. Detection of HCV RNA predicts the response to therapy but neither the prognostic marker nor disease severity.

   Presence of anti-HCV in absence of HCV RNA by RT-PCR confirms the patient as "cured".
   8. Detection of core antigen or nucleocapsid protein alone or in combination with anti-HCV. It has following advantages:
      - It is simpler to use than molecular assay.
      - It has 99% specificity in testing blood donor.
      - It has 97% sensitivity in detecting HCV RNA positive or anti-HCV negative specimens in seroconverted persons following acute infection.

Treatment of HCV Infection

Primary goal of HCV therapy is sustained virological response (SVR); it can be defined as HCV RNA reduction to undetectable level as measured by RT-PCR when it is measured ≥24 weeks after completion of therapy. It is generally associated with: (1) Normalization of liver enzymes, (2) Improvement or regression of necroinflammation or fibrosis of liver, (3) Improvement of liver function, (4) Reduction of liver-related mortality, (5) Reduction of risk of HCC, and (6) Clearance of HCV in cirrhotic patients, but here mortality may not be reduced as these patients may suffer from metabolic syndrome or obesity or concurrently HBV positive. Previously IFN-based therapy started to cure HCV from the blood and hepatocytes. It was administered subcutaneously thrice weekly for 6 months but SVR is achieved only <10% which was increased to 20% by doubling the duration of therapy not the dose. Then SVR of 40% can be achieved by addition of daily dose of ribavirin. This combination can increase SVR in genotype 1 and 4 to >40% and in genotype 2 and 3 to >80%. Histological improvement occurs in absence of biochemical or virological response. In case of chronic hepatitis infection treatment will precipitously reduce ALT and virological response in early phase. Two types of IFN are available. These are PEG IFN-α2b and PEG IFN-α2a.

Dose of PEG IFN-α2a is 180 μg and PEG IFN-α2b is 1.5 μg/kg.

Ribavirin dose—for genotype 1, it is 1,000 mg (<75 kg patient) and 1,200 mg (>75 kg patient), for genotype 2 and 3, it is 80 mg. Recommended duration of treatment is 48 weeks for genotype 1 and 24 weeks for genotype 2 and 3. But full duration of treatment should be 48 weeks in patients with advanced hepatic fibrosis or cirrhosis or very high level of HCV RNA in the blood. Since after 2013, a number of antivirals have been introduced and replaced PEG IFN-based treatment. These drugs are:

- **a.** Orally administered
- **b.** Well-tolerated
- **c.** Highly efficacious
- **d.** High barrier of resistance
- **e.** Simple dosing
- **f.** Pill burden will be low.
- **g.** Duration of treatment is 8–12 weeks.

There are three classes of drugs:

- **a.** NS3/4 protease inhibitors: These will cleave single HCV polyprotein into structural and nonstructural proteins.
- **b.** NS5B nucleoside and nonnucleoside polymerase inhibitors: These prevent viral RNA synthesis by interfering RNA-dependent RNA polymerase.
- **c.** NS5A inhibitors: These interfere with membrane-associated phosphoprotein which is essential for HCV RNA complex.

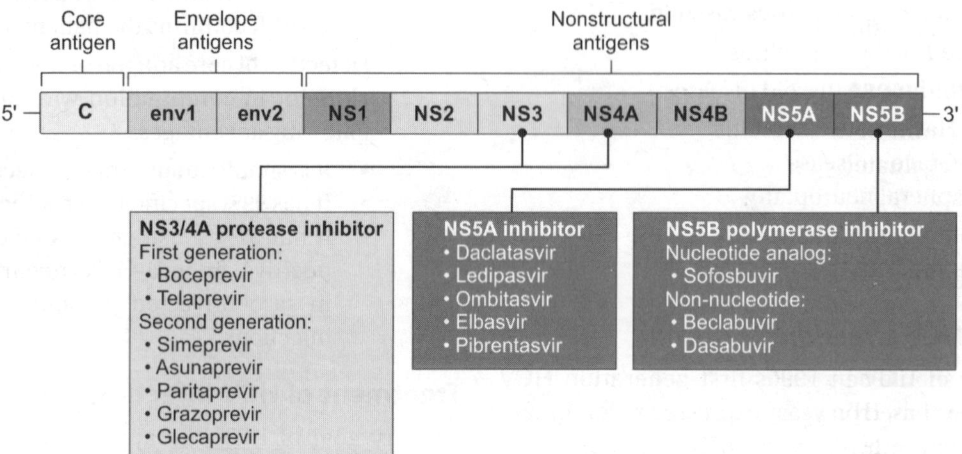

Standard Indications of Therapy

- **a.** All chronic HCV-infected patients having detectable HCV RNA with or without elevated ALT.
- **b.** Any stage of hepatic fibrosis with highest priority for advanced fibrosis (METAVIR 2 or 3) or METAVIR 4 cirrhosis.
- **c.** Previously refractory to IFN-based therapy (patients with HIV-HCV coinfection, renal insufficiency), IL-28B non-C genotype, insulin resistance, obese patients, decompensated (Child–Pugh B or C), and compensated liver disease (Child–Pugh A)
- **d.** Patients with extrahepatic manifestations, such as vasculitis, mixed cryoglobulinemia, HCV immune complex-mediated nephropathy, or non-Hodgkin lymphoma
- **e.** Recurrence of HCV after transplantation
- **f.** Rapid evaluation of liver disease in patient with stem cell recipients
- **g.** Individual at risk of transmitting HCV

Contraindication to Therapy

- **a.** Use of cytochrome P450/P-gp-inducing drugs, such as phenytoin and carbamazepine, is contraindicated as these drugs will reduce the concentration of these drugs leading to virological failure.
- **b.** HCV protease inhibitors, such as grazoprevir, glecaprevir, and voxilaprevir, are contraindicated in patients with decompensated cirrhosis (Child–Pugh B or C)

End point of HCV Therapy

a. After 12 (SVR12) to 24 (SVR24) weeks after the completion of therapy HCV RNA will not be detectable with lower limit of detection of <15 IU/mL.
b. After 12 (SVR12) to 24 (SVR24) weeks after the completion of therapy undetectable HCV RNA level in the blood who had HCV core antigen prior to commencement of therapy.
c. After 12 (SVR12) to 24 (SVR24) weeks after the completion of therapy undetectable HCV RNA level in the blood using qualitative RNA assay having lower limit of detection of ≤1,000 IU/mL; it can be used as end point of therapy where sensitive HCV RNA assay is not available.
d. In patient with advanced fibrosis (METAVIR stage 3) or cirrhosis (METAVIR stage 4) surveillance for HCC must be continued as it may reduce but not abolish the possibility.

Pretherapeutic Assessment

a. Consumption of alcohol and substance abuse must be evaluated and quantified as it requires counseling.
b. Extrahepatic manifestation of HCV should be searched.
c. Renal function, such as creatinine and eGFR, should be assessed.
d. Patients should be evaluated for current and past HBV infection, HIV, and HAV infection.
e. In case of nonimmune patients HBV and HAV vaccinations should be proposed.
f. Influence of comorbidities in the progression of liver disease must be evaluated.

Assessment of Severity

a. Assessment of severity of liver disease must be assessed.
b. In case of advanced fibrosis (F3 or F4) post-treatment surveillance of HCC should be done.
c. Some treatment regimens must be adjusted if cirrhosis is identified.
d. Fibrotic stage must be initially assessed by following methods, such as measurement of liver stiffness, serum biomarkers—APRI and FIB-4 that are inexpensive.
e. In case of uncertainty of etiologies liver biopsy should be served.
f. To assess the fibrotic stage after therapy noninvasive method is used.

Treatment of Chronic Hepatitis C Patients without Cirrhosis or Compensated Cirrhosis

a. Fixed dose combination: Sofosbuvir 400 plus valpatasvir 100 mg in single tablet daily
b. Fixed dose combination: Glecaprevir 300 mg plus pibrentasvir 120 mg in 3 tablets each containing glecaprevir 100 mg plus pibrentasvir 40 mg
c. Fixed dose combination: Sofosbuvir 400 mg plus valpatasvir 100 mg plus voxilaprevir 100 mg in a single tablet once daily.
d. Fixed drug combination: Grazoprevir 100 mg plus elbasvir 50 mg in a single tablet once daily in genotype 1b.
e. In case of HIV-coinfected patients same drug combinations are used but in case of interactions with retroviral drugs dose or drug can be altered.

Simplified Genotyping- or Subtyping-free Treatment of HCV with Pangenotypic Drugs in Compensated Cirrhotic Patients

a. The use of pangenotypic drugs can increase global cure rate where genotyping or subtyping of HCV is not available.
b. Pretreatment assessment by detection of HCV RNA or core antigen or noninvasive methods of cirrhosis is not available.
c. Drug-to-drug interaction has to be carefully checked.
d. Treatment-native patients should be treated with fixed drug combinations of sofosbuvir plus valpatasvir for 12 weeks or glecaprevir plus pibrentasvir for 12 weeks and treatment experienced patients fixed drug combination of sofosbuvir plus valpatasvir or glecaprevir plus pibrentasvir for 12 weeks.
e. In case of adherence SVR testing can be omitted 12 weeks after treatment.

Genotype-based Treatment in Case of Compensated Cirrhotic Patients

<table>
<tr><th>Type of treatment</th><th>Genotype</th><th>Status of cirrhosis</th><th>Prior treatment experience</th><th>Sofosbuvir/ Velpatasvir</th><th>Glecaprevir/ Pibrentasvir</th><th>Sofosbuvir/ Velpatasvir/ Voxilaprevir</th><th>Grazoprevir/ Elbasvir</th></tr>
<tr><td rowspan="12">Genotype/ subtype determination-based treatment</td><td rowspan="4">1a, 1b, 2, 4, 5 and 6</td><td rowspan="2">No cirrhosis</td><td>Treatment-native</td><td rowspan="4">12 weeks</td><td rowspan="3">8 weeks</td><td rowspan="4">NO</td><td rowspan="4">12 weeks
For 1b only</td></tr>
<tr><td>Treatment experienced</td></tr>
<tr><td rowspan="2">Compensated cirrhosis</td><td>Treatment-native</td></tr>
<tr><td>Treatment experienced</td><td>12 weeks</td></tr>
<tr><td rowspan="4">3</td><td rowspan="2">No cirrhosis</td><td>Treatment native</td><td rowspan="2">12 weeks</td><td>8 weeks</td><td rowspan="2">NO</td><td>NO</td></tr>
<tr><td>Treatment experienced</td><td>12 weeks</td><td>NO</td></tr>
<tr><td rowspan="2">Compensated cirrhosis</td><td>Treatment native</td><td rowspan="2">12 weeks with weight-based ribavirin</td><td>8–12 weeks</td><td rowspan="2">12 weeks</td><td>NO</td></tr>
<tr><td>Treatment experienced</td><td>16 weeks</td><td>NO</td></tr>
<tr><td rowspan="4">Subtype 1, 4r, 3b, 3g, 6u, or any other subtypes harboring one or several NS5A RASs</td><td rowspan="2">No cirrhosis</td><td>Treatment native</td><td rowspan="4">Unknown</td><td rowspan="4">Unknown</td><td rowspan="4">12 weeks</td><td rowspan="4">NO</td></tr>
<tr><td>Treatment experienced</td></tr>
<tr><td rowspan="2">Compensated cirrhosis</td><td>Treatment native</td></tr>
<tr><td>Treatment experienced</td></tr>
</table>

Other Types of Treatment Formulation

Pangenotypic direct-acting drug formulations:

Drugs	Formulation	Drugs
NS5B polymerase inhibitor (Sofosbuvir) + (NS5A inhibitor) Daclatasvir	• Sofosbuvir 600 mg • Daclatasvir 60 mg	1 tablet daily
NS5B polymerase inhibitor (Sofosbuvir) + (NS5A inhibitor) Velpatasvir	• Sofosbuvir 600 mg • Velpatasvir 100 mg	1 tablet daily
NS5B polymerase inhibitor (Sofosbuvir) + (NS5A inhibitor) Velpatasvir + (NS3/4 A protease inhibitor) Voxilaprevir	• Sofosbuvir 600 mg • Velpatasvir 100 mg • Voxilaprevir 100 mg	1 tablet daily
(NS3/4 A protease inhibitor) Glecaprevir + (NS5A inhibitor) Pibrentasvir	• Glecaprevir 100 mg • Pibrentasvir 40 mg	3 tablets daily

Genotypic specific direct-acting agent combinations:

Drugs	Formulations	Dosages
Sofosbuvir + Ledipasvir (for genotype 1, 4, 5, and 6)	Sofosbuvir 400 mg + Ledipasvir 90 mg	1 tablet daily
Elbasvir + Grazoprevir (1, 4, and 6)	Elbasvir 50 mg + Grazoprevir 100 mg	1 tablet daily

In case of patient without cirrhosis or compensated cirrhosis in HCV positive patients:

Genotype	Regimen	Dosage
Genotype 1 or 4	Elbasvir (50 mg) + Grazoprevir (100 mg)	12 weeks
	Glecaprevir (400 mg) + Pibrentasvir (120 mg)	8 weeks
	Sofosbuvir (400 mg) + Ledipasvir (90 mg)	12 weeks
	Sofosbuvir (400 mg) + Velpatasvir (100 mg)	12 weeks
Genotype 2 or 3	Glecaprevir (400 mg) + Pibrentasvir (120 mg)	8 weeks
	Sofosbuvir (400 mg) + Velpatasvir (100 mg)	12 weeks
Genotype 5 and 6	Glecaprevir (400 mg) + Pibrentasvir (120 mg)	8 weeks
	Sofosbuvir (400 mg) + Ledipasvir (90 mg)	12 weeks
	Sofosbuvir (400 mg) + Velpatasvir (100 mg)	12 weeks

Treatment of Chronic Hepatitis in Pregnant Women

A. Treatment should not be recommended in absence of safety and efficacy data.

B. In case of conception during treatment a thorough discussion should be done as case to case basis and its risk during therapy.

C. Breast-feeding is not contraindicated except in case of cracked nipple or bleeding.

Treatment of HCV Infection in Case of Renal Impairment or in Case of Hemodialysis

A. Patients with end-stage renal disease (ESRD) on hemodialysis with HCV infection should be treated with same drugs without any dose adjustment.

B. Fixed dose combination of glecaprevir plus pibrentasvir, and for infected with genotype 1b patients only, fixed dose of grazoprevir and elbasvir are preferred in case of severe renal impairment and patients with ESRD requiring hemodialysis.

C. Decompensated cirrhotic patients with mild to moderate renal impairment should be treated with fixed drug combination of 400 mg sofosbuvir and 100 mg velpatasvir and 600 mg ribavirin to start with followed by dose adjustment according to tolerance and hemoglobin levels for 12 weeks.

D. Decompensated cirrhotic patients with mild to moderate renal impairment should be treated with fixed drug combination of sofosbuvir and velpatasvir for 24 weeks.

E. Patients with eGFR $\geq$ 30 mL/min/m^2 do not require any dose modification.

Treatment of HCV Infection in Case of Coinfection with HBV

A. Patient should be tested for HIV also.

B. The patient should be treated with same anti-HCV regimen with same dose.

C. HBsAg positive patients should receive nucleoside analog anaphylaxis until 12 weeks of post HCV therapy and should be monitored at monthly interval if treatment of HBV is stopped.

D. In case of anti-HBc positive but HBsAg negative patients serum ALT has to be monitored.

Retreatment is required in the following cases:

A. Relapse

B. Partial responder or nonresponders after previous course of IFN-based therapy

C. Partial responder or nonresponders after previous course of direct-acting antiviral therapy

Recent guidelines of hepatitis virus infection:

Condition of the patient	Recommended regimen	Duration of treatment
Without cirrhosis	Sofosbuvir/Velpatasvir	12 weeks
	Glecaprevir/Pibrentasvir	8 weeks
With compensated cirrhosis	Glecaprevir/Pibrentasvir	8 weeks
	Sofosbuvir/Velpatasvir	12 weeks

Extrahepatic features of HCV infection:

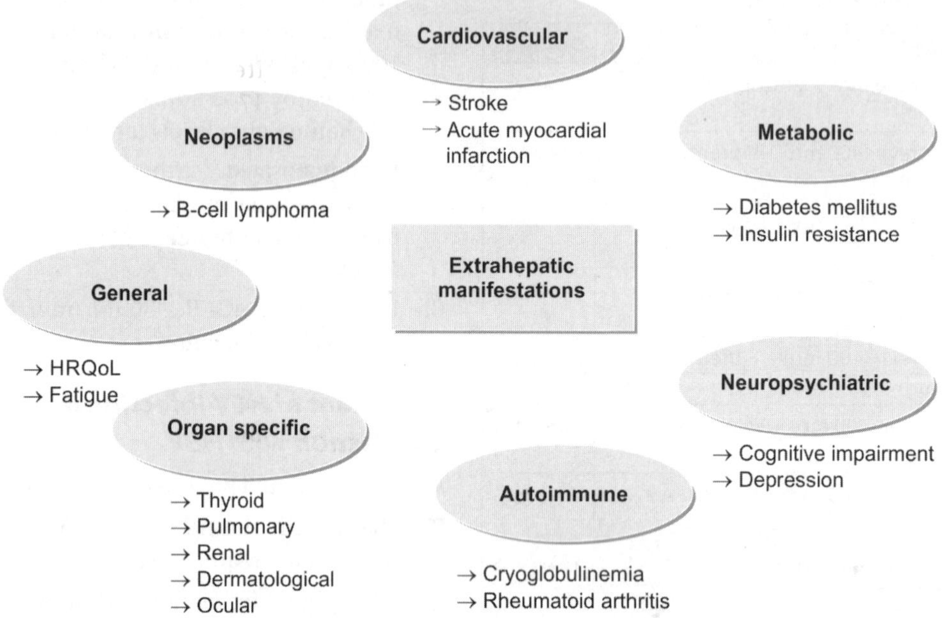

Cardiovascular manifestations:

A. Acute coronary syndrome

B. Myocarditis

C. Dilated cardiomyopathy

D. Hypertrophic cardiomyopathy

Immunologic manifestations:

A. Mixed cryoglobulinemia due to involvement of medium or small sized blood vessels presenting with the triad of purpura, arthralgia and weakness.

B. Lymphoproliferative disorders:

- **a.** Non-Hodgkin lymphoma
- **b.** Monoclonal gammopathy of undetermined significance

C. Autoimmune phenomenon:

- **a.** ITP
- **b.** Positivity of RA factor, ANA

Neurological manifestations:

A. Cognitive decline

B. Guillain–Barré syndrome

C. Peripheral neuropathy

Renal manifestations:

A. Membranous nephropathy

B. Membranoproliferative glomerulonephritis

Endocrine manifestations:

A. Autoimmune thyroiditis

B. Graves' disease

C. Insulin resistant type 2 diabetes mellitus

Dermatological manifestations:

A. Lichen planus

B. Porphyria cutanea tarda

C. Leukocytoclastic vasculitis

Psychiatric manifestations:

A. Anxiety

B. Depression

Q19. Drug-induced hepatitis.

MGR/MAR2010/MDII (6)

Drug induced liver injury.

KERALA UNI, 2022 (10)

Antibiotic alternatives in hepatic and renal dysfunction.

SAURASHTRA UNI, 2022 (20)

Drug induced hepatitis.

MGR UNIVERSITY, TAMIL NADU, 2020 (10)

Drug induced liver injury.

NTR UNI OF HEALTH SC, 2020 (10)

Hepatotoxicity of the drugs.

RAJIV GANDHI UNI OF HEALTH SC, KARNATAKA, 2018 (10)

Drug induced liver injury.

RAJIV GANDHI UNI OF HEALTH SC, KARNATAKA, 2018 (10)

Discuss the approach to a case of anti-tubercular drug induced hepatitis.

MAHATMA UNIVERSITY, 2022 (10)

ANSWER

Usually, drugs are water-insoluble but become water-soluble to excrete through kidney or bile; they have to pass through two reactions:

a. Phase I reaction by microsomal mixed-function oxygenase and cytochrome 450
b. Phase II reaction by glucuronidation, sulfation, and inactivation by glutathione

Most of the hepatotoxicity occurs in phase I toxic metabolite. There are two types of hepatotoxicity:

A. Direct injury:
  a. It is dose-dependent.
  b. Latent period is short but clinical manifestation will be delayed.
  c. Toxic injury is characteristic of different toxic metabolite:
    1. Centrilobular zonal necrosis—carbon tetrachloride and trichloroethylene
    2. Periportal injury—Yellow phosphorus
    3. Massive hepatic necrosis—hepatotoxic octapeptide of amanita phalloides, lethal dose is 10 mg.

B. Idiosyncratic injury:
  a. It is dose-independent.
  b. Latent period is short or variable.
  c. Hepatotoxicity of following types usually occurs:
    1. Chronic or autoimmune hepatic injury—minocycline, hydralazine, and nitrofurantoin
    2. Morphologic pictures typical of viral hepatitis, necrosis in liver lobule with infiltration of lymphocytes—isoniazid (INH) and ciprofloxacin
    3. Portal hypertension without cirrhosis—vitamin A and arsenic intoxication, polyvinyl chloride
    4. Hepatic adenoma or HCC or hepatic vein occlusion—oral contraceptives
    5. Drug-induced mild, moderate, or severe cholestasis:
      - Bland cholestasis along with limited hepatocyte injury—estrogen, 17α-substituted androgen
      - Inflammatory cholestasis—oxacillin, erythromycin, and amoxicillin-clavulanic acid
      - Sclerosing cholangitis—intrahepatic infusion of chemotherapeutic agent floxuridine given to treat secondaries
      - Ductopenic cholestasis or disappearance of bile duct—in case of carbamazepine and levofloxacin
      - Binding of ducts in the membrane transporters of canaliculi resulting canalicular pump defect

Methods of Liver Cell Injury

1. Here toxic metabolite directly produces peroxidation of membrane lipid.
2. By activation innate or adaptive immune response followed by stimulation of apoptosis
3. Interference with pumps of biliary canaliculi allowing endogenous bile acids and injures the liver cells, as a result there is:
   - Necrosis of hepatocytes
   - Bile duct injury leading to cholestasis
   - Blocking of lipid movement pathways
   - Inhibition of protein synthesis.
   - Impairment of mitochondrial oxidation of fatty acids
   - Intracellular accumulation of triglyceride resulting microvascular steatosis

First diagnosis regarding drug toxicity has to be diagnosed then following treatment to be provided:

A. Removal of offending drugs
B. Otherwise supportive management except acetaminophen where N-acetylcysteine has to be given.
C. In case of hepatocellular failure urgent liver transplantation should be done.
D. Following drugs can be given in specific conditions:
  a. Steroids for allergic hepatotoxicity
  b. Silibinin for hepatotoxic mushroom poisoning
  c. Ursodeoxycholic acid—cholestatic drug toxicity

Differentiation between cholestatic and hepatocellular injury can be done by observing the ratio of ALT and ALP (R) value:

1. R value >5.0—indicates hepatocellular injury

2. E value <2—indicates cholestatic injury
3. R value between 2 and 5—indicates mixed hepatocellular-Cholestatic injury

Morphological Alteration in the Liver Injury

1. Bridging hepatic necrosis—methyldopa
2. Hepatic granuloma—sulfonamides
3. Macrovesicular or microvesicular steatohepatitis—reverse transcriptase inhibitor for treatment of HIV, it is usually reversible.
4. Affection of sinusoidal lining cells—high-dose melphalan, cyclophosphamide prior to liver transplantation resulting veno-occlusive disease.
5. Nodular regenerative hyperplasia—results from vascular injury to endothelium of portal vein—systemic chemotherapy oxaliplatin.

Antibiotic Alternatives in Hepatic Dysfunction

A. Safe antibiotics in liver dysfunction:
   a. Beta-lactam antibiotics like penicillin, cephalosporin, and carbapenem are administered safely because they are excreted in urine.
   b. Piperacillin and tazobactam can be given because it is required in sepsis and no dose adjustment is not required.
   c. Meropenem also can be administered because it is generally excreted through the urine.
   d. Fluoroquinolone like norfloxacin, ofloxacin, levofloxacin can be administered safely.

B. The following drugs are not hepatotoxic:
   a. Daptomycin as this drug is excreted through the urine.
   b. Linezolid can be given but should be administered cautiously as the chronic liver disease already produces thrombocytopenia and over and above linezolid also produces thrombocytopenia.
   c. Colistin can be administered safely.

C. Following drugs should be administered cautiously as these drugs are metabolized in the liver:
   a. Macrolide groups like erythromycin, azithromycin
   b. Doxycycline can be administered but tetracycline should be avoided because it is metabolized in the liver.

Drugs in renal dysfunction has been written in nephrology chapter in question number 37.

Q20. Define hepatopulmonary syndrome. Describe its pathogenesis, diagnosis and management.

DNBII/JUN2012 (10)

Pulmonary manifestation of chronic liver disease.

MGE/MAR2008/MDIV (6)

Hepatopulmonary syndrome.

NTR UNI OF HEALTH SC, VIJAYAWADA, 2020 (10)

ANSWER

Pulmonary Manifestation of Chronic Liver Disease

The main problem in case of cirrhosis is abnormalities in gas exchange leading to development of respiratory symptoms secondary to following various causes:

A. Related to intrinsic lung causes:
   a. Interstitial lunge disease
   b. Congestive cardiac failure
   c. Pneumonia
   d. Chronic obstructive lung disease
   e. Asthma

B. Related to liver disease:
   a. Association with specific liver diseases
   b. Ascites
   c. Hepatic hydrothorax
   d. Muscular wasting
   e. Specific abnormalities in the lung
   f. α-1 antitrypsin deficiency leading to pan acinar emphysema
   g. Associated with cirrhosis with or without portal hypertension
   h. Hepatopulmonary syndrome
   i. Portopulmonary hypertension

Hepatopulmonary Syndrome

Definition

This syndrome can be defined as a triad of:

A. Hepatic dysfunction or portal hypertension
B. Widened alveolar-arterial oxygen gradient in patient breathing room air
C. Presence of intrapulmonary vasodilatation (IPVD)

About 40–60% of cirrhotic patients have detectable IPVD. 30% patients develop significant functional limitations due to impaired oxygen transfer.

It occurs in the following diseases:

A. Cirrhosis with or without portal hypertension

B. Noncirrhotic portal hypertension (NCPH)

C. Nodular regenerative hyperplasia

D. Congenital hepatic fibrosis

E. Hepatic venous flow obstruction

F. Metastatic carcinoid tumor due to liberation of vasoactive substances

G. Congenital cardiac anomaly

Pathogenesis

As a result of hepatic injury due to cirrhosis with portal hypertension, following substances are released:

A. Cytokines (TNF-α)

B. Inflammatory mediators (endotoxin)

C. Vasoactive mediators (endothelin-1)

D. Genetic factor:

- **a.** Endothelin-1 is released into circulation. It acts on vascular endothelial B receptor and activates nitric oxide synthetase (eNOS) to produce nitric oxide.
- **b.** There is accumulation of vascular monocyte in the vascular lumen. Monocyte firstly adheres to endothelial cell wall by activating the CXCL1 and produces nitric oxide from inducible nitric oxide synthetase (iNOS). It also releases carbon monoxide from heme oxygenase 1 (HO-1). Both nitric oxide and carbon monoxide produce IPVD.

Mechanism of hypoxemia: In case of true anatomical shunt 100% oxygen administration cannot recover the patient but HPS can recover. According to recent hypothesis capillary is grossly dilated but oxygen molecules cannot enter in the center of the capillary as it is filled up with streams of erythrocytes which contain hemoglobin, so there is inadequate oxygenation of hemoglobin leading to systemic hypoxemia which can be overcome by oxygen supplementation.

Clinical Feature

A. May be asymptomatic

B. Progressive dyspnea

C. Dyspnea mainly on standing position and relieved in lying down position (platypnea)

D. Increasing dyspnea in standing position (orthodeoxia)

E. Signs:

- **a.** Spider angioma
- **b.** Clubbing
- **c.** Cyanosis
- **d.** Other features of portal hypertension

Investigations

A. Chest X-ray: Normal or interstitial changes in the lower lobe.

B. Pulse oximetry: It measures saturation of oxygen indirectly to screen hypoxemia. Value of 96% is 100% sensitive and 88% specific.

C. Contrast echocardiography:

- **a.** Two-dimensional method using agitated saline as contrast agent demonstrates microbubbles in the left cardiac chambers after more than 3 cardiac cycles. But if it is visualized immediately after injection then it proves intracardiac shunting. Transesophageal method is more sensitive.
- **b.** It can assess cardiac function.
- **c.** It can estimate pulmonary arterial systolic pressure.

D. Radionuclide lung perfusion scanning with technetium 99m-labeled macroaggregated albumin with particle size of 20 μm in size has to be administered intravenously. Normal diameter of capillary is 7–15 μm. So, normally all the particles will be trapped in the pulmonary microvasculature. But in HPS due to IPVD these particles will pass the capillaries.

E. Calculation of shunt fraction by quantitative imaging of the lung and brain—if shunt fraction is >6%, it indicates HPS.

F. Pulmonary angiography: It is invasive. It detects two types of lesions:

- **a.** A diffuse spongiform pulmonary vessel during arterial phase—type 1
- **b.** Small discrete arteriovenous communications—type 2

G. HRCT:

- **a.** Dilated pulmonary vessels
- **b.** Intrapulmonary shunting

Treatment

A. No medical therapy is established till now. Following drugs are tried:

- **a.** Somatostatin
- **b.** Almitrine
- **c.** Indomethacin

d. Nebulization of NG-nitro-L-arginine methyl ester
e. Aspirin
f. Pentoxifylline, a phosphodiesterase inhibitor
g. Plasma exchange

B. Orthotropic liver transplantation is only the effective treatment.

Q21. Bridging necrosis.
MGR/SEP2008 (5)/MGR/OCT2011 (5)

ANSWER

Bridging Necrosis

It occurs due to submassive necrosis of zone 3 which involves:

A. Death of entire zone of hepatocytes or more of the hepatic acini leading to confluent necrosis.
B. Lysis of the necrotic tissue
C. Collapse of surrounding stroma

This necrosis usually involves zone 3 entirely around the terminal hepatic venule called centrilobular necrosis but may sometimes involve zone 2 and 1. It may extend to adjacent hepatic acini around terminal venule to the edge of porta. If there is associated collapse of surrounding intact reticulin framework, it will extend in between the vascular structures. This collapse is due to loss of hepatocytes. As a result the adjacent necrotic lobules are interlinked producing bridging necrosis. There may be approximation of portal areas. There are different types of bridging:

A. Linkage between portal areas with terminal hepatic venules—portal to central bridging
B. Linkage between two or more terminal hepatic venules—central to central bridging

In the necrotic and collapsed area there is infiltration of chronic inflammatory cells including lymphocytes, plasma cells, and lesser number of eosinophils.

There may be associated endophlebitis of central vein, hypertrophy of Kupffer cell containing lipofuscin in their cytoplasm. Hepatic acinus demonstrates proliferation of putative hepatic stem cells forming ductules as well as ductular hepatocytes in zone 1.

Causes of Bridging Necrosis

A. All types of acute viral hepatitis
B. Drugs
C. Toxins
D. Autoimmune hepatitis

Q22. Acute intermittent porphyria—causes, clinical features and management.
DNB/JUNE 2011 (10)

Acute intermittent porphyria.
MGR/SEP2007/MDI (5)/MGR/MAR2006/MDVI (5)
BF/MAY2009/MDIII (10)

Outline the heme biosynthetic pathway and classify porphyria. Discuss the etiology, clinical features and management of acute intermittent porphyria.
MGR/MAR2007/MDI (20)

Acute porphyrias.
MUGS/MAY2012/MDIII (10)

Porphyrin metabolism.
MGR/SEP2008/MDI (5)

Discuss heme biosynthesis with reference to porphyrias.
BF/MAY2009/MDI (25)

Acute intermittent porphyria.
MGR UNI, TAMIL NADU, 2022, (10)
MGR UNI, TAMIL NADU, 2021 (10)
RAJASTHAN UNIVERSITY, 2019 (11)

ANSWER

Acute Porphyria

Biosynthesis of heme: It is a member of the group of compounds; tetrapyrroles are composed of four pyrrole rings being attached with one carbon atom-bridge arranged into a larger ring, nitrogen atom in each pyrrole ring is orientated toward the center of the larger ring. Chemical properties of this central nitrogen atom help this ring to be attached to the iron (producing heme), magnesium (producing chlorophyll), cobalt (producing vitamin B12)—these are very crucial to the living organism.

In case heme iron has six coordinates, four are attached with the nitrogen atoms of four pyrrole ring, other two being attached with the protein of solvent or solute molecules.

Synthesis of Heme

There are eight steps in heme synthesis. Defect in each synthesis is responsible for different types of porphyria.

A. Step 1: Glycine reacts with succinyl-CoA to form δ-aminolevulinic acid (ALA) catalyzed by ALA synthetase in mitochondrial matrix. ALA diffuses into hepatic cytoplasm.

B. Step 2: In the cytoplasm two molecules of ALA are condensed to form porphobilinogen, reaction will be catalyzed by ALA dehydratase. Deficiency of this enzyme is known as ALA dehydratase deficiency.

C. Four molecules of porphobilinogens displace four amino acid groups and attached from head to tail to form linear tetrapyrrole hydroxymethylbilane with the help of the enzyme porphobilinogen deaminase or hydroxymethylbilane synthetase (*HMBS*), the deficiency of which will produce acute intermittent porphyria (AIP). Hydroxymethylbilane will be spontaneously transformed to uroporphyrinogen I. Porphyrinogens is composed of four tetrapyrrole rings joined by methylene groups nonenzymatically.

D. Uroporphyrinogen I will be converted into uroporphyrinogen III with the help of uroporphyrinogen synthetase III (cosynthatase). Deficiency of this enzyme leads to development of congenital erythropoietic porphyria.

E. Uroporphyrinogen III will be converted into coproporphyrinogen III catalyzed by uroporphyrinogen carboxylase—deficiency of this enzyme produces porphyria cutanea tarda and hematopoietic porphyria.

F. In this sixth step propionate side chain at R2 and R4 positions of coproporphyrinogen III will be oxidized and decarboxylated to form protoporphyrinogen IX catalyzed by coproporphyrinogen oxidase located in between inner and outer membrane of mitochondria—deficiency of this enzyme leads to hereditary coproporphyria.

G. Protoporphyrinogen IX will be converted into protoporphyrin IX in presence of protoporphyrinogen oxidase present in the inner mitochondrial membrane, deficiency of which will lead to disease called variegate porphyria.

H. Last step is the insertion of ferrous iron atom into protoporphyrin IX to form heme, this will be catalyzed by ferrochelatase—deficiency of this enzyme will lead to protoporphyria.

Metabolism of Heme in the Liver

In the liver heme synthesis is controlled by regulatory heme pool through the initiating enzyme ALA synthetase activity by negative feedback mechanism. Two forms of ALA synthetase, euthyroid and nonthyroid—both are encoded by different genes.

Heme controls this enzyme by two mechanisms:

A. Repression of the synthesis of this enzyme by decreasing the ALA synthase messenger RNA

B. Inhibition of its transport from cytoplasm into the mitochondria.

Heme after its synthesis will efflux into the hemoprotein pool in the cytoplasm with the help of heme-binding protein from mitochondria. In the cytoplasm following binding proteins are found:

a. Microsomal cytochrome P450 system

b. Cytochrome b5

c. Catalase

In the hepatocytes and Kupffer cells heme oxygenase under oxidative stress breaks and opens heme-releasing iron and carbon monoxide to produce green pigment biliverdin which in turn will be catabolized by biliverdin reductase into bilirubin.

Heme that will be excreted into the bile will not enter into enterohepatic circulation as it is metabolized by microsomal enzymes present in the intestinal mucosal cell.

Excretion of Porphyrin and its Precursors

Urinary excretion is determined by their water solubility as only water-soluble product is excreted in urine.

A. ALA and porphobilinogen are water soluble and thus excreted in urine.

B. Uroporphyrin, due to its eight carboxyl group, is water soluble and excreted in urine.

C. Protoporphyrin having two carboxyl groups is not water soluble hence excreted in the bile.

D. Coproporphyrin containing four carboxyl groups excreted both in bile and urine. Coproporphyrin I is mainly excreted in the bile. But in hepatobiliary diseases its biliary excretion decreases but urinary excretion increases—hence is known as secondary porphyrinuria.

E. Porphyrinogens follow their symmetrical porphyrins during excretion, only coproporphyrinogen excretes more in urine as compared to coproporphyrin.

In healthy individual, coproporphyrin is predominantly excreted in bile, negligible amount of uroporphyrin in bile and protoporphyrin only in feces. Choate in the bile acids increases the biliary excretion of protoporphyrin than chenodeoxycholate and ursodeoxycholate. This biliary excretion of protoporphyrin is linked to secretion of phospholipid.

Acute Intermittent Porphyria

It is most common type of porphyria in USA (1 in 10,000 to 20,000).

The enzyme responsible for AIP is porphobilinogen deaminase which converts porphobilinogen to hydroxymethylbilane resulting increased excretion of ALA as well as porphobilinogen in urine. It is autosomal dominant disease.

Pathogenesis

Pathogenesis behind neurological dysfunction in acute attack is nuclear but there are several factors responsible for this attack:

A. Blood and urinary levels of ALA are high in acute attack with neurological manifestation than without neurological crises. In case of lead intoxication and hereditary tyrosinemia similar elevation of ALA can be found with neurologic features.

B. Due to the structural similarity between GABA, a major inhibitory neurotransmitter and ALA, ALA acts as a potent GABA receptor agonist produces neurologic attack.

C. In experimental animal ALA inhibits neural Na^{+}/K^{+}-ATPase activity leading to breakdown of membrane anion gradient.

D. Impaired heme synthesis decreases intracellular hemoprotein which depresses the cellular respiration in the nervous tissue. Hepatic metabolism is also impaired as a consequence of abnormal heme synthesis.

E. There is elevation of serotonin occurs due to deficiency of tryptophan pyrrolase which usually degrades tryptophan as a first step. This elevated serotonin can produce neurological manifestation in acute porphyria.

Clinical Features

Women are frequently affected suggestive of role for estrogen or progestins. Precipitating factors are:

A. Drugs:

- **a.** Analgesic, such as antipyrine and pentazocine
- **b.** Anesthetics, such as halothane, chloroform, and lignocaine
- **c.** Antimicrobials, such as antifungals, sulfonamide, trimethoprim, and doxycycline
- **d.** Cardiovascular drugs, such as nifedipine, amiodarone, and verapamil
- **e.** Antihypertensive, such as furosemide, clonidine, enalapril, and thiazides
- **f.** Sedatives
- **g.** Alcohol ingestion

B. Periods of fasting or low-calorie diet for weight loss

C. Just before menses probably due to progesterone, but pregnancy is well tolerated due to ameliorating the effect of high progesterone level, but there is increased frequency of miscarriage.

In case of heterozygous for *HMBS* mutations most of the patients remain asymptomatic along with normal excretion of precursor of porphyrin half-normal activity of HMBS that is sufficient to perform near normal function of heme synthesis provided heme synthesis activity of liver is not increased.

Severity of the attack depends upon the extent of neurological damage prior to institution of treatment.

A. Signs of autonomic dysfunction:

- **a.** Abdominal pain is usually colicky, poorly localized with absent bowel sound, may be associated with nausea and vomiting, if associated leukocytosis—can be diagnosed as acute abdomen leading to laparotomy.
- **b.** Tachycardia, hypertension, and postural hypotension
- **c.** Fever
- **d.** Disturbed sweating
- **e.** Distension of bladder and dysuria

B. Peripheral nervous system: It involves both sensory and motor dysfunction due to axonal degeneration.

- **a.** Upper limb and proximal muscles are mainly affected.
- **b.** Respiratory muscles may be involved leads to respiratory paralysis requiring ventilatory support.
- **c.** In early case deep tendon reflexes are normal but later on lost progressively. But ankle jerk is preserved selectively.
- **d.** Diffuse pain in extremities, chest, and back.
- **e.** Dysesthesias and paresthesias

C. Central nervous system involvement:

- **a.** Increased irritability
- **b.** Insomnia
- **c.** Anxiety
- **d.** Behavioral changes
- **e.** Psychiatric evaluation demonstrates hallucination, paranoia, and severe depression
- **f.** Seizure
- **g.** Progressive somnolence leading to coma

D. Other features:

- **a.** Hyponatremia due to syndrome of inappropriate antidiuretic hormone (SIADH)—may be due to hypothalamic lesion and sodium loss due to vomiting, diarrhea inadequate salt intake.

Mortality in AIP requiring hospital admission is three times higher than general population in last 50 years.

Biochemical Features

In AIP, ALA and porphobilinogen are found in urine in increased quantities. Fecal porphyrin level will be within normal limit. But in case of heterozygous form ALA and porphobilinogen levels are within normal limit.

Porphobilinogen level in urine is 50–200 mg/day (normal level is 0–4 mg/day).

ALA level in urine is 20–100 mg/day (normal level is 1–7 mg/day).

In AIP, the level may remain high even after resolution of symptoms hence diagnosis of AIP is always based on clinical features only.

But, specific for AIP is erythrocyte porphobilinogen deaminase activity which will be low.

Management

A. If the patient is able to take orally, 400 g of glucose should be given orally. If the patient is not able to take orally, intravenous 10% glucose has to be given as glucose suppresses the effect of ALA synthetase activity.

B. Intravenous fluid has to be given as normal saline at 2 L/day.

C. Monitoring should be done in following respects:

- **a.** Monitoring of sodium and potassium
- **b.** Monitoring the progression of neuropathy
- **c.** Respiratory function in the form of vital capacity, forced expiratory volume

D. Hematin: It will suppress the ALA synthetase activity. At a dose of 3–4 mg/kg intravenously for 4 days can reduce the serum ALA and porphobilinogen. It will also improve antipyrine metabolism—it suggests that apoproteins of cytochrome P450 will be reconstituted with this therapy. Mixing it with albumin prevents its degradation. The hematin can be administered in different forms:

- **a.** Heme arginate
- **b.** Heme albumin

Complications:

- **a.** Thrombophlebitis—which can be prevented by administration of solution for 15–30 minutes as free flow method.
- **b.** Transient coagulopathy by breakdown product of hematin. Hence, it should be administered as soon as possible after making its aqueous preparation.

E. Other medications:

- **a.** Pain can be prevented by narcotics.
- **b.** Nausea and vomiting can be prevented by ondansetron.
- **c.** Agitation can be controlled by chlorpromazine and chloral hydrate.
- **d.** Autonomic manifestations, such as tachycardia and hypertension can be corrected by 20–200 mg/day propranolol.
- **e.** Seizures can be controlled by phenytoin, barbiturates, clonazepam, or newer drug gabapentin.
- **f.** Status epilepticus can be treated by 10 mg intravenous diazepam, 8–10 mL paraldehyde per rectally or 0.5 mg to 1 g/h as intravenous infusion.

F. Avoidance of the porphyrinogenic drugs, alcohol, and fasting.

G. In menstruating females attack is due to endogenous progesterone. It can be treated by gonadotropin-releasing hormone. Oral contraceptive pill (OCP) should be avoided.

H. Orthotopic transplantation of liver: It is done in following cases:

- **a.** Refractory to hematin therapy
- **b.** Intractable severe disabling attacks

Results of transplantation:

- **a.** Improvement of neuropathic manifestations
- **b.** Normalization of urinary level of ALA and porphobilinogen

I. Newer treatment:

- **a.** Liver-directed gene therapy: It prevents drug-induced biochemical attacks.
- **b.** Clinical trial of transfer of adeno-associated virus vector—*HMBS* gene—till now no effectiveness is found.
- **c.** Phase 1 clinical trials of hepatic-targeted RNA interference therapy directed against hepatic ALA synthetase mRNA in patients having high level of ALA and porphobilinogen in urine—it demonstrated lowering of the two chemicals.

Long-term complications:

A. There may be risk of hypertension in the long run leading to chronic kidney disease—it may require renal transplantation.

B. There is increased risk of HCC, hence yearly imaging is required.

C. Chronic pain

D. Neuropathy

E. Depression/anxiety

Q23. Define spontaneous bacterial peritonitis. Describe its pathogenesis, clinical features and managements.

DNBIII/DEC2011 (10)

How do you diagnose spontaneous bacterial peritonitis and how do you treat it?

DNB (DEC2020) (6)

Spontaneous bacterial peritonitis.

AIIMS, BHU, 2020 (10)

BHARATI VIDYAPEETH DEEMED UNI, 2018 (10)

Diagnosis and management of spontaneous bacterial peritonitis.

WBUHS, 2020 (10)

ANSWER

Definition

Spontaneous bacterial peritonitis: It can be defined as infection of ascitic fluid in absence of any one of these:

- **a.** Infections from contiguous source, such as intestinal perforation and intra-abdominal abscess
- **b.** Intra-abdominal inflammatory focus, such as acute pancreatitis and cholecystitis

Organisms are:

- **a.** 50% gram-negative organisms; most common are *Escherichia coli*, remaining are aerobic gram-positive organisms mainly streptococcal species.
- **b.** Antibiotic-resistant organism as a result of inappropriate antibiotic use or widespread use of antibiotic.

Epidemiology

It is most common in hospitalized patients with cirrhosis and occurs in 25% of patients. But it is less common in case of outpatients.

Pathogenesis

Most important predisposing factors are:

- **a.** Intestinal bacterial overgrowth due to delayed intestinal transit
- **b.** Impaired phagocytic function
- **c.** Low serum and ascitic fluid complement level
- **d.** Decreased activity of reticuloendothelial system

As a result bacterial translocation into mesenteric lymph nodes, from there the bacteria enter into systemic circulation resulting bacteremia, and from there bacteria enter into the ascitic fluid.

Risk Factors

- **a.** Decompensated cirrhosis
- **b.** Low complement level
- **c.** Decreased hepatic synthetic functions
- **d.** Prolonged PT
- **e.** Patient with protein in ascitic fluid of <1 g/dL is 10-fold increased risk of SBP.

Clinical Features

- **a.** May be completely asymptomatic in 30% of patients.
- **b.** Fever with chill in 80% of patients
- **c.** Diffuse abdominal pain
- **d.** Diarrhea
- **e.** Absent bowel sounds
- **f.** Worsening or new onset of renal failure: It may be due to decreased effective circulating blood volume due to cytokine-mediated vasodilatation such as sepsis along with depressed cardiac function.
- **g.** Worsening of ascites
- **h.** Diffuse abdominal tenderness
- **i.** Features of hepatocellular failure
- **j.** Tachycardia and hypotension

Diagnosis

Ascitic fluid analysis:

- **a.** Cell count >500/µL—sensitivity 86%, specificity 98% and >250/µL—sensitivity 94%, specificity 84%.
- **b.** In case of hemorrhagic ascites when RBC count is >10,000/µL, one polymorph has to be subtracted for every 250 RBCs.
- **c.** Detection of leukocyte esterase for rapid diagnosis
- **d.** Ascitic fluid lactate level >25 mg/dL—100% sensitive and specific.
- **e.** pH < 7.35
- **f.** Culture of the fluid—positive

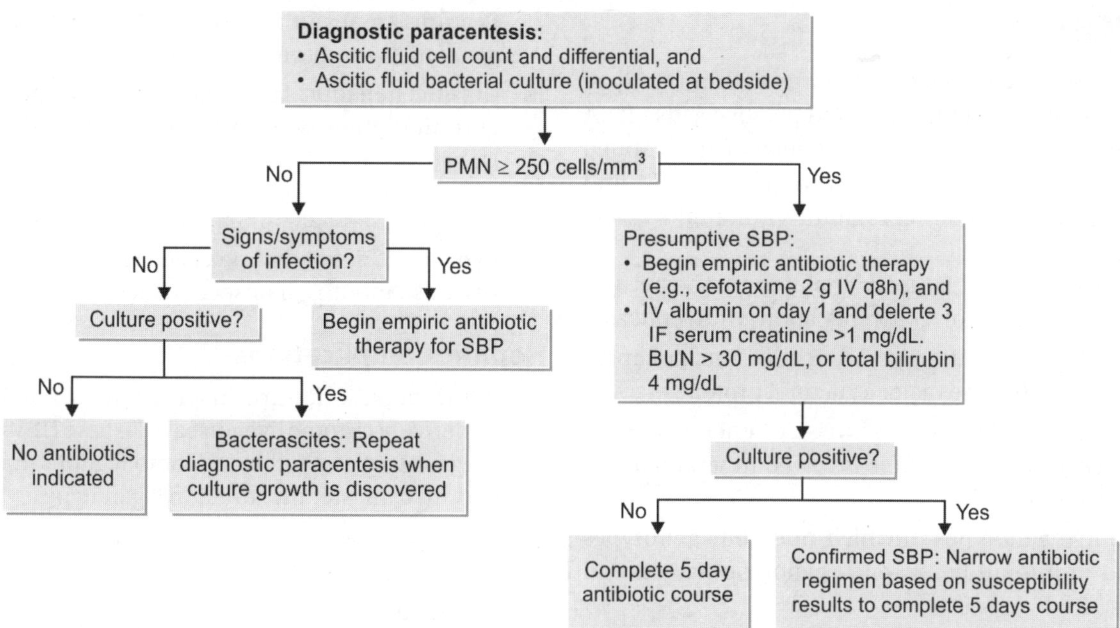

(PMN: polymorphonuclear)

Treatment

A. Empirically broad-spectrum antibiotic which may be beta-lactam antibiotic if not recently exposed to it. Third-generation cephalosporin especially cefotaxime 2 g 6–8 hourly intravenously. But in following conditions alternative to cefotaxime ofloxacin can be used:

a. Vomiting

b. Grade II encephalopathy

c. Shock

d. Serum creatinine > 3 mg/dL

If the ascitic fluid count is >500/μL—antibiotic has to be started at the earliest without waiting for culture report. But if cell count is <250/μL—antibiotic should be given according to culture report. If cell count is 250–500/μL, then empirical antibiotic followed by sensitivity specific antibiotic has to be given.

Antibiotic failure may occur in case of hospitalized patient infected with multidrug-resistant organisms. In that case piperacillin-tazobactam or carbapenem antibiotics can be administered.

After therapy of 5 days polymorph count should be decreased to <250/cc. In case of responded patient oral antibiotic therapy has to be started.

Therapy of worsening of renal function: Administration of albumin 1.5 g/kg in first 6 hours followed by 1 g/kg of body weight on the third day to maximum 100 g/day. Following patients get benefit from albumin infusion:

a. Blood urea nitrogen (BUN) > 30 mg/dL

b. Creatinine > 1 mg/dL

After 48 hours of commencement of therapy follow-up diagnostic paracentesis should be done to:

a. Assess the response of therapy

b. Initiate investigation of secondary peritonitis

Prophylaxis

If the patient survives from SPB there is higher recurrence of SBP within a year (70% per year). So in that case 400 mg/day norfloxacin orally has to be given till death or until transplantation of liver or disappearance of ascites. In cirrhosis with ascites, malnourished hospitalized patient with upper gastrointestinal bleeding and altered sensorium, intravenous cefotaxime should be started but for others norfloxacin is of choice. In following conditions also norfloxacin prophylaxis can be given:

a. Ascitic fluid protein < 1.1 g/dL

b. Advanced liver failure:

  1. Child–Pugh score ≥ 9

  2. Serum bilirubin ≥ 3 mg/dL

c. Evidence of circulatory dysfunction:

  1. Serum creatinine ≥ 1.2 mg/dL

  2. BUN ≥ 25 mg/dL

  3. Serum sodium ≤ 130 mEq/L

Q24. Hepatitis E.

MJPRU/2015/MDII (10)

NTR UNI OF HEALTH SC, VIJAYAWADA 2019 (10)

ANSWER

Hepatitis E virus belongs to hepavirus within family of Hepeviridae. HEV is single-stranded positive sense RNA consisting of short 5' noncoding region which is capped with 7-methylguanosine, three overlapping ORFs, and the other end 3' noncoding region terminated by poly adenosine.

a. ORF 1 is the largest, encodes nonstructural proteins. It involves in replication (viral replicase)
b. ORF 2 is middle sized, encodes nucleocapsid protein. It is the major structural protein.
c. ORF 3 is the smallest in size, encodes small structural protein. It is involved in viral particle secretion.

It has five genotypes of which only four genotypes are found in human being, each genotype has several serotypes:

a. HEV1: Five serotypes—1a, 1b, 1c, 1d, and 1e
b. HEV2: Two serotypes—2a and 2b
c. HEV3: Ten serotypes—3a, 3b, 3c, 3d, 3e, 3f, 3g, 3h, 3i, and 3j
d. HEV4: Seven serotypes—4a, 4b, 4c, 4d, 4e, 4f, and 4g

Genotypes 1 and 2 are found in developing countries and are more virulent.

Genotypes 3 and 4 are found in developed countries and China respectively, they are more attenuated and responsible for subclinical infection.

Name of the animal reservoir of viruses: Camel, rats, deer, rabbit, and swine.

No genomic homology is found between HEV and HAV and other picornaviruses.

Incubation period is about 40 days.

It is transmitted through contaminated water; virus is detected in bile, stool, and liver. It is excreted in stool in late incubation period and during infection.

There are two types of antibodies: IgM HEV antibody develops during acute infection and IgG HEV antibody is found for sometimes after acute episode protecting against further infection.

The prevalence of HEV is low in children; it will start rising in adolescent and young adult.

Spectrum of Infection of HEV Hepatitis

A. Acute hepatitis: Clinical features include malaise, abdominal pain, nausea, vomiting, fever, tender hepatomegaly, and raised transaminases with hyperbilirubinemia—returns to normal within 6 weeks. Features are severe in genotype 1 and 2. But in case of genotype 3 symptoms are mild.
B. Chronic hepatitis: HEV 3 genotype is responsible for chronic hepatitis in immunosuppressed patients, HIV-infected patients with CD4 T-cell count <250/cc, and patients suffering from hematological malignancy receiving chemotherapy. Chronic HEV infection is defined as persistence of HEV replication beyond 3 months of onset of infection.

Hepatic Complications

A. Acute hepatic failure in pregnant women and in underlying chronic liver disease. In case HEV-infected pregnant women following complications may occurs in third trimester due to 1 and 2 genotypes:
   a. Eclampsia
   b. Hemorrhage
   c. Stillbirth
   d. Acute fulminant hepatic failure
B. In older adult males acute hepatic failure or decompensation of chronic liver disease.

Extrahepatic Complications

A. Impaired renal function from glomerular disease by genotype 1 and 3. These are membranoproliferative and membranous glomerulonephritis.
B. Neurologic complications: Guillain–Barré syndrome, meningoencephalitis, myositis, mononeuritis multiplex, transverse myelitis, and vestibular neuritis
C. Hematologic complications: Aplastic anemia, thrombocytopenia, cryoglobulinemia, and lymphopenia
D. Other complications: Acute pancreatitis, myocarditis, arthritis, and autoimmune thyroiditis.

Diagnosis

A. Viral RNA will be detectable in late incubation period and in early infectious period in stool, blood, and other sites. This is estimated by RT-PCR.
B. Serum ALT starts rising during incubation period and gradually reaches its peak as HEV antibody appears in the serum.
C. There are two types of antibodies:
   a. IgM HEV antibody: It starts appearing from the second week, gradually peaks during 6th week and lasts for 12 weeks.
   b. IgG HEV antibody: It will appear nearly second week of infection and lasts for years and prevents further infection.

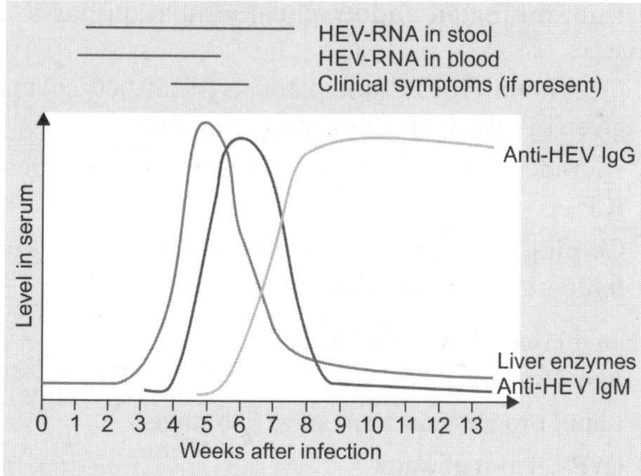

Treatment

In case of acute hepatitis there is no specific treatment for HEV, so treatment is mainly conservative.

There is no antiviral therapy discovered against HEV, hence in case of HEV-associated chronic hepatitis other causes of immunosuppression and HIV treatment have to be considered.

Prophylaxis

Recombinant genotype 1 vaccines have been developed and is given for protection against all genotypes in endemic areas of world. Chinese HEV vaccine lasts long.

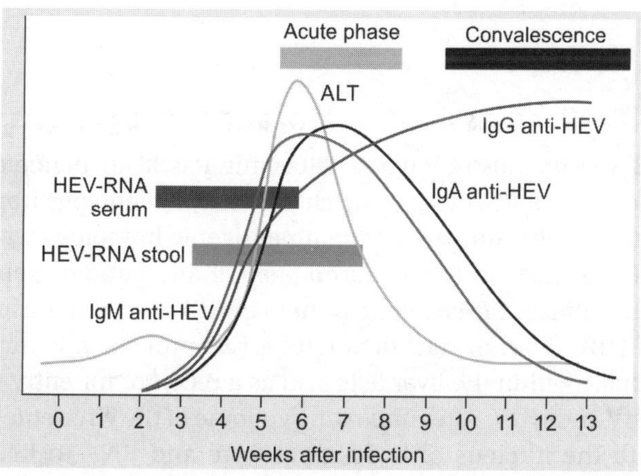

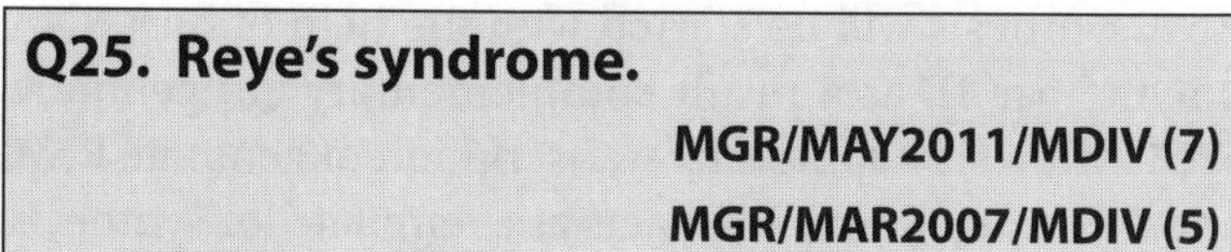

Q25. Reye's syndrome.

MGR/MAY2011/MDIV (7)

MGR/MAR2007/MDIV (5)

ANSWER

Definition

It is a serious condition that mostly occurs in children recovering from viral infections, such as flu or chickenpox characterized by features due to swelling of brain and liver.

Pathogenesis

It may be precipitated by intake of aspirin for myalgia or fever.

There may be inborn error if enzyme is responsible for fatty acid oxidation.

Medium chain acyl-CoA dehydrogenase deficiency will predispose the patient to exposure to toxin, such as insecticides, herbicides, etc.

In case of viral infection there is mitochondrial injury leading to dysfunction disrupting oxidative phosphorylation as well as fatty acid beta-oxidation in the virus-infected cells in patients with inborn error of metabolism or mitochondrial disorder.

Histologically:

- **a.** Fatty vacuolization in the hepatocyte cytoplasm
- **b.** Edema of astrocyte with neuron loss in the brain
- **c.** Fatty degeneration of the proximal lobules of the kidneys

Clinical Features

Initial clinical features for children younger than 2 years of age:

- **a.** Diarrhea
- **b.** Rapid breathing

Initial clinical features for older children and teenagers than 2 years of age:

- **a.** Lethargy and unusual sleepiness
- **b.** Protracted and continuous vomiting

Additional features are:

- **a.** Irritability, aggressive behavior
- **b.** Disorientation, confusion
- **c.** Weakness of both extremities
- **d.** Excessive lethargy
- **e.** Lowered level of consciousness
- **f.** Seizures
- **g.** Complete loss of consciousness

Centers for Disease Control and Prevention (CDC) classification of stages of Reye syndrome:

- **A.** Stage 0: Alert, no clinical feature but history and laboratory features suggest this syndrome.
- **B.** Stage 1: Vomiting, lethargy, and sleepiness
- **C.** Stage 2: Restlessness, irritability, disorientation, delirium, tachycardia, hyperventilation, dilated pupil with sluggish response, hyperreflexia, and positive Babinski response

D. Stage 3: Obtunded, comatose, decorticate rigidity, and inappropriate response to noxious stimuli

E. Stage 4: Deep coma, decerebrate rigidity, fixed and dilated pupil, and oculovestibular reflexes loss

F. Stage 5: Seizures, flaccid paralysis, absent deep tendon jerk, and respiratory arrest

Complications

A. Status epilepticus
B. Herniation of brain
C. Aspiration pneumonia
D. Cardiac arrhythmias
E. Respiratory failure
F. Myocardial; infarction
G. Pancreatitis
H. Gastrointestinal bleeding
I. Acute renal failure
J. SIADH
K. Sepsis
L. Death

Diagnosis

The CDC diagnostic criteria include:

A. Acute noninflammatory encephalopathy with altered level of consciousness.

B. Hepatic dysfunction with fatty metamorphosis without inflammation or necrosis in liver biopsy or >3-fold rise in ALT, AST, or ammonia level.

C. No other explanation for cerebral edema or hepatic abnormality.

D. In cerebrospinal fluid (CSF) white blood cell count of 8/cc, but lumbar puncture is not possible in hemodynamically unstable patient or raised ICP.

E. Brain biopsy finding of cerebral edema without inflammation or necrosis.

Treatment

A. Intravenous fluid: Intravenous glucose and electrolyte has to be given in stage 1. If pH is <7–7.2, sodium bicarbonate 0.5–2 mEq/Kg/day should be given to correct it.

B. In stage 2: Hyperammonemia is corrected by sodium phenylacetate—sodium benzoate in patient with encephalopathy. If patient fails to respond hemodialysis is of choice.

C. Stage 3–5: Continuous monitoring of:

  a. Central venous pressure (CVP)
  b. Arterial pressure
  c. End-tidal carbon dioxide

If not intubated endotracheal intubation has to be done.

Vitamin K, FFP, and platelets (if <50,000/cc) to be given in case of bleeding manifestation.

D. Diuretics: It has to be given intravenously to decrease ICP.

E. Cooling of blanket: It is given to maintain body temperature at normal level.

Risk of increased mortality in the following cases:

A. Age < 5 years
B. Rapid progression from stage 1 to stage 3
C. CVP < 6 mm of water
D. Ammonia > 45 μg/dL
E. Glucose level < 60 mg/dL
F. Hypoproteinemia refractory to FFP and vitamin K
G. Muscle involvement
H. Previous diarrheal illness

Q26. Delta virus hepatitis infection.
MGR/SEP2008/MDI (5)

Hepatitis D infection.
RAJIV GANDHI UNI OF HEALTH SC, KARNATAKA, 2020 (10)

ANSWER

HDV Virus, its Replication, and Pathogenesis

HDV virus is also known as delta virus. It is 36 nm diameter incomplete RNA virus particle and has 8 genotypes from 1 to 8. Delta antigen having no antigenic homology with HBsAg exists in two isoforms—small and large protein. HDV utilizes the envelope protein of HBV such as parasite of HBV. Sodium taurocholate, a receptor for bile acid uptake within the liver acts also as a receptor for entry of HBV and HDV. After uncoating genome of the virus enters into the nucleus of host hepatocyte and RNA to RNA replication without DNA intermediates via RNA-directed RNA synthesis will be started with the help of host RNA polymerase II, as a result complementary antigenomic RNA synthesis happens by transcription of genomic RNA and this antigenomic RNA acts as a template for synthesis of subsequent genomic RNA with the help of host RNA polymerase I. HDV RNA contains only one ORF and a protein HDAg which exists in two forms:

  a. One is small and is involved in facilitating in RNA replication
  b. Larger one is required for assembly of antigen to form virion but suppress replication.

Hepatitis delta virus antigen combines with RNA polymerase II stimulating transcription. The complete virion with the help of HBV starts injury to liver but intracellular replication occurs without HBV.

HDV infects hepatocytes by two methods:

a. It infects with HBV simultaneously (coinfection).
b. It can infect the liver already infected with HBV (superinfection)

If HDV infection will transmit from donor of one subtype of HBsAg to recipient of other subtype of HBsAg, it assumes the recipient's subtype of HBsAg. Duration of HBV infection will determine the duration of HDV infection because HDV completely rely on HBV. Again, HDV suppresses the replication of HBV.

Hepatitis delta virus antigen can be detected in the serum occasionally and anti-HDV IgM can be found 30–40 days after appearance of symptoms.

In case of self-limited infection this antibody is transient and in low titer and remains detectable beyond the clearance of both antigens, HBsAg and HDV.

In case of chronic infection both anti-HDV IgM and IgG are clearly detected and during replication of HDV, in the liver HDV antigen and in the serum HDV RNA are detected.

Epidemiology

There are two epidemiologic patterns that seen:

A. In case of endemic infection transmission occurs through nonpercutaneous route.
B. In case of nonendemic infection transmission occurs through percutaneous route by blood and blood products, intravenous drug users, and hemophiliac.

Clinical Features

Hepatitis delta virus produces both acute and chronic infection but duration of HBV infection can limit the HDV infection.

In case of coinfection with HBV the clinical and biochemical features are indistinguishable from HBV infection alone but may be severe in few coinfected cases.

If there is superinfection in case of chronic HBV hepatitis or in case of unresolving HBV hepatitis, HDV replication will be started indefinitely thus HDV superinfection will produce clinical exacerbation or acute viral hepatitis in already developed chronic hepatitis leading to clinical deterioration of the patient.

Laboratory Diagnosis

A. Presence of HDV antigen in the hepatocyte nuclei
B. Brief appearance of circulating HDV antigen
C. In case of coinfection: HBsAg, HBV DNA, and Anti-HBs IgM along with HDV RNA
D. In case of superinfection anti-HBs IgG can differentiate acute from chronic hepatitis.

Summary of diagnostic tests in case of hepatitis D evaluation:

Test	Interpretation	Comments
Serum HDAg	Acute infection	It will disappear quickly
Anti HDV IgG antibody	Ongoing infection or previous infection	First screening test and it has to be performed in all HBV patients
Anti HDV IgM antibody	• Acute infection • Chronic infection with disease activity	It determines disease activity
HDV RNA qualitative	• Replication of HDV • Active infection	Gold standard for determining HDB infection
HDV RNA quantitative	Blood level of HDV RNA	It is useful for setting of treatment to predict response
Genotyping of HDV	HDV genotype	Different clinical course for different genotype

Complications

A. In case of simultaneous infection with HBV, HDV may increase the severity of hepatitis.
B. In case of superinfection mild chronic hepatitis may progress into:
    a. Fulminant hepatic failure
    b. Progressive chronic hepatitis
    c. Chronic active hepatitis
    d. Cirrhosis
    e. Hepatocellular failure

Treatment

No specific treatment is given in case of acute hepatitis D. Treatment of HBV infection is required in case of chronic hepatitis.

Prophylaxis

This infection can be prevented by HBV vaccination as there is no prophylaxis available for HDV to prevent superinfection. So, percutaneous exposure should be avoided. Contact with the infected person also should be avoided.

Q27. Bile acids.

MGR/MAY2011/MDI (5)

ANSWER

Bile Acids

Daily production in the body and loss from the body is between 250 and 500 mg, loss occurs from the feces with daily maximal excretion 4–6 g. Bile acids are mainly stored in gallbladder and synthesis is under negative feedback control. There are two primary bile acids (60–90% of total bile acids), these are:

a. Cholic acid
b. Chenodeoxycholic acid

Three secondary bile acids are:

a. Deoxycholic acid
b. Lithocholic acid
c. Ketolithocholic acid

Two tertiary bile acids are:

a. Sulfolithocholic acid
b. Ursodeoxycholic acid

Synthesis of Bile Acids

Cholesterol is synthesized from acetyl CoA with the help of hydroxy-glutaryl-CoA reductase. There are two pathways of production of bile acids from cholesterol; these are classical and alternate pathways.

A. In the classical pathway there is 7 hydroxylation of cholesterol via CYP7A1 to form 7-α hydroxycholesterol which in turn is converted to chenodeoxycholic acid by CYP7A1 and to cholic acid via CYP8B1.
B. In the alternate pathway 27-α hydroxylation to (25R)-26 hydroxycholesterol via CYP7A1 and then to chenodeoxycholic acid via CYP7B1.

C-7α hydroxylase and C-27-α hydroxylase are found in endoplasmic reticulum and mitochondria, respectively. Carboxyl group of bile acids are conjugated with glycine and taurine with the help of enzyme in the cytoplasm that produces following four conjugated bile acids:

a. Glycocholic acid
b. Taurocholic acid
c. Glycochenodeoxycholic acid
d. Taurochenodeoxycholic acid

Bile acids are secreted into the bile and from there it is secreted into the intestine. In the ileum and cecum bile acids are deconjugated into cholic acid and chenodeoxycholic acid which in turn after 7-dehydroxylation produces three hydrophilic bile acids, these are:

a. Deoxycholic acid
b. Lithocholic acid
c. Ketolithocholic acid

The above bile acids are absorbed from the intestine and are again conjugated with glycine and taurine in hepatocytes and again secreted into biliary canaliculi.

Lithocholic acid will be sulfolithocholic acid in the liver and ketolithocholic acid to ursodeoxycholic acid in liver and intestine. Ursodeoxycholic acid is returned into liver through cholehepatic shunt and it also acts as inhibitory feedback mechanism over 3-hydroxy-3-methylglutaryl (HMG) CoA reductase as well as 7-α hydroxylase. In advanced age bile acid production will be reduced, so biliary excretion of cholesterol is increased. Bile acids circulate in the body 3–10 times per day through excretion in bile into intestine followed by absorption into intestinal mucosa followed by recirculation. There are several transport systems which will help in absorption against concentration gradient:

A. Bile acids uptake at sinusoidal membrane by Na^+ dependent and Na^+ independent gradient
B. Through MRP2, an ATP driven carrier glycoprotein helps to release bile acids at the surface of biliary membrane.
C. Na^+ dependent carrier system in the ileal and colonic mucosa

Functions of Bile Acids

A. Helps in emulsification of fat-soluble vitamins
B. It stimulates intestinal motility.
C. Control the bile flow through osmotic water movement
D. Digestion and resorption of dietary fat by:
    a. Through micelle formation
    b. Stabilize and activate several enzymes, such as pancreatic lipase, cholesterol esterase, and phospholipase A_2
E. It helps in metabolism of cholesterol by:
    a. Reducing excess cholesterol by stabilization and degradation to bile acids.
    b. Reduction of synthesis of cholesterol in the liver
    c. Regulation of cholesterol output into the bile

Q28. Blood supply to liver.

MGR/MAR2010/MDI (5)

ANSWER

Blood Supply to the Liver

Hepatic vascular supply includes the following:

Hepatic artery:

A. Common hepatic artery

B. Phrenic artery

C. Splenic artery

D. Left gastric artery

Sometimes second hepatic artery originates from:

A. In 10% of cases from superior mesenteric artery

B. In 18% cases from gastroduodenal artery

Hepatic artery runs close to portal vein or sometimes coils around the portal vein in the porta hepatis and will be divided into two branches:

A. Right hepatic artery—from this branch cystic artery arises.

B. Left hepatic artery—from this branch occasionally middle hepatic artery arises.

There is a sphincter prior to its division into interlobar arteries which again divide into intralobar arteries supplying nutrients to hepatic lobules. From there arterial blood enters into sinusoids through their terminal branches.

Hepatic artery supplies the following regions:

A. Portal interstitium

B. Peribiliary biliary plexus as greatest compartment of arteriole

C. Vasa vasorum of hepatic vein

D. Vasa vasorum of portal vein

Pressure:

A. In hepatic artery: 100 mm Hg

B. In hepatic arteriole: 30–40 mm Hg

Hepatic arterial flow:

A. In men: 1,200 mL/min

B. In women: 1,800 mL/min

Blood volume in liver is 10–15% of total blood volume in case of normal adult. Consumption of oxygen by the liver is 6 mL/100 g of wet weight of the liver. But this oxygen supply varies in different zones of lobule of the liver:

A. Zone 1: This acinoperipheral region receives best oxygen supply so based on aerobic metabolism.

B. Zone 2: This centroacinar region receives lowest supply of oxygen so is based on anaerobic metabolism.

C. Zone 3: This zone is in between two above zones.

Blood supply to liver is decreased in following conditions:

A. Sleep

B. Elderly

C. Standing condition

D. Fasting condition

Sinusoidal blood supply is influenced by the following factors:

A. Neural factors:

- **a.** Dopaminergic receptor
- **b.** Adrenergic receptor

B. Vasoactive factors:

- **a.** Endothelin
- **b.** Adenosine
- **c.** Carbon monoxide

C. Anatomical mechanisms by the sphincters

Internal anatomy of liver

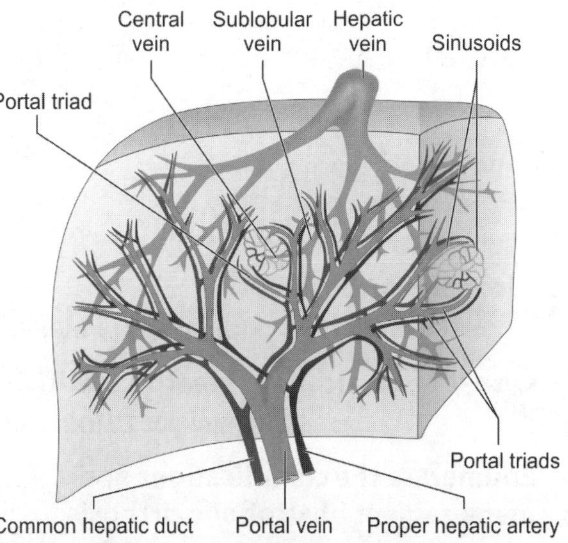

Anatomy of veins and arteries of the liver

Portal vein: Superior mesenteric vein and splenic vein join posterior to isthmus to form portal vein. Near the origin of portal vein inferior mesenteric vein joins the splenic vein. After its formation portal vein runs along the hepatoduodenal ligament to reach porta hepatis and divides into two, right and left branches.

Right portal branch takes two veins:

A. Two veins from caudate lobe

B. Cystic vein

Left branch will flow with paraumbilical vein.

Each branch of portal vein extends along the portal tract and merge with interlobular veins and divides into:

A. Venulae interlobulares

B. Conductor veins: It will be divided into distributor veins which continue ultimately as terminal branches.

So, blood flowing in the portal vein will pass through periportal limiting plate via hepatocytic venular inlets to reach hepatic sinusoids. Hepatic arterial terminal branches will also enter into sinusoids.

So, hepatic sinusoids contain:

A. 75% of portal blood

B. 25% of hepatic arterial blood

Blood from hepatic sinusoids enters into hepatic vein through venous capillaries.

Hepatic vein: This vein originates in the center of hepatic lobule from central hepatic vein which runs at acute angles as sublobular veins. These sublobular veins join to form collecting veins. Collecting veins fuse to form following five venous trunks:

A. Left superior hepatic vein

B. Right superior hepatic vein

C. Left hepatic vein

D. Right hepatic vein

E. Middle hepatic vein

Above veins run intersegmentally and receive branches from adjacent segments. Superior group of hepatic veins will join with inferior vena cava below the diaphragm at the posterior surface of the liver but group of inferior hepatic veins varies regarding their draining sites.

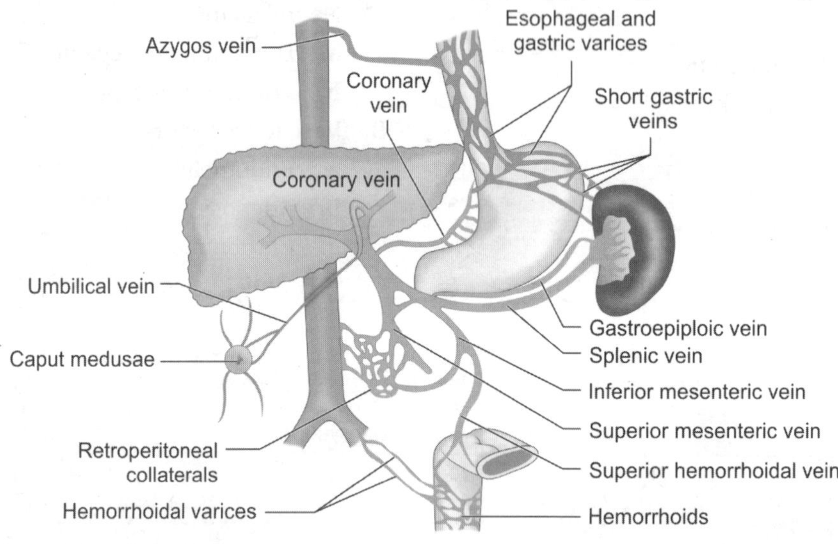

Q29. Alcoholic cirrhosis.

MGR/APR2013/MDI (5)

Cytokines in alcoholic steatohepatitis.

SNMC/MAY2001/MDIII (10)

Enumerate the complications and management of alcoholic cirrhosis.

DNB (DEC2019) (6)

Describe the pathogenesis, clinical features, laboratory findings, prognosis and treatment of alcoholic liver disease.

NTR UNI OF HEALTH SC, VIJAYAWADA, 2020 (10)

Write briefly about the current management of alcoholic hepatitis.

WBUHS, 2023 (10)

ANSWER

Introduction

Excessive alcohol ingestion is a major cause of liver disease. There are three distinct forms of liver disease seen in alcohol ingestion; these are fatty liver, alcoholic steatohepatitis, and alcoholic cirrhosis. Fatty liver is present in 90% of binge alcoholic, 20% alcoholic develop alcoholic steatohepatitis and 10% patients develop cirrhosis.

Risk Factors in Alcoholic Liver Disease

A. Quantity of alcohol: Threshold in case of men—>14 drinks per week and >7 drinks per week 1 beer, 4 ounces of wine or 1 ounce of 80% spirit—contain 12 g of alcohol.

B. Gender: Women are more susceptible to alcoholic liver disease. In case of women >20 g/day whereas in men it is 40–80 g/day produces fatty liver and ≥160 g/day for 10–20 years develops cirrhosis.

C. Hepatitis C: In case of alcoholic liver disease coinfection with HCV progresses it toward decompensation, failure, HCC, and ultimately to death.

D. Genetics: There is association of PNPLA3 and alcoholic liver disease.

E. Fatty liver: Obesity, insulin resistance, nonalcoholic fatty liver disease, and malnutrition are the risk factor in case of alcoholic liver disease.

Pathogenesis

Liver is the main site of alcohol metabolism. Alcoholic steatosis is attributed to increased NADH (reduced nicotinamide adenine dinucleotide) and metabolic stress. Alcohol in the hepatocyte produces following effects to develop steatosis:

a. Mitochondrial fatty acid β-oxidation will be suppressed.

b. Free fatty acid uptake of hepatocytes from the circulation will be enhanced.

c. Increased synthesis of fatty acids and triglyceride in the liver

d. Derailment of synthesis and secretion of lipoprotein

e. Defect in methionine cycle leading to glutathione synthesis

f. Changes in the profile of transfer factors responsible for lipid homeostasis

g. Decreased activity of PPAR-α leading to suppression of mitochondrial as well as peroxisomal fatty acid oxidation and catabolic lipid metabolic pathways.

h. Enhanced lipid synthesis due to increased activity of sterol regulatory element-binding protein-1c and 2 (SREBP-1c and 2)

i. Changes in NAD-redox state in the liver as a result of inhibition of deacetylase sirtuin-1

j. Inhibition of AMP-activated protein kinase (AMPK).

Mechanism of Development of Fatty Liver

Consumption of alcohol:

A. Upregulates SREBP-1c and downregulates PRAR-α activity by different factors leading to fatty acid synthesis side by side and inhibition of fatty acid β-oxidation.

B. Reduces activation of AMPK at the same time attenuates acetyl-CoA carboxylase activity, on the other hand decreases carnitine palmitoyltransferase activity leading to increased synthesis of fatty acid activity and decreases fatty acid β-oxidation.

C. Increase $NADH/NAD^+$ ratio which is followed by inhibition of β-oxidation in mitochondria.

D. Activates several factors, such as C3, C1qa, PKCe, and iNOS.

All the above mechanisms lead to development of alcoholic steatosis.

Pathogenesis of Alcoholic Steatohepatitis

In this state following inflammatory cells are found in the liver, such as polymorphs, activated Kupffer cells, T cells, NK cells, and activated macrophages.

Neutrophils Activation

It is the hallmark of alcoholic hepatitis.

A. It releases reactive oxygen species (ROS) and damages hepatocytes.

B. It promotes repair of liver by:

- **a.** Secretion of growth factors
- **b.** Removing dead cell debris

C. Infiltration of neutrophils promotes generation of liver cells and suppresses bacterial infection.

There are several mechanisms responsible for infiltration of neutrophils in alcoholic liver disease:

A. Due to intestinal overgrowth of bacterial leads to overproduction of bacterial toxin which permeate through the intestinal wall as a result of increased permeability and enter into the liver. In the liver these toxins damage the hepatocytes releasing cellular debris and nucleic acids which ultimately induce neutrophil activation.

B. Several factors, such as elevated production of chemokines, adhesion molecules, and chemokine receptors induce neutrophil infiltration.

C. Chronic with recurrent binge eating may increase neutrophil infiltration due to elevation of hepatic E-selectin and activation of hepatic NK T cells.

Kupffer Cells Activation and Macrophage Infiltration

A. In the liver there are large number of Kupffer cells which after being activated by bacterial endotoxins play an active role in liver cell injury through increased production of proinflammatory mediators and ROS.

B. There is also recruitment of infiltrating macrophages; these are of two subtypes: $Ly6C^{high}$ which is tissue damaging and proinflammatory phenotype and $Ly6C^{low}$ which is tissue protective and anti-inflammatory phenotype. In case of chronic low alcohol intake $Ly6C^{low}$ concentration will be high but in case binge eating the ratio of $Ly6C^{high}$ to $Ly6C^{low}$ leading to hepatocyte damage.

Natural Killer T-cells Activation

These are heterogeneous group of cells having receptors for both NK cells and T cells and thus recognize glycolipid antigen, it is presented by nonclassical class I major histocompatibility complex such as molecule CD1d. These NK T cells act as bridge between innate and adaptive immunity. In case of chronic binge alcohol intake these cells are activated leading to direct killing of injured hepatocytes, promotion of neutrophil infiltration, and production of various inflammatory mediators which perpetuate further hepatic injury.

Adaptive Immunity Activation

In case of chronic and binge alcohol intake as a result of oxidative stress is induced resulting generation of products of lipid peroxidation, malondialdehyde as well as 4-hydroxynonenal which produce antibodies against them and thus elevating T cells in the liver and activating the adaptive immunity.

Inflammatory Mediators

A large number of inflammatory mediators act synergistically or additively induce inflammation in liver targeting nonparenchymal and parenchymal cells and various types of inflammatory cells in liver. There is evidence of LPS-Kupffer cells-TNF-α axis which acts in a best pathogenic way to produce hepatocyte injury. Other mediators are complements, IL-8, IL-1, IL-17, LPS, chemokines, and C-X-C motif.

Dysfunction of Microbiota in the Intestine

Intestinal luminal environment is maintained by gastric acidic pH, motility of the gut, immunogenic defense mechanisms, bile salts, colonic pH, and lastly competition for the intestinal binding sites and nutrients between gut bacteria. In case chronic ethanol intake luminal environment will be altered leading to decreased concentration of Bacteroides and Firmicutes and increased concentration of actinobacteria and Proteobacteria and thus increased production of endotoxin. Now, metabolic product of alcohol, acetaldehyde along with alcohol, will disrupt the tight junction in the intestinal wall and endotoxins permeate through the intestinal wall to reach the liver and induce TNF-α and other inflammatory mediators' production. Few bacterial derived toxins, such as flagellin and peptidoglycans, may impact toll-like receptor signaling as well as proinflammatory cytokine production. Again, chronic alcohol intake itself increases toll-like receptor and thus sensitizing the hepatocytes to cytokine mediated injury.

Complications of Alcoholic Cirrhosis

A. Portal hypertension:
- **a.** Esophageal and gastric varices
- **b.** Spontaneous bacterial peritonitis
- **c.** Ascites
- **d.** Hepatorenal syndrome

B. Hepatic encephalopathy

C. Hepatopulmonary syndrome—it consists of triad of liver disease, hypoxemia and intrapulmonary vascular dilatation that leads to respiratory distress.

D. Different types of coagulopathy and bleeding disorders due to:
- **a.** Thrombocytopenia
- **b.** Decreased synthesis of factor II, VII, XI and X
- **c.** Disseminated intravascular coagulation

E. Endocrine and metabolic complications:
- **a.** Gynecomastia
- **b.** Testicular atrophy
- **c.** Malnutrition
- **d.** Sarcopenia
- **e.** Impaired neoglucogenesis leading to hypoglycemia
- **f.** Electrolyte disturbances:'
  - Hypokalemia due to use of diuretics
  - Hyponatremia

F. Acute on chronic liver failure due to sudden decompensation of the liver or due to excess alcohol consumption

Management of alcoholic cirrhosis:

Diseases	Treatment
Alcohol dependence	• Absolute abstinence from alcohol • Counseling • Cognitive behavioral therapy • To reduce the craving from alcohol: • Disulfiram—it is alcohol dehydrogenase inhibitor • Naltrexone—it is opioid receptor antagonist • Acamprosate—to restore glutamate balance.
Malnutrition	• High protein diet • High calorie diet • Supplementation of vitamin: o Thiamine—to prevent Wernicke-Korsakoff syndrome o Folate to reduce macrocytic anemia o Vitamin B12 to replenish the deficiency o Zinc—to improve the immune function
Portal hypertension	• Nonselective beta blockers • Variceal sclerotherapy • Variceal banding
Ascites	• Orally fluid restriction • Diuretics—spironolactone as 1st line and loop diuretics as 2nd line of therapy • Large volume paracentesis under cover of 20% salt poor albumin
Spontaneous bacterial peritonitis	• Empirical antibiotics • Infusion of 20% salt poor albumin to prevent renal failure and Hepatorenal syndrome • As long term prophylaxis—norfloxacin or ciprofloxacin
Hepatic encephalopathy	• Avoid protein intake in large amount • Administration of lactulose to lower the level of ammonia • Rifaximin to reduce the formation of ammonia by gut bacteria • Correction of the precipitating factors like gastrointestinal complication • Infection • Electrolyte imbalance
Hepatorenal syndrome	• Administration of vasoconstrictors like terlipressin or midodrine • Intravenous infusion of 20% salt poor albumin • Liver transplantation

Alcoholic hepatitis can be diagnosed when the following criteria are fulfilled:

A. Onset of jaundice within 60 days of consumption of heavy alcohol (more than 50 g daily for a minimum of 6 months).

B. Serum level of bilirubin of more than 3 g/dL

C. Increase in the serum SGPT of >50–400 U/L

D. Ratio of AST:ALT of >1.5

E. No other cause of hepatitis

Alcoholic steatohepatitis is the histological diagnosis whereas alcoholic hepatitis is clinical diagnosis.

Evaluation

A. Liver function test demonstrates raised AST but normal ALT.

B. Most reliable marker of alcoholism is carbohydrate deficient transferrin.

C. Elevation of CRP is the good marker of alcoholic hepatitis.

Management of Alcoholic Hepatitis

Alcoholic hepatitis can be subdivided into mild to moderate and severe alcoholic hepatitis.

Severe alcoholic hepatitis leading to high mortality is characterized by:

A. MDF score greater than 32.

B. MELD score greater than 20

C. ABIC score category C

D. Glasgow alcoholic hepatitis score of 9.

The drug of choice is prednisolone because it does not require hepatic metabolism. If the patient is unable to take it orally, in that case intravenous methylprednisolone 32 mg daily. If the patient fails to respond to steroids as evidenced by the little score of greater than 0.45. If the score is less than 0.45, in that case steroid should be continued for another 3–4 weeks. Steroid increases the expression of the anti-inflammatory gene leading to promotion of anti-inflammatory activity.

Contraindications to steroid administration are:

A. Active gastrointestinal bleeding

B. Active infection

C. Renal failure

D. Uncontrolled diabetes

E. Severe pancreatitis

Patient having contraindications to steroid should be managed by 400 mg pentoxifylline orally thrice daily for 28 days.

Commonest cause of death in this is hepatorenal syndrome. Response of steroid can be graded in the following manner:

A. Complete response—little score of less than 0.16
B. Partial response—little score of between 0.16 and 0.56
C. Null response—if little score is greater than 0.56
D. Little score of more than 0.45 after 1 week of steroid therapy indicates 75% mortality in 6 months.

Patient with alcoholic hepatitis are at risk of alcohol withdrawal, so in that case lorazepam or oxazepam should be the choice. Daily calorie intake should be 2,000 kcal.

Liver transplantation should be considered in the patient is not responsive to steroids with MELD score of greater than 26.

If the patient develops hepatorenal syndrome, in that case nephrologist should be consulted.

Following are the complications of alcoholic hepatitis:

A. Hepatic encephalopathy
B. Variceal hemorrhage
C. Ascites
D. Thrombocytopenia
E. Coagulopathy
F. Spontaneous bacterial peritonitis
G. Iron overload

Q30. Discuss etiopathology, serological and viral markers of acute viral hepatitis.

MUHS/MAY2011/MDIII (25)

HBV in Question no 10.
HCV in Question no 18.
HEV in Question no 24.
HDV in Question no 26.

ANSWER

HAV or Hepatitis A Virus

Hepatitis virus, previously known as *Enterovirus* type 72, is 27 nm, heat, ether, and acid resistant nonenveloped virus containing positive sense RNA genome. Its unique features are:

a. Internal ribosomal entry site
b. Truncated VP4 capsid protein which is lack of N-terminal myristoylation
c. C-terminal pX extension of VP1
d. VP2 late domains which is involved in envelopment by membrane
e. Cis-acting replication element within the sequence of 3Dpol.

This virus has four genotypes: I, II, III, and IV, again each genotype has two subtypes, A and B. Other three genotypes: V, VI, and VII are present in primates. Genotype I is very common in human being.

Mode of Transmission

a. Fecal-oral route, contaminated water
b. Male homosexuals
c. Personal contact in daycare center and household contact
d. Illicit drug use rarely

Pathogenesis

HAV activates cytotoxic T cells leading to injury of hepatocytes through cellular immunity. In the HAV-infected liver CD8+ cells lyse infected liver cells leading to cascade of inflammatory response involving inflammatory mediators, Kupffer cells, TNF-α, lymphokine activated killer cells, and IL-6. Ultimately apoptosis of hepatocytes, activation of coagulation cascade, oxygen-free radicle formation, and activation of inflammation lead to necrosis of liver cells thus fulminant hepatic failure or multiorgan failure can develop.

Serologic markers:

a. HAV RNA is excreted in the stool soon after increase of ALT and just before appearance of detectable anti-HAV IgM in the blood. In saliva HAV RNA persists for an average of 60 days after onset of clinical presentation.
b. Anti-HAV IgM is detectable 5–10 days after exposure, present in the symptomatic phase and it will persist for 4–6 months, but test cannot detect the lowest level of IgM. If anti-HAV IgM is detected in absence of total anti-HAV, it is called as false anti-HAV IgM, it is more common in females.
c. Anti-HAV IgG can be detected at the disease onset but persists for many years as marker of prior infection.

Q31. Acute hepatitis—gross structure and microscopic appearance.

MGR/OCT2012/MDI (5)

ANSWER

The gross structures in case of acute hepatitis are: Liver is grossly enlarged, yellowish, and greasy with shining Glisson's capsules surrounding it.

In all types of viral hepatitis histological features of liver are:

A. Panlobular infiltration of mononuclear cells:
 a. Small lymphocytes
 b. Plasma cells
 c. Occasionally eosinophils

B. Damage of hepatocytes:
 a. Degeneration of hepatocytes
 b. Necrosis of hepatocytes
 c. Cell dropout
 d. Ballooning of cells
 e. Acidophilic degeneration of hepatocytes—called Councilman or apoptotic bodies
 f. Large hepatocytes containing ground glass cytoplasm within which there may be presence of HBsAg diagnosed histochemically by orcein or aldehyde stain.

C. Variable degree of cholestasis

D. Kupffer cell hyperplasia

E. Hepatic cell regeneration:
 a. Numerous mitotic figures
 b. Multinucleated cells
 c. Rosette or "Pseudoacinar" formation

F. In uncomplicated case there is preservation of reticulin framework.

In case of hepatitis C, special histologic features are:

A. Paucity of inflammation

B. Activation of sinusoidal lining cells

C. Aggregates of lymphoid tissue

D. Presence of accumulation of fat linked with increased incidence of fibrosis which is more in case of genotype 3.

E. Piled up of biliary epithelial cells without interruption of basement membrane.

In case of hepatitis D, there is increased evidence of microvascular steatosis

In case hepatitis E, there is marked evidence of marked cholestasis

In case of hepatitis A, slowly resolving cholestatic variant may be seen.

In more severe lesion:

A. Bridging necrosis or confluent necrosis or interface hepatitis. Bridging results from:
 a. Large areas of hepatocyte dropout
 b. Collapse of reticulin framework

 Bridge consists of:
 a. Condensed reticulin fibers
 b. Degenerating liver cells
 c. Inflammatory debris

 Bridge spans from portal to portal areas connecting portal to central vein, central to central vein. Bridging necrosis is of some prognostic significance as the patient may die within several weeks to months.

B. Massive hepatic necrosis or acute yellow atrophy in fulminant hepatitis. The striking features are:
 a. Small shrunken soft liver
 b. Histologically:
  1. Massive hepatocyte death
  2. Dropout of hepatocytes from most of the lobules
  3. Extensive collapse of hepatic architecture
  4. Condensation of reticulin framework.

Drug-induced Acute Hepatitis

Morphologic features are indistinguishable from acute viral hepatitis ranging from spotty necrosis in the lobule of the liver with predominant lymphocytic infiltration to bridging necrosis in case of methyldopa or hepatic granuloma in sulfonamide or microvascular steatosis or steatohepatitis due to mitochondrial dysfunction or lipid peroxidation in case of retroviral therapy. There may be damage of sinusoidal lining cells due to high dose of chemotherapy.

Q32. Write short notes on portal circulation. Discuss etiopathogenesis of non-cirrhotic portal hypertension.

MUZ/MAY2016/MDI (30)

Portal circulation Question no 28.

Non-cirrhotic portal hypertension.

NTR UNI OF HEALTH SC, VIJAYAWADA, 2021 (21)

Portal circulation.

NTR UNI OF HEALTH SC, VIJAYAWADA, 2020 (10)

Sites of portosystemic shunts.

MGR UNIVERSITY, TAMIL NADU, 2018 (5)

Write shortly about the recent guidelines of anticoagulant therapy in portal vein thrombosis in a cirrhosis of liver patient.

MANIPUR UNIVERSITY, 2020 (10)

ANSWER

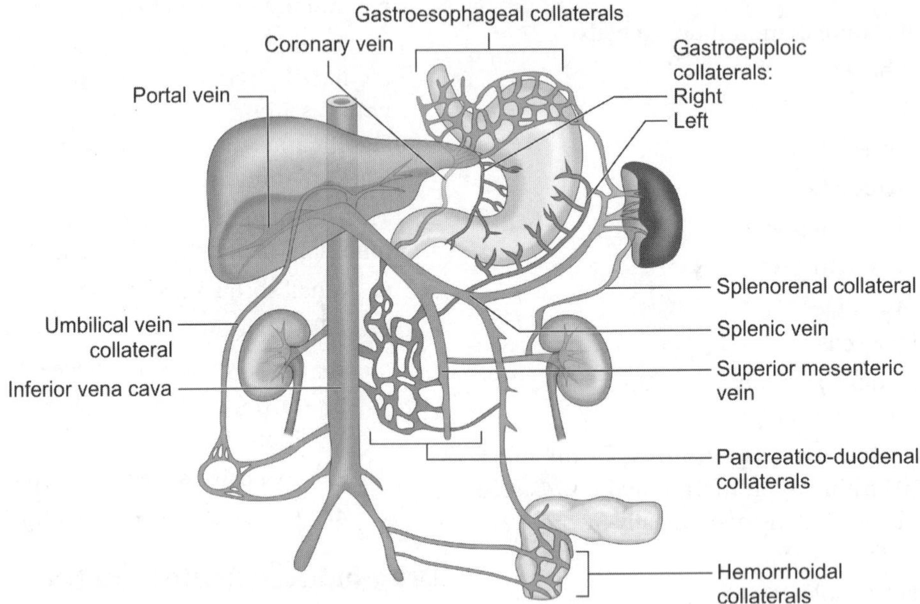

Portal Hypertension

Etiopathogenesis of noncirrhotic portal hypertension: Portal hypertension can be defined as a disorder where portal venous pressure gradient between inferior vena cava and portal vein is >5 mm Hg. Portal hypertension may be cirrhotic where hepatic venous pressure gradient (HVPG) is elevated due to increased sinusoidal resistance whereas in case of NCPH HPVG will be normal or mildly elevated.

Classification of NCPH

A. Prehepatic causes [normal free hepatic venous pressure (FHVP), normal right atrial pressure (RAP), normal wedged hepatic venous pressure (WHVP), normal HVPG, normal portal venous pressure (PVP), and normal intrasplenic pressure (ISP)]:
- **a.** Extrahepatic portal venous obstruction (EHPVO)
- **b.** Splenic venous thrombosis
- **c.** Portal vein thrombosis
- **d.** Splanchnic arteriovenous fistula
- **e.** Massive splenomegaly:
  1. Storage disease
  2. Myeloproliferative disorders
  3. Lymphoma

B. Hepatic causes [normal FHVP, normal RAP, high WHVP, normal or high HVPG, high PVP, and high ISP]:
- **a.** Presinusoidal causes:
  1. Congenital causes:
     - Congenital hepatic fibrosis
     - Arteriovenous fistula
     - Adult polycystic diseases
  2. Biliary causes:
     - Sclerosing cholangitis
     - Primary biliary cirrhosis
     - Toxic vinyl chloride
     - Autoimmune cholangiopathy
  3. Neoplastic causes:
     - Chronic lymphocytic leukemia
     - Lymphoma
     - Epithelial malignancies
  4. Granulomatous lesions:
     - Sarcoidosis
     - Schistosomiasis
     - Hepatic sclerosis
     - Partial nodular transformation
     - Idiopathic portal hypertension
     - Noncirrhotic portal fibrosis
- **b.** Sinusoidal causes:
  1. Sinusoidal fibrosis:
     - Alcohol
     - Toxins
     - Drugs—methotrexate and amiodarone
     - Metabolic—nonalcoholic fatty liver disease
     - Inflammatory—Q fever, viral hepatitis, and cytomegalovirus

2. Collapse of sinusoids:
   - Acute necroinflammatory diseases
   - Defenestration of sinusoids
   - Early cases of alcoholic liver diseases
3. Infiltration of sinusoids:
   - Gaucher's disease
   - Mastocytosis
4. Compression over the sinusoids:
   - Enlarged Kupffer cells
   - Enlarged fat-laden hepatocytes

c. Postsinusoidal causes:
1. Veno-occlusive diseases due to toxins, drugs, and irradiation
2. Phlebosclerosis of hepatic veins due to hypervitaminosis A, irradiation, and alcohol
3. Primary vascular malignancies
4. Granulomatous causes
5. Hepatic venous outflow obstruction—Budd-Chiari syndrome, prothrombotic states

C. Posthepatic causes (high FHVP, normal or high RAP, high WHVP, normal or high HVPG, high PVP, and high ISP):
a. Constrictive pericarditis
b. Inferior venacaval obstruction by web, tumor, and thrombus
c. Tricuspid regurgitation
d. Severe right-sided heart failure

There are various theories regarding the pathogenesis of NCPF. In case of young adult a major thrombotic event involving major pulmonary vein and in later life multiple and repeated thrombotic events occurring in multiple small and medium branches of portal veins may produce NCPF.

In the liver increased intrahepatic resistance in case of portal hypertension is controlled by two types of cells, fenestrated sinusoidal cell which maintains and facilitate transport of macromolecules across the space of Disse and the other one is hepatic stellate cell. These cells maintain vasoregulatory function in hepatic circulation by vasoregulatory molecules—canonic vasodilator, nitric oxide and canonic vasoconstrictor, endothelin. In case of liver injury these cells are activated, proliferate, migrate, and deposit collagen.

Dual theory: Increased splenic blood flow and intrahepatic obstruction of portal venules generate nitric oxide from various NOS isoforms, such as iNOS and eNOS in sinusoidal endothelial cells and will diffuse into hepatic stellate cells where these activate guanylate cyclase/kinase and promote relaxation leading to dilatation of splenic sinuses and increased splenic venous inflow.

Endothelial mesenchymal transition theory: Endothelial cells of portal venous radicle acquire myofibroblastic features which can be evidenced by reduced expression of CD34, a vascular endothelial cell marker and increased expression of S100A4, COL1A1 and α-SMA as well as pSmad2. Tumor growth factor alpha acts as potent inducer of this transition. After transformation these cells will synthesize collagen which will lead to perisinusoidal portal hypertension and obliterative portal venopathy.

There are two mechanisms by which nitric oxide production is increased: One is increased production of vascular endothelial growth factor (VEGF) and the other is mechanical stress which stimulates endothelial cells to generate nitric oxide.

Endothelins: These are potent vasoconstrictor. They act on two different types of receptors on endothelial cells:

A. When ET_A receptors are activated it will lead to vasoconstriction.
B. When ET_B receptors are activated it will lead to vasodilatation through the release of nitric oxide. In the liver endothelin binds to hepatic stellate cells leading to contraction of vascular endothelial cells and thus increase the resistance in hepatic microcirculation.

If the portal blood flow will be decreased there is compensatory increase in hepatic arterial flow to maintain total hepatic blood flow at constant level. It indicates that there is hyperdynamic hepatic arterial flow at splanchnic and systemic arterial beds.

Extrahepatic portal venous obstruction occurs due to intravascular thrombosis. Here inherited and acquired prothrombotic states in children occur due to tetrahydrofolate reductase deficiency, prothrombin gene mutation, and in adult due to myeloproliferative disorders with or without Janus kinase 2 and JAK2 mutation. In acute portal vein thrombosis this type of extravenous portal vein obstruction will go unnoticed and ultimately becomes organized. Within 6–20 days multiple collateral develop around the portal vein to form cavernoma and ultimately terminate in middle-sized intrahepatic portal venous branches to compensate total hepatic blood flow. So there is formation of varices or hemorrhoids at the site of communication of systemic and portal veins.

Clinical Features

All the signs and symptoms are related to portal hypertension. These are the following:

A. Splenomegaly may lead to cytopenia.
B. Variceal bleeding from esophageal or gastric varices.
C. Presence of ascites but it may be low as compared to ascites due to cirrhosis of liver.

Investigations

A. Complete blood count reveals cytopenia especially thrombocytopenia in case of hypersplenism.
B. Liver function test will be normal until the later stage, absence of hypoalbuminemia.
C. Doppler ultrasonography demonstrates:
   a. Dilated portal vein
   b. Slow blood flow through the portal vein
   c. Presence of collaterals
D. Hepatic venous pressure gradient: It can assess the severity and differentiates noncirrhotic portal hypertension from cirrhotic portal hypertension. In this case the pressure will be normal but in case of cirrhotic portal hypertension it will be high.
E. Liver biopsy: It can detect the following features:
   a. Obliterative portal venopathy, Or
   b. Nodular regenerative hyperplasia
   c. Exclude cirrhotic picture

Management

A. Treatment of variceal bleeding.
B. Management of ascites
C. Splenomegaly with hypersplenism, splenectomy or partial splenic embolization
D. In case of portal venous thrombosis and if there is no active bleeding from the varices, anticoagulant can be started.
E. If the patient is refractory to the treatment or progressive liver damage, liver transplantation is of choice.

Recent Guidelines of Anticoagulant Therapy in Portal Vein Thrombosis in a Cirrhosis of Liver Patient

Thrombosis occurs in the main portal vein or its intrahepatic branches and it can extend up to superior mesenteric vein or splenic vein. Portal vein thrombosis occurs in cirrhosis or malignancy, acute pancreatitis or abdominal sepsis in absence of liver cirrhosis. Pathophysiology of portal vein thrombosis occurs may be associated with following two major conditions:

A. Inherited thrombophilia:
   a. Mutations of factor V
   b. Protein S or protein C deficiency
   c. Mutation of prothrombin G20210
   d. Antithrombin deficiency
   e. Elevated level of factor VIII
   f. Mutation of gene of tetrahydrofolate reductase
B. Major causes of acquired thrombophilia:
   a. Cirrhosis
   b. Acute pancreatitis
   c. Abdominal sepsis
   d. IBD related
   e. PNH
   f. Following endoscopic sclerotherapy
   g. Pregnancy

Treatment of Portal Vein Thrombosis

A. Anticoagulation: It is indicated in the following conditions:
   a. Impending intestinal ischemia
   b. Decompensated liver disease awaiting liver transplantation
   c. Newly diagnosed hepatic cirrhosis with acute portal vein thrombosis
   d. Risk of cavernous transformation
   e. Extension into mesenteric vein.

Option of Anticoagulants

A. Low molecular heparin: It is preferred as initial treatment of choice. In case of renal impairment dose of it has to be modified.
B. Vitamin K antagonist can be used as long-term therapy with target INR in between 2 to 3.
C. Direct oral anticoagulant like apixaban, rivaroxaban or edoxaban can be used in Child–Pugh A and B but not in case of Child–Pugh C and active variceal bleeding.

Duration of Therapy

It should be minimum 3–6 months. But in following conditions duration should be increased:

A. Ongoing prothrombotic risk as in case cancer.
B. Progressive thrombosis
C. Awaiting for transplantation of liver.

Thrombolysis: It can be done by:

A. Indirect intra-arterial infusion of
   a. Tissue plasminogen activator
   b. Urokinase
   c. Streptokinase
B. Direct infusion into superior mesenteric artery through portal vein either by transhepatic or transjugular approach.

Thrombectomy either surgical or mechanical process by percutaneous trans-hepatic approach.

Transvenous intrahepatic portosystemic shunt if can be done in the setting of portal vein thrombosis it can either recanalize or disrupt thrombus.

Q33. Liver transplantation.

RGUHS/APR2001/MDII (10)

Discuss liver transplantation.

BF/MAY2012/MDIV (20)

Indications, contraindications and postoperative management of liver transplantation.

DNB (DEC2019) (10)

Deceased donor organ transplantation in India—challenges and solutions. Live donor liver transplantation.

DNB (OCT2024) (10)

Indications and assessment of patient for liver transplantation.

DR. YSR UNI OF HEALTH SC, VIJAYAWADA, ANDHRA, 2022 (10)

ANSWER

Liver transplantation is a replacement of native diseased organ with whole or a portion of healthy liver from another healthy donor. The most preferred approach is orthotopic transplantation where the donor organ is transplanted in the same location. It has been started in 1960 by Thomas Starzl in the University of Colorado. Indications of liver transplantation:

A. Adult causes:

- **a.** Fulminant hepatitis
- **b.** Autoimmune hepatitis
- **c.** Primary biliary cirrhosis
- **d.** Secondary biliary cirrhosis
- **e.** Cryptogenic cirrhosis
- **f.** Alcoholic cirrhosis
- **g.** Chronic viral hepatitis
- **h.** Primary HCC: In this case the patient who can fulfill the Milan criteria can be selected for transplantation.

  Milan criteria are:

  1. Single HCC nodule <5 cm
  2. <3 lesions each being <3 cm

  If patient presents with the size of tumor beyond the Milan criteria, in that case with the help of radiofrequency ablation or TACE tumor size has to be reduced so that the patient can into Milan criteria.

  Other than number and tumor size following surrogate markers also reflect the tumor biology, these are:

  - Level of AFP and protein induced by vitamin absence
  - Neutrophilic-lymphocyte ratio >5
  - Radiological response to locoregional ablative therapies
  - Histologically proved lack of micro-vascular invasion
- **i.** Hepatic vein thrombosis
- **j.** NASH
- **k.** Familial amyloid polyneuropathy
- **l.** Caroli's disease
- **m.** In case of decompensated hepatic failure if Child–Pugh score is >7.

B. Causes in childhood:

- **a.** Biliary atresia
- **b.** Congenital hepatic fibrosis
- **c.** Alpha-1 antitrypsin deficiency
- **d.** Neonatal hepatitis
- **e.** Byler's disease
- **f.** Inherent disorder of metabolism:
  1. Crigler–Najjar Disease
  2. Tyrosinemia
  3. Wilson's disease
  4. Glycogen storage disease
  5. Familial hypercholesterolemia
  6. Familial hyperoxaluria type 1

King's criteria in acute liver failure for acetaminophen toxicity:

- Acidosis (pH < 7.3) or,
- PT INR > 6.5, creatinine > 3.4 mg/dL

For other causes of acute liver failure:

PT INR > 6.5

Or,

Any three of the following:

- Age < 10 years or >40 years
- Non-A non-B hepatitis or drug-induced liver disease
- Duration of jaundice before encephalopathy >7 days
- INR > 3.5
- Bilirubin 17.5 mg/dL

Contraindications

A. Absolute contraindications:
   a. Acute on controllable sepsis
   b. Alcohol or active substance abuse
   c. Advanced cardiovascular disease
   d. AIDS
   e. Cholangiocarcinoma
   f. Uncontrollable life-limiting congenital anomalies
   g. Uncontrollable extrabiliary infection
   h. Extrahepatobiliary malignancy
   i. Life-threatening systemic diseases
B. Relative contraindications:
   a. Age > 70 years
   b. Severe malnutrition with wasting
   c. Portal vein thrombosis
   d. Severe morbid obesity
   e. Renal failure attributable to liver disease
   f. Medical noncompliance
   g. Prior extensive hepatobiliary surgery
   h. HIV seropositivity with CD4 count <100/μL
   i. Intractable sepsis
   j. Severe hypoxemia right to left intrapulmonary shunt with PO_2 < 50 mm Hg
   k. Uncontrollable psychiatric disorders

Selection of Cadaver Donor

Donor should be victim of head trauma, brain-dead having age of 60 years in case the patient will fulfill following criteria:

A. Adequate oxygenation
B. Hemodynamic stability
C. Absence of fungal or bacterial infection
D. Absence of hepatic dysfunction
E. Absence of trauma in abdomen
F. Negative for HBV, HCV, and HIV—but liver from HBV or HCV positive donor can be used if the recipient is HBV or HCV positive, respectively. In case of urgent transplantation, liver from donor with antibodies against HBV core antigen can be used but with prophylactic antiviral treatment.

ABO compatible with organ size between donor and recipient should be matched but in urgency ABO incompatible and split liver can be used. Whole liver graft from the donor can be split into three segments:

A. Left lateral segment in case pediatric donor
B. Right extended segment in case of adult donor
C. Right and left segment for 2 adult donor

This procedure is known as split liver transplant.

Tissue typing for HLA matching is not required. After perfusion of the organ with cold electrolyte solution the liver will be packed in ice, reasonable cold ischemic time is 12 hours. Recipient with severe disease will get highest priority, but priority has to be balanced with the posttransplant outcome.

Recently, MELD score has been used as:

A. It decreases waiting list mortality.
B. It reduces waiting time.
C. It will predict posttransplant mortality.
D. It satisfies that medical need should be decisive determinant.

The MELD score of <15 is associated with higher posttransplant mortality. But in few cases disease-specific MELD exceptions are there; these are:

A. Hepatocellular carcinoma
B. Hepatopulmonary syndrome
C. Portopulmonary hypertension
D. Primary hyperoxaluria
E. Cystic fibrosis liver disease
F. Highly selected cases of cholangiocarcinoma
G. Familial amyloid polyneuropathy

Selection of Living Donor

Right lobe of liver from healthy donor can be given to recipient usually but in case of extreme shortage of cadaveric donor left lobe can be transplanted and now more or less one-third of healthy donor transplant is being done from left lobe.

Advantage of Living Donor

A. Reduction of waiting time
B. Reduction of cold ischemic time
C. It can be done as elective procedure.
D. It is life-saving for the recipient.

Disadvantages of Donor

A. Medically disable for at least 10 weeks
B. Biliary complications
C. Wound infection
D. Incisional hernia
E. Small-bowel obstruction
F. Vascular complications

Requisites for the Donor

A. Age should be 10–60 years
B. ABO compatible
C. No chronic medical problems
D. No history of major abdominal surgery

E. Donor should be genetically and emotionally related to the recipient.

F. He must pass extensive series of clinical, biochemical, and serological evaluations.

Immunosuppressive Therapy

A. Cyclosporine, a calcineurin inhibitor by the process of calcium-dependent transduction pathway, blocks the T cells from preventing their action on T-cell receptors leading to inhibition of activation of lymphokine gene as well as block TNF-α, IL-2, IL-3, and IL-4 and other lymphokines. This drug also inhibits the function of B cells without involving the division of rapidly dividing cells in the bone marrow. Side effect is mainly dose-dependent renal tubular injury which can be reversed by reducing the dose. It can also produce nephrotoxicity by direct vasospasm of renal artery. Other side effects are: seizures, tremor, hirsutism, glucose intolerance, gingival hyperplasia, hyperkalemia, and hypertension.

B. Tacrolimus, macrolide lactone antibiotic: Its mechanism of action is same as of cyclosporine but it is 10–100 times more potent. Incidence of acute, chronic, and refractory rejection is less with this drug. Advantages of this drug are:

a. Oral absorption is predictable.
b. Episodes of rejection are minimum.
c. Reduction of need of additional steroid
d. Reduction of incidence of bacterial and cytomegalovirus infection

Side effects are:

a. Neurotoxicity—hallucinations, tremor, seizures, psychoses, and coma
b. Nephrotoxicity
c. Gingival hyperplasia
d. Glucose intolerance
e. Lymphoproliferative disorders

Both the above drugs are metabolized by hepatic cytochrome 450 IIIA systems.

So inducers of the above cytochrome 450, such as phenytoin, carbamazepine, and phenobarbital, reduce the concentration of cyclosporine and tacrolimus.

Drugs that inhibit this enzyme, such as erythromycin, ketoconazole, and clotrimazole, increase the concentration of cyclosporine and tacrolimus.

Due to the overlapping toxicities of cyclosporine and tacrolimus these drugs are not used together.

C. Mycophenolic acid: It is nowadays used as immunosuppressive in case liver transplantation but its side effects are gastrointestinal complaints and suppression of bone marrow.

D. Antithymocyte globulin and monoclonal antibodies to T cells, OKT3, are helpful in reversal of acute rejection in post-transplant period. These drugs are given as intravenous infusion but side effects are fever, chill, myalgia, diarrhea and pulmonary edema, opportunistic infection, and lymphoproliferative disorders.

E. Sirolimus: It will block the T-cell activation, approved in kidney transplantation but now it has been approved in case of liver post-transplant. It can be used in patient with current history of malignancy, like HCC. Side effects are oral ulcers, peripheral edema, hyperlipidemia, and interstitial pneumonitis.

F. Everolimus: It can be used in association with low dose of tacrolimus to protect successfully against acute rejection.

In case of hepatitis C pulse dose of glucocorticoid or OKT3 will accelerate recurrent allograft hepatitis.

Post-transplant Complications

A. Nonhepatic complications:

a. Cardiovascular:
1. Arrhythmias
2. Congestive cardiac failure
3. Cardiomyopathy

b. Infection: Bacterial, fungal, and viral infections

c. Renal:
1. Drug-induced nephrotoxicity
2. Prerenal azotemia

d. Pulmonary:
1. Fluid overload
2. Pneumonia
3. Permeability in the pulmonary capillary

e. Neuropsychiatric:
1. Depression
2. Seizures
3. Metabolic encephalopathy

f. Hematologic:
1. Anemia
2. Hemolytic anemia
3. Thrombocytopenia

g. Malignancy:
    1. Post-transplantation B cell lymphoma
    2. De novo malignancy mainly squamous cell carcinoma

B. Hepatic complications after major surgery:
  a. Prehepatic:
    1. Hemolysis
    2. Collection of blood—hematoma
  b. Intrahepatic:
    1. Hypoperfusion
    2. Benign postoperative cholestasis
    3. Hepatotoxic drugs
    4. Transfusion hepatitis
    5. Aggravation of primary hepatic disease
  c. Posthepatic:
    1. Biliary obstruction
    2. Decreased renal clearance of conjugated bilirubin

C. Hepatic complications unique to transplantation of liver:
  a. Vascular compromise:
    1. Portal vein thrombosis
    2. Hepatic artery thrombosis
    3. Anastomotic leak
  b. Rejection of transplant
  c. Primary disease recurrence
  d. Biliary duct: Bile duct obstruction, stenosis, and biliary leak—it is more frequent with living donor transplantation where there are multiple ducts in the donor.
  e. Small-for-size syndrome: In this liver dysfunction occurred predominantly in living donor liver transplant where the quantity of grafted liver is inadequate to supply the demand required by the recipient. It mainly occurs when the graft to recipient weight ratio is <0.7. Its diagnosis is based on the following parameters:
    1. Persistent bilirubin level > 5.85 mg/dL
    2. INR > 2
    3. Grade 3–4 encephalopathy
    4. Massive ascites in the first week in absence of vasculobiliary, infective, or immunological problem
  f. Post-transplant steatosis: Risk factors are:
    1. Pre- and post-transplant obesity
    2. Alcoholic cirrhosis
    3. Post-transplant diabetes mellitus
    4. Hyperlipidemia
    5. Hypertension
    6. Pretransplant graft steatosis
    7. Administration of tacrolimus
  g. Recurrence of hepatitis B and C
  h. Post-transplant metabolic bone disease

Q34. Endoscopic ultrasonography.

BF/MAY2012/MDIV (10)

Endoscopic ultrasound.

MLB/MAY2009/MDI (20)

ANSWER

Fiberoptic endoscopy was started in 1911, ultrasound in 1956 but in 1980 both facilities were merged to form endoscopic ultrasound (EUS) to visualize the structures near gastrointestinal tract. EUS can be done by either radial or linear view. There are both diagnostic and therapeutic indications of EUS.

Diagnostic Indications

A. Pancreatic disorders:
  a. Pancreatic carcinoma: Pancreatic carcinoma of >2 mm in size can be diagnosed with 90–95% accuracy. EUS associated with fine needle aspiration cytology (FNAC) improves the diagnostic yields. But sensitivity will decline in presence of chronic or acute pancreatitis.
  b. In case of gallstone-induced acute pancreatitis bile duct stones or sludge can be detected by EUS in case of failure with USG or ERCP or MRCP.
  c. Other causes of acute pancreatitis are pancreatic divisum or small pancreatic tumor undetected by CT or MRI.
  d. Pancreatic fluid collection: According to revised Atlanta classification fluid collection are of four types:
    1. Acute peripancreatic fluid collection in case of acute edematous pancreatitis
    2. Pancreatic pseudocyst occurring as a delayed complication of (>4 weeks) interstitial edematous pancreatitis
    3. Collection of acute necrotic fluid in case of necrotizing pancreatitis
    4. Walled-off necrosis having radiologically identifiable capsule (>4 weeks)

Surgical or percutaneous drainage of pancreatic or peripancreatic fluid is done. Disadvantages:

1. Longer hospital stay
2. High cost
3. Increased morbidity
4. Discomfort of external catheters

Complications of drainage:

1. Bleeding
2. Perforation
3. Infection

e. Chronic pancreatitis: Technological advances in EUS, such as contrast-enhanced harmonics and elastography, improve the diagnostic accuracy.

f. Pancreatic cystic neoplasm: Differentiation between benign and malignant nonmucinous cyst can be done by EUS-associated FNAC.

B. Gallbladder and other biliary disorders:

a. Choledocholithiasis: Sensitivity of EUS in diagnosing CBD stone is very high as compared to other modalities of investigation.

b. Obstructive jaundice: It may be due to benign or malignant causes. Due to its close proximity to stomach and duodenum EUS is the method of choice for diagnosing it. In case of malignant lesion FNAC also has to be done. Again biliary drainage can also be done through EUS. Complications are perforation and biliary leak.

c. Cholecystitis: In case of calculus or acalculous cholecystitis in patients with high surgical risk percutaneous cholecystostomy can be done by EUS to decompress the gallbladder.

C. Gastrointestinal tract lesions:

a. Esophagus:

1. Submucosal esophagogastric tumor
2. FNAC in case of subepithelial esophagogastric solid lesion
3. Staging of malignant tumor
4. High-grade malignant esophageal stricture

b. Stomach:

1. In case of linitis plastica marked thickening of gastric wall can be visualized by EUS if required FNAC.
2. Gastrointestinal stromal tumor in stomach can be diagnosed by EUS-guided FNAC.
3. It can distinguish benign lesions, such as pancreatic rest, leiomyoma, and granular cell tumor, and neuroendocrine tumor, schwannoma from malignant lesions, such as primary and secondary tumors.

c. Retroperitoneal masses: In case of intra-abdominal masses EUS-guided FNAC for accurate diagnosis. Other retroperitoneal masses, such as adrenal metastases, paraganglioma, and leiomyosarcoma can also be diagnosed by EUS.

D. Mediastinal adenopathy and nonsmall cell cancer:

a. Posterior and inferior mediastinal lesions can be diagnosed by EUS-guided FNAC for histological diagnosis.

b. Staging of lung cancer

c. It can evaluate metastasis involving adrenal glands.

E. Colonic lesion: FNAC-based diagnosis, staging of colorectal cancer along with glandular staging can be done by EUS.

Injection: Injection of alcohol and phenol (neurolysis) can be given in celiac plexus in case of chronic pancreatitis or pancreatic cancer.

Tattooing: Administration of carbon particle into the pancreatic lesion can be performed by EUS-guided tattooing.

Alcohol ablation: Alcohol can be injected into pancreatic lesion, metastases, and neuroendocrine tumors through EUS guidance in case of surgically unfit patient.

Radiotherapy: 3–5 mm radiopaque metal marker, Fiducials, can be placed into the tumor under EUS guidance by 19-gauge FNA needle as external beam radiation therapy.

Endoscopic ultrasound can act as guide for injection of seeds for brachytherapy.

Chemotherapy: Chemotherapeutic agents, paclitaxel along with alcohol ablation, can be given in case of pancreatic neoplasm or cyst or esophageal cancer.

Photodynamic therapy: Photosensitizing drugs can be given under EUS guidance.

Surgery: Natural orifice transluminal endoscopic surgery (NOTES) can be done through EUS guidance.

Vascular access:

A. Angiography:

a. Under EUS celiac branches of hepatic vein can be accessed.

b. In case of portal hypertension portal venous pressure can be measured through EUS.

B. Control of bleeding: This EUS can be used to control following bleeding:
  - **a.** Variceal bleeding
  - **b.** Portosystemic shunt
  - **c.** Arterial embolization
  - **d.** Application of coil
  - **e.** Control of pseudoaneurysm

C. 3D reconstruction: Three-dimensional ultrasound is done in case of gynecological cases.

Molecular marker analysis: Specimen can be obtained by EUS-guided FNAC for DNA analysis and microdissection-based genotyping.

Endoscopic ultrasound-guided transgastric ERCP can be done in patient with Roux-en-Y gastric bypass.

> **Q35. What liver function tests are affected in acute and chronic liver disease? Give an account of causes.**
>
> **Clinical features, complications and management of fatty liver.**
>
> **MLB/MAY2009/MDI (20)**

ANSWER

Acute Viral Hepatitis

A. Rise in transaminases to a variable degree: It may precede the rise of bilirubin, then it is called as anicteric hepatitis. Transaminases may rise to 400–4,000 IU/L and gradually diminishes progressively during the period of recovery. But it does not correlate with the severity of liver damage.

B. Patient can be diagnosed as icteric when serum bilirubin level will rise >2.5 mg/dL. It may rise up to 20 mg/dL in case of severe disease. Total bilirubin is divided into direct or conjugated and indirect or unconjugated bilirubin. In early phase of hepatitis direct component will be more than the indirect component. But if the patient suffers from underlying hemolytic anemia, in that case rise in bilirubin >30 mg/dL is not associated with poor prognosis because this level is due to superimposed hemolysis.

C. Alkaline phosphatase is raised in early phase of acute hepatitis.

Chronic Viral Hepatitis

A. Serum bilirubin level will be near normal or mildly raised depending upon the degree of decompensation.

B. Serum aminotransferases will be within normal limit.

C. Serum albumin level will be low or low normal depending upon the loss of synthetic capacity of liver. Globulin level will be gradually increased with ratio of albumin to globulin will be reversed.

Alcoholic Hepatitis

A. Serum aminotransferases—ALT and AST. AST will be increased up to seven-fold and greater than AST. AST level will be increased up to several fold. ALT:AST ratio will be >2.

B. Serum bilirubin will be markedly increased despite only modest elevation of ALP.

C. In case of advanced liver injury albumin level will be decreased.

Drug-induced Hepatitis

A. Aminotransferases are raised.

B. Ratio of ALT to ALP:
  - **a.** R value if >5—hepatocellular injury
  - **b.** R vale if <2—cholestatic injury
  - **c.** If R value between 2 and 5—hepatocellular-cholestatic injury

Fatty liver disease has been discussed in Q17.

> **Q36. Microscopic structure of liver.**
>
> **MGR/OCT2012/MDI (5)**
>
> **Hepatic lobular structure and function. Etiopathogenesis of chronic liver disease.**
>
> **SCB MED COL, 2021, (20)**
>
> **Discuss the microanatomy of liver and the histological changes in cirrhosis of liver.**
>
> **WBUHS, 2024 (10)**
>
> **Discuss the microanatomy of liver and the histological changes in cirrhosis of liver.**
>
> **WBUHS, 2024 (10)**

Histology of liver in cirrhosis has been described in question number 39.

Etiopathogenesis and histopathological changes of cirrhosis described in question number 38.

ANSWER

Microscopic structure consists of the following:

A. Acinus: It contains:

- **a.** Portal tract at the center
- **b.** At the periphery terminal hepatic venules.

This structural unit has been divided into three zones:

- **a.** Zone 1: It is present adjacent to limiting lamellae. It has highest supply of substrates and oxygen.
- **b.** Zone 2: This intermediate zone has less blood supply, and has no functional boundaries. This zone has two imaginary halves that can be added to zone 3 and 1.
- **c.** Zone 3: This zone is present nearer to center and it has very low blood supply and thus it has least regenerative capacity.

B. Hepatic lobule:

- **a.** Portal vein lobule: Main characteristic of it is the glandular character of the liver. Here the flow direction is centrifugal—blood flows from the center toward periphery but biliary flow is just the reverse, i.e., centripetal—bile flows from periphery toward center.
- **b.** Central vein lobule: This is hexagonal structure having portal tract at the corners. It contains 15–25 hepatocytes arranged radially and placed in between limiting lamellae as well as central vein. In between the plates there are hollow spaces called space of disk and sinusoids.

C. Portal tract: It originates at the hilum and passes in branching pattern. Structures within the portal tract are the following:

- **a.** Bile duct
- **b.** Bile ductules
- **c.** Portal vein
- **d.** Hepatic artery
- **e.** Lymphatic nerves
- **f.** Nerve fibers
- **g.** Inflammatory cells
- **h.** Supporting connective tissue consisting of type 1 collagen

D. Hepatocytes: These are polygonal cells having six or more faces. Life span of hepatocyte is 150–200 days and these cells as oncocytes. Contoured cell membrane of hepatocyte has been divided according to morphological and functional cellular polarization into three compartments:

- **a.** 37% of external area of cell membrane of hepatocyte is sinusoidal surface having numerous microvilli which increase the absorptive and secretary function of these cells.
- **b.** 12% of outer membrane consists of canalicular surface—it is secretary pole of the cell.
- **c.** 50% of external membrane consists of smooth intercellular fissure which is connected with disk space. This fissure is separated from canaliculi by tight junctions—zonula occludens.

E. Sinusoidal lining cells: Through the sinusoids blood flows from portal tract to hepatic venules. Sinusoids are lined by Kupffer cells and endothelial cells. Kupffer cells are irregular with cytoplasmic extension, belong to macrophage phagocytic system. Endothelial cells are fenestrated plate-like cells which allow easy exchange between hepatocyte and blood. There are liver-associated lymphocytes present in the sinusoidal lining. These lymphocytes are in contact with Kupffer cells and endothelial cells, they are also present in the space of disc, and these have NK cell phenotype.

F. Space of disk: This is the space present in between endothelial cells and hepatocytes; it contains micro-environment for exchange between hepatocytes and blood. This space contains:

- **a.** Plasma
- **b.** Type 3 connective tissue which forms reticulin frame work
- **c.** Hepatic stellate cells called Ito cells: These belong to myofibroblast which is closely related to small nerve endings. It controls blood flow through the sinusoids, and controls fibrogenesis and stores vitamins.

G. Vasculatures: Hepatic artery terminates as terminal hepatic arteriole and plexuses in the smallest tract around portal vein and bile duct. Portal vein terminates into portal venules, now both portal and arterial blood flows through the sinusoids into terminal hepatic venules which combine to form segmental veins and to lobar hepatic veins which ultimately drain the blood to inferior vena cava. Lymph forms in the space of Disse and drain into portal lymphatic vessels.

H. Bile duct and ductules: These are lined by cuboidal to columnar epithelium, they anastomose to form larger bile duct and exit at the hilum.

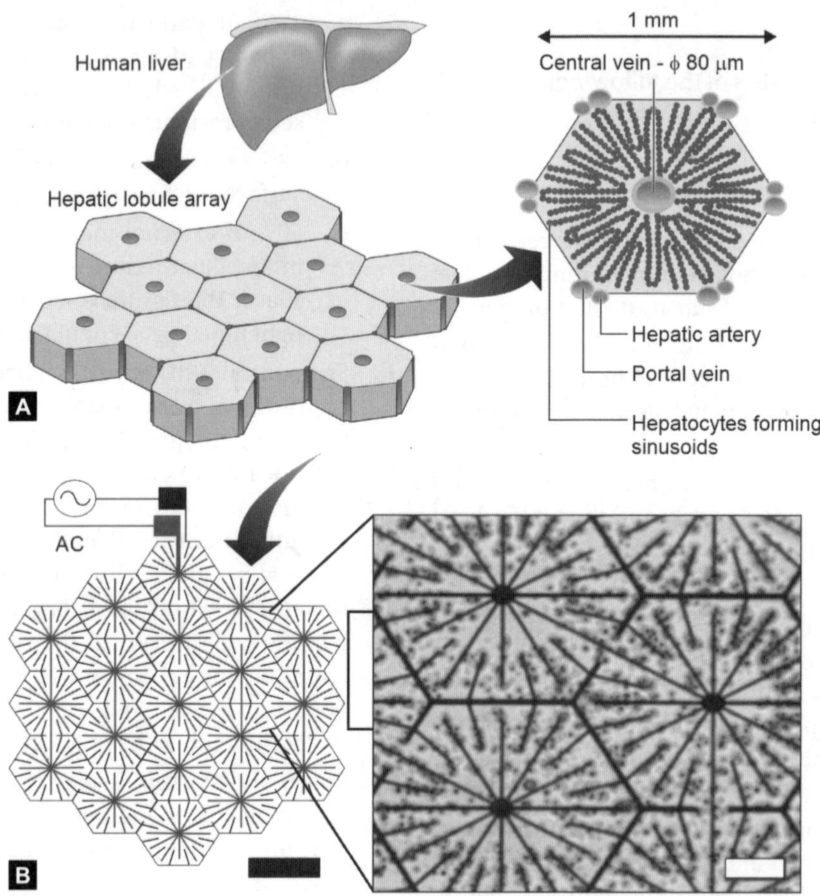

Histology of Liver in Cirrhosis

A. Hepatic fibrosis:

- **a.** Bridging of the portal tract with the other adjacent portal tracts—Portal to portal tract bridging
- **b.** Bridging of the portal tract with central veins—portal to central bridging.
- **c.** Disruption of the normal hepatic lobular architecture.
- **d.** Fibrous septa contains blood vessels, bile ductules and the chronic inflammatory cells like lymphocytes, macrophages and plasma cells.

B. Regeneration of the nodules:

- **a.** Within the fibrous septa there is proliferation of the hepatocytes.
- **b.** Regenerative nodules are surrounded by the fibrous septa not containing portal triads as well as central veins.
- **c.** There is loss of vascular architecture leading to hepatic dysfunction.

C. There is loss of normal hepatic lobular architecture leading to portal hypertension.

D. In case of biliary cirrhosis there is proliferation of the bile ductules.

Q37. Development of spleen.

MGR/OCT2014/MDI (5)

Spleen.

MGR/SEP2008/MDI (5)

Tropical splenomegaly.

MGR/SEP2010/MDII (6)

MGR/APR2014/MDIII (7)

ANSWER

Introduction

It is a shoe-shaped reddish purple colored organ present in the left hypochondrium in relation to 9th to 11th ribs between fundus of the stomach and left dome of diaphragm.

Development

In the sixth week of intrauterine life from cephalic part of dorsal layer of mesogastrium a number of nodules arise which fuse ultimately to form lobulated spleen. Its notch in the upper border of spleen proves its multiple origin.

Gross Anatomy

It has two ends:

A. Anterior end: It expands forward and downward like border to reach left midaxillary line.

B. Posterior end: This rounded end extends upward and backward to rest on upper pole of left kidney.

It has three borders:

A. Superior border: It is notched at its anterior end.

B. Inferior border: It is rounded.

C. Intermediate border: It is directed toward right.

It has two surfaces:

A. Diaphragmatic surface: It is smooth rounded, convex

B. Visceral surface: It is concave having impressions:

- **a.** Largest concave gastric impression: It is for fundus of the stomach.
- **b.** Renal impression: It is for left kidney present in between intermediate and inferior border of spleen.
- **c.** Colonic impression: It is for splenic flexure of colon, from this flexure phrenocolic ligament it extends like a horizontal fold and forms upper end of paracolic gutter.
- **d.** Pancreatic impression: It is for the tail of the pancreas present in between hilum and colic impression.

Hilum: It is present on the inferomedial part of gastric impression. Here following structures are present:

A. Splenic artery

B. Splenic vein

C. Nerves

D. Attachment of two ligaments:

- **a.** Lienorenal ligament extending from the hilum to anterior surface of left kidney.
- **b.** Gastrosplenic ligament extending from spleen to the greater curvature of stomach.

Vascular supply: Splenic artery after arising from celiac trunk enters the spleen through lienorenal ligament and divides into different straight branches, such as penicillin, ellipsoids, and arterial capillaries. Splenic circulation is adapted to separate and store RBCs. It has two vascular segments—superior and inferior segments separated by avascular plane. Other branches of splenic artery are 5–7 short gastric arteries and left gastroepiploic artery.

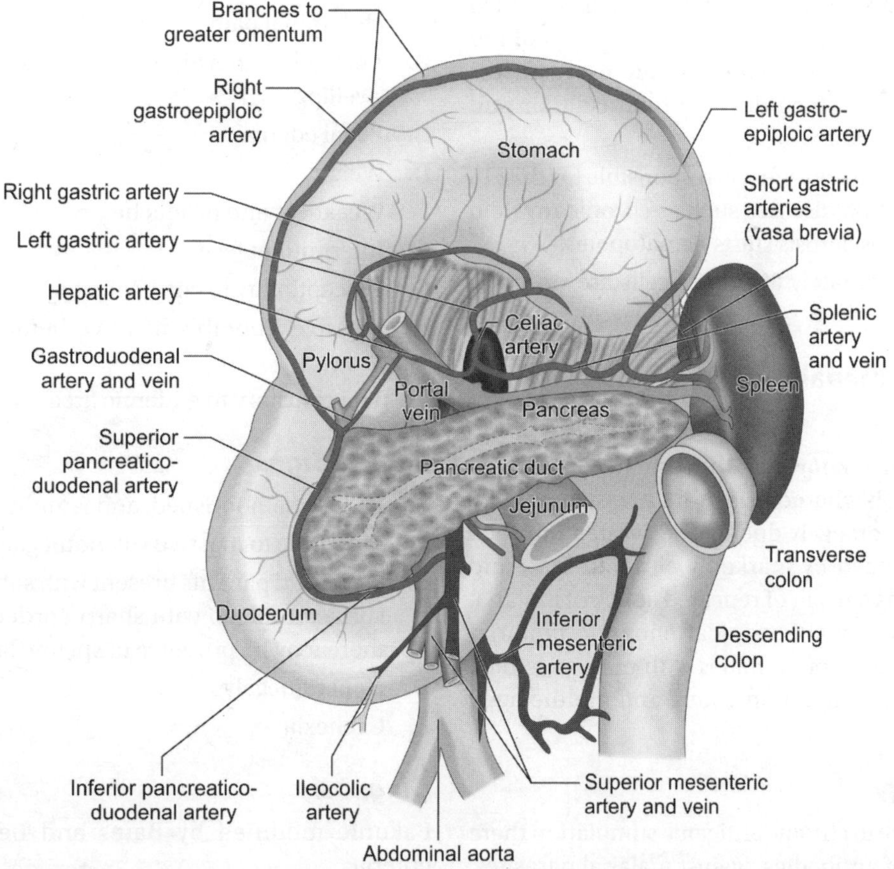

Venous drainage: Splenic vein runs behind the pancreas to join superior mesenteric vein to form portal vein behind the neck of the pancreas. Its tributaries are:

A. Short gastric vein
B. Inferior mesenteric vein
C. Pancreatic vein
D. Gastro-omental vein

Nerve supply: Sympathetic fibers arise from celiac plexus.

Microanatomy: It has three compartments:

A. White pulp: It is formed by lymphatic nodules and formed around the Malpighian corpuscle.
B. Red pulp: It is formed by collection of lymphocytes, blood cells, and fixed and free macrophages present in between the sinusoids. These lymphocytes ultimately transform into plasma cells and immunoglobulin.
C. Supporting tissue: It is fibroblastic tissue and forms coarse trabeculae, capsule, and reticulum.

Functions of Spleen

A. In response to antigen in the body it produces both humoral response leading to antibody production and cellular immunity leading to lymphopoiesis.
B. Phagocytosis: Reticuloendothelial systems of spleen consists of phagocytes such as reticular cells, modified reticular cells of ellipsoids, and macrophages of red pulp. They phagocytize red cells, micro-organisms releasing antigen which develop both cellular and cellular immunity.
C. Hematopoiesis: In fetal life it is responsible for this. In adult life in certain diseases such as chronic myeloid leukemia, myelosclerosis starts hematopoiesis.
D. Storage: Approximately 8% of red cells are stored in spleen.

Tropical Splenomegaly

Introduction

This condition is also known as "hyperreactive malarial syndrome" which is characterized by massive splenic enlargement, hepatomegaly due to exaggerated immune response as evidenced by markedly elevated IgM, and malarial antibody as a result of repeated attack of malaria. It is more common in the tropical endemic malarial region. It is more common in males with male to female ratio 2:1. It is more common in young and middle aged adults.

Pathophysiology

In endemic area due to chronic antigenic stimulation there will be high level of antibodies against malarial parasites. These antigens stimulate polyclonal B lymphocytes leading to excessive and uncontrolled production of IgM, which being polyclonal is not specific for any particular malarial parasite. Other factors are responsible for development of tropical splenomegaly. Patient with sickle cell trait is relatively protective from malaria. But patient with sickle cell disease if develops splenomegaly will be functionally asplenic and not get any benefit from expansion of marginal B cell as well as macrophages in enlarged spleen. Malarial parasitemia by unknown mechanism is responsible for defective immunoregulatory control of B lymphocytes by cytotoxic T cells or suppressor cells, as a result there is uncontrolled proliferation of B lymphocytes along with infiltration of T cell in hepatic and splenic sinusoids. So, serum cryoglobulin, antibody, and immune-complexes levels will be high. The results will be:

A. Anemia
B. Deposition of immune complexes in the Kupffer cells in liver and spleen is high.
C. Hyperplasia of reticuloendothelial cells
D. Increase in plasma level of IL-10 and IFN-gamma
E. Hepatosplenomegaly

Clinical Symptoms

A. Chronic abdominal swelling—wax and wanes, abdominal pain
B. Abdominal hernia due to pressure by abdominal swelling
C. Pedal edema
D. Weight
E. Weakness and headache
F. Intermittent fever
G. Susceptibility to chest infections
H. Massive Coomb's positive hemolysis preceded by fever
I. Travel history to endemic area

Clinical Signs

A. Pallor, malnourished, and jaundice
B. Moderate to massive splenomegaly
C. One-third patients present with soft, tender smoothed surfaced spleen with sharp border. On auscultation, there may be presence of splenic bruit.
D. Hepatomegaly
E. Cachexia

Diagnosis

Fakunle modified by Bates and Bedu-Addo refined criteria:

A. Major criteria:
- **a.** Gross splenomegaly 10 cm or more below the costal margin in adult for which no other cause found
- **b.** Elevated serum IgM level 2 standard deviations or more above the local mean
- **c.** Clinical as well as immunological response to antimalarial therapy
- **d.** 40% reduction in splenomegaly by 6 months after start of therapy
- **e.** High level of antibodies to plasmodium species

B. Minor criteria:
- **a.** Hepatic sinusoidal lymphocytosis
- **b.** Hypersplenism
- **c.** Normal cellular and humoral response
- **d.** Lymphocytic proliferation
- **e.** Familial occurrence

Hematological manifestations:
- **a.** Normochromic normocytic anemia
- **b.** Increased reticulocyte count reflecting erythroid hyperplasia
- **c.** Leukopenia with lymphocytosis
- **d.** Thrombocytopenia

  Thrombocytopenia and leukopenia may be due to trapping by spleen.
- **e.** No malarial parasite in peripheral blood smear

Other tests:
- **a.** High titer of antimalarial antibodies
- **b.** Titer of rheumatoid factor, cold agglutinin, cryoprotein, ANA may be raised but C3 may be reduced.
- **c.** Detection of parasitemia is not the criterion for diagnosis.
- **d.** Detection of parasitic nucleic acid by PCR is more sensitive than direct microscopy.
- **e.** Antibody detection by ELISA (enzyme-linked immunosorbent assays) or by IFA (immunofluorescence assays)
- **f.** Phytohemagglutination test can differentiate tropical splenomegaly from chronic myeloid leukemia (CML) and lymphoma.

Treatment

Antimalarial treatment is the corner stone of this disease but selection of drugs depends upon the resistance of drugs in that endemic area and treatment has to be continued regularly for months to years. Response can be detected with months of treatment but discontinuation will relapse the disease.

This drug will clear the antigenic stimulus helps to return the immune system to normal. Weekly chloroquine or daily proguanil may be affective. Pyrimethamine may be an alternative drug.

Effective antimalarial treatment or chemoprophylaxis is associated with:

A. Reduction in the splenic size

B. Correction of anemia and lymphocytosis

C. Decrease in serum level of IgM

Q38. Portal hypertension.

MGR/APR2014/MDI (5)

Discuss portal hypertension and management of its complications.

MUHS/NOV2013/MDIII (25)

Bleeding from esophageal varices.

SNMC/MAY2013/MDIV (15)

Portal hypertension evaluation.

SCB MED COL, 2019 (20)

Management of portal hypertension.

MGR UNI, TAMIL NADU, 2021 (10)

Discuss classification and pathogenesis of portal hypertension. Describe medical management of bleeding esophageal varices.

MGU, 2024 (20)

Describe Porto-systemic anastomosis and write the management of portal-hypertensive bleed.

MANIPUR UNIVERSITY, 2019 (10)

ANSWER

Definition of Portal Hypertension

Normal portal venous pressure is 5–10 mm Hg and it should not be >5 mm Hg than the pressure in inferior vena cava or hepatic vein.

Difference of pressure between hepatic vein and portal vein as measured by HVPG > 6 mm Hg is known as portal hypertension if it is >10 mm Hg it is associated with increased risk of complications.

It can be measured from the following formula:

Hepatic venous pressure gradient (HVPG) = Wedged hepatic venous pressure (WHVP) – Free hepatic venous pressure (FHVP)

Sites of Portosystemic Anastomosis

Collateral circulation: There are four main groups of collaterals where portal systems anastomose with systemic veins.

A. Group 1: Here protective epithelium joins absorptive epithelium through following methods:

- **a.** At the cardiac end of stomach:
  - **1.** Portal system consisting of:
    - Short gastric vein
    - Posterior gastric vein
    - Left gastric veins
  - **2.** Systemic veins consisting of:
    - Intercostal veins
    - Azygos minor veins
    - Diaphragmatic esophageal veins

  Result: Varicose veins develop in the submucosal layer at the lower end of esophagus and fundus.
- **b.** At the site of anus:
  - **1.** Portal system consists of superior hemorrhoidal vein.
  - **2.** Systemic system consists of middle and inferior hemorrhoidal veins.

  Results: Development of rectal varices.

B. Group 2: Paraumbilical veins in the falciparum ligament with the relics of umbilical veins in fetal life.

C. Group 3: Here collateral circulation will be developed where abdominal organs are in contact with retroperitoneal tissues:

- **a.** Collateral veins run from liver to diaphragm
- **b.** In the lienorenal ligament and omentum, the involved veins are:
  - **1.** Lumbar veins
  - **2.** Veins in the scar of previous operations
  - **3.** Veins of small or large bowel stomas

In women especially there are communications between ovarian and iliac veins.

D. Group 4:

- **a.** Portal blood from:
  - Splenic vein
  - Diaphragmatic vein
  - Pancreatic vein
  - Gastric vein
- **b.** Systemic collateral from left renal vein.

Classification of Portal Hypertension

A. Presinusoidal:

- **a.** Extrahepatic causes:
  - **1.** Portal vein:
    - Thrombosis
    - Invasion of portal vein
    - Compression by the tumor
  - **2.** Splenic vein:
    - Thrombosis
    - Invasion of portal vein
    - Compression by the tumor
  - **3.** Increased blood flow:
    - Tropical splenomegaly syndrome
    - Arteriovenous fistula
    - Idiopathic
- **b.** Intrahepatic causes:
  - **1.** Involvement of portal vein:
    - Early primary biliary cirrhosis
    - Schistosomiasis
    - Chronic active hepatitis
    - Congenital hepatic fibrosis
    - Sarcoidosis
    - Idiopathic portal hypertension
    - Toxins—vinyl chloride, copper, and arsenic

B. Hepatic causes:

- **a.** Sinusoidal:
  - **1.** Cirrhosis
  - **2.** Noncirrhotic portal fibrosis
  - **3.** Acute alcoholic hepatitis
  - **4.** Cytotoxic drugs
  - **5.** Intoxication with vitamin A
- **b.** Postsinusoidal:
  - **1.** Veno-occlusive disease
  - **2.** Alcoholic central hyaline necrosis

C. Posthepatic causes:

- **a.** Hepatic veins:
  - **1.** Thrombosis
  - **2.** Web
  - **3.** Tumor
  - **4.** Invasion
- **b.** Inferior vena cava:
  - **1.** Web
  - **2.** Tumor
  - **3.** Thrombosis
  - **4.** Invasion
- **c.** Heart: Constrictive pericarditis

Pathophysiology of Portal Hypertension

Vascular bed plays main pathogenic role in the development of portal hypertension which includes:

A. Intrahepatic circulation: Changes in this is the main impetus in the development of portal hypertension.

B. Splanchnic circulation: It allows greater blood flow in the portal circulation.

C. Portosystemic collateral circulation: As the portal pressure increases the expansion of collateral circulation can decompress the portal pressure at the expense of a number of complications.

Increased Hepatic Vascular Resistance

There are two components:

A. Structural component: Mechanical obstruction due to external compression by regenerative hepatic nodules and distorted architecture of liver due to collagen deposition leading to fibrosis, constriction of sinusoids, and altered sinusoidal structure all of which are irreversible component.

B. Dynamic component: It is reversible component. It is caused by contraction of vascular smooth muscle cell.

In case of cirrhosis there is profound endothelial dysfunction both in systemic and intrahepatic vessels resulting intrahepatic vasoconstriction and it is mediated by following mechanisms:

A. Decreased activity of endothelial nitric oxide synthetase activity (eNOS) and decreased nitric oxide production. Activity of hepatic eNOS is decreased due to impairment of Akt-mediated eNOS phosphorylation (it can be reversible by statins) and increased expression of cavolin especially in case of folate deficiency.

B. Decreased availability of nitric oxide as it is utilized for nitrosylation reactions due to oxidative stress.

C. Endothelins are a group of vasoconstrictors binds to following two different types of receptor:

  a. ET_A presents on the vascular smooth muscle cells and is responsible for vasoconstriction.

  b. ET_B presents on the endothelial cells and is responsible for release of nitric oxide which leads to vasodilatation.

  Endothelin also binds to hepatic stellate cells leading to contraction and increase in pressure in hepatic microcirculation.

D. Angiotensinogen

E. Eicosanoids

Hepatic stellate cell interspersed within hepatic sinusoids become activated in response to hepatic injury which is characterized by proliferation, migration, and capacity of collagen deposition. Structure and functions of sinusoidal cells will be changed to act as effector cells for sinusoidal endothelial cells-derived molecules.

Peribiliary fibroblast also activates to myofibroblast and acts as hepatic stellate cells. According to one theory epithelial cells transactivate into myofibroblast through the process of epithelial-mesenchymal transactivation.

As a result pool of effector contractile cells will be increased.

In the cirrhotic liver due to reduction of portal blood flow there is compensatory increase in blood flow through hepatic artery with the aim of maintaining the consistency of hepatic blood flow. This can theoretically increase the intrahepatic resistance leading to portal hypertension.

Other vascular changes in cirrhotic liver are:

A. Remodeling of vasculature of sinusoids induces increased mass effect of hepatic stellate cells around endothelial cell tube.

B. Angiogenesis of endothelial cells.

  a. Thus these cells dedifferentiate with loss of fenestrae and development of basement membrane—called "capillarization."

  b. Presence of "scar vessels" that run through the scar and supply metabolic as well as oxygen needs for progress of the scar. This is intimately linked to fibrotic process.

Increased Splanchnic Blood Producing Hyperdynamic Circulatory State

In cirrhosis it acts as propagator of portal hypertension which is triggered by increased intrahepatic vascular resistance and it is associated with significant portal hypertension. Again in cirrhosis total blood flow through portal venous system is not equal to total blood entering into the liver because due to increase portal pressure will divert a significant amount of blood into portosystemic collaterals.

Due to resistance in the portal circulation hepatic blood flow will decline but it is partially maintained by hepatic arterial flow. Again, due to increased portal pressure large amount of blood will be diverted into portosystemic collaterals decreasing vascular resistance in the splanchnic vessels which leads to development of hyperdynamic circulation which in turn portal pressure further in spite of opened collaterals. So increasing amount of portal blood enters into collaterals and the hepatocytes will be deprived of portal blood leading to acceleration of liver disease. This hyperdynamic circulation is also responsible for portopulmonary, hepatorenal syndrome, cardiomyopathy, and ascites. This hyperdynamic circulatory state is produced by nitric oxide overproduction due to VEGF and hemodynamic force-induced mechanical stress.

Portosystemic Collaterals

It is seen and will increase in association with the rise in portal pressure and associated with significant morbidity and mortality. But these collaterals will try to minimize the rate of rise in pressure. These collaterals are formed by following distinct and inter-related processes:

A. Vasodilatation of existing collateral vessels

B. Remodeling of existing vessels

C. Angiogenesis

Above processes are being controlled by following factors:

A. Changes in the level of VEGF

B. Mechanical factors related to increased portal pressure

Varix formation and its rupture: As a result of increased portal venous pressure nearly 90% of portal blood will be diverted into portosystemic collaterals and back to heart leading to flow-mediated remodeling vessel enlargement catalyzed by VEGF, platelet-derived growth factor (PDGF), and NO-driven VEGF type II receptor. These vessels are commonly present in gastroesophageal junction producing esophageal and gastric varices. Development of varix depends upon following factors:

A. Size of the varix: Once the varices develop its rate of progression increases 5–10% every year with rapid worsening of liver disease and with continued alcohol abuse. Small varix bleeds 7% in 2 year whereas, large varix 30% in 2 years.

B. Thickness of vessel wall

C. Pressure gradient between variceal and esophageal limen

D. Wall tension: When it will exceed the variceal wall elastic limit it ruptures.

Normal HVPG is 3–5 mm Hg. When HVPG is ≥10 mm Hg varices will form and it is the transition from compensated to decompensated state and when it is >12 mm Hg it may rupture and if it is >20 mm Hg there will be continued bleeding resistant to medical therapy. Variceal wall tension can be defined by Frank's modification of Laplace's law.

E. Variceal blood flow: It is driven by the portal hypertension.

Most superficial varices are present at gastroesophageal junction hence the wall will be thinnest and is liable to invariable rupture.

Varices

A. Esophageal varices: Combination of low platelet count, spleen diameter, and liver stiffness as measured by fibroscan can identify which patient will develop large varices. It occurs in 30–40% compensated cirrhotic patients and 60% patients with ascites. Bleeding stops spontaneously because resultant hypovolemia produces splanchnic vasoconstriction and lowering of portal pressure. In 80–90% patients medical and endoscopic therapies reduce bleeding but failure of controlling bleed occurs due to following:

a. HPVG is >20 mm Hg

b. Active bleeding at endoscopy

c. Infection

d. Advanced Child–Pugh score

e. Portal venous thrombosis complicating cirrhosis

Blood supply of esophageal varices:

A. Anterior branch drains into azygos vein

B. Posterior branch communicates with the varices below the esophageal junction.

Rebleeding occurs in one-third patients within 6 weeks after initial bleed. The factors responsible are:

a. HPVG is >20 mm Hg

b. Renal insufficiency

c. Active bleeding from gastric varices

d. MELD score of >18

Gradation of esophageal varices:

a. Grade 1: Varices extend just above the mucosal level.

b. Grade 2: Varices project by one-third of luminal diameter that cannot be compressed with air insufflation.

c. Grade 3: Varices project up to 50% of luminal diameter and are in contact with each other.

B. Gastric varices: These are of four types according to SARIN classification:

a. Type 1 isolated gastric varix: This is present in gastric fundus and will never extend to esophagus or cardia

b. Type 2 isolated gastric varix: It is ectopic gastric varix present in the other part of stomach.

c. Type 1 gastroesophageal varices: These will extend over the cardia and lesser curvature of the stomach ultimately end in gastric fundus.

d. Type 2 gastroesophageal varices: These will extend ahead of cardia toward greater curvature of stomach and ultimately ends in cardia. Bleeding is more common in these varices.

These are supplied by short gastric veins draining into deep intrinsic veins in the esophageal mucosa.

C. Ectopic varices:

a. Duodenal varices

b. Anorectal varices

c. Rectal varices: These are developed in association with splanchnic thrombosis.

d. Peristomal varices are seen in the patient with IBD or progressive sclerosing cholangitis and undergone proctocolectomy.

Diagnosis of Portal Hypertension

A. Bleeding from esophageal or gastric varices: Hematemesis, melena, or hematochezia

B. Ectopic varices present with melena and hematochezia.

C. Patient may present with features of chronic liver disease or in some case there may not be any feature of liver disease. But other causes of bleeding have to be ruled out such as Mallory Weiss tear, ulcer disease.

D. Presence of splenomegaly—suggests portal hypertension

E. Caput medusa—suggest patent umbilical vein hence pointing toward intrahepatic portal hypertension.

F. Bruit:

a. It may be heard in left upper quadrant of abdomen indicating splenic arteriovenous fistula.

b. It may be heard over the liver—in patient with hereditary hemorrhagic telangiectasia.

G. Venous hum:

a. It is usually heard xiphoid process and/or umbilicus.

b. Venous hum can be heard over the collaterals like inferior mesenteric vein.

H. Arterial murmur—alcoholic cirrhosis, primary liver cancer

I. Palpation of liver:

a. Soft liver—extrahepatic portal hypertension

b. Firm liver—cirrhosis

c. Nodularity:

1. Micronodular—alcohol-related

2. Macronodular—viral

d. May not be palpable.

J. Rectum: For detection of rectal varices in 44% of patients.

K. Ascites: In case of cirrhosis it indicates portal hypertension.

L. Laboratory features of portal hypertension:

a. Thrombocytopenia

b. Hypoalbuminemia

c. Hyperbilirubinemia

d. Prolongation of PT

M. X-ray chest:

a. Enlarged azygos vein due to collaterals around azygos vein

b. Widened paravertebral shadow—due to dilated hemiazygos vein

c. Massive dilatation of paraesophageal collaterals produces a shadow of retrocardiac posterior mediastinal mass.

N. Abdominal imaging: Confirm—

a. Splenomegaly

b. Abnormal configuration of liver suggestive of cirrhosis

c. Obstruction of portal venous system

d. Presence of venous collaterals

O. Upper gastrointestinal endoscopy:

Appearance of esophageal varices:

a. Varices are white and opaque

b. Red color due to blood flow through subepithelial or communicating veins—it occurs in large varices.

c. Cherry-red spot and red wheal markings on the top of varices—due to dilated subepithelial veins

d. Hemocystic spots: It is 4 mm in diameter due to flow of blood from deep intrinsic veins directly straight outward through communicating veins to subepithelial veins.

Appearance of gastric varices:

a. It is seen in the fundus of the stomach as worms along the gastric folds.

b. It is looking like lobulated mass in the fundus.

Appearance of portal hypertensive gastropathy (PHG):

a. It usually occurs in antrum or fundus or involve throughout the stomach mucosa.

b. Description of lesions:

1. Small polygonal reddish areas surrounded by whitish yellow depressed border

2. Red point lesion
3. Cherry-red spot
4. Black-brown spot—due to intramucosal hemorrhage

P. Endoscopic ultrasound:

a. Assess gastroesophageal varices
b. EUS is better than endoscopy for gastric varices diagnosis.
c. It can evaluate the anatomy of collaterals and perforating veins.

Q. Capsule endoscopy: It is the method of choice when patient is not willing to do invasive procedure or PHG where endoscopy is contraindicated.

R. Hepatic venous portal gradient:

a. Normal 3–5 mm Hg
b. >5 to <10 mm Hg—compensated cirrhosis
c. ≥10 to <12 mm Hg—varices with transformation of compensated to decompensated cirrhosis
d. >12–20 mm Hg—bleeding from esophageal varices
e. >20 mm Hg—bleeding from esophageal varices refractory to therapy

S. Transient elastography:

a. >20 kPa with platelet count >150,000/cc—<5% chance of having high risk varices

T. Doppler ultrasound: It can demonstrate:

a. Portal vein:

1. Patency—echogenic debris or thrombus
2. Spontaneous centrifugal flow in portal, splenic, and superior mesenteric veins—its presence indicates:
   - Tendency toward hepatic encephalopathy
   - Severity of cirrhosis
3. Anatomical abnormalities of intrahepatic portal vein
4. Acute flow changes
5. Demonstration of portal-systemic shunt, patency of shunt, and direction of flow like surgical shunt, TIPS, and intrahepatic portal-systemic shunt.

b. Hepatic artery:

1. Post-transplant patency
2. Anatomical abnormalities

U. CT arteriography: It can detect:

a. Arteriovenous shunt
b. Collateral circulation
c. Focal lesion

V. Magnetic resonance arteriography: It can detect:

a. Patency of portal vein
b. Portal vein morphology
c. Portal blood flow velocity

W. Portal venography:

a. Patency, anatomy, and filling defect of portal vein
b. Presence of collaterals
c. Space-occupying lesions in the liver
d. Intrasplenic pulp pressure

Treatment of Portal Hypertension

General Measures

A. Initial step is assessment of blood volume and its rapid correction. 25% loss of blood volume may not produce tachycardia and hypotension. But blood pressure and heart rate measurement both in supine and standing position have to be done. In case of moderate to severe loss of blood volume replacement is required as because varices will be collapsed in severe hypotension and endoscopy fails to detect the esophageal varices. During the interval of blood grouping and cross matching normal saline has to be transfused, but excess saline cannot be given as it may increase edema and ascites. If glucose is transfused there is chance of hyponatremia. Due to splanchnic vasodilatation there is increased pooling of blood in the splanchnic bed which leads to decreased central venous pressure. Hence measurement of central venous pressure or pulmonary capillary wedge pressure may provide false impression of fluid loss resulting overcorrection of plasma volume. RBCs should be transfused when hemoglobin level will come down to 7 g/dL as this is associated with decreased incidence of mortality in patients with Child–Pugh class A and B cirrhosis. Again, overtransfusion of blood may be associated with severe variceal bleeding.

B. Administration of prophylactic antibiotic: Bacterial infection is very common in cirrhosis and in 20% patients with variceal bleeding in the form of pneumonia, spontaneous bacterial peritonitis, and urinary tract infection. Hence following antibiotics have to be administered for 7 days irrespective of presence or absence of ascites:

a. Norfloxacin 400 mg twice daily for or
b. Ciprofloxacin 500 mg twice daily or
c. Levofloxacin 500 mg or
d. Ceftriaxone 1 g twice daily intravenously. It is also a preferred choice if the patient has been suffering from advanced cirrhosis and is on norfloxacin prophylaxis.

C. Recombinant activated factor VII can be given in case of coagulopathy but there is no evidence of benefit in control of bleeding other than only few day decrease in mortality from this factor. It is not recommended for following reasons:
   a. Exorbitant requirement of this factor
   b. Potential for thromboembolic disease
   c. Lack of demonstrated efficacy

Main Aims of Treatment

A. Control of acute variceal bleeding
B. Prevention of first variceal bleed
C. Prevention of rebleed

The drugs are classified according to following headings:

A. The drugs responsible for reducing the portal blood flow:
   a. Vasopressin or its analog
   b. Somatostatin or its analog
   c. Beta blockers
B. Drugs reducing the intrahepatic vascular resistance:
   a. Alpha-adrenergic blocking agents
   b. Angiotensin receptor blockers
   c. Simvastatin
   d. Nitrates

Vasopressin and its Analog

A. Vasopressin, an endogenous peptide hormone, produces splanchnic vasoconstriction leading to decrease in portal venous pressure. It is not currently used for its serious side effects, such as negative ionotropic and chronotropic effect on myocardium which leads to bradycardia and low cardiac output and systemic vasoconstriction resulting bowel necrosis.
B. Terlipressin or triglycl-lysine-vasopressin, long-acting vasopressin analog, produces splanchnic vasoconstriction leading to reduction of portal pressure and systemic vasoconstriction leading to systemic hypertension. Single dose of terlipressin decreases splanchnic blood flow by 20% leading to drop of portal pressure within 30 minutes. Dose is:
   a. Initial 48 hours 2 mg intravenously 4 hourly till the control of bleeding
   b. Maintenance dose is 1 mg intravenously 4 hourly for 5 days to prevent rebleeding

Side effects are less common but may produce myocardia or intestinal ischemia.

Somatostatin Analog

This group of drugs inhibits glucagon-mediated postprandial increase in portal blood flow thus decreasing the portal pressure. The drugs are:

A. Somatostatin, 14 amino acid residue: Its half-life is 3 minutes. Dose is initial 250 μg as bolus intravenously and it can be repeated in case of rebleeding, this is followed by 250–500 μg/h up to 5 days.
B. Octreotide: Initial intravenous bolus dose of 50 μg which can be repeated in case of ongoing bleeding, this is followed by continuous intravenous infusion of 50 μg/h to prevent rebleeding up to 5 days. Half-life is 80–120 minutes.
C. Vapreotide: Initial 50 μg intravenously followed by 50 μg/h intravenous infusion for 5 days.

Beta-adrenergic Blocking Drugs

Here nonselective beta blockers are used because β_1 blocker decreases cardiac output and β_2 blocker decreases portal blood flow thus reducing the portal pressure. Nonselective beta blockers are nadolol, propranolol, and timolol. Most effective beta blocker decreases HVPG to <12 mm Hg.

A. Timolol are not used in clinical practice.
B. Nadolol being less lipid soluble has fewer side effects of central nervous system like depression and nightmares. It is excreted through kidney. Starting dose 40 mg/daily, in case elderly 20 mg/day.
C. Propranolol: Goal of treatment is reduction of heart rate between 55 and 60 beats/min or 25% from baseline. The dose can be increased every 3–5 days.

Combined alpha and beta blockers: Carvedilol in addition to its beta blocking agent, also block alpha receptor producing vasodilatation as well as decreasing intrahepatic vascular resistance leading to decrease in portal pressure. In addition it has antiproliferative and antioxidant effect.

Nitrates: These drugs decrease intrahepatic resistance by producing venodilatation and decreases the portal flow by reflex splanchnic vasoconstriction. The drugs are:

A. Short-acting nitrate nitroglycerin
B. Long-acting nitrate isosorbide mononitrate

Drugs Responsible for Decreasing Intrahepatic Resistance

The ideal action of these drugs is to reduce intrahepatic resistance without worsening systemic vasodilatation or splanchnic vasoconstriction. The drugs are:

A. Alpha-1 adrenergic blocker—prazosin: It is associated with sodium retention and ascites.

B. Combined alpha and beta blocker—carvedilol
C. Angiotensin-2 receptor type-2 antagonist—losartan: It may worsen renal function.
D. Endothelin receptor blocker—decreases portal pressure
E. Liver selective nitric oxide donor
F. Serotonin antagonist—ketanserin: It is used to reduce HVPG by 14%.
G. Simvastatin decreases intrahepatic resistance and maintain hepatic blood flow, at the same time decreases portal pressure.

Endoscopic Therapy

A. Sclerotherapy:
 a. Agents are sodium 1% tetradecyl sulfate, 5% ethanolamine oleate and sodium morrhuate
 b. Site of injection is intravariceal or paravariceal or combination of both.
 c. Dose is 2 mL per injection but not >4 mL per injection.
 d. Interval in between injections are 1–4 weeks until total or near total obliteration of varices.
 e. Complications:
  1. Ulcerations
  2. Bleeding
  3. Stricture
  4. Perforation
  5. Postsclerotherapy dysphagia: It is due to combination of esophageal dysmotility and stenosis.
 f. Proton-pump inhibitors with sucralfate decreases the sclerotherapy-induced bleeding.
B. Endoscopic variceal ligation by banding: It is universally accepted. Complications are less severe as compared to sclerotherapy but following complications may occur:
 a. Postbanding ulcer
 b. Hemorrhage
 c. Slipping of band
 d. Esophageal stricture
C. Cyanoacrylate glue injection: Gastric varices are obliterated by polymers of cyanoacrylate glue. It has to be diluted with lipiodol to delay polymerization. But upon contact with weak bases like blood it will polymerize to form cast. Immediate effect is subtotal occlusion and late effect is total occlusion. Site of administration is:
 a. Isolated gastric varices
 b. Type 2 gastroesophageal varices

 Caution:
 a. In presence of spontaneous lienorenal shunt it should be avoided because of risk of pulmonary embolism.
 b. In case of HRS or intracardiac shunt there is risk of cerebral embolism.
D. Detachable snares and clips: It can be used to ligate gastric varices but during traction there is risk of traction-induced bleeding.

Radiological procedures:
A. Transjugular intrahepatic portosystemic shunt:
 a. Indications:
  1. Mainly for prevention of rebleeding
  2. When endoscopic and pharmacologic therapy have been failed.
  3. As salvage therapy when two sessions of endoscopic therapy within 24 hours to control acute variceal bleeding have been failed.
  4. There is high risk of rebleeding.
  5. For better control and prevention of gastric variceal bleeding.
  6. Other causes such as refractory ascites, hepatic hydrothorax, Budd–Chiari syndrome, and HRS
 b. Type of operation: Side-to-side shunt by covered stent to make bridge between right hepatic vein and right portal vein.
 c. Aim of treatment:
  1. Reduction of portocaval pressure gradient to <12 mm Hg
 d. Advantage: Frequency of shunt stenosis is reduced.
 e. Procedure-related mortality is 1–2% due to:
  1. Pulmonary edema
  2. Intra-abdominal bleeding
 f. Long-term mortality is due to:
  1. Shunt occlusion: It can be detected by following:
   - Recurrence of portal hypertension
   - Portal venography to demonstrate stenosis
   - Portocaval pressure gradient >12 mm Hg
  2. Hepatic encephalopathy
  3. Pulmonary hypertension
 g. Markers of high mortality following TIPS:
  1. Serum bilirubin > 3 mg/dL
  2. Serum ALT is > 100 U/L

3. Previous history of hepatic encephalopathy
4. Patient with high Child-Turcotte-Pugh score

B. Balloon-occluded retrograde transvenous obliteration of varices:

a. Indications:

1. In case of refractory encephalopathy secondary to spontaneous lienorenal shunt
2. Embolization of gastric varices

b. Postprocedure following can be aggravated:

1. Increase in HVPG
2. Ascites
3. Splenomegaly

C. Balloon tamponade:

a. Indications: Acute variceal bleeding refractory to endoscopic and pharmacologic treatment until TIPS is carried out.

b. Types of tube:

1. Sengstaken-Blakemore tub: It has three lumen:
   - One tube for aspirating gastric content
   - One tube for gastric balloon with 200–400 mL in volume
   - One tube will lead to esophageal balloon.
2. Minnesota tube: It is modified Sengstaken-Blakemore tube:
   - Tube leading to gastric balloon has volume of 500 mL.
   - One lumen for esophageal aspiration
3. Linton-Nachlas tube:
   - Gastric balloon has 600 mL volume
   - Lumen for aspirating gastric and esophageal contents

c. Duration of keeping in the esophagus is 24–48 hours

d. Complications:

1. Aspiration of esophageal content
2. Pressure ulceration

Surgical Management of Portal Hypertension

The following are the broad groups of operative procedure:

A. Decompressive shunt:

a. Total: In this procedure entirely total portal venous system is decompressed thus there is significant loss of portal blood flow to the liver.

Example is portocaval shunt—both side-to-side and end-to-side shunt. But side-to-side is currently used.

Indications:

1. Treatment of variceal bleeding at the same time for controlling ascites
2. With the aim to increase hepatic venous flow and also to reduce portal pressure

Complications:

1. Recurrent variceal bleeding in 10% of patients
2. Hepatic encephalopathy in 40% of patients
3. Increased mortality and mortality in patients undergoing liver transplantation. Hence in case of candidates for liver transplantation portocaval shunt should be avoided.

b. Selective: In this procedure of lienorenal shunt selectively gastroesophageal junction and spleen are decompressed without decompressing mesenteric and portal venous system thus maintaining portal hypertension. To decompress gastroesophageal junction prior to anastomosis between left renal and splenic vein following procedures have to be done:

1. Portoazygous disconnection
2. Ligation of left adrenal vein
3. Mobilization of entire length of pancreas.

Ascites also persists as because hepatic sinusoids are not decompressed. There is low incidence of rebleeding and hospital mortality.

c. Partial: In this procedure of portosystemic shunt where by the process of graft placement between portal vein and inferior vena cava varices are decompressed but maintaining the portal blood flow to the liver. There is low incidence of rebleeding and hospital mortality. But ascites also persists as because hepatic sinusoids are not decompressed.

B. Nonshunt procedure: It was previously used for controlling acute bleeding but very little used today.

C. Mesentericoportal venous bypass:

a. Indications:

1. Extrahepatic portal venous thrombosis but patent intrahepatic portion of portal vein
2. Thrombosis of portal vein which is developed after liver transplantation.

b. Advantages:

1. Early restoration of portal blood flow to the liver
2. No risk of hepatic encephalopathy
3. No risk of learning disability in case of children

c. Site of operation:

Graft is jugular vein will anastomose between superior mesenteric vein and intrahepatic portion of left portal vein in Rex recess where it will divide to supply 3rd and 4th segment of the liver.

D. Liver transplantation

Q39. Liver dialysis.

Describe various modalities of artificial liver transport support system and enumerate their advantages and disadvantages.

DNB (DEC2018) (10)

ANSWER

Definition

Liver dialysis is an extracorporeal temporary method which will detoxify and provide artificial support liver between liver transplantation and acute or acute-on-chronic liver failure.

Role of Liver Dialysis in the Pathogenesis of Acute on Chronic Liver Failure

A. "Cytokine burst" with accumulated low-molecular weight toxins, different types of cytokines, and vasoactive substances are responsible for hepatocellular injury.

B. Endotoxins released from the gut bacteria not only potentiates hepatocyte injury but also deprives the proper environment for regeneration.

C. Released toxins are also responsible vital organ dysfunction by following mechanisms:

a. Systemic inflammation

b. Loss of innate as well as adaptive immunity

Artificial liver support devices perform three key functions:

A. Detoxification

B. Synthesis of important proteins

C. Facilitation of regeneration of liver cells

Liver support devices can be divided into two groups:

A. Artificial liver support device

B. Bioartificial liver support device

Comparisons between two devices:

Item	Artificial liver support device	Bioartificial liver support device
Cost	Less	High for its design, operation, and manage
Cellular component such as primary hepatocyte and hepatic cell line	Absent, it is purely mechanical	Present
Function on liver	Detoxification	• Oxidative detoxification • Biotransformation • Excretion • Synthesis
Efficacy	Limited	Very high and promising
Ease to use	Simple	Complex due to presence of cellular components

There are two types of toxic substances in human being:

A. Water-soluble: AAAs, creatinine, interleukin-6, ammonia, urea, GABA, and tryptophan.

B. Albumin bound: Bilirubin, bile acids, middle-chain and short-chain fatty acids, cytokines, nitric oxide, furancarboxylic acid, benzodiazepines, and proto-porphyrin.

Extracorporeal liver-assisted devices, such as hemodialysis, hemofiltration, charcoal perfusion, and plasma exchange, can remove water-soluble toxins and only minor amount of albumin bound toxins. Hence albumin has been used as an adsorbent of protein bound toxins to remove them in Molecular Adsorbent and Recirculation System (MARS) or simple Pass Albumin Dialysis (SPAD).

Other approach is to use large pore filters that will retain cellular component separating plasma protein including albumin in fractional plasma separation and adsorption (FPSA-Prometheus) and Selective Plasma Filtration Technology (SEPET).

Artificial liver support devices:
A. MARS
B. SPAD
C. SEPET
D. FPSA-Prometheus

Bioartificial liver support devices:
A. HepatAssist
B. Extracorporeal liver assist device
C. Bioartificial liver support system
D. Molecular extracorporeal liver support

Artificial Liver Support System

MARS

It is a combination of convention dialysis and hemodialysis but here dialysate is albumin solution and membrane is albumin impermeable.

It consists of two circuits:
A. Blood circuit: It passes the blood of the patients through high flux dialyzer over one side of albumin impermeable membrane.
B. Secondary circuit where on opposite side of the membrane there is 600 mL of 20% albumin. Albumin is refreshed by activated charcoal and ion exchange resin in the secondary circuit.

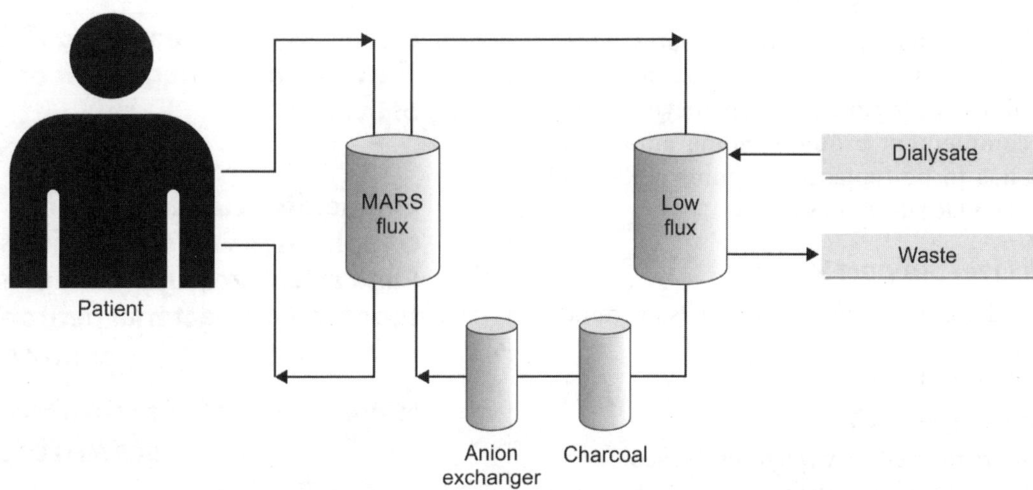

Activity of MARS:
A. Improve the bilirubin level
B. Improve encephalopathy
C. May worsen coagulopathy
D. Causes hypoglycemia
E. Alters pharmacokinetics of drugs

Prometheus System

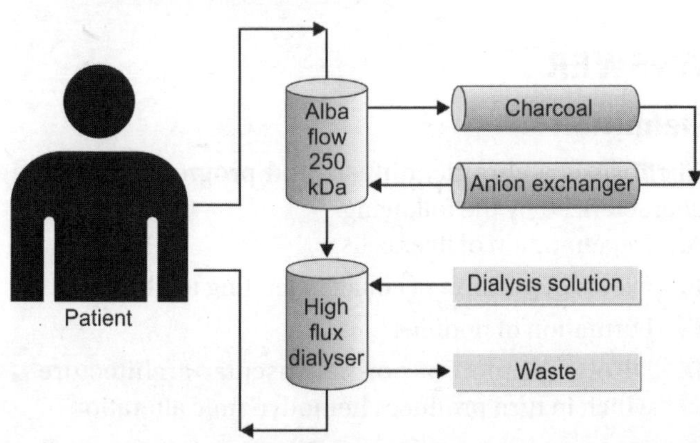

Here albumin bound toxins will diffuse across the albumin permeable membrane, then the filtrate returns to the patient after passing through the two column of activated charcoal and ion exchange resin. It provides high clearance of most of the liver toxins.

Albumin is clear of toxins, here no exogenous oxygen is used.

Single Pass Albumin Dialysis (SPAD)

Here concentration of albumin is 5% instead of 20%. Here albumin will be discarded after single counter-current pass through the dialyzer against blood of the patient.

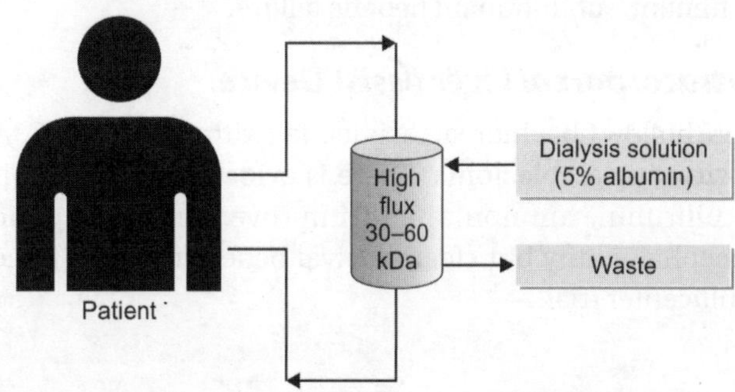

Selective Plasma Filtration Therapy

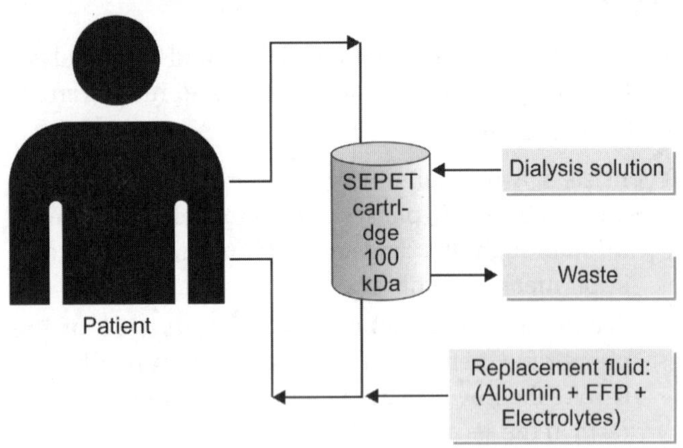

It uses hollow fiber having membrane pores which allow the passage of <100 kDa molecules but preserves immunoglobulin, clotting factors, hepatocyte growth factors and complement proteins. Some amount of albumin lost has to be replaced. Albumin, FFP, and electrolytes will replace the removed fluid.

Bioartificial Liver Support System

Here widespread use of human hepatocyte is prevented due to following causes:

A. Lack of widespread availability

B. They cannot be generated in vitro.

C. During culture their efficacy will be decreased.

Hence following other cell lines are used as cell mattresses for stimulating cell-to-cell interaction:

A. C3A human hepatoblastoma cell line as it has a capacity of unlimited expansion in vitro. But these cells do not express normal metabolic profile like ureagenesis. But as compared to normal hepatocyte they have inferior metabolic activity.

B. Porcine hepatocytes

HepatAssist

It uses hollow fiber extracorporeal bioreactor which is loaded with porcine hepatocytes which is cryopreserved. There is evidence of survival benefit in patients with fulminant/subfulminant hepatic failure.

Extracorporeal Liver Assist Device

Here hollow fiber bioreactor is loaded with cell lines of C3A human hepatoblastoma. There is evidence of reduction of bilirubin, ammonia, and improvement of hepatic encephalopathy but clear survival benefit requires large multicenter trial.

Modular Extracorporeal Liver Support System

Here hollow fibers contain fresh porcine hepatocytes. According to some studies it acts as bridge to transplant. But its use is a bit complex and highly costly.

Bioartificial Liver Support System

Here hollow fiber utilizes porcine hepatocytes. Phase II/ III trial are going on.

Amsterdam Medical Center Bioartificial Liver

It utilizes porcine hepatocytes which is bound to spiral-shaped polyester fabric integrated with hollow fiber. Though primary study demonstrated encouraging results but large trial is needed.

Q40. Discuss etiology, pathology, clinical features and management of cirrhosis of liver.

MGR/OCT2012/MDII (15)

Enumerate acute and chronic complications of liver cirrhosis. Clinical features and management of spontaneous bacterial peritonitis.

DNB (DEC 2018) (10)

Management of liver cirrhosis.

SCB MED COL, 2017 (20)

Pathology of cirrhosis.

MGR UNI, TAMIL NADU, 2019 (5)

Describe etiopathogenesis, clinical features, diagnosis and management of chronic active hepatitis.

VEER NARMAD SOUTH GUJARAT UNI, 2019 (25)

SBP part has been written in the question number 23.

ANSWER

Definition

Cirrhosis is a chronic, diffuse, and progressive disease characterized by the following:

A. Degeneration of liver cells

B. Excess deposition of collagen leading to fibrosis

C. Formation of nodules

D. Disorganization of normal vascular architecture—which in turn produces hemodynamic alteration

The inciting events produces parenchymal inflammation and necrosis followed by fibrosis by following mechanisms:

A. Directly
B. Indirectly by immunological mechanisms

Causes of nodule formation with or without fibrosis:

A. Fibrosis without nodule formation—congenital hepatic fibrosis
B. Fibrosis with nodule formation—cirrhosis
C. Nodule formation without fibrosis—partial nodular transformation

Etiology of Cirrhosis

A. Viral causes—HAV, HBV, HCV, HEV, and HDV
B. Alcohol
C. Nonalcoholic fatty liver
D. Metabolic:
    a. Iron overload hemochromatosis
    b. Copper overload—Wilson's disease
    c. Alpha-1 antitrypsin deficiency
    d. Galactosemia
    e. Tyrosinemia
    f. Type IV collagen formation
E. Primary biliary cirrhosis
F. Primary sclerosing cholangitis
G. Hepatic venous outflow obstruction:
    a. Budd-Chiari syndrome
    b. Heart failure
H. Autoimmune hepatitis
I. Toxins:
    a. Amiodarone
    b. Methotrexate

Cofactors for the development of cirrhosis:

A. Alcohol: Large number of people take large amount of alcohol but only small proportion develop cirrhosis
B. Obesity: Nonalcoholic steatohepatitis will develop in a small proportion of obese patients.
C. Genetic factors: Patient with Alpha-1 antitrypsin deficiency may develop cirrhosis.
D. Age
E. Sex
F. Immunological status: Diabetic obese patients with insulin resistance may develop cirrhosis if he or she is immunosuppressed.
G. Patient with hepatitis C will develop cirrhosis if the infection occurs at old age.

Classification of Cirrhosis

Cirrhosis has been classified according to the size of the nodules:

A. Micronodular cirrhosis: Here the nodule size is <3 mm in diameter and all the lobules are involved in etiology:
    a. Alcoholic
    b. Hemochromatosis
    c. Cholestasis
    d. Hepatic venous outflow obstruction
B. Macronodular cirrhosis: Here the diameter of the nodule is >3 mm and presence of normal lobule in larger nodule. Cause is viral hepatitis.
C. Mixed nodular cirrhosis: Here there is transition between micronodular and macronodular cirrhosis. So alcoholic micronodular cirrhosis may transform into macronodular cirrhosis with the advance of liver damage.

Reversible Cirrhosis

Normally, cirrhosis is irreversible but in the following diseases if the inciting events can be removed fibrosis may revert:

A. Hepatitis C
B. Iron overload
C. Obesity
D. Biliary obstruction

Histological Changes in Cirrhosis

A. Formation of fibrous septa from the portal tract to central vein leading to distortion of the liver lobular architecture.
B. Proliferation of the hepatocytes leading to formation of regenerative nodules which are surrounded by the fibrous tissue.
C. Loss of normal hepatocytes due to apoptosis and/or necrosis.
D. Rupture of the architecture of sinusoids due to polarization of the sinusoid as a result of deposition of fibrous tissue in the basement membrane.
E. Proliferation of the bile ductules at the edges of the fibrous septa.
F. Portal and periportal infiltration of lymphocytes and plasma cells.

G. In case of alcoholic or nonalcoholic liver damage there is microvascular or macrovascular deposition of fat.

Clinical Features

A. Constitutional symptoms such as weakness, anorexia, fatigue, weight loss, dyspepsia, and low-grade fever

B. Symptoms related to liver disease:

- **a.** Spontaneous bleeding from gums
- **b.** Easy bruising
- **c.** Loss of axillary and pubic hair
- **d.** Loss of libido in males
- **e.** In females menstrual abnormalities
- **f.** Gynecomastia
- **g.** Jaundice
- **h.** Arterial spider
- **i.** Pruritus
- **j.** Spider nevi
- **k.** Enlarged parotid
- **l.** Edema
- **m.** Bleeding from gastrointestinal tract

C. Symptoms related to nervous system:

- **a.** Drowsiness
- **b.** Irritability
- **c.** Stupor
- **d.** Coma

D. Symptoms related to kidney:

- **a.** Oliguria
- **b.** Raised urea and creatinine

E. Associated diseases:

- **a.** Diabetes
- **b.** Peptic ulcer
- **c.** Symptoms related to gallstones
- **d.** Psychiatric abnormalities

Physical findings in cirrhosis:

A. Hepatocellular failure—it comprises of:

- **a.** Skin lesions:
  1. Palmar erythema: It is distributed in the area of superior venacaval distribution in face, necklace area, forearms, and dorsum of the hands. It is a central arteriole from which there are numerous radiating vessels. Size is pinhead to 0.5 cm in diameter.
     - It may disappear with improvement of the condition.
     - Appearance of fresh lesion indicates progression of liver disease.
     - Multiple spider with clubbing—HPS
- **b.** Hand findings:
  1. Palmar erythema
  2. Dupuytren's contracture—flexion deformity of the little and ring and sometimes middle fingers due to thickening and shortening of palmar fascia. There may be knobs and knots formation under the skin.
  3. Asterixis: Rhythmic bilateral tremor of wrist on dorsiflexion found in hand and tongue.
- **c.** Disorder of protein metabolism—muscle wasting, atrophy of thenar and hypothenar eminence, ascites, and edema
- **d.** Splenomegaly
- **e.** Ascites
- **f.** Abdominal collaterals
- **g.** Pulmonary complications
- **h.** Esophageal varices
- **i.** Parotid enlargement
- **j.** Nail changes:
  1. Leukonychia: Presence of white spots or white lines on the nails
  2. Azure lunula: Whitish appearance on the two-thirds of the nails and bluish colored lunule—it is found in Wilson's disease
  3. Muehrcke's nails: Horizontal white bands separated by normal colored across the skin.
  4. Clubbing
- **k.** Testicular atrophy
- **l.** Gynecomastia

B. Eye sign:

- **a.** Lid retraction
- **b.** Lid lag in absence of thyroid disease

C. Muscle cramps

D. Nutrition: Muscle wasting

E. Fetor hepaticus: Sweetish slightly fecal smell of breath just like freshly opened corpse or mice.

Extrahepatic manifestations:

A. Autoimmune hemolytic anemia

B. Thyroiditis

Laboratory Tests

A. Hematology:

- **a.** Normally normocytic normochromic anemia
- **b.** In alcoholic patient macrocytic anemia
- **c.** In case of bleeding microcytic hypochromic anemia
- **d.** In case of infection—leukocytosis

e. In hypersplenism—leukopenia with or without thrombocytopenia

f. Prolonged PT—refractory vitamin K deficiency

g. Bone marrow demonstrate:

 1. Macronormoblastic
 2. Increased number of plasma cells due to hypergammaglobulinemia

h. Liver enzymes:

 1. Serum bilirubin:
    - Conjugated bilirubin is normal in compensated cirrhosis.
    - Raised in severe liver disease
 2. ALT: It is a screening test for detection of metabolic injury or drug-induced injury.
 3. AST/ALT ratio:
    - >2—alcoholic liver disease
    - <1—chronic hepatitis or chronic cholestatic syndrome
    - >1—nonalcoholic cirrhosis
 4. Serum albumin—decreased in case advanced liver disease
 5. Serum globulin level—increased due to:
    - Poor reticuloendothelial function
    - Increased blood level of bacterial product
 6. GGT: It is raised in alcoholic liver disease, barbiturate, and phenytoin poisoning.
 7. Serum ALP:
    - Nearly twice of normal—noncholestatic liver disease
    - >2 times normal—primary biliary cirrhosis and primary sclerosing cholangitis

Cholesterol and triglyceride:

A. Raised in biliary obstruction

B. Low in nonbiliary advanced cirrhosis

Other tests to detect the synthetic function of the liver:

A. Ceruloplasmin

B. Ferritin

C. Alpha-1 antitrypsin

D. Lipoproteins

Serological tests for viral hepatitis:

A. HBsAg

B. HBeAg

C. Anti-HAV

D. Anti-HEV

E. Anti-HBc antibody

F. HBV DNA

G. HCV RNA

Autoantibody profile:
There are two types of AIH—characterized by specific type of autoantibodies:

A. Antismooth muscle cell antibody, ANA, antiactin antibody, and/or perinuclear antineutrophil cytoplasmic antibody for detection type-1 AIH.

B. Anti-LKM-1 antibodies and anti-liver cytosol antibodies—detect type 2 AIH.

For patient suffered from hemochromatosis:

A. Fasting transferrin saturation 45%

B. Serum ferritin level:

 1. >300 ng/mL for men
 2. >200 ng/mL for women

C. Analysis of *HFE* gene mutation

D. Liver biopsy to confirm diagnosis

For patient of <45 years with family history of cirrhosis:

A. Serum ceruloplasmin level is low (<20 mg/mL)

B. High basal 24 hours urinary copper secretion >100 µg (normal 10–80 µg)

C. Low serum copper level (normal 60–80 µg/mL)—suggest Wilson's disease

D. Increased copper content in liver biopsy (250 µg/g of dry weight)

For alpha-1 antitrypsin deficiency: It is useful in chronic hepatic injury in neonates.

Radiological Investigation

A. In case of cirrhosis ultrasound demonstrates following features:

 a. Altered echo pattern
 b. Nodular irregular surface
 c. Nodular liver edges
 d. Collateral vessels related to portal hypertension
 e. Grades of steatosis: Bright echo pattern with fibrosis—indicates fatty liver as a cause of cirrhosis
 f. Mass in the liver

B. Doppler ultrasound demonstrates:

 a. Vascularization of the lesion
 b. Blood flow in the hepatic veins
 c. Direction of blood flow in the portal vein—whether centripetal or centrifugal
 d. Patency of portal vein and hepatic vein
 e. Localization and states of collaterals

C. Contrast-enhanced CT scan: It will differentiate between benign lesion and dysplastic nodule or HCC.

D. MRI assesses:
 a. Volume and direction of flow of portal vein
 b. Iron overload
 c. Portal vein thrombosis

Treatment of Cirrhosis

Basic Goals of Treatment

A. Treatment of the etiology to prevent further progression of liver disease
B. Prevention of intake of substances which is harmful to liver
C. Prevention of complication of cirrhosis
D. Control of symptoms of cirrhosis
E. Prioritization of patient for liver transplantation

Treatment of the Etiology

A. To treat hepatitis C—pegylated IFN, ribavirin, sofosbuvir, velpatasvir, and daclatasvir
B. To treat hepatitis B—tenofovir, entecavir, and adefovir
C. In case of autoimmune etiology—steroids, immunosuppressive drugs
D. In case of Wilson's disease—D-penicillamine and trientine
E. Avoidance of substances which are harmful to the liver:
 a. Alcohol abuse
 b. Over-the-counter drugs
 c. Dose of vitamin A—25,000 IU/day
 d. NSAIDs
F. Following immunization should be required:
 a. Vaccination of HAV
 b. Vaccination of HBV
 c. Vaccination against influenza and pneumococcus
G. Nutrition requirement:
 a. Generally low sodium, low fat, high protein, and carbohydrate diet. Energy requirement is 25-35 kcal/kg/day
 b. In malnourished patient:
  1. Energy requirement 35–40 kcal/kg/day
  2. Protein requirement 1–1.2 g/kg/day
 c. Cirrhotic patient in ICU or associated complications: Protein requirement 1.5 g/kg/day
 d. Other supplements are iron, vitamin K, B12, and zinc
H. Treatment of pruritus in cholestatic cirrhosis:
 a. It can be treated by antihistaminics.
 b. Cholestyramine: It is bitter in taste.
 c. Other medications to get relief from pruritus: Ursodeoxycholic acid, rifampin, naltrexone, ondansetron, and gabapentin.
 d. In severe pruritus: Ultraviolet therapy or plasmapheresis
I. To treat hepatic encephalopathy: Lactulose and rifaximin
J. To treat edema:
 a. Low-sodium diet
 b. Spironolactone and furosemide combination to reduce excess salt
 c. Patient with refractory ascites: Total paracentesis with 20% albumin
 d. Albumin infusion at 1.5 g/kg/day to reduce hyponatremia
K. To treat HRS:
 a. Vasoconstrictor and albumin
 b. TIPS
 c. Extracorporeal albumin dialysis—molecular adsorbents recirculating system—in type 1 syndrome
 d. Liver transplantation
L. Treatment of hypogonadism: Topical testosterone preparation
M. Cirrhotic patient may develop osteoporosis so these patients may get benefit from calcium and vitamin supplementation.
N. To prevent bleeding from esophageal varices nonselective beta blocker can be administered to reduce the heart rate 25% from baseline.
O. Surgical treatment: All the operations in cirrhotic patients carry high risk and high mortality because of following reasons:
 a. Low serum albumin
 b. Presence of infection
 c. Increased PT

Following operations carry bad prognosis:

A. Biliary tract operation
B. Colonic resection
C. Operation for peptic ulcer

Q41. Enumerate the differences between type 1 and type 2 Crigler–Najjar syndromes.

DNB (DEC2020) (5)

ANSWER

Features	Type 1 Crigler-Najjar disease	Type 2 Crigler-Najjar disease
Genetic basis	Autosomal recessive	Autosomal recessive or dominant
Enzyme deficiency	Complete deficiency of UDP-glucuronosyltransferase	Partial deficiency of UDP-glucuronosyl-transferase
UDP-glucurono-syltransferase	Less than 10% of the activity	10 to 30% Of the normal activity
Level of bilirubin	More than 20 to 50 mg%	Less than 20 mg%
Kernicterus	Very high risk	Low risk
Administration of phenobarbital	No response	Decrease the level of bilirubin
Disease onset	Neonatal period	Late childhood
Line of treatment	Phototherapy Liver transplantation	Administration of phenobarbital Phototherapy
Prognosis	Worse even with liver transplantation	Good response to drug

Q42. Diagnosis and management in a case ascites.

DNB (DEC2020) (4)

Ascites etiopathogenesis and its evaluation.

SCB MED COL, 2019, 2020 (20)

ANSWER

Approach to a Patient with Ascites

Definition

Accumulation of free fluid in abdomen is called ascites. It produces progressive increase in size of the abdomen. Distension of abdomen which may mimic ascites are:

A. Flatus (gaseous distension) may be due to intestinal obstruction—which may be generalized or localized

B. Feces—localized

C. Fat—obesity - generalized

D. Fetus—Pregnancy - generalized

E. Filthy tumor or organomegaly - usually localized

F. Abdominal malignancy:

- **a.** Patient usually complains of increase in clothing size, feeling of abdominal tightness, or pulling.
- **b.** Low back pain
- **c.** Early satiety
- **d.** At least 500 mL of free fluid should be present to detect abdominal shifting dullness.
- **e.** At least 1500 mL of free fluid should be present to defect fluid thrill.
- **f.** Ultrasonography can detect ascites with at least 50 mL of free fluid is present in abdomen.

Causes of Ascites

A. *Hepatic*

- **a.** Cirrhosis
- **b.** Hepatocellular carcinoma
- **c.** Alcoholic hepatitis
- **d.** Hepatic Veno—occlusive disease (Budd-Chiari Syndrome)

B. *Cardiac cause*

- **a.** Congestive cardiac failure
- **b.** Constrictive pericarditis
- **c.** Tricuspid in competence

C. *Renal cause*

- **a.** Nephrotic syndrome

D. *Peritoneum*

- **a.** Tuberculosis
- **b.** Neoplastic—Primary mesothelioma
- **c.** Spontaneous bacterial peritonitis

E. *Malignant disease*

- **a.** Carcinomatosis
- **b.** Abdominal or pelvic tumor
- **c.** Pseudomyxoma peritonei

F. *Venous obstruction*

- **a.** Veno-occlusive disease
- **b.** Hepatic portal vein obstruction
- **c.** Inferior vena caval obstruction

G. *Gastrointestinal causes*:

- **a.** Pancreatitis
- **b.** Malabsorption
- **c.** Bile ascites

H. *Other cause chylous ascites*:

- **a.** Due to surgical trauma to cistern chili
- **b.** Obstruction to lymphatic by tumor

Evaluation from History

A. History of Jaundice, hematemesis, wasting right upper quadrant pain—*cirrhosis*

B. History of alcoholism, jaundice, hematemesis, washing—*alcoholic cirrhosis*

C. Past history hepatitis with evidence of HBsAg positivity or HBs antibody having ongoing cirrhosis for several years suddenly develop hepatic decompensation & pain in right upper quadrant, pruritus, progressively increasing jaundice—suggest *hepatocellular carcinoma*

D. History of breathlessness, cough, palpitation, swelling of legs—suggest *congestive cardiac failure.*

E. History of symptoms referable to gastrointestinal tract e.g., Dyspepsia, anorexia, postprandial abdominal fullness, symptoms of low cardiac output e.g., fatigue wasting, less frequently dyspnea or orthopnea—*constrictive pericarditis*

F. History of palpitation, results of venous congestion producing fatigue, anorexia, loose motion, fatigue—exclude tricuspid valve disease—because no obvious significant history suggestive of cardiac origin—is present is *tricuspid incompetence*

G. Sudden onset of ascites suggests decompensated *cirrhosis, malignancy—portal or splenic vein thrombosis and Budd-Chiari syndrome.*

H. Swelling of whole body starting from face, diminished urine volume, headache—suggest *nephritic syndrome.*

I. Low grade fever gradual swelling of abdomen with pain all over abdomen—suggest *tuberculosis*

J. History of cancer from breast, ovarian, prostate, testicular tissue, hematological malignancies or any malignancy in abdomen suddenly develops rapid tender swelling of abdomen—*malignant peritonitis.*

K. History of Central or epigastric severe abdominal pain, radiating to back, with nausea vomiting fever—*acute pancreatitis.*

L. History of biliary tract operation—laparoscopic or endoscopic (ERCP)—develop suddenly abdominal distension, tenderness evidence of shown—*bile ascites.*

M. Cirrhosis may result from iron storage disease or Wilsons disease or primary biliary cirrhosis so in these cases—we have to diagnose the cause of cirrhosis.

Evaluation from Physical Examination

To diagnose evidence of ascites—two methods are mainly required:

A. Shifting dullness

B. Fluid thrill

From Inspection

A. Presence of jaundice, spider nevi, gynecomastia palmar erythema, caput medusa—cirrhosis

B. Triad of palmar erythema gynecomastia, Dupuytren's contracture—alcoholic liver disease

C. Elevated jugular venous pressure, cardiac etiology

- **a.** Prominent 'v' ware in Jugular venous wave—tricuspid regurgitation
- **b.** Inspiratory elevation in JVP—constrictive pericarditis.

D. Cullen sign—(periumbilical ecchymoses), Grey Turner sign (Flank ecchymoses)—acute pancreatitis

E. Facial puffiness—Nephrotic syndrome

From Palpation

In case of ascites—abdominal organs should be palpated by dipping method

A. hepatomegaly splenomegaly—*cirrhosis, primary biliary cirrhosis Hematological malignancy.*

B. Tender hepatomegaly, splenomegaly—HCC

C. Cardiomegaly, apex beat displacement. Tachycardia, pedal edema—*congestive cardiac failure*

D. Jaundice, edema, hepatomegaly—*cirrhosis*

E. Tender abdomen all over:

Primary malignant peritonitis:

- **a.** HCC
- **b.** Tuberculosis
- **c.** Spontaneous bacterial peritonitis

F. Associated parietal edema:

- **a.** Nephrotic syndrome
- **b.** Any cause producing hypoproteinemia

G. Edema—Cirrhosis, congestive cardiac failure, malabsorption, lymphatic obstruction, nephrotic syndrome

Percussion

Dullness in right or left lung bases:

- Pleural effusion due to tuberculosis, secondary to ascites, malignancy in genital organ, HCC, collagen vascular disease (polyserositis)

Auscultation

A. *Auscultation of abdomen* after paracentesis—bruit on liver—*HCC, nodular regeneration on cirrhotic liver.*

B. *Auscultation of chest*:

- **a.** Rapid heart rate with gallop rhythm (S2S3S4) fine crepitations at bases (pulmonary edema)—*congestive cardiac failure.*
- **b.** Murmur of TI or murmur of M1 suggests CCF due to tricuspid or mitral regurgitation respectively.
- **c.** Distort or muffled heart sound may be due to *pericardial effusion or constrictive pericarditis.*

Internal Examination

A. per rectal examination—ulcerative mass in rectum—suggestive of rectal carcinoma

B. Per vaginal examination.

Important Points to be Remembered

A. Triad findings of hepatomegaly, ascites, and increased venous collateral or the anterior abdominal walls—presence of portal hypertension.

B. Triad of findings of parotid enlargement gynecomastia and Dupuytren's contracture—indicates alcoholic cirrhosis.

C. Diagnosis of cirrhosis can be made on the basis of two physical findings + two laboratory findings:

Two physical findings are:

- Asterixis
- Ascites

Two laboratory findings are:

- Hypoalbuminemia, (<2.8 g/dL)
- Prolongation of prothrombin time (international normalized ratio > 1.6)

Evaluations on the Basis of Laboratory Investigation

Most useful parameter to classify ascites is serum—ascitic fluid albumin (SAAG) gradient—it can be calculated by:

Subtracting the peritoneal fluid albumin concentration from serum albumin concentration, value i.e., albumin Serum/albumin Ascites

The value which is the main bar is 1.1 g/dL

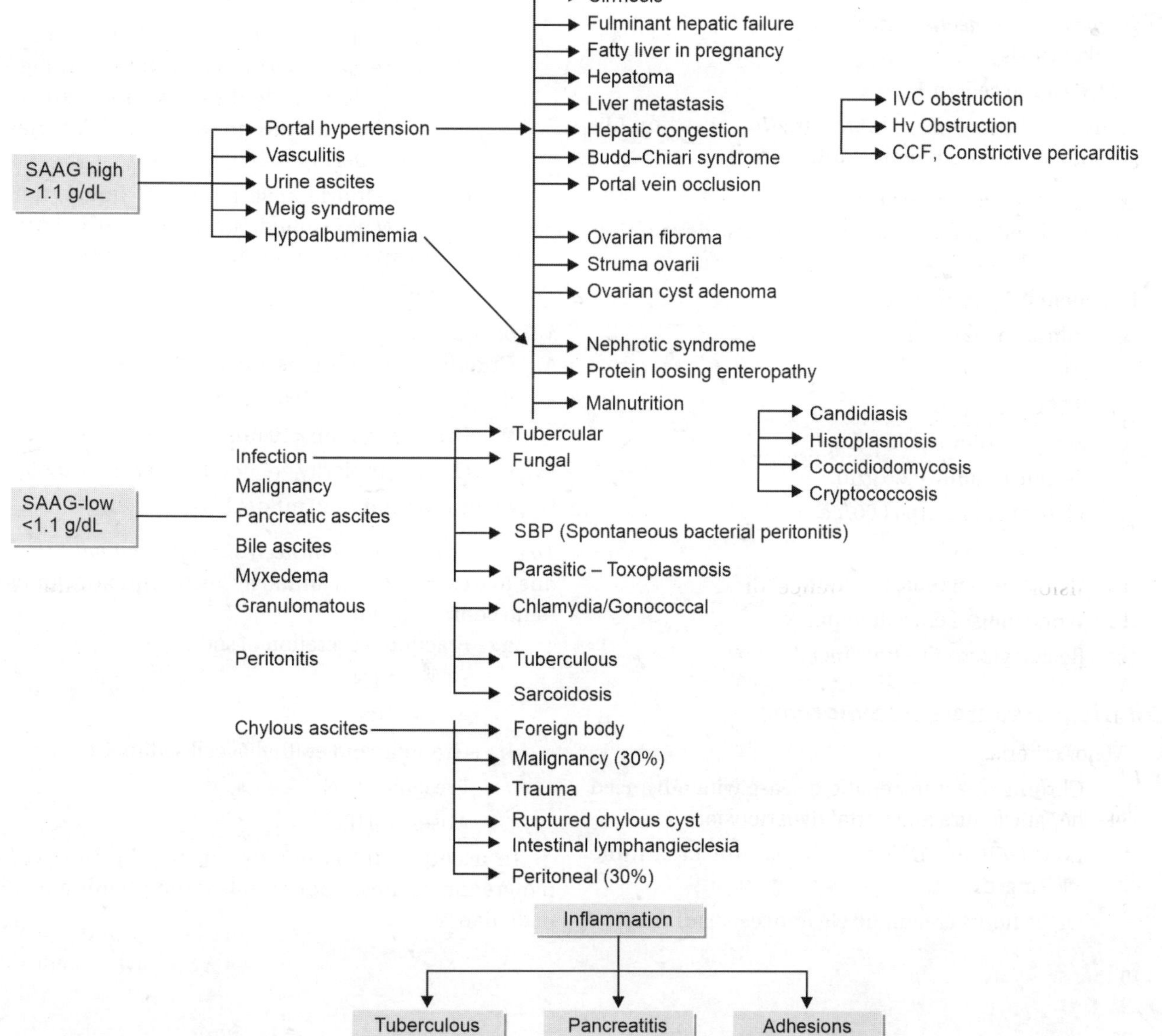

Characters of Paracentesis Fluid

Etiology	Color	RBC (10^6/L)	WBC (10^6/L)	Cytology	Other
Cirrhosis	Straw	Few	<250	×	×
Tuberculosis	Clear Hemorrhagic Turbid	Many	>1000 75% lymphocytes	×	Acid-fast stain Culture ADA >40
Cardiac failure	Straw	0	<250	×	×
Pancreatic ascites	Turbid hemorrhagic	variable	variable	×	Amylase >20,000 somogyi units
Lymphatic obstruction	White	0	0	×	Fat globules on Sudan III stain
Neoplastic peritonitis	Straw Hemorrhagic Mucinous	Variable	Variable	Malignant cells	×

To diagnose fungus as etiological agent:

A. KOH preparation.

B. Culture

To diagnose spontaneous bacterial peritonitis:

A. Leukocytosis

B. PMN's > 250 cells/mL

C. Culture shows—*E. coli, Klebsiella*, occasionally streptococci, infrequently staphylococci

Predictors of first episode of SBP:

A. Hospitalized patient having cirrhosis, developing abdominal pain.

B. Biochemical parameters:

- **a.** Bilirubin: >2.5 mg/dL
- **b.** PT > 1.6 (INR)
- **c.** SAAG <1.1 g/dL
- **d.** Serum sodium <130 mEq/L
- **e.** Serum albumin <2.6 g/dL
- **f.** Platelet count <100,000/cc

C. Associated signs of:

- **a.** Worsening of renal function
- **b.** Worsening of encephalopathy
- **c.** Recent gastrointestinal bleed

Criteria of Hepatorenal Syndrome

A. Major criteria:

- **a.** Chronic or acute hepatic disease with advanced hepatic failure and portal hypertension
- **b.** Low GFR as indicated by serum creatinine >1.5 mg/dL
  Or, 24 hours creatinine clearance <40 mL/min
- **c.** No shock, ongoing bacterial infection, sepsis, SBP, renal fluid loss due to diuretics, ongoing breathing problem or treatment for toxic drugs (NSAID, ASA)
- **d.** No improvement in renal function (i.e., decrease in serum creatinine <1.5 mg/dL) after diuretic withdrawal and expansion of plasma volume with 1.5 L of plasma expander.
- **e.** Proteinuria <500 mg for 24 hours, normal renal ultrasound, (no evidence of obstructive uropathy or chronic renal parenchymal disease)

Minor criteria:

A. Criteria frequently present:

- **a.** Urine volume <500 mL/day
- **b.** Urinary sodium <10 mEq/dL
- **c.** Urine osmolarity greater than serum osmolarity

B. Serum sodium <130 mEq/dL

To exclude acute tubular necrosis in patient with cirrhosis due to treatment with aminoglycoside antibiotic or use of radio contrast agent:

- **a.** Fractional excretion of sodium:
  > 2%—ATN
  <2%—HRS
- **b.** Granular and epithelial cell sediment
  Present—ATN
  Absent—HRS

In ascetic fluid is bloody—it may be tuberculosis pancreatic ascites, abdominal trauma, endometriosis, malignancy.

To Diagnose Malignancy

a. Ratio of ascetic fluid LDH to serum LDH >0.6—suggestive of malignancy, but in 15% of non-malignant cirrhotic patient it is >0.6.
b. Carcinoembryonic antigen (CEA) is raised in ascetic fluid in half of the cases of malignancy producing ascites.

Pancreatic amylase may be raised in patient with pancreatic disease related to alcohol or abdominal trauma.

SBP can be differentiated from secondary peritonitis due to rupture viscous—by culture of ascetic fluid single organism present in 78 to 88% of SBP patient.

But multiple organisms are always cultured in secondary peritonitis.

Increased triglyceride in ascetic fluid—*chylous ascites*

General investigations to diagnose the etiology:

A. *Blood count*:
   a. Raised WBC—infectious etiology
   b. Raised Polymorphonuclear leukocytes—Bacterial infection
B. *Urine examination*:
   a. Strongly positive for blood in dipstick method in case of nephritic syndrome—if protein strongly +ve >3.5 g/24 hours—nephrotic syndrome.
   b. Urinary sodium <10 mEq/L, Fractional excretion of sodium <1%—HRS (N sediment in urine)
   c. Urine osmolarity is more than serum osmolarity—HRS
C. Blood:
   a. LFT—derange with hypoalbuminemia and reversal of alb: globulin ratio—cirrhosis
   b. α-fetoprotein raised in HCC
   c. Tumor marker
   d. ANA, anti SMA, anti LKM antibody—to diagnose autoimmune etiology.
D. *Chest X-ray*:
   a. Cardiomegaly, upper venous distribution of blood, Kerley's Blinds—*congestive cardiac failure*
   b. Pleural effusion—Tuberculosis Vasculitis, malignancy, cirrhosis
   c. Bilateral plural effusion—vasculitis, malignancy congenital connection with pleural and peritoneal cavity.
   d. Small heart with evidence of calcification in pericardial wall—constrictive pericarditis, calcification in pericardium—suggests tubercular etiology. Calcified pericardium—does not always suggest constriction.
E. *Ultrasonography*:
   a. Small shrunken, heterogenic liver with fatty infiltration—*cirrhosis*
   b. Presence of nodule or large SOL in cirrhotic liver or normal liver—*HCC*
   c. Enlarged spleen in *cirrhosis with portal hypertension*
   d. Thrombosis of portal vein or hepatic run:
      - Budd-Chiari syndrome
      - Hepatic venous obstruction
   e. Enlarged pancreas—*pancreatitis*
   f. Evidence of *genital malignancy* in women
F. Abdominal X-ray—gas under diaphragm—*perforated viscous*

Echocardiography:

A. Echo free space between left ventricle and pericardium—*pericardial effusion*
B. Calcification on the wall of pericardium, pericardial knocking, normal or small cardiac chambers with preserved left ventricular ejection fraction in patient with heart failure—*constrictive pericarditis.*
C. Characteristic feature—septal bounce—a shuttering motion of the septum during diastole—*constrictive pericarditis*
D. Right ventricular volume overload, paradoxical septal motion, diastolic fluttering of inter ventricular septum, right atrial enlargement, systolic turbulence in right atrium—*Tricuspid regurgitation*

   Liver biopsy: To diagnose—chronic liver disease

   Renal biopsy: To diagnose cause of nephritic syndrome

   Portal venography: To diagnose—venous outflow tract obstruction in suspected:

   - Budd-Chiari syndrome
   - Veno-occlusive disease

Algorithm

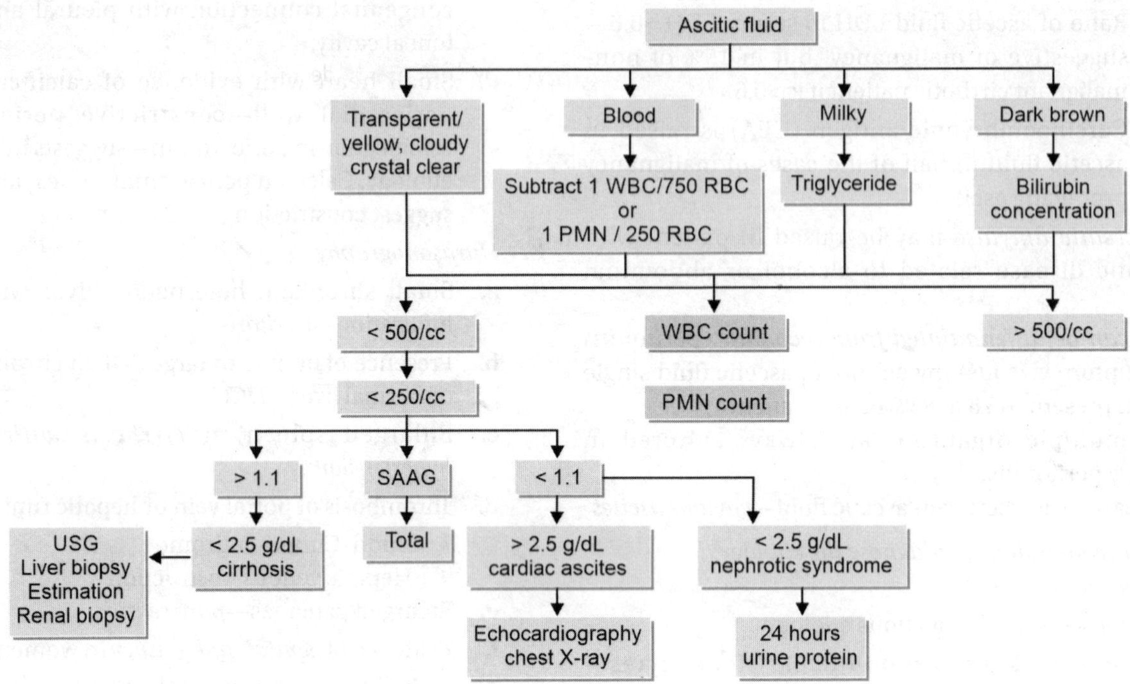

WBC count

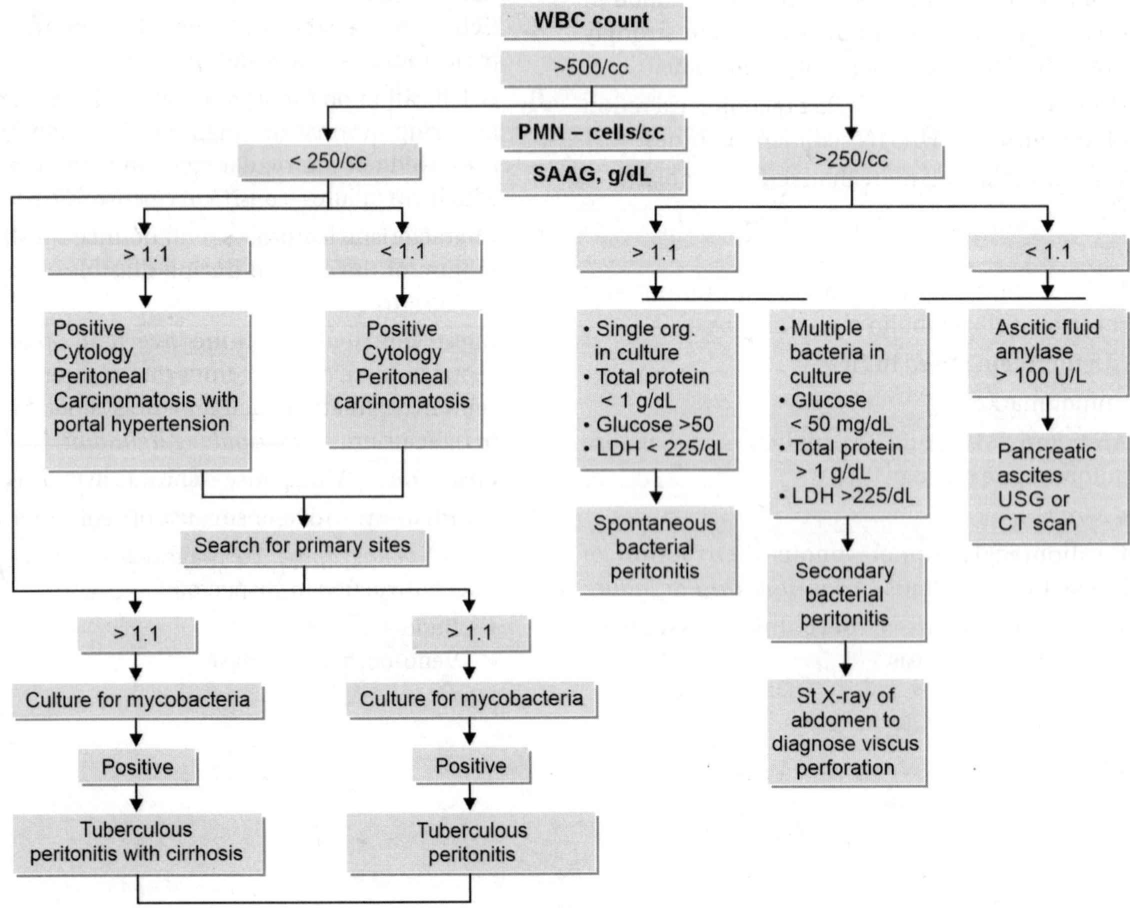

Management of ascites:

Method	Intervention	Indications	Clinical implications
General measures	• Dietary sodium restriction to ≤ 2 g/day • If serum sodium is <125 mEq/L, fluid restriction • If there is history of alcohol addiction, it should be stopped	In case of any patient with ascites	It will decrease the fluid accumulation. It will increase the response to diuretics
Administration of diuretics	• Furosemide 40–160 mg/day • Spironolactone 100–400 mg/day	In case of diuretics responsive ascites	• The aim is to reduce the body weight to 0.5 g/day in absence of edema • Reduction of body weight to 1 kg/day in case of ascites • Electrolyte level monitoring should be done
Large volume paracentesis	Under cover of 20% salt poor albumin intravenous infusion, 3 to 4 L of free fluid can be drained	• Refractory ascites • Tense ascites	• Albumin prevents post drain hypotension • It will reduce the abdominal pressure
Spontaneous bacterial peritonitis	• Intravenous 2 g cefotaxime 8 hourly or 2 g ceftriaxone intravenously twice daily • Infusion of albumin if serum creatinine more than 1 mg/dL or blood urea nitrogen is >30 mg/dL or total bilirubin >30 mg/dL • Secondary prophylactic treatment is 400 mg daily oral norfloxacin	If Ascitic fluid neutrophil is ≥ 250/cc	It will decrease the acute kidney injury or mortality
Refractory ascites	• Diuretics along with α-agonist Midodrine • Transjugular intrahepatic porto-systemic shunt • Transplantation of liver if diuretics fail	Diuretic resistant ascites	TIPS can increase the chance of hepatic encephalopathy
Secondary ascites	• In case of tubercular ascites—anti-tubercular treatment • In case of malignant ascites—palliative chemotherapy. In case of chylous ascites—Modification of diet with octreotide	Non cirrhotic ascites	Underlying ascites should be screened
Nutrition	• Protein intake adequate • Monitoring for hyponatremia, renal function	In all ascites	Prevent sarcopenia

Q43. Jaundice in pregnancy.

DNB (DEC2019) (5)

Jaundice in pregnancy.

SARDAR PATEL UNIVERSITY, 2019 (10)

ANSWER

Causes of Jaundice in Pregnancy

A. Pregnancy related causes:

a. Benign intrahepatic cholestasis in pregnancy:

- It is most common disorder
- It occurs due to impaired flow of bile secondary to genetic and hormonal factors.
- There is evidence of pruritus, conjugated hyperbilirubinemia, and increased concentration of bile acids.
- Fatal complications like stillbirth, or preterm birth may occur.

b. HELLP syndrome:

- In case of severe preeclampsia the liver may be affected.
- There is history of right upper abdominal pain, jaundice, nausea and vomiting and thrombocytopenia.

- Increased incidence of maternal and fetal mortality.

c. Acute fatty liver in pregnancy:
- It occurs due to defective oxidation of fatty acids.
- There are evidences of coagulopathy, hypoglycemia, jaundice and multiorgan failure.
- It is very dreadful condition requiring early delivery of the baby.

B. Pregnancy unrelated causes:
a. Viral hepatitis due to hepatitis A, B, C, D and E.
b. Cholecystolithiasis and choledecholitiasis due to estrogen mediated supersaturation of bile acids.
c. Hemolytic anemia
d. Following drugs may induce liver injury:
- Anti-tuberculous drugs
- Antiretroviral drugs

e. Autoimmune hepatitis
f. Chronic liver disease

Q44. Congenital hyperbilirubinemia.

MGR UNI, TAMIL NADU, 2022 (5)

Gilbert syndrom.

BHARATI VIDYAPEETH, JHELUM 2018 (10)

ANSWER

Unconjugated Hyperbilirubinemia

A. Gilbert syndrome:
a. It is autosomal recessive disorder commonly associated with homozygous polymorphism of A(TA)7TAA in the promotor region of Uridine diphosphoglucuronate glucuronosyltransferase (UDPT1A1) leading to significant reduction in the glucuronidation of bilirubin.
b. Only homozygous with the promotor region when associated with the other factors sex factor will develop Gilbert syndrome.
c. This disease develop in adolescence with male preponderance (3:1) as compared to female.
d. There is increased incidence of pigment gall stones.
e. Liver enzymes are normal only bilirubin content is up to 5 mg/dL.
f. Following drugs are responsible for developing this disease are:
- NSAIDs
- Statin
- Acetaminophen
- Tyrosine kinase inhibitors
- Oxazepam
- Lorazepam
- Cyclosporine A
- Menthol
- Tocilizumab

g. Serum unconjugated bilirubin is less than 4 mg/dL. Complete blood count, reticulocyte count, serum LDH do not support hemolysis. Ultrasonography of liver will be normal.
h. Prolonged 72 hours fasting or administration of rifampin, phenobarbital nicotinic acid will lead to increase in the level of serum bilirubin.
i. Treatment is symptomatic. No drugs are required. But provocative medication should not be given.

B. Crigler-Najjar syndrome—It has been discussed in question number 40.

Conjugated Bilirubinemia

A. Dubin Johnson syndrome:
a. It is autosomal recessive disorder resulting from mutation of ATP binding cassette subfamily C member (*ABCC2*) gene.
b. There is defect in the MRP2 protein i.e., multiple resistance protein 2.
c. Classic feature is reversal of the ratio of the by product which will be generated during synthesis of heme i.e., level of urinary coproporphyrin 1 is increased as compared to coproporphyrin III.
d. This rare disease manifests in adolescence or early adulthood.

e. May present with upper abdominal pain, jaundice bot never develop pruritus because serum bile acid will be normal.

f. Serum bilirubin level is usually 2–5 mg/dL, but rarely >25 mg/dL. But liver enzymes, LDH, complete blood count reticulocyte count will be within the normal limit.

g. Usually no treatment is required.

B. Rotor syndrome:

a. It is rare type of autosomal recessive disorder due to homozygous mutation of both SLCO1B1 and SLCO1B3 on the chromosome 12 consisting of mixed conjugated and unconjugated hyperbilirubinemia doe to chronically elevated conjugated bilirubin to more than 50% due to impaired storage of conjugated bilirubin that is leaking into bilirubin canaliculi.

b. Absence of dark melanin like pigmentation on liver biopsy which is present in Dubin–Johnson syndrome.

c. Asymptomatic patient with generalized non-pruritic jaundice presenting from birth or early childhood.

d. Mild jaundice from yellow orange tinge in the skin or sclera and mucous membrane under the tongue.

e. Analysis of urine coproporphyrin can distinguish Dubin–Johnson syndrome from Rotor syndrome which demonstrates ratio of urine coproporphyrin 1 and 3 is high in both these conditions but amount of coproporphyrin 1 is more that 90% in Dubin–John syndrome and less in Rotor syndrome.

f. Plasma level of bromosulfophthalein after its injection will be delayed with absence of secondary rise is not present in this Rotor syndrome which will be present in Dubin–Johnson syndrome.

g. Treatment is not required as this jaundice will remain life-long.

Q45. Write briefly about the hepatic segments. Write briefly about the liver function test.

DR YSR UNI OF HEALTH SC, VIJAYAWADA, ANDHRA, 2022 (10)

Liver function evaluation has been describe in question number 9.

ANSWER

Hepatic Segments

A. Segment I—caudate lobe.

a. It is bounded posteriorly by fossa of inferior vena cava, anteriorly by ligamentum venosum, inferiorly by porta hepatis.

b. Blood supply from both right and left portal veins.

c. It drains directly to inferior vena cava.

B. Segment II and III—both are left to left hepatic vein and falciform ligament, but segment II is superior to portal plane and segment III is inferior to portal plane.

C. Segment IV:

a. It is present in between the left and middle hepatic vein.

b. It is subdivided into superior and inferior subsegments:
- 4a is above the portal plane
- 4b is below the portal plane.

c. It is quadrate lobe.

D. Segment V: It is in between middle and right hepatic vein and below the portal plane.

E. Segment VI: It is right to right hepatic vein and below the portal plane.

F. Segment VII: It is right to right hepatic vein and above the portal plane.

G. Segment VIII: It is in between the middle and right hepatic vein and above the portal plane.

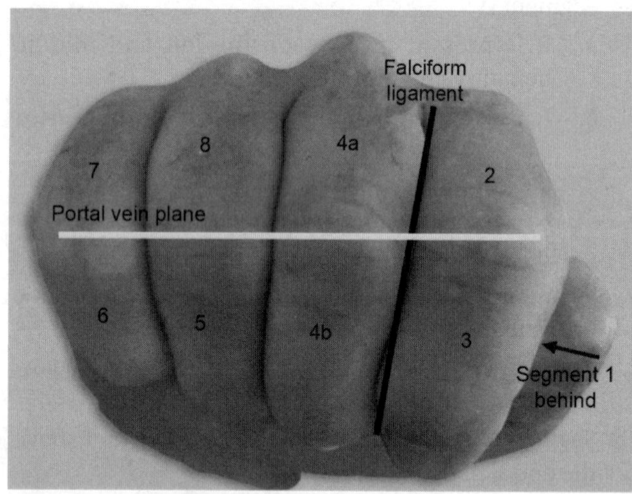

Q46. Hepatitis vaccines.

TEERTHANKER MAHAVEER UNI, 2020 (10)

ANSWER

Hepatitis B Vaccine

This vaccine is the non-infective subunit of the virus that develops active immunity against all the genotypes starting from A to H of this virus. The antibody targets the outer membrane protein or surface antigen.

This vaccine should be given to the following patients having high risk factors and can develop complications from this disease:

A. Persons with high risk for STD
B. Positive hepatitis C patients.
C. Intravenous drug users
D. Incarcerated persons
E. If the sex partners of the patient is hepatitis B positive
F. Persons having positive for HIV
G. If the traveler will go to the HBV endemic countries
H. Homosexuals
I. Dialysis patients
J. Health care workers
K. If household contact is HBsAg positive.
L. Diabetic patient having age between 19 to 59 years.

Administration of this vaccine:

Age	Dose	Volume	Schedule
Dose at birth	5–10 mcg	0.5 mL	0, 1, 6 months
Children and patient less ≤ 19 years	5–10 mcg	0.5 mL	0, 1, 6 months
Adult	10–20 mcg	1 mL	0, 1, 6 months

Continued

Continued

In special cases			
Preterm infant of less than 2 kg	5–10 mcg	0.5 mL	0, 1, 2, 6 months
Healthcare workers	10–20 mcg	1 mL	0, 1, 6 months
Hemodialysis patient	40 mcg	2 mL	0, 1, 2, 6 months
Immunocompromised patients	40 mcg	2 mL	0, 1, 2, 6 months
Post exposure prophylaxis in case of needle stick injury	Hepatitis B immunoglobulin plus standard dose of vaccine		0, 1, 6 months

Contraindications:

A. Any anaphylactic reaction previously to this vaccine

B. Yeast hypersensitivity

Adverse effects:

A. Reaction and pain at the site of injection.

B. Fever

Hepatitis A Vaccine

This vaccine is available in the following forms:

A. Inactivated monovalent hepatitis A vaccine

B. Combination of hepatitis A and B vaccine

Dose schedule:

Patient group	Dose	Volume	Schedule
Children from ≥12 months to 18 years	720 EUSA units	0.5 mL	0, 6–12 months
Adult	1449 EUSA units	1 mL	0, 6, 12 months
Combination of hepatitis A and B vaccine			
Adult ≥18 years	720 EUSA units hepatitis A + 20 mcg hepatitis B	1 mL	0, 1, 6 months Or in accelerated schedule, 0, 7 days, 21 days and 12 months

Q47. Biliary cirrhosis.

RAJIV GANDHI UNI OF HEALTH SCIENCE, KARNATAKA, 2020 (10)

Primary biliary cirrhosis.

TEERTHANKER MAHAVEER UNIVERSITY, 2018 (10)

ANSWER

Definition

Primary biliary cirrhosis, recently known as primary biliary cholangitis is an autoimmune disorder resulting destruction of the intrahepatic biliary canaliculi leading to periportal inflammation which ultimately forms cirrhosis with portal hypertension.

Etiopathogenesis

Main pathophysiology of this disease is the interaction between the genetic factors and the environmental triggers. There is high incidence of incidence in the 1st degree relatives. There are association between the HLA allele with this disease, these are:

A. DRB1

B. DR3

C. DPB1

D. DQA1

E. DQB1

The protective HLA allele against this disease is HLA DRB1*11.

The environmental triggers are the following:

A. Toxic waste

B. Cigarette smoking

C. Hair dye

D. Nail polish

E. Various xenobiotics

- **a.** *Escherichia coli*
- **b.** *Mycobacterium gordonae*
- **c.** *Novosphingobium aromaticivorans*

These environmental factors in the genetically susceptible subjects produce autoimmune reactions against intracytoplasmic antigens presence of highly specific anti-mitochondrial antibody and T lymphocyte involvement in the destruction of biliary canaliculi.

Again, via molecular mimicry bacterial lipolyted protein reacts with cellular lipolyted protein.

Following antibodies are found in this disease:

A. Antimitochondrial antibody found in 85% patients binds with lipoic acid containing E2 component of pyruvate dehydrogenase present in the inner side of the mitochondrial membrane.

B. Antinuclear antibodies

C. Anti-multiple nuclear dot antibodies

D. Anti-centromere antibodies

E. Antinuclear envelope antibodies

Antinuclear antibodies and anti-multiple nuclear dot antibodies are the surrogate markers of this disease in absence of antimitochondrial antibody positivity.

Clinical Symptoms

A. The patient may be asymptomatic—in this case abnormal results of liver function test may be the pointer to the diagnosis.

B. Jaundice—cholestasis

C. Pruritus—it may be due to retained bile salts. According to recent theory, it may be due to increased serum level of lysophosphatidic acid, it is product of circulating phospholipase and autotoxin. Pruritus will be increased at night time and in humid weather.

D. Vague right upper quadrant pain

E. Mild cognitive impairment

Signs are:

A. Dry skin

B. Hyperpigmentation

C. Xanthelasma

D. Xanthoma

E. Jaundice

F. Dermographism

G. At the later stage of the disease hepatomegaly

H. Splenomegaly

I. Stigmata of chronic liver disease

J. Evidences of other autoimmune conditions:
- **a.** Hashimoto thyroiditis
- **b.** CREST syndrome
- **c.** Rheumatoid arthritis
- **d.** Celiac disease
- **e.** Telangiectasia

K. Other diseases associated are:
- **a.** Osteoporosis
- **b.** Renal tubular acidosis
- **c.** Discoid lupus
- **d.** Pemphigoid

Evaluation of this Disease

Diagnostic criteria for this disease includes:

A. Absence of other liver disease

B. No evidence of extra-hepatic biliary obstruction on imaging

C. Associated 2 of the following three:
- **a.** Alkaline phosphatase level is 1.5 times upper limit of normal
- **b.** Presence of anti-mitochondrial antibody in the titer of 1:40
- **c.** Histopathological evidences of primary biliary cirrhosis like "florid duct lesion" and destruction of the interlobular bile ducts surrounded by infiltration of lymphocytes.

Treatment

The goal is to prevent the progression of the disease along with the management of the complications related to cholestasis.

A. Ursodeoxycholic acid: This hydrophilic bile salt stabilizes the membrane of the hepatocytes against the bile salts thereby inhibiting the cellular apoptosis and fibrosis. The recommended dose is 13 to 15 mg/kg/day orally.

B. If the patient is refractory or not responding this Ursodeoxycholic acid, in that case obeticholic acid—it is farnesoid X receptor agonist, due to its antifibrotic and choleretic properties it will reduce the alkaline phosphatase, GGT and transaminases levels.

C. The ultimate goal of treatment in this disease is liver transplantation.

Treatment of the complications of chronic cholestasis:

A. Fat soluble vitamin levels should be checked at regular interval and should be replenished.

B. With the progression of this disease, LDL level increases and HL level decreases, so statin should be administered

C. Cholestyramine, naltrexone, UDCA can be given to reduce pruritus.

D. Proper cause of steatorrhea should be evaluated as this disease may be associated with celiac disease and should be treated accordingly.

Complications in this disease:

A. Osteoporosis

B. Malabsorption

C. Hyperlipidemia

D. Renal tubular acidosis

E. Liver cancer

F. Esophageal motility disorder

G. Hypoglycemia

H. Autoimmune thrombocytopenia

I. Myelopathy

Q48. Paraneoplastic manifestations in case of hepatocellular carcinoma.

KERALA UNIVERSITY, 2020 (10)

ANSWER

A. *Endocrinological manifestations:*
   a. Excessive production of insulin like growth factor-1 by the tumor cells leading to hypoglycemia.
   b. Excessive production of erythropoietin like substances leading to polycythemia.
   c. Due to ectopic production of parathyroid hormone related protein there is evidence of hypercalcemia.

B. *Rheumatological manifestations:*
   a. Dermatomyositis and polymyositis
   b. Hand-foot syndrome

C. *Neurological manifestation:*
   a. Myasthenia gravis
   b. Eton-Lambert syndrome
   c. Due to hyperammonemia and increased production of cytokines paraneoplastic encephalopathy

D. *Hematological manifestations:*
   a. Due to increased thrombopoietin production from the tumor, there is thrombocytosis.
   b. As a result of increased procoagulant activity of the tumor cells disseminated intravascular coagulation

E. *Metabolic manifestations*:
   a. Immune complex glomerulopathies
   b. Hypercholesterolemia

Q49. Refractory ascites.

NTR UNI OF HEALTH SCIENCE, VIJAYAWADA, 2020 (10)

ANSWER

Definition

It can be defined as the recurrent accumulation of free fluid in the peritoneal cavity shortly after therapeutic paracentesis in spite of strict restriction of sodium and treatment with diuretics.

Causes of Refractory Ascites

Diagnostic Criteria of Refractory Ascites

A. Lack of response to maximal dose of diuretic for at least 1 week.
B. Diuretic induced complications in the absence of other precipitating factors
C. Early recurrence of ascites within 4 weeks of fluid mobilization
D. Persistent ascites despite sodium restriction
E. Mean weight loss of <0.8 kg over 4 days.
F. Excretion of urinary sodium less than intake of sodium.

Pathophysiology

There are three theories relating to the formation of refractory ascites. These are:

A. Overflow theory: According to this theory, expansion of the extracellular volume is due to
   a. Increased sodium reabsorption from the proximal and distal tubules.
   b. Activation of the renin-angiotensin-aldosterone system
   c. Activation of the sympathetic nervous system

B. Underflow theory: According to this theory, splanchnic vasodilatation due to increased portal pressure in the background of portal hypertension leading to splanchnic vasodilatation resulting
   a. Accumulation of fluid in the peritoneal cavity.
   b. Decrease in the arterial blood volume
   c. Activation of the baroreceptors

   Above result lead to:
   a. Activate central nervous system causing vasoconstriction of the arteries
   b. Activation of RAAS

   The end result is retention of sodium.

Clinical Features

A. Progressive distention of the abdomen
B. In spite of administration of diuretics, there is weight gain.
C. As the abdominal fluid increases there is shortness of breath mainly in lying down position which can be relieved by sitting down position
D. Pedal edema
E. Pleural effusion
F. Features of hepatocellular failure
G. Signs of secondary infection like spontaneous bacterial peritonitis.

Laboratory Diagnosis

A. Analysis of ascitic fluid:
   a. Serum ascitic albumin gradient:
      - If it is ≥ 1.1 g/dL—cirrhosis, Budd-Chiari syndrome, chronic heart failure

- If it is ≤ 1.1 g/dL—tuberculosis, nephrotic syndrome, malignancy

b. Total protein:
- If it is less than 2.5—cirrhosis related ascites
- If it is more than 2.5—Malignancy, tuberculosis, chronic heart failure

c. Neutrophil count—if it is ≥ 250/cc—subacute bacterial peritonitis

B. Blood investigations:

a. Liver function test
b. Blood urea, creatinine
c. Serum electrolytes
d. Complete blood count—leukocytosis—subacute bacterial peritonitis

Treatment: Treatment should be as per decompensated cirrhosis, subacute bacterial peritonitis.

Q50. Diagnostic criteria of acute on chronic liver failure.

KERALA UNIVERSITY, 2019 (10)

ANSWER

EASL-CLIF Criteria

Acute on chronic liver failure is diagnosed when organ failure will be started in patient suffering from acute decompensated cirrhosis. Severity can be classified based on the number of organ failure:

A. ACLF-1: Single organ failure with renal dysfunction or non-renal organ failure with high level of serum lactate.

B. ACLF-2: Failure of 2 organs

C. ACLF-3: There are evidences of 3 or more organ failure.

Mortality is high 28 days varies with the severity.

APASL Criteria

It is characterized by acute hepatic insult (jaundice with encephalopathy) in a patient suffering from chronic liver disease leading to high mortality due to hepatic failure.

Diagnostic criteria:

A. Acute insult to the liver by the drugs, infections or alcohol

B. Bilirubin ≥ 5 mg/dL

C. INR ≥ 1.5 or prolonged prothrombin time.

D. Any grade of hepatic encephalopathy

E. Presence or absence of ascites

Presence of cirrhosis is not essential as it may occur in case of chronic liver disease.

Q51. Serum Ascites Albumin gradient.

BABA FARID UNI OF HEALTH SC, 2019 (10)

ANSWER

This gradient determine the cause of ascites and can differentiate ascites related to portal and non-portal hypertension.

Calculation of this gradient: (Serum albumin—Ascitic fluid albumin)

Interpretation of results:

A. If ≥ 1.1 - Portal hypertension - Causes are:

a. Cirrhosis
b. Alcoholic cirrhosis
c. Budd-Chiari syndrome
d. NAFLD
e. Heart failure
f. Portal vein thrombosis

B. If ≤ 1.1—Non-portal hypertension - peritoneal Causes

a. Tuberculosis
b. Malignancy
c. Nephrotic syndrome
d. Pancreatic ascites

Advantages:

A. It is more accurate as compared to total protein as it can determine the etiology

B. It is cost effective

C. It can be easily interpreted

Q52. A 38 years old male presented with pain right upper abdomen with fever and chills for last 1 week. On examination, tender hepatomegaly and pleural rub on right side infra-axillary and infra-mammary area was present.

Reason out the differential diagnosis and investigations to reach the diagnosis and management of this patient.

SRI GURU RAM DAS UNI OF HEALTH SC, AMRITSAR, 2022 (10)

ANSWER

The differential diagnosis are:

A. Acute viral hepatitis
B. Amebic liver abscess
C. Acute alcoholic hepatitis
D. Right sided empyema

All the diseases are described in this Hepatology chapter. You should write accordingly.

Q53. Write short notes on sarcopenic obesity.

MAHATMA UNIVERSITY, 2022 (10)

ANSWER

Definition

Sarcopenic obesity can be defined as loss of loss of skeletal muscle mass ad function in the face of increased content of fat seen in the elderly and metabolically unhealthy people.

Etiology

A. In case aging due to natural loss of gradual loss of anabolic hormones growth hormone, insulin like growth factor-1, testosterone and estrogen.
B. Development of chronic inflammation leading to loss of muscle mass ad insulin resistance due to increased level of cytokines like interleukin-6 and TNF-α.
C. Inadequate intake of protein and micronutrients leading to loss of muscle mass.
D. Decreased physical activity leading to loss of muscle mass along with increased fat content.
E. Obesity and altered metabolism lead to
  a. Insulin resistance
  b. Imbalance of adipokines
  c. Deposition of ectopic fat
F. Endocrine disorders:
  a. Cushing's syndrome
  b. Diabetes mellitus
  c. Hypothyroidism

Pathophysiology

A. There is fat infiltration of the muscles leading decrease in the quality and strength of the skeletal muscle mass.
B. There is reduced synthesis of the protein in the muscle in spite of increased protein intake due to anabolic resistance.
C. There is presence of low grade inflammation in the muscles.
D. Insulin resistance leads to decreased uptake of glucose and reduced synthesis of protein.

Clinical Features

A. Muscle weakness leading to reduced grip strength, decreased ability
B. Features of diabetes mellitus
C. Features of metabolic syndrome
D. Increased risk of falls and frailty.

Evaluations

A. Muscle mass can be measured by:
  a. Dual energy X-ray absorptiometry
  b. Bioelectrical impedance analysis
B. Muscle strength can be measured by:
  a. Handgrip dynamometry
    - Less than 27 kg in case of men
    - Less than 16 kg for women
C. Physical performance:
  a. Gait speed: Less than 0.8 m/s
  b. Short physical performance battery
D. Assessment of obesity:
  a. BMI: Less than 30 k/m^2
  b. Waist circumference:
    - More than 102 cm for men
    - More than 88 cm for women

Treatment

A. Resistance exercise at a rate of 2–3 times/week to improve muscle mass and muscle strength.
B. Aerobic exercise weekly to steady weight loss and improve cardiometabolic health.
C. Protein content at 1.2–1.5 g/kg/day—it includes increased leucine containing diet.
D. Vitamin D supplementation to improve to function of the muscles.
E. Pharmacological agents like myosin inhibitors, testosterone.
F. Management of comorbidities.

Q54. Elaborate on the clinical perspective of the national viral hepatitis program.

WBUHS, 2025 (10)

ANSWER

According to WHO, in 2015, 1.34 million death occurred due to viral hepatitis which is comparable to tuberculosis, Worldwide.

40 million death due to hepatitis B
6–12 million deaths due to hepatitis C.

Aim

A. Combat hepatitis and achieve country-wise elimination of Hepatitis C by 2030.

B. Achieve significant reduction in the number of infected population, morbidity, mortality associated with hepatitis B and C viz. Cirrhosis and hepatocellular carcinoma.

C. Reduce the risk, morbidity, mortality due to hepatitis A and E.

Key Objectives

1. Enhance community awareness of hepatitis and lay stress on preventive measures among general especially high risk groups and hospitals.
2. Provide early diagnosis and treatment of viral hepatitis at all the levels of health care.
3. Develop standard diagnostic and treatment protocols for the management of viral hepatitis and its complications.
4. Strengthen infrastructural facilities, building capacities of existing human resources, where required for providing comprehensive services for the management of viral hepatitis and its complications I all the districts of the country.
5. Develop linkage with the National program towards awareness, prevention, diagnosis & treatment of viral hepatitis.
6. Develop a Web based "Viral hepatitis information and management system" to maintain a registry of persons affected with viral hepatitis and its sequelae.

Component of the Program

A. Preventive component which is the cornerstone of National Viral hepatitis Control Program, it includes:
   - **a.** Generation of awareness
   - **b.** Immunization of hepatitis B to high risk groups, children and healthcare workers.
   - **c.** Safety blood and blood products
   - **d.** Safety of injection
   - **e.** Safe socio-cultural practices.
   - **f.** Safe drinking water, hygiene and use of safe sanitary toilets.

Diagnosis and Treatment

A. Screening of the pregnant woman for HBsAg to be done in areas where Institutional deliveries are <80% to ensure their referral for Institutional delivery for birth dose of hepatitis B vaccination.

B. Free screening, diagnosis and treatment for both hepatitis B and C would be made available at all levels of health care in a phased manner.

C. Provision of linkages, including with the private sector and not for profit Institutions for diagnosis and treatment.

D. Engagement with community/peer support to enhance and ensure adherence to treatment and demand generation.

Monitoring and Evaluation

A. Surveillance and Research Effective linkages to the surveillance system would be established and operational research would be undertaken through the department of health research.

B. Standard framework would be developed and an online web based system established.

Training and Capacity Building

A. This would be a continuous process and will be supported by national centre of disease control, ILBS and State tertiary care Institute and coordinated by NVHCP.

B. The Hepatitis induction and update program for all levels of health care worker would be made available using both, the traditional cascade model of training through the master trainers and variable platform available for enabling electronic, e-learning and e-courses.

C. *The purpose of this control program is to educate the health care practitioner and the public about the importance of vaccination against hepatitis A and B and the importance of testing and treatment of hepatitis B and C.*

Two ways to prevent hepatitis are:

- Ensuring good hygiene
- Avoidance of contact with the body fluids of the diseased person.

In New Delhi, Hepatitis awareness month 2024,

- Annual Awareness day held in May to raise awareness about viral hepatitis and its impact in the individual, communities and health care system.

There are 3 units:

1. National viral hepatitis management unit
2. State viral hepatitis management unit
3. District viral management unit

National Action Plan Combating Viral Hepatitis in India

- Target viruses are B and C
- Location: India
- WHO region: South East Asia
- Geographical level: Country
- Source: Ministry of Health & Family welfare Government in India
- Year of viral elimination: 2030
- Published: 2019

Following are the hindrances towards reaching the goal of National Viral Hepatitis Control Program in INDIA:

A. *Limited awareness and stigma*:

a. Many people are unaware about the hepatitis types, routes of transmissions and treatment

b. Social stigma deter the people from doing investigations and treatment.

c. In some case people is confused with the HIV due to overlapping risk factors.

B. *Inadequate screening and diagnosis*:

a. Poor access to the diagnostic services mainly in the rural and underserved areas.

b. Lack of routine screening in the high risk groups mainly in pregnant and IV drug users.

C. *Weak health infrastructure*:

a. Inconsistent supply of the antiviral drugs, diagnostic kits and trained personnel.

b. Limited lab capacity for confirmatory testing like viral load and genotyping.

D. *Financial constraints*:

a. Limited Government funding for sustained awareness, diagnostics and treatment.

b. Out-of-pocket expenses are still high despite the program being free in public settings.

E. *Lack of data and surveillance*:

a. Poor data surveillance system results in underreporting and incomplete epidemiological data.

b. Difficult to track outcomes or measure the program impact without robust monitoring.

F. *Vaccine hesitancy and coverage issue*:

a. Low uptake of hepatitis B vaccine in the remote village areas and in unaware people.

b. Missed opportunities for catch-up vaccination in adults or in high risk groups.

G. *Policy and operational gaps*:

a. Delay in decentralizing the services in primary health care.

b. Inconsistent training and motivation of the health care workers on hospital protocols.

With Special Reference to Hepatitis C Viruses

A. Asymptomatic nature of early infection:

a. HCV causes no symptoms until advanced liver disease sets in leading to underdiagnosis due to late diagnosis thereby reducing the opportunity of early treatment.

B. Limited awareness and health literacy:

a. Many people are unaware of transmission route like blood transfusion, unsafe injection, tattoo and IV drug users.

b. In rural and underdeveloped areas, there is misconception regarding its curability.

C. There is risk of reinfection among the people who inject drugs or are in prison settings, so it is common if the harm in the reduction measures are weak or absent.

D. In case of older person, who received blood transfusion before screening HCV or dialysis patient who are on routine dialysis in any machine are supposed to become HCV positive in future.

Section 2 Hematology

Q1. Etiological factors, pathophysiology, laboratory findings, and treatment of disseminated intravascular coagulation (DIC).

DNBI/JUN2010 (10)

Define DIC. Enumerate the causes of DIC and discuss the clinical approach to its management.

DNBI/DEC2012 (10)

Management of DIC.

RGUHS/MDIV (10)

Causes and management of DIC.

MGR/APR2012/MDIII (7)

Diagnostic criteria and management of disseminated intravascular coagulation.

DNB 2022 (5)

Describe etiopathogenesis of DIC.

NTR UNI of Health SXC, Vijayawada, Andhra, 2022 (10)

Causes and management of disseminated intravascular coagulation.

NTR UNI of Health SC Vijayawada, Andhra, 2022 (10)

Describe the coagulation mechanism in human being. Describe etiopathogenesis, clinical features, diagnosis, and management of disseminated intravascular coagulation.

WBUHS, 2025 (10)

ANSWER

Coagulation mechanism has been written in question number 32 in this chapter.

Definition

Disseminated intravascular coagulation can be defined as uncontrolled bleeding as a result of activation of coagulation factors due to various underlying systemic disorders. It may be localized or diffuse, acute or chronic, and may be associated with thrombosis or bleeding.

Causes of DIC

Causes	Subetiologies
Tissue damage	Burns, trauma, and head injury
Shock	Cardiogenic
Sepsis	Gram-negative or -positive bacterial, viral, and rickettsial infections
Pregnancy	Abruption previa, retained fetal tissue in uterine cavity (HELLP syndrome), fatty liver of pregnancy, amniotic fluid embolism, and pre-eclampsia
Dysfunction of organ	Acute necrotizing pancreatitis
Fat embolism	Fracture of femur
Malignancy	Adenocarcinoma, acute promyelocytic leukemia (APL), and tumor of brain
Vascular stasis	Abdominal aortic aneurysm
Neonatal causes	Hereditary protein S and C deficiency, necrotizing enterocolitis, and birth asphyxia
Toxic reactions	Snakebite and recreational drugs
Immunological	Transfusion reaction and post-transplant reactions
Other causes	Acute respiratory distress syndrome (ARDS) and near-drowning

Pathophysiology

A. Due to vascular, hypoxic, and cellular injury, there is release of tissue factors.

B. Presence of exogenously and exogenously activated procoagulant molecules such as production of bacterial lipopolysaccharide by neoplastic cells.

The result is inappropriately systemic activation of coagulation thus, consumption of clotting factors and platelets leading to uncontrollable bleeding.

In case of chronic and low-grade DIC used, clotting factors and platelets will be replenished in such a way that features of hypercoagulability may occur. So, there is damage of end organ from hypoperfusion from either hemorrhage or thrombosis.

Clinical Features

A. Features of hemorrhage:
   a. Localized: At the insertion sites, vascular catheters from the surgical insertion sites
   b. Involvement of the organs such as:
      1. Central nervous system (CNS)—hemorrhage
      2. Lung—hemoptysis
      3. Gastrointestinal system—hematemesis, melena, and hematochezia
      4. Urinary system—hematuria
      5. Skin—ecchymoses, bruise, or petechiae. In case of meningococcal infection, there are petechiae in the trunk and extremities known as purpura fulminans
      6. Mucosal bleeding from nose, gum, and mouth

B. Features of thrombosis: Due to tissue hypoxia in different organs:
   a. Heart
   b. Kidney
   c. Liver

Diagnosis

Single test cannot diagnose DIC. Following tests are required to diagnose DIC:

A. Activated partial thromboplastin time (APTT), thrombin clotting time, and prothrombin time (PT) are increased—suggest consumption of clotting factors, fibrinogen.

B. Serum fibrinogen is low—suggests increased consumption of fibrinogen.

C. Serum fibrinogen degradation product—it occurs as a result of cleavage between fibrinogen and fibrin. D-dimer assay can detect the fibrin degradation product (FDP), which has been cross-linked with activated factor XIII.

D. Platelet count—decreased because it will be cleared from the circulation due to activation and aggregation of platelets. But, in case of chronic DIC due to malignancy, platelet count will be increased.

E. Presence of schistocytes in the peripheral blood smear—occurs due to microvascular hemolysis.

F. Factor VIII is elevated in coagulopathy of liver disease.

There is scoring system of the International Society on Thrombosis and Haemostasis (ISTH) for overt DIC.

	Point			
Parameters	**0**	**1**	**2**	**3**
Platelet K/μL	>100	<100	<50	
Elevated FDP	No increase		Moderately increased	Severely increased
Prolonged PT	<3 s	>3 s but <6 s	>6 s	
Fibrinogen	>1 g/dL	<1 g/dL		

If the score ≥5—compatible with overt DIC. In this case, score should be repeated daily.

If the score <5—suggest nonovert DIC. Here, this score has to repeat in 1–2 days.

Treatment

A. Treatment of the causes:
   a. In case of sepsis—antibiotic administration
   b. Repair of the aneurysmal dilatation
   c. Treatment of ARDS
   d. Treatment of malignancy
   e. In case of abortion, removal of conception and placenta
   f. Treatment of other causes

   Blood or blood products should not be administered in acute DIC:
   a. No evidence of significant bleeding
   b. If the risk of bleeding is not so high such as evidence of thrombocytopenia in case of major trauma

B. Platelet transfusion:
   a. If the platelet count is 20,000/cc to 30,000/mL
   b. More than 50,000/cc with evidence of intracranial hemorrhage
   c. Higher count with major surgery

C. Cryoprecipitate: It can be given, if fibrinogen level is <80–100 mg/mL.

D. Fresh frozen plasma: It can be given in case of prolonged PT and APTT.

E. Heparin: It can be given in case of acute DIC where bleeding continues in spite of proper treatment. It is preferred over low-molecular-weight heparin due to its short half-life. Heparin should not be given where:

a. Unless platelet count will be ≥50,000/cc
b. Unless there is no bleeding from CNS and gastro-intestinal tract

Dose of heparin is 6–10 units/kg/h infusion without no bolus dose.

Signs of improvement: Elevation of fibrinogen and platelet.

Contraindications:

a. In case of placental abruption
b. Other obstetrical conditions requiring surgical management

F. Fibrinolytic inhibitor: It can be given:
   a. In case of severe and profuse bleeding who failed to respond to other treatment
   b. Where FDP fails to inhibit platelet

   Risk: There is a risk of thrombosis.

G. Recombinant factor VIIa:
   a. Indication: There is evidence of persistent bleeding in spite of transfusion of blood product
   b. Dose: 20 μg/kg
   c. Risk—thrombosis
   d. Associated conditions: Acidosis, hypothermia, and thrombocytopenia have to be corrected prior to starting of this drug

H. Activated protein C is not at all recommended associated with DIC, but it can be given purpura fulminans, if it is due to homozygous or acquired protein C deficiency.

Monitoring: Every 6 hours in case of acute DIC:

A. Prothrombin time
B. Activated partial thromboplastin time
C. Fibrinogen level
D. Platelet count

Q2. Describe the clinical features, diagnosis, and management of chronic myeloid leukemia (CML).

DNBIII/DEC2013 (10)

Classify chronic MPD. Describe chromosomal findings and treatment of CML.

DNBIIA/DEC2013 (10)

Chronic myeloid leukemia.

MGR/MAR2010/MDI (5)
MGR/MAR2009/MDI (5)

Management of chronic granulocytic leukemia.

MUHS/NOV2013/MDIII (10)

Management of CML.

BF/NOV2012/MDIII (10)

Clinical features, diagnosis, and treatment of CML.

DNB 2019 (10)

Clinical stages of CML and management in each stages.

DR YSR UNI of Health SC, Vijayawada, Andhra, 2022 (10)

Describe etiopathogenesis, clinical features, diagnosis, and management of CML.

Veer Narmad South Gujarat UNI, 2021 (20)

Chronic myeloid leukemia.

MGR University, Tamil Nadu, 2020 (5)

ANSWER

Definition

Chronic myeloid leukemia can be defined as uncontrollable proliferation of all cells of myeloid lineage involving erythroid, granulocytic, and megakaryocytic cells, but not the lymphocytic cells.

Pathophysiology of CML

A. Leukemic transformation starts in multipotent stem cells: There are two hypotheses demonstrate BCR-ABL1 translocation in multipotent cell lineage, except T cells.
   a. According to one hypothesis, these multipotent stem cells cannot differentiate into T cells.
   b. According to other hypothesis, uncontrolled proliferation of BCR-ABL1-positive stem cells leads to massive production and expansion of granulocytic series leading to leukocytosis.

B. Clonal dominance: At the time of diagnosis in bone marrow, there are mixed population of Ph-positive and Ph-negative cells, but with disease progression

BCR-ABL1-positive CML stem cells outnumber the normal population because of autocrine production as well as less requirement of growth factor by these cells.

C. Molecular basis of CML: BCR-ABL1, an oncoprotein activates tyrosine kinase, which phosphorylates different intermediate molecules in the following pathways leading to development of leukemic phenotype:

   a. Cell proliferation
   b. Cell maturation
   c. Development of resistance to apoptosis
   d. Cell adhesion

D. Genomic instability: CML usually starts as benign disorder, but evolves into accelerated phase where it is very difficult to control along with abnormalities of additional chromosomes. Ultimately, it enters into blast phase where it will be transformed into acute myeloid leukemia or B myelocytic leukemia.

Clinical Features

About 30% of patients are asymptomatic and they can be diagnosed after complete blood picture. Other patients may present with:

A. Lassitude, fatigue, weight loss, and night sweat
B. Early satiety due to massive splenomegaly
C. Left hypochondrial pain due to recurrent splenic infarction
D. Symptoms of granulocyte dysfunction—bacterial or fungal infection, but it is rare as the function of neutrophil is usually preserved
E. Symptoms of platelet dysfunction—subcutaneous or submucosal bleeding and thrombosis
F. Present with leukostatic manifestations:

   a. Vaso-occlusive diseases
   b. Cerebrovascular accident
   c. Venous thrombosis
   d. Myocardial infarction
   e. Priapism
   f. Visual disturbances
   g. Pulmonary infarction

G. Progressive and massive splenomegaly
H. Mild hepatomegaly
I. Course of chronic phase varies:

   a. Few patients enter into accelerated or blast phase within months after diagnosis.
   b. Some patients may take a decade to progress to next phase.
   c. Some patients may be in accelerated phase during presentation. In this case, it is very important to distinguish between Ph-positive acute myeloid leukemia (AML) and Ph-negative AML because treatment schedule is different.

Progression to accelerated phase or blast phase is characterized by:

A. Significant weight loss
B. Joint pain, bleeding, thrombosis, and infection
C. Secondary to histamine release—pruritus, diarrhea, and flushing
D. Persistent splenomegaly in spite of continued therapy
E. Chloroma
F. Bruising or petechiae

Diagnosis

A. Complete hemogram:

   a. More than 30×10^9/L to 300×10^9/L, occasionally 700×10^9/L.
   b. Predominantly mature and immature granulocytes.
   c. Basophilia often exceeding 1×10^9/L, occasionally eosinophilia.
   d. There is leftward shift of <5% blast cells—these are myelocytes, metamyelocytes, and band forms, occasionally nucleated red blood cells (RBCs).
   e. Platelet count is normal or elevated, but sometimes giant form of platelets is also seen.
   f. Normochromic and normocytic anemia
   g. Decreased erythrocyte sedimentation rate (ESR) in absence of infection

B. Biochemistry:

   a. Neutrophil alkaline phosphatase (ALP) is low.
   b. Lactate dehydrogenase (LDH) and uric acid levels are increased. Histamine level is increased due to basophilia.

C. Bone marrow trephine biopsy:

   a. It is hypercellular with complete effacement of fat spaces.
   b. Hyperplasia of neutrophil, eosinophil, and basophil series.
   c. Megakaryocytes are normal or increased in number.
   d. Sea-blue histiocytes are seen.
   e. Blast cells are <10% in chronic phase, 10–19% in accelerated phase, and >20% in blast phase.
   f. It assesses fibrosis in marrow stained by reticulin.

D. Chromosomal analysis:

  a. There is evidence of translocation of t(9;22)(q34;q11).

  b. Other variants are: there is translocation of chromosome numbers 9, 22, 11, and 19.

  c. Duplication of Ph chromosome indicates very advanced stage.

  d. Fluorescence in situ hybridization (FISH) technique can detect Ph chromosome directly in blood and bone marrow because it does not depend upon dividing cells.

E. Molecular diagnosis: About 95% of CML patients are Ph positive, only 5% patients are Ph negative cryptically, in that case BCR-ABL1 may be positive by polymerase chain reaction (PCR).

Accelerated phase of CML can be defined as one or more of the following:

A. Progressively increasing anemia

B. Cytogenetic clonal evolution

C. Bone marrow and peripheral blood cells >10–19%

D. Peripheral basophil ≥20%

E. Platelet count <100,000/cc

F. Progressively increasing organomegaly

G. Leukocytosis, basophilia, thrombocytosis, or thrombocytopenia in patient controlled by therapy

H. Myelofibrosis with tear drop cells in blood smear and increased bone marrow fibrosis

Blast phase of CML can be characterized by following:

A. Features of acute leukemia

B. Bone marrow blast cells >20%

C. Hypersegmented neutrophil may appear

D. Cytochemical and immunologic features

E. Blast cells can be classified as myeloid, erythroid, or undifferentiated cells

Prognosis

A. Sokal score: It is based on spleen size, age, platelet count, and percentage of blast cells in the blood. It can identify patient's prognosis.

  a. Low risk <0.8

  b. Intermediate risk 0.8–1.2

  c. High risk >1.2

B. Based on interferon-alpha treatment, Ashford calculation has been developed. It demonstrates the effect of basophilia and eosinophilia during diagnosis with above Sokal score.

Treatment

Initial treatment aims at: (1) Reduction of disease bulk; and (2) Obtaining hematological remission.

Subsequent treatment aims to cure residual minimal disease.

Monitoring the Response of Treatment

A. Hematologic response:

  a. Every 2 weeks complete blood count (CBC) until complete response.

  b. Then, maintenance of this response in subsequent occasions.

B. Cytogenetic response:

  a. Every 6 months bone marrow aspiration for analysis of at least 20 metaphases for Ph chromosome. 0% means complete response indicating prolonged remission.

  b. Two successive demonstrations at 12 months apart for similar response are required.

C. Major molecular response: Every 3 months quantitative PCR estimation of BCR-ABL1 transcripts. Reduction of transcripts by ≥3 logs below the standardized value indicates major molecular response.

Choice of Therapy

Tyrosine kinase inhibitor—imatinib—400–600 mg/day in chronic phase. It signals transduction inhibitor having target BCR-ABL1 fusion gene and other tyrosine kinase.

Response

(1) 96% hematological response, (2) 87% major cytogenetic response, (3) 76% complete cytogenetic response, and (4) 50% major molecular response.

Side Effects

Edema, nausea, rash, cramps, fatigue, diarrhea, headache, and abnormal liver function test (LFT).

Caution

A. Granulocyte-stimulating factor to maintain neutrophil count to >1,000/cc.

B. If platelet count <50,000/cc, administer platelet or dose of imatinib should be reduced.

C. In case of anemia, imatinib dose should be reduced or stopped and erythropoietin (EPO) can be added.

D. In case of disturbed LFT, imatinib dose should be reduced or stopped.

E. In case of rash, administration of topical or systemic corticosteroid should be reduced or stopped.

In case of intolerance or resistance to imatinib, second drugs of choice are dasatinib 100 mg/day orally and nilotinib 400 mg/twice daily.

Here, food restriction is required before and after administration of these drugs.

Complications are: (1) Pleural effusion in dasatinib; and (2) Sudden death in case of nilotinib.

Suboptimal Response

- **A.** Clonal cytogenetic abnormalities having Ph-positive chromosome
- **B.** In 3 months less than partial cytogenetic response
- **C.** In 3 months BCR-ABL1 >10%
- **D.** No major molecular response in last 12 months
- **E.** In 6 months BCR-ABL1 1–10%
- **F.** No evidence of complete cytogenetic response in 6 months

Failure of Response

- **A.** No hematologic response in last 3 months
- **B.** No cytogenetic response in last 6 months
- **C.** BCR-ABL1 is >1% in last 12 months
- **D.** BCR-ABL1 is >10% in last 6 months
- **E.** No complete cytogenetic response (absence of Ph) in last 12 months
- **F.** No cytogenetic response (Ph > 95%) in last 3 months
- **G.** Evolvement of tyrosine kinase inhibitor-resistant mutations

Other drugs are:
Hydroxycarbamide—It is used in elderly. Effects are:

- **A.** It controls leukocytosis and thrombocytosis
- **B.** It will normalize full blood count
- **C.** In chronic phase, it reduces the size of spleen

Side effects are rash, mouth ulcers, and diarrhea.

Dose is 1–1.5 g once daily.

Interferon: Dose is 3 million units subcutaneously thrice weekly.

Side effects are malaise, febrile reaction, anorexia, and weight loss.

Allopurinol: 300 mg daily orally to prevent tumor lysis syndrome.

Hydroxyurea: 1–2 mg daily orally in patients with high leukocyte count 100,000/cc along with massive splenomegaly.

Treatment of Accelerated Phase

- **A.** Imatinib—600–800 mg/day
- **B.** Allogeneic stem cell transplantation from fully- or partially-matched sibling donors
- **C.** In case of imatinib-resistant cases, dasatinib and nilotinib can be given
- **D.** Alternatively, interferon-alpha subcutaneously in combination with cytosine arabinoside can achieve disease control

Treatment of Blast Crisis

- **A.** Small proportion of patients responds to 600–800 mg imatinib daily. But, duration of response is <10 months. So, stem cell transplantation should be advisable.
- **B.** In case of imatinib-refractory patients, dasatinib or nilotinib may be given.

In Case of Blast Crisis of AML Type

- **A.** Daunorubicin 50 mg/m^2 for 2–3 days
- **B.** Cytosine arabinoside 200 mg/m^2 for 5–7 days

For ALL Types of Blast Crisis of Acute Lymphoblastic Leukemia (ALL) Type

- **A.** Prednisolone
- **B.** Vincristine
- **C.** Daunorubicin

In case of leukostasis—it suggests that leukocyte count is >300,000/cc. Treatment is:

- **A.** Large-volume apheresis to lower the leukocyte count. It should be associated with:
  - **a.** High-dose hydroxyurea up to 4 mg/day
  - **b.** Cytosine arabinoside along with allopurinol
- **B.** Adequate hydration is required
- **C.** Imatinib can be started in low dose, once leukocyte will be under control

Allogeneic Stem Cell Transplantation

- **A.** Stem cell transplantation from human leukocyte antigen (HLA)-matched sibling donor is the treatment of choice <45 years.
- **B.** Treatment-related mortality is 20%.
- **C.** Disease-free survival:
  - **a.** In case of early phase of CML—50%
  - **b.** In case of late phase of CML—20%

Q3. Define bone marrow failure syndrome. Describe its management.

DNBI/DEC2010 (10)

Differential diagnosis of pancytopenia. Outline the clinical features and treatment of aplastic anemia.

DNBIIA/JUN2016 (10)

Describe the etiology, clinical features, diagnosis, and management of aplastic anemia.

MGR/SEP2009/MDII (20)

Bone marrow failure.

MGR/MAR2010/MDIV (6)

Management of aplastic anemia.

BF/MAY2013/MDII (10)

BF/MAY2012/MDIII (10)

Aplastic anemia.

KUHS/MAY2013/MDIII (10)

Define aplastic anemia. Discuss its pathophysiology and treatment.

DNBIIIA/DEC2013 (10)

Differential diagnosis and investigation of pancytopenia.

KUHS/MAY2013/MDI (10)

How would you manage a patient with aplastic anemia?

MGR/APR2013/MDII (7)

Discuss the etiopathogenesis, clinical features, diagnosis, and management of a patient presenting with pancytopenia.

MGM UNI Tamil Nadu, 2022 (15)

Diagnosis and treatment of aplastic anemia.

DR YSR UNI of Health SC, Vijayawada, Andhra, 2022 (10)

Approach to pancytopenia.

NTR UNI of Health SC, Vijayawada, 2021 (10)

ANSWER

Definition

Bone marrow failure syndrome can be defined as decreased production of all three cell lines leading to reduced number of RBCs, white blood cells (WBCs), and platelets. To start with marrow, failure occurs against single lineage and ultimately it involves all the three lines.

Etiology

A. Constitutional:

- **a.** Telomerase reverse transcriptase (TERT) and telomerase RNA (TERC) mutation in case of dyskeratosis congenita—aplastic anemia occurs in later life. Here, accelerated erosion of chromosomes during each cell division ultimately develops marrow failure. So, measuring the length of telomere is required to make decision for treatment.
- **b.** Mutation of germline *GATA2* gene is associated with wart and mycobacterial infections and markedly reduced B cells, natural killer (NK) cells, and monocytes.

B. Acquired causes:

- **a.** Pancytopenia with hypocellular marrow:
  1. Some myelodysplastic syndromes (MDS)
  2. Some ALL
  3. Some lymphomas of bone marrow
- **b.** Pancytopenia with cellular marrow:
  1. Primary bone marrow disease
     - Paroxysmal nocturnal hemoglobinuria (PNH)
     - Myelodysplasia syndrome
     - Myelofibrosis
     - Hairy cell leukemia
  2. Secondary to systemic disease:
     - Alcoholism
     - Vitamin B12 and folic acid deficiency
     - Overwhelming infections
     - Brucellosis
     - Hypersplenism
     - Sarcoidosis
     - Tuberculosis
- **c.** Hypocellular bone marrow with or without cytopenia:
  1. Mycobacteria
  2. Q fever

3. Legionnaires' disease
4. Toxoplasmosis
5. Hypothyroidism
6. Anorexia nervosa
7. Drugs:
   - Allopurinol
   - Antibiotics
   - Cardiovascular drugs
   - Sulfonamide
   - Gold
   - Indomethacin

Clinical Features

Symptoms

A. Features of anemia:
  a. Headache
  b. Lassitude
  c. Fatigue
  d. Exertional dyspnea
  e. Chest pain
  f. Weakness

B. Features of low WBC:
  a. Increased incidence of infection

C. Features of thrombocytopenia:
  a. Bleeding from mucosa, like gum, teeth, gastrointestinal tract, retina, and nasal mucosa. But, these bleeding are not brisk from low platelet count.
  b. Bleeding from skin such as petechiae and bruise.
  c. Most dreaded complication is intracranial bleeding.

D. Dark urine in PNH.

E. Constitutional symptoms, like weight loss, malaise, and anorexia are absent usually.

F. Sometimes, it can be accidentally detected during preoperative blood tests.

Physical Examination

A. Anemia detected in lower palpebral conjunctiva, palmar crease, and dorsum of tongue.

B. Evidence of bleeding such as ecchymosis, petechiae, epistaxis, retinal hemorrhage, and subconjunctival and retinal hemorrhage.

C. Short stature, hyper- or hypopigmented skin, abnormal hands, and thumb—Fanconi anemia.

D. Oral leukoplakia and dystrophy of nails—dyskeratosis congenita.

Diagnosis and Differential Diagnosis

A. Peripheral blood slide—platelet, WBC count are low and RBC may be normal or low.

B. Marked pancytopenia involves two or three cell lines.

C. Evidence of peripheral destruction, like microspherocytes and giant platelets is absent.

D. Bone marrow examination:
  a. Less than 30% cellularity excluding lymphocytes occasionally with pocket of normal cellularity—known as "hot spots"
  b. Myeloblast is not increased
  c. Megakaryocytes are always absent
  d. Marrow cytogenetics demonstrate:
    1. Trisomy 6 or 8
    2. Loss of Y or del20q

In case of pancytopenia secondary to underlying diseases:

A. History of intake of drugs

B. History of infections anywhere in the body

C. History or stigmata of liver disease

D. History of hypothyroidism

E. Family of Fanconi anemia

F. Family history of telomeropathy having history of hematologic malignancy or cirrhosis or pulmonary fibrosis

G. Features suggestive of Fanconi anemia—short stature, anomalies of upper limb or thumb, and café au lait spots

H. Features of oral leukoplakia and dystrophy of nails—dyskeratosis congenita

I. In case of myelodysplasia:
  a. In 20% cases—hypocellular
  b. Extreme changes in megaloblast
  c. Myeloid precursors are increased
  d. Megakaryocyte is preserved and poorly granulated with leftward shift
  e. Cytogenetic abnormalities may be found

J. In case of PNH: Flow cytometry is diagnostic.

K. In children with ALL and elderly with AML—lymphadenopathy with hepatomegaly in children and massive splenomegaly with hepatomegaly in elderly with pancytopenia and hypocellular bone marrow.

L. In myelofibrosis—hepatosplenomegaly, leukoerythroblastic blood picture, and dry tap in bone marrow biopsy are common.

M. Large granular lymphocytosis—less frequent anemia and thrombocytopenia along with prolonged neutropenia and large granular lymphocytes in peripheral blood, here marrow is normocellular. Flow cytometry and molecular evidence of T-cell receptor rearrangement are diagnostic.

N. Diagnosis of abnormal cells may require following investigations:
 - **a.** Bone marrow aspiration biopsy
 - **b.** Cytogenetic testing by FISH of the peripheral blood or bone marrow.
 - **c.** Flow cytometry of the peripheral blood or bone marrow.
 - **d.** Molecular studies:
   - **1.** Mutation analysis
   - **2.** Gene expression profiling
 - **e.** Level of vitamin B12 and folic acid

Severe aplastic anemia can be characterized by the following:

A. White blood cell count—<500/cc

B. Platelet count—<20,000/cc

C. Automated reticulocyte count—<60,000/mL

Management

A. Hematopoietic stem cell transplantation (HSCT):
 - **a.** It is used in HLA-matched sibling donors.
 - **b.** Better results are found in children and people <40 years.
 - **c.** Survival rate is 65–90%.
 - **d.** Short-term toxicity:
   - **1.** Infection—pneumonitis
   - **2.** Graft-versus-host disease (GVHD): Here, leukocyte-depleted platelets or erythrocytes decrease the risk of graft rejection
   - **3.** Veno-occlusive disease
 - **e.** Long-term effects:
   - **1.** Hematologic cure
   - **2.** Increased risk of solid tumor
   - **3.** Secondary organ dysfunction

B. Transplantation from matched unrelated donor (MUD)—result is as half good as that of HLA-matched donor. In this case, donor selection should be started by the younger age group who can be available as MUD. MUD can be offered in following types of patients:
 - **a.** Failed in a course of immunosuppression
 - **b.** In adult who are refractory to multiple courses of antithymocyte globulin, eltrombopag, or androgens

C. Immunosuppression: It is usually given in patients with severely depressed neutrophil count.
 - **a.** Horse antithymocyte globulin (ATG)—40 mg/kg/day for 4 days
 - **b.** Rabbit ATG—3.5 mg/kg/day for 5 days
 - **c.** Intravenous methylprednisolone—1 mg/kg/day for first 2 weeks to get relief from serum sickness

Hematologic response in case of horse ATG is 68% as compared to rabbit ATG where it is 37%.

In case of relapse or the patient is refractory to initial dose of ATG:
 - **a.** Second course of rabbit ATG can be given with hematologic response about 30–40%.
 - **b.** Cyclosporin A: Dose is 10 mg/kg in adult, but dose has to be adjusted to maintain blood level of 200–400 ng/mL. It has to be continued for 6–12 months followed by regular tapering with constant monitoring of blood count. Side effects are:
   - **1.** Nephrotoxicity needs continuous monitoring of the functions
   - **2.** Hepatotoxicity needs constant monitoring of liver functions
   - **3.** Gingival hypertrophy
   - **4.** Hypertension
   - **5.** Tremulousness
 - **c.** Alemtuzumab: Toxicities:
   - **1.** It can activate latent infection with herpes simplex virus
   - **2.** It increases cytomegalovirus (CMV) and Epstein–Barr virus (EBV) in the circulation

Toxicities of ATG:
 - **a.** Allergic reaction: In this case, proper hydration, antihistaminic for urticaria, and meperidine for associated rigors
 - **b.** Serum sickness
 - **c.** Transient depression of blood count
 - **d.** Rarely anaphylaxis

D. Thrombopoietin receptor agonist, eltrombopag, in case of patient refractory to ATG—daily dose is 150 mg/day with hematologic response of 40–50%. It can be given as a single agent. If the platelet level is less 10,000/cc, transfusion of platelet should be given to prevent intracranial bleeding.

E. Eltrombopag, if combined with ATG and cyclosporin as first line of therapy, demonstrates increased bone marrow cellularity with increased progenitor cells suggesting the effect of former drug on primitive hematopoietic cellular component.

F. Danazol, a male hormone, can be effective in patient with constitutional bone marrow failure having underlying telomeropathy.

G. Other therapies include:
- **a.** Growth factor combination of granulocyte colony-stimulating factor (G-CSF) and EPO
- **b.** Androgen
- **c.** High-dose cyclophosphamide

Causes of Pancytopenia

A. Decreased production (central type): It has been discussed in the bone marrow failure syndrome.

B. Infiltration of the bone marrow:
- **a.** Malignancies like lymphoma, leukemia, metastatic deposits, and multiple myeloma
- **b.** Granulomatous diseases
- **c.** Storage disorders

C. Increased destruction (peripheral type)
- **a.** Autoimmune disorders like SLE, rheumatoid arthritis
- **b.** Sequestration in the spleen like:
  1. Alcoholic liver disease
  2. HIV
  3. Tuberculosis
  4. Malaria

D. In case of COVID-19 pandemic pancytopenia is due to respiratory syndrome coronavirus 2.

E. Idiopathic pancytopenia of unknown significance.

Clinical features and diagnosis are described in the above parts in this question.

Q4. Describe clinical features, investigations, and management of multiple myeloma (MM).

DNBII/DEC2011 (10)

Discuss the clinical manifestations, diagnosis, and management of MM.

DNBIII/JUN2013 (10)

Clinical features, complications, and chemotherapy regimens used in treatment of MM.

DNBIIA/DEC2014 (10)

Multiple myeloma.

MGR/MAR2010/MDI (5)

Chemotherapy of MM.

MGR/MAY2011/MDII (7)

Diagnosis and treatment of MM.

MUHS/MAY2012/MDIII (10)

PGI/APR2014/MDIII (10)

Describe the clinical features, diagnosis, and management of MM.

DNB 2021 (10)

Multiple myeloma.

MGR UNI, Tamil Nadu, 2022 (5)

Discuss diagnostic criteria, clinical features, investigations, and treatment of MM.

Veer Narmad South Gujarat UNI, 2022 (25)

ANSWER

Definition

Multiple myeloma can be defined as proliferation of clone of plasma cells. Before 2014, in multiple myeloma, "end-organ damage" according to CRAB criteria is hypercalcemia, renal insufficiency, anemia, and bone disease which will direct the therapy. But, after 2014, according to the International Myeloma Working Group, three additional biomarkers such as:

A. ≥60% plasmacytosis

B. Involved/uninvolved serum-free light chain ratio ≥100 with involved serum-free light chain >100 mg/L

C. MRI detectable more than focal lesion

It confers 80% chance of progression to symptomatic MM within next 2 years.

In few cases, MM is preceded by monoclonal gammopathy of undetermined significance (MGUS) or smoldering myeloma. Annual progression from MGUS and smoldering MM to frank MM is 0.5–1% and 10%, respectively.

Pathophysiology

A. Evidence of somatic mutation in the antigen-binding region of clonal immunoglobulin proves that transformation occurs in the plasma cell or postgerminal center of B cell.

B. Most common abnormality is seen in the heavy chain of chromosome number 14.

C. There may be abnormality seen in the chromosome number 13, which denotes poor prognosis.

Clinical Features

Clinical features result from following insults:

A. Infiltration of bone marrow by malignant clone
B. Secretion of cytokines and osteoclastic-activating factors
C. Presence of high level of circulating immunoglobulin
D. Free light chains
E. Depressed immunity

Symptoms/Signs:

A. Asymptomatic which can be detected on routine tests
B. Weakness
C. Fatigue
D. Recurrent infections
E. Bone pain in 60% of patients in the form of back pain, pathological fracture, kyphosis with loss of height, compression fractures in the vertebrae, or extensive destruction of bones
F. Renal insufficiency in the form of oliguria, polyuria, pedal edema, and thirst
G. Features of hypercalcemia in 20% of patients
H. Evidence of hyperviscosity syndrome as evidenced by neuropathy, amyloidosis, coagulopathy, visual upset, purpura, and retinal hemorrhage

Diagnostic Criteria

According to the World Health Organization (WHO):

A. Major criteria:
- **a.** Bone marrow plasmacytosis >30%
- **b.** Biopsy demonstrates plasmacytoma
- **c.** Presence of monoclonal protein in serum and urine:
  - **1.** Serum immunoglobulin G (IgG) > 3.5 g/dL
  - **2.** Serum immunoglobulin A (IgA) > 2 g/dL
  - **3.** Bence Jones protein in urine >1 g/24 h

B. Minor criteria:
- **a.** Plasmacytosis in bone marrow 10–30%
- **b.** Evidence of lytic bone lesions
- **c.** Serum immunoglobulin to <50% of normal

Diagnosis requires:

A. One major and one minor criteria
B. Three minor criteria, which include presence of lytic bone lesion and presence of M protein

In case of MM:

A. In 60% of patients, IgG immunoglobulin
B. In 20% of patients, light chain only can be detected by presence of Bence Jones protein
C. In 17% of patients, IgA immunoglobulin
D. In 2% of patients, IgD immunoglobulin
E. In 1% of patients, biclonal proteins

According to the International Myeloma Working Group (IMWG):

A. Bone marrow- or biopsy-proven plasmacytoma consisting of ≥10% of plasma cells
B. Myeloma defining events attributable to plasma cell disorder:
- **a.** Hypercalcemia calcium level >1 mg/dL higher than upper limit of normal (11 mg/dL)
- **b.** Anemia—hemoglobin level <20 g/L below the normal limit of normal
- **c.** Bone lesion—≥1 lesions in X-ray, CT, or positron-emission tomography (PET)-CT
- **d.** ≥2 focal lesions on MRI of the spine
- **e.** Ratio of involved/uninvolved free light chain in the serum ≥100 mg/dL with involved free light chain in the serum ≥100 mg/dL

Staging of Multiple Myeloma

Durie–Salmon System

Items	Stage 1	Stage 2	Stage 3
Tumor mass	Low	Medium	High
	All of the following	Not fitting stage 1 or 3	One or more of the following
Monoclonal IgG (g/L)	<50		>70
Monoclonal IgA (g/L)	<30		>50
Bence Jones protein secretion	<4		>12
Hg (g/dL)	>10		<8.5
Serum calcium (mmol/L)	≤2.6		>2.6

Continued

Continued

Items	Stage 1	Stage 2	Stage 3
Lytic lesion	None or one		Advanced
Stage A: Serum creatinine	<175 μM/L		
Stage B: Serum creatinine	≥175 μM/L		

Bataille Staging System

Serum β2-microglobulin (β2M) is a powerful prognostic factor for measuring tumor bulk and C-reactive protein (CRP) is the surrogate marker of interleukin-6 (IL-6). It signifies aggression of tumor.

Low risk	Both	β2M < 6 mg/L and CRP < 6 mg/L	Median survival of 54 months
Medium risk	Either	β2M or CRP ≥ 6 mg/L	Median survival of 27 months
High risk	Both	β2M ≥ 6 mg/L and CRP ≥ 6 mg/L	Median survival of 6 months

Diagnosis

Tests	Features
Full blood count	• Normocytic, normochromic anemia • Increased rouleaux formation due to hypergammaglobulinemia • TLC is normal or low. Neutropenia with relative lymphocytosis • In minority of cases, leukoerythroblastic blood picture • Platelet count is normal or low • Raised ESR due to increased rouleaux formation
Packed cell volume	Increased
Urea and creatinine	May be increased, if >2 mg/dL—it is one of the diagnostic criteria of PCM
Uric acid	Increased
Serum albumin	Low
Serum calcium	Increased >1 mg/dL above the upper limit of normal or 11 mg/dL
Serum ALP	Normal or mildly increased, it can differentiate it from hyperparathyroidism or metastatic carcinoma where it is very high
Serum protein electrophoresis with immunofixation	Sharply defined M band is present in 80% of patients, mostly located in gamma-globulin region, and it can migrate to β or α2 regions
Serum immunoglobulin	It can detect immunoparesis
Serum-free light chain	• It can detect light chain unbound to immunoglobulin. Normal ratio of κ to λ is 0.26 to 1.65 • If it is <0.26—suggestive of monoclonal λ-free light chain • If ratio is >1.65—suggestive of monoclonal κ-free light chain • If involved/uninvolved free light chain ratio is ≥100—it is suggestive of one of myeloma defining events • It can predict response in monoclonal gammopathy, smoldering myeloma, light chain multiple myeloma, AL amyloidosis, and solitary plasmacytoma
Urinalysis	Proteinuria
Urine electrophoresis	In case of absence of M-band, it can detect Bence Jones protein in 22% of cases
24 hours urine test	To detect creatinine and protein clearance
X-ray of bones	Lytic lesions and pathological fractures
Diagnosis	
Radiological survey of skeleton	Lytic lesions, osteoporosis, and pathological fractures

Continued

Continued

Tests	Features
Bone marrow aspirates	Monotonous sheets of mature looking plasma cells to immature plasma cells. Immature cells are larger in size and large eccentrically or centrally located nucleus containing finely dispersed chromatin and one to two prominent nucleoli. Characteristics of neoplastic plasma cell are nuclear cytoplasmic dissociation (deep basophilic cytoplasm), immature nucleus, and pleomorphism. Characteristics of plasmablastic myeloma cells are high nuclear-cytoplasmic ratio, small nucleoli, and dispersed chromatin
	Different types of morphological features of plasma cells are: • Numerous grape-like cytoplasmic inclusions (Mott cells) • Pale-stained single larger intranuclear inclusions (Dutcher bodies) • Cytoplasmic round hyaline inclusions (Russell bodies)
	In case of IgA-secreting myeloma: • Cell with red cytoplasmic margin (flaming plasma cell) • Markedly pleomorphic multinucleated cells • Cells with fragmented and frayed cytoplasm
Immunofixation of paraprotein and densitometry	It can characterize and quantify type of immunoglobulins (IgG 55–60%, IgA 15–20%, light chain in 20–25%, rarely biclonal, and only 1% is nonsecretary myeloma)
Following tests can estimate tumor burden	
Serum CRP	It can measure IL-6, which can correlate with tumor progression
Serum β2-microglobulin	• It can measure tumor burden and renal function • If it is >5.5 mg/L—suggest high tumor mass and shorter survival • Serial estimation assesses growth rate in MM
Serum LDH	• It measures tumor aggression • It is increased in plasmablastic MM
Serum albumin	Hypoalbuminemia can correlate with poor prognosis
Bone marrow trephine biopsy	• It can demonstrate light chain restriction • It can demonstrate extent of marrow infiltration • It can detect hematopoietic reserve • Pattern of infiltration: Focal, interstitial, and diffuse. In case of former, two types of hematopoiesis will be preserved, but in last one hematopoiesis will not be preserved
Immunophenotyping	• CD38, CD138, CD19, and CD45 are positive for plasma cells and CD56, CD117, and CD200 are negative for plasma cells. K:λ is 1–2:1 • Neoplastic plasma cells are positive for CD38 and CD138, but negative for CD19
Immunohistochemistry	• Accurately identifies plasma cells when interstitially distributed in bone marrow • It can identify monoclonal or polyclonal nature of proliferation of plasma cells • It can confirm plasmacytic lineage in case of poor differentiation • It can differentiate poorly differentiated myeloma from metastatic tumors and lymphoma
Bone marrow cytogenetics	• T(4;14): Poor prognosis, bortezomib overcomes it in newly diagnosed and relapsed MM • T(14;16): Poor prognosis • T(11;14): In new MM, it has better prognosis • del(17p): Powerful poor prognostic factor • del(13): Poor prognostic factor when associated with t(4;14) or del(17p)
Following tests useful in few patients	
MRI	• In case of cord compression • In staging of plasmacytoma of bone to exclude occult disease • To clarify ambiguous CT findings

Continued

Continued

Tests	Features
CT	• Can detect localized site of disease, vertebrae, skull, ribs, and proximal areas in the long bones • Extraosseous plasmacytoma • In case of suspected cord compression • To clarify ambiguous radiologic finings • In symptomatic patient with negative radiologic findings • To take guided biopsy
PET-CT	Useful in case of solitary plasmacytoma
Fluorodeoxyglucose (FDG)-PET scan	• To detect extent of extramedullary disease • To identify local recurrence of disease • To identify focal extramedullary disease • To detect persistent positive post-therapy early relapse
Bone marrow flow cytometry	• It confirms plasma cell infiltration and aberrant phenotype • It is useful when bone marrow plasma cells are <10%
Plasma cell labeling index	It can predict prognosis
Fat pad biopsy for amyloid	In case of suspected amyloidosis
Tissue biopsy	Confirm solitary plasmacytoma in bone or extraosseous tissues
Bone densitometry	It will provide baseline in case of osteoporosis

Treatment

General Management

A. Management of pain:

- **a.** For mild pain—paracetamol 650 mg three times daily
- **b.** For moderate pain—dihydrocodeine 30–60 mg 4–6 hourly
- **c.** For severe pain—fentanyl patch
- **d.** Nonsteroidal anti-inflammatory drug (NSAID) can be used with caution in case of renal impairment
- **e.** 8–30 Gy radiotherapy locally sometimes extremely effective
- **f.** Neuropathic pain can be relieved by amitriptyline, gabapentin, or carbamazepine

B. In case of renal dysfunction:

- **a.** 3–4 L fluid per day to raise the urine output to >3 L/day
- **b.** Dialysis in the form of peritoneal or hemodialysis may be done
- **c.** In case of cast nephropathy, plasmapheresis can be of choice
- **d.** After rehydration, dexamethasone-based regimens can be given in case of plasma blood stem cells harvest

C. Hypercalcemia:

- **a.** Vigorous rehydration with 3–6 L/day intravenous (IV) saline with closed monitoring
- **b.** Loop diuretics increase calcium excretion and maintain fluid balance
- **c.** Intravenous bisphosphonate—pamidronate 30–90 mg over 2 hours or zoledronic acid 4 mg over 5 minutes
- **d.** In refractory cases corticosteroids

D. Bone disease:

- **a.** Local radiotherapy
- **b.** Fracture fixation followed by radiotherapy
- **c.** In case of persistent back pain—vertebroplasty or kyphoplasty

E. Infection:

- **a.** Intravenous vigorous broad-spectrum antibiotics such as aminoglycoside should be avoided.
- **b.** *Annual influenza, Haemophilus influenzae*, or pneumococcus vaccination is recommended.
- **c.** In first 2 months of therapy, prophylactic trimethoprim-sulfamethoxazole can be given.

F. Anemia:

- **a.** Blood transfusion can be given with caution due to risk of hyperviscosity syndrome.
- **b.** Erythropoietin in case of persistently low hemoglobin once weekly.

G. Hyperviscosity syndrome:

a. Plasmapheresis

H. Cord compression:

a. Local radiotherapy

b. Oral dexamethasone

c. In case of spinal instability surgery

Specific Therapies

General Considerations

A. Stem cell collection should be done after four cycles of chemotherapy to prevent stem cell cytotoxicity.

B. For frail and unfit patients, dose reduction is necessary.

C. During selecting the regimen, following cautions are required:

a. Patient's age

b. Current comorbidities

c. Ease of administration

d. Availability of drugs in the country

e. Balance between efficacy and toxicity of the drugs

f. Functional status of kidneys, heart, lung, and liver

Drugs are the following:

A. Bortezomib:

a. It is a first-generation reversible proteasome inhibitor.

b. It inhibits the cellular ability to degrade protein product, which leads to myeloma tumor death.

c. It is used intravenously or subcutaneously 1.5 mg/m^2 weekly or 1.3 mg/m^2 twice weekly.

d. Side effects: Gastrointestinal toxicity, peripheral neuropathy, activation of shingles, and thrombocytopenia.

e. It is used in disease associated with renal dysfunction and newly diagnosed MM in combination with lenalidomide and dexamethasone.

B. Carfilzomib:

a. It is an irreversible proteasome inhibitor.

b. It acts on chymotrypsin domain of proteasome complexes.

c. Dose is twice weekly IV infusion of 20/27 mg/m^2 to 20/56 mg/m^2.

d. Side effects: Decreased blood cell count, gastrointestinal, cardiac, and renal toxicities.

e. It is used in case of refractory and relapsed MM and patient with one or more prior treatment.

C. Lenalidomide:

a. It is an immunomodulating agent.

b. It binds with a protein cereblon, which regulates degradation of Ikaros and Aiolos that are responsible for lymphoid cell development.

c. It is used orally 5–25 mg daily.

d. Side effects: Rash, fatigue, diarrhea, cytopenias, and risk of thromboembolism.

In patients who can receive transplant: Two to four cycles of following three-drug regimens:

A. Bortezomib + Lenalidomide + Dexamethasone

B. Bortezomib + Cyclophosphamide + Dexamethasone

C. Bortezomib + Doxorubicin + Dexamethasone

D. Carfilzomib + Lenalidomide + Dexamethasone

E. Bortezomib + Thalidomide + Dexamethasone

After collection of stem cells from the patient, conditioning therapy with high dose of melphalan is given.

After giving autologous stem cell transplantation, maintenance therapy with thalidomide and lenalidomide is given.

In case of nontransplant patients:

A. Melphalan + Dexamethasone + either Bortezomib or Lenalidomide

B. Lenalidomide + Dexamethasone

C. Bortezomib + Cyclophosphamide + Dexamethasone

D. Carfilzomib + Lenalidomide + Dexamethasone

Maintenance therapy should be given with the following drugs: Lenalidomide: But with this drug, there is an increased risk of secondary primary malignancies.

Salvage therapy can be given by following:

A. Pomalidomide:

a. It is thalidomide analog

b. Daily dose is 1–4 mg

c. It is approved for those patients:

1. Who already received two or more prior lines of therapies

2. Who shows progression of disease within 60 days of completion of therapies

B. Ixazomib:

a. It is orally active reversible proteasome inhibitor

b. It is given weekly 4 mg along with lenalidomide and dexamethasone

C. Panobinostat:

a. It is deacetylase inhibitor.

b. It is given in MM with at least two prior lines of bortezomib and ixazomib.

c. Starting dose is 20 mg thrice weekly.
d. Side effects are vomiting, diarrhea, anorexia, and cytopenias.
e. It can be kept ready in case of:
   1. Refractory to ixazomib and proteasome inhibitors
   2. Patients who cannot tolerate newer monoclonal proteins

D. Daratumumab:
   a. It is CD38 monoclonal antibody (MAB).
   b. It can be given in following conditions:
      1. Patients formerly treated with three or more prior lines of therapy
      2. Double refractory to PI
   c. It is approved for giving with lenalidomide or bortezomib who received therapy.
   d. Side effects are fatigue, thrombocytopenia, and anemia
   e. Dose is 16 mg/kg infusion.

E. Elotuzumab:
   a. It is MAB having target for SLAMF7 or CS1 glycoprotein antigen present on NK cells and plasma cells.
   b. Dose is 10 mg/kg weekly for two cycles followed by every 2 weeks.
   c. Minimally activated, if administered isolated; hence, coadministration of dexamethasone and lenalidomide is required.

Q5. Causes, diagnostic algorithm, and management of a patient with thrombocytopenia.

DNBII/JUNE2010 (10)

Describe clinical features, laboratory findings, and treatment of idiopathic thrombocytopenic purpura (ITP).

DNBIII/JUN2012 (10)

Discuss the etiology, clinical features, and management of immune thrombocytopenic purpura.

DNBII/JUN2013 (10)

Thrombocytopenia.

MGR/MAR2010/MDII (6)

Immune thrombocytopenic purpura in children.

MGR/OCT2015/MDIV (7)

Management of ITP.

MGR/SEP2006/MDIII (6)

Describe the functions of platelet. Describe the etiology, clinical features, diagnosis, and treatment of ITP.

RGUHS/NOV2001/MDII (25)

Enumerate the causes of thrombocytopenia. How will you manage a case of ITP?

MJPRU/2016/MDI (25)

Describe recent advances in management of adult ITP.

BF/NOV2013/MDIV (10)

Approach and treatment of ITP.

DNB 2019 (6)

Describe the physiology of platelet function. Discuss diagnostic evaluation and management of functional disorders of platelets.

WBUHS 2022 (10)

Thrombocytopenia etiology and management.

Saurashtra UNI 2022 (20)

Discuss the physiology of platelet functions and will you investigate a case of ITP.

WBUHS, 2025 (10)

Describe the platelet biology and its role in coagulation. Narrate the mechanism of action of different NOAC agents and its therapeutic applications.

WBUHS, 2024 (10)

ANSWER

Role of coagulation has been described in question number 32. NOAC has been described in question number 27.

Functions of Platelets

A. Platelets adhere with the exposed collagen in the vessel wall after injury via Von Willebrand factor, thereby become activated to change its shape releasing granules like ADP and thromboxane A2.
B. Platelet contracts via interaction with actin-myosin to shrink the clot thereby stabilizing it.
C. Platelet seal the microvascular injuries if any in the capillaries and venules.
D. It will maintain the vascular integrity and barrier function.
E. Platelets interact with the vascular endothelium and leukocytes to release proinflammatory cytokines and chemokines in the area of inflammation.
F. Platelets interact with the pathogens by expressing the toll-like receptors thereby contributing to the innate immune response.
G. Platelet releases growth factors, platelet derived growth factor and vascular endothelial growth factor promoting angiogenesis and helps in tissue repair.
H. Membrane of the platelets provide surface phospholipid to assemble coagulation factors.

Causes of Thrombocytopenia

A. Decreased production of platelets:
   a. Bone marrow failure:
      1. Congenital causes: Fanconi syndrome, dyskeratosis congenita, and thrombocytopenia-absent radius syndrome
      2. Acquired causes: Aplastic anemia and amegakaryocytic thrombocytopenia
   b. Myelodysplastic syndrome
   c. Infiltration of the marrow:
      1. Infections: Tuberculosis and ehrlichiosis
      2. Neoplasia: Leukemia, lymphoma, and myeloma
   d. Irradiation: By direct toxicity on megakaryocytes
   e. Chemotherapy: Myelotoxic drugs but resolves slowly as compared to neutropenia and anemia
   f. Cyclic thrombocytopenia: It occurs cyclically every 3–6 weeks
   g. Nutritional deficiencies:
      1. Folic acid
      2. Vitamin B12
      3. Iron deficiency
   h. Alcoholism
B. Causes of increased clearance of platelets:
   a. Immune thrombocytopenia
   b. Heparin-induced thrombocytopenia
   c. Hemolytic uremic syndrome
   d. Thrombotic thrombocytopenic purpura (TTP)
   e. Post-transfusion purpura
   f. Disseminated intravascular coagulation
   g. Von Willebrand disease
   h. Cyclic thrombocytopenia
   i. Mechanical destruction of platelets—aortic valve dysfunction
C. Increased destruction of platelets: Hypersplenism
D. Other causes:
   a. Hemophagocytosis
   b. Drugs
   c. Human immunodeficiency virus (HIV) associated
   d. Sepsis
   e. Wiskott–Aldrich syndrome

Pathophysiology of Immune Thrombocytopenia

Antiplatelet antibodies bind with platelet glycoprotein complexes such as IIb/IIIa and Ib/IX. These antibody-coated platelets, bind to Fc receptors on macrophages, are destroyed in the reticuloendothelial system in spleen and liver. As a result, the life span of the platelets will be decreased to 2–7 days. But, compensatory increase in platelets is not increased due to following:

A. Binding of antiplatelet antibodies with megakaryocytes in the bone marrow
B. Lack of compensatory increase in thrombopoietin production

This GPIIb/IIIa is the sites of fibrinogen binding during platelet aggregation, which is also blocked by antiplatelet antibody.

Causes of Immune Thrombocytopenia

A. Adult-onset primary: It is idiopathic and chronic
B. Secondary:
   a. Lymphoproliferative disorder:
      1. Leukemia
      2. Lymphoma

b. Infections:
   1. Human immunodeficiency virus
   2. Tuberculosis
c. Immune degranulation: Systemic lupus erythematosus (SLE)
d. Drugs

C. In children: Viral infection. It will resolve spontaneously without treatment

Clinical Features

Newly diagnosed ITP: All the cases are diagnosed within first 3 months from diagnosis.

Persistent ITP: These are the cases between 3 and 12 months from diagnosis.

There is wide spectrum of clinical presentation: It may be completely asymptomatic and can be detected accidentally or it may present moderate-to-severe features of thrombocytopenia.

A. Acute ITP:
   a. Mainly children of 2–6 years of age
   b. Sex ration of 1:1
   c. It follows respiratory tract infection or vaccination after an interval of 2–6 weeks
   d. It occurs in winter and spring season
   e. Bleeding occurs from skin in the form of ecchymoses, bruises, and purpuric spot
   f. Bleeding can occur from mucous membrane from gum, nose, gastrointestinal tract, urinary tract, and rarely in the CNS but it is fatal
   g. Spleen tip may be palpable, but massive splenomegaly is rare
   h. This disease is self-limited with spontaneous remission within 2–6 weeks
   i. Recurrence is rare

B. Chronic ITP:
   a. It occurs in young females
   b. Male:Female is 1:3
   c. Onset is insidious and may be asymptomatic detected during routine blood examination
   d. Patient may present with iron deficiency anemia
   e. Bleeding may occur from skin or mucous membrane. Menorrhagia is common presentation
   f. Spontaneous remission is rare
   g. No seasonal variation
   h. It persists for many years with remissions and exacerbations

Laboratory Features

A. Peripheral blood examination:
   a. In case of acute ITP:
      1. Platelet count is <20,000/cc
      2. Hemoglobin may be reduced
   b. In chronic ITP:
      1. Hemoglobin is reduced
      2. Platelet count is moderately low, nearly around 50,000/cc
      3. Morphologically, platelet is frequently large—megathrombocytes
      4. Bleeding manifestation is mild due to presence of hyperactive large giant platelets in circulation
   c. Blood film should be examined to rule out—aplastic anemia, myelodysplasia, leukemia, megaloblastic anemia, and inherited thrombocytopenia

B. Bone marrow examination:
   a. Megakaryocytes are increased in number
   b. Morphological changes are:
      1. Hypergranularity
      2. Vacuolization
      3. Lack of platelet budding
      4. Hypolobulation of nucleus

C. Coagulation profile:
   a. Bleeding time is prolonged
   b. Coagulation time is normal
   c. Clot retraction time is deficient

D. Platelet antibodies: Platelet-associated immunoglobulin is increased in 90% of cases.

E. Screening for hepatitis B, C, and HIV infections.

F. In few patients, antiphospholipid antibodies, antinuclear antibodies, and serology for *Helicobacter pylori* should be done.

Treatment

In case of mild-to-moderate thrombocytopenia, absence of active bleeding or surgery should not get any treatment. But, adult with platelet count of <20,000/cc with or without bleeding should be actively treated.

Initial Therapy

A. Prednisolone orally 1 mg/kg/day for 7–10 days or alternatively pulse prednisolone 40 mg daily for 4 days. Platelet count should be measured to see increase in platelet count if it is increased within 3–7 days. If there is positive response, prednisolone should be tapered to 20 mg/day followed by gradual tapering by 5 mg alternate week for four cycles or every month for 6 months.

B. If the platelet count is <5,000–10,000/cc, along with corticosteroid as described above, intravenous immunoglobulin (IVIg) at a dose of 1 g/kg/day has to be given for 1–2 days as it decreases antibody-coated platelets from the circulation.

C. In case of contraindication to corticosteroids, only IVIg can be given.

D. 75 μg/kg/dose of IV anti-D from Rh-positive nonanemic patients is more effective in case of intact spleen and response will start within 3–5 days of administration.

E. In case of severe bleeding, platelet transfusion can be given but it will be cleared very rapidly by antiplatelet antibodies but it will temporarily help in hemostasis.

F. Prior to prolonged immunosuppressive therapy or splenectomy, vaccination should be done against:
   - **a.** Meningococcus
   - **b.** Pneumococcus
   - **c.** *Haemophilus influenzae*

Second-line Treatment

In case of adults, in spite of initial response, many patients will relapse after discontinuation or reduction of initial therapy. In these chronic ITP cases, second line of therapy is required.

A. Intravenous anti-D immunoglobulin should be readministered every 1–3 weeks

B. Thrombopoietin receptor antagonist:
   - **a.** Eltrombopag: To start with 50 mg orally or 25 mg orally in case of Asian decent
   - **b.** Romiplostim: Starting dose is 1 μg/kg subcutaneously every week

   Platelet response is >50,000/cc and drug is well tolerated.

   Complications:
   - **a.** Thrombocytosis
   - **b.** Thrombosis
   - **c.** Reticulin deposition in the bone marrow

C. Rituximab:
   - **a.** It is monoclonal anti-CD20 antibody and dose is 375 mg/m^2
   - **b.** Initial response occurs in 50% of patients and long-term response in 25% of patients

D. Splenectomy: It produces immediate as well as durable response. But that, patient must receive vaccinations against encapsulated organisms at least several weeks prior to splenectomy.

In case of secondary ITP treatment, underlying predisposing conditions have to be treated.

Pregnancy Associated with ITP

Indications for Treatment

A. During second or third trimester, platelet count is <30,000/cc

B. Platelet count is <10,000/cc

C. Bleeding in any trimester

Treatment of Choice

A. Intermittent infusion of IVIg

B. Prednisolone at alternate day schedule

C. Splenectomy can be considered in following cases:
   - **a.** In first or second trimester where IVIg and steroid treatment have been failed
   - **b.** Platelet count is <10,000/cc in continuously bleeding patients

D. Transfusion of platelets: Prophylactic transfusion can be given in case of:
   - **a.** Platelet count is <10,000/cc
   - **b.** Mucocutaneous bleeding near the delivery time

Adequate platelet count is >50,000/cc prior to cesarean section.

Q6. Indications for blood transfusion and discuss complications of massive blood transfusion and its management.

DNBIII/JUN2011 (10)

Discuss the blood transfusion-associated reactions and their management.

DNBIII/DEC2012 (10)

Massive blood transfusion: definition, indications, complications, and their prevention and management.

DNBIIB/JUN2015 (10)

Blood transfusion in perioperative and intensive care setting.

PGI/APR2013/MDII (10)

Complication of blood transfusion.

BF/OCT2011/MDII (13)

Name various immune and non-immune mediated adverse reactions following blood transfusion. Write short notes on transfusion related acute lung injury.

DNB 2020 (10)

Transfusion related acute lung injury.

MGR UNI, Tamil Nadu, 2022 (10)

Maharashtra UNI of Health SC, Vijayawada, 2022 (10)

Adverse reactions to blood transfusion.

Kerala University, 2021 (10)

Describe blood transfusion related reaction and sequelae.

WBUHS, 2020 (10)

ANSWER

Indications of Blood Transfusion

A. For whole blood:
- **a.** Severe hypovolemia with red cell loss
- **b.** For massive transfusion
- **c.** For exchange transfusion

B. Packed RBC:
- **a.** In asymptomatic patient having hemoglobin level of <7 g/dL.
- **b.** Patients with high risk of bleeding, pulmonary as well as cardiac compromise. Usually requiring higher hemoglobin.

C. Platelets:
- **a.** Thrombocytopenia: In this regard, prophylactic transfusion is required depending on the patient's underlying condition:
    1. Platelet count <10,000/cc with bleeding from any site as it prevents mortality in stable cancer patient and no other hemostatic defect undergoing chemotherapy
    2. Platelet count >50,000/cc is required prior to any invasive procedure or immediate post-operative period
    3. Platelet count >100,000/cc in case of high-risk patients with cerebral leukostasis and underlying any neurosurgical procedure

D. Granulocyte:
- **a.** In patient with absolute neutrophil count of <500/cc with evidence of antibiotic refractory bacterial and fungal infection.
- **b.** In case of infants with bacterial sepsis with absolute neutrophil count of <300/cc and postmitotic neutrophils comprising <10% of nucleated marrow cells.

E. Fresh frozen plasma (FFP):
- **a.** In case of clotting factor deficiency in ongoing bleeding patient or prior to invasive procedure
- **b.** In consumptive coagulopathy
- **c.** Deficiency of coagulation factors in case of liver disease
- **d.** In case of massive transfusion, dilutional coagulopathy to prevent
- **e.** Replacement of fluid for plasma exchange
- **f.** Replacement of single congenital factor deficiency in absence of any virus-safe fractionated product availability
- **g.** Reversal of warfarin overdose

F. Cryoprecipitate:
- **a.** Dysfibrinogenemia
- **b.** Acquired fibrinogen deficiency
- **c.** Factor XIII deficiency
- **d.** Disseminated intravascular coagulation
- **e.** To correct platelet defect in uremic bleeding rarely

Massive Blood Transfusion

Massive blood transfusion can be defined as replacement of:

A. More than one volume of blood in 24 hours

B. More than 50% of blood volume in 4 hours in an adult having blood volume of 70 mL/kg

C. In children >40 mL/kg whose blood volume is approximately 40 mL/kg

Massive transfusion protocol has a predicted ratio of RBC, FFP/cryoprecipitate, and platelets at 1:1:1 or 2:1:1.

Total volume of blood components, if it is equal to or exceed to the total blood volume of the patient over 24 hours period, is called as massive blood transfusion. It is equivalent to 10 or more units of whole blood or 20 units of packed RBC component in case of adult.

After transfusing one or more units, group O Rh-positive or Rh-negative blood, initially RBC, has to be collected from the patient for cross-matching, after that transfusion of properly cross-matched blood has to be done.

In some cases, initially blood volume and blood pressure have to be maintained by colloids such as albumin, fractionate plasma protein, or crystalloid such as normal saline.

In case of loss of >25–30% blood loss, transfusion of packed RBCs can be given in following cases:

A. Low oxygen status of the patient

B. Low tissue perfusion

C. Increased rate of blood loss

Complications of Massive Blood Transfusion

A. There will be dilution or consumption of different components of blood, hence platelet, APTT, PT, and fibrinogen level should be measured at frequent interval.

B. Replacement therapy will be warranted if:

- **a.** Platelet count is <50,000/cc
- **b.** Prothrombin time >1.5
- **c.** Activated partial thromboplastin time >1.5
- **d.** Serum fibrinogen level is <100 mg/dL

C. Hypocalcemia, hyperthermia, acidosis, and hyperkalemia may occur. Hence, serum electrolytes should be monitored.

D. If the blood is transfused at 100 mL/h, especially in case of renal and liver dysfunction, citrate will chelate serum calcium leading to hypocalcemia

E. Coagulopathy, if associated with trauma, is highly lethal and can be managed by aggressive blood component therapy

F. Massive blood transfusion may be complicated by DIC. It is more complicated when associated with trauma. Hence, following measures are to be taken:

- **a.** If fibrinogen level is below 100 mg/dL, cryoprecipitate or fibrinogen concentrate should be administered.
- **b.** In case of severe bleeding, platelet transfusion should be given.
- **c.** Underlying disorders should be corrected as transfusion is secondary to maintain the life of the patient.
- **d.** In case of consumption of multiple factors, plasma factor can be normalized above 30% by 10–20 mL/kg FFP.

Complications of Blood Transfusion

Classification of blood transfusion reaction:

A. Immune mediated reaction:

- **a.** Acute hemolytic transfusion reaction due to ABO blood group incompatibility.
- **b.** Delayed hemolytic transfusion reaction due to reaction with minor blood group antigens.
- **c.** Febrile non-hemolytic transfusion reaction due to various leukocyte antigen or presence of cytokines.
- **d.** Acute transfusion related lung injury due to activation of leukocytes due to anti-leukocyte antibodies leading to capillary leak.
- **e.** Allergic reaction due to appearance of urticarial as a result of severe anaphylactic reaction in presence of IgA deficiency.
- **f.** Purpura due to thrombocytopenia as a result of allogenic antibodies against platelets.
- **g.** Graft-versus-host disease occurring in immunocompromised patient where viable T lymphocytes of donor react with tissue of the recipients.

B. Non-immune mediated reaction:

- **a.** Bacterial sepsis due to introduction of organisms like *Yersinia* or *Pseudomonas* with the blood transfusion.
- **b.** Multiple blood transfusion leading to iron overload.
- **c.** Hypothermia due to transfusion of rapid transfusion of cold blood.
- **d.** Cardiac arrhythmias due to binding of citrate with the blood calcium leading to hypocalcemia.
- **e.** There may be hyperkalemia due transfusion of stored blood.
- **f.** There may be chance of physical hemolysis due to mechanical damage of the stored blood.

Description of Blood Transfusion Reaction

A. Acute hemolytic transfusion reaction: It may occur after as little as 10 mL of incomplete blood transfusion due to ABO blood group incompatibility between RBC and plasma.

- **a.** Mechanism: It occurs as a result of destruction of RBC by already formed anti-A or anti-B IgM isohemagglutinin in the plasma or recipient.
  1. Hemolysis: Intravascular due to complement fixation of IgM antibodies and it leads to hemoglobinemia and hemoglobinuria.
  2. Hemolysis results from hemolysis.
  3. Histamine and serotonin released from complement activation produce chest pain, breathlessness, and gastrointestinal symptoms.

   b. Presentations: Fever, chill, rigor, flank pain, chest pain, and dyspnea leading to hypotension, renal failure, and death.
   c. Management:
      1. Maintain blood pressure and renal blood flow to maintain urine flow at 1 mL/kg/h
      2. Stop further transfusion
      3. Monitoring of coagulation status
      4. If DIC develops, it should be treated

B. Delayed hemolytic transfusion reaction: It develops within weeks, months, or even years after transfusion who are immunized by transfusion or by pregnancy.
   a. Mechanisms: In case of previously alloimmunized patients who have already developed antibody may develop anamnestic reaction by repeat infusion.
   b. Presentation: Anemia, jaundice, and chills
   c. Management:
      1. Close monitoring of the patient's hemoglobin for continued hemolysis and supportive therapy
      2. Eculizumab can be given with sickle cell disease or indirect complement-induced hemolysis

C. Other types of hemolysis:
   a. Drug-induced hemolysis: It may be extravascular or intravascular presenting with anemia, raised LDH, bilirubin, and positive direct antiglobulin test.
   b. Hemolysis—results from:
      1. Saline
      2. Hypotonic saline
      3. 5% dextrose water
   c. Mechanical hemolysis due to:
      1. Prosthetic heart valves
      2. Intravascular device
   d. Thermal hemolysis results from exposure of the RBC to cold between 1 and 6°C or high temperature > 42°C.

D. Anaphylactic reaction: It occurs at the start of infusion.
   a. Mechanisms:
      1. Immunoglobulin E (IgE)-mediated response to transfused proteins.
      2. In patients with IgA-deficient patient having IgA antibody are susceptible to anaphylactic reaction.
   b. Clinical features: Urticaria, vomiting, diarrhea, coughing, laryngeal edema followed by hypotension, angioedema, stridor, respiratory distress, and shock.
   c. Management:
      1. Transfusion has to be discontinued.
      2. Treatment of anaphylaxis—epinephrine, steroids, and circulatory support.

E. Acute lung injury:
   a. It is associated with transfusion of plasma containing different blood components.
   b. Mechanisms:
      1. Donor-derived HLA class I/II antibodies or antineutrophil antibodies to corresponding antigen of the recipients deposit and react in the pulmonary vasculature, which leads to endothelial damage.
      2. Two-hit theory: It suggests interaction between primed neutrophil in lung and biologically active response modifiers, lipid, and cytokines during transfusion.
      3. Multiparous females are likely to be alloimmunized.
   c. Clinical features: Acute respiratory distress producing tachycardia, hypotension, oxygen desaturation, fever with chill, and rigor. These features occur within 6 hours of transfusion.
   d. Management:
      1. Discontinue transfusion
      2. Circulatory support and respiratory support

F. Circulatory overload:
   a. It is associated with raised central venous pressure leading to pulmonary edema and cardiac failure. Mainly elderly with compromised heart, kidney, and lung are susceptible to expansion of plasma volume.
   b. Presentation: Cough, dyspnea, orthopnea, cyanosis, crepitations, headache, engorged neck vein, and tachycardia.
   c. Management:
      1. Discontinuation of transfusion
      2. Administration of oxygen and administration of diuretics, if required phlebotomy

G. Graft-versus-host disease:
   a. It is a worst outcome of transfusion and universally fatal. The risk factors are:
      1. Immunocompromised patients
      2. Malignancies such as neuroblastoma, lymphoma, and sarcoma
      3. Premature infants

b. Mechanisms: Donor's immunocompetent lymphocytes react with patient's antigen and initiate immune response.
c. Clinical features: Diarrhea, rash, hepatitis, and pancytopenia
d. Management: Supportive therapy. It can be prevented by:
    1. Irradiation of blood components with irradiation dose of 2,500 cGy.

H. Bacterial contamination and sepsis:
a. It occurs shortly within 2 hours after commencement of transfusion.
b. Mechanisms:
    1. Bacteria that can thrive iron of RBC and cold are *Yersinia* and *Pseudomonas*.
    2. Platelets are susceptible to bacterial overgrowth and bacteria involved are staphylococci, streptococci, and *Propionibacterium*.
    3. Highest mortality is associated with endotoxin producing gram-negative bacteria.
c. Presentation: Chills with fever and fever may be less marked due to use of antipyretics. Other features are vomiting, abdominal cramps, bloody diarrhea leading to hypotension, renal failure, shock, and DIC.
d. Management:
    1. Discontinuation of transfusion
    2. Blood samples from the patient and donor should be sent for culture

I. Post-transfusion purpura:
a. It occurs from transfusion of any blood components or whole blood.
b. Mechanisms: Antibodies of patients who have previously transfused or as a result of pregnancy will react with platelet-specific antigen from donor that produces thrombocytopenia (bystander effect). It will resolve within 2–3 weeks.
c. Management:
    1. Intravenous immunoglobulin is the treatment of choice.
    2. Severe purpura will not resolve spontaneously or the patient is refractory to IVIg, plasma therapy has to be started.

J. Hypotension:
a. Transfusion-related hypotension—which can be resolved spontaneously after discontinuation of treatment.
b. Mechanisms:
    1. It is caused by activation of bradykinin
    2. It is associated with use of bedside leukoreduction filter as well as apheresis procedure
    3. Patient under angiotensin-converting enzyme (ACE) inhibitor is mainly susceptible as this drug blocks the normal metabolism of bradykinin.
c. Management: Other reactions, like anaphylaxis and acute hemolytic reaction have to be evaluated.

K. Febrile reaction:
a. It can be defined as rise in 1°C temperature for which no other cause is found. Risk factors are:
    1. Age
    2. Type of blood components
    3. Variety of donors
    4. Donor factors
    5. Platelets, RBC, FFP, or older blood components and leukocyte-reduced blood components
b. Mechanisms:
    1. Recipient antibodies against donor platelets or RBC resulting in release of cytokines
    2. Stored cytokines during storing of cellular components
c. Management: Same as that of hemolytic reaction.

L. Hemosiderosis: It occurs in chronically transfused patients.
a. Accumulation of iron in the liver, skin, heart, and endocrine organ.
b. Clinical features: Bronzing of the skin, hepatomegaly, hepatic fibrosis with features of hepatic dysfunction, diabetes, cardiac failure, and other dysfunction of other endocrine organ.
c. Management:
    1. Chelation of 50 units of red cell burden
    2. Apheresis for red cell exchange

M. Transfusion-transmitted infections: Following tests should be done prior to release of blood components:
a. Antibodies to HIV-1 and 2, hepatitis C virus (HCV), hepatitis B core antigen, human T-lymphotropic virus type I (HTLV-I) and II, *Trypanosoma cruzi*, and *Treponema pallidum*
b. Hepatitis B surface antigen (HBsAg)
c. Polymerase chain reaction testing for HIV, West Nile virus, HCV, and Zika virus.

Q7. Define febrile neutropenia. Describe its pathogenesis, diagnostic evaluation, and management.

DNBIV/DEC2011 (10)

Febrile neutropenia.

MUHS/NOV2013/MDIII (10) GMC/2015/MDIII (10)

MGR/SEP2006/MDI (5)

Management of febrile neutropenia.

PGI/NOV2013/MDIII (10) BF/NOV2013/MDII (10)

MUZ/MAY2016/MDIV (8)

Diagnosis and treatment of febrile neutropenic patients.

MLB/MAY2013/MDIII (25)

Acute febrile neutropenia.

NTR UNI of Health SC, Vijayawada, 2021 (10)

Febrile neutropenia.

Teerthanker Mahaveer UNI, 2020 (10)

Write short notes on febrile neutropenia and management of DHF.

WBUHS, 2024 (10)

ANSWER

DHF has been discussed in infectious disease chapter.

Definition

According to the Infectious Diseases Society of America (IDSA), neutropenia can be defined as absolute neutrophil count of 500/cc or <1,000/cc with an anticipated decline to <500 cells/cc within 48 hours.

Other definition is <500/cc or 1,000/cc as severe or moderate neutropenia, respectively.

Febrile neutropenia is neutropenia associated with single tympanic membrane or oral temperature ≥101°F or equal to 100.4°F for at least 1 hour.

Causes

A. Hematologic malignancies:
- **a.** Acute leukemia
- **b.** Myelodysplastic syndrome

B. Following chemotherapy

C. Following radiation

D. Infections:
- **a.** Gram-negative organisms:
  1. *Klebsiella*
  2. *Pseudomonas aeruginosa*
  3. *Escherichia coli* (*E. coli*)
  4. *Acinetobacter* species
  5. *Stenotrophomonas maltophilia*
- **b.** Gram-positive organisms:
  1. *Staphylococcus* species
  2. *Streptococcus* species
  3. *Enterococcus* species
- **c.** Polymicrobial infections:
  1. *Candida*
  2. *Aspergillus*
- **d.** Fungal infections

E. Use of broad-spectrum antibiotics

F. No obvious cause

Pathology

A. There is release of cytokines from the epithelial cells during neutropenia that produces fever.

B. Introduction of organisms occurs due to damage of host barriers during chemotherapy and radiotherapy.

C. There is access of organisms through central venous lines.

But in case of barrier damage whether the sustained inflammatory response due to release of cytokines or infecting organism plays a role in production of fever is unknown.

Clinical Features

Fever and many typical symptoms and signs are masked by neutropenia. Possible symptoms include the following:

A. Diarrhea

B. Pain in abdomen or in rectum

C. Nausea with or without vomiting

D. Chills

E. Change in cough or new cough

F. Shortness of breath

G. Nasal congestion

H. Burning pain during micturition

I. Unusual vaginal discharge or irritation

J. Frequent micturition

K. New onset of pain

L. Stiff neck

Signs are according to involvement of organs, but perineal area and oral cavity must be examined. In all patients, risk categorization is must which will determine the following:

A. Mortality and morbidity

B. Treatment setting whether in outpatient or inpatient basis

C. Empiric antibiotic therapy whether it will be oral or IV form

D. Duration of antibiotic therapy

Evaluation and Treatment of Patient

The Multinational Association of Supportive Care in Cancer (MASCC) risk index score was instituted to detect the risk of medical complications.

Multinational Association of Supportive Care in Cancer Risk Index

Characteristics	Points
Burden of illness: A. No or mild symptoms B. Moderate symptoms	 5 3
No hypotension	5
No chronic obstructive lung disease	4
Solid tumor or hematologic malignancy with no previous fungal infection	4
No dehydration	3
Outpatient status	3
Adult age <60 years	2

Clinical Index of Stable Febrile Neutropenia

Performance status ≥2 (Eastern Cooperative Oncology Group)	2
Stress-induced hyperglycemia	2
Chronic obstructive pulmonary disease	1
Chronic cardiovascular disease	1
Grade ≥2 mucositis	1
Monocytes <200/cc	1

Low risk: 0 point, moderate risk: 1–2 points, and high risk: ≥3 points.

Initial Assessment for the Patient of Febrile Neutropenia

Low risk of mortality (no high-risk factor and most of the following factors):

A. The Multinational Association of Supportive Care in Cancer risk index score of ≥21

B. At the time of development of fever, patient is of outpatient status

C. No evidence of concomitant comorbid illness

D. No evidence of hepatic and renal insufficiency

E. Anticipated short duration of severe neutropenia, i.e., absolute neutrophil count ≤100/cc for fewer than 7 days

F. Good performance status (Eastern Cooperative Oncology Group 0–1)

High risk of mortality (any of the following factors listed below):

A. Multinational Association of Supportive Care in Cancer risk index score is <21

B. At the time of development of fever, the patient is inpatient status

C. Allogeneic HSCT

D. Significant medical comorbidity or the patient is clinically unstable.

- **a.** Pneumonia
- **b.** Hypotension
- **c.** Neurological changes
- **d.** New-onset abdominal pain

E. Anticipated prolonged severe neutropenia, i.e., absolute neutrophil count ≤100/cc for ≥7 days

F. Hepatic insufficiency (five times upper limit of aminotransferase)

G. Renal insufficiency (creatinine clearance <30 mL/min)

H. Uncontrolled/progressive cancer:

- **a.** Leukemia is not in complete remission (CR)
- **b.** Patient without leukemia with evidence of disease progression after more than two courses of chemotherapy

I. Pneumonia or other complex infection at clinical presentations.

J. Treatment with alemtuzumab

K. Grade 3–4 mucositis

Guideline of treatment is followed according to the IDSA.

The Multinational Association of Supportive Care in Cancer score should be calculated according to following criteria:

A. Tumor type and solidity or liquidity of tumor

B. Burden of illness

C. Presence or absence of hypotension

D. History of chronic obstructive lung disease

E. History of fungal illness

F. Volume status

G. Age of the patient

In case of low-risk patient (MASCC score ≥ 21): Patient should be selected carefully for oral antibiotics as outpatient with close careful monitoring for clinical deterioration. The antibiotics of choice are:

A. Fluoroquinolone monotherapy such as moxifloxacin or ciprofloxacin

B. Ciprofloxacin 750 mg twice daily with amoxicillin and clavulanic acid 875 mg thrice daily × 7 days

C. In case of penicillin allergic patient, clindamycin is used instead of amoxicillin and clavulanic acid

D. If patient is already on fluoroquinolone therapy, he should not take fluoroquinolone therapy

If the patient remains febrile for 48 hours after commencement of antibiotics, broad-spectrum antibiotics should be started along with hospital admission.

In case of high-risk patient: This patient has to be admitted to hospital. For culture: two samples from two lumens of central line and one sample from peripheral line. In absence of central line, two samples from peripheral line.

Chest X-ray, high-resolution CT scan of the chest, culture of urine, and sputum have to be done.

Antipseudomonas beta-lactam agent such as cefepime, piperacillin-tazobactam, imipenem-cilastatin, or meropenem has to be administered as it should be the main target in case of empiric therapy. But, empiric coverage against gram-positive organisms is usually not given unless any evidence is present. Vancomycin is administered in case of gram-positive soft-tissue infection, catheter-related infection, severe sepsis with or without hypotension, pneumonia, or hemodynamically unstable patient. After commencement of this antibiotic, no evidence of bacterial infection is found and this antibiotic should be stopped.

Urine output should be maintained at 0.5 mL/kg/h and defervescence of fever should be expected within 2–5 days.

Common therapeutic regimen is: cefepime, imipenem-cilastatin and meropenem, ceftazidime, and Zosyn.

Dual therapy includes aminoglycoside in addition to the above.

Treatment of Resistant Pathogens

Organisms	Antibiotics to be used
Methicillin-resistant *Staphylococcus aureus*	Vancomycin, linezolid, and daptomycin
Vancomycin-resistant *Staphylococcus aureus*	Linezolid and daptomycin
Extended-spectrum beta-lactamases	Carbapenem
Klebsiella pneumoniae carbapenemases	Colistin and tigecycline

If hemodynamically stable patient remains febrile for >4 days in spite of antibiotic treatment, absolute neutrophil count has to be evaluated.

A. If there is myeloid recovery, antibiotic should not be changed

B. If there is no myeloid recovery, CT scan of the chest and sinus and lung should be done

If the fever persists for >4 days, antifungal prophylaxis with fluconazole should be started. In case of fluconazole-resistant *Candida krusei*, *Candida glabrata*, or in case of *Aspergillus* infection, echinocandin such as caspofungin should be recommended. In addition to antibiotic, myeloid growth factor has to be added.

Product	Route of administration
Filgrastim	Intravenous or subcutaneous administration
Filgrastim-Sndz	Subcutaneous injection
Tbo-filgrastim	Subcutaneous injection

Q8. Tumor lysis syndrome (TLS).

DNBII/JUN2011 (10)

Enumerate oncologic malignancies. Discuss the clinical features, diagnosis, and management of TLS.

DNBII/DEC2012 (10)

Classify and enumerate the oncologic emergencies, clinical manifestations, and management of TLS.

DNBIIA/JUN2016 (10) PGI/APR2013/MDI (10)
KUHS/MAY2013/MDIII (10)

Explain the clinical features, laboratory abnormalities, and management of TLS.

MGR/APR2013/MDII (7)

Discuss tumor lysis in case of malignancy.

MUHS/MAY2013/MDIII (25)

Tumor lysis syndrome.

DNB 2022 (5) Kerala UNI 2022 (10)
MGR UNI, Tamil Nadu, 2021 (10)

ANSWER

Definition

Tumor lysis syndrome is a constellation of metabolic abnormalities as evidenced by hyperuricemia, hyperkalemia, hyperphosphatemia, and hypocalcemia due to lysis of malignant cells leading to release of intracellular content into the circulation at a rate exceeding the clearance capacity of the kidney.

Etiopathogenesis

Causes are:

A. High-grade lymphoma, mainly Burkitt lymphoma
B. Acute leukemia
C. Kinetically active solid tumor
D. Other modalities of treatment:
- **a.** Ionizing radiation
- **b.** Radiofrequency ablation
- **c.** Treatment with glucocorticoids
- **d.** Embolization
- **e.** Therapy with MAB
- **f.** Interferon
- **g.** Hematopoietic stem cell transplantation

Risk Factors

A. Advanced age with reduced glomerular filtration rate
B. Patient with volume depletion
C. Cancer patient with anorexia and nausea with or without vomiting
D. Patients on drugs affecting renal function:
- **a.** Nonsteroidal anti-inflammatory drugs
- **b.** Angiotensin-converting enzyme inhibitor
- **c.** Angiotensin receptor blockers (ARBs)

E. Comorbid conditions:
- **a.** Cardiac disease
- **b.** Renal disease
- **c.** Diabetes mellitus

There are three risk groups:

A. High-risk group:
- **a.** Burkitt lymphoma/acute leukemia at early stage of disease with raised level of LDH
- **b.** Acute lymphocytic leukemia with ≥100,000/cc or less WBC count, if LDH level > twice than normal
- **c.** Acute myeloid leukemia with WBC count ≥100,000/cc
- **d.** Diffuse large B-cell lymphoma (DLBCL) with LDH level > two times normal

B. Intermediate-risk group:
- **a.** Acute myeloid leukemia with WBC count between 25,000 and 100,000/cc
- **b.** Acute lymphocytic leukemia with WBC count <100,000/cc and LDH level < 2 times normal
- **c.** Early stage of Burkitt lymphoma/leukemia with LDH level < 2 times normal
- **d.** Diffuse large B-cell lymphoma with LDH level >2 times normal

C. Low-risk group:
- **a.** Indolent lymphoma
- **b.** Chronic lymphocytic leukemia (CLL)
- **c.** Chronic phase of CML
- **d.** Acute myeloid leukemia with WBC count <25,000/cc and LDH level < 2 times normal
- **e.** Multiple myeloma
- **f.** Solid tumor

Clinical Features

Clinical features are fairly nonspecific. It appears within 12–72 hours after initiation of chemotherapeutic treatment.

A. Features of hyperkalemia present with weakness, muscle cramps, nausea with or without vomiting, paresthesia, and diarrhea.
B. Features of hyperphosphatemia present with renal failure, secondary hypocalcemia presenting with muscle cramps, muscle twitching, paresthesia, carpopedal spasm, tetany, nephrocalcinosis, changes in mental status, and seizures rarely.
C. Hyperuricemia presenting with renal failure as evidenced by decreased urine output along with volume overload.

Laboratory Diagnosis

A. Complete blood count
B. Urinalysis and urine microscopy
C. Biochemistry:
- **a.** Hyperuricemia
- **b.** Hyperkalemia
- **c.** Hyperphosphatemia
- **d.** Hypocalcemia.

D. Electrocardiogram (ECG) manifestations:

  a. Prolongation of QT interval in hypocalcemia

  b. Narrow T waves, prolonged PR interval, prolonged QRS interval, and sine wave configuration—suggestive of hyperkalemia

E. Ultrasound of kidney

Cairo and Bishop classify laboratory and clinical diagnosis according to different grades:

Laboratory TLS for adult:

Items	Values	Change from baseline value
Uric acid	≥8 mg/dL	25% increase
Potassium	≥6 mEq/L	25% increase
Phosphorus	≥4.5 mg/dL in adult and ≥6.5 mg/dL in children	25% increase
Calcium	≤7 mg/dL	25% decrease

Clinical TLS grading for adult:

Variables	Grade 0	Grade 1	Grade 2	Grade 3	Grade 4	Grade 5
Creatinine	None	• 1.5 times of ULN • Rise is not due to chemotherapeutic agents	• >1.5–3 times of ULN • Rise is not due to chemotherapeutic agents	• >3–6 times of ULN • Rise is not due to chemotherapeutic agents	• >6 times of ULN • Rise is not due to chemotherapeutic agents	Death
Cardiac arrhythmias	None		• Nonurgent medical intervention needed • Cardiac arrhythmia is not due to chemotherapeutic agents	• Symptomatic, medically incompletely controlled or controlled with device • Cardiac arrhythmia is not due to chemotherapeutic agents	• Life-threatening arrhythmias, hypotension, heart failure, syncope, and shock • Cardiac arrhythmia is not due to chemotherapeutic agents	Death
Seizures	None		One brief generalized seizure, well controlled by anticonvulsant, and focal motor seizures not interfering with ADL	• Seizures in which consciousness is altered • Poorly controlled seizure with breakthrough generalized seizures despite anticonvulsant	Any kind of seizure but prolonged, repetitive, and difficult to control (status epilepticus, intractable epilepsy)	Death

(ADL: activities of daily living; ULN: upper limit of normal)

Treatment

Low-risk patients are monitored, but intermediate- and high-risk groups have to be treated prophylactically.

A. In intermediate- and high-risk group patient, hydration with normal saline or Ringer's lactate solution should be done at a rate of 150–200 mL/h or to maintain urine output 2 mL/kg/h to minimize acute kidney injury. These fluids correct hypovolemia and hyponatremia. But, normal saline produces hyperchloremic metabolic acidosis and Ringer's lactate solution worsens hyperkalemia. Overhydration sometimes produces volume overload, which can be corrected by loop diuretics; it also improves hyperkalemia.

B. Correction of hyperuricemia: Allopurinol 100 mg thrice daily for 2–3 days prior to commencement of chemotherapy or radiotherapy to reduce the incidence of urate nephropathy and has to be continued for 3–7 days after the uric acid becomes normalized. In patients with inheritance of HLA-B*58.01 allele, there is chance of severe cutaneous eruption. Other adverse effects are acute kidney injury and elevated liver transaminases level. In case of renal disease, allopurinol has to be given in reduced dose; in that case, febuxostat can be given without any dose adjustment. Allopurinol inhibits xanthine oxidase inhibitor, hence it prevents further uric acid synthesis does not reduce preexisting serum uric acid level, thus it takes 48–72 hours to reduce the serum level. In that case, rasburicase can be given in intermediate- or high-risk groups of TLS as it will improve the serum level within 4 hours at a dose of 0.2 mg/kg/day in high-risk groups and 0.15 mg/kg/day in intermediate-risk groups having uric acid level of ≤7.5 mg/dL. Rasburicase degrades the uric acid. Duration of treatment is 5–7 days.

C. Hyperkalemia:

- **a.** Patient is asymptomatic but level is >6 mmol/L:
  - **1.** Limitation of intake
  - **2.** Sodium polystyrene sulfonate 15–30 g orally 6 hourly. It will bind potassium in the intestine. In case of enema, 50 g of this drug have to be mixed with soap water. But, it should not be used in case of paralytic ileus or intestinal obstruction, intestinal necrosis, or ischemia.
  - **3.** Electrocardiogram monitoring
- **b.** Severe hyperkalemia (serum potassium level >7 mmol/L):
  - **1.** Above treatment
  - **2.** Regular insulin 10 units + 100 mL 50% dextrose in patient with blood glucose <250 mg%, whereas if blood level is >250 mg%, 50% dextrose administration is not necessary.
  - **3.** Albuterol 10–20 mg in 4 mL nebulized saline over 20 minutes.
  - **4.** Dialysis in case of refractory hyperkalemia.
  - **5.** 1 g calcium gluconate or 500 mg to 1 g calcium chloride intravenously.
  - **6.** 45–50 mEq sodium bicarbonate slow IV infusion to be given over 5–10 minutes—it will push potassium into the cells in exchange of hydrogen. But, it is not the sole agent for reducing the serum potassium. But there are two disadvantages:
    - i. Alkalization of serum further decreases the free serum calcium due to its increased binding with serum albumin.
    - ii. Alkalization of urine aggravates the deposition of calcium phosphate in the kidney
  - **7.** Electrocardiogram monitoring

D. Hypocalcemia:

- **a.** Asymptomatic patient—no treatment is usually required.
- **b.** Symptomatic patient—10% of 10 mL calcium gluconate to be given slowly intravenously with continuous ECG monitoring.
- **c.** Correction of hyperphosphatemia.

E. Hyperphosphatemia:

- **a.** In moderate cases:
  - **1.** Limitation of intake
  - **2.** Administration of phosphate binders—calcium carbonate, sevelamer, lanthanum, and aluminum hydroxide. It should be taken with each meal and it prevents absorption of phosphate from the intestine.
- **b.** In severe cases or refractory cases: Hemodialysis.

Q9. Define Waldenstörm macroglobulinemia (WM). Describe its clinical feature, diagnostic evaluation, and treatment.

DNBII/DEC2010 (10)

Waldenstörm macroglobulinemia

MGR/APR2014/MDII (7) MGR/APR2014/MDIV (7)

ANSWER

Definition

Waldenström macroglobulinemia is an uncommon indolent B-cell lymphoproliferative disorder characterized by lymphoplasmacytic cells infiltration of the bone marrow along with paraproteinemia, mainly immunoglobulin M (IgM) variety.

Pathophysiology

A. This disorder arises from memory B cells, which is arrested after somatic hypermutation before terminal differentiation to plasma cells in the germinal center; as a result, there is absence of IgH rearrangement in these cells due to defect in initiation of normal switching process.

B. Most frequent chromosomal abnormality is deletion of 6q21-23. There is no evidence of putative tumor suppressor gene.

C. There is upregulation of IL-6 as evidenced by raised IL-6 and CRP.

D. Clinical features are due to infiltration of WM cells in the bone marrow, spleen, and liver.

E. Evidence of hyperviscosity due to increased serum level of IgM.

Clinical Features

A. Occasionally, the patient is asymptomatic; it can be diagnosed during routine blood examination.

B. Symptoms: Features of anemia, shortness of breath, weight loss, infection, and epistaxis.

C. Symptoms of hyperviscosity syndrome such as congestive cardiac failure, headache, dizziness, disturbance in vision, ataxia, stupor, and unconsciousness.

D. Signs:

- **a.** Evidence of sensory or sensory-motor distal symmetrical slowly progressive lower extremity neuropathy
- **b.** Hepatomegaly
- **c.** Splenomegaly
- **d.** Lymphadenopathy

e. Evidence of cryoglobulinemia such as arthralgia, purpura, and skin ulcers
f. Hemorrhagic features such as easy bruising and epistaxis—due to defect in coagulation and platelet function
g. Autoimmune disorders due to paraproteinemia—glomerulonephritis, angioedema, and acquired von Willebrand syndrome

Investigations

A. Complete blood count:
 a. Normochromic, normocytic anemia
 b. Occasionally lymphocytosis
 c. Pancytopenia
 d. Increased rouleaux formation
B. Raised ESR—>100 mm/h
C. Viscosity: Increased
D. Serum biochemistry:
 a. Uric acid—increased
 b. Lactate dehydrogenase—increased
 c. β2-microglobulin—increased
E. Serology:
 a. C-reactive protein—raised
 b. Immunoglobulin—increased IgM
F. Serum protein electrophoresis, immunofixation, and densitometry—it will characterize and quantify IgM. It shows reactivity against heavy chain μ activity chain along with any one light chain κ or λ. Concentration of IgM is >3 g/dL.
G. Urine protein electrophoresis—in 50% cases, Bence Jones protein.
H. Bone marrow: Infiltration by lymphoplasmacytic cells and variable differentiation of mast cells (MCs) distributed in interstitial, nodular, diffuse, or paracellular areas.
I. Immunophenotyping:
 a. It shows CD19+ and CD20+
 b. Cytoplasmic cells show IgM, CD5-, CD10-, CD23-, and CD103-
 c. Plasma cells show CD38+ and CD138+
J. Genetic analysis: There is mutation in primary response gene 88 on chromosome 3p22.2
K. Tests for hemostasis:
 a. Bleeding time increased due to coating of platelet by IgM
 b. Defective platelet aggregation
 c. Prolonged thrombin time as a result of inhibition of polymerization of fibrin monomer
L. Biopsy of lymph node:
 a. Paracortical infiltration of lymphocytes, plasmacytoid lymphocytes, and plasma cells
 b. Dilated open sinuses
M. CT scan of the chest, abdomen—organomegaly, lymphadenopathy

Prognostic Factors

Predictors of Early Progression in Asymptomatic WM

A. IgM > 30 g/L
B. Hb < 11.5 g/dL
C. β2-microglobulin ≥ 3 mg/L

Predictors of Shorter Survival in WM

A. Age ≥ 60 years
B. High β2-microglobulin
C. Hemoglobin < 10 g/dL
D. Other less identifiable factors:
 a. White blood count <4,000/cc
 b. Neutrophil < 1,800/cc
 c. Platelet < 150,000/cc
 d. Decreased serum albumin
 e. Male sex

Treatment

Indications of Therapy

A. Constitutional symptoms
B. Platelet < 100,000/cc
C. Hemoglobin < 10 g/dL
D. Symptoms of hyperviscosity
E. Severe peripheral neuropathy
F. Symptomatic cryoglobulinemia
G. Cold agglutinin disease

Drugs

Alkylating Agents

A. Chlorambucil 0.1 mg/kg/day for 14 days + Prednisolone 0.1 mg/kg/day for 7–14 days in 28 days cycle. Duration of therapy is not established. Duration of response is 2–4 years.

Purine Analogs

A. Fludarabine: 40 mg/m^2 orally for 5 days, monthly for 4–6 cycles, and duration of response is 40–50 months.

B. Cladribine: 0.1 mg/kg continuous infusion monthly for two to four cycles.

Two above drugs are cross-resistant.

Monoclonal Antibody

A. Rituximab: It is monoclonal CD20 antibody 375 mg/m^2 IV for 4 weekly cycles. Duration of response is 9–16 months

B. Bortezomib

C. Thalidomide

D. Alemtuzumab

Plasmapheresis

Indication: In case of hyperviscosity syndrome, 1–1.5 volume exchange reduces plasma viscosity. It reduces IgM by 80% plasma viscosity by 50%. One to two sessions reduce viscosity to near normal for several weeks.

Q10. Classify tumor markers and describe their roles in various medical conditions.

DNB/DEC2011 (10)

Name the biomarkers of internal malignancies and mention their importance.

MGR/APR2013/MDIV (7)

Biological markers in malignancy.

MGR/APR2013/MDI (5)

Tumor markers.

MGR/SEP2007/MDI (5) MGR/MAR2002/MDI (10)
MUHS/MAY2012/MDI (10)
MUHS/MAY2009/MDI (10)
BF/MAY2010/MDIII (10)

Tumor markers in clinical practice.

MGR/OCT2003/MDIII (5)

Role of tumor markers.

BF/NOV2013/MDII (10)

Cancer biomarkers.

BF/MAY2009/MDIII (10)

Enumerate tumor markers in relation to medicine and discuss their clinical applications and limitations.

DNBIV/JUN2010 (10)

ANSWER

Definition

Tumor markers are measurable biochemical markers associated with cancer either derived from tumor cells or response of the body to tumor cells and released into the circulation. It is not the primary modality for diagnosis of malignancy rather than support to the diagnosis.

A. It is not the screening test to detect hidden cancer, but it can monitor the success or failure of the progress of treatment

B. It can detect the progress of the disease

C. It can detect the extent of the disease

D. Rising titer of markers may be alarm of progression of the disease

Advantages of Cancer Biomarkers

A. Help in the diagnosis of cancer: In most of the cases, cancers are diagnosed by biopsy not by biomarkers. But, it can help whether the particular cancer diagnosis is likely in that patient. It can help in detecting the origin of the primary cancer in case of widespread metastasis.

B. Screening and early detection of cancer: Screening means early and accidental detection of cancer in absence of any symptom. But, very few markers have been shown to be helpful as it cannot detect very early cancer in asymptomatic patient.

C. Response to therapy: The level of the biomarkers, prior to and during the treatment, demonstrates the decreasing trend—suggests positive response to chemotherapy. On the other hand, increasing level of markers proves no response to therapy.

D. Prognostic indicator: Some newer markers indicate the aggressiveness and progress of the disease.

E. Detection of relapse: It can detect relapse after initial response to treatment. Following markers are useful after completion of treatment without any residual cancer in the body:

- **a.** Prostate-specific antigen (PSA) for prostate cancer
- **b.** Cancer antigen 125 (CA-125): For epithelial ovarian tumor
- **c.** Human chorionic gonadotropin in case of gestational trophoblastic tumor

Disadvantages of Cancer Biomarkers

A. Standardization of sample regarding sample collection, sample storage, and sample handling leads to biochemical and analytical variation in the measurement.

B. In case of early cancer, very small concentration of marker may not be detected by different methods.

C. Lack of variability.

D. It may not be present in the early stage of cancer.

E. It may be present in many noncancerous conditions as normal cells can also produce cancer biomarkers.

F. In some cases, very high biomarkers cannot confirm the presence of cancer.

G. Among the individuals, proteins and modified proteins vary in different types of cells and sometimes same cells in different disease states. So, it is very difficult to obtain accurate value.

Characteristics of Ideal Markers

Characteristics	Remarks
Highly specific	It can detect only one specific type of cancer
Highly sensitive	It cannot detect benign tumor or cannot present in physiologic conditions
Long lead time	There will be sufficient time for alteration the course of the disease
Short half-life	Frequent serial monitoring of the markers
Simple and cheap	It is used for screening test
Easily obtainable specimen	Acceptability in the populations
Correlation between the tumor burden and level of the marker	It acts as prognostic marker

Classification Scheme of Tumor Markers

Categories	Subcategories	Examples
Hormones		Catecholamines, calcitonin, and β-hCG
Oncofetal antigen		α-fetoprotein (AFP) and carcinoembryonic antigen
Metabolites		VMA and HIAA
Glycoproteins		CA-19.9, CA-125, CA-72.4, CA-15.3, and PSA
Tumor-associated markers	Enzymes	LDH, ALP, pteridines, and pterins
	Acute phase protein	Ferritin and CRP
Tumor-associated antigens	MHC-related antigens	H-2K antigen
	Viral-specific antigens	Polyoma and SV-40
	Oncogenic products	c-myc and c-erbB2
	Cytogenic products	Philadelphia chromosome
	Different proteins	β2-microglobulin and immunoglobulins
Ultrastructural components	Intermediate filament components	Vimentin and desmin

(β-hCG: β-human chorionic gonadotropin; HIAA: hydroxyindoleacetic acid; MHC: major histocompatibility complex; VMA: vanillylmandelic acid)

Common Markers in Different Malignancies

Malignancies	Tumor markers	Roles
Breast	CA-15.3 and CA-27.29	Monitor and recurrence of tumor
	ER, PR, and HER2/neu	Response to therapy
Adrenal carcinoma	Catecholamines and steroids	Diagnosis
Carcinoid tumor	HIAA	Diagnosis
Choriocarcinoma	β-hCG	Diagnosis, monitoring, and prognosis
Colorectal, gastric, and pancreatic carcinoma	CEA and CA-19.9	Prognosis and monitoring
Hepatoma	AFP	Screening, diagnosis, prognosis, and monitoring
Germ cell tumor	AFP and β-hCG	Monitoring, diagnosis, and prognosis
	LDH and placental alkaline phosphatase (PLAP) (seminoma)	Prognosis and monitoring
Lymphoma	LDH	Diagnosis and prognosis
	Cytogenic alteration	Diagnosis
Myeloma	Immunoglobulins	Diagnosis and prognosis
Melanoma	Tyrosinase	Diagnosis
Prostate	PSA	Diagnosis, prognosis, monitoring, and screening

Continued

Continued

Malignancies	Tumor markers	Roles
Ovarian tumor	CA-125	Monitoring, diagnosis, and recurrences
Sarcoma	Cytogenetic alterations	Diagnosis
Thyroid	Thyroglobulin	Screening and monitoring
	Calcitonin (medullary carcinoma)	Screening, monitoring, and prognosis

Following markers are associated with nonmalignant conditions:

Markers	Nonmalignant conditions
AFP	Inflammatory bowel disease, viral hepatitis, pregnancy, and liver injury
Carcino-embryonic antigen (CEA)	Inflammatory bowel disease, smokers, cirrhosis, pancreatitis, hepatitis, and gastritis
CA-125	Endometriosis, peritoneal irritation, hepatitis, pregnancy, and pelvic inflammatory disease
PSA	Benign prostatic hypertrophy and prostatitis
β-hCG	Pregnancy, testicular failure, and marijuana smokers

Q11. Discuss etiology, diagnosis, and management of acute myeloid leukemia (AML).

ERA/MAY2012/MDIV (25)

Discuss the clinical features, staging, diagnosis, and management for AML.

MUHS/MAY2010/MDIII (25)

Classify leukemias. Give an account of the clinical presentation, prognostic factors, and therapy of AML.

MGR/OCT2003/MDIII (15) MGR/SEP2010/MDIV (20)

Acute myeloid leukemia.

MGR/MAR2008/MDI (5)

How acute myeloid leukemia is diagnosed? What are the genetic abnormalities in AML that are associated with favorable outcomes, if appropriately treated?

DNB 2020 (10)

Classify AML. Add a note on its management.

NTR UNI of Health SC, Vijayawada, Andhra, 2022 (10)

ANSWER

Definition

Acute leukemia can be defined as a malignant clonal disorder of hematopoietic stem cells leading to uncontrolled proliferation of poorly differentiated blast cells in the bone marrow, which, if untreated, develops rapidly progressive fatal course.

Classification of Acute Leukemias

French–American–British (FAB) cooperative group classification of acute leukemias:

A. Acute lymphoblastic leukemias:
- **a.** Acute lymphoblastic leukemia—L1 type
- **b.** Acute lymphoblastic leukemia—L2 type
- **c.** Acute lymphoblastic leukemia—L3 type

B. Acute myeloid leukemias:
- **a.** Acute minimally differentiated myeloblastic leukemia (M0)
- **b.** Acute myeloblastic leukemia without maturation (M1)
- **c.** Acute myeloblastic leukemia with maturation (M2)
- **d.** Hypergranular promyelocytic leukemia (M3):
  - **1.** Hypogranular or microgranular promyelocytic leukemia (M3 variant)
- **e.** Acute myelomonocytic leukemia (M4):
  - **1.** Acute myelomonocytic leukemia with bone marrow eosinophilia.
- **f.** Acute monocytic leukemia (M5):
  - **1.** Undifferentiated, i.e., monoblastic leukemia (M5a)
  - **2.** Well differentiated, i.e., promonocytic-monocytic leukemia (M5b)
- **g.** Acute erythroleukemia (M6)
- **h.** Acute megakaryocytic leukemia (M7)

WHO classification of acute leukemias:

A. Acute myeloid leukemia with recurrent genetic abnormalities:
- **a.** Acute myeloid leukemia with t(8;21)(q22;q22)

b. Acute myeloid leukemia with abnormal bone marrow eosinophils and inv(16)(q13;q22)

c. Acute promyelocytic leukemia with t(15;17)(q22;q12)

d. Acute myeloid leukemia with 11q23 [mixed-lineage leukemia (MLL)] abnormalities

B. Acute myeloid leukemia with multilineage dysplasia:

a. Following MDS/myeloproliferative disorder (MPD)

b. Without preceding MDS/MPD, but without dysplasia in at least 50% of cells involving at least myeloid lineages

C. Acute myeloid leukemia and MDS therapy related

Acute Myeloid Leukemia

Definition

It is a heterogeneous group of disorders caused by uncontrolled myeloid lineage blast cell proliferation leading to gradual replacement of normal hematopoietic cells in the bone marrow by variably immature hematopoietic cells.

Etiology

A. Environmental factors:

a. Benzene
b. Ionizing radiation
c. Smoking

B. Genetic disorders:

a. Fanconi anemia
b. Bloom syndrome
c. Down syndrome
d. Ataxia telangiectasia
e. Kostmann syndrome
f. Klinefelter syndrome

C. Preexisting hematologic abnormalities:

a. Myelodysplastic syndrome
b. Aplastic anemia
c. Myeloproliferative disorders

D. Treatment associated:

a. Radiotherapy with or without chemotherapy
b. Topoisomerase II inhibitors: AML without preceding incidence of myelodysplasia:

1. Shorter latency period
2. Exhibits monocyte morphology
3. Change in the long arm of chromosome 11

c. Alkylating agents: AML usually arises from MDS:

1. Long latency period
2. Associated with deletion of chromosome 5 or 7

Clinical Features

Patients usually present with features of:

A. Anemia—fatigue, shortness of breath, and weakness

B. Leukopenia—focal bacterial infection and disseminated infections

C. Thrombocytopenia—bleeding from different sites such as gum, petechiae, bruise, and meninges

D. Disseminated intravascular coagulation—striking bruising and life-threatening hemorrhage—it usually occurs in promyelocytic leukemia.

E. Features of hyperviscosity syndrome or leukostasis occurs, if the blast cell count is >100,000/μL. This can manifest as visual problem, confusion, shortness of breath due to hemorrhage in retina, brain, lungs, etc.

F. Rare manifestations are:

a. Sweet syndrome characterized by skin rash due to infiltrates of neutrophils
b. Chloromas characterized by tumors of myeloid blast cells

G. Extramedullary leukemic infiltrations:

a. Bone pain producing tenderness
b. Moderate splenomegaly
c. Infiltration of CNS
d. Visual involvement such as retinal hemorrhage, papilledema, and retinal involvement

Laboratory Diagnosis

A. Hematologic:

a. Normocytic normochromic anemia
b. Low reticulocytes
c. Total leukocyte is low or raised
d. Blast cells:

1. Type 1, 2, and 3 myeloblasts
2. Monoblasts
3. Megakaryoblasts

e. Blast equivalent:

1. Granular or hypogranular promyelocytes suggest APL
2. Pronormoblast containing atypical cytoplasmic vacuoles suggests pure erythroid leukemia

f. Morphologic abnormalities in neutrophils:

1. Pelger-Huët cells
2. Hypogranular form

g. Thrombocytopenia with large and bizarre platelets

h. Fibrin degradation product increased—DIC

B. Biochemistry:

a. Hyperuricemia—due to high cell turnover and it will be worsened during chemotherapy

b. Increased blood urea nitrogen and creatinine—urate nephropathy

c. Hyperkalemia, hyperphosphatemia, and hypocalcemia suggest TLS

d. Lactic acidosis from leukostasis with high LDH

e. Renal tubular dysfunction due to released muramidase from blast cells produces hypokalemia

f. High cellular metabolic activity produces hypokalemia, hypoglycemia, and hypoxemia

C. Bone marrow examination:

a. ≥20% blast cells

b. Marrow is hypercellular but in case of old patients are hypocellular; here, bone marrow interstitium demonstrates blast cells

c. Severely depressed normal hematopoietic elements

d. There may be significant myelodysplasia—associated with poor prognosis

D. Cytochemistry:

a. Acute myeloid leukemia of M1 to M4 stains with myeloperoxidase stain—which in early phase demonstrates in the perinuclear area

b. Nonspecific esterase activity is positive for AML of M4 and M5

c. In AML of M6, there is granular positivity with periodic acid-Schiff (PAS) stain in erythroblast

d. In AML of M7, there is presence of platelet peroxidase demonstrated by electron microscopy

E. Immunophenotyping: Flow cytometry should be performed in all cases of AML.

a. Precursor cells—CD34 and CD117

b. T lymphoid cells—cytoplasmic CD3

c. Erythroid—glycophorin A and hemoglobin A

d. Megakaryocytes—CD41, CD42b, CD61, and von Willebrand factor (VWF)

F. Cytogenetic analysis: It is common in AML. The WHO classification is also based on this cytogenetic analysis.

G. Imaging studies:

a. CT scan of the chest to demonstrate chest infiltration and intracranial hemorrhage in hyperviscosity syndrome

b. MRI can demonstrate thickened nerve sheaths

Treatment

Emergency Treatment

A. Cardiovascular and respiratory resuscitation in case of massive hemorrhage or septic shock

B. In case of neutropenic sepsis, empirical broad-spectrum antibiotic has to be started

C. Leukapheresis in following cases:

a. Peripheral blast cell count is high

b. If there is leukostasis

D. To prevent TLS, intensive hydration with or without alkalinization of urine

Supportive Treatment

A. Cytomegalovirus-negative products for potential stem cell transplant recipient

B. In case of patients treated with purine analog irradiated blood product

C. Platelet transfusion is required to maintain platelet count 100,000/cc

a. If the patient is not septic and is on antibiotic

b. Patient has hemorrhagic abnormality

D. Hydration to maintain urine output >100 mL/h

E. To prevent hyperuricemia (when WBC count is >100,000/cc) allopurinol or rasburicase has to be started

F. Insertion of central venous catheter has to be done

Chemotherapy

It has been divided into two phases:

Induction of remission therapy:

A. In case of patients younger than 60 years of age:

a. Cytarabine 100–200 mg/m^2/day IV infusion or twice daily in bolus doses × 7 days

b. Anthracycline derivative such as daunorubicin 45–60 mg/m^2 intravenously × 3 days

This 7+3-day therapy demonstrates complete hematological response in 60–85% of patients.

Addition of 5 mg/m^2 cladribine improves remission rate.

c. Fludarabine, cytarabine, G-CSF and idarubicin (FLAG) is effective in doing remission in younger than 60-year-old patients.

B. In older patients with no morbidities may do better with intensive therapy.

C. In case of patients with presence of comorbidities are unable to get benefit from intensive therapy.

Consolidation therapy:

A. In case of <60-year-old patients:

a. Patient responded to induction therapy has residual disease, which may relapse without treatment. So, relapse can be done by high-dose cytarabine (2–3 g/m^2 twice daily on first, third, and fifth day or twice daily for 6 days with or without homologous stem cell transplantation). It is required in following patients:

1. Younger than 60 years of age
2. Better risk cytogenetics
3. Those with core-binding factor mutations t(8:21) and inv(16)

But choice of treatment depends upon risk of relapse.

b. Patients older than 60 years may not benefit from cytarabine therapy.

Stem Cell Transplantation

A. Allogeneic stem cell transplantation is offered to younger patients of <60 years of age with poor risk of acute myelocytic leukemia in first complete response. But, few patients with poor risk of AML beyond first complete response benefit from this type of transplantation.

B. Sibling donor stem cell transplantation is offered in patients with intermediate-risk acute myelocytic leukemia.

Following genetic abnormalities in AML are associated with favorable outcome if treated:

A. t(8;21) due to fusion of RUNX1 and RUNX1T1 occurring in younger patients.

B. inv(16) or t(16;16) due to fusion of CBFB-MYH11.

C. t(15;17) due to fusion of PML-RARA found in acute promyelocytic leukemia

D. Mutation of NPM 1 without FLD3-ITD due to mutation of nucleoplasm - favorable prognosis due to low allelic burden.

E. Mutation of Biallelic CEBPA due to mutation of both the alleles of CEBPA or enhancer binding protein.

Q12. Henoch–Schönlein purpura.

MGR/OCT2015/MDII (7)

MGR/APR2015/MDIV (7)

BF/MAY2011/MDII (13)

ANSWER

Definition

It is an acute IgA-mediated disorder producing small vessel vasculitis in the small intestine, skin, kidney, joints, rarely lungs, and CNS, most common in children and gradually decreasing in adult.

Clinical Features

Symptoms

A. Fever

B. Headache

C. Anorexia

D. Joint pain

E. Hematuria

F. Cramping abdominal pain and nausea

G. Hematochezia and bloody diarrhea

H. Rashes

I. Confusion or unconsciousness

Signs

A. Skin: Erythematous, macular, and palpable papular rashes present in the dependent areas in the body

B. Kidney: Hematuria

C. Gastrointestinal system: Frank blood in the stool

D. Joints: Deformed

E. Genital system:

a. Priapism

b. Penile edema

c. Orchitis

F. Central nervous system: Intracranial hemorrhage

Diagnosis

According to the European League against Rheumatism (EULAR)—presence of palpable purpura or petechiae with predominance of lower limb in absence of thrombocytopenia and coagulopathy along with at least one of the following:

A. Acute-onset diffuse abdominal pain

B. Acute arthritis or acute arthralgia involving any joint

C. Kidney involvement (any hematuria or proteinuria) along with IgA deposition

D. Any sample of biopsy demonstrating leukocytoclastic vasculitis or kidney biopsy in patients with atypical purpura distribution demonstrating rapidly progressive glomerulonephritis predominantly with IgA deposition

Imaging Modalities

A. Abdominal, scrotal, or testicular ultrasonography

B. Radiography:

- **a.** Chest X-ray to see the presence and extent of pulmonary hemorrhage
- **b.** Abdominal plain X-ray to see the extent of obstruction
- **c.** Contrast radiography of small intestine to see the thickened mucosal fold, small barium flecks, and thumb printing
- **d.** Barium enema to detect intussusception, ischemic colitis, thickened mucosa, and thumb printing

C. MRI of the brain to detect posterior reversible encephalopathy syndrome—bilateral gray and white matter abnormalities, which suggests edema in the posterior region of cerebral hemispheres

D. CT scan of the brain and abdomen

Endoscopy of upper or lower gastrointestinal tract from stomach to anal mucosa to see any purpuric lesion.

Kidney biopsy to examine any deposition of IgA and C3. Absence of C4 and C1q will exclude other causes of immune complex nephritis.

Following tests can exclude other diseases:

A. Complete blood count, differential count, and platelet count

B. Blood urea nitrogen and creatinine

C. Prothrombin time

D. Activated partial thromboplastin time

E. Lipase level

Treatment

A. Adequate hydration

B. Immediate discontinuation of any antigenic exposure

C. In the first month follow each month, alternate week for the second month and then monthly

Complications

A. Acute abdomen—small bowel infarction and perforation

B. Acute scrotum

C. Acute kidney injury

Q13. Von Willebrand disease.

BF/MAY2011/MDIII (10)

RGUHS/APR2001/MDII (10)

ANSWER

Definition

It is an inherited disorder of deficiency of VWF in the circulation leading to evidence of bleeding from the mucous membrane.

Pathophysiological Classification

Von Willebrand factor, a large multimeric glycoprotein, is synthesized by endothelial cells and megakaryocytes. In case of primary hemostasis at the site of injury of arteriole, platelets attach to subendothelial collagen matrix and also attach to other platelets. VWF binds to glycoprotein Ib (GPIb) receptor present on the platelets.

Von Willebrand factor also attaches with the factor VIII and, thus, prevents its clearance from the circulation. There are three types of VWF:

A. Type 1 von Willebrand disease: It is an autosomal dominant disease, present in 75–80% of patients, and most of them do not have the mutation in the chromosome number 12. It is mainly quantitative defect.

- **a.** 15% of type 1 patients demonstrate increased clearance of VWF. These patients show initial increased response to desmopressin acetate (DDAVP) followed by decrease after 4 hours.

B. Type 2 von Willebrand disease: It is a qualitative defect and present in the adulthood. These are of four types:

- **a.** Type 2A: Here the defect is either in intracellular transport or it makes the factor susceptible to proteolysis.
- **b.** Type 2B: Here the defect is abnormal structure in the binding sites of the platelet GPIb and produces "gain-of-function" defect leading to spontaneous bleeding. These patients also present with thrombocytopenia due to removal of aggregates of VWF-bound platelets.
- **c.** Type 2N: Here due to mutation of VWF there is decrease ability to bind thereby decreased ability to protect factor VIII from clearance from the circulation. So that factor VIII will be cleared from the circulation very rapidly. As a result factor VIII will be reduced in the circulation. Here the patient presents with soft tissue and joint bleeding. Here serum factor VIII will be low but VWF is normal.
- **d.** Type 2M: Here there is mutation of A1 domain of VWF and rare variety. Defect is decreased binding of platelets to VWF.

C. Type 3 von Willebrand disease: Here there are mutations including deletions of VWF. Bleeding is present in the childhood. Factors VIII and VWF are low.

Clinical Features

A. Most common sites of bleeding are gastrointestinal, nasal, oral, and uterine sites.

B. In case of marked abnormalities of VWF, bleeding starts in early life. In type 3 VWF disease, bleeding occurs in childhood.

C. Bleeding can occur from operative sites.

D. In case of type 2N VWF, there will be bleeding in the joints and soft tissue.

Diagnosis

A. History of bleeding from different sites.

B. Personal and family history of bleeding.

C. Serum level of VWF antigen by enzyme-linked immunosorbent assay (ELISA): It is low.

D. Von Willebrand factor activity by ristocetin cofactor assay: In this test, 1.2 mg/mL of ristocetin is added to mixture of patient's plasma (source of VWF) and washed normal platelet. Ristocetin is added to VWF allowing to bind with platelets at GPIb receptors on the membrane leading to aggregation of platelets.

E. In type 2N VWF disease, factor VIII is low but VWF is normal.

F. Secondary testing of VWF multimers detects distribution of multimers. In types 2A and 2B, there is absence of large and intermediate multimers. In type 3 disease, there is few or no multimer.

G. Von Willebrand factor levels: It is usually low but in some other diseases, this factor may be abnormal:

- **a.** Menstruation: In first 4 days of menstruation, this factor will be lowest.
- **b.** Stress, acute illness, and estrogen increase the serum level of VWF.

Treatment

A. Desmopressin acetate: It is responsible for the release of VWF and factor VIII from vascular endothelium. Dose is 0.3 μg/kg IV infusion that will increase the two factors in the blood to two- to sevenfolds after 6–12 hours. In case of nonresponders, second dose can be applied. Within the span of 12 hours, second dose should be avoided as there is an increased risk of hyponatremia and tachyphylaxis.
It is effective in type 1 and 2 disease.

B. Administration of VWF: In case of continuous bleeding, in spite of DDAVP administration, it can be given:

- **a.** As prophylaxis
- **b.** Clinically significant bleeding in type 3 patients

Cryoprecipitate should not be recommended because of its lack in viral inactivation.

C. Antifibrinolyic drugs: The drugs are:

- **a.** Epsilon-aminocaproic acid
- **b.** Topical agents such as gel foam, topical thrombin, and fibrin sealant

Contraindications:

- **a.** Hematuria
- **b.** Increased risk of thrombosis

D. Avoidance of following drugs:

- **a.** Aspirin
- **b.** Antiplatelet medications

Q14. Burkitt's lymphoma (BL).

MGR/MAR2006/MDI (5)
ERA/MAY2011/MDIII (10)

ANSWER

Definition

It is a highly selective non-Hodgkin lymphoma (NHL) resulting from degranulation and translocation of *Myc* gene present in the chromosome number 8 and involves multiple organs in the body.

Types

There are three types of BL:

A. Sporadic type:

- **a.** It is observed commonly in the pediatric population around the age of 10 years in USA and Western Europe. It represents <1% of NHL in adult.
- **b.** It is associated with EBV.
- **c.** Most common site of involvement is intestine in abdomen.

B. Endemic type:

- **a.** It is found in Equatorial Africa and New Guinea.
- **b.** It is 50% of all childhood cancer.
- **c.** Nearly all cases are associated with EBV.
- **d.** Most common presentation is facial tumor.

C. Immunodeficiency type:

- **a.** It is most common in HIV-associated patients with CD4 count >200 cells/μL.
- **b.** Majority demonstrates EB virus positivity.
- **c.** Most common sites of involvement are CNS, lymph nodes, and bone marrow.

Pathology

All the subtypes arise from B cells at different stages of development. It depends upon MYC expression encoding for c-Myc protein, a transcription factor located in chromosome 8q24—it regulates the process of proliferation, differentiation, and apoptosis. In this disease, inappropriately high level of c-Myc develops by following mechanisms:

A. Translocation of long arm in chromosome 8

B. Translocation of heavy chain gene in chromosome 14

Overexpression of c-Myc is responsible for uncontrollable proliferation and rapid doubling time of malignant cells.

There is also evidence of two flowing phenomena seen in DLBCL:

A. Double-hit DLBCL—there is presence of both MYC and BCL2 rearrangement

B. Triple-hit DLBCL—there is presence of MYC, BCL2, and BCL6 rearrangement

Histology

Among the background of abundant basophilic and homogeneous tumor cells, there is "starry sky" with benign histiocytes containing clear cytoplasm. There is evidence of high rates of apoptosis of the tumor cells.

Clinical Features

A. Most common presentation is:

- **a.** Abdominal pain with mass in the right iliac fossa from:
  1. Intussusception
  2. Distention
  3. Nausea and vomiting
  4. Gastrointestinal bleeding
- **b.** Next common sites are neck and head.
  1. Involvement of nasopharynx
  2. Tonsils
  3. Oropharynx
  4. Sinuses
  5. Jaw swellings
  6. Periorbital swellings
  7. Hepatomegaly
  8. Splenomegaly
- **c.** Rare presentation sites are:
  1. Skin
  2. Testes
  3. Breast
  4. Thyroid gland
  5. Central nervous system—15% of patients present with sudden paraplegia and incontinence
  6. Mediastinum

Cytogenetics and Molecular Studies

There is evidence of translocation in following areas:

A. t(8;14)(q24;q32) in 70–80% of patients

B. t(2;8)(p12;q24) and t(8;22)(q24;q11) in 20% of patients

Staging of Burkitt's Lymphoma

St Jude/Murphy Staging System

A. Stage 1:

- **a.** A single tumor (extranodal) or single anatomical area (nodal) excluding mediastinum or abdomen.
- **b.** A single tumor (extranodal) with single regional node involvement on same side of diaphragm.

B. Stage 2:

- **a.** A single tumor (extranodal) with single regional node involvement
- **b.** On the same side of diaphragm
  1. Two or more nodal areas
  2. Two single extranodal tumors with or without regional node involvement
- **c.** A primary gastrointestinal tract tumor (usually ileocecal) with or without associated with involvement of mesenteric node, grossly completely resected.

C. Stage 3:

- **a.** On both sides of diaphragm:
  1. Two or more nodal areas
  2. Two single extranodal tumor
- **b.** All primary intrathoracic tumors (mediastinal or pleural thymic)
- **c.** All extensive primary intra-abdominal disease, unresectable abdominal disease, even if only in one area
- **d.** All primary paraspinal or epidural tumors, irrespective of other sites

D. Stage 4:

- **a.** Any of the above with initial CNS or bone marrow involvement (only <25% of the marrow is composed of Burkitt cells).

Diagnosis

Imaging Studies of Abdomen

Ultrasonography can detect:

A. Most frequently, small bowels are involved due to increased concentration of lymphoid tissue present there. Segmental wall thickening, focal masses along with dilatation of abdomen, and there may be communication of masses with lumen of the bowel identified as "dirty shadowing."

B. Signs of intussusception include:

- **a.** Target sign—alternate echogenic and hypoechoic bands of bowel layers on transverse view.
- **b.** Pseudokidney sign—it corresponds in longitudinal view.

C. CT scan assesses the benign and malignant features of the lymph nodes. Malignant node includes:

- **a.** Echogenic hilum
- **b.** Asymmetric cortical thickening
- **c.** Intranodal vascular architectural distortion
- **d.** Amputated short subcapsular vessels

D. CT scan demonstrates:

- **a.** "Telescoping bowel associated with mesenteric vessels and fat"
- **b.** Enlarged mesenteric nodes grow in conglomerate masses compressing biliary, urinary, and bowel obstruction
- **c.** Ascites
- **d.** Peritoneal nodules

Imaging Study of Chest

A. Mediastinal widening

B. Pleural effusion

C. Mediastinal and hilar lymphadenopathy

D. Pericardial involvement

E. Myocardial involvement

F. Pleural nodules or masses

Imaging of Head, Neck, and CNS

A. Jaw masses

B. Osteolytic lesion in the mandible with invasion of orbit

C. Involvement of Waldeyer's ring including palatine tonsil, lingual tonsil, and adenoids of nasopharynx

D. Thyroid nodule

E. Masses in CNS or leptomeningeal thickening in spinal cord

Treatment

A. Treatment protocols:

- **a.** Short or long duration, intensive multiagent regimens: Doxorubicin, alkylators, vincristine, and etoposide
- **b.** Less intense regimen (CHOP-based therapies)
- **c.** In the second cycle, rituximab can be started to minimize the adverse effect
- **d.** Central nervous system prophylaxis with intrathecal methotrexate or cytarabine can be given in high risk of CNS involvement

B. Surveillance and refractory cases:

- **a.** Regular physical examination
- **b.** Laboratory studies including CBC, LDH, and biochemical examination
- **c.** Imaging studies such as chest X-ray and PET-CT to detect any relapse

C. In case of relapse, autologous stem cell transplantation

D. Treatment-related complications:

- **a.** Tumor lysis syndrome
- **b.** Interstitial or airspace infiltrate in case of methotrexate
- **c.** Hemorrhagic cystitis in case of cyclophosphamide
- **d.** Neutropenic colitis

Q15. Discuss hematological indications for bone marrow transplantation and complications of allogeneic bone marrow transplantation.

DNBIII/JUN2011 (10)

What is autologous bone marrow transplantation? What are its indications? Complications of bone marrow transplantation.

DNBI/APR2016 (10)

Bone marrow transplantation.

MGR/MAR2008/MDIV (6)

Describe indications of procedure, complications, and outcome of bone marrow and peripheral blood stem cell transplant.

GMC/2015/MDIV (25)

Autologous blood transfusion.

MGR/SEP/MDIII (6)

Hematopoietic stem cell transplantation: Mechanisms, indications and complications.

DNB 2019 (5)

ANSWER

Definition

Bone marrow transplantation is procedure where normal hematopoietic stem cells from the appropriate donor are transfused intravenously to patients having diseased marrow or defective marrow to generate normal hematopoiesis.

Classification

There are three types of bone marrow transplantation:

A. Allogeneic HSCT: In this method, hematopoietic stem cells from HLA-matched or -unmatched related or unrelated donor will be transfused into another individual.

B. Autologous HSCT: In this method, hematopoietic stem cells obtained from the own bone marrow of the patient and will be transfused back to the same individual after administration of conditioning regimen.

C. Synergic HSCT: In this method, stem cells are collected from genetically identical one person to another person such as identical twins.

Allogenic HSCT: Here stem cells are best collected from HLA-matched sibling donor. *HLA* gene is present in the chromosome number 6 and it follows Mendelian pattern of inheritance, so there is 1:4 chance of complete HLA matching.

Indications of Allogeneic HSCT

A. Hematologic malignancy:
- **a.** Acute myeloid leukemia
- **b.** Acute lymphocytic leukemia
- **c.** Myelodysplastic syndrome
- **d.** Non-Hodgkin lymphoma
- **e.** Tyrosine kinase inhibitors
- **f.** Chronic myeloid leukemia
- **g.** Chronic lymphocytic leukemia

B. Nonmalignant conditions:
- **a.** Potentially curable by HSCT: Aplastic leukemia
- **b.** Immunodeficiency syndrome:
  - **1.** Chediak–Higashi disease
  - **2.** Severe combined immunodeficiency syndrome
- **c.** Congenital disorders of congenital disorders:
  - **1.** Thalassemia
  - **2.** Sickle cell anemia
- **d.** Inborn error of metabolism: Mucopolysaccharidoses

Indications of Autologous Bone Marrow Transplantation

A. Plasma cell myeloma after induction of chemotherapy

B. Mantle cell lymphoma in first remission

C. Relapsed aggressive NHL

D. Relapsed NHL

E. In second remission of AML in case of nonavailability of allogeneic HSCT

F. Solid tumor with metastasis:
- **a.** Breast
- **b.** Ovarian
- **c.** Lung cancer

Procedure of Allogeneic HSCT

A. Conditioning of the patients: High-dose chemotherapy with cyclophosphamide alone or combined with total body irradiation is given for over 1 week:
- **a.** To eradicate malignant cells
- **b.** To ablate marrow of the patients
- **c.** To create space for marrow graft
- **d.** To produce immunosuppression to prevent rejection of graft

B. Transplantation: 1 day after conditioning phase, stem cells are to be harvested from peripheral blood or bone marrow of selected donor and have to be infused into the blood of the recipient. Due to the phase of conditioning, patient may be susceptible to frequent infections.
- **a.** Barrier nursing, necessary in filtered environment, is required.
- **b.** Prophylactic antibiotic is to be administered routinely.

C. Stage of engraftment: 7–21 days following transplantation, stem cells start producing blood cells in the bone marrow.

D. Stage of prevention of GVHD: T lymphocytes of donor recognize host tissue as foreign leading to GVHD, which increases morbidity as well as mortality. It can be prevented by routine administration of methotrexate and cyclosporine as immunosuppressive therapy for 6 months post-transplant.

E. Follow-up care: It is usually done for managing chronic GVHD and other long-term side effects.

Complications of Allogeneic HSCT

A. Complications as a result of conditioning regimen: It consists of:

- **a.** Early complications occur in <100 days post-transplant.
  1. Alopecia
  2. Pancytopenia
  3. Diarrhea
  4. Hemorrhagic cystitis
  5. Oropharyngeal mucositis
  6. Cardiomyopathy
  7. Hepatic veno-occlusive disease
  8. Interstitial pneumonitis
- **b.** Late complications occurring >100 days post-transplant.
  1. Cataract due to total body irradiation
  2. Sterility
  3. Endocrine abnormalities
  4. Osteopenia
  5. Osteoporosis
  6. Early menopause
  7. Secondary cancers in the skin

B. Graft rejection: Here immunocompetent T cells of the recipient will do this in presence of:

- **a.** Human leukocyte antigen incompatibility
- **b.** Insufficient immunosuppression
- **c.** Previously sensitized to HLA antigens by previous blood transfusion

It occurs mainly in case of aplastic anemia.

Prevention can be done by transplantation of T-cell depleted graft as it increases survival rate.

C. Graft-versus-host disease: Here reaction occurs as a result of recognition of recipient tissue as foreign antigen by immunocompetent T lymphocytes present in the transplanted donor graft. It is of two types:

- **a.** Acute GVHD:
  1. It occurs within 100 days of transplantation
  2. It is more common in unrelated or HLA-mismatched HSCT
  3. Organ affected with variable severity:
     - Skin: Maculopapular skin rash
     - Liver: Cholestatic hepatitis
     - Gastrointestinal tract: Nausea, vomiting, diarrhea, and ileus
  4. It can be prevented by:
     - Immunosuppressive therapy with methotrexate and cyclosporine
     - Transplantation of T cells-depleted marrow

     Complications of above method of prevention:
     - It will increase the rate of graft rejection
     - Loss of graft versus leukemic effect
  5. Treatment:
     - Corticosteroids
     - Antithymic globulin
     - Monoclonal antibodies against lymphocytes
- **b.** Chronic graft-versus-host disease:
  1. It occurs in 10% patients after transplant
  2. It resembles autoimmune disorders such as SLE, scleroderma, Sjögren's syndrome, and primary biliary cirrhosis
  3. Treatment: Immunosuppressive therapies

D. Infections:

- **a.** It is major complications of GVHD.
- **b.** During early neutropenic period: Bacterial, herpes simplex, and fungal infections.
- **c.** After engraftment, infection with life-threatening CMV and pneumonia
- **d.** Late infections with varicella zoster and encapsulated bacteria few months after transplant

E. Recurrence of malignancy: Recurrence of leukemia—it is a cause of graft failure. It is less likely to occur when it is done during first remission.

Procedure of Autologous HSCT

A. Stage of harvest of stem cells: Stem cells are obtained from the patients in CR.

B. Stage of process and storage: After collection, the stem cells are processed to remove the malignant cells present and then it will be frozen and stored in liquid nitrogen.

C. Stage of conditioning: Conditioning regimen has to be started within few days to weeks of harvesting the marrow cells with high-dose chemotherapy. But, as compared to allogeneic HSCT:

- **a.** Conditioning intensity will be less
- **b.** Restoration of immunity will be quicker
- **c.** There is no potential for GVHD

D. 1 day after completion of conditioning, stem cells have to be rapidly thawed and transfused intravenously.

E. Length of hospital stay will be less as compared to allogeneic HSCT.

Complications of Autologous HSCT

A. Most common complications:

- **a.** Relapse of underlying malignant disease due to contamination of the graft stem cells with tumor cells.

B. Other complications:

- **a.** Graft-versus-host disease
- **b.** Graft rejection
- **c.** Graft versus leukemic effect
- **d.** Development of secondary malignancies

C. Disadvantages:

- **a.** It cannot be used in case of genetic disorders

D. Advantages:

- **a.** Donor lymphocytes recognize the malignant lymphocytes in the recipient's blood as foreign and, thus, causing destruction of residual leukemic cells

Q16. Paroxysmal nocturnal hemoglobinuria.

MGR/SEP2010/MDI (5)

MUHS/MAY2014/MDIII (10)

MUHS/NOV2010/MDIII (10)

Classify hemolytic anemia. Write clinical features, diagnosis, and management of paroxysmal nocturnal hemoglobinuria.

DNB 2021 (10)

ANSWER

Classification of hemolytic anemia has been described in question number 21.

Definition

It is a clonal disease of bone marrow characterized by:

A. Aplastic anemia

B. Intravascular hemolysis

C. Venous thrombosis

Etiopathology

Mutation of PIG-A [phosphotidylinositol glycan complementation class A gene occurring in hematopoietic stem cell responsible for synthesis of glycolipid moiety called glycosylphosphatidylinositol (GPI) anchor]

↓

Lack of surface protein of large family of GPI-linked proteins on RBC membrane CD55 and CD59

↓

Red blood cell is susceptible to complement

↓

Intravascular hemolysis

This PIG-A mutant cells are usually present in bone marrow. But, in case of PNH, this clone will expand, especially in aplastic anemia and MDS, cell size being from small to large. The cause is unknown.

Clinical Features

A. Evidence of intravascular hemolysis: Dark urine in the morning, sometimes patient may unnotice or suppress it.

B. Features of anemia: Fatigue, lethargy, shortness of breath, and ringing in the ear

C. Venous thrombosis:

- **a.** Hepatic vein—Budd-Chiari syndrome
- **b.** Portal vein—portal hypertension
- **c.** Intracranial vein—intracranial venous thrombosis
- **d.** Mesenteric vein—mesenteric venous thrombosis

D. Marrow failure—frank aplastic anemia or poor function of marrow

Diagnosis

Laboratory Investigations

A. Red blood cells:

- **a.** Normocytic or macrocytic anemia
- **b.** Mean corpuscular volume—increased (macrocytosis)—denotes reticulocytosis
- **c.** Reticulocyte count is 20% (400,000 cells/μL)
- **d.** In case of chronic urinary blood loss through hemoglobinuria, cell size will be microcytic

B. White blood cells—neutropenia

C. Platelet—thrombocytopenia

D. Blood biochemistry:

- **a.** Unconjugated bilirubin—raised
- **b.** Lactate dehydrogenase—markedly elevated
- **c.** Haptoglobin—undetectable
- **d.** Urine:
  1. Hemoglobinuria—it is the telltale sign of intravascular hemolysis. Since hemoglobinuria will vary from day to day or hour to hour, so serial sample of urine is required to confirm it.

E. Bone marrow: Normocellular with massive erythroid hyperplasia. But, later on, marrow becomes hypocellular.

F. Definite diagnosis:

   a. To see the hemolysis of the clone of RBC deficient in CD55 and CD59 on the surface membrane of RBC because they are very sensitive to complement. Gold standard test is flow cytometry—it can be carried out on RBC and granulocytes. Bimodal distribution of cells with discrete population of CD55 and CD59 is the diagnostic of PNH.

Treatment

A. Supportive treatment:

   a. Transfusion of RBCs in the form of packed RBCs to raise the hemoglobin level.
   b. Folic acid supplementation at a dose of 3 mg/day is mandatory.
   c. Iron supplementation is appropriate. Secondary hemochromatosis is prevented by loss of hemoglobin due to intravascular hemolysis.
   d. In case of chronic hemolysis, steroid can be given at a dose of 30–50 mg alternate day to control hemolysis
   e. Marrow failure due to associated aplastic anemia should be treated by homologous stem cell transfusion. It can be considered in case of:
      1. Younger patients with severe marrow failure
      2. Thrombotic complications
   f. Coumadin prophylaxis is effective, but long-term anticoagulation may lead to hemorrhagic complications.

B. Definite treatment:

   Eculizumab: It is MAB, which is approved by DDA for the PNH treatment as:

   a. It will block intravascular hemolysis
   b. It will reduce the incidence of thrombotic complications

   Cautions:

   a. It is mandatory to give meningococcal vaccine 14 days prior to administration of eculizumab.
   b. Prophylactic antibiotic should be maintained.

   Long-term results:

   a. It will change the life expectancy of the patients
   b. It will change the natural history of the disease

   Dose: 1,200 mg every 2 weeks.

Q17. Iron deficiency anemia.

MGR/SEP2009/MDIII (6)

Discuss the etiopathogenesis, clinical features, investigation, and management of iron deficiency anemia.

MGR/APR2012/MDIV (15)

Refractory iron deficiency anemia.

PGI/APR2014/MDIII (10)

Evaluation and management of refractory iron deficiency anemia.

PGI/APR2013/MDIII (10)

Give causes of anemia seen in India. Discuss management of iron deficiency anemia in pregnancy.

ERA/MAY2011/MDII (10)

Newer diagnostic tools for assessment of iron stores.

DNB 2022 (5)

Describe the iron-metabolism. What is the role of hepcidin in iron metabolism?

WBUHS, 2023 (10)

Describe iron metabolism with special reference to IDA and anemia of chronic disease.

WBUHS, 2025 (10)

ANSWER

Iron Metabolism

Iron is present in the oxidized form like ferric form. To be absorbed from duodenum, proximal jejunum, iron will reduce to ferrous form. In the brush border of proximal duodenum, ferric reductase will reduce the ferric form of iron into ferrous form in presence of gastric acid, thereby gastric acid takes an important role in the iron homeostasis. Hence proton pump inhibitor reduces the iron absorption.

Ferrous form of iron will be absorbed from the apical membrane of the enterocytes with the help of a protein, divalent metal cation transporter 1. Level of this protein will be upregulated in case of hypoxic environment of the intestinal mucosa by hypoxia inducible factor-2.

A. Enhancer of gastric pH dependent iron absorption:

- **a.** Ascorbic acid: It will overcome all dietary inhibitory factors. It will form a chelate with ferric form of iron in the gastric low pH and persist and will be soluble in the duodenal alkaline environment.

B. Inhibitors of iron absorption are:

- **a.** Phytate: It demonstrates dose dependent iron absorption.
- **b.** Polyphenol: It inhibits non-heme iron absorption.
- **c.** Calcium inhibits both heme and non-heme iron absorption at the point of iron absorption site.
- **d.** Animal proteins:
  1. Egg white
  2. Whey
  3. Casein
  4. Soy protein
- **e.** Oxalic acids are present in the beans, chards, spinach and nuts which bind iron from the diet.

In the enterocytes, iron either is stored as ferritin or transported into the systemic circulation bounded with ferroportin.

Ferritin is a spherical protein containing 24 amino acids that potentiates and regulates the body iron store thereby regulating the serum iron in the body. Within the ferritin iron is stored in the ferric state through the incorporation of it into the solid crystalline mineral ferrihydrite.

Ferroxidase activity of the monomers of ferritin mobilizes ferrous iron out of ferrihydrite allows subsequent efflux of ferrous iron into the enterocytes. Ferroportin is the only efflux route that is regulated by Hepcidin levels as Hepcidin binds ferroportin leading to internalization and degradation of resulting shunting of the cellular iron into the ferritin.

Hepcidin potentiates the excretion of iron through the sloughing of the enterocytes into the feces.

In case of low Hepcidin level and downregulation of ferroportin ferrous form of iron is released from the enterocytes and oxidized into the ferric form to bind with carrier protein transferrin present in the plasma.

Two copper containing enzymes, ceruloplasmin in the plasma and hephaestin present on the basolateral membrane of the enterocytes catalyze the oxidation of ferrous iron and its subsequent binding with transferrin in the plasma. Main action of the transferrin is to make iron available for future incorporation into the hemoglobin and prevents formation of reactive oxygen species.

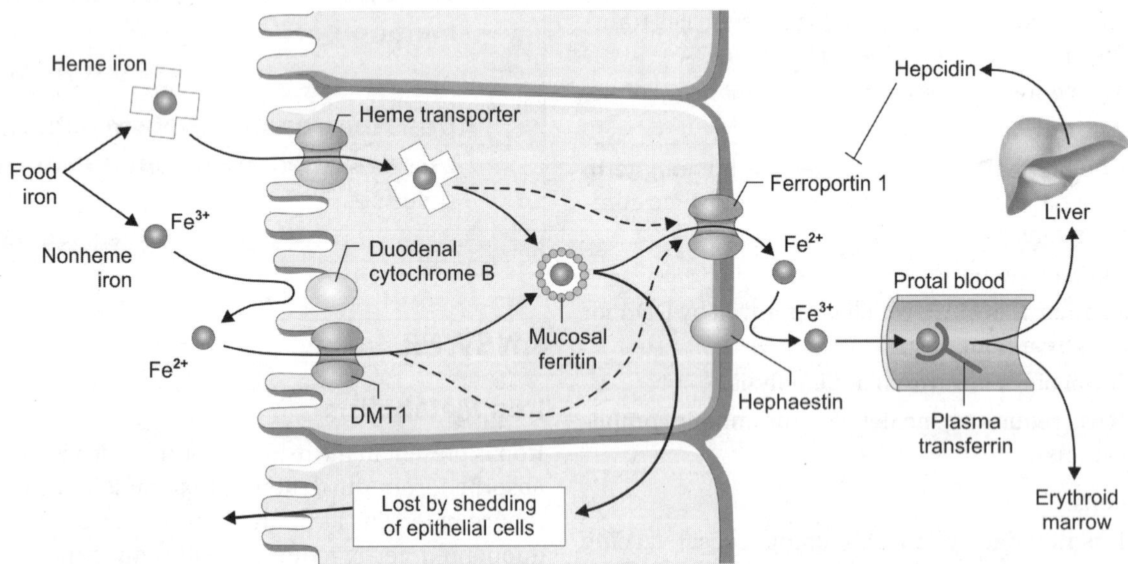

Causes of Anemia

A. Reduced proliferation of precursors:

- **a.** Iron deficiency anemia
- **b.** Anemia of chronic disorders:
  1. Infections
  2. Collagen diseases
  3. Malignancy
- **c.** Reduced EPO production: Renal disease
- **d.** Reduced oxygen requirement:
  1. Hypopituitarism
  2. Hypothyroidism

e. Reduced oxygen affinity of hemoglobin
f. Primary disease of bone marrow:
   1. Aplastic anemia:
      - Primary
      - Secondary due to drugs, irradiation, chemicals, and toxins
g. Pure red cell aplasia
h. Infiltrative disorders:
   1. Leukemia
   2. Lymphoma
   3. Myelofibrosis
   4. Secondary carcinoma

B. Defective maturation of the precursors:
a. Defective nuclear maturation:
   1. Vitamin B12 deficiency
   2. Folate deficiency
   3. Erythroleukemia
b. Defective cytoplasmic maturation:
   1. Iron deficiency
   2. Defective in globin synthesis
   3. Disorder of heme and/or globin metabolism
   4. Disorder in porphyrin metabolism
c. Other mechanisms:
   1. Congenital dyserythropoietic anemia
   2. Myelodysplastic syndrome
   3. Infections
   4. Toxins
   5. Chemicals

Causes of Iron Deficiency Anemia

A. Gastrointestinal tract: Any type of bleeding from stomodeum to proctodeum—ulcer, polyp, cancer, and congenital arteriovenous malformation
B. Malabsorption: Celiac disease, atrophic gastritis, and gastrectomy
C. Physiological—growth spurts and pregnancy
D. Dietary—vegans, elderly
E. Genitourinary system—hematuria and hemodialysis
F. Others—surgery, PNH, and blood donation
G. Worldwide: Hookworm infestation

Pathogenesis

A. Increased demand:
a. Physiological state:
   1. Pregnancy
   2. Childhood
b. Blood loss:
   1. Menorrhagia
   2. Inflammatory bowel disease
   3. Peptic ulcer disease
   4. Gastrointestinal blood loss
   5. Blood donation

B. Decreased availability:
a. Poor intake:
   1. Vegans
   2. Vegetarian
b. Poor absorption:
   1. Gastric bypass surgery
   2. Gastroesophageal reflux disease
   3. Gastritis
   4. Infection with *Helicobacter pylori*
   5. Antacid/Proton pump inhibitor (PPI) use
   6. Celiac disease
   7. High caffeine ingestion
   8. Parasitic infestation

Evaluation of Iron Deficiency Anemia

A. From history:
a. Clinical history: Review of potential sources of blood loss, especially gastrointestinal loss, trauma, and blood donation
b. Menstrual loss
c. Other sources of blood loss—hemoptysis, hematuria, and epistaxis
d. Drug history—intake of NSAIDs and corticosteroids may cause gastrointestinal bleeding
e. Past history of gastric surgery (malabsorption)
f. In children—poor attention and retardation of behavior
g. Pica—craving for eating unusual substances such as clay, starch, and hair
h. In elderly—restless legs syndrome

B. Examination:
a. Assessment of mucous membrane—pallor, glossitis, and stomatitis
b. Search for possible sources of blood loss
c. Abdominal examination—tenderness and lump
d. Rectal examination—seek for source of bleeding
e. Per vaginal examination to look for source of bleeding
f. Hair loss—may be consequence of low ferritin
g. Spoon-shaped nails—koilonychia

h. Retinal hemorrhage and exudate in severely anemic (Hb < 5 g%) patients
i. Mucosal atrophy in laryngopharynx leads to web formation in the postcricoid region producing dysphagia (Plummer-Vinson syndrome or Paterson-Kelly syndrome)

Laboratory Examination

Hematology

A. Hemoglobin—low (men < 13.5 g% and women—11.5 g%)
B. Mean corpuscular volume (MCV)—<76 fl
C. Mean corpuscular hemoglobin concentration (MCHC)—low (32.5 ± 2.5 g/dL)
D. Red cell distribution width (RDW)—increased (>14.5%)
E. Serum ferritin—in absence of chronic inflammation <20 ng/mL
But, in chronic inflammation < 100 ng/mL (it is the cutoff value)
F. Soluble transferrin assay—it is useful where ESR is raised (rheumatoid arthritis and chronic disease)
G. Serum iron <50 μg/L
H. Red blood cell is hypochromic and percentage will be increased in iron deficiency anemia
I. Reticulocyte count will be raised
J. Red blood cell count <4 × 10^6/mm^3

Treatment

Following medications retard the iron absorption from gastrointestinal tract:

A. Antacids
B. Proton pump inhibitors
C. H2 blockers
D. Bisphosphonates
E. Doxycycline
F. Tea
G. Cholestyramine
H. Dairy products

Following factors enhance the iron absorption:

A. Citrus food and tomatoes
B. Vitamin C
C. Nonenteric iron tablets
D. Fasting state

Oral Iron Therapy

A. Ferrous gluconate or ferrous fumarate and iron sulfate.
B. Daily supplementation of 200 mg of elemental iron taken in fasting state will provide marrow to increase the hemoglobin concentration 0.25 g/dL/day in severely affected patients.
C. Elemental iron:
   a. In ferrous fumarate—106 mg
   b. In ferrous gluconate—38 mg
   c. In iron sulfate—65 mg
D. Side effects in 10-25% of patients: Gastrointestinal intolerance, constipation, abdominal pain, nausea, and vomiting
E. Response to treatment:
   a. Rise in hemoglobin—2 g/dL over 3 weeks
   b. Mean corpuscular volume will be raised
   c. Reticulocyte count will be raised initially in 3–4 days
F. How much iron absorption occurs after administration of oral iron can be estimated by:
   a. 8–12 fasting serum iron level will be estimated
   b. Serum iron level has to be estimated after 1 hour
   c. If the level of serum iron is 100 μg/mL more than baseline—it suggests adequate iron absorption
G. Duration of treatment:
   a. Generally, 6 months
   b. After normalization of hemoglobin level and MCV treatment should be continued for at least 3 months
H. Failure of response:
   a. Diagnosis may be wrong; in that case, chronic anemia may be the diagnosis
   b. Any additional complicating illness
   c. Is blood loss is being continued?
   d. Is there any associated continued malabsorption?
   e. Is the dose being correct or adequate?
   f. Are there any associated vitamin B12 or folate deficiencies?

Intravenous Iron Therapy

A. Indications:
   a. Intolerance to oral iron therapy
   b. Problem with compliance
   c. Need to replace the store rapidly
   d. Prior to major surgery
B. The drugs are:
   a. Ferric gluconate—125 mg/h (12.5 mg/mL elemental iron)

b. Iron sucrose (ferric hydroxide with sucrose): 100–400 mg in 15 minutes to 4 hours (20 mg/mL elemental iron)
c. Iron dextran (ferric hydroxide with dextran)

C. These can be administered in two ways:
a. Administration of total dose of iron required to correct hemoglobin deficit and provide the total iron stores of 500 mg in any patient.
b. Administration of repeated small dose of parenteral iron over a protracted period—it is common in dialysis.

D. The amount to be given to any patient according to his need can be calculated from the following formula:
Body weight (in kg) × 2.3 × [15 – patient's hemoglobin (in g/dL)] + 500 or 1,000 mg (for stores)

E. Response to iron therapy:
a. Within 3–4 days, peripheral reticulocyte count increases
b. Within first week, hemoglobin begins to rise

F. Complications of newly developed preparations:
a. Arthralgia
b. Low-grade fever
c. Skin rash

G. Method of administration: Iron dextrose has to be dissolved in 5% dextrose or 0.9% sodium chloride (NaCl) and to be given in 60–90 minutes.

Newer Diagnostic Tools for Assessment of Iron Stores

Diagnostic tools	Markers	Interpretations
Soluble transferrin receptors	It will indicate cellular demand for the iron	It is increased in iron deficiency anemia
Soluble transferrin receptor/Log of ferritin index	Combine result of both	It is specific for mixed anemia
Hepcidin	It is gate keeper iron homeostasis	It is decreased in iron deficiency anemia It is decreased in chronic anemia
Percentage of hypochromic red blood cells.	It indicates red blood cells with low hemoglobin content.	It indicates functional iron deficiency anemia.
Reticulocyte hemoglobin content.	Content of hemoglobin in red blood cell	It will detect early iron restricted erythropoiesis
Zinc erythropoiesis	It will accumulate in iron deficient erythropoiesis	Functional iron status

Q18. Diagnosis of infectious mononucleosis.
MGR/APR2013/MDIII (7)

Infectious mononucleosis—complications and management.
MGR/OCT2011/MDIII (7)

Infectious mononucleosis.
MGR/APR2003/MDIII (10)
MUHS/NOV2013/MDII (10)

ANSWER

Definition

It is an acute infectious disorder due to Epstein–Barr virus (EBV) characterized by fever, lymphadenopathy, and pharyngitis along with atypical lymphocytes in the peripheral blood.

Etiopathogenesis

A. Epstein–Barr virus is a double-stranded deoxyribonucleic acid (DNA) virus related to family of herpesvirus.

B. Transmission:
a. From kissing through saliva from infected persons to the susceptable individual's oropharynx.
b. Through blood to other B-lymphoid sites.

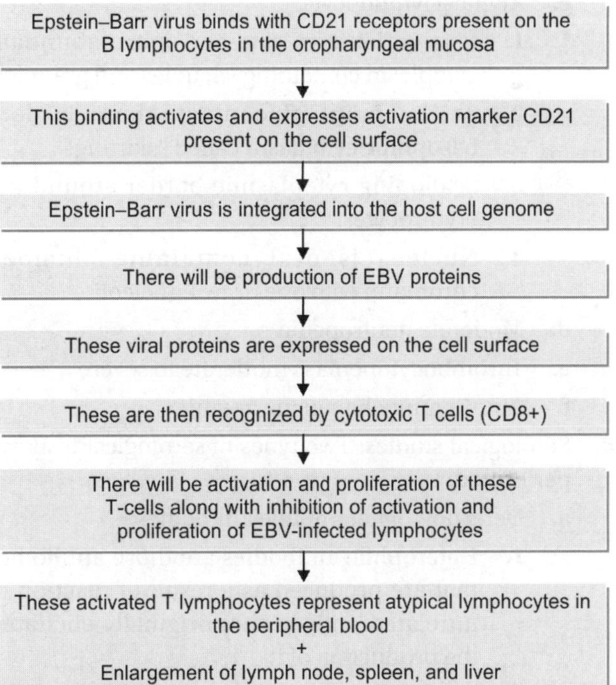

Clinical Features

A. Incubation period is 3–8 weeks

B. Symptoms: Fever—Pel-Ebstein type, sore throat, malaise, and backache

C. Examinations:

- **a.** Enlarged tonsil
- **b.** Congested pharynx
- **c.** Palatal petechiae
- **d.** Splenomegaly in 50% of cases
- **e.** Skin rash

Complications

A. Guillain-Barré syndrome

B. Encephalitis

C. Splenic rupture

D. Bell's palsy

E. Myocarditis

F. Pericarditis

G. Tonsillar hyperplasia producing airway obstruction

H. Pneumonia

Laboratory Features

A. Peripheral blood examinations:

- **a.** Leukocyte count is raised due to absolute lymphocytosis.
- **b.** Differential count demonstrates >50% cells are lymphocytes along with >10% cells are atypical.
- **c.** Atypical lymphocyte:
  1. It is variable in size and more abundant cytoplasm containing vacuoles and granules.
  2. At the point of contact, there is dark basophilic cytoplasm called "skirting."
  3. Scalloping cytoplasmic border around the erythrocytes.
  4. Nucleus is oval containing clumped chromatin with one or two nucleoli.
- **d.** Moderate neutropenia
- **e.** Thrombocytopenia is moderate to severe
- **f.** Autoimmune hemolytic anemia

B. Serological studies: Two types of serological tests are performed.

- **a.** Detection of heterophile antibodies:
  1. Heterophile antibodies are those antibodies that are produced as a result of reaction of unrelated antigen that originally elicitated the production of it
  2. It is of IgM class
  3. It becomes detectable during second week of illness and it will persist for 2 months

  Paul-Bunnell test: In this test, patient's serum will agglutinate sheep's erythrocytes.

  1. In case of normal individual, the agglutination titer is ≤1:56
  2. In case of infectious mononucleosis, titer will be ≥1:224
  3. These antibodies are seen also in following diseases:
     - Serum sickness
     - Lymphomas
     - Leukemias

  Paul-Bunnell-Davidsohn test: Heterophile antibodies in infectious mononucleosis absorb beef red cells but not guinea pig red cells, whereas, in other patients, antibodies absorb guinea pig red cells but not beef red cells. Based on this theory:

  - Firstly, beef red cells have to be absorbed with heterophile antibodies present in patient's serum
  - Secondly, sheep red cells then are allowed to be absorbed by rest of the heterophile antibodies in patient's serum
  - If there is no clumping—it suggests positive for infectious mononucleosis

  Rapid slide test: It is most widely used test for diagnosis.

- **b.** Epstein-Barr virus-specific antibodies:
  1. It detects antibodies IgM against following antigens:
     - Viral capsid antigen (VCA)
     - Early antigen D means diffuse form of EA
     - Epstein-Barr nuclear antigen (EBNA)
     - Presence of anti-VCA IgM antibodies or anti-D IgM antibodies in absence of anti EBNA antibodies are the diagnostic of infectious mononucleosis.

C. Lymph node biopsy:

- **a.** Hyperplasia of paracortical zones
- **b.** Varying size of lymphocytes from lymphoblast to small atypical lymphocytes
- **c.** Sinuses filled up with varying size of lymphocytes

D. Other features:

- **a.** Varying types of autoantibodies resulting from polyclonal B cell stimulation:
  1. Cold reactive autoantibodies
  2. Antinuclear antibodies

Treatment

A. Supportive treatment

B. Symptomatic treatment such as antipyretics, intravenous fluid, and vitamins

Q19. Pathophysiology and management of APL.

PGI/NOV2012/MDIV (10)

Treatment of promyelocytic anemia (PML).

KUHS/NOV2013(S)/MDIII (10)

Promyelocytic leukemia.

MGR UNIVERSITY, 2020 (10)

ANSWER

Definition

Promyelocytic leukemia is characterized by uncontrollable heterogeneous proliferation of myeloid progenitor cells replacing normal hematopoiesis in the bone marrow.

Pathogenesis

According to FAB classification, it is in M3 variety.

Risk factors for developing PML:

A. Environmental factors: Smoking, radiation, and benzene

B. Genetic factors

C. Preexisting hematologic disorders: MDS and aplastic anemia

Treatment

Acute promyelocytic leukemia is an entity with:

A. Distinct epidemiology

B. Characteristic morphology

C. Life-threatening coagulopathy

Acute promyelocytic leukemia requires separate treatment because:

A. Risk of DIC prior and during initial therapy due to release of thromboplastin from leukemic cells—is an indication for urgent treatment.

B. Rapid confirmation of PML-RARA fusion protein by PML—immunofluorescence test and FISH analysis predict favorable response with all-trans retinoic acid (ATRA) and arsenic trioxide (ATO).

C. Variant PLZF-RARa fusion protein confers resistance.

Drugs are: Noncytotoxic chemotherapeutic agents are ATRA and arsenic trioxide ATO.

It is the most curable subtype of AML with long-term disease-free survival of >90%.

Because of associated coagulopathy, there is high risk of mortality in the initial phase of treatment and it should be accepted and treated as medical emergency.

All-trans retinoic acid should be started as soon as the disease will be suspected even before performing confirmatory test.

Mode of Action of ATRA

A. It will act against leukemogenic event, i.e., translocation of chromosome t(15;17), thereby helps in differentiation of abnormal clone of cells and improve outcome.

B. It reduces the risk of DIC.

Mode of Therapy

In Induction Period

ATRA + cytarabine—70% of patients can be cured.

In Consolidation Phase

Cytarabine therapy.

Since bleeding is the most common complication and the cause of death, hence coagulopathy should be treated with:

A. Cryoprecipitate to maintain the fibrinogen level 150 mg/dL

B. Fresh frozen plasma and platelets to maintain the platelet level >50,000/cc

Complications of ATRA Therapy

Acute ATRA differentiation syndrome is characterized by:

A. Fever

B. Dyspnea

C. Hypoxemia

D. On examination:

- **a.** Pulmonary infiltrate
- **b.** Pleural effusion
- **c.** Pericardial effusion

E. White blood cell count >10,000/cc

It can be treated by:

A. 10 mg dexamethasone twice daily

B. Discontinuation of ATRA treatment

In case of relapse (persistence of abnormal PML-RARa fusion protein)—ATO should be given for second control of CR.

In patient on ATO therapy, ECG monitoring is done to see any prolongation of QT interval and measurement of electrolytes.

Now, only in case of high-risk disease with WBC count >10,000/cc, anthracycline chemotherapy for 3–4 days.

Stem cell transplantation has limited role in the treatment of PML, but it can be given in patient with second CR. Autologous HSCT is given in PCR-negative CR2 PML and allogeneic HSCT is given in PCR-positive CR2 PML.

Q20. Tropical eosinophilia

MGR/APR2016/MDIII (7)
KUHS/MAY2014/MDIV (10)
MGR/MAR2009/MDIII (6)
MGR/SEP2008/MDIII (6)

Diagnostic and management approach for a patient with eosinophilia.

PGI/NOV2013/MDIII (10)

Causes and consequences of eosinophilia.

PGI/APR2013/MDI (10)

Pulmonary eosinophilic syndrome.

MGR/MAR2010/MDII (6)

Define hypereosinophilic syndrome. Describe its etiopathogenesis, clinical spectrum, and management.

DNBI/JUN2012 (10)

Tropical pulmonary eosinophilia (TPE).

MGR/OCT2013/MDIII (7)

Discuss tropical eosinophilia.

Kerala UNI 2022 (10)

Discuss the approach in a case of hypereosinophilia.

WBUHS, 2024 (10)

ANSWER

Definition

Eosinophilia can be defined as count of eosinophil in peripheral blood >500/cc. It may be graded as:

A. Mild eosinophilia as absolute eosinophil count of 500–1,500/cc

B. Moderate eosinophilia as absolute eosinophil count of 1,500–5,000/cc

C. Severe eosinophilia as absolute eosinophil count of >5,000/cc

Hypereosinophilia

Eosinophil count in the 1,500/cc in blood in two examinations (interval > 1 month) and/or tissue hypereosinophilia defined by the following:

A. Eosinophil percentage in bone marrow exceeds 20% of all nucleated cells

B. Extensive infiltration of tissue by eosinophil based on pathologic report

C. Marked deposition of eosinophil granule proteins (in absence or presence of major tissue infiltration by eosinophils)

Hypereosinophilic Syndrome

It is a myeloproliferative disorder characterized by persistent eosinophilia associated with different organ damage. Following three features for diagnosis of hypereosinophilic syndrome:

A. Sustained eosinophillic count >1,500/cc for >6 months

B. No identifiable cause of eosinophilia

C. Features of organ involvement

Differential diagnosis of hypereosinophilic syndrome includes the following:

A. Familial eosinophilia

B. Acquired eosinophilia

- **a.** Secondary eosinophilia
- **b.** Clonal eosinophilia
- **c.** Idiopathic eosinophilia

Pathogenesis

Differentiation of eosinophil production is controlled by several factors:

A. Cytokines like IL-3 and IL-5, IL-5 is the most important one for differentiation into eosinophils

B. Granulocyte-macrophage colony-stimulating factor

Survival of eosinophil is several weeks due to sustained presence of cytokines but in absence of cytokines, survival is only 48 hours.

Granules in the eosinophils are toxic cationic proteins, primary mediators of tissue damage. These are:

A. Major basic protein

B. Eosinophilic-derived neurotoxin is ribonuclease

C. Eosinophil peroxidase produces free radicals

D. Eosinophilic cationic protein is ribonuclease

These free radicals and respiratory burst oxidative pathways of infiltrating eosinophils produce tissue damage.

Several mechanisms responsible for pathogenesis of hypereosinophilic syndrome:

A. Overproduction of eosinophilopoietic cytokines

B. Enhanced activity of eosinophils

C. Defects in the normal suppressive regulation of eosinophilopoiesis

Organ damage in case of eosinophilic syndrome is due to following:

A. Infiltration of eosinophils in the tissues

B. Release of mediators from the eosinophilic granules

Eosinophils secrete following chemoattractants, which amplify inflammatory cascade and recruit more eosinophils:

A. Platelet-activating factors

B. Eotaxin

C. RANTES (regulated upon activation, normal T cell expressed and secreted) cytotoxin

Cardiac system is most frequently involved organ as damage occurs in three stages:

A. Initial acute necrosis, but no clinical symptoms

B. Thrombotic phase

C. Endomyocardial fibrosis

Most serious complication of hypereosinophilic syndrome is involvement of the heart due to severe endocardial fibrotic thickening either or both ventricles resulting in:

A. Cardiac fibrosis

B. Chronic heart failure

C. Death

Clinical Features

Symptoms

A. Hematologic manifestations:

- **a.** Anemia producing fatigue
- **b.** Left upper quadrant pain due to splenomegaly
- **c.** Thrombotic events due to hypercoagulability

B. Neurologic symptoms:

- **a.** Embolic or thrombotic strokes or transient ischemic attack
- **b.** Blurring of vision
- **c.** Slurring of speech
- **d.** Peripheral neuropathy
- **e.** Encephalopathy producing CNS dysfunction

C. Respiratory manifestations:

- **a.** Recurrent angioedema
- **b.** Bronchospasm or asthmatic symptoms
- **c.** Rhinitis
- **d.** Breathlessness due to heart failure
- **e.** Evidence of pulmonary fibrosis
- **f.** Chronic nonproductive persistent cough

D. Gastrointestinal manifestations:

- **a.** Nausea
- **b.** Abdominal pain
- **c.** Diarrhea
- **d.** Small bowel necrosis due to microthrombi
- **e.** Evidence of sclerosing cholangitis

E. Dermatologic manifestations:

- **a.** Pruritus
- **b.** Dermographism
- **c.** Angioedema

Physical Findings

A. Cardiac features:

- **a.** Splinter hemorrhage
- **b.** Murmur
- **c.** Features of restrictive heart disease

B. Neurologic features:

- **a.** Features of ischemic cerebral attack
- **b.** Features of symmetric or asymmetric sensory and motor or mixed neuropathy
- **c.** Mononeuritis multiplex
- **d.** Generalized weakness

C. Pulmonary manifestations:

- **a.** Features of fibrosis
- **b.** Evidence of pleural effusion

D. Rheumatologic features:

- **a.** Joint effusion
- **b.** Digital necrosis
- **c.** Raynaud's phenomenon

E. Less common dermatologic manifestations:

- **a.** Mucosal ulceration
- **b.** Erythroderma
- **c.** Erythema gyratum repens
- **d.** Erythema annulare centrifugum

Laboratory Studies

A. Hematologic studies:

- **a.** Eosinophil count >1,500/cc
- **b.** Platelet count normal
- **c.** Neutrophil count normal
- **d.** Hemoglobin may be low

e. Hypergranularity or hypogranularity and hypersegmentation of WBC

f. Features of MPDs with thrombocytopenia or thrombocytosis and teardrop cells nucleated RBC

g. Leukocytosis ≥90,000/cc—bad prognostic sign

B. Other blood studies:

a. Increased serum tryptase suggests FIP1L1-PDGFRA mutation—it is characteristic of systemic mastocytosis and hypereosinophilic syndrome

b. Immunophenotyping of MCs demonstrates CD117 with CD25 and/or CD2

c. Interleukin-5 will be raised

d. Immunoglobulin E may be elevated

e. Serum B12 will be elevated

C. Bone marrow studies:

a. Reticulin stain to see myelofibrosis

b. Tryptase stain in case of increased tryptase level

c. Features of myelofibrotic disorders

d. Molecular genetic studies by FIP1L1-PDGFRA mutation in case of systemic mastocytosis and hypereosinophilic syndrome

e. Normal karyotyping

Treatment

A. As far today, there is no specific treatment for hypereosinophilic syndrome as the treatment is also not without any risk. Asymptomatic patient is continuously monitored with serum troponin level every 3–6 months and pulmonary function test (PFT) and echocardiography every 6–12 months.

B. Hypereosinophilic syndrome with MPDs with FIP1L1-PDGFRA mutation should be treated aggressively.

C. In patients with absence of FIP1L1-PDGFRA mutation, they should be treated with glucocorticoids as first line of therapy. Those who will not respond to steroid should be treated with hydroxyurea and interferon-alpha.

D. If the patients will not respond to first and second line of therapy, they can respond to high-dose imatinib.

E. FIP1L1-PDGFRA-negative patients can respond to mepolizumab, humanized MAB specific for IL-5.

F. Hypereosinophilic syndrome refractory to usual treatment can respond to chlorambucil, etoposide, vincristine, and cytarabine.

G. Patient refractory to imatinib therapy should be treated with HSCT to reverse the organ dysfunction.

H. There is no documentation of administration of aspirin or warfarin in absence of documented thrombi.

I. To control symptoms of leukocytosis, leukopheresis can be done.

Secondary (Reactive) Eosinophilia

Causes

A. Parasitic infestation:

a. Trichinosis

b. Strongyloidiasis

c. Ascariasis

B. Drugs:

a. Antibiotics:

1. Penicillin

2. Cephalosporin

b. Nonsteroidal anti-inflammatory drugs:

1. Aspirin

2. Ibuprofen

c. Allopurinol

d. Phenytoin

C. Atopy:

a. Allergic rhinitis

b. Food allergy

D. Eosinophilic esophagitis

E. Hypereosinophilic syndrome

F. Eosinophilic granulomatosis

G. Acute myeloid leukemia, variety of eosinophilic leukemia

Clonal Eosinophilia

It can be diagnosed by histology and cytogenetics and molecular genetics of the bone marrow. Causes are the following:

A. Acute leukemia:

a. Pre-B AML

b. M4 type AML with bone marrow eosinophilia

B. Chronic myeloid disorder

On the molecular basis, this disorder includes:

a. BCR-ABL CML

b. PDGFRβ rearranged eosinophilia

c. KIT-mutated systemic mastocytosis

d. PDGFR rearranged eosinophilia

Clinicopathologically assigned disorder includes:

A. Myelodysplastic syndrome

B. Myeloproliferative disorder—classical (polycythemia) and atypical (chronic eosinophilic leukemia, systemic mastocytosis, and chronic myelomonocytic leukemia)

Idiopathic eosinophilia is a diagnosis of exclusion when secondary and clonal causes of eosinophilia.

Tropical Pulmonary Eosinophilia

Definition

It is a distinct syndrome characterized by wheeze, fever, nocturnal cough, and eosinophilia due to immunological hyperresponsiveness to filarial parasites such as *Wuchereria bancrofti* and *Brugia malayi.*

Epidemiology

Male to female ratio 4:1 and occurs in third decade of life. It is endemic in tropical and subtropical regions.

Pathology

Three types of histopathological reactions seen in this disease:

A. Perivascular, peribronchial, and interstitial infiltrates containing histiocytes

B. Presence of eosinophilic infiltrates in peribronchial, perivascular, and interstitial tissues

C. Mixed cellular infiltrates consisting of lymphocytes, histiocytes, and eosinophils with well-marked interstitial fibrosis

Pathogenesis

Adult filarial parasite in the lymphatic tissue releases microfilariae, which are trapped in the pulmonary circulation. These will degenerate and release their antigenic materials into the circulation and trigger local inflammatory reaction. These antigenic materials also release into systemic circulation leading to extrapulmonary manifestations. Eosinophilic degranulation products such as eosinophil-derived neurotoxin, eosinophilic cationic protein, and major basic protein have also role in tropical eosinophilic pneumonia.

Bm2325, an antigen responsible for production of IgE, is released from infective stage 3 larvae. *Brugia malayi* is detected in patient with TPE and there is mimicry between this antigen and human gamma-glutamyltransferase (GGT), which are present on the pulmonary epithelium.

Clinical Features

A. Systemic symptoms: Fever, weight loss, and fatigue

B. Respiratory symptoms: Paroxysmal cough, breathlessness, cough, wheezing, and chest pain. It is usually present at night due to the activity of microfilariae. Occasionally, severe cough may produce fracture of the ribs

C. Sputum is scanty, viscous, and mucoid

D. On examination, there will be rhonchi and crepitations in both the lung fields

E. Extrapulmonary manifestations:
- **a.** Hepatomegaly
- **b.** Splenomegaly
- **c.** Lymphadenopathy
- **d.** Pericarditis
- **e.** Pericardial effusion
- **f.** Cor pulmonale
- **g.** Central nervous system manifestations
- **h.** Gastrointestinal manifestations

Tests

Sputum

Sputum contains eosinophils and Charcot–Leyden crystals.

Chest X-ray

A. Reticulonodular shadows in the mid and lower zones

B. Miliary mottling bilaterally, sometimes honeycomb appearance

C. In 20% of patients, normal lung fields

D. Other features are:
- **a.** Pleural effusion
- **b.** Cavitation
- **c.** Consolidation
- **d.** Air trapping
- **e.** Interstitial fibrosis

Pulmonary function test:

A. Reduction in single breath transfer factor for carbon dioxide.

Criteria for Diagnosis of Tropical Pulmonary Eosinophilia

A. Appropriate history of exposure in the endemic area

B. History of breathlessness and paroxysmal nocturnal cough

C. Leukocytosis in the blood

D. Evidence of pulmonary infiltrations in chest radiograph

E. Raised IgE level in the serum

F. Peripheral blood eosinophil >3,000/cc

G. Elevated antifilarial antibodies IgG and IgE in the serum

H. Clinical response to diethylcarbamazine (DEC)

Treatment

A. Oral DEC citrate 6 mg/kg of body weight in three divided doses for 3 weeks.

Most of the patients respond symptomatically and radiologically after 1 month of treatment, a mild alveolitis may persist after treatment.

B. Corticosteroids will reduce lower respiratory tract infection and release of oxidants.

C. Persisted interstitial lung disease may respond to repeated course of DEC at 2–3 monthly intervals for 1–2 years may be useful.

D. According to the WHO, treat the populations at risk of lymphatic filariasis by yearly combination of two drugs of 400 mg of albendazole and 6 mg/kg of DEC to cover the reproductive life span of adult parasite for 4–6 years.

Q21. Etiology, clinical features, and management of autoimmune hemolytic anemia.

DNBI/JUN2011 (10)

Hemolytic anemia.

MGR/MAR2010/MDI (5)

Classify hemolytic anemias. Describe the hemolytic mechanism and recognition of hemolysis.

RGHUS/APR2003/MDII (25)

Autoimmune hemolytic anemia.

RGUHS/MDIII (10)

Classify hemolytic anemia and discuss the laboratory diagnosis.

DNB 2020 (10)

Classify hereditary hemolytic anemia. Management of beta thalassemia.

DR YSR UNI of Health SC, Vijayawada, Andhra, 2022 (10)

Classify hemolytic anemia. Explain the diagnostic approaches of identifying various causes.

WBUHS, 2024 (10)

ANSWER

Etiology of Hemolytic Anemia

A. Intrinsic hemolytic anemia:

- **a.** Abnormal hemoglobin:
  1. Alpha- and beta-thalassemia
  2. Other hemoglobinopathies
  3. Unstable hemoglobin
- **b.** Membrane defect:
  1. Hereditary spherocytosis
  2. Hereditary elliptocytosis
  3. Hereditary acanthocytosis
  4. Hemolytic uremic syndrome
  5. MacLeod syndrome
  6. Paroxysmal nocturnal hemoglobinuria
- **c.** Enzyme defect:
  1. Glucose-6-phosphate dehydrogenase (G6PD) deficiency
  2. Pyruvate kinase deficiency
  3. Hexokinase deficiency

B. Extrinsic hemolytic anemia:

- **a.** Immune hemolytic anemia:
  1. Transfusion-induced alloantibody
  2. Hemolytic disease of the newborn
  3. Autoimmune syndrome
- **b.** Infection:
  1. Babesosis
  2. Malaria
  3. *Clostridium perfringens*
  4. Bartonellosis
- **c.** Chemicals:
  1. Snake venom
  2. Oxidants
  3. Lead
  4. Arsenic
- **d.** Fragmentation:
  1. Prosthetic heart valves
  2. Hemolytic uremic syndrome
  3. Thrombotic thrombocytopenic purpura
  4. Burns
  5. Hemodialysis
  6. Malignant hypertension
  7. Drowning
  8. March hemoglobinuria

e. Other causes:
 1. Liver disease
 2. Hypersplenism

Classification of Autoimmune Hemolytic Anemia

A. Warm antibody IgG hemolytic anemia (antibody is maximally active at 37°C):
 a. Primary (idiopathic)
 b. Secondary causes:
  1. Autoimmune causes such as SLE
  2. Drug induced
  3. Malignancy:
   - Malignant lymphoma
   - Chronic lymphocytic anemia
   - Carcinoma
   - Teratoma
  4. Immunodeficiency disorders:
   - Hypogammaglobulinemia
   - Acquired immunodeficiency syndrome (AIDS)

B. Cold antibody hemolytic anemia (antibody maximally active between 0 and 4°C):
 a. Cold agglutinin disease IgM type:
  1. Primary cause
  2. Secondary causes:
   - Infections:
    ○ *Mycoplasma pneumoniae*
    ○ Epstein–Barr virus
    ○ Cytomegalovirus
    ○ Malaria
   - Autoimmune disorders
   - Malignancy: Lymphoproliferative disorders
 b. Paroxysmal cold hemoglobinuria IgG type:
  1. Primary cause
  2. Secondary causes:
   - *Treponema pallidum*
   - Viruses

C. Mixed type warm and cold antibody type

D. Transplant-associated hemolytic anemia:
 a. Hematopoietic stem cell transplantation (ABO group incompatibility)
 b. Solid organ transplant (Passenger lymphocyte syndrome)

Causes of Intravascular and Extravascular Hemolysis

Intravascular Hemolysis	Extravascular Hemolysis
Immune: • PCH • PNH • Drug-induced immune hemolytic anemia • Acute hemolytic transfusion reactions *Thrombotic microangiopathies*: • HUS • TTP • DIC *Mechanical trauma*: • Arteriovenous malformations • Burns *Infections*: • Malaria (blackwater fever) • *Clostridium perfringens*	*Intrinsic RBC defects*: • Hemoglobinopathies (e.g., sickle cell, thalassemia) • Enzyme deficiencies (e.g., G6PD deficiencies) • Membrane defects (e.g., hereditary spherocytosis) *Immune*: • Warm AIHA • CHAD • Drug-induced immune hemolytic anemia • Delayed hemolytic transfusion reactions

Initial Laboratory Tests for Intravascular Hemolysis

Test	Finding in hemolysis	Cause
Haptoglobin	Decreased	Binds free hemoglobin
Lactate dehydrogenase	Elevated	Released from lysis of red blood cells
Peripheral blood smear	Abnormal red blood cells	Based on cause of anemia
Reticulocyte count	Increased	Marrow response to anemia
Unconjugated bilirubin	Increased	Increased hemoglobin breakdown
Urinalysis	Urobilinogen, positive for blood	Free hemoglobin and its metabolites

Difference between intravascular and extravascular hemolysis are:

- Macrophages of liver and spleen
- Fc receptor mediated
- Moderate reduction of haptoglobin
- No hemoglobinuria, e.g., warm type autoimmune hemolytic anemia
- Splenomegaly
- Usually less dramatic (unless massive)
- Intravascular compartment

- Sheer stress/oxidant stress
- Absent haptoglobin
- Plasma hemoglobinemia
- Hemoglobinuria
- Hemosiderinuria, e.g., paroxysmal cold, hemoglobinuria, microangiopathic hemolysis, etc.
- Backache, muscle spasms, cola colored urine, etc.

Diagnostic Clues for Hemolytic Anemia

History and physical examination findings	Suggested diagnosis
Diarrhea	Hemolytic uremic syndrome
Family history of hemolytic anemia	Sickle cell disease, hereditary spherocytosis, thalassemias, G6PD deficiency
Fever	Autoimmune hemolytic anemia, disseminated intravascular coagulation, hemolytic uremic syndrome, infection
Hematuria	Paroxysmal nocturnal hemoglobinuria, intravascular hemolysis
Medications (Table 4)	Drug-induced thrombotic microangiopathic anemia, drug-induced immune hemolytic anemia, G6PD deficiency
New-onset jaundice	Any hemolytic anemia
Personal history of cancer	Warm autoimmune hemolytic anemia
Personal history of mononucleosis or *Mycoplasma pneumoniae* infection	Cold autoimmune hemolytic anemia
Recent transfusion history	Hemolytic transfusion reaction

(G6PD: glucose-6-phosphate dehydrogenase)

Pathophysiology of Warm Antibody IgG Hemolytic Anemia

As warm antibodies are panagglutinins, hence they will react with all the red cells in the diagnostic panel.

A. If the red cells are coated lightly with IgG, they do not activate complement and taken up by the macrophages in the spleen only because the circulation in the spleen is sluggish but not by the liver macrophages as the circulation in the liver is fast.

B. If the red cells are heavily coated with IgG antibodies, they activate complement and will be taken up by the spleen as well as liver macrophages because the macrophages possess receptor for both IgG antibody and complement C3b.

Macrophages completely destroy the red cell membrane or part of the red cell membrane. In latter case, due to loss of surface membrane, microspherocyte will be developed and escaped into the circulation. But, being rigid, they will be sequestered and destroyed in the spleen. There is a direct relationship between severity of hemolysis and spherocytes number with IgG1 and IgG3 subclass of immunoglobulin.

Clinical Features of Warm Antibody IgG Hemolytic Anemia

A. Mild-to-moderate anemia

B. Mild jaundice

C. On examination splenomegaly

D. Features of parent disease responsible for anemia

Laboratory Features

A. Peripheral blood examinations:

- **a.** Spherocytes—it is smaller in size with lack of central pallor and densely hemoglobinized
- **b.** Fragmented red cells
- **c.** Polychromasia
- **d.** Nucleated RBCs
- **e.** Neutrophilic leukocytosis
- **f.** Platelet count—thrombocytopenia (it is called Evans syndrome)

B. Biochemical tests:

- **a.** Decreased haptoglobin
- **b.** Increased LDH

C. Antiglobulin Coombs' test: It is done based on immunological basis. Two types of tests are:

- **a.** Direct antiglobulin test: It is based on antibodies already attached with RBCs in vivo. If these red cells are mixed with Coomb's antisera, then antibodies present in the sera combine with red cells to produce clumping of red cells.
- **b.** Indirect antiglobulin test: Here the patient's serum is mixed with donor red cells in vitro where antibodies are attached with donor red cells. Now if Coomb's antisera are mixed with these sensitized red cells, then specific antibodies combine with red cells to produce clumping of red cells.

First polyspecific antiglobulin reagent consisting of IgG and complement anti-C3 antibodies are mixed with already sensitized red cells—if there is clumping of red cells, it means presence of IgG or C3 in the red cell membrane.

Then, monospecific antisera containing either IgG or C3 complement are mixed with sensitized red cells. If there is clumping of red cells seen in any test—it suggests either IgG or C3 is the antibody attached with red cells.

Treatment

A. Treatment of the parent diseases

B. Corticosteroid at a dose of 1 mg/kg of body weight can be administered as it reduces phagocytosis and synthesis of antibodies by spleen.

C. If the patient does not respond to corticosteroid, splenectomy is the procedure of choice to reduce destruction of red cells.

D. In unresponsive cases, MAB against CD20 antigen, rituximab or chemotherapeutic agents—azathioprine, cyclosporine, and cyclophosphamide can be tried.

E. Blood transfusion can be given when it is absolutely essential. As because antibody developed in the patient is panagglutinin, hence it may react with the red cells of the donor.

If the patient already received blood transfusion or was pregnant previously, he or she will develop alloantibodies; during cross-matching, autoantibody conceals these alloantibodies and these patients may develop hemolytic transfusion reaction after transfusion. So, in these cases, autoadsorption of autoantibodies should be done to reveal the alloantibodies for testing.

Pathogenesis of Cold Antibody-induced Hemolytic Anemia

Cold antibody IgM is usually present in low titer in human sera due to immunologic reaction to infection by certain microorganisms such as *Mycoplasma pneumoniae*, EBV, and lymphoproliferative disorders such as large cell lymphoma hence, they are clinically insignificant. These cold agglutinins are directed against antigens present on the red blood cells. Hemolysis by cold agglutinin depends upon:

A. Titer of cold agglutinin

B. Thermal amplitude—it is the highest temperature at which the red cells agglutinate with antibody

In cold agglutinin disease in cooler peripheral circulation, cold agglutinin reacts with antigen present on the red cells to:

A. Form aggregation of red cells in the peripheral circulation

B. Via classical pathway activation of complement

Regulatory inhibitors on the red cell surface inhibit activation of C3b stage, thus in cold circulation IgM and C3b are attached on the red cell surface. But, as the blood becomes warmer, IgM becomes dissociated from the red cell surface leaving only C3b. Red cells coated with C3b are only phagocytized by the liver. Now, C3b inactivator rapidly converts C3b to C3dg which is resistant to hemolysis by macrophages present in the liver as they have no receptor for C3dg. Once C3dg is formed, complement activation will be terminated. As further membrane attack, complex will not be generated hence, intravascular hemolysis will not occur. Hence, in cold agglutinin disease, hemolysis is extravascular.

Clinical Features

Clinical features depend upon the temperature amplitude.

A. In case of high temperature, hemolysis is chronic hence, mild anemia and icterus.

B. In exposure to cold, hemolysis will be acute and patient may present with icterus along with Raynaud's phenomenon and acrocyanosis.

If the patient suffers from infection, hemolysis occurs after 2–3 weeks after infection.

Laboratory Features

A. Hemoglobin level—low

B. Spurious elevation of MCH, MCHC, and MCV by agglutinated RBC

C. Evidence of agglutinate in the peripheral blood. This may ocuur in the following conditions:

  a. Immunoglobulin M paraproteinemia

  b. Paroxysmal cold hemoglobinuria

D. Direct antiglobulin test with anti-C3 can detect C3dg-coated red cells.

Cold agglutinin antibody agglutinates all the red cells and hinders in blood grouping. Hence, at 37°C, blood sample should be washed in normal saline to remove the IgM autoantibodies. Again, alloantibodies should be screened in the method at 37°C.

Treatment

A. Exposure to cold should be avoided

B. Treatment of the underlying cause

C. Here steroid and splenectomy are not helpful

D. In case of primary disease, MAB rituximab can be given

E. Plasmapheresis has to be done to reduce the antibody as a temporary measure

F. Transfusion can be given when it is absolutely essential

Mechanism of Hemolysis

In Case of Membrane Defect

There are two linkages by which lipid bilayer of red cell is anchored with the underlying skeleton.

A. First one involves ankyrin and spectrin of skeleton with band 3 in the bilayer

B. Second one is glycophorin C and protein 4.1 of skeleton with the bilayer

Any defect in these interactions produces weakness in the bilayer in the form of vesicles where there is loss of support of the skeleton resulting in loss of surface cell wall leading to formation of spherocytes.

These rigid and less deformable spherocytes cannot pass from splenic cords into splenic sinuses via narrow slit-like openings. Due to stuck in the splenic cords, there is formation of unsuitable environment in the form of reduced pH and low glucose. As a result of metabolic deprivation, red cells will be more spherical and more cellular dehydration occurs resulting from loss of intracellular potassium. Few microspherocytes release into the circulation and they are osmotically fragile. These cells will be destroyed in the splenic pulp by macrophages.

In Case of Sickle Cell Anemia

In the β-globin chain, there is substitution of thymine in place of adenine in the sixth codon, which results in substitution of amino acid valine for glutamic acid at position 6 of β-polypeptide chain.

Ultrastructurally, bundle of fibers are arranged along the long axis of the red cell and each bundle being composed of 14 filaments arranged in pairs. On deoxygenation, HbS molecules aggregate to form polymer of critical size. Later on, aggregation of additional HbS will form well-aligned fibers.

Initially, sickling is reversible. But, on oxygenation in lung, there is rapid dissociation of polymerized HbS (viscous state) to depolymerized state (fluid state). But, repeated sickling-unsickling will lead to permanent damage of RBC wall thereby, formation of irreversibly sickled cells. These cells never return to normal in shape upon oxygenation in lung.

Following factors influencing sickling:

A. Intracellular concentration of HbS with or without other hemoglobin: There is direct relationship between concentration of HbS and propensity to sickling. In presence of other hemoglobin, these cells will sickle in presence of very low concentration of HbS.

B. Association with thalassemia: This disease will be milder in presence of HbA.

C. Temperature: Cold temperature increases sickling through vasoconstriction.

D. Low pH: Acidic pH (acidosis) increases sickling producing deoxy state of hemoglobin.

E. Low oxygen tension: Amount of deoxygenation depends upon the amount of HbS. So, in case of homozygous sickle cell anemia, arterial oxygen tension at 40 mm Hg will produce sickling whereas in case of heterozygous sickle cell anemia, critical value of oxygen tension may be as low as 15 mm Hg.

F. Mean corpuscular hemoglobin concentration: Increased MCHC will enhance the intermolecular contact between HbS.

G. Coexistence of fetal hemoglobin: It will produce milder manifestation.

Pathogenesis of Vaso-occlusion

A. Depletion of nitric oxide by free heme released as a result of hemolysis leading to:
   - **a.** Slowing of blood flow
   - **b.** Upregulation of adhesion molecules
   - **c.** Alteration of vascular tone

B. Adhesion of young deformable cells to the vascular endothelium leading to:
   - **a.** Leukocyte activation
   - **b.** Release of inflammatory cytokine during infection

C. Increased blood viscosity by sickle formed RBC

Pathogenesis of Warm Antibody and Cold Antibody Autoimmune Hemolytic Anemia

Already written in this question.

Laboratory Diagnosis of Recognition of Hemolytic Anemia

A. Signs of excessive red cell destruction:
   - **a.** Survival of erythrocytes:
      1. Life span of red cell can be measured by random labeling with chromium-51.
      2. Bilirubin: Absence of bilirubin does not exclude hemolytic anemia. Serum unconjugated bilirubin 1–4 mg/dL suggests hemolytic anemia.
      3. Lactate dehydrogenase: LDH2 increases in hemolytic anemia, but LDH1 increases in megaloblastic anemia.
      4. Haptoglobin level: After hemolysis, released hemoglobin binds to haptoglobin and hepatocyte removes the complex. In case of extravascular hemolysis such as sickle cell

anemia, hereditary spherocytosis, hereditary elliptocytosis, pyruvate kinase deficiency, and intravascular hemolysis, haptoglobin will be low in the serum.

5. Decrease in glycosylated hemoglobin falls below 3.9%, normal being 6.5%.
6. Signs of intravascular hemolysis:
   - Hemoglobinuria
   - Methemoglobinemia
   - Hemosiderinuria

B. Signs of accelerated erythropoiesis:

a. Peripheral blood:

1. Reticulocytosis: Uncorrected count >5%—hemolysis suspected and >10%—hemolysis likely
2. Polychromasia
3. Basophilic stippling
4. Macrocytosis
5. Nucleated RBCs
6. Thrombocytosis
7. Leukocytosis

b. Bone marrow: Erythroid hyperplasia (in the bone marrow aspirate, 20–25% are normoblast)

C. Laboratory findings specific for differential diagnosis:

a. Specific morphology of RBC:

1. Spherocytes:
   - Hereditary spherocytosis
   - Autoimmune hemolytic anemia
   - Alloimmune hemolytic anemia
   - Acute and delayed transfusion reaction
   - Bartonellosis
   - Snakebite
   - Paroxysmal nocturnal hemoglobinuria
2. Elliptical cells—hereditary elliptocytosis
3. Stomatocyte—hereditary stomatocytosis
4. Sickle-shaped cell—sickle cell anemia
5. "Bite cell" or "keratocyte"—G6PD deficiency
6. Blister cells
7. Microspherocytes—significantly reduced in size with hyperchromatic:
   - Spherocytosis
   - Microangiopathic hemolytic anemia
     - Pregnancy-associated hypertension
     - Disseminated cancer
     - Chronic DIC
   - Burns
8. Schistocytes—trauma
9. Heinz bodies—refractile red cell inclusion eccentrically located adhered to cell membrane:
   - Hemolytic anemia due to G6PD deficiency
   - Drugs and toxins
   - Unstable hemoglobinopathies
   - Thalassemia

b. Laboratory investigations of abnormal hemoglobin and thalassemia:

1. Initial tests:
   - Complete blood count
   - At pH 9.2 electrophoresis
   - Test for solubility and sickling
   - Quantification of A2 and HbF
2. If abnormal is found in above tests, following tests are recommended:
   - At 6–6.2 electrophoresis
   - Globin chain separation
   - Isoelectric focusing
   - Heat stability
   - Isopropanol stability for detection of unstable HbS or HbS with altered oxygen affinity
   - Direct and indirect antiglobulin test for autoimmune hemolytic anemia
   - Osmotic fragility test to measure the resistance of erythrocytes to hemolysis by osmotic stress. Increased osmotic fragility is seen in hereditary spherocytosis

Q22. Sickle cell anemia.

LB/MAY2013/MDII (20) MGR/SEP2009/MDII (6)

Crisis in sickle cell disease.

KUHS/MAY2014/MDIII (10)

MGR/SEP2006/MDI (5)

Classify hemoglobinopathies. Diagnosis and treatment of sickle cell syndrome.

DNB 2019(10)

Clinical features and management of sickle cell anemia (including crises)

DNB 2018 (5)

ANSWER

Classification of Hemoglobinopathies

A. Structural hemoglobin variants due to point mutation in the globin gene.
   a. HbS
   b. HbC
   c. HbD
   d. HbE
B. Thalassemia due to qualitative defect in the globin chain synthesis
   a. Alpha thalassemia
   b. Beta thalassemia—major, intermediate, and minor
C. Hereditary persistence of fetal hemoglobin
   a. Deletional
   b. Non-deletional
D. Unstable hemoglobin due to instability of globin chain
   a. Hemoglobin Köln
   b. Hemoglobin Zürich
E. Methemoglobinemia related hemoglobin due to oxidation of iron in the heme:
   a. Hemoglobin M Boston
   b. Hemoglobin M Milwaukee
F. Hemoglobin having high or low oxygen affinity:
   a. Hemoglobin Chesapeake (high oxygen affinity)
   b. Hemoglobin Kansas (low oxygen affinity)
G. Combined hemoglobinopathies due to coinheritance of structural and thalassemic trait.
   a. Hemoglobin S/β thalassemia
   b. Hemoglobin E/β thalassemia

Definition

It is a condition where red cells become sickle in shape when they are subjected to low oxygen tension.

Sickle cell anemia is a homozygous state where gene for sickle cell is inherited from both parents. So, here the genotype is $\beta^s\beta^s$.

Epidemiology

It is frequent in equatorial Africa, Middle East, and Central and Southern India. Where malaria is common, there is high prevalence of sickle cell anemia in that area. From that point of view, there is protection in case of sickle cell heterozygote.

Pathogenesis

In the β-globin chain, there is substitution of thymine in place of adenine in the sixth codon which results in substitution of amino acid valine for glutamic acid at position 6 of β-polypeptide chain.

Ultrastructurally, bundle of fibers are arranged along the long axis of the red cell and each bundle being composed of 14 filaments arranged in pairs. On deoxygenation, HbS molecules aggregate to form polymer of critical size. Later on, aggregation of additional HbS will form well-aligned fibers.

Initially, sickling is reversible. But, on oxygenation in lung, there is rapid dissociation of polymerized HbS (viscous state) to depolymerized state (fluid state). But, repeated sickling-unsickling will lead to permanent damage of RBC wall, thereby formation of irreversibly sickled cells. These cells never return to normal in shape upon oxygenation in lung.

Following factors influencing sickling:

A. Intracellular concentration of HbS with or without other hemoglobin: There is direct relationship between concentration HbS and propensity to sickling. In presence of other hemoglobin, these cells will sickle in presence of very low concentration of HbS.
B. Association with thalassemia: This disease will be milder in presence of HbA.
C. Temperature: Cold temperature increases sickling through vasoconstriction.
D. Low pH: Acidic pH (acidosis) increases sickling producing deoxy state of hemoglobin.
E. Low oxygen tension: Amount of deoxygenation depends upon the amount of HbS. So, in case of homozygous sickle cell anemia, arterial oxygen tension at 40 mm Hg will produce sickling whereas in case of heterozygous sickle cell anemia, critical value of oxygen tension may be as low as 15 mm Hg.
F. Mean corpuscular hemoglobin concentration: Increased MCHC will enhance the intermolecular contact between HbS.
G. Coexistence of fetal hemoglobin: It will produce milder manifestation.

Pathogenesis of vaso-occlusion:

A. Depletion of nitric oxide by free heme released as a result of hemolysis leading to:
   a. Slowing of blood flow
   b. Upregulation of adhesion molecules
   c. Alteration of vascular tone

B. Adhesion of young deformable cells to the vascular endothelium leading to:

- **a.** Leukocyte activation
- **b.** Release of inflammatory cytokine during infection

C. Increased blood viscosity by sickle formed RBC.

Clinical Features

A. Retardation of growth and development

B. Splenomegaly: In early life, splenomegaly occurs due to hyperplasia of reticuloendothelial system. But, in later life due to repeated splenic infarction, spleen becomes fibrotic and nonpalpable.

C. Infections: Children of <5 years are susceptible to fulminant infection by organisms such as *Streptococcus pneumoniae* producing sepsis and meningitis, *Salmonella* producing osteomyelitis, *E. coli, Haemophilus influenzae,* and *Shigella*—all are due to functional splenectomy as a result of impaired phagocytic function of spleen.

D. Ischemic stroke due to vaso-occlusion by deformed RBC. Recurrence of stroke is also common.

E. Genitourinary system:

- **a.** Renal medulla is very prone to ischemic injury due to its hypertonic, acidic, and anoxic milieu.
- **b.** Papillary necrosis producing hematuria.
- **c.** Proteinuria and nephrotic syndrome leading to renal failure.
- **d.** Persistent, painful, prolonged, or short-lived priapism due to obstruction in venous return of corpora cavernosa.
- **e.** Impotence due to damage of vascular endothelial system.

F. Skeletal system:

- **a.** Widening of medullary cavity
- **b.** Dactylitis—painful, tender, and swollen joints
- **c.** Avascular necrosis of humeral heads
- **d.** *Salmonella* osteomyelitis

G. Pregnancy:

- **a.** In case of mother and fetus:
  1. Spontaneous abortion
  2. Stillbirth
  3. Intrauterine growth retardation
- **b.** In case of mother only:
  1. Incidence of infection
  2. Chest syndrome
  3. Postpartum hemorrhage

H. Respiratory system:

- **a.** Acute chest syndrome characterized by:
  1. Fever
  2. Cough
  3. Wheezing
  4. Respiratory distress
  5. Chest pain—pleuritic type
  6. New lung infiltrate involving at least one segment in chest X-ray
- **b.** Repeated chest infection may lead to chronic lung disease with lung fibrosis
- **c.** Pulmonary hypertension

I. Iron overload from repeated blood transfusion

J. Chronic leg ulcers on the medial aspect of ankle

K. Proliferative retinopathy

L. Hepatobiliary system:

- **a.** Hepatic damage due to:
  1. Transfusion-related hepatitis
  2. Infarction in the liver
- **b.** Gallstones—bilirubin stones may develop in patients having variant of UGT1A1 that also causes Gilbert syndrome.

M. Sickle cell crises: It is an episodic event. There are two major types of crises:

- **a.** Vaso-occlusive crises: It occurs from ischemia and infarction in the area of distribution of obstructed artery by stiff sickled RBC. Precipitating factors are:
  1. Exposure to cold
  2. Physical stress
  3. Emotional stress
  4. Unidentifiable factor

  Effects:
  1. Avascular necrosis of head of the femur
  2. Dactylitis
  3. Hand-foot syndrome
- **b.** Hematologic crises: It is characterized by sudden severe anemia leading to cardiac failure and death, if untreated. It consists of following types:
  1. Aplastic crisis: There is extravascular hemolysis of abnormal RBC due to its shortened life span. So, if over and above, there is decreased erythropoiesis, which may be due to parvovirus infection infecting erythroblast. It usually persists for 7–10 days.

In the blood smear, there is disappearance of polychromatic cells and nucleated RBCs.

2. Megaloblastic crises: It results from folate deficiency occurring during pregnancy or intercurrent infections.
3. Hemolytic crisis: There is sudden fall in hemoglobin level with increase in unconjugated bilirubin level due to increased RBC destruction over chronic hemolytic state. There may be associated G6PD deficiency or oxidant stress. Presence of ghost cells in the blood smear suggests hemolytic crisis.
4. Splenic crisis: In children with sickle cell anemia or in adult with sickle beta-thalassemia, sudden accumulation of blood in the spleen over several hours leads to destruction of RBC along with decrease in circulating blood volume, fall in hemoglobin and platelet, and, ultimately, circulatory failure. Peripheral blood demonstrates increase in reticulocyte, nucleated RBC, and polychromatic cells.

Laboratory Features

A. Peripheral blood examinations:
- **a.** Anemia—hemoglobin level 6–9 g/dL and RBC is normocytic and normochromic
- **b.** Red cell distribution width increased
- **c.** Different shapes: Anisopoikilocytosis and sickle-shaped and boat-shaped cells (crescent-shaped cells without pointed ends)—highly pathognomonic. Basophilic stippling, polychromatic cells, nucleated cells, and irreversibly sickled cells are also present
- **d.** Increased reticulocyte count—10–20%
- **e.** Platelet—it may be increased due to loss of splenic trapping. In case of vaso-occlusive crisis, it may be decreased

B. Other tests:
- **a.** Erythrocyte sedimentation rate increased
- **b.** Factor VIII raised
- **c.** Fibrinogen level increased
- **d.** Unconjugated bilirubin increased

C. Identification of HbS can be detected by slide test by using 2% sodium metabisulfite

D. Hemoglobin electrophoresis

E. Estimation of HbF by alkali denaturation test to detect the severity of sickle cell anemia

F. Neonatal screening for sickle cell anemia:
- **a.** Prenatal diagnosis in early pregnancy for HbS carrier state by two methods:
  1. Fetal blood analysis
  2. Fetal DNA analysis

Treatment

A. Prevention of crises by:
- **a.** Early detection and treatment of infections
- **b.** Avoidance of exposure to cold, hypoxia, dehydration, and stress
- **c.** Routine vaccination for *Neisseria meningitidis, Haemophilus influenzae,* influenza, and hepatitis B virus

B. Treatment of vaso-occlusive crises by analgesic, adequate fluid intake, keeping the patient warm and partial exchange transfusion to reduce the sickle cell burden

C. During pregnancy, supplement of folic acid and iron closes antenatal supervision

D. Oral contraceptive pill should be avoided as there is an increased risk of thrombosis

E. Prior to surgery, exchange transfusion to reduce vaso-occlusive crisis

F. During surgery, hypoxia, circulatory stasis, and dehydration should be avoided

G. Radiographic contrast media increases MCHC and dehydration of RBC—it should be avoided by proper hydration

H. In case of cerebrovascular accident, exchange transfusion is required to reduce the HbS burden

I. In acute chest syndrome, adequate analgesia, oxygenation, exchange transfusion, and broad-spectrum antibiotic should be administered

J. Drug of choice is hydroxyurea: It has certain benefits:
- **a.** It increases the HbF production and reduces the severity
- **b.** It reduces WBC count thus, anti-inflammatory effect
- **c.** It will increase RBC volume and hydration and reduce sickling
- **d.** It will decrease the adhesiveness of RBC and leukocytes
- **e.** It will release nitric oxide leading to vasodilatation
- **f.** It reduces incidence of painful crises, transfusion requirement, and acute chest syndrome

K. Hematopoietic stem cell transplantation: It is the only treatment, which may cure this disease. But, it should be reserved as ultimate resort.

L. Transfusion therapy:

a. Benefits: It will rise HbA concentration and reduce HbS concentration by:

1. Temporary suppression of erythropoiesis

2. Dilution of donor RBCs

b. Types of transfusion:

1. Packed RBC to improve oxygen carrying capacity in crises

2. Regular chronic infusion therapy: It is usually given to reduce the burden of HbS

3. Partial exchange transfusion

Q23. Non-Hodgkin lymphoma.

MGR/SEP2010/MDI (5) MGR/MAR2008/MDI (5)

Discuss the etiopathogenesis, clinical features, investigations, and management of NHL.

MGR/OCT2012/MDIV (15)

Diagnosis of NHL.

SNMC/MAY2013/MDIV (10)

Treatment of NHL.

KUHS/MAY2014/MDIII (10)

Non-Hodgkin lymphoma.

MGR UNI, Tamil Nadu, 2022 (5)

ANSWER

Definition

Non-Hodgkin lymphoma can be defined as a transformation of heterogeneous group of cells of T, B, or NK cell of origin.

Etiopathogenesis

Risk Factors

A. Infections: EBV, HCV, HIV, HTLV-I, *Chlamydia*, and *Campylobacter jejuni*

B. Drugs: Phenytoin, methotrexate, tumor necrosis factor (TNF) agonists, and immunosuppressive agents

C. Environmental factors: Radiation and occupational exposure

D. Congenital: Ataxia telangiectasia, Bloom syndrome, X-linked agammaglobulinemia, and SCI

E. Acquired syndrome: HSCT, solid organ transplantation, inflammatory bowel disease (IBD), Hashimoto's thyroiditis, and SLE

Antigen-independent normal B-cell development requires rearrangement of immunoglobulin genes in the progenitor cells in the bone marrow which consists of:

A. Somatic recombination of variable (V), joining (J), and diversity (D) segments of immunoglobulin heavy chain genes

B. Variable (V) and joining (J) of light chain genes

Naïve "B" cells that migrate to germinal centers in the lymphoid tissues express IgD and IgM on their surface. Variable region genes in these cells are unmutated due to nonexposure to antigen, but after exposure to an antigen in the germinal center mutation occurs in the variable region of B cells with production of antibodies toward targeted antigen. These sensitized B cells will survive as memory cells and may switch to IgG, IgA, and IgE classes. These mutated cells produce plasma cells. These mutations occur in majority of B-cell lymphoma such as Burkitt cell lymphoma and follicular cell lymphoma—it indicates their origin either from germinal or postgerminal center B cells. Inciting antigen *Helicobacter pylori* may be responsible for gastric malt lymphoma and HCV in case of splenic marginal zone lymphoma.

Translocation of chromosomes involving immunoglobulin heavy chain genes is responsible for several types of B-cell lymphoma, which may occur from following errors:

A. Variable, diversity, and joining recombination

B. Somatic hypermutation in the germinal centers

C. Switching of classes

Genes involving translocation regulates:

A. Cell proliferation such as MYC

B. Apoptosis such as BCL2

These are responsible for producing NHL.

Constitutive expression of MYC increases proliferation of cells. In case of follicular lymphoma, there is reciprocal translocation between BCL2 from chromosome 18 and IgH of chromosome 14, thus there is overexpression of BCL2 that protects the lymphocyte from apoptosis and prolonged survival of the abnormal cells.

In case of BL, similar translocation occurs in MYC oncogene from chromosome 8 to chromosome 14 leading to overexpression of MYC oncogene which is a transcription factor which is responsible for controlling growth regulating genes.

In case of mantle cell lymphoma, cyclin D gene present on the chromosome number 11 will be placed to transcriptionally active immunoglobulin heavy chain gene. Cyclin D is a regulator of G1 phase cycle, so its overexpression will dysregulated the cycle.

Clinical Features of Non-Hodgkin Lymphoma

A. Painless peripheral lymphadenopathy involving cervical or supraclavicular region

B. Following features distinguishes from HL are:

- **a.** Involvement of multiple lymph nodes
- **b.** With or without hepatosplenomegaly
- **c.** Extranodal diseases involving head, neck, and gastrointestinal tract involving most common sites such as stomach followed by small intestine, colon and esophagus, skin, CNS, thyroid gland, and testes.
- **d.** Disseminated involvement in the bone marrow in small lymphocytic, plasmacytoid lymphocytic, follicular small-cleaved cell, and lymphoblastic lymphoma. Bone marrow involvement means stage IV disease and it occurs in 50% of NHL.

C. Other manifestations are:

- **a.** Mediastinal mass in case of lymphoblastic lymphoma
- **b.** Jaw tumor in case of African BL
- **c.** Nodules and plaques known as mycosis fungoides

There are different types of presentations:

A. Patient may present with low-grade lymphoma with slow progression of disease in long run.

B. Disease may be limited to nodes only or only in extranodal locations.

C. Patients may present with high-grade lymphoma and rapid progression, which often prove fatal.

Laboratory Diagnosis

A. Peripheral blood smear examination to rule out leukemia and lymphoma mimics such as infectious mononucleosis.

B. Trephine biopsy of bone marrow is better than bone marrow examination and site will be posterior iliac crest. Patterns of infiltration are following:

- **a.** Focal paratrabecular infiltration—infiltration along the bony trabeculae
- **b.** Focal nonparatrabecular infiltration—here nodules of lymphoma cells do not completely fill up the intertrabecular space
- **c.** Interstitial pattern—here small groups of neoplastic cells will infiltrate in between the hematopoietic elements
- **d.** Diffuse pattern—complete replacement of full intertrabecular space by neoplastic cells

  Focal paratrabecular and nonparatrabecular infiltration are seen in case of low-grade follicular, small cleaved, and small lymphocytic lymphoma. Diffuse infiltration is seen in high-grade lymphoblastic and small noncleaved cell lymphoma.

C. Lymph node excision biopsy from the cervical or axillary node rather than inguinal node because of repeated chronic nonspecific inflammation followed by fibrosis. Following studies are performed from the excised node:

- **a.** Morphological examination of types of cells.
- **b.** Immunophenotyping for subclassification of B- and T-cell lymphoma: It can identify surface, nuclear, and cytoplasmic antigen by specific antibodies. It is useful in the following:
  1. It can differentiate neoplastic from non-neoplastic proliferation of lymphocytes
  2. It can differentiate lymphoma from undifferentiated neoplasm
  3. It can identify T- or B-cell lineage
  4. It can differentiate stages of neoplastic cells
  5. It can assess the prognosis as well as survival of certain lymphomas
- **c.** Cytogenetic analysis to detect chromosomal abnormalities
- **d.** Gene rearrangement studies by complementary DNA probes to detect:
  1. Rearrangement of immunoglobulin gene, which is indicative of B-cell nature
  2. Rearrangement of T-cell receptor gene, which is indicative of T-cell nature

  Uses of gene rearrangement studies:
  1. It can differentiate neoplastic from non-neoplastic proliferation of lymphocytes
  2. It can differentiate undifferentiated neoplasm from lymphoma
  3. It can identify T- or B-cell lineage
  4. It is also helpful in those cases where surface antigen analysis by specific antibodies fails to establish clonality of the disease

Staging of NHL

Lugano Staging System

Stage	Description	Extranodal status
I	Single lymph node region	Single extranodal lesions without nodal involvement
II	Two or more lymph node regions on the same side of the diaphragm	Stage I or II by nodal extent with limited contagious extranodal involvement

Continued

Continued

Stage	Description	Extranodal status
II bulky	II as above with bulky disease	Not applicable
III	Nodal regions on both sides of the diaphragm or nodal involvement above the diaphragm plus involvement of spleen	Not applicable
IV	Diffuse or disseminated involvement of one or more extralymphatic organ: bone marrow, brain, and liver involvement	Not applicable

Management

A. For follicular lymphoma with heavy tumor burden:

R-CHOP: Rituximab + Cyclophosphamide + Vincristine + Doxorubicin + Prednisolone

It is less toxic and improves disease-free survival. A newer first-line treatment option includes lenalidomide along with rituximab.

In case of relapse or refractory to treatment:

a. Chemoimmunotherapy regimen, single-agent rituximab, or radioimmunotherapy in the form of targeted radiotherapy directed to tumor tissues by conjugating a radioisotope with anti-CD20 antibody.

b. Recently, phosphatidylinositol-3-kinase delta inhibitor, idelalisib, has been approved as monotherapy who has already received at least two systemic therapies.

B. Lymphoplasmacytoid lymphoma:

a. Single-agent rituximab

b. Chemoimmunotherapy regimens such as BR and rituximab in combination with bortezomib and dexamethasone. But, serum viscosity has to be observed as rituximab is prone to develop hyperviscosity syndrome. Hence, plasmapheresis prior to rituximab therapy is strongly recommended.

c. MYD88 mutations result in increased nuclear factor-κB (NF-κB) signaling—it is the rationale for the use of inhibitors of Bruton's tyrosine kinase (BTK) that can treat the disease.

C. Marginal zone lymphoma: It occurs in gastrointestinal tract, salivary gland, lungs, ocular adnexa, and breast. Treatment includes:

a. Therapeutic approach follows follicular lymphoma.

D. Diffuse large B-cell lymphoma:

a. R-CHOP is the standard therapy of choice for stages I and II—three cycles plus involved field radiotherapy will result in 5 years survival rate in 77% of patients.

b. In case of relapse within 12 months of initial R-CHOP therapy, prognosis is poor with survival rate is <12 months.

c. In case of relapse, autologous stem cell transplantation can cure 50% of patients.

d. For HIV-associated lymphoma:

1. DA-EPOCH: Rituximab + Etoposide + Doxorubicin + Vincristine + Prednisolone + Cyclophosphamide

Each cycle has to be repeated every 21 days.

E. B-cell acute lymphoblastic leukemia:

a. Rituximab is the standard method of treatment in case of adult.

b. Three cycles of CODOX-M for low-risk disease

c. Three cycles of CODOX-M and IVAC for high-risk disease

CODOX-M: Cyclophosphamide + Vincristine + Doxorubicin + Cytarabine + Methotrexate

IVAC: Etoposide + Ifosfamide + Mensa + Cytarabine

Treatment of Refractory B-cell Lymphoma

A. In aggressive NHL, 40–50% of patients fail to achieve CR with conventional chemotherapy hence, these patients receive salvage therapy.

B. Grades I and II are not curable hence, high-dose chemotherapy with ASCT is of choice.

Principle of Salvage Therapy

High dose of chemotherapy along with ASCT may produce substantial benefit.

High-dose chemotherapy:

- R-DHAP: Rituximab + Cisplatin + Cytarabine + Dexamethasone
- R-ESHAP: Rituximab + Etoposide + Methylprednisolone + Cytarabine + Cisplatin
- R-ICE: Rituximab + Etoposide + Carboplatin + Ifosfamide

Reduced intensity of stem cell transplantation produces immunologic effect against tumor cells without risk of high-dose chemotherapy.

T-cell Lymphoma

A. T-cell lymphoma has poorer prognosis than aggressive B-cell lymphoma. Systemic anaplastic large cell lymphoma (ALCL) can be treated by doxorubicin-based treatment such as brentuximab vedotin approved by the Food and Drug Administration (FDA).

B. Corticosteroids, alkylating agent, bexarotene for topical use along with ultraviolet A (UVA) or ultraviolet B (UVB), and total skin electron beam therapy are of choice.

C. Histone deacetylase (HDAC) inhibitors are the treatment of choice in cutaneous lymphoma.

Q24. Hodgkin's disease.

MGR/SEP2009/MDI (5)

Stages of lymphoma.

MJPRU/2015/MDIII (6) MJPRU/2015/MDIII (6)

Pathology of Hodgkin's lymphoma.

MGR/APR2016/MDI (5)

Enumerate the Ann-Arbor staging for lymphoma.

DNB 2020 (5)

Pathology of Hodgkin's lymphoma.

Kerala University, 2021 (10)

ANSWER

Definition

Lymphoma is a heterogeneous group of disorder characterized by malignancy of lymph nodes and other lymphoid tissues. It has been divided into two types: (1) Hodgkin's lymphoma and (2) NHL.

Hodgkin's lymphoma, histologically, is characterized by Reed–Sternberg (RS) giant cells in the background of reactive cells, like plasma cells, lymphocytes, eosinophils, and fibroblasts representing the immune reaction of the host against the tumor cells.

Etiopathogenesis

Reed–Sternberg cells originate from B cells in the germinal center of lymph nodes hence, called Hodgkin's lymphoma. Classically, immunoglobulin genes of RS cells have undergone somatic mutation and rearrangement of heavy chain—it indicates that the origin of this lymphoma is from B cells in the germinal center or postgerminal center. NF-κB is the transcription factor, which is activated by c-REL proto-oncogene on 2p chromosome; this NF-κB is expressed in RS cells leading to proliferation, survival, and inhibition of apoptosis of cells.

Role of EBV: On the basis of the identification of EBV DNA in the lymph nodes and elevated titer of antibody to EBV, it has been determined as a cause of infectious mononucleosis. EBV latent membrane protein-1 is strongly expressed in 75% of nodular cellularity of Hodgkin's lymphoma. In case of AIDS, there is significant association of Hodgkin's lymphoma; these cases are also universally associated with EBV.

Cytokines are also released from RS cells and lymphocyte is responsible for B symptoms of Hodgkin's lymphoma.

Clinical Features

A. Age: Bimodal age distribution:
   - **a.** Highest peak in younger adult (20–30 years)—mainly nodular sclerosis variety
   - **b.** Older age of >50 years of age—mainly mixed cellularity variety

B. Sex: Males are predominant but in case of nodular sclerosis, both sexes are equal

C. Involvement of lymph nodes:
   - **a.** Site: Mainly cervical lymph nodes and axillary nodes—all are supradiaphragmatic. Inguinal nodes are infradiaphragmatic in site.
   - **b.** Character: Painless, rubbery, discrete, freely mobile, firm, and alcohol-induced pain in the node.
   - **c.** According to histological involvement of lymph nodes:
     1. In case of nodular sclerosis—lower cervical, supraclavicular, and mediastinal nodes
     2. In case of mixed cellularity—involvement of nodes on both sides of diaphragm in stages III and IV and B symptoms
     3. In case of lymphocytic depletion—it is more common in adult and older age

D. B symptoms: Fever with night sweats and >10% of weight loss in last 6 months.

E. Organ involvement: Hepatomegaly and splenomegaly. Bone marrow is mainly involved with both sides of involvements.

Pathology

Reed–Sternberg cell is the classical cell in the midst of inflammatory cells that are the diagnostic of Hodgkin's lymphoma.

Features of RS Cell

A. It is giant cell containing two nuclei or two nuclear lobes appearing as mirror images

B. Each nuclear lobe has accentuated membrane and pale chromatin containing prominent eosinophilic nucleolus looking like viral inclusion surrounded by clear zone (owl eye-like appearance)
C. Cytoplasm is eosinophilic or amphophilic
D. In mononuclear form of RS cells have single nucleus
E. In case of degenerative changes in RS cell, cytoplasm is basophilic and chromatin is condensed—it is called "mummified" cells

Variants of RS Cell

A. Lacunar cells: It is large cell with abundant clear to slightly eosinophilic cytoplasm containing a multilobar nucleus with multiple small nuclei and coarse chromatin.
B. Popcorn cell or lymphocytic predominant cell: It is large folded multilobed nucleus containing small nucleoli.

Classification of RS Cells

A. Nodular lymphocytic predominant: There is loss of architecture of node replaced by nodules composed of:
   a. Lymphocytes
   b. Histiocytes
   c. Epithelioid histiocytes
   d. Dispersed lymphocyte predominant called popcorn cells. These cells are large containing scanty cytoplasm and single multilobed nucleus having basophilic multiple nucleoli
B. Nodular sclerosis classical Hodgkin's lymphoma:
   a. It is cellular nodules with areas of necrosis or microabscesses surrounded by birefringent collagen.
   b. There is presence of lacunar cells in sheets or scattered in clusters but classical RS cells are rare.
   c. Background cells are lymphocytes, eosinophils, neutrophils, macrophages, and fibroblasts.
C. Mixed cellularity classical Hodgkin's lymphoma:
   a. Architecture is diffusely obliterated by mixed population of lymphocytes, plasma cells, histiocytes, and eosinophils.
   b. Reed–Sternberg cells are dispersed frequently throughout the node.
   c. Histiocytes form granuloma and demonstrate epithelioid features.
D. Lymphocyte-rich classical Hodgkin's lymphoma:
   a. Small number of RS cells is dispersed in nodular or diffuse background of small lymphocytes, but neutrophils and eosinophils are absent.
   b. Germinal centers are eccentrically placed and regressed.
   c. Reed–Sternberg cells resemble lymphocytic predominant classical Hodgkin's lymphoma.
   d. There is presence of groups of epithelioid cells also.
E. Lymphocytic-depleted classical Hodgkin's lymphoma: It is two types:
   a. Diffuse fibrosis subtype: It demonstrates:
      1. Reticulin fibers
      2. Reed–Sternberg cells
      3. Sparse heterogeneous background population of cells
   b. Reticular subtype:
      1. Sheets of neoplastic RS cells showing anaplastic pleomorphic features.

Staging of Hodgkin's Lymphoma

A. Stage I: Involvement of single lymph node region or lymph node structure (spleen, Waldeyer's ring, and thymus) or of a single extralymphatic site (IE).
B. Stage II: Involvement of two or more lymph node regions on the same side of diaphragm (II), which may be accompanied by localized contagious involvement of an extralymphatic organ or site (IIE). The number of anatomic sites may be indicated by numeric subscript.
C. Stage III: Involvement of lymph node regions on both sides of diaphragm (III), which may also be accompanied by localized involvement of an associated extralymphatic organ or sites (IIIE) by involvement of spleen (IIIS) or both (IIIE + S).
D. Stage IV: Disseminated involvement of one or more extralymphatic organ with or without associated lymph node involvement or isolated extralymphatic organ involvement with distant (nonregional) nodal involvement.

Treatment of Hodgkin's Lymphoma

Evaluation Prior to Treatment

A. Echocardiography to evaluate left ventricular ejection fraction prior to anthracycline therapy
B. Pulmonary function test prior to bleomycin therapy

C. Cessation of smoking should be counseled
D. Counseling regarding fertility for preservation of sperm and ovum

Management

A. Early stage of disease combined modality of treatment with chemotherapy and radiotherapy or chemotherapy alone in highly selected cases.
B. In advanced case, chemotherapy alone is considered.
C. In few advanced cases following full course of chemotherapy radiation, consolidation can be given in PET-positive areas who are poor candidates for intensive second-line chemotherapy.

Principles of Chemotherapy

A. Standard chemotherapy of 28 days cycle:
   a. A: Doxorubicin 25 mg/m^2/dose IV days 1 and 15
   b. B: Bleomycin 10 units/m^2/dose IV days 1 and 15
   c. C: Vinblastine 6 mg/m^2/dose IV days 1 and 15
   d. D: Dacarbazine 375 mg/m^2/dose IV days 1 and 15

This regimen is associated with less myelosuppression and less risk of leukemia.

According to German Hodgkin Lymphoma Study Group, following extended regimen are:

A. Dose-escalated BEACOPP of every 3 weeks:
   a. Bleomycin on the day 8
   b. Etoposide on days 1–3
   c. Doxorubicin on the day 1
   d. Cyclophosphamide on the day 1
   e. Vincristine on the day 8
   f. Procarbazine on days 1–7
   g. Prednisolone on days 1–14
   h. Filgrastim (G-CSF) support is required

Principles of Radiotherapy

After the development of effective combination of chemotherapy, only radiation therapy involved areas based on imaging is given to treat disease-bearing in the node.

According to the National Comprehensive Cancer Network (NCCN), unfavorable prognostic factors in early stage of disease with any of the following features:

A. Involvement of >3 nodal areas
B. Presence of B symptoms
C. Erythrocyte sedimentation rate > 50 mm/first hour
D. Bulky disease: Mass > 10 cm in diameter or mediastinal mass ratio exceeding one-third of maximum intrathoracic diameter

In case of advanced stage of disease, following are the adverse prognostic factors:

A. Stage IV disease
B. Age > 45 years
C. Male sex
D. White blood cell count ≥15,000/cc
E. Hemoglobin < 10.5 g/dL
F. Albumin level < 4 g/dL

Q25. Acute lymphoblastic leukemia.

MGR/SEP2009/MDI (5)

ANSWER

Definition

Acute lymphoblastic leukemia is a malignant disorder arising from precursor lymphoid cells in the bone marrow.

Classifications

Morphology	L1	L2	L3
Blast cell size	Small	Large and heterogeneous	Large and heterogeneous
Cytoplasm	Scanty	Moderate	Intensely basophilic
Nuclear/ Cytoplasmic ratio	High	Low	Lower
Vacuoles in cytoplasm	±	±	Prominent
Nuclear membrane	Regular	Irregular	Regular
Nucleoli	Indistinct	Prominent	Prominent (one to two)

Clinical Features

B cell-related ALL occurs in childhood with peak age of 2–5 years.

T cell-related ALL occurs in adolescents and young adults.

Onset is acute and short in duration.

Features

A. Fatigue, weakness, and pallor due to anemia
B. Bruise and ecchymoses in thrombocytopenia
C. Fever and intercurrent infection in case of leukopenia
D. Bone or joint pain due to periosteal involvement
E. Organ involvement:
   a. Lymphadenopathy

b. Hepatomegaly
c. Splenomegaly
d. Testis
e. Eye
f. Gastrointestinal tract

F. On chest X-ray—anterior mediastinal mass due to leukemic infiltration of thymus. It may produce superior vena cava syndrome by impairing venous drainage from upper part of the body
G. Pericardial and pleural effusion
H. Compression over the trachea
I. Patient presents with headache, vomiting, and papilledema. By cerebrospinal fluid (CSF) examination, CNS disease can be divided into four types:
  a. CNS1: In CSF, there is no detectable leukocyte with blast cells
  b. CNS2: In CSF, <five leukocytes with blast cells
  c. CNS3: In CSF, ≥five leukocytes with blast cells
  d. TLP+: Traumatic LP with ≥10 RBC/μL with blast cells
J. Bone marrow status:
  a. M1: <5% blast cells
  b. M2: 5–25%
  c. M3: >25%

Risk Factors

Clinical features	Standard risk	High risk	Very high risk
Age (years)	1–9	10–35	<1 and >35
WBC/μL	<30,000	≥30,000	
CNS	Negative	Positive	
Ploidy	Hyperploidy	Hypoploidy	
Response to treatment	Rapid early responder	Slow responder	
Chromosomes	t(12;21)	11q23	
Postinduction minimal residual disease	<0.01	0.01–0.1	

Treatment

Treatment includes induction phase, consolidation phase, CNS sterilization, intensification, and maintenance phase. Total duration is 2–3 years.

Initial induction therapy begins with three to five drugs given in 28 days cycle.

Three-drug regimen: Prednisolone + Vincristine + Pegylated L-asparaginase with intrathecal methotrexate

Four-drug regimen: Addition of doxorubicin

Five-drug regimen: Addition of cyclophosphamide

Evaluation of Drug Response

Day 14: Bone marrow:

M1: Rapid early responder.

M2 or M3: Slow early response.

Day 29: Bone marrow:

M1: Remission.

M3: If there is induction failure, salvage reinduction is required.

Postinduction Regimen

Pretreatment criteria:

a. Absolute neutrophil count is more than equal to 750/cc, platelet count is more than equal to 75,000/cc.
b. Alanine transferase level is <2 times upper limit of normal and direct bilirubin is normal for age.
c. No active infection or life-threatening organ dysfunction is noted.

Consolidation Phase (Week 5)

Cyclophosphamide + Mercaptopurine + Vincristine + Cytarabine with intrathecal methotrexate.

Maintenance/Continuation Regimen

Repetition of cycles to complete 24–36 months of total treatment:

Prednisolone + Vincristine + Mercaptopurine + Methotrexate with intrathecal methotrexate

Supportive Care

A. Antiemetic
B. Treatment of TLS by proper hydration and allopurinol
C. Prophylaxis of infections by antibiotics
D. Nutritional support
E. Transfusion of platelets, packed RBC, leukodepleted platelet, or RBC

Q26. POEMS syndrome.

BF/MAY2010/MDIII (10)
MGR/MAY2011/MDIV (7)

ANSWER

Definition

POEMS syndrome is rare paraneoplastic syndrome as a consequence of plasma cell disorder characterized by polyneuropathies, organomegaly, endocrinopathies, monoclonal plasma cell disorders, and skin changes.

Criteria for the Diagnosis of POEMS Syndrome

A. Mandatory major criteria:
- **a.** Typically demyelinating polyneuropathy
- **b.** Monoclonal plasma cells proliferative disorders

B. Other major criteria (one required):
- **a.** Castleman disease
- **b.** Sclerotic bone lesions
- **c.** Elevation of vascular endothelial growth factor

C. Minor criteria:
- **a.** Organomegaly (hepatomegaly, splenomegaly, or lymphadenopathy)
- **b.** Extravascular volume overload (edema, pleural effusion, or ascites)
- **c.** Endocrinopathies (adrenal, thyroid, pituitary, pancreatic, gonadal, and parathyroid)
- **d.** Skin changes (hyperpigmentation, hypertrichosis, glomeruloid hemangioma, plethora, white nails, flushing, and acrocyanosis)
- **e.** Papilledema
- **f.** Thrombocytosis/Polycythemia

D. Other symptoms and signs: Clubbing, weight loss, hyperhidrosis, pulmonary hypertension, restrictive lung disease, diarrhea, thrombotic diathesis, and low vitamin B12 values

Diagnosis of POEMS Syndrome

Both mandatory major criteria plus one of the three major criteria plus one of the three minor criteria are present.

Laboratory Investigations

A. Complete blood count
B. Clotting profile
C. Renal function test
D. Liver function test
E. Endocrine screen
F. Level of vascular endothelial growth factor
G. Imaging: 99mTc-HMDP bone scintigraphy
H. Paraprotein screen: Serum protein electrophoresis, immunofixation, and serum-free light chain along with Bence Jones protein

Bone histology: Histologically, reactive lymphoid aggregates containing T and B cells containing plasma cell rim mostly λ restricted—unique of POEMS syndrome.

Within osteosclerotic lesion, infiltration of atypical plasma cells within normal marrow with sclerosis of bony lamellae.

I. Lymph node biopsy
J. Nerve biopsy

Management of POEMS Syndrome without Bone Marrow Involvement

In patient with single isolated bone lesion without clonal plasma cells found on iliac crest biopsy, recommended therapy is radiation—it will improve the symptoms over 3–36 months and it can be curative.

Management of POEMS Syndrome with Bone Marrow Involvement

Once the bone marrow is involved, even the percentage of plasma cells are low, radiation is not the curative therapy. If the bony lesion is considerably large, radiation is considered as primary therapy. Next, this is to follow the symptoms, serum M-protein, and vascular endothelial growth factor over 6–12 months, and then systemic therapy has to be added.

Drug of choice is melphalan with or without autologous stem cell transplantation (ASCT). Other drugs are lenalidomide and bortezomib, a reversible proteasome inhibitor.

Bevacizumab, a MAB targeting vascular endothelial growth factor, can be given.

Q27. Newer antiplatelet drugs.

MUZ/MAY2016/MDIV (8)
MGR/MAR2002/MDIII (10)
MGR/OCT2011/MDI (5)
MJPRU/2015(S)/MDIV (10)
MUHS/MAY2012/MDIV (10)

ANSWER

Platelet is the main prothrombotic element interconnected by fibrin in the development of thrombosis and responsible for >10 million of cases of ischemic stroke, heart disease, and peripheral gangrene. This action is counteracted by aspirin, the first-line antiplatelet drug and this is followed by invention of newer antiplatelet drugs.

In the areas of endothelial damage or site of rupture of atherosclerotic plaque, there will be adhesion, activation, and aggregation of platelet mediated by numerous adhesive proteins, which ultimately occlude the vascular flow leading to ischemia or infarction of the involved organ.

A. Aspirin: It is cyclooxygenase inhibitor:

- **a.** It irreversibly inhibits COX1
- **b.** Prostaglandin A2 is blocked
- **c.** Bioavailability is 60%
- **d.** Thromboxane A2 cannot synthesize, so there will be no activation of platelet and, thus, no platelet aggregation
- **e.** Dose is 75 mg/day orally. It is equivalent to impact of large dose (300 mg). Bleeding risk is also less in low dose
- **f.** Coadministration of other nonselective COX2 inhibitor may impair the efficacy
- **g.** Plasma protein binding is strong
- **h.** After aspirin withdrawal, adverse event results from rebound platelet activation
- **i.** Genetic polymorphism (COX1, COX2, and platelet glycoprotein receptor) or increased turnover of platelet reduces the effect of aspirin
- **j.** Recommended period of withdrawal prior to surgery is at least 5 days

B. P2Y12 receptor antagonists: These are the receptors present on the surface of thrombocytes that can be blocked chemically. Activations of these receptors lead to change in configuration, aggregation, emergence of platelet pseudopodia, and interaction with other cellular and plasma components. The drugs are:

- **a.** Clopidogrel:
  1. It is a prodrug; its 15% are activated by cytochrome P3A4/3A5 to active metabolite and combines irreversibly with P2Y12.
  2. For rapid onset of action, loading dose is necessary.
  3. Proton pump inhibitor can reduce its effect.
  4. Genetic polymorphism and altered intracellular signaling pathways may be responsible for inadequate platelet activation.
  5. Causes of inadequate platelet inhibition are:
     - Inadequate intake
     - Discontinuation of drug intake
     - Noncompliance
     - Lack of access to clopidogrel
- **b.** Prasugrel:
  1. It is a prodrug, which will be converted to active metabolite by cytochrome P450.
  2. It will bind to P2Y12 and irreversibly inactivate platelet.
  3. Onset of action is more rapid than clopidogrel.
  4. Genetic polymorphism will not influence the metabolism of prasugrel.
- **c.** Ticagrelor:
  1. It is a nonthienopyridine antiplatelet agent than directly reversibly and noncompetitively blocks P2Y12 receptor thereby preventing ADP from binding to it.
  2. Its active metabolite is platelet-inhibiting agent.
  3. After 24 hours of drug intake, antiplatelet activity will be declined by 50%.
  4. Drug interactions:
     - Serum concentration of statins is increased
     - Concomitant use of CYP3A4 inhibitors or inducers should be avoided
- **d.** Cangrelor:
  1. It is a nonthienopyridine antiplatelet agent that reversibly and noncompetitively blocks P2Y12 receptor thereby preventing binding of ADP to it.
  2. After 18–24 hours of infusion, steady concentration will be achieved without loading dose.
  3. This drug will be inactivated by plasma enzymes within 1 hour of stopping the infusion.
  4. It is a good agent for bridging the high-risk patient in perioperative setting.

C. Glycoprotein IIb/IIIa inhibitors: These receptor proteins are most numerous present on platelet surface. This receptor activation is the final step of platelet activation, cross-linking between platelet-fibrinogen complexes. Inhibitor of these receptors will block the adhesion of fibrinogen with activated platelets thus, preventing the formation of interplatelet bridges.

It will prevent the adhesion of VWF, fibronectin, and vitronectin. The drugs are the following:

- **a.** Abciximab:
  1. It is a humanized monoclonal mouse antibody.
  2. It will block the thrombocytes by binding with it within 1 minute after administration.
  3. It will block >80% receptor after loading dose.
  4. It has long biological half-life but short plasma half-life.

b. Tirofiban and eptifibatide:
   1. These are synthetic reversible competitive receptor inhibitors by competing with fibrinogen for occupying the same receptor.
   2. Their plasma concentration determine:
      - Receptor occupancy
      - Extent of inhibition of platelets

D. Other antiplatelet agents:
   a. Cilostazol and dipyridamole: These are phosphodiesterase inhibitors:
      1. They interfere with degradation of cyclic adenosine monophosphate and cyclic guanosine monophosphate.
      2. They produce vasodilatation due to their effect on vascular smooth muscles.
   b. Protease-activated receptor-1 antagonists: Vorapaxar and atopaxar:
      1. They inhibit aggregation of platelet through alternative route, which includes thrombin-mediated platelet aggregation.
   c. Other platelet surface proteins such as glycoprotein VI, Ib, and prostaglandin E are the potential target for inhibitory drugs, which are under investigation.

Q28. Hairy cell leukemia.

MGR/MAR2006/MDIV (5)
MUHS/NOV2014/MDIII (10)

ANSWER

Definition

It is a chronic lymphoproliferative disease of B-cell origin characterized by pancytopenia, splenomegaly, and presence of hairy cells in the peripheral blood, bone marrow, and splenic pulp.

Pathogenesis

It occurs due to activating mutation of *BRAF* gene.

Clinical Features

Patient is asymptomatic and can be diagnosed accidentally. It will not occur in children, but middle-aged persons are involved.

Symptoms

Symptoms are tiredness, abdominal distension, easy fatigability, bruisability, and repeated infections.

Signs

Splenomegaly, hepatomegaly, and no peripheral lymphadenopathy. But, there may be retroperitoneal or abdominal lymphadenopathy.

Laboratory Diagnosis

A. Peripheral blood examination:
   a. Red blood cells:
      1. Anemia mild-to-moderate
      2. Size is normochromic and normocytic
   b. White blood cells:
      1. Leukopenia hairy cell is difficult to find
      2. Neutropenia
      3. Monocytopenia—it is a helpful clue to the diagnosis and is present in almost all the cases.
      4. In case of leukocytosis, hairy cells can be easily found.
      5. Mild-to-moderate thrombocytopenia.
   c. Features of hairy cell:
      1. Size is larger than twice that of small lymphocyte
      2. Cytoplasm: Clear and lightly basophilic
      3. Presence of small hair-like broader projection from the surface of the cell
      4. Nucleus is round, oval, or may be indented
      5. Chromatin dispersed or reticular
      6. Nucleoli are inconspicuous

B. Examination of bone marrow: Due to reticulin fibrosis of the bone marrow, trephine biopsy is required for definitive diagnosis. It demonstrates:
   a. Mononuclear cellular infiltration in the interstitium, loosely arranged with widely spaced nuclei from each other looking like "fried egg" appearance whereas in case of other leukemia or lymphoma, nuclei are close.
   b. Reticulin demonstrates fibrosis of the bone marrow surrounding individual cells.
   c. Trichome stain demonstrates collagen fibrosis.

C. Cytochemistry: Anti-TRAP antibody is used to demonstrate TRAP enzyme reactivity in hairy cell.

D. Immunophenotypic analysis: Flow cytometry of peripheral blood and bone marrow aspirate demonstrate:
   a. B cell nature of hairy cells (CD19+, CD20+, and CD22+)
   b. Hairy cell expresses SmIg, CD11c, CD25, CD103, CD123, and HC2

c. Bone marrow shows positivity of hairy cells for B cell markers such as CD79a and CD19

E. Molecular genetic analysis:
   a. Mutation of BRAF V600E—it is an oncogene located on chromosome 7q24. Mutation of this gene leads to activation of mitogen-activated protein kinase pathway.

F. Histology of spleen:
   a. Infiltration of red pulp by hairy cells
   b. Formation of splenic pseudosinuses lined by hairy cells
   c. Broadening of splenic cords
   d. Atrophy of white pulp

G. Complications:
   a. Vasculitis
   b. Infiltration in the bone, mainly femur
   c. Infections due to reduction of granulocytes and monocytes

H. Treatment:
   a. A small number of patients having no manifestation of cytopenia need not require any treatment, but only require regular observation.
   b. Patients having cytopenia at the time of diagnosis require treatment.
   c. Currently available therapies are:
      1. Purine nucleoside analogs—cladribine and pentostatin—these are the first line of therapy for hairy cell leukemia with prolonged duration of remission
      2. Alpha-interferon
      3. Splenectomy
      4. If patient does not respond to purine nucleoside analogs:
         - Monoclonal antibodies such as rituximab
         - Anti-CD22 antibody immunotoxin
      5. Inhibitor of BRAF—vemurafenib

Q29. Sideroblastic anemia.

MGR/MAR2009/MDII (6) MGR/SEP2008/MDII (6)

ANSWER

Sideroblasts are iron containing granules stained by Prussian blue. There are three types of sideroblasts:

A. Type 1 sideroblast:
   a. It is normal, iron containing granules that are present in cytoplasm, scanty in number, and these granules represent aggregates of ferritin.
   b. These constitute 30–50% of erythroblasts in the bone marrow.
   c. Number of ring sideroblast varies with the percentage of saturation of transferrin.
   d. They are reduced in:
      1. Iron deficiency anemia
      2. Anemia of chronic disease

B. Type 2 sideroblast:
   a. It is abnormal sideroblast and its cytoplasm contains numerous iron containing large granules.
   b. These cells are present in:
      1. Hemolytic anemia
      2. Iron overload

C. Type 3 sideroblast:
   a. Here nonferritin containing granules present in the mitochondria are arranged around the nucleus like complete ring.
   b. Size of the granules is large and multiple.
   c. If ring sideroblasts are ≥15% of marrow fibroblast—it is called sideroblastic anemia.

Definition

Sideroblastic anemia can be defined as dimorphic anemia or hypochromic microcytic anemia with bone marrow containing ring sideroblast and ineffective erythropoiesis.

Causes

A. Hereditary type:
   a. It is an X-linked, autosomal recessive.
   b. There is reduced activity of enzyme in the heme biosynthetic pathway delta-aminolevulinic acid (ALA) synthase.
   c. Moderate-to-severe anemia with features of iron overload.
   d. Serum iron increased with increased percentage of transferrin saturation.
   e. Bone marrow contains ring sideroblasts with erythroid hyperplasia.

B. Acquired type:
   a. Primary:
      1. It is refractory anemia with ring sideroblast.
      2. It occurs in middle-aged and elderly patients.
      3. Anemia is typically dimorphic such as microcytic, hypochromic, and macrocytic.
      4. Neutrophil shows hypergranular form or Pelger-Huet abnormality.

5. Bone marrow—dyshematopoietic features, megaloblastic maturation, and ring sideroblast.
6. There may be progression to AML in 1–2% of cases.

b. Secondary causes:

1. Alcoholism—folate deficiency and malnutrition produce dimorphic anemia.
2. Lead poisoning—associated with abdominal colic, blue line in the gum, motor neuropathy, impaired growth, low IQ, peripheral blood basophilic stippling, and bone marrow show ring sideroblasts. Anemia occurs due to heme synthetase deficiency and ALA dehydratase deficiency.
3. Drugs—isoniazid, pyrazinamide, chloramphenicol, and cycloserine.
4. Hematologic malignancies—MPDs, MM, and M6 AML.

Pathogenesis

A. There is impaired heme synthesis in the mitochondria, but this uptake is regulated partially by intracellular concentration of heme.

B. There is associated increased uptake of iron due to feedback mechanism.

C. There is reduced availability of protoporphyrin.

The result is accumulation of excess iron in the mitochondria.

Q30. Discuss the hematological changes and management of children with thalassemia.

BF/JUN2016/MDI (10)

Discuss clinical genetics in thalassemic disorders.

BF/NOV2013/MDIII (10)

Thalassemia.

RGUHS/MAR2008/MDII (6)

MGR/MAR2007/MDIV (5)

Management of α-thalassemia.

MGR/APR2013/MDIII (7)

Classify α thalassemia syndrome.

DNB 2020 (5)

Thalassemia.

MGR University, 2021 (10)

Beta thalassemia.

MGR University, Tamil Nadu, 2020 (10)

ANSWER

Definition

Thalassemia is a group of disorders of hemoglobin synthesis characterized by defective synthesis of hemoglobin.

Classification of Thalassemia

Thalassemia can be classified according to following heads:

A. According to defect in globin synthesis:

- **a.** α-thalassemia
- **b.** β-thalassemia
- **c.** δβ-thalassemia
- **d.** γδβ-thalassemia

B. According to clinical severity:

- **a.** β-thalassemia can be subdivided into three types:
  1. β-thalassemia major
  2. β-thalassemia intermedia
  3. β-thalassemia minor
- **b.** α-thalassemia can be subdivided into four types:
  1. α-thalassemia silent carrier
  2. α-thalassemia trait
  3. Hemoglobin H disease
  4. Hemoglobin Bart's hydrops fetalis syndrome

C. According to transfusion requirements:

- **a.** Nontransfusion-dependent thalassemia:
  1. α-thalassemia silent carrier
  2. α-thalassemia trait
  3. β-thalassemia trait
- **b.** Transfusion occasionally required:
  1. β-thalassemia intermedia
  2. Mild-to-moderate β-thalassemia
  3. Hemoglobin H disease
- **c.** Transfusion dependent:
  1. β-thalassemia major
  2. α-thalassemia major

Clinical Genetics of α-thalassemia

In each chromosome pair 16, there are two α-genes. Since human is diploid hence, there are 4α genes. So, normal haplotype is αα and genotype can be written as αα/αα.

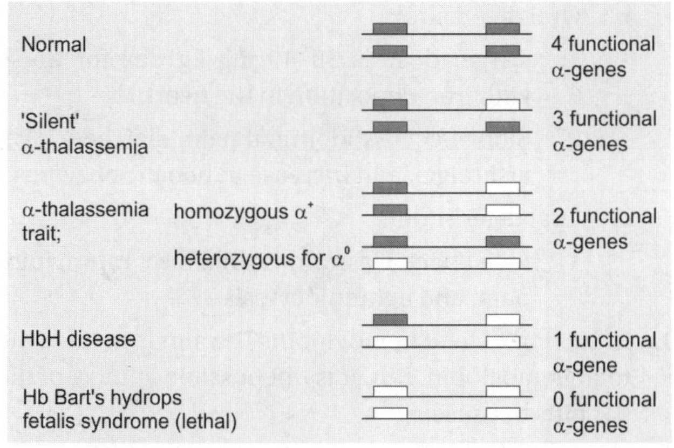

A. If there is loss of one gene, there are three functional genes (α/--)(α/α)—it is known as silent α-thalassemia.

B. If there are loss of two α genes, there are two types of α-thalassemic traits:

  a. Homozygous α^+ trait (α/--) (α/--)

  b. Heterozygous α^0 trait (α/α) (--/--)

C. If there is loss of three functional genes and only one functional gene:

Hemoglobin H disease (α/--) (--/--)

D. In there is loss of all four genes:

Hemoglobin Bart's hydrops fetalis syndrome (--/--) (--/--)

Clinical Features

In Hemoglobin Bart's Hydrops Fetalis Syndrome

Absolute deficiency of α gene results in formation of γ^4, i.e., tetramer of γ in fetal RBCs. It is incompatible with life and the affected fetus will be still born.

Hemoglobin H Disease

As a result of marked deficiency of α chain, tetramer of β4 is formed. Patient may be asymptomatic, there may be episodic anemia often requiring blood transfusions. This anemia is due to combination of ineffective erythropoiesis and hemolysis. Hemolysis may be increased by increased oxidant stress, sepsis and several medications. On physical examination, there is hepatosplenomegaly, jaundice, premature biliary tract disease, variable bony changes, leg ulcers.

Laboratory Diagnosis

Blood film demonstrates: Anisocytosis, microcytosis, and inclusion bodies in the RBCs due to precipitation of HbH when blood is incubated with oxidizing dye or when stained by methyl violet target cells. MCV, MCH and MCHC are low. There is indirect hyperbilirubinemia, raised LDH and decreased haptoglobin.

Hemoglobin electrophoresis demonstrates:

A. Cord blood in newborn—10–40% of Hb Bart

B. In infancy to adult—HbH will be increased

Globin chain synthesis study demonstrates α/β 0.2–0.4.

Alpha-thalassemic Trait

Patient is asymptomatic, so it can be detected during routine hematological studies or during family studies.

Laboratory studies demonstrate: Microcytic anemia, low MCV, MCH, and there may be inclusion bodies in the hemoglobin.

Hemoglobin electrophoresis demonstrates 5–15% Hb Bart in newborn, which gradually disappears in first few months after birth.

Alpha-thalassemia Silent Carrier

There is no symptom.

Laboratory Diagnosis

There may be mild decrease in MCV or MCH.
α:β ratio is 0.8.

Complications

In absence of blood transfusion, hemolytic anemia and severe tissue hypoxia result in:

A. Bone marrow expansion

B. Skeletal and metabolic derangements

C. Bony deformities

D. Extramedullary hematopoiesis

E. Increased iron absorption from gastrointestinal tract

F. Due to red cell membrane damage, activation of vascular endothelium and platelet as well as abnormal levels of inhibitors of coagulators, there is an increased risk of thromboembolism

G. Development of pigment stones in gallbladder

H. Chronic leg ulcers

I. Folate deficiency

J. Mental retardation is rare in case of α-thalassemia

Therapy

A. Blood transfusion improves as well as expectancy of life. In case of infancy and childhood, transfusion depends upon impact of anemia on the following of the child:

  a. Fatigue

  b. Skeletal dysmorphism

  c. Velocity of growth will be reduced

d. Weight gain will be poor
e. Organomegaly

After commencement of transfusion, target of hemoglobin to be maintained will be 9–10 g/dL hence, blood transfusion has to be given every 2–4 weeks and continued through adulthood.

To avoid alloimmunization, major and minor blood group typing for AB, Rh, Duffy, Kidd, and Kell.

B. Splenectomy: Indications:
 a. Inadequate transfusion
 b. Worsening of anemia
 c. Red cell alloimmunization

In case of nonsplenectomized patient, weekly drop of hemoglobin is 1.5 g/dL and in case of postsplenectomized individual, weekly drop of hemoglobin is 1 g/dL and it will be higher in case of hypersplenism. But, splenectomy will improve the hematological parameter. But, prior to splenectomy, following vaccinations are required in children older than 5 years of age:
 a. *Streptococcus pneumoniae*
 b. *Haemophilus influenzae*
 c. *Neisseria meningitidis*

C. Iron overload and chelation: Chronic blood transfusion results in iron overload when:
 a. Ferritin 1,000 ng/L
 b. Transfusion of 20 units
 c. Within 18 months from the commencement of transfusion

Areas of deposition:
 a. Heart: In the cardiac myocyte leading to cardiac arrhythmias and sudden cardiac death.
 b. Liver: It will lead to hepatic inflammation and hepatic dysfunction leading to fibrosis.
 c. Endocrine gland: It leads to delayed puberty or arrest; hypoparathyroidism leading to hypocalcemia, osteoporosis, and diabetes.

Drugs:
 a. Intravenous or subcutaneous deferoxamine:
  1. 20–60 mg/kg/day over 8–12 or 24 hours and to be started from 2.5 years of age.
  2. Toxicities: Impaired vision or hearing, motor sensory neuropathy, renal dysfunction, pulmonary dysfunction, joint pain, and growth retardation.
 b. Oral deferasirox:
  1. Target dose is 30–40 mg/kg/day for those with iron deposition in the heart.
  2. Side effects: Abdominal pain, diarrhea, rash, arthralgia, and increase in hepatic enzymes.
 c. Oral deferiprone:
  1. Side effect: Gastrointestinal discomfort, joint pain, and agranulocytosis.

D. Induction of fetal hemoglobin: The aim is to raise the total hemoglobin. But, it is not possible in most of the patients because:
 a. Loss of HbF due to blood transfusion
 b. Certain mutations, which are resistant to HbF induction

E. Inducers of HbF such as decitabine or HDAC inhibitors can also be considered.

Q31. Plasmapheresis: Indications and complications.
PGI/APR2013/MDI (10)

Plasmapheresis in medical disorders.
BF/JUN2016/MDIII (10)

Plasmapheresis.
MJPRU/2015/MDIV (10)

Plasmapheresis in medical disorders.
Sourashtra UNI 2022 (20)

Plasmapheresis.
MGR University, Tamil Nadu, 2022 (10)

ANSWER

Plasmapheresis

In this procedure, in which plasma after harvesting from the donor, all the cellular components are returned to the donor. There are two ways by which plasmapheresis can be done:

A. Occasional plasmapheresis: It is done once in every 12 weeks. Criteria of collection are same as that of blood donor.

B. Frequent plasmapheresis: Here plasmapheresis is done more than once in every 12 weeks. Here donor testing is done prior to every procedure with hemoglobin level ≥ 12 weeks and serum protein ≥ 6 g/dL.

Volume of plasma for a donor having weight ≥ 55 kg should not be >500 mL.

Indications of Plasmapheresis

A. Category I:
   a. Antineutrophil cytoplasmic antibody (ANCA) associated rapidly progressive glomerulonephritis
   b. Focal glomerulosclerosis
   c. Acute inflammatory demyelinating polyradiculoneuropathy
   d. Chronic inflammatory demyelinating polyradiculoneuropathy
   e. Cryoglobulinemia
   f. Anti-GBM antibody disease
   g. Myasthenia gravis
   h. Sydenham's chorea
   i. Thrombotic thrombocytopenic purpura
   j. Hyperviscosity with monoclonal gammopathy
   k. Demyelinating polyneuropathy
   l. Homozygous familial hypercholesterolemia
   m. Antibody-induced rejection in renal transplantation
B. Category II:
   a. ABO incompatible allograft
   b. ABO incompatible hematopoietic progenitor cell or marrow transplantation
   c. Demyelinating disease
   d. Familial hypercholesterolemia
   e. Lambert–Eaton myasthenic syndrome
   f. Myeloma with acute renal failure
   g. Cryoglobulinemia with polyneuropathy
   h. Phytanic acid storage disease and rheumatoid arthritis—refractory (immunoadsorption)

Contraindications to Plasmapheresis

A. Severe hypersensitivity reaction
B. Patient who cannot tolerate central vein placement
C. Patients who are on ACEI are advised to stop the medication for at least 24 hours prior to plasmapheresis

Different Techniques of Plasmapheresis

A. Centrifugation technique:
   a. Continuous flow technique: In this method, blood is withdrawn continuously into the bowl from which different components are separated into different layers and remaining part is returned into the patient with replacement fluid. Procedure is faster and complete.
   b. Intermittent technique: In this method, blood is drawn by venipuncture, centrifuged, and kept it separated. It will be returned in alternating steps through same venipuncture. It takes at least 4 hours to complete one cycle.
B. Membrane filtration technique: It is alteration to centrifugation technique. Here the patient's blood will be pumped through parallel plate or hollow fiber at a rate of 50–200 mL/min and pore of the membrane is sufficient to allow plasma but not the cells. Average time required for membrane filtration is <3 hours. Plasma can be removed at a rate of 30–50 mL/min and large vein catheter is required.

Complications of Plasmapheresis

A. Drop in blood pressure
B. Infection
C. Bleeding due to use of anticoagulant
D. Allergic reaction to solution
E. Temporary suppression of immune system
F. Patients are at risk of worsening of hypocalcemia because of use of citrate to prevent clotting
G. Electrolyte abnormalities
H. Seizures

Q32. Coagulation cascade.

KUHS/MAY2014/MDI (10)
MGR/APR2014/MDI (5)
MGR/SEP2009/MDI (5)

Define hemostasis. Discuss in detail the normal homeostasis and fibrinolysis.

BF/MAY2010/MDI (25)

Coagulants and anticoagulants.

MGR/SEP2009/MDI (5)

Describe coagulation pathways.

DNB 2019 (4)

Coagulation pathways.

Kerala UNI, 2022 (10)

Coagulation cascade. Discuss etiology, investigation and management of hypercoagulable state.

Saurashtra UNI 2022 (20)

Describe the clotting factors and sequence of clotting mechanism.

DR YSR UNI of Health SC, Vijayawada, Andhra, 2022 (10)

Write about clotting mechanism. Write briefly about thrombolytic agents.

DR YSR UNI of Health SC, Vijayawada, Andhra, 2022 (10)

Recombinant tissue plasminogen activator.

MGR UNI, Tamil Nadu, 2021 (5)

Hypercoagulable state has been discussed in question number 34.

Thrombolytic agents are described in questions number 27, 35.

Coagulation pathways.

NTR UNI of Health SC, Vijayawada, 2021 (10)

Coagulation cascade

NTR UNI of Health SC, Vijayawada, Septem, Andhra, 2020 (10)

Rajiv Gandhi UNI of Health SC, Karnataka, 2020 (10)

ANSWER

Definition

Homeostasis can be defined as a complex mechanism by which the loss of blood from the blood vessel following vessel injury is strictly and tightly controlled by complex interactions between platelets, vascular endothelial wall, and plasma proteins. There are two stages of hemostasis:

A. Primary hemostasis where platelets will interact with the vascular wall to limit the blood loss from the vessel.

B. Secondary stage: In this stage, stable fibrin clot is ultimately formed due to interactions of coagulation factors through intrinsic or extrinsic pathways and finally a common pathway.

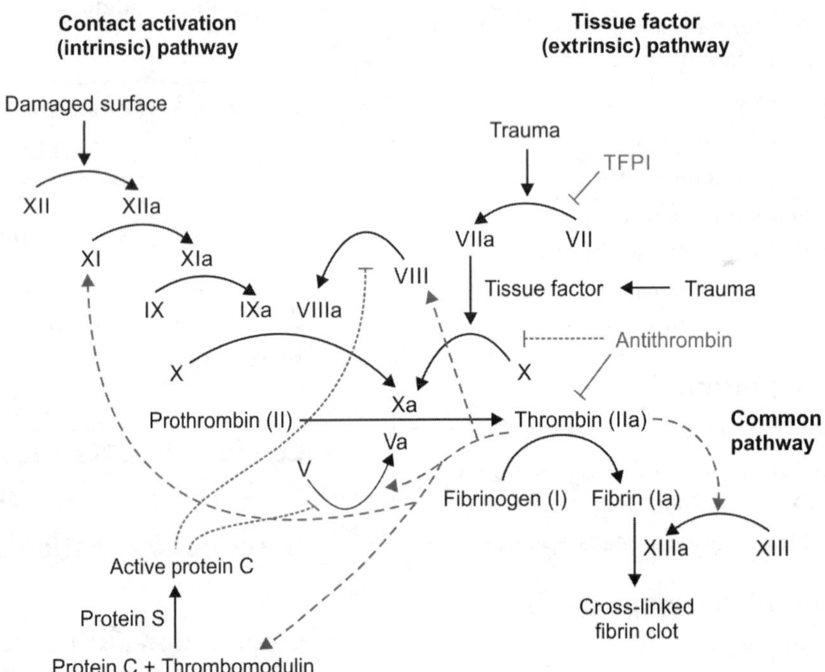

(TFPI: tissue factor pathway inhibitor)

Coagulation Cascade

It includes formation of fibrin clot through the activation of coagulation factors. It involves:

A. Contact pathway or extrinsic pathway: Contact factor will be activated at the site of tissue injury, which will convert factor XII to activated factor XII, which, in turn, activates sequentially factor XI to activated factor XI and factor IX to activated factor IX. Now, activated IX complexes with activated factor VIII, calcium, and platelet to form tenase complex.

B. Tissue injury pathway or intrinsic pathway: After tissue injury, factor VII will be activated to form activated factor VII, which will combine with tissue factor to form activated VII-TF complexes.

Now, activated factor tenase complex and activated VII-TF complexes activate factor X to form activated factor X, which, in turn, complexes with platelet and activated factor V and calcium cleave factor II (prothrombin) to form activated factor II (thrombin).

C. Common pathway: Now thrombin (activated factor II) cleaves fibrinogen (factor I) to fibrin, which will cross-link via activated factor XIII.

Fibrinolysis

It is a process of dissolution of blood clot that is very essential to maintain the free flow of blood through the vessel. Main enzyme that initiates fibrinolysis is plasmin, which will be generated from plasminogen activators by following methods:

A. Tissue plasminogen activators synthesized by endothelial cells

B. Kallikrein, which is formed from prekallikrein with the help of activated factor XII

The conversion of plasminogen to plasmin occurs on the surface of fibrin. Plasmin digests insoluble cross-linked fibrin to produce fibrin degradation product, which will be cleared by mononuclear phagocyte system from the circulation.

Plasmin firstly initially attacks α chains of fibrinogen molecule to remove small fragments designated as A, B, and C from C terminal of A α chain which is followed by degradation of B β chain with removal of 42 amino acids leading to formation of large fragment X retaining fibrinopeptide A.

Now, rest of all the chains are involved in the next cleavage leading to release of fragment D, fragment Y (molecular weight 15,000 kDa), the last one will be rapidly degraded by plasmin into fragment D (molecular weight 90,000 kDa), and fragment E (molecular weight 50,000 kDa).

Fibrin degradation products are different due to presence of covalent bonding, hence fragments are:

A. Oligomers of X and Y

B. D-dimer

C. D2E complex

D. YD complex

Due to presence of cross-linkage, degradation of fibrin is slower.

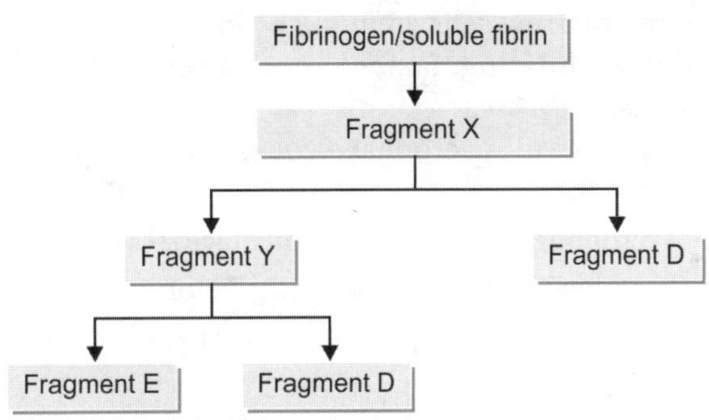

Tissue Plasminogen Activators

These are classified as serine protease which cleaves peptide bonds in the proteins, so it is an essential component of dissolution of blood clot. Its main function is to catalyze the conversion of plasminogen to plasmin thereby dissolution of blood clot.

Indications for the use of this protein are the following:

A. In case of ischemic stroke if there is treating facility within 3 days.

B. In myocardial infarction if there is delay of more than 1 to 2 hours prior to PTCA

C. Thrombolysis in case of DVT

D. Massive pulmonary embolism leading to severe instability due to high pressure in the heart.

Rest of the part of the answers are present in the cardiology chapter.

Q33. Colony-stimulating factors.
BF/OCT2011/MDI (9)

ANSWER

Definition

Colony-stimulating factors are glycoproteins bind to the specific receptors on the surface of the hematopoietic stem cells activating intracellular signaling pathways leading to proliferation as well as differentiation of specific kinds of WBCs.

Pathophysiology

In case of any type of infection, granulocytes and macrophages, as a part of innate immunity system, protect the body and are continuously replaced by the new cells present all over the bone marrow and are under tight regulatory control. According to the demand, the control and coordinated production of specific granulocytes from scattered marrow cells are done by four glycoproteins—colony-stimulating factors, commonly referred as cytokines, these are:

A. Granulocyte-macrophage colony-stimulating factor (GM-CSF)

B. Macrophage colony-stimulating factor (M-CSF)

C. Granulocyte colony-stimulating factor

D. Multipotential colony-stimulating factor (interleukin-3)

Cerebrospinal fluid has short half-life of few hours, but after stimulation of bacterial cell wall component and endotoxin, it will increase up to 1,000-fold locally and systematically.

Actions of CSF

Cerebrospinal fluid acts on specific membrane receptors on the target cells in picomolar concentrations.

A. Two receptors (G-CSF and M-CSF) are homodimers and M-CSF has tyrosine kinase activity.

B. Two other receptors are heterodimers sharing common signaling β chain.

There are five major actions of CSF on granulocyte-macrophage cells:

A. They maintain the viability of progenitor cells and mature progeny by blocking apoptosis.

B. They stimulate cell division and their concentration determine the
   - **a.** Cell-to-cell cycle time
   - **b.** How many cells are produced by per progenitor cells?

C. Cerebrospinal fluid can also influence the lineage commitment, i.e., one progenitor cell can produce only granulocyte or macrophage progenitor cells.

D. Cerebrospinal fluid also directs the process by which one cell can produce ultimate mature cell.

E. Cerebrospinal fluid also enhances the function of the mature cells, i.e., phagocytic activity or production of cytokines by neutrophils or macrophages.

Pharmacokinetics

In case of subcutaneous injection, it has short half-lives, i.e., 3–12 hours. In case of human beings after injection of G-CSF or M-CSF, progenitor cells mobilize from the bone marrow to the peripheral blood and it will reach as high as in the bone marrow.

Loss of GM-CSF reduces the mature cell functional activity and reduction of function of macrophage cells will lead to accumulation of surfactant in the lung.

Granulocyte-macrophage Colony-stimulating Factor and Immune Response to Cancer

Granulocyte-macrophage colony-stimulating factor is especially involved in the immune response in cancer. This cytokine is mainly involved in the formation and the enhancement of activity of dendritic cells. It has also been incorporated into the vaccinia virus to enhance the activity of dendritic cells.

Granulocyte-macrophage Colony-stimulating Factor and Myeloid Leukemia

It is common conception that these agents, if administered for prolonged periods, can stimulate the proliferation of cell populations and, thus, acting as a cofactor for cancer development. It is a well-established factor for development of cancer tissues producing hormones. Continuous activation of GM-CSF or IL-3 in continuous cell lines can transform these cells into leukemogenic cells; in that respect, these *CSF* genes can be called as oncogenes. It has been demonstrated in vitro that the human CML or AML proliferation is the resultant effect of stimulation of CSF in the same dose as given for normal progenitor cells.

However, long-term use of GM-CSF is non-leukemogenic in chronic neutropenic patients, but some of them may be at risk of AML—it proves the chronic overstimulation by GM-CSF that may be leukemogenic.

Q34. Discuss the clinical and laboratory approach to hypercoagulable states.

BF/MOV2013/MDIII (10)

Hypercoagulable states.

MGR/FEB2005/MDIII (5)

Investigation of thrombophilia.

MGR/OCT2013/MDII (7)

ANSWER

Introduction

There are three risk factors for development of thrombosis. These are:

A. Reduction in the blood flow

B. Damage to the vessel wall

C. Alteration of blood components

Homeostasis depends upon complex actions of different components of blood such as:

A. Platelets

B. Wall of the vessel

C. Coagulation factors

D. Inhibitors of coagulation

Any disturbance between the coagulation factors or their components and fibrinolysis leads to chance of formation of thrombosis, i.e., hypercoagulable state or prothrombotic state. So, it is a coagulation disorder with shifting of balance toward procoagulation forces. Body can counteract initial thrombotic process by inactivating coagulation esterase with the help of physiologic inhibitors such as protein S, protein C, and antithrombin III. So, reduced activities of these factors will lead to propensity for thrombus formation.

Classification of Hypercoagulable State

A. Primary hypercoagulable states:

- **a.** Protein C deficiency
- **b.** Protein S deficiency
- **c.** Antithrombin III deficiency
- **d.** Prothrombin gene mutation
- **e.** Dysfibrinogenemia
- **f.** Resistance to activated protein C due to mutation of factor V gene

B. Acquired or secondary hypercoagulable states:

- **a.** Antiphospholipid syndrome (APS): This is found in 50% of SLE patients after administration of certain drugs and infection. Antibodies are directed against β2 glycoprotein I, a phospholipid-binding protein called anticardiolipin antibodies, and some antibodies will prolong phospholipid-dependent clotting reaction called lupus anticoagulant. Origin of these antibodies may be infection or cellular injury.
- **b.** Due to thrombogenic stimuli, following causes are:
  1. Pregnancy
  2. Postpartum period
  3. Use of estrogen
  4. Advancing age
  5. Postoperative states
  6. Injury
  7. Immobilization
- **c.** Some clinical disorders:
  1. Malignancy
  2. Congestive cardiac failure
  3. Nephrotic syndrome

C. Mixed hypercoagulable states: Hyperhomocysteinemia: There is an increased incidence of arterial or venous thrombosis. The level of homocysteine is determined by genetic and environmental factors such as both dietary intake and absorption of vitamin B12, vitamin B6, and folic acid.

Screening of Laboratory Tests for Hypercoagulable States

A. Functional assay of:

- **a.** Protein C
- **b.** Protein S
- **c.** Antithrombin III

B. Genetic tests for:

- **a.** Factor V
- **b.** Prothrombin gene mutation

C. Immunological assay of:

- **a.** Total and free protein S

D. Immunological and functional assay of:

- **a.** Fibrinogen
- **b.** Thrombin time

E. Clotting assay for lupus anticoagulant

F. Measurement of total homocysteine level in serum

G. Serological tests for antiphospholipid antibodies

Criteria of Antiphospholipid Antibody Syndrome

Following one clinical and one laboratory criteria can diagnose APS. Persistent positivity of laboratory test is very important.

Clinical Criteria

A. Vascular thrombosis: One or more episodes of arterial, venous, or small blood vessel thrombosis involving any organ or tissue.

B. Pregnancy morbidity: Evidence of one or more unexplained death of a morphologically normal fetus or premature birth of morphologically normal neonate due to severe preeclampsia or eclampsia or recognized features of insufficiency of placenta or three or more unexplained consequences of spontaneous abortions.

Laboratory Criteria

A. Presence of lupus anticoagulant in plasma on two or more occasions at least 12 weeks apart.

B. Presence of anticardiolipin antibody IgM and/or IgG in serum or plasma in medium or high titer on two or more occasions at least 12 weeks apart, which is measured by standardized ELISA.

C. Presence of anti-2 glycoprotein I antibody IgM and/or IgG in serum or plasma in medium or high titer on two or more occasions at least 12 weeks apart, which is measured by standardized ELISA.

Molecular Markers of Coagulation Activation in the Assessment of Prothrombotic State

Coagulation system is activated locally at the site of vascular injury or in the entire blood volume, which ultimately leads to activation of coagulation by variety of mechanisms culminating DIC syndrome. Following assays can reflect the activation of coagulation:

A. Test for generation of thrombin, which is responsible for formation of fibrin from fibrinogen.

B. Measurement of prothrombin fragments 1 + 2 released during conversion of prothrombin to thrombin.

C. Interaction of thrombin and its inhibitor can be measured by thrombin-antithrombin complexes.

D. Detection of soluble fibrin is fibrin monomer units by procoagulation and precipitation assay and advantageous because of its longer half-life in the circulation.

E. Measurement of fibrin degradation product.

F. Fibrin digestion product of cross-linked fibrin, D-dimer assay: It is a marker of fibrin turnover, which will be increased in prothrombotic state.

G. Plasma fibrinogen level: It is a strong predictor of clinical ischemic event such as arterial thrombosis.

Q35. Newer anticoagulants.

GMC/2016/MDII (5)

Describe newer developments in oral anticoagulants.

BF/MAY2013/MDIV (10)

Coagulants and anticoagulants.

MGR/SEP2009/MDI (5)

Newer oral anticoagulants.

Kerala University, 2021 (10)

Parenteral direct thrombin inhibitors. Add a note newer oral anticoagulants.

NTR UNI of Health SC, Vijayawada, Andhra, 2020 (10)

ANSWER

Advantages of Newer Oral Anticoagulant

A. No need of fixed dosing for monitoring

B. No drug interactions

C. There is wide therapeutic window, which will counteract with their current drawback

D. Rapid onset and offset of action

E. Short half-life

F. Predictable pharmacokinetics and pharmacodynamics

Disadvantages

A. Lack of effective antidote

B. High cost

C. Limited use in case of chronic kidney disease

D. Sometimes, short half-life and rapid offset can be considered as disadvantages

E. No enough experience

F. These drugs can be initiated without low-molecular-weight heparin due to their onset of action.

There are two classes of oral anticoagulants: These drugs will block only one step in the coagulation cascade unlike vitamin K antagonists that will block factors such as II, VII, IX, and X.

A. Oral direct thrombin inhibitors—dabigatran

B. Oral direct-activated factor X—apixaban, rivaroxaban, and edoxaban

Recently, dabigatran, rivaroxaban, and apixaban are accepted as treatment of thromboembolism by the FDA.

According to the European Society of Cardiology

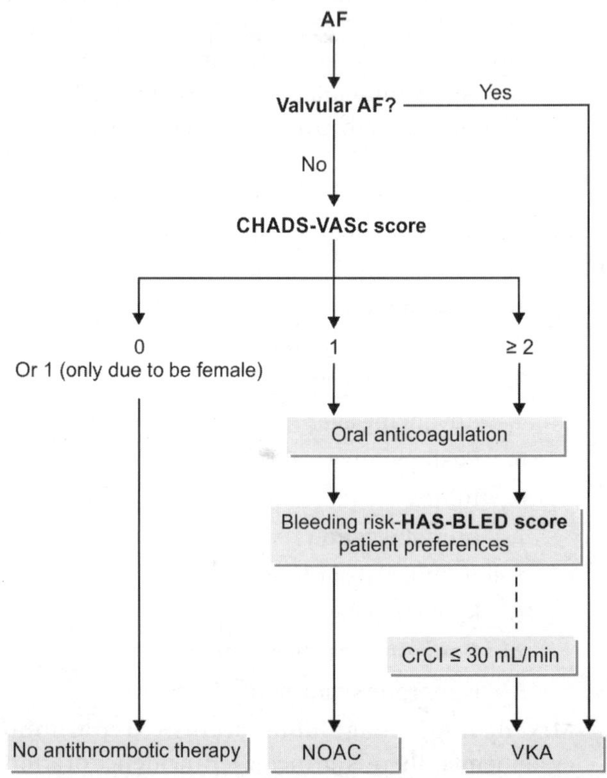

(AF: atrial fibrillation; CrCl: creatinine clearance; NOAC: nonvitamin K antagonist oral anticoagulants; VKA: vitamin K antagonist)

A. Dabigatran:
   a. It is a direct thrombin inhibitor, which inhibits conversion of fibrinogen to fibrin thus, prevents formation of clot in the vessels.
   b. This synthetic prodrug, hirudin analog after ingestion, will be converted into active metabolite after hepatic processing.
   c. It shows univalent binding in only one of the two binding sites.
   d. Its oral bioavailability is low; after oral administration, it is rapidly absorbed.
   e. Plasma concentration of this drug increases in dose-dependent manner.
   f. Half-life of this drug is 12–14 hours.
   g. It does not inhibit cytochrome 450; hence, drug-to-drug interaction is low.
   h. Primary route of elimination of this drug is kidney.
   i. Dose is 110 mg twice daily.
B. Rivaroxaban:
   a. It is a oxazolidinone derivative and selective direct inhibitor of activated factor X as activated factor X acts in the rate-limiting step of thrombin formation in both intrinsic and extrinsic pathways.
   b. Bioavailability is 60–70%.
   c. Renal excretion is 70% with 30% unchanged.
   d. Dose is 2.5 mg twice daily.
C. Apixaban:
   a. It is a reversible direct inhibitor of activated factor X.
   b. It is 25% excreted in urine.
   c. Bioavailability is 66%.
   d. Dose is 5 mg twice daily.
D. Edoxaban:
   a. It is a direct specific inhibitor of activated factor X.
   b. 35% is excreted in urine.
   c. Bioavailability is 58%.

Indications of Oral Anticoagulants

A. Treatment of deep venous thrombosis (DVT) with pulmonary thromboembolism.
B. Prevention of DVT and pulmonary embolism (PE).

Contraindications

A. Clinically significant active bleeding
B. Hepatic disease with coagulopathy
C. Use of NSAIDs
D. Use of platelet inhibitors
E. In case of creatinine clearance < 30 mL/min, dabigatran is contraindicated. If it is <15 mL/min, rivaroxaban and apixaban are contraindicated.

Q36. Pure red cell aplasia.

MJPRU/2015(S)/MDIII (10)

ANSWER

Definition

Pure red cell aplasia can be defined as anemia due to absent reticulocyte in peripheral blood and erythroid precursor cells in bone marrow.

Etiopathogenesis

A. Constitutional: Diamond-Blackfan syndrome due to inherited mutation of ribosomal protein.
B. Acquired: Immunologically mediated:
   a. Collagen vascular disease
   b. Myasthenia gravis
   c. Thymoma in 10% of cases
   d. Large granular lymphocytic leukemia
   e. Chronic lymphocytic leukemia
C. Myelodysplastic syndrome
D. Parvovirus B19 infection producing erythema infectiosum. It occurs in children. Patient suffers from aplastic crises along with underlying hemolysis. There is development of antiviral neutralizing antibodies. But, in following immunodeficient conditions, parvovirus infection B19 will continue:
   a. Congenital immunodeficiencies (Nezelof's syndrome)
   b. Human immunodeficiency virus-induced immunodeficiency
   c. Immunosuppressive drugs
   d. Chemotherapy

Clinical Features

A. Anemia
B. Features of fifth disease due to parvovirus infection

Laboratory Diagnosis

A. Reticulocyte count—very low or absent
B. Red blood cell count is very low, but WBC and platelet count are normal
C. Bone marrow demonstrates:
   a. Few normoblast

b. Giant pronormoblast signals parvovirus B19
c. 5q- syndrome indicating uninuclear micromegakaryocytes

D. CT scan to detect thymoma
E. Serology:
a. In case of persistent parvovirus infection, either viral antibodies are absent or IgM-specific antibodies are present.
b. Virus can be detected by PCR.

Treatment

A. In case of Diamond–Blackfan syndrome, corticosteroid is the drug of choice but in case of relapse, steroid may not be effective.
B. In case of acquired cases, moderate dose of corticosteroids along with either cyclosporine or antithymic globulin or other cytotoxic drugs such as cyclophosphamide and azathioprine may be effective.
C. Thymoma can be surgically removed.
D. Large granular lymphocytic leukemia is alemtuzumab responsive.
E. In case of persistent parvovirus B19 infection, immunoglobulin 0.4 g/kg intravenously should be given for 5–10 days. In HIV infection with high viral load, periodic treatment is necessary.

Q37. Anti-TNF biological agents.

GMC/2015/MDI (10)

ANSWER

Mechanism of Action

Tumor necrosis factor is made by activated macrophages intracellularly. TNF-converting enzyme will produce soluble TNF from TNF precursor, which, in turn, oligomerizes to form biologically active homotrimer TNF. There are two types of TNF:

A. TNF-α
B. TNF-β

Both types of TNF react with two types of receptor type I and type II, which are present in cell types, except erythrocytes. This reaction will activate several signaling pathways such as:

A. Transcription factor activation
B. Activation of proteases (caspases)
C. Activation of protein kinases (c-Jun N-terminal kinase)

As a result of activation of above signaling pathways, there will be activation of target cells such as macrophages, T cells, and B cells leading to release of proinflammatory cytokines like IL-1, IL-6, and chemokines such as IL-8, RANTES, and apoptotic pathways. There is also expression of adhesion molecules such as intercellular adhesion molecule-1 (ICAM-1), E-selectin, regulatory T-cells inhibition, and upregulation of RANK ligands expression.

Structures and Mechanism of Actions of Various TNF Agents

Name	Mechanism of actions	TNF binding and actions
Etanercept	Human recombinant fusion protein	• Binds both TNF-α and -β with high affinity • It can bind two cell bound or circulating TNF molecules • It will not produce apoptosis of TNF-expressing cells
Infliximab	Chimeric mouse human MAB	• Binds TNF-α with high affinity • It can bind two cell bound or circulating TNF molecules • It will produce apoptosis of TNF-expressing cells
Golimumab	Fully humanized IgG1k monoclonal anti-TNF antibody	• Binds TNF-α with high affinity • It can bind two cell bound or circulating TNF molecules • It will produce apoptosis of TNF-expressing cells
Adalimumab	Fully humanized IgG1k monoclonal anti-TNF antibody	• Binds TNF-α with high affinity • It can bind two cell bound or circulating TNF molecules • It will produce apoptosis of TNF-expressing cells
Certolizumab pegol	400 kDa PEG moiety combines with Fab fragment of fully humanized monoclonal anti-TNF antibody	• Binds TNF-α with high affinity • It can bind two cell bound or circulating TNF molecules • It will not produce complement- or antibody-mediated cytotoxicity

Contraindications

A. Hypersensitivity reaction to these agents
B. Presence of infection or sepsis
C. New York Heart Association (NYHA) class III and IV heart failure
D. Use of other biological immunosuppressive agents

Adverse Effects

A. Headache
B. Reaction at the administered sites
C. Anemia
D. Transaminitis
E. Sinusitis
F. Cough
G. Pharyngitis
H. Abdominal pain and diarrhea
I. Serious side effects:
   a. Infections: Bacterial, fungal (blastomycosis, histoplasmosis, and coccidioidomycosis), viral, and protozoal infections in patients using other immunosuppressive agents.
   b. Risk of malignancies: Lymphoma is common mainly in patients with rheumatoid arthritis. In some cases, nonmelanoma skin cancers may occur.
   c. Congestive cardiac failure: There may be worsening of heart failure in patients with rheumatoid arthritis.
   d. Drug-induced lupus—rash, thrombocytopenia, leukopenia, and hypocomplementemia, rarely hemolytic anemia.
   e. Demyelinating disorders—optic neuritis, multiple sclerosis, myelitis, encephalitis, and transverse myelitis.
   f. Skin reactions—local skin reactions, urticaria, hypersensitivity vasculitis, and new-onset psoriasis
   g. Pregnancy and lactations: This drug has been labelled as class B pregnancy risk factor.

Monitoring of the Following Prior to Commencement of Drugs

A. Active and latent tuberculosis
B. Hepatitis B and C virus infection
C. Complete blood count
D. Liver function test
E. Antinuclear antibody
F. Anti-dsDNA antibody

Q38. Role of monoclonal antibodies in hematology.

MUHS/MAY2012/MDIV (10)
DNB 2022 (5)
DR YSR UNI of Health SC, Vijayawada, Andhra, 2022 (10)

ANSWER

Introduction

Antigen is a molecule or a part of a molecule, which can be recognized as foreign body by the immune system of the body and combat in two ways:

A. Production of antibody against new antigenic epitopes, which is expressed by genetic constituents shuffling and reshuffling.
B. Mutated paratope encoding genes of the antibody bind strongly with the epitope or antigenic determinants of the antigen with greater affinity and specificity.

But monoclonal antibodies are specific type of identical clone of B cells produced against single-specific antigen that can be generated by use of hybridoma formed by fusion of B cells with specific and single clonal lineage containing single antibody gene.

Specific characteristics of MAB:

A. Specificity of binding
B. Homogeneity
C. Ability of reproducibility in unlimited quantities
D. Mixture of antigens can be used to produce specific type of antibody
E. They are also capable to produce specific antibody from a mixture of antibody population with purified antigen

Polyclonal antibodies can identify antigen from different orientations, i.e., multiplicity of the epitopes but in case of MAB only single-specific antigen will be detected. Polyclonal antibodies are very cheap to produce in short term. It can be recovered in large volume due to use of large animals. But, polyclonal antibodies may not produce antibody in same titer. Monoclonal antibodies are formed in following ways:

A. Stage of immunization: Here different immunogens such as multiple antigenic synthetic peptides and short peptide linked to carrier protein are introduced into ice to remove antigenically responding B cells from spleen to get viable cells for hybridization.
B. Stage of fusion and selection: This process involves fusion of histocompatible hypoxanthine guanine

phosphoribosyltransferase devoid of myeloma cells with murine splenic B cells, the fusion agent being polyethylene glycol. These hybridomas are plated in "hypoxanthine-aminopterin-thymidine" (HAT). Viable hybridomas are scanned under inverted microscope.

C. Stage of screening: It includes:
   - **a.** Primary analysis hybridoma present in the culture
   - **b.** Expansion of selected hybridoma in tissue culture
   - **c.** Selected hybridoma will be re-evaluated
   - **d.** Selected hybridomas have to be cryopreserved

D. Stages of characterization:
   - **a.** Isotope has to be determined.
   - **b.** Cloning and cryopreservation to be done.
   - **c.** Then, these hybridoma has to be purified and specificity against antigen. This will be followed by profiling of reactivity as well as mapping of epitopes.
   - **d.** Then, these have to be validated with other reagents.
   - **e.** After confirmation, bulk production has to be started.

E. Stage of further development: It is used for following developments:
   - **a.** Different applications like analysis of probes
   - **b.** Application in diagnostic kits:
     1. Biosensors
     2. Microarrays
   - **c.** Commercial distribution of single MAB
   - **d.** Therapeutic applications:
     1. Cancer therapy:
        - Rituximab—NHL—target CR20 on B lymphocytes.
        - Gemtuzumab—relapsed case of AML—target myeloid cell surface antigen CD33 on leukemic cells.
        - Alemtuzumab—β-cell leukemia—target is anti-CD52 on I and B lymphocytes.
        - Bevacizumab—colorectal cancer—it inhibits vascular endothelial growth factor.
     2. Infectious diseases—palivizumab
     3. Rejection of transplant—muronomab—CD3
     4. Inflammatory disease:
        - Infliximab—rheumatoid arthritis and inflammatory bowel disease—it will inhibit anti-TNF-alpha signaling.
        - Etanercept—rheumatoid arthritis
        - Omalizumab—moderate-to-severe allergic asthma—it inhibits human IgE
        - Eculizumab—PNH
        - Belimumab—SLE
     5. Cardiovascular diseases—abciximab
     6. Macular degeneration—ranibizumab
   - **e.** Future applications: Fight against bioterrorism

Side Effects of Monoclonal Antibodies

A. Common side effects are the following:
   - **a.** Allergic reactions at the site of injection
   - **b.** Fever
   - **c.** Chill
   - **d.** Nausea with or without vomiting
   - **e.** Diarrhea
   - **f.** Lowering of blood pressure

B. Other side effects are usually related to the antigen:
   - **a.** Bevacizumab—kidney damage, rising of blood pressure, bleeding, and poor wound healing
   - **b.** Raxibacumab used against inhalation anthrax—extreme pain and drowsiness

Disadvantages are:

A. As a result of advancement of genetic engineering, the newer MABs are highly costly.

Q39. Discuss biomarkers in prostate cancer.
AMU/2011/MDIII (10)

ANSWER

Prostate cancer is the second most common cancer-related death in male in the world. There are several biomarkers that recognize the prostate cancer. These are the following:

A. Prostate-specific antigen: It is a serine protease (kallikrein-3) secreted by prostatic epithelial cells and secreted into the prostatic duct and contributes the seminal fluid. But, in cancer of prostate due to disruption of basal layers, this will be released into the circulation leading to elevation of serum level of PSA. Its related gene is encoded in the chromosome 19.

   But serum PSA level can be raised in following conditions:
   - **a.** Prostatitis
   - **b.** Benign prostatic hypertrophy
   - **c.** Dietary alterations
   - **d.** Medications

False-positive test may overdiagnose the case, which may culminate in unnecessary surgery.

Defect:

a. It cannot detect the stages of prostatic cancer

b. It cannot detect the metastasis

There is false positivity in case of PSA testing. If PSA is >4 ng/mL, prostatic biopsy will be indicated but it misses 20–40% cases of cancer. It can identify 40% of indolent prostatic cancer cases and are unnecessarily treated. Radical prostatectomy will reduce the mortality for men with PSA level >10 ng/mL with high-risk tumor. 10-year mortality in case of modern radical prostatectomy is 77%, but there may be complications such as incontinence and erectile dysfunction.

To increase the accuracy of PSA, following methods of measuring PSA have been developed:

a. Monitoring personal PSA changes over time (PSA velocity)

b. Ratio of PSA to prostatic volume (PSA density) as determined by transrectal to biopsy specimen.

B. Refined PSA test: It will increase the diagnostic accuracy. Total PSA refers to total PSA (bound) plus bound PSA (complexed to α-antichymotrypsin). Rate of increase in total PSA can be defined as total PSA velocity—it is important from diagnostic and prognostic point of view.

C. Free PSA is now approved in case of men because PSA in the serum is bound to α2-microglobulin, α1-antitrypsin, and α1-protease inhibitor as:

a. It helps to discriminate between benign prostatic hypertrophy and prostatic cancer.

b. It is better than total PSA alone as a predictor of prostate biopsy.

D. Gleason score: It is accepted as best predictor of outcome. Here the pathologist will look for the most prominent cell type (primary Gleason grade) and second most prominent type of cell (secondary Gleason grade). The grade is 1–5. Gleason score = Primary grade plus secondary grade. If it is >7—it suggests:

a. Extraprostatic extension

b. Recurrence after therapy

E. Human glandular kallikrein-1 (hKLK2): It is a serine protease enzyme from kallikrein family that shows 80% homology with PSA, but its enzymatic activities may differ. This will correlate with:

a. Progression of prostatic cancer

b. Volume of the tumor

c. Prognostic indicator of biochemical recurrences in patient with PSA level ≤ 10 ng/mL

F. Prostatic cancer antigen: It is specifically expressed in prostate and highly expressed in 90% of the tumors. PCA3 is detected in urine and prostatic fluid. PCA3: PSA ribonucleic acid (RNA) is also known as PCA score—it along with clinical examination will help to give decision regarding repeat biopsy in ≥50 years of aged male whose previous biopsy is negative.

G. Prostatic health index (PHI): It can be calculated from the following formula:

$$[(p2PSA/fPSA) \times \sqrt{tPSA}]$$

Patient with high p2PSA and tPSA but with low fPSA indicates prostatic carcinoma.

H. Homeobox-containing transcription factor engrailed-2 (EN-2): It encodes homeodomain-containing protein. It will secrete PCA in the urine, which can be detected by simple ELISA test or Western blot test from supernatant part of urine. This EN-2 oncogene is found in breast cancer, lung carcinoma, and astrocytoma.

I. ETS-related gene: It is discovered in the urine in patients with prostatic cancer. Urine assay measures transmembrane protease serine 2 (TMPESS2) to PSA RNA.

J. Urinary biomarkers:

a. α-hepatocyte growth factor (αHGF)

b. Insulin-like growth factor-binding protein 3 (IGFBP3)

c. Osteopontin (OPEN)

These are directly secreted into the urinary tract hence, can be detected by ELISA. They have a role in prostatic cancer initiation, progression, adhesion, angiogenesis, migration, invasion, and proliferation of prostatic cancer cells. OPEN has a role in tumerogenesis and angiogenesis.

K. Circulating endothelial cells and circulating endothelial progenitors: These functionally and phenotypically different biomarkers for prediction of prognosis and treatment evaluation response to cancer.

L. Circulating tumor cells: These cells will shed into the bloodstream and in case of distant metastases also.

M. Transforming growth factor-β: It is overexpressed in case of prostatic carcinoma to detect its grade and metastasis.

N. Autoantibodies against alpha-methylacyl-CoA racemase (AMACR) in the level of 4–10 ng/mL can stratify prostatic carcinoma from noncancer.

O. Circulating nucleic acids in PCA:
- **a.** Hypermethylation event
- **b.** Microsatellites: It is found in increased frequency in case of metastatic prostate cancer
- **c.** mtDNA: It is of great prognostic value in prostatic cancer serum/plasma
- **d.** Circulating mRNA: It has a potential role in prostate cancer
- **e.** Circulating microRNA: It functions as oncogenes and encourages tumor growth or tumor suppressor

Q40. Philadelphia chromosome.

MGR/SEP2006/MDIV (5)

2BCR ABL

MJPRU/2015(S)/MDIV (5)

ANSWER

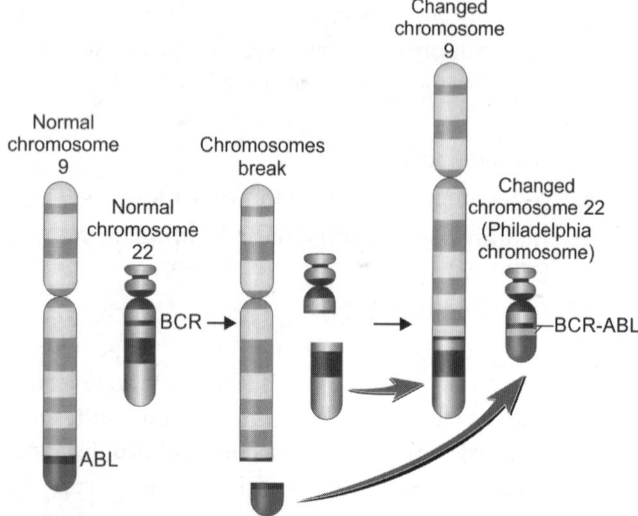

(ABL: Abelson; BCR: breakpoint cluster region)

Definition

There is reciprocal translocation of long arm of chromosome numbers 9 and 22 that produce Philadelphia chromosome—which is the inciting event in the diagnosis of CML and in some case chronic lymphoblastic leukemia.

Transfer

Transfer of *ABL* gene 1 present on chromosome number 9 to the BCR on the chromosome number 22 leading to formation of fusion gene BCR-ABL gene which is an oncogene.

Domain

Domain of BCR

- **A.** CC domain: It is responsible for activation of *ABL1* gene and it is closely associated with sensitivity to tyrosine kinase inhibitor.
- **B.** Ser/Thr kinase domain
- **C.** Rho/GEF kinase domain: It is important in activating differentiation in the proto-oncogene-induced leukemogenesis

Domain of ABL1

- **A.** SH domain: It is responsible for activation and deactivation of gene—it is the site of pharmacologic intervention.
- **B.** Proline-rich domain
- **C.** DNA- and actin-binding domain

Effect of Oncogene

BCR-ABL 1 fusion gene is responsible for activation of tyrosine kinase. This translocation decreases the requirement of growth factor and provides complete freedom from regulation of control of growth.

There is uncontrolled proliferation, inhibition of cell differentiation, and death of granulocytes, especially neutrophils, sometimes eosinophils, and basophils at various maturation stages.

Characters of Oncogene

In most of the patients suffering from CML, this gene is present. The weight of oncoprotein is 210 kDa, but <10% expresses 230 kDa or 190 kDa oncoprotein. The variations in molecular oncoprotein may be due to:
- **A.** Change in the breakpoint
- **B.** Different mRNA slicing

Testing: It can be detected by cytogenetic testing or reverse transcriptase PCR testing, which can demonstrate BCR-ABL transcript.

Definition of response of treatment with any tyrosine kinase inhibitor:

Item	Warnings	Failure	Optimal response
Baseline	High-risk CML or clonal abnormalities	Not applicable	Not applicable
3 months	BCR-ABL1 > 10% with/without Ph+ 36–95%	Ph+ > 95%	BCR-ABL1 ≤ 10% with/without Ph+ ≤ 35%

Continued

Continued

Item	Warnings	Failure	Optimal response
6 months	BCR-ABL1 1–10% with/ without Ph+ 1–35%	Ph+ > 35% with/ without BCR-ABL > 10%	BCR-ABL < 1% with/without Ph+ 0%
12 months	BCR-ABL > 0.1–1%	Ph+ > 0% with/ without BCR-ABL > 1%	BCR-ABL ≤ 0.1%
Then and at any time	Clonal abnormalities	Loss of any aforementioned response	BCR-ABL ≤ 0.1%

Q41. Describe the dermatological manifestations of internal malignancies.

DNBIII/DEC2011 (10)

BF/NOV2012/MDII (12)

Cutaneous manifestations of internal malignancy.

MGR UNI, Tamil Nadu, 2022 (10)

Dermatological manifestations of hematological malignancies.

Kerala University, 2021 (10)

ANSWER

A. Metastasis to skin:

a. Breast cancer:

1. Erythematous patches or plaques having active border affecting breast
2. Telangiectatic papules due to accumulation of blood in vascular channels
3. En cuirasse—morphea-like diffuse induration
4. Multiple ulcerated papulonodules
5. Painless well-demarcated pinkish oval well-demarcated alopecia—alopecia neoplastica
6. Paget's disease—well-demarcated scaling plaque on nipple or areola—cutaneous infiltration
7. Histiocytoid nodule over the eyelid—painless eyelid swelling along with induration

b. Lung cancer: Metastases on the chest wall, posterior abdomen, anal area, and toes

c. Gastrointestinal cancers: Metastases occur in abdominal wall and perineal area

d. Melanoma: Most are multiple pigmented or erythematous or apigmented nodules

e. Renal cell carcinoma, bladder, prostate, or testicular cancer produces skin metastases

f. Subungual metastases:

1. Lesions from distinct primary site—lung cancer, breast, genitourinary, head and neck cancers as well as sarcomas
2. From hematopoietic or lymphoreticular malignancy

g. Umbilical metastasis: Sister Mary Joseph nodule—from stomach, ovarian, and gynecologic cancer

B. Cutaneous paraneoplastic syndrome:

a. Acanthosis nigricans: Hyperpigmented, velvety plaques present in the neck, groin, axilla, and antecubital fossa—adenocarcinoma of gastrointestinal tract.

b. Amyloidosis in the skin—multiple myeloma and Waldenström macroglobulinemia. Lesions seen in the paranasal skin, flexural areas, and anogenital regions. It is seen around the eyes and neck region.

c. Bazex syndrome: Psoriasiform lesions in ears, nose, hands, elbows, and knees are produced by cancer of upper aerodigestive tract, hepatocellular carcinoma (HCC), lymphoma, and bladder carcinoma.

d. Dermatomyositis: Breast, lung, and ovarian cancer produces violeceous flat-topped papules around the eyes, periungual telangiectasia, and patchy discoloration of skin.

e. Ectopic Cushing syndrome: Small cell and nonsmall cell carcinoma, bronchial carcinoid tumor, thymoma, islet cell tumor, and pheochromocytoma secrete adrenocorticotropic hormone (ACTH).

f. Erythema gyratum repens: Lung cancer, less commonly breast and esophageal cancer, produces erythematous, scaly, ring-forming, and rapidly progressing eruptions in body, but spares hands and feet.

g. Exfoliative erythroderma: Cutaneous T-cell lymphoma and AML produce erythematous pruritic lesions and generalized lymphadenopathy.

h. Hypertrichosis lanuginosa acquisita: Lung and colonic cancer produces unpigmented fine hair localized to head and neck.

i. Ichthyosis: Hodgkin lymphoma

j. Multicentric reticulohistiocytosis: Gastric, breast, cervical, ovarian, and hematologic malignancy produces pink, brown, and gray papules.
k. Necrolytic migratory erythema: In glucagonoma, irregular erythematous lesions with central bulla are seen, which erode subsequently with hyperpigmentation.
l. Paget's disease: Either contagious or distant cancer present in apocrine gland-bearing areas.
m. Pachydermoperiostosis: Thickened skin and new skin creations seen in scalp, lid, ears, and face looking-like leonine facies may be seen in cancer.
n. Papillomatosis: Keratotic papules develop in hands, wrists, and then to face and body and commonly found in gastric carcinoma.
o. Palmoplantar hyperkeratosis: It is seen in Hodgkin's lymphoma, breast, gastric cancer, and lymphoma.
p. Pemphigus: It is seen in NHL, CML, and Castleman disease.
q. Pityriasis rotunda: Round, scaly, and hyperpigmented lesion in buttock, thigh, and trunk present in HCC and stomach cancer.
r. Pyoderma gangrenosum: It is seen in Waldenström macroglobulinemia, Hodgkin's and NHL, myeloma, and myeloid leukemia.
s. Sweet syndrome: It is common in AML presented as erythematous tender nodule or papule.
t. Urticaria pigmentosa: Hyperpigmented macules or papules with positive Darier sign in systemic mastocytosis.
u. The sign of Leser–Trélat—it is ominous sign of malignancy found in lymphoproliferative disorders, cancers, and gastrointestinal malignancies.
v. Vitiligo: In case of malignant melanoma hypopigmented macule.
w. Others are:
    1. Alopecia mucinosa: In case of lymphoreticular malignancies, mucinous degeneration of collagen hair follicle as well as sebaceous glands.
    2. Circinate erythema: Lymphoma and other visceral cancer produce circular elevation of skin, erythema annulare centrifugum to start with followed by central clearing surrounding erythematous area.
    3. Erythromelalgia: Myeloproliferative disorders produce erythematous painful warm extremities.
    4. Porphyria cutanea tarda: HCC and metastatic liver tumors produce blistering disease.
    5. Tripe palms: Lang, gastric, and genitourinary cancers produce thickened skin in palm with exaggerated dermatoglyphics.

C. Inherited malignancy-associated syndromes:
a. Ataxia telangiectasia: Autosomal recessive disorder and there is risk of Hodgkin's and NHL and leukemia.
b. Cowden disease: It is multiple hamartoma—neoplasia syndrome, autosomal dominant, and there is risk of breast, thyroid, endometrial, and thyroid cancers.
c. Cronkhite–Canada syndrome: It is acquired nonfamilial gastrointestinal polyposis syndrome and there is risk of gastric, colonic, and rectal carcinoma.
d. Gardner syndrome: It is familial adenomatous polyposis having extracolonic symptoms. This patient may be at risk of developing colonic and desmoid tumors.
e. Howel–Evans syndrome: It may be early manifestation esophageal cancer.
f. Muir–Torre syndrome: It is rare genodermatosis and there is risk of colonic and genitourinary cancer.
g. Peutz–Jeghers syndrome: It is autosomal dominant disorder and this patient is at risk of gastrointestinal adenocarcinoma.
h. Von Recklinghausen disease: It is autosomal dominant disorder. There is an increased risk of malignancy of peripheral nerve sheath tumors, pheochromocytoma, astrocytoma, urogenital rhabdomyosarcoma, and brainstem glioma.
i. Werner syndrome: It is autosomal recessive disorder and the patient is at risk of sarcoma.
j. Wiskott–Aldrich syndrome: It is sex-linked immunodeficiency syndrome and the patient is at risk of B-cell lymphoma.

Q42. Discuss the etiopathogenesis of anemia of chronic kidney disease (CKD) and outline its management.

DNBII/JUNE2013 (10)

Anemia in CRF.

MGR/OCT2011/MDII (7)

Newer therapy in CKD.

RGUHS/MDIV (10)

ANSWER

Etiopathology of Anemia in Chronic Kidney Disease

Decreased production of EPO from kidney:

A. Hypoxia stimulates production of erythrocytes through interaction of hypoxia-inducible factor (HIF) system. EPO is secreted by:

- **a.** Interstitial cells of peritubular capillaries of kidneys
- **b.** Hepatocytes
- **c.** Tissue macrophage system

Hypoxia triggers extrarenal source of EPO. It is inactivated in liver and mainly excreted in urine.

Hypoxia of kidney will release erythrogenin, a renal erythropoietic factor. It will act on plasma substrate, erythropoietinogen to form EPO. It will reach its peak within 24 hours of stimulus.

Its functions:

- **a.** It will differentiate erythropoietic stem cells to mature erythrocytes.
- **b.** It will also increase the release of reticulocytes from bone marrow.
- **c.** It will increase the heme synthesis by increasing the synthesis of DNA, RNA, globin, and ferritin.

B. Due to microvascular disease in diabetic or hypertensive patients, it producing breakdown of RBCs

C. Increased oxidative stress

D. Blood loss from hemodialysis

E. Blood loss from gastrointestinal tract due to peptic ulcer disease or intestinal angiodysplasia.

F. Functional iron deficiency: Here, there is bone marrow mismatch in iron supply demand in presence of normal or elevated iron stores and low transferrin saturation index (TSI). It occurs in presence of inflammation, liver disease, malignancy, and infection. Regulation and maintenance of homeostasis of iron are regulated by hepcidin. It is produced in liver. It will degrade the ferroportin in enterocytes, hepatocytes, and macrophages, thus prevents absorption as well as use of iron. Again, cytokines released as a result of inflammation-induced transcription of hepcidin and its level will be increased in chronic kidney disease.

G. Hexose monophosphate shunt pathway is impaired in chronic renal failure. As a result, hemoglobin is prone to oxidant damage by any drug and chemical. There is also subnormal activity of ATPase, which acts as fuels for Na^+-K^+ pump present on the RBC membrane. Both these processes are responsible for shortening of RBC survival.

Clinical Consequences

A. Due to reduced oxygen capacity: Fatigue, insomnia, and headache

B. Left ventricular hypertrophy

C. Progression of CKD

D. Mortality will be increased, if hemoglobin level will be ≤8 g%

E. Progression of hypoxia of peritubular cells in kidney due to anemia-induced hypoxia that leads to injury to renal tubulointestinal system

F. There is also an increased oxidative stress

Diagnosis

A. Red blood cell:

- **a.** Normochromic and normocytic, occasionally hypochromic and microcytic
- **b.** Presence of bull cell—regularly placed projections on the surface of RBC

B. Reticulocyte count—normal or slightly increased

C. Ferritin level is normal or increased

D. Transferrin saturation index is low

E. Blood urea nitrogen is increased

F. Platelet function is defective:

- **a.** Bleeding time is increased
- **b.** Platelet aggregation test to epinephrine, adenosine diphosphate (ADP), and collagen is impaired

G. Bone marrow—normocellular with normal sequence of maturation

H. Erythropoietin concentration is lower as compared with anemia

Treatment

Goal

A. In stage 1 and 2 of CKD: Serum ferritin level and TSI are normal.

B. In stage 3 and 5 but not on dialysis, serum ferritin and TSI will be kept higher than 100 ng/mL and 20%, respectively.

C. In patient on dialysis, serum ferritin and TSI will be kept above 200 ng/mL and >20%, respectively.

D. Iron supplement should be stopped when serum ferritin and TSI are >500 ng/mL and >30%, respectively.

Methods of Treatment

A. Erythropoietin: It is the drug of choice. After commencement of EPO, there will be expected rise of hemoglobin around 1 g/dL in the first month. If this rise occurs within 2 weeks, 25–50% dose reduction will be required.

  a. If the hemoglobin level is <10 g/dL—it clearly benefit.

  b. If hemoglobin level >13 g/dL, there is an increased risk.

  c. So, hemoglobin level should be maintained between 10 and 11.5 g/dL—there is benefit without increased risk.

  d. Dose is 4,000–5,000 unit biweekly or 10,000 unit weekly subcutaneously postdialysis.

B. Human recombinant EPO (epoetin): It can be given in subcutaneous or IV route. But subcutaneous dose is better because of its slow absorption and longer half-life.

  a. In case of IV administration, 50 units/kg of body weight thrice weekly.

  b. In case of subcutaneous administration, 30 units/kg of body weight thrice weekly in patient on dialysis.

  c. In case of subcutaneous administration, 100 unit/kg once weekly in predialysis patient or in case of peritoneal dialysis.

  d. Monthly administration of methoxy-pegylated epoetin beta is effective and is approved by the FDA due to its longer duration of action and subcutaneous administration.

C. Darbepoetin alfa: It is an EPO analog with two extra carbohydrate side chains and has longer duration of action.

  a. Dose is 0.45 μg/kg weekly or 0.75 μg/kg biweekly in dialysis patient in IV and subcutaneous route and maintenance dose vary according to its serum concentration.

  b. Adverse events are cardiovascular and cerebrovascular events, if hemoglobin level >11 g/dL. There is chance of pure red cell aplasia due to development of antibodies against this EPO analog, which also cross-react with endogenous EPO. It occurs exclusively in case of subcutaneous administration.

  c. Anemia resistant to proper dose of erythropoietin-stimulating agent (ESA) in presence of adequate iron store may be due to the following:

    1. Acute or chronic inflammation

    2. Malignancy

    3. Chronic infection

    4. Inadequate dialysis

    5. Severe hyperparathyroidism

    6. Chronic blood loss

D. Hypoxia-inducible factor stabilizer (roxadustat):

  a. It inhibits prolyl hydroxylase thus, stabilizing HIF. It is the main determinant in response to physiological stress due to tissue hypoxia. This stabilization of HIF leads to stimulation of endogenous EPO production and as compared to EPO analog, its level will be low and cardiovascular access thrombosis is low with this factor stabilizer.

  b. It also reduces hepcidin level thus, increasing the iron absorption from the intestine.

  c. It also increases release of iron from macrophages to transferrin.

E. Oral iron therapy: Orally iron can be given but due to poor iron absorption and gastrointestinal intolerance, IV iron therapy should be initiated.

F. Intravenous iron therapy:

  a. Prior to ESA therapy, adequate iron store in the form of ferritin and immediate availability of iron should be kept by IV iron supplementation.

  b. 1 g intravenously administered iron can elevate serum hemoglobin by 1 g/dL in CKD patients with iron deficiency anemia.

  c. In CKD with iron deficiency and nondialysis patient intolerant to oral iron therapy—larger dose of IV iron should be given.

  d. In CKD with iron deficiency and dialysis patient, small and frequently repeated transfusion of iron is required.

Q43. Erythropoiesis.

MGR/OCT2014/MDI (5) MGR/APR2013/MDI (5)

Erythropoiesis and its regulation.

MGR/SEP2009/MDI (5)

Erythropoiesis.

MGR UNI, Tamil Nadu, 2022 (5)

ANSWER

Erythropoiesis

Hematopoietic stem cells are 0.5% of total hematopoietic precursor cells and they will proliferate and differentiate into three lineages of cells. To start differentiation, they will enter into hematopoietic progenitor cells compartment, which comprises 3% of total precursor cell population. These progenitor cells will differentiate into two cells lineages, which are common myeloid progenitor cells and common lymphoid progenitor cells, among which former progenitor cells will be further divided into two progenitor cells:

A. Megakaryocyte erythroid progenitor cells

B. Granulocyte monocyte progenitor cells

Megakaryocyte erythroid progenitor cells again will be divided into two:

A. Burst-forming unit erythroid (BFU-E)

B. Burst-forming unit megakaryocyte (BFU-MK)

Burst-forming unit erythroid further differentiates into following cells serially: Colony-forming unit erythroid (CFU-E).

It will differentiate into proerythroblasts arranged in the form of islands—these cells are large with fine and uniform chromatin containing one or nucleoli present in dark blue cytoplasm.

Proerythroblast will mature into next cell basophilic normoblast or early normoblast—these cells are small in size with coarser chromatin with visible nucleoli in the midst of basophilic cytoplasm.

These cells will transform into intermediate of polychromatic normoblast—it contains smaller nuclei containing clumped chromatin. Polychromasia results from admixture of blue RNA and pink-colored hemoglobin.

It will be transformed into orthochromatic normoblast—it contains small dense pyknotic eccentrically nucleus. They are orthochromatic because stain of cytoplasm is similar to that of erythrocytes.

Orthochromatic normoblast will enter into the stage of reticulocyte where the nucleus will be extruded outside, but it still contains remnants of ribosomal RNA. It will stay 1–2 days in bone marrow and 1–2 days in peripheral blood and ultimately becomes mature pink staining erythrocyte.

Control of Erythropoiesis

Erythropoiesis is controlled by two types of factors:

A. Hypoxia: It is the most potent stimulus of bone marrow mediated by EPO, which increases red cell production. EPO is secreted by:

- **a.** Interstitial cells of peritubular capillaries of kidneys
- **b.** Hepatocytes
- **c.** Tissue macrophage system

Hypoxia triggers extrarenal source of EPO. It is inactivated in liver and mainly excreted in urine.

Hypoxia of kidney will release erythrogenin, a renal erythropoietic factor. It will act on plasma substrate, erythropoietinogen to form EPO. It will reach its peak within 24 hours of stimulus.

Its functions:

- **a.** It will differentiate erythropoietic stem cells to mature erythrocytes.
- **b.** It will also increase the release of reticulocytes from bone marrow.
- **c.** It will increase the heme synthesis by increasing the synthesis of DNA, RNA, globin, and ferritin.

B. Special maturation factors:

- **a.** Dietary factors:
  1. Protein—it will help in globin synthesis
  2. Manganese, iron, cobalt, copper, and nickel—it will help in heme synthesis
  3. Calcium—it will increase absorption of iron from intestine
  4. Vitamin B12, vitamin C, and folic acid—it will help in synthesis of nucleic acid
- **b.** Castle's intrinsic factors: This glycoprotein is secreted by parietal cells of stomach, hence it is decreased in case of gastric cancer, big gastric ulcers, and gastrectomy. It will bind to vitamin B12 producing IF-B12 complex. This complex binds to ileal receptor and B12 will be split off from intrinsic factor and released into portal blood.
- **c.** Extrinsic factors: These are foods containing vitamin B12 and folic acid.

Q44. Parvovirus infection and anemia.
MUHS/MAY2013/MDIII (10)

ANSWER

Introduction

Parvovirus B19 is a single-stranded DNA virus of Parvoviridae family. Though it usually causes infection in animals, but it was discovered in the normal donor blood in the blood bank. There is close association between aplastic crises and Parvovirus infection.

Pathophysiology

Incubation period is 4–21 days. Parvovirus is highly tropic to erythroid progenitor cells. P antigen on the surface of the red cell acts as a receptor (also known as globoside) for parvovirus hence, those human being lacking in P antigen is resistant to this virus infection. After entering the cell, virus immediately enters into the nucleus where 3′ end of DNA will fold back on itself to produce hairpin-like band and it will act as self-primer for replication of virus. As the virus is highly toxic to host cells, it due to its tropism attaches with rapidly multiplying erythrocyte precursors such as proerythroblasts and normoblasts and suppresses the erythropoiesis during severe infection. Reticulocytes cannot replace the damaged erythrocytes because they are phagocytosed by reticuloendothelial system. In case of patients with hemoglobinopathies, this virus infection can decrease the hemoglobin to 2–6 g/dL but in case of healthy children it can decrease only 1 g/dL. Though occasionally, this virus can infect leukocytes, especially neutrophil, but it does not affect megakaryocytes. It may produce pancytopenia, but it is rare.

If the nonimmune pregnant patient will be affected by this virus within 20 weeks of pregnancy, hydrops fetalis may develop with evidence of 2–6% of fetal death. In 13–16 weeks of pregnancy, there is highest rate of hematopoiesis in fetus hence that may be affected by this viral infection.

Development of Crisis

In patients with hemoglobinopathies with shortened red cell survival and 0–1% reticulocyte count, transient aplastic crises may be precipitated which is characterized by severe and sudden anemia due to sudden temporary stop in RBC production from the bone marrow as well as removal of remaining abnormal RBC by reticuloendothelial cells in spleen. In 80% of patients with sickle cell anemia, parvovirus infection produces aplastic crisis. During this crisis, bone marrow is devoid of erythroid precursors with presence of giant pronormoblasts.

In case of immunocompromised host, chronic parvovirus infections produce chronic anemia and pure red cell aplasia and it will persist until the clearance of this virus from the circulation.

It is common in school-aged children and young, but there is no sex predilection. Transmission of this viral infection occurs from children to their parents.

Diagnosis

A. Anti-parvovirus antibody IgM and IgG by ELISA test: IgM may be detectable starting from third day of illness and persists for months, but IgG remains detectable throughout the life.

B. Polymerase chain reaction of parvovirus B19—it may be detected 4–5 months in serum after acute infection. There is high level of viremia during aplastic crisis.

C. Hematological examination:
- **a.** Reticulocyte count is 0–1%
- **b.** In case of aplastic crisis, hemoglobin level may drop to 2 g/dL
- **c.** In immunodeficient chronically infected patient, pure red cell aplasia is characterized by very low or absent antibody levels; in this case, PCR for viremia should be of choice.

In case of pregnant women who is exposed to parvovirus infection, serology should be done:
- **a.** If IgG is positive but IgM is negative—past infection and no risk for fetus
- **b.** If IgG and IgM are both positive—infection was within 7–120 days and possible risk for fetus.
- **c.** IgG is negative and IgM is positive—acute infection and there is high risk to fetus.
- **d.** If both IgG and IgM are negative—mother is neither immune nor acutely infected, in that case repeat tests should be done after 3 weeks, if IgM positive at that time—it suggests acute infection.

Treatment

A. Acetaminophen can be given in case of fever but most of the cases do not require antipyretic treatment.

B. Intravenous immunoglobulin can be given in case of pure red cell aplasia, but patients should be monitored for viremia.

C. Packed RBCs can be given in case of aplastic crises.

D. If the patient is receiving immunosuppressive drugs, its dose should be reduced to enable the body's immune system to produce large amount of immunoglobulin to eradicate parvovirus infection as well as to provide lifelong protection.

E. In case of HIV-infected patient, potent antiretroviral therapy should be introduced to restore immune function of that patient so that that patient can eradicate parvovirus infection.

Q45. Critical analysis of CBC.

MLB/MAY2013/MDIII (25)

ANSWER

A. Analysis of RBCs: Number of erythrocytes per cc. Normal level in males is 4.6–5.9 million/cc and normal level in females is 4.1–5.4 million/cc.
- **a.** Increased number of RBC along with increased number of WBC and platelets is known as polycythemia.

b. Decreased number of RBC is known as anemia.

c. To classify anemia, following parameters have to be estimated:

1. Mean corpuscular volume: Average size of RBC. Normal value is 80–100 f.

2. Mean corpuscular hemoglobin concentration: Average weight of hemoglobin per RBC. Normal value is 28–33 pg.

3. Mean corpuscular hemoglobin concentration: Average concentration of hemoglobin per erythrocyte. Normal vale is 32–36%.

4. Red cell distribution width: It estimates uniformity of individual size of cell. Normal value is 11.5–14.5%. It can be calculated as (standard deviation of MCV/mean MCV) × 100. In case of microcytic anemia:

- In thalassemia, small RBC is of uniform size so RDW is normal.
- In case of iron deficiency anemia, RDW is large.

Large RDW is also found in vitamin B12 deficiency anemia or dimorphic anemia.

B. Estimation of hemoglobin: In case of male, it is 14–18 g/dL and in females, it is 12–16 g/dL. So, according to hemoglobin content, there are two types of anemia:

a. Hypochromic anemia—red cell is pale in color

b. Normochromic anemia—red cell is normal in color

C. Different types of inclusions in RBC:

a. Basophilic stippling: Coarse blue dots in RBC—lead poisoning, 5'-nucleotidase deficiency, ineffective erythropoiesis, and hemoglobinopathies.

b. Howell-Jolly bodies—it is nuclear remnants—defective function of spleen.

c. Nuclei: Here RBC will be released from the marrow prematurely prior the extrusion of nuclei—myelophthisic anemia or vigorous response to hemolytic anemia.

d. Parasites—malaria or babesia and bartonellosis.

e. Polychromatophilia—cytoplasm of RBC has bluish hue due to persistence of ribosome.

f. Heinz bodies: Precipitation of hemoglobin—it is found in G6PD deficiency, thalassemia, unstable hemoglobin, and drug-induced oxidant injury.

D. Different shapes of RBC: Varying shapes of RBC are known as poikilocytosis. Different shapes are following:

a. Spherocytes: It is found in:

1. Hereditary spherocytosis
2. Other causes of spherocytosis
3. Clostridial sepsis

b. Dacrocytes: Teardrop cells: It is found in:

1. Hemolytic anemia
2. Thalassemia
3. Myelofibrosis
4. Myelodysplastic syndrome

c. Schistocytes: These are helmet-shaped cells found in:

1. Microangiopathic hemolytic anemia
2. Friction against artificial heart valves
3. Genetically determined disorders such as thalassemia and congenital dyserythropoietic anemia
4. Acquired red cell formation disorders such as megaloblastic or dyserythropoiesis
5. Thermal injury

d. Echinocytes: Evenly spaced spikes on the surface of RBC and it is found in:

1. Abnormal drying on the blood smear
2. Renal failure
3. Reversible malnutrition

e. Acanthocytes: Irregularly and irreversibly spaced spikes on the surface of red cells and it is found in:

1. Liver disease
2. Asplenia
3. Glucose-6-phosphate dehydrogenase deficiency
4. Abetalipoproteinemia
5. McLeod syndrome
6. Lecithin cholesterol acyltransferase deficiency
7. Choreoacanthocytosis

f. Elliptocytosis:

1. Inherited membrane defect
2. Iron deficiency anemia
3. Megaloblastic anemia
4. Thalassemia
5. Myelodysplastic syndrome
6. Glycophorin C deficiency

g. Stomatocytosis: Here the area of central pallor takes the shape of round-shaped slit-like space and it is found in:
   1. Inherited membrane defect
   2. Alcoholism
h. Keratocytes: Here one or two pairs of spicules are present on the surface of erythrocyte membrane resulting from removal of a Heinz body. These are also known as helmet cells or bite cells.
i. Leptocytosis: These cells look like ring due to presence of hemoglobin attached with the wall of the cells. It is present in:
   1. Iron deficiency anemia
   2. Thalassemia
j. Target cell: In this cell, there is central and peripheral round-stained area separated by an area of lightly stained cytoplasm. They are present in:
   1. Thalassemia
   2. Hemoglobin C, E, and H disease
   3. Sickle cell disease
   4. Sickle beta-thalassemia
   5. Postsplenectomy
   6. Some patients with hemoglobin C and E trait
   7. Hypobetalipoproteinemia
k. Sickle cell: It is present in homozygous sickle cell disease, but absent in neonates with high hemoglobin F content

E. Inclusion bodies:
   a. Hemoglobin SC crystals: In homozygous hemoglobin C disease, straight edged crystals of hemoglobin C may be present.
   b. Howell–Jolly bodies: Small round purple-colored cytoplasmic inclusions are present within the RBC. It is found in:
      1. Postsplenectomy
      2. Splenic atrophy
      3. Pernicious anemia
      4. Celiac disease with splenic atrophy or megaloblastosis
   c. Pappenheimer bodies: These are peripherally situated basophilic erythrocyte inclusion bodies composed of hemosiderin. It corresponds to siderotic granules of siderocytes. It is present in:
      1. Sideroblastic anemia
      2. Hyposplenism

F. Increased rouleaux formation: It is found in myelomatosis.

G. Changes in case of compensatory increased erythropoiesis:
   a. Polychromasia: It means red cells are stained with many colors. If red cells are stained bluish gray—it is reticulocytes. So, blue shades called "blue polychromasia" means young reticulocytes. These occurs:
      1. In response to intense drive for erythropoiesis
      2. In case of extramedullary erythropoiesis as in case of carcinomatosis or myelofibrosis

      If polychromasia is absent, it suggests bone marrow failure in case of pure red cell aplasia or aplastic anemia.
   b. Erythroblastemia: These are present in following conditions:
      1. Extramedullary hematopoiesis in case of:
         - Hemolytic disease of the newborn
         - Myelofibrosis
         - Carcinomatosis
      2. More common in case of newborn
      3. Sickle cell anemia with painful crises
      4. Cord blood of normal infants
      5. Cyanotic heart failure
      6. Septicemia

H. White blood cell:
   a. Total count: Normal range is 3,400–10,000/cc. It may be increased in following conditions:
      1. Neutrophilic leukocytosis:
         - Infection
         - Inflammation
         - Extremely low birth weight babies (<1 kg) and leukemoid reaction (neutrophil >30,000/μL)
         - Administration of prostaglandin E1 (PGE1) in case of neonate with patent ductus arteriosus (PDA) produces reversible leukocytosis
         - Myeloproliferative disorders
         - Lithium administration
         - Heparin
         - Familial cold autoinflammatory syndrome
         - Decreased egress from the circulation in case of splenectomy and corticosteroid administration
         - Decreased migration of neutrophils in case of exercise, administration of steroids, and other stressful conditions

- Increased release of neutrophils from the bone marrow as in case of trauma, stress, and hypoxia
- Mutation of *CSF3R* genes

2. Lymphocytosis: Normal count is <4,000/cc. If it is >4,000/cc, it is known as lymphocytosis. Causes are:
   - Pertussis infection
   - Viral infection
   - Chronic lymphocytic leukemia
3. Eosinophilia: Normal count is <500/cc. If it is >500/cc, it is known as eosinophilia. Causes are:
   - Allergy
   - Drug hypersensitivity
   - Infection with parasites
   - Skin diseases: Dermatitis herpetiformis and erythema multiforme
   - Recovery phase of scarlet fever
   - Hypereosinophilic syndrome
   - Viral infection
4. Monocytosis: If the monocyte count is >950/cc, it is called monocytosis. Causes are:
   - Bacterial infection: Tuberculosis, brucellosis, bacterial endocarditis, and syphilis
   - Recovery phase of infection
   - Autoimmune diseases, vasculitis, and SLE
   - Sarcoidosis
5. Basophilia: Normal count is 100–150/cc. If it is >100–150/cc, it is called basophilia. Causes are:
   - Chronic myelogenous leukemia

b. Leukopenia: When the leukocyte count is <4,000/cc, it is called leukopenia. Causes are:

1. Bone marrow diseases: CML, myelofibrosis, and MDS
2. Depression of bone marrow by drugs, chemicals, toxins, and radiation
3. Autoimmune diseases: SLE and rheumatoid arthritis
4. Severe infection
5. Immunodeficiency disease
6. Hypersplenism
7. Other conditions: Hypothyroidism and aplastic anemia
8. In case of early phase of infection, there is margination of leukocytes at the sites of infection leading to apparent decrease in leukocyte count. It is called pseudoleukopenia.

c. Appearance of neutrophils:

1. Neutrophil is usually three lobed connected by chromatin bands, but in few cases lobes may be increased up to five lobes. <8% are found in band forms.
2. Leukoagglutination: Sometimes, red cells may adhere to leukocytes due to immune hemolytic anemia.
3. Phagocytosed RBC in the neutrophil in case of paroxysmal cold hemoglobinuria

d. Granules in the neutrophils:

1. Densely stained and increased number of granules—toxic granules are seen in bacterial infection and acute liver failure after administration of G-CSF and neutrophil leukomoid reaction.
2. Hypodense and agranular neutrophil is seen in MDS and myeloid leukemia.
3. In case of Alder–Reilly anomaly, neutrophilic granules are large, deeply stained discrete but functionally normal.
4. In case of Chediak–Higashi syndrome, giant scanty azurophilic granules containing neutrophil are functionally defective, hence this patient is prone to infection.

e. Vacuoles: It is present in following conditions:

1. Associated with toxic granules in severe sepsis
2. Alcoholic toxicity
3. Acute liver failure
4. As artifact in case of prolonged standing
5. Very rarely in case of severe meningococcal or pneumococcal infection, bacteria may be seen in the phagocytic vacuole
6. In case of premature infant, staphylococcal sepsis bacteria may be present
7. In endemic areas, ehrlichiosis and anaplasmosis can be diagnosed by detection of bacteria in neutrophils

f. Other inclusion bodies: Bilirubin crystal, cryoglobulin, and malarial pigment

g. Döhle bodies: These are small, oval or round, and blue-gray pale bodies peripherally situated in the neutrophil and composed of endoplasmic reticulum and ribosomes. These are found in:

1. Bacterial infection
2. Inflammation
3. Burns
4. Administration of G-CSF

5. Neutrophilic leukomoid reaction
6. Pregnancy
7. In case of May–Hegglin anomaly, these inclusion bodies are morphologically same but are larger and present in all types of leukocytes, except lymphocytes

h. Nuclei: Normally, it is three lobed.
1. But leftward shift with band forms, metamyelocyte or myelocyte may be seen in sepsis, but it is associated with toxic granules
2. Leftward shift with band forms is seen in pregnancy
3. Promyelocyte and myeloblast are seen in leukemia or leukoerythroblastic anemia
4. Hypersegmented nuclei: It can be defined as six or more lobes of nuclei attached with chromatin or >3% of neutrophils contain >five-lobed nuclei. It is found in:
   - Megaloblastic anemia
   - Treatment with cytotoxic or anti-metabolite drugs such as methotrexate and hydroxycarbamide as these drugs induce megaloblastosis
5. Pelger–Huet cells: Nuclei of these cells are bilobed connected by chromatin bridge. It may be associated with hyposegmentation of nuclei of eosinophils and basophils. It is autosomal dominant disease.
6. Pseudo Pelger anomaly: In this acquired disorder, neutrophil is hypogranular with irregular nuclear pattern. It is found in:
   i. Myelodysplastic syndrome
   ii. Acute myeloid leukemia with dysplastic maturation
   iii. Chronic myelogenous leukemia

i. Pyknotic neutrophils: These cells are apoptotic cells and dying cells are round, featureless nuclei, and dark pink cytoplasm—it is found in infection

I. Lymphocytes:
a. Turk cells containing round nucleus having large nucleolus and abundant basophilic cytoplasm—found in bacterial viral infections
b. Formation of plasmacytoid lymphocytes or plasma cells—MM
c. Lymphocyte with slightly larger nuclei, open chromatin, and abundant cytoplasm—infectious mononucleosis
d. Small lymphocytes with larger nucleated cells—CML
e. Larger than small lymphocytes with more cytoplasm and larger distinct nucleolus—prolymphocytic leukemia
f. In different types of lymphoma, different types of lymphoma cells are seen:
1. Lymphoma cells are irregular lobed with cleaved or indented nuclei and scanty agranular varying degree of basophilic cytoplasm in follicular lymphoma
2. Pleomorphic lymphocytes in mantle cell lymphoma
3. Lobulated lymphocytes are features of T-cell leukemia or T-cell lymphoma

Platelets

A. Larger platelet seen: It is seen in hyposplenism and severe immune thrombocytopenia
B. Very high platelet count with extreme anisocytosis of platelet is seen in MPDs
C. Thrombocytosis is seen in acute inflammatory stress
D. In Bernard–Soulier syndrome, giant platelet with defective response to ristocetin
E. In gray platelet syndrome, platelet contains decreased cytoplasmic granules and ghost-like appearance
F. In May–Hegglin anomaly, platelet size is large with thrombocytopenia.
G. In case of ethylenediaminetetraacetic acid (EDTA) containing blood, there is platelet clumping leading to pseudothrombocytopenia. Here, platelet function is normal.

Q46. Discuss etiology, genetics, pathology, clinical features, and management of hemophilia.

MGR/OCT2012/MDII (15)

Hemophilia

MGR UNI, Tamil Nadu, 2021 (10)

ANSWER

Definition

Congenital deficiency of factor VIII produces hemophilia A, i.e., classical hemophilia and deficiency of factor IX produces hemophilia B, also called Christmas disease.

Genetics

Hemophilia A is sex-linked recessive inheritance. Gene for factor VIII is present on the long arm of X chromosome.

A. This disease is manifested in males because of absence of complementary normal X chromosome.

B. But female is carrier but cannot manifest because of presence of normal complementary X chromosome. So, positive family history can be obtained from maternal side.

C. Now, if carrier female marries normal male, there is 50% chance of obtaining affected male and 50% chance of obtaining carrier female.

D. If affected male marries normal female, all males are normal and all the daughters are carrier.

E. Carrier female does not suffer from hemorrhagic diathesis but in following circumstances, hemophilia occurs in carrier female:

  a. Lyonization of predominantly normal X chromosome

  b. Homozygosity of hemophilic gene in female offspring of carrier females

  c. Hemizygosity of hemophilic gene in case of chromosomal abnormalities as in case of Turner syndrome

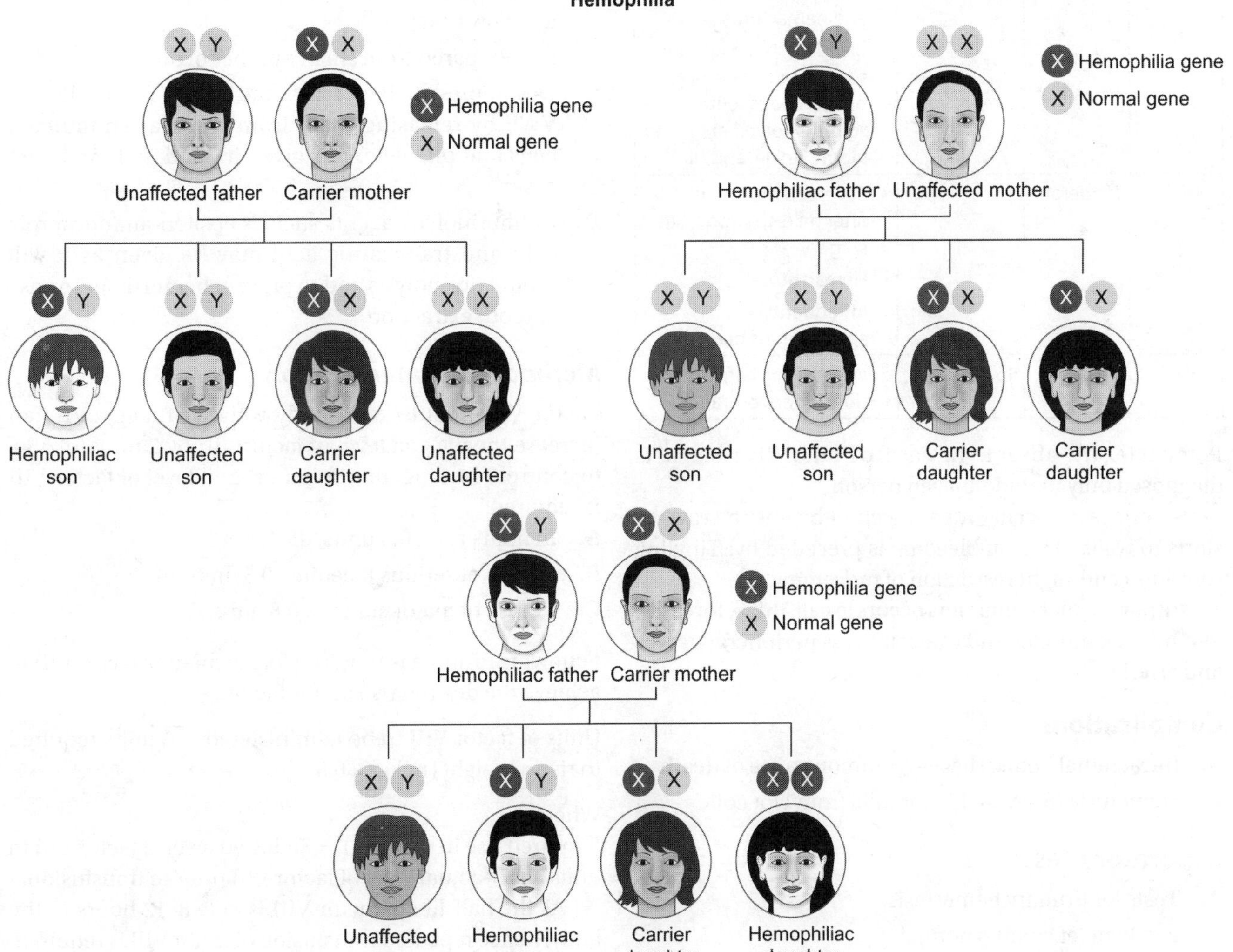

Pathogenesis

Tissue factor and factor VII complexes activate factor IX, which, in turn, generate thrombin in limited amount on tissue injury. Through feedback mechanism, thrombin activates factor IX and factor VIII of intrinsic pathway and increases the amount of thrombin. In case of deficiency of factor VIII:

A. Inadequate amount of thrombin is produced

B. Increased amount of thrombin is required, which can activate thrombin activatable fibrinolysis inhibitor, which is also not possible in case of factor VIII deficiency

So, factor VIII deficiency is responsible for firstly, insufficient clot formation, and, secondly, rapid clot removal.

Clinical Features

Factor VIII level	Grade	Percentage (%)	Clinical features
<1%	Severe	70	• Spontaneous and infrequent hemorrhage and hemarthrosis • Bleeding in the lips and tongue or after eruption of deciduous teeth. Joints involved are knee, elbow, ankle, and hips
1–5%	Moderate	15	• Severe hemorrhage after mild-to-moderate surgery • Hemarthrosis • Infrequently spontaneous bleeding
>5%	Mild	15	Severe hemorrhage after major surgery or trauma

Petechiae are absent. In case of mild disease, it is diagnosed only in middle-aged person.

Severe cases occur when the child begins to crawl or starts to walk. Onset of bleeding is preceded by: Tingling sensation and slight restriction of movement.

Intramuscular hematoma occurs in calf, thigh, forearm, and buttock muscles and can compress peripheral nerves and arteries.

Complications

A. Intracranial hemorrhage—common cause of death

B. Hematuria in severe hemophilia from clot colic

Laboratory Tests

A. Tests for primary hemostasis:
- **a.** Platelet count—normal
- **b.** Bleeding time—normal

B. Extrinsic and common pathway of coagulation—prothrombin time—normal

C. Intrinsic and common pathway of coagulation:
- **a.** Activated partial thromboplastin time—abnormal
- **b.** Clotting time—increased

Treatment

A. Factor VIII concentrate: This is of two types:
- **a.** Plasma-derived factor VIII concentrate: It is obtained from pooled plasma from multiple donors and available in the form of freeze-dried powder.
- **b.** Recombinant factor VIII—it is prepared by genetic engineering. Advantages are:
  1. It can be produced in large scale
  2. It is free from infectious agent

B. Cryoprecipitate: It has high concentration of factor VIII, fibrinogen, VWF, fibronectin, and factor XIII. Advantages are:
- **a.** Low cost
- **b.** Prepared from small number of donor

C. Desmopressin: It increases the level of factor VIII and VWF by releasing them from vascular endothelial cells and platelets. It is given in mild and moderate cases.

D. Antifibrinolytic agents such as epsilon-aminocaproic acid and tranexamic acid may be given as it will inhibit fibrinolysis and to prevent hemorrhage in case of tooth extraction.

Methods of Administration

Factor VIII: 1 unit/kg of body weight of factor VII can increase the plasma level of factor VIII by 2 units/dL. So, to control bleeding, minimum desired level of factor VIII is required:

A. In mild cases: 0.3 units/dL

B. In case of serious bleeding: 0.5 units/dL

C. In case of major surgery: 0.8 units/dL

Following formula is required for calculating factor VIII to achieve the desired rise of this factor:

Units of factor VIII to be administered = % units required to rise × Weight (in kg) × 0.5

Where,
Required rise in units/mL = Required level of factor VIII in units/mL—actual level of factor VIII prior to transfusion.

As the half-life of factor VIII is only 8–12 hours in the body, hence repeated transfusion of factor VIII is required.

Prophylactic therapy with factor VIII is required every 2–3 days to maintain the level at desired limit to prevent serious hemorrhage.

Following should be avoided:

A. Unnecessary trauma

B. Administration of aspirin

C. Avoidance of intramuscular injection

Complications of replacement therapy:

A. Inhibitors antibodies against factor VIII: It occurs in 10–15% of severe hemophiliac patients receiving multiple transfusions. These antibodies will inactivate the factor VII making the patient resistant to factor VIII. There are two types of inhibitors:
   - **a.** One type will rise in low titer
   - **b.** Other type demonstrates anamnestic and rise to high titer after administration of factor VIII.

   Both the inhibitors can be measured by Bethesda method.

   Treatment: High titer of antibodies treatment is difficult. But following products are given:
   - **a.** Porcine factor VIII concentrate
   - **b.** Prothrombin complex concentrates
   - **c.** Activated factor VIII.

B. Transmission of infection:
   - **a.** Hepatitis B
   - **b.** Hepatitis C
   - **c.** Human immunodeficiency virus

Q47. Classify polycythemia with causes of high hemoglobin.

MGR/APR2012/MDIV (7)

Polycythemia.

RGUHS/MAR2008/MDII (6)

Clinical approach to diagnosis in a patient with polycythemia.

BF/MAY2013/MDIII (10)

Discuss polycythemia under the following headings: Definition, causes, and approach to diagnose patient.

WBUHS, 2024 (10)

ANSWER

Definition

It refers to increase in absolute RBC mass characterized by increase in hematocrit and hemoglobin according to age and sex.

Reference Level

A. In case of males, RBC mass is 36 mL/kg and in case of females, RBC mass is 32 mL/kg

B. In case of healthy adult male, hemoglobin is 16 g% ± 2 g% and hematocrit is 47% ± 6%

C. In case of menstruating female, hemoglobin is 13 g% ± 2 g% and hematocrit is 40% ± 6%

Classification of Polycythemia

A. Spurious polycythemia: It occurs in case of volume contraction without increase in RBC mass.
   - **a.** Severe dehydration due to fluid loss in vomiting and diarrhea
   - **b.** Gaisbock syndrome is seen in obese hypertensive males; contributory factors are being smoking, alcohol, and diuretic use

B. True polycythemia:
   - **a.** Based on EPO level in the serum:
     1. Low serum EPO level:
        - Primary congenital and congenital polycythemia
        - Polycythemia rubra vera
     2. Secondary polycythemia with raised serum EPO level:
        - Congenital cyanotic heart disease with right-to-left heart shunt
        - Respiratory disorders:
          - ◊ Chronic obstructive lung disease
          - ◊ Pickwickian syndrome
        - High altitude
        - Kidney disease:
          - ◊ Renal artery stenosis
          - ◊ Bartter syndrome
          - ◊ Focal sclerosing glomerulonephritis
        - In smoker due to raised carboxyhemoglobin level
        - Hemoglobinopathies:
          - ◊ Methemoglobinemia
          - ◊ Hemoglobin Yakima
        - Erythropoietin-secreting tumor:
          - ◊ Uterine leiomyoma
          - ◊ Hepatoma
          - ◊ Cerebellar hemangioma
        - Iatrogenic causes:
          - ◊ Anabolic steroids
          - ◊ Erythropoietin administration
          - ◊ Testosterone replacement therapy

Epidemiology

Male:female ratio is 2:1. Median age of presentation is 60 years. But, polycythemia due to congenital cyanotic heart disease and hemoglobinopathies occur in younger age.

Pathophysiology

A. Erythropoietin secretion will be increased from the renal peritubular capillary lining cells and hepatic cells in response to cellular hypoxia leading to action on erythroid progenitor cells during erythropoiesis.

B. In case of low EPO level, there is acquired mutation in exon 14 and occasionally exon 12 of tyrosine kinase JAK2. As a result, there is loss of autoinhibition of pseudokinase domain of JAK2 leading to constitutive activation resulting in EPO independent erythroid colony formation.

There are two phases of polycythemia:

A. Proliferative polycythemic phase: It is characterized by proliferation of erythroid cells producing increased RBC mass.

B. "Spent" or postpolycythemic phase: It is characterized by:
- **a.** Cytopenias
- **b.** Extramedullary hematopoiesis
- **c.** Hypersplenism
- **d.** Myelofibrosis

From History

A. Constitutional symptoms: Fatigue, malaise, backache, headache, and dizziness due to increased blood viscosity.

B. Pruritus after bathing in warm water shower.

C. Left hypochondrial pain suggestive of splenomegaly.

D. Bleeding—epistaxis, hematemesis, and melena.

E. Evidence of unexplained thrombotic complications such as Budd-Chiari syndrome or infarct in the digits.

F. History suggestive of chronic smoking, congenital cyanotic heart disease, chronic obstructive lung disease, or kidney disease.

G. History of administration of EPO, anabolic steroid, or testosterone.

H. Family history of hemoglobinopathy.

From Physical Examination

A. Abnormal ruddiness of the face and blurring of vision.

B. Evidence of thrombosis in coronary arteries, cerebrovascular and peripheral arteries, or portal, mesenteric, or hepatic veins.

C. Warm and painful and burning sensation of hands and feet is called erythromelalgia.

D. Splenomegaly—it excludes secondary polycythemia. Marked splenomegaly suggests "spent" phase.

Laboratory Analysis

A. Red blood cells:
- **a.** Normocytic and normochromic or microcytic and hypochromic as iron store will be depleted due to production of excess RBCs.
- **b.** In "spent" phase, teardrop cells, anisocytosis, poikilocytosis, and leukoerythroblastic blood picture are present.

B. White blood cell count: 10,000–20,000/cc

C. Platelet count rarely >100,000/cc

Biochemical Investigations

A. Neutrophil ALP: Normal or increased

B. Blood gas analysis is normal

Other Tests

A. Platelet function test—reduced primary and secondary aggregation in response to ADP.

Histopathology

In case of clinical suspicion of polycythemia with absence of Janus kinase 2 (JAK2) mutation, bone marrow findings are:

A. Hypercellular marrow

B. Erythroid hyperplasia

C. Atypical megakaryocytes

D. Trilineage hyperproliferation

World Health Organization Diagnostic Criteria

Major Criteria

A. Raised hemoglobin concentration: >16.4 g/dL in male and >16 g/dL in women

Raised hematocrit: >49% in men and >48% in women

Increased red cell mass >25% above mean predictive value.

B. Bone marrow biopsy trilineage hyperplasia (erythroid, granulocytic, and megakaryocytic) with mature and pleomorphic megakaryocytes of different sizes.

C. JAK2 V617F or JAK2 12 mutation.

Minor Criteria

A. Estimation of serum EPO

B. Genetic testing—JAK2 V617F mutation

Treatment

Goals of Treatment

A. Clinical features due to elevated RBC mass

B. Decrease in risk of thrombosis
C. Prevention of leukemic transformation

Following modes of therapy:

A. Phlebotomy to lower packed red cells along with low-dose aspirin to maintain hematocrit to <45% in men, 42% in women, and <37% in late pregnancy. It may paradoxically increase the incidence of thrombosis.
B. Myelosuppressive therapy, which can control the RBC reduction.
   a. Janus kinase inhibitor, ruxolitinib, is used to treat this patient refractory to hydroxyurea.
   b. Interferon-alpha is used in younger patient and in pregnant patient to reduce red cell mass.
   c. In case of elderly, busulfan or P32 is used who are unable to tolerate hydroxyurea or ruxolitinib.
   d. Hydroxyurea and interferon-alpha can alleviate cytopenias and splenomegaly in case of fibrotic transformation of bone marrow.
C. Other therapies:
   a. Aspirin in low dose can reduce microvascular sequelae.
   b. Pruritus can be cured by: Use of antihistaminics and reduction of water temperature. Selective serotonin reuptake inhibitors such as paroxetine 20 mg/day or fluoxetine 10 mg/day can be given to relieve pruritus.
   c. Splenectomy may give some relief from symptoms.
   d. Allogeneic stem cell transformation in case of advanced disease and can be curative.

Q48. Paraneoplastic visual syndrome.

MGR/MAY2011/MDII (7)

Paraneoplastic syndrome.

MUHS/MAY2012/MDIII (10)

SNMC/MAY2013/MDI (10)

ANSWER

Definition

It is a rare clinical manifestation due to altered immune system in a patient already suffering from underlying malignancy due to development of antibodies, cytokines, hormones, or peptides affecting various systems in the body. These symptoms may manifest prior to appearance of hidden malignancy and can affect the ultimate outcome of the patient.

Etiologies

A. Lung cancer
B. Prostate cancer
C. Breast cancer
D. Medullary carcinoma of the thyroid
E. Gynecological malignancies

Pathophysiology

As tumor cells are immunogenic, these can activate both humoral and cell-mediated immunity. Cytotoxic T cells, after recognition of antigen, are present on the tumor cells and attack these cells or develop antibodies against these tumor cells. On the other hand, body's own immune system recognizes similar antigen present on the normal cells and develops symptoms. Paraneoplastic syndrome involves immunologic and nonimmunologic mechanisms.

Immunologic mechanisms involve:

A. Cell-mediated immunity where T cells attack antigens present on the tumor cells and normal cells.
B. Paraneoplastic antibodies or onconeural antibodies develop against onconeural antigens leading to development of following antibodies:
   a. Type 1 antineuronal nuclear antibodies
   b. Type 2 antineuronal nuclear antibodies
   c. Type 1 Purkinje cell cytoplasmic antibody
   d. Antiamphiphysin antibody
   e. Antibipolar cell of the retina
   f. N-methyl-D-aspartate receptor antibodies
   g. Acetylcholine receptor antibodies
   h. Collapsing response mediator protein 5
   i. Acetylcholine receptor antibodies
   j. Antigamma aminobutyric acid A antibodies

Nonimmunologic mechanisms involve production of cytokines and hormones leading to development of:

A. Hyponatremia due to production of antidiuretic hormone (ADH)
B. Hypercalcemia due to parathormone-like peptide
C. Peripheral neuropathy due to involvement of peripheral nervous system by hematologic malignancies

Clinical presentations are based on organs:

A. Central nervous system:
   a. Panencephalitis or encephalomyelitis producing:
      1. Seizures
      2. Different types of psychosis such as hallucinations, personality changes, and somnolence

3. Autonomic dysfunction
4. Endocrine dysfunction due to hypothalamic involvement

b. Subacute cerebellar degeneration is associated with cancer of lung, ovary, and Hodgkin's lymphoma. It is manifested by ataxia, diplopia, dysphagia, dysarthria, dizziness, nausea, and vomiting.

c. Opsoclonus-myoclonus syndrome: It is clinically characterized by:
1. Uncontrolled eye movements
2. Ataxia
3. Hypotonia
4. Body jerk
5. Irritability

It commonly affects children of 4 years. Opsoclonus is common in children, but ataxia is common in adult.

B. Involvement of myoneural junction:

a. Myasthenia gravis:
1. It occurs in patients with thymoma.
2. Clinically involvement of voluntary muscles and diaphragmatic muscles.
3. Patient is positive for antiacetylcholine receptor positive.
4. Decremental response on repetitive stimulation on electromyography.

b. Lambert–Eaton syndrome:
1. It occurs in any stage of small cell lung cancer.
2. Autoantibodies to presynaptic membrane at the neuromuscular junction lead to impairment of voltage-gated calcium channels (VGCCs), so secretion of acetylcholine will be reduced.
3. Evidence of weakness of proximal muscles of thigh and pelvic girdle, which is gradual in onset and gradually progressive.
4. Autonomic symptoms such as dry mouth, constipation, and decreased sweating.
5. Positive deep tendon reflexes.
6. Blood is positive for VGCC antibodies.

c. Peripheral nervous system:
1. Autonomic neuropathy:
   - It is present in small cell lung cancer and thymoma.
   - It involves sympathetic, parasympathetic, and enteric nervous system.
   - Features are dry mouth, bowel and bladder dysfunction, altered pupillary reflexes, and orthostatic hypotension.
   - Chronic pseudo-obstruction leading to nausea, vomiting, constipation, and abdominal distension.
2. Subacute sensory neuropathy: It is characterized by paresthesia, decreased sensation, and depressed deep tendon reflexes affecting both upper and lower extremities.
3. Affection may be asymmetric or symmetric and multifocal.

C. Endocrine involvement:

a. Cushing syndrome: It occurs due to secretion of ectopic ACTH secretion by tumor cells.

b. Syndrome of inappropriate antidiuretic hormone (SIADH):
1. It occurs due to ectopic secretion of ADH from small cell carcinoma of lung.
2. Features are weakness, fatigue, confusion, seizures, respiratory depression, and coma.
3. Laboratory features are hyponatremia, plasma hypo-osmolarity, and urine hyperosmolarity.

c. Hypercalcemia:
1. It is associated with renal cell carcinoma, lung cancer, and MM.
2. Mechanisms are:
   - Ectopic production of parathormone-like peptide
   - Local osteolytic hypercalcemia
   - Excess extrarenal vitamin D
3. Clinical features are altered mental status, bradycardia, hypertonia, and acute renal failure.

D. Rheumatologic manifestations:

a. Paraneoplastic migratory asymmetric nonerosive polyarthritis.

b. Polymyalgia rheumatica involving shoulder girdle and hip girdle—it occurs with MDS.

c. Hypertrophic osteoarthropathy manifested by digital clubbing, joint pain, and swelling.

d. Multicentric reticulohistiocytosis is featured by papules, nodules, and destructive polyarthritis.

E. Dermatological manifestations:

a. Acanthosis nigricans:
1. Gastric carcinoma is associated with it
2. Hyperpigmented skin

b. Sweet syndrome or acute febrile neutrophilic dermatoses are characterized by fever, neutrophilia, and painful erythematous plaques, papules, or nodules.
c. Leukocytoclastic vasculitis is characterized by painful purpura of lower extremities.
d. Paraneoplastic pemphigus:
    1. It occurs in B-cell lymphoproliferative disorders.
    2. It is characterized by blistering of trunk, palms as well as soles and mucosal erosions.
e. Dermatomyositis: It is characterized by Gottron's papules on phalangeal joints, heliotropic rash on upper eyelids, and erythematous rashes on neck, back, chest, and shoulder.

F. Renal manifestations:
    a. Electrolyte imbalance producing nephropathy.
    b. Ectopic production of ACTH and ADH producing acid-base imbalance.
    c. Nephrotic syndrome.

Q49. Cancer cachexia.

MUHS/MAY2013/MDI (10)

ANSWER

Definition

The word cachexia is derived from the Greek word "kakos" and "hexia"—means bad condition—it is the key sign of cancer. Cancer cachexia is a multifactorial condition characterized by loss of adipose tissue and skeletal muscle mass, which may be compounded by increased basal energy expenditure, anorexia, and dysregulated metabolic rate, which can never be corrected by conventional metabolic support. Loss of >5–10% of body weight can be defined as cachexia and it has a great impact on prognosis and performance status of the patient. Ultimately, patient will die when >30% of body weight will be lost.

Pathophysiology

Stage one: It is the stage of host-tumor interaction:

A. Tumor factors:
    a. Proinflammatory factors: It is found in urine from pancreatic, colon, lung, ovary, breast, and liver cancer patients. Another tumor-related factor such as parathyroid hormone-related peptide is associated with lowering of albumin and transferrin levels.
    b. Procachectic factors: These are proteolysis-inducing and lipid-mobilizing factors. Lipid-mobilizing factors will sensitize the adipose tissue to lipolytic stimuli through increased CAMP production and it also increases the expression of G protein.

B. Host-tumor interaction: Proinflammatory cytokines such as IL-6, IL-1, TNF, and proteolysis-inducing factor increase both:
    a. Degradation of body protein through ubiquitin-proteasome pathway
    b. Decrease the protein synthesis through phosphorylation of eukaryotic initiation factor 2 alpha

C. Host-response factors:
    a. Acute phase protein response: It is a systemic response to inflammation and can be assessed by measuring the CRP. It is associated with hypermetabolism. In case of pancreatic cancer, resting energy expenditure is high and energy intake is reduced. Prognosis can be assessed by the Modified Glasgow Prognostic Scale:

Biochemical measurements	Score
CRP ≤ 10 mg/L + Serum albumin ≥ 35 g/L	0
CRP ≤ 10 mg/L + Serum albumin < 35 g/L	0
CRP > 10 mg/L	1
CRP > 10 mg/L + Serum albumin < 35 g/L	2 (bad)

    b. Neuroendocrine factors: In cancer dysregulation, neuroendocrine factors as a result of systemic inflammatory response will lead to:
        1. Insulin resistance
        2. Elevated cortisol
        3. Reduced metabolic activity
        4. Endogenous production of anabolic growth factors is also responsible for cachexia
        5. Testosterone or its derivatives are responsible for increase in muscle mass
        6. Insulin-like growth factor 1 will be reduced

Stage 2: Metabolic derangements:

A. Protein catabolism
B. Increased lipolysis
C. Increased resting energy expenditure

Stage 3: Clinical endpoints:

A. Weight loss: It is the consequence of loss of appetite and reduced intake of energy leading to cancer cachexia.

B. Survival: Weight loss is the main determinant of survival. Again, weight loss depends upon the following factors such as site and size, stage and histological type of tumor, and age of the patient.

  a. Increased incidence of weight loss is seen in solid tumors such as gastric, pancreatic, lung colorectal, and head and neck cancer and lower risk in breast and hematological cancers. There is an increased incidence of complications from chemo- or radiotherapy in case of increased weight loss.

C. Quality of life: Cachexia is associated with increased fatigability, poor physical performances, and weakness.

D. Physical activity: It is a novel objective and functional outcome, which is seriously impaired in cachexia.

Diagnostic Criteria of Cachectic Syndrome

Weight loss of at least 5% in 12 months or less [or body mass index (BMI) < 20 kg/m^2]		
Any three of five	1. Decreased muscle strength	
	2. Fatigue	
	3. Anorexia	
	4. Low fat-free mass index	
	5. Abnormal biochemistry	Increased inflammatory markers (CRP and IL-6)
		Anemia (hemoglobin < 12 g/dL)
		Serum albumin < 3.2 g/dL

Fatigue is defined by mental and physical weariness as a result of exertion.

Anorexia can be defined by total calorie intake of <20 kcal/kg/day or poor appetite.

Low fat-free mass index denotes lean tissue depletion, i.e., midarm circumference < 10th percentile for age and sex.

Pharmacological Management of Cachexia

Primary endpoint of treatment is:

A. Improvement in:

  a. Lean body mass
  b. Resting energy expenditure
  c. Fatigue
  d. Anorexia
  e. Performance status
  f. Quality of life
  g. Survival

B. Decreased production of cytokines

Clinically endpoint of evaluation of intervention in cancer cachexia:

A. Gastrointestinal symptoms
B. Nutritional status
C. Dietary tolerance
D. Infections
E. Survival

Biochemical endpoint for evaluation of intervention in cancer cachexia:

A. Composition of plasma fatty acids
B. Measurement of proinflammatory cytokines
C. Acute phase reactant proteins measurement

Parent compound	Agent	Effect	Mechanisms
Anabolic drugs	Corticosteroids	Short-lasting and well-tolerated improvement in anorexia and weakness	May inhibit metabolism of prostaglandin
	Insulin	Increases carbohydrate intake and whole body fat	Not established
	Oxandrolone	No published data	Not established
	Nandrolone	Decrease in weight loss	Not established
	ATP	Increases intake of energy and stabilization of weight loss	Not established
Appetite stimulants	Progesterone: Megestrol acetate (MA)	Improves appetite, weight but not lean body mass and improves calorie intake	• MA: Increase central appetite stimulant neuropeptide • YMP: Reduces production of serotonin and cytokine
	Cannabinoids	No obvious benefit	

Continued

Continued

Parent compound	Agent	Effect	Mechanisms
Cytokine inhibitors	Cyproheptadine	Weight gain not improved	Serotonin antagonist
	Thalidomide	• Lean body mass increased • Attenuates weight loss	Immunomodulatory
	Melatonin	Improves cachexia	Immunomodulatory
Anti-inflammatory	NSAIDs	• Reduces inflammation • Reduces expenditure of resting energy	Downregulate systemic inflammatory response

Potential therapeutic targets:

A. Melanocortin-4 receptor inhibitor: It increases lean body mass and decreases basal metabolic rate.

B. Ghrelin: It regulates appetite, induces growth hormone secretion, and harbors anti-inflammatory properties. Phase 1 trial demonstrated it.

C. Myostatin inhibitor and IL-6 inhibitor: Phase 1 trial is being continued.

Q50. Discuss hematopoiesis in the bone marrow. Discuss the WHO classification of lymphoid malignancy and prognostic markers and treatment of CLL.

GMC/2015/MDI (25)

Chronic lymphocytic leukemia.

MJPRU/2016/MDIII (15)

ANSWER

Hematopoiesis

Hematopoietic stem cells are 0.5% of total hematopoietic precursor cells and they will proliferate and differentiate into three lineages of cells. To start differentiation, they will enter into hematopoietic progenitor cells compartment, which comprises 3% of total precursor cell population. These progenitor cells will differentiate into two cells lineages, which are common myeloid progenitor cells and common lymphoid progenitor cells, among which former progenitor cells will be further divided into two progenitor cells:

A. Megakaryocyte erythroid progenitor cells

B. Granulocyte monocyte progenitor cells

Megakaryocyte erythroid progenitor cells again will be divided into two:

A. Burst-forming unit erythroid

B. Burst-forming unit megakaryocyte

Erythropoiesis

Burst-forming unit erythroid further differentiates into following cells serially:

Colony-forming unit erythroid: It will differentiate into proerythroblasts arranged in the form of islands—these cells are large with fine and uniform chromatin containing one or nucleoli present in dark blue cytoplasm.

Proerythroblast will mature into next cell basophilic normoblast or early normoblast—these cells are small in size with coarser chromatin with visible nucleoli in the midst of basophilic cytoplasm.

These cells will transform into intermediate of polychromatic normoblast—it contains smaller nuclei containing clumped chromatin. Polychromasia results from admixture of blue RNA and pink-colored hemoglobin.

It will be transformed into orthochromatic normoblast—it contains small dense pyknotic eccentrically nucleus. They are orthochromatic because stain of cytoplasm is similar to that of erythrocytes.

Orthochromatic normoblast will enter into the stage of reticulocyte where the nucleus will be extruded outside, but it still contains remnants of ribosomal RNA. It will stay 1–2 days in bone marrow and 1–2 days in peripheral blood and ultimately becomes mature pink-staining erythrocyte.

Megakaryopoiesis

It has been divided into four stages:

A. Stage I: Megakaryoblast—it is derived from colony-forming unit (CFU) megakaryocyte. It contains oval- or kidney-shaped nucleus with multiple nucleoli in basophilic agranular cytoplasm.

B. Stage II or promegakaryocyte: Size is larger than megakaryoblast containing lobulated or horseshoe-shaped nucleus in basophilic cytoplasm containing azurophilic granules.

C. Stage III or granular megakaryocyte: It contains large multilobed nucleus and coarse chromatin in abundant mildly basophilic cytoplasm containing multiple azurophilic granules.

D. Stage IV or mature megakaryocyte: It contains multi-lobed pyknotic nucleus in acidophilic cytoplasm and cytoplasmic granules are arranged in "platelet fields." It extends long and slender cytoplasmic processes called proplatelets in between the endothelial cells of sinusoids and they are released by the fragmentation of these processes. As a result, each megakaryocyte will produce 1,000–5,000 platelets, but "bare" nucleus will remain which will be removed by macrophages.

So, during maturation from megakaryoblast to megakaryocytes, there will be:

A. Gradual increase in cell size
B. Gradual increase in nuclear lobes
C. Increase in red pink granules
D. Gradual decrease in cytoplasmic basophilia

Thrombopoietin binds to cell surface receptors c-Mpl and, thereby, directs the growth and development of megakaryocytes.

Markers of megakaryocytic differentiation are CD41 (GPIIb), CD42 (GPIb), and CD61 (GPIIIa).

Granulopoiesis

Common myeloid progenitor will be converted into granulocyte monocyte progenitor, which, in turn, will be divided into CFU, MCs, basophil (Ba), eosinophil (Eo), granulocyte (G), and monocyte (M).

CFU-MC will be directed to form MCs.

Sequence of maturation of granulopoiesis is:

A. Myeloblast: It is the earliest cells of maturation stage, large oval nucleus containing two to five nucleoli, and fine chromatin in small amount of basophilic cytoplasm.
B. Promyelocyte: This is second stage of maturation, size is larger than myeloblast, and nucleus contains nucleoli with slightly condensed chromatin. Azurophilic granules appear.
C. Third stage is myelocyte stage: It is small cell containing round to oval eccentrically nucleus, condensed chromatin but absence of nucleoli, greater amount of cytoplasm containing primary and secondary granules. Secondary granules are neutrophilic, eosinophilic, or basophilic. It is the last cell, which can divide.
D. Stage IV or metamyelocytes: Here nucleus is indented and kidney shaped, more coarse chromatin, primary and secondary granules in cytoplasm, and tertiary granules being synthesized in this stage.
E. Stage V or band stage: Here, the nucleus is band shaped with constant diameter throughout the nucleus and more condensed chromatin.
F. Stage VI or segmented neutrophil: Here, nucleus is deep purple containing two to five lobes connected by thin bands and coarse chromatin is present in pink cytoplasm.

In neutrophil, there are four types of granules:

A. Primary granules contain:
  - **a.** Proteases:
    - **1.** Elastase
    - **2.** Cathepsin G
  - **b.** Acid hydrolases
  - **c.** Antimicrobials:
    - **1.** Lysozyme
    - **2.** Myeloperoxidase
    - **3.** Defensins

B. Secondary granules:
  - **a.** Lactoferrin
  - **b.** Collagenase
  - **c.** Transcobalamin 1
  - **d.** Plasminogen activator

C. Tertiary granules: Gelatinase

D. Secretory vesicles:
  - **a.** LAP
  - **b.** Cytochrome b558
  - **c.** CD35

Eosinophil: Size is larger than neutrophil, bilobed nucleus, and cytoplasm contains three types of bright orange granules:

A. Primary granules contain:
  - **a.** Charcot–Leyden crystal protein

B. Secondary granules contain:
  - **a.** Major basic protein
  - **b.** Eosinophil cationic protein
  - **c.** Eosinophil peroxidase
  - **d.** Eosinophil-derived neurotoxin

C. Small granules:
  - **a.** Arylsulfatase enzyme
  - **b.** Acid phosphatase enzyme

Cytokine responsible for differentiation to eosinophil and basophil is interleukin-5 and interleukin-3, respectively.

Basophil: It is small oval to round cells containing deep purple granules containing multilobed nucleus, condensed chromatin, and granules containing histamine, peroxidase, heparin, cathepsin G, and major basic protein.

Monocyte: It will originate in the bone marrow under the action of interleukin-3, GM-CSF, and M-CSF into monoblast, which, in turn, divides into promonocytes and finally into monocyte; it is a large cell containing oval or clefted nucleus and fine delicate chromatin in the midst of abundant blue-gray ground-glass cytoplasm containing azurophilic granules. These granules contain lysozyme, myeloperoxidase, and nonspecific esterase.

Monocytes after circulating in the blood for 3 days ultimately will settle down in tissues in the form of macrophages.

Lymphocytes: There are two types of lymphocytes—T lymphocytes are larger, nucleus is clefted or round, but abundant cytoplasm, few azurophilic granules, and constitute 60–70% of total lymphocytes. It originates in bone marrow from progenitor cells followed by maturation in thymus from where it will transport in the circulation to secondary lymphoid organ such as paracortex of lymph nodes and periarteriolar lymphoid sheath present in the spleen to differentiate into T-helper cells, cytotoxic T cells, and regulatory T cells.

B lymphocytes are smaller, cytoplasm is small, and constitute 10–15% of total lymphocytes. B lymphocytes initially developed in the bone marrow, primary lymphoid organ. Later on, further maturation occurs in lymph nodes and spleen through antigenic stimulation into plasma cells and memory cells.

Classification of Lymphoid Malignancy According to the World Health Organization

A. Pre B- and T-cell neoplasm:
- **a.** Precursor B lymphoblastic leukemia/lymphoma
- **b.** Precursor T lymphoblastic leukemia/lymphoma

B. Mature B-cell neoplasm:
- **a.** Chronic lymphocytic leukemia/small lymphocytic lymphoma
- **b.** Monoclonal B-cell lymphocytosis
- **c.** B-lymphocytic leukemia
- **d.** Hairy cell leukemia variant
- **e.** Splenic marginal zone lymphoma
- **f.** Splenic B-cell lymphoma/leukemia, unclassifiable
- **g.** Lymphoplasmacytic lymphoma/Waldenström macroglobulinemia
- **h.** Monoclonal gammopathy of undetermined significance, IgM
- **i.** Solitary plasmacytoma of bone
- **j.** Plasma cell myeloma
- **k.** Extraosseous plasmacytoma
- **l.** Monoclonal immunoglobulin deposition disease
- **m.** Extranodal marginal zone lymphoma of mucosa-associated tissue lymphoma
- **n.** Nodal marginal zone lymphoma
- **o.** Follicular lymphoma
- **p.** Pediatric-type follicular lymphoma
- **q.** Large B-cell lymphoma with IRF4 rearrangement
- **r.** Primary cutaneous follicle center lymphoma
- **s.** Mantle cell lymphoma
- **t.** Diffuse large B-cell lymphoma
- **u.** T-cell/histiocyte-rich large B-cell lymphoma
- **v.** Primary DLBCL of the CNS
- **w.** Primary cutaneous DLBCL, leg type
- **x.** Epstein–Barr virus, DLBCL, and NOS

Prognostic Factors of Chronic Lymphocytic Leukemia

A. Clinical staging: It can determine the prognosis and time of initiation of treatment. Anemia and thrombocytopenia due to bone marrow infiltration adversely affect prognosis as compared to autoimmune destruction of RBC and platelets.

B. *IgV* genes: Patients with somatic mutations of *V14* genes have better prognosis as compared to unmutated *V14* genes.

C. Infiltration pattern in bone marrow: Nodular and interstitial pattern of bone marrow involvement has better prognosis as compared to diffuse pattern of involvement.

D. CD38 expression on the chronic lymphoid cells is associated with poor prognosis than absent expression.

E. Chromosomal abnormalities:
- **a.** Presence of del(11q) and/or del(17p) is associated with limited progression-free survival.
- **b.** Presence of del(13q) is associated with favorable prognosis.
- **c.** Complex karyotype with more than two unrelated chromosomal abnormalities in >1 stimulated CLL cells also signifies unfavorable prognosis.

F. Lymphocyte doubling time of <12 months suggests unfavorable prognosis.

G. Elevated serum β2-microglobulin level is another bad prognostic factor.

Management

Indications of Instituting the Therapy

A. Persistence or progression of constitutional symptoms such as fever, weight loss, fatigue, and sweat

B. Enlarged lymph gland producing mechanical obstruction or dysfunction of end organ

C. Lymphocyte doubling time is rapid

D. Immune destruction of thrombocytes and platelets

E. Replacement of bone marrow with lymphocytes in stage III or IV disease

F. Progressive enlargement of spleen, liver, and lymph node

Treatment Options

A. Nucleosides: Drugs are fludarabine, cladribine and pentostatin. These drugs are the drug of choice. Fludarabine is used because:

- **a.** It is superior to alkylating agent
- **b.** It is associated with increased complete response
- **c.** Increases the duration of response

Adverse effects are:

- **a.** Marked immunosuppression
- **b.** Increased risk of opportunistic infection
- **c.** Increased chance of autoimmune hemolysis
- **d.** Myelodysplasia

B. Alkylating agents: Drugs are chlorambucil, cyclophosphamide, and bendamustine.

- **a.** Chlorambucil can be given as palliative therapy.
- **b.** Cyclophosphamide can be given in combination with nucleoside analog and anti-CD20 antibody.

C. Monoclonal antibodies:

- **a.** Rituximab:
  1. It is anti-CD20 chimeric monoclonal antibody.
  2. Overall response rate is 50%, but CR is low.
  3. It can be administered in patients with low performance status and substantial comorbidities.
  4. Dose is 375 mg/m^2 infusion in first week and then 500 mg/m^2 thereafter.
  5. Infusion-related release of cytokine during first infusion.
- **b.** Obinutuzumab: It is humanized type 2 glyco-engineered anti-CD20 antibody having superior efficacy with chlorambucil.
- **c.** Ofatumumab: It is CD20 fully humanized monoclonal antibody and can be effective as single agent.
- **d.** Alemtuzumab:
  1. This humanized anti-CD20 monoclonal antibody expresses its antigen on >95% of both mature B and T lymphocytes.
  2. It eliminates leukemic cells from blood, bone marrow, and spleen, but not from lymph nodes.
  3. Adverse reactions:
     - Cytokine release syndrome
     - Profound immunosuppression
     - Neutropenia
     - Opportunistic infection—for this, trimethoprim/sulfamethoxazole and acyclovir can be administered as prophylactic agent.

D. Immunomodulatory agents: Drug is lenalidomide.

- **a.** It has higher CR rate and higher overall response rate in older patients with 11q abnormality.
- **b.** Toxicities: Neutropenia, anemia, and thrombocytopenia with fever.

E. B-cell receptor signaling inhibitors:

- **a.** Ibrutinib:
  1. It is a reversible inhibitor of BTK inhibitor. Dose is 420 mg/day orally.
  2. It will rapidly improve the adenopathy and it will early mobilize lymphocytes into the blood.
  3. It is effective in refractory patients or in previously treated but relapsed patients.
- **b.** Idelalisib:
  1. It is orally active phosphoinositide-3 kinase inhibitor delta isoform.
  2. In case of refractory CLL, it can be given in combination with rituximab and there is improved overall survival.
  3. Toxicities: Hepatotoxicity, pneumonitis/pneumonia, diarrhea, rash, and CMV reactivation.

Consideration of Treatment Choice

A. Age—elderly

B. Renal function

C. Hepatic function

D. Selection of patient having del(17q)—these patients should be treated with cytotoxic therapy

E. Selection of patients having del(11q) as these patients need alkylators for therapy.

Treatment of Relapsed or Refractory Cases

A. Ibrutinib continuous dosing chemotherapy

B. Combination of rituximab and idelalisib

C. Retreatment with chemoimmunotherapy mainly in those patients who already received chemoimmunotherapy with durable response

Radiation Therapy

A. Local radiation therapy:

- **a.** To reduce the lymph node masses to prevent vital organ dysfunction
- **b.** That responds poorly to chemotherapy

B. Splenic radiation: It will improve the signs of hypersplenism temporarily.

Surgery: It is indicated in case of immune thrombocytopenia or immune hemolytic anemia who are refractory to IVIg, corticosteroid, or rituximab.

Etiology

A. Genetic factors: 8–10% of patients with CLL have family history of CLL. There may be history of dominant inheritance. Genetic studies identified the chromosome 2q21.2 as association with CLL.

B. Immunologic factors: Inherited and acquired immunodeficiency results in malignant cells proliferation as well as increased susceptibility to leukemogenic viruses.

C. Enhanced exposure to radiation and cytotoxic therapy increases the susceptibility to CLL.

D. Molecular and cytogenic aberrations: There is incidence of mutation in the germinal center of lymphoid follicles in response to antigenic exposure such as IgV14 hypermutation and seen in approximately half of CLL cases. There are chromosomal abnormalities such as del(11q), del(13q), and del(17q).

Immunoglobulin Abnormalities

A. Hypogammaglobulinemia: They are prone to suffer from encapsulated bacterial pathogens

B. Monoclonal paraprotein, mainly IgM

C. Coombs-positive warm antibody hemolytic anemia

D. Skin cancers

E. Elevated number of T cells by two to four times of normal, but contracted T-cell repertoire with monoclonal or oligoclonal subsets

Clinical Features

A. Reduced tolerance to exercise chronic fatigue

B. Fever, weight loss, and bruising

C. Physical signs:

- **a.** Lymphadenopathy
- **b.** Splenomegaly
- **c.** Hepatomegaly
- **d.** Pedal edema due to lymphatic obstruction
- **e.** Thrombophlebitis

Clinical Course

A. Renal manifestations—uncommon in CLL, but may occur in case of TLS in the form of autoimmune nephropathy and hyperuricemia.

B. Pulmonary manifestation occurs in late course of the disease.

C. Dermatological involvement and osteolytic lesions are unusual.

D. Transformation into diffuse large cell lymphoma and prolymphocytic leukemia occurs in <5% of patients with CLL.

E. Progressive disease: It is associated with depressed humoral and cell-mediated immunity as evidenced by progressive pancytopenia and persistent fever.

Laboratory Studies

A. Erythrocytes: Normochromic and normocytic anemia due to following:

- **a.** Infiltration of bone marrow with lymphocytes
- **b.** Hypersplenism
- **c.** Immune-mediated destruction

B. Lymphocytes:

- **a.** Absolute count may rise to 500,000/cc and cells are mature with scanty cytoplasm and clumped chromatin.
- **b.** During preparing, smear cells are damaged producing "smudge" cells or "basket" cells.

C. Granulocytes: Normal till late phase

D. Platelet: Thrombocytopenia may be due to:

- **a.** Bone marrow infiltration by lymphocytes
- **b.** Hypersplenism
- **c.** Immune destruction

E. Reticulocyte count

F. Direct antiglobulin test

G. Haptoglobin level

H. Fractionated bilirubin level

Other Studies

A. Molecular analysis—it can detect variable region maturation status
B. Biologic markers of the disease—del(11q), del(17q), and del(13q)
C. Flow cytometry by CD38 and ZAP70 expression
D. Renal function test
E. Liver function test
F. Serum protein electrophoresis
G. Hepatitis B profile

Radiological Studies

Different sites of lymph node enlargement such as retroperitoneal, mediastinal, pelvis, and abdominal sites can be delineated by CT scan, PET scan, and MRI scan.

Bone Marrow Study

It should be done in following conditions:

A. Coombs-negative unexplained anemia
B. Unexplained thrombocytopenia

Lymph Node Biopsy

It will demonstrate malignant lymphoma of small lymphocyte type. It can be done if in case of CLL, there is suspicion of Richter transformation.

Q51. What is myelofibrosis? Discuss its causes and management.

BF/MAY2013/MDI (10)

ANSWER

Definition

Bone marrow fibrosis is the nonspecific manifestation of various diseases involving either reticulin or collagen fibers or it is mediated by different types of cytokines released from:

A. Macrophages
B. T cells
C. Monocytes
D. Megakaryocytes
E. Bone marrow stromal cells

Reticulin fibrosis: It occurs in response to infection and inflammation involving bone marrow.

Collagen fibrosis: It commonly occurs in case of carcinoma and lymphomatous conditions infiltrating marrow.

Causes of Myelofibrosis

A. Hematologic causes:
   a. Acute myeloid leukemia
   b. Myelodysplastic syndrome
   c. Hairy cell leukemia
   d. Multiple myeloma
   e. Acute lymphatic leukemia
   f. Chronic myeloid leukemia
   g. Hypereosinophilic syndrome
B. Nonhematologic causes:
   a. Tuberculosis
   b. Histoplasmosis
   c. Leishmaniasis
   d. Human immunodeficiency virus
   e. Hyper- or hypothyroidism
   f. Renal osteodystrophy

Pathophysiology

Primary myelofibrosis (PMF) can be defined as a clonal myeloproliferative neoplasm characterized by:

A. Trilineage proliferation with predominantly involving granulocytic and megakaryocytic lines in the bone marrow
B. Reactive fibrosis of the bone marrow
C. Extramedullary hematopoiesis in the spleen

Triggering factors for bone marrow fibrosis: Stimulation of fibroblast as well as synthesis of collagen is done by following factors synthesized by abnormal megakaryocytes—

A. Platelet-derived growth factor
B. Transforming growth factor-β

"Driver mutations" developed in primary myelofibrosis are:

A. JAK2V617F in 50% of cases
B. CLAR in 30% of cases
C. MPL in 10% of cases

They produce persistent activation of JAK/signal transducer and activator of transcription (STAT) signaling pathway when cytokine pathway is absent.

If above three mutations are absent, it is called triple-negative PMF.

There are two phases of PMF:

A. Prefibrotic phase:
   a. Bone marrow is hypercellular
   b. Minimal or absence of fibrosis
   c. Peripheral thrombocytosis

B. Thrombotic phase:

- **a.** Marked bone marrow fibrosis
- **b.** Extramedullary hematopoiesis
- **c.** Peripheral leukoerythroblastic blood picture and teardrop cells

Clinical Pictures

A. Age—median age is 65 years
B. Sex incidence—equal
C. Constitutional symptoms: Fever and night sweat
D. Right and left upper quadrant pain
E. Symptoms of anemia, weakness, and fatigue
F. Weight loss
G. Evidence of bleeding
H. Signs:

- **a.** Hepatomegaly
- **b.** Splenomegaly
- **c.** Peripheral edema
- **d.** Tenderness over the spleen from splenic infarction

Laboratory Features

A. Peripheral blood pictures:

- **a.** In prefibrotic stage:
    1. Thrombocytosis or thrombocytopenia
    2. Leukocytosis or leukopenia with shift to left
- **b.** Fibrotic stage:
    1. Leukoerythroblastic blood picture
    2. Leukopenia
    3. Thrombocytopenia

B. Bone marrow:

- **a.** Prefibrotic stage:
    1. Granulocytic and megakaryocytic hyperplasia
    2. Pleomorphic and bizarre appearances of megakaryocytes
- **b.** Fibrotic stage:
    1. Dry tap in the bone marrow
    2. Trephine biopsy demonstrates:
        - Decreased cellularity
        - Increased number of abnormal megakaryocytes
        - Osteosclerosis
        - Dilated marrow sinuses with intrasinusoidal hematopoiesis

C. Cytogenetic analysis demonstrating chromosomal abnormalities
D. Molecular genetic analysis

Prognostic Factors

A. Advanced age
B. Hemoglobin < 10 g/dL
C. White blood cell count < 4,000/cc or >30,000/cc
D. Hypercatabolic symptoms
E. Abnormal cytogenetics or abnormal circulating blasts cells

Treatment

Treatment is mostly palliative. Symptomatic anemic patients can be treated by:

A. Combination of androgen:

- **a.** Oxymethalone 50 mg four times/day
- **b.** Fluoxymesterone 10 mg three times/day
- **c.** Prednisolone 30 mg/day

B. Blood transfusion

Response is very brief.

Treatment of thrombocytosis, leukocytosis, or organomegaly is treated by:

A. Hydroxyurea: 20–30 mg/kg twice or thrice weekly

Thalidomide and prednisolone in case of anemia

To relief the symptoms of splenic size reduction, JAK2 inhibitors such as ruxolitinib are used in case of intermediate or high risk of fibrosis.

Curative treatment in case of PMF is allogeneic stem cell transplantation as successful transplantation may resolute fibrosis.

Q52. Discuss the approaches to bleeding disorder and its management.

MGR/APR2016/MDII (15)

Outline the coagulation cascade and describe the formation of homeostatic plug.

Discuss the investigation of bleeding disorders.

MGR/MAR2007/MDIV (15)

Approach to a case of bleeding disorders.

Kerala University, 2021 (10)

A 65 years old gentle man presents to you with multiple ecchymoses and a significant muscle bleed. How would you approach to diagnose and manage him.

WBUHS, 2021 (10)

ANSWER

Coagulation Cascade: Written in Question in Investigation of Bleeding Disorder

Laboratory investigations can be divided into two headings:

A. Screening tests for primary hemostasis: It includes following tests:

a. Platelet count: Normal range is 150,000–400,000/cc. So, thrombocytopenia results when platelet count is <150,000/cc.

1. Mild thrombocytopenia: Platelet count 50,000–<1,500,000/cc
2. Moderate thrombocytopenia: Platelet count 20,000–<50,000/cc
3. Severe thrombocytopenia: Platelet count <20,000/cc

Common causes are:

1. Hematologic malignancies
2. Ingestion of certain drugs
3. Disseminated intravascular coagulation
4. Immune thrombocytopenic purpura (ITP)
5. Aplastic anemia
6. Megaloblastic anemia
7. Connective tissue diseases
8. Platelet count <40,000/cc occurs in: inflammation and MPDs

b. Platelet distribution width: It is normal in reactive thrombocytosis; in essential thrombocytopenia, it is decreased.

c. Mean platelet volume: It differentiates causes of thrombocytopenia due to peripheral destruction where it is increased from thrombocytopenia due to impaired platelet production where platelet volume is normal or low.

d. Presence of reticulated platelets which are analog to reticulocytes: It is increased in ITP whereas lower values are seen in aplastic anemia.

e. Complete blood count:

1. Cytopenia: Anemia, leukopenia, and thrombocytopenia
2. Red cell abnormalities: Fragmented red cells in DIC
3. Abnormal WBCs—leukemia
4. Abnormal platelet:
   - Thrombocytopenia
   - Giant platelet—MPDs and Bernard-Soulier syndrome
   - Isolated discrete platelet without clumping in smear obtained from finger prick

f. Bleeding time: It will assess the formation of primary hemostatic plug following puncture of skin as it depends on adequate function of platelets. There are three methods and these are Ivy's, Duke's, and template method. Normal range in Ivy method is 2–7 minutes. It is increased in:

1. Thrombocytopenia
2. Inherited coagulation disorders—von Willebrand disease and afibrinogenemia
3. Disordered function of platelets: Glanzmann's thrombasthenia, Bernard-Soulier syndrome, and mild-to-moderately prolonged defect in storage pool
4. Vascular disorders

g. Closure time by platelet function analyser-100: In this machine after aspiration of small amount of citrated blood, the suction aperture has to be coated with adenosine monophosphate or epinephrine. After exposure of blood under shearing stress to platelet agonists, there will be serial event such as VWF binding, adhesion of platelet, and platelet activation followed by aggregation. As a result, there will be occlusion of aperture. This closure time will be prolonged in platelet function disorders and von Willebrand disease.

B. Screening tests for secondary hemostasis:

a. Prothrombin time: Here in platelet-poor plasma, tissue thromboplastin and calcium are added followedbywatchingofclottingtimeofthatmixture as this mixture measures extrinsic and common pathways. It measures the activity of factors VII, X, V, prothrombin, and fibrinogen. Normal PT is 11–16 seconds. Causes of prolonged PT:

1. Vitamin K deficiency
2. Disseminated intravascular coagulation
3. Inherited deficiency of factors II, V, VII, and X
4. Oral anticoagulant therapy

b. Activated partial thromboplastin time: Here platelet-poor plasma is put into incubator followed by addition of phospholipid and calcium and clotting time is noted. Here activator such as kaolin, celite, silica, and ellagic acid has to be added. APTT measures the clotting time through intrinsic and common pathways. Normal value of

APTT is 30–40 seconds. It is increased in following cases:

1. Disseminated intravascular coagulation
2. Liver disease due to reduced synthesis of coagulation factors
3. Vitamin K deficiency
4. Inherited deficiency of factor VIII or IX
5. Circulating inhibitors: Specific inhibitor is usually directed against specific factor

c. Thrombin time: Here in platelet-poor plasma, thrombin reagent is added followed by recording of clot formation. Normal range is 8–12 seconds. Prolonged thrombin time occurs in following cases:

1. Chronic liver disease
2. Fibrinogen/fibrin degradation products
3. Heparinization in plasma
4. Disorders of fibrinogen:
   - Afibrinogenemia
   - Hypofibrinogenemia (<100 mg/mL)
   - Dysfibrinogenemia

C. Specific tests for primary hemostatic disorders:

a. Platelet aggregation studies: Here special machine aggregometer is used. Common aggregating agents used are ADP, epinephrine, collagen, ristocetin as well as arachidonic acid.

1. Defective or absent aggregation with ADP, epinephrine, collagen, and arachidonic acid due to congenital absence of receptors on platelet GPIIb/IIIa, which is required for binding of fibrinogen during aggregation, but normal activity with ristocetin.
2. Defect in aggregation with ristocetin but not with ADP, epinephrine, collagen, and arachidonic acid—occurs in Bernard–Soulier syndrome and von Willebrand disease.

b. Verify/Now test: This test uses whole blood to assess the level of inhibition of platelet by antiplatelet agents such as clopidogrel and aspirin.

c. Flow cytometry: It is widely used for:

1. Demonstration of reduced expression of platelet integrin αIIbβ3—it can diagnose Glanzmann's syndrome.
2. Absent expression of GPIb-IX-V—it can diagnose Bernard–Soulier syndrome.

d. Platelet secretion test or release of ristocetin by platelet: Indirect evidence of release reaction is secondary wave of aggregation with ADP or epinephrine. For direct testing of assessing release reaction, following tests are available:

1. Quantitation of serotonin can be assessed by dense granule secretion
2. Firefly bioluminescence technique of adenosine triphosphate (ATP) concentration can be measured
3. Hypercoagulable tests can measure platelet factor 4 and β-thromboglobulin, which are released from α-granules

e. Detection of abnormalities in arachidonic acid metabolism: Quantitation of thromboxane B2 (TXB2), malondialdehyde, and other intermediate products of arachidonic acid metabolism as these are required for its metabolism. Arachidonic acid activates platelet by generating thromboxane A2. So, abnormal estimation of any of the above leads to deficiencies of cyclooxygenase, thromboxane synthase, and phospholipases.

f. Tests for procoagulant activity: It can be estimated by prothrombin consumption test as it estimates the amount of residual prothrombin after clotting of whole blood—it may be due to deficiency of coagulation factors or platelet phospholipid.

g. Clot retraction test: This test estimates the recalcification of citrated platelet-rich plasma—this test depends upon the number and function of platelets.

D. Specific tests for coagulation phase:

a. Mix study based on PT and APTT: Here PT and APTT is repeated by using 50:50 mixture of patient's normal plasma and to see whether normalization of previously prolonged test can be found or not.

50:50 mixing results	Causes
Correction of previously abnormal test	Deficiency of factors
No correction of result	Lupus anticoagulant
Correction done immediately but after incubation there will be prolongation	Inhibitor of factors

b. Thromboplastin generation test (TGT): In this two-stage test—in the first stage, adsorbed plasma, serum, calcium, and phospholipid are incubated together. Serum provides factors IX and X. Adsorbed plasma provides factors V and VIII and both provide factors XI and XII. Result is the generation of prothrombinase complex (activated factor X-V-calcium-phospholipid).

In the second stage, adequacy of prothrombinase generation is estimated by assessing its ability to clot normal plasma.

Patient's history	Coagulation studies	TGT	Inferences
Bleeding	• PT—normal • APTT—prolonged	Defect in plasma	Factor VIII deficiency
Bleeding	• PT—prolonged • APTT—prolonged	Defect in plasma	Factor V deficiency
Bleeding	• PT—normal • APTT—prolonged	Defect in serum	Factor IX deficiency
Bleeding	• PT—prolonged • APTT—prolonged	Defect in serum	Factor X deficiency
Bleeding	• PT—normal • APTT—prolonged	Defect in both plasma and serum	Factor XI deficiency
No bleeding	• PT—normal • APTT—prolonged	Defect in both plasma and serum	Factor XII deficiency

c. Estimation of fibrinogen: It may be deficient in case of hypofibrinogenemia, dysfibrinogenemia, and DIC. Transient hypofibrinogenemia occurs in:
   1. Myocardial infarction
   2. Neoplasia
   3. Trauma
   4. Inflammatory disorders

d. Coagulation factor assay

e. Quantitative assay of factor XIII: In case of factor XIII deficiency, all other screening tests of hemostasis are normal.

f. Paracoagulation test: It is done to detect soluble fibrin monomer in plasma. In this test, protamine is added to platelet-poor plasma to watch the formation of gel. If the test is positive, it indicates:
   1. Intravascular coagulation
   2. Liver disease
   3. Lobar pneumonia
   4. After major surgery

g. Reptilase time: In this test, snake venom, reptilase, is added to patient's serum to note the clotting time. This test is done, if the thrombin time is elevated. This test will be normal in presence of heparin; in other cases where thrombin time is prolonged, reptilase time is also elevated.

h. Ecarin time: Here ecarin, a venom obtained from a saw-scaled snake viper, activates directly prothrombin to form clot. It is used to monitor the antithrombin drug dabigatran.

E. Tests for fibrinolysis:

a. Detection of fibrinogen and fibrin degradation product (FDP): After exclusion of presence of heparin, plasma fibrinogen and FDP estimation will be done.
   1. If FDP is high and fibrinogen is low—it suggests DIC
   2. If FDP is normal but fibrinogen level is low—it suggests:
      - Hypofibrinogenemia
      - Dysfibrinogenemia
      - Afibrinogenemia

b. D-dimer test: It is the smallest end product of FDP, which is cross-linked by plasmin. It is elevated in:
   1. Venous thromboembolism: Negative test rule out this disease
   2. Pulmonary embolism
   3. Arterial thrombosis
   4. Disseminated intravascular coagulation
   5. Pregnancy
   6. Postoperative state
   7. Liver disease
   8. Cancer

F. Thromboelastography: It can assess both whole blood coagulation and fibrinolysis. Its main uses are in the following:

a. Liver transplantation
b. Cardiac surgery
c. Trauma care unit

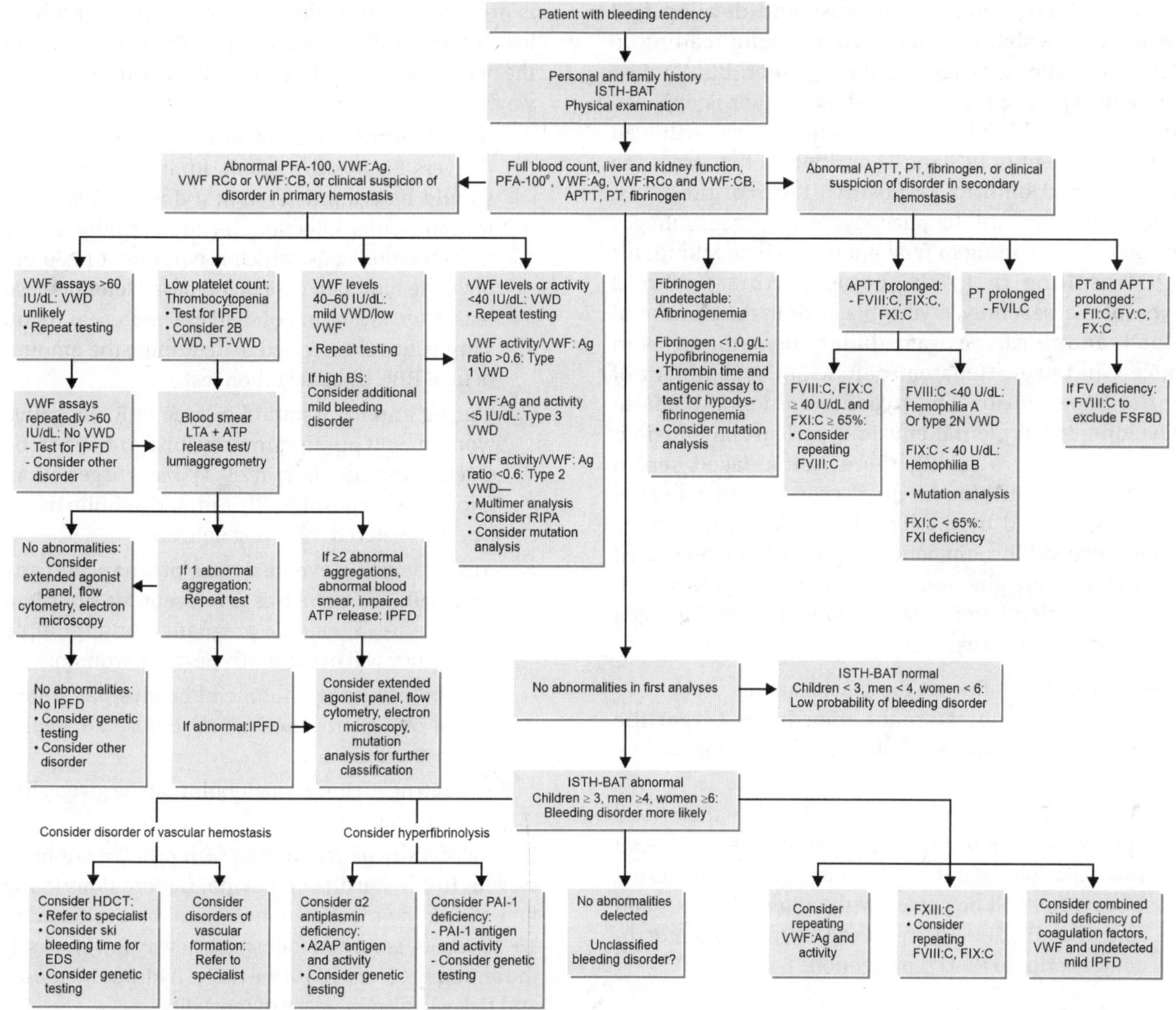

Q53. Discuss the pathophysiology and management of Rh isoimmunization.

BF/JUN2016/MDI (10)

ANSWER

Definition

Rh isoimmunization is the development of IgG antibodies against antigen present on the fetal RBCs resulting in hemolytic disease of the newborn characterized by severe fetal anemia, generalized fetal edema, and hemolysis.

Pathophysiology

Rhesus system consists of following antigens such as D, C, c, E, and e, of which D is most common; presence of D antigen signifies Rh positivity and absence of D antigen produces Rh negativity. Most common causes of sensitization of Rh-negative mother are:

A. Previous pregnancy
B. Previous Rh-positive blood transfusion
C. Abortion
D. Amniocentesis
E. Medical termination of pregnancy
F. Ruptured ectopic pregnancy
G. Accidental hemorrhage
H. Abdominal trauma
I. Lower segment cesarean section

During pregnancy, the most common cause of Rh isoimmunization is fetomaternal hemorrhage during separation of placenta at the time of delivery. It will induce primary immune response and develop IgM antibodies, which will not cross placenta leading to development of sensitization during labor. But, in next and subsequent pregnancies when mother is exposed to Rh-positive blood, slight fetomaternal leak will lead to development of IgG anti-D antibodies that cross the placenta and bind to Rh-positive RBCs of the fetus. This coated RBC will be phagocytized by macrophages in the spleen leading to fetal anemia, which stimulates EPO resulting in firstly, bone marrow erythroid hyperplasia, secondly, erythroblastosis in the peripheral blood, and thirdly, extramedullary hematopoiesis in spleen and liver. Hepatomegaly with development of portal hypertension and hypoalbuminemia leads to development of pleural effusion, pericardial effusion, and ascites. As a result, there is increased serum bilirubin in fetal blood, which crossed the placenta and metabolized by the liver in mother. After birth, unconjugated bilirubin concentration will be increased due to immature glucuronyl transferase enzyme, which crosses the blood–brain barrier to reach basal ganglia producing kernicterus.

Following factors influence the sensitization:

A. Amount of fetomaternal hemorrhage: Larger the amount of hemorrhage, risk of sensitization will be better.

B. ABO incompatibility between fetus and mother: It will reduce the risk of Rh D sensitization because ABO incompatible fetal RBC after entering into maternal circulation will be coated with maternal anti-A and anti-B antibodies and removed by maternal macrophages prior to Rh D sensitization.

Status of zygosity of father:

A. If father is homozygous for Rh D (DD), then all his offsprings will be Rh positive

B. If father is heterozygous for Rh D (Dd), then 50% of offsprings are Rh positive

Management

A. In case of Rh-negative mother having paternal ABO blood group, Rh status has to be determined. If the father is Rh positive, zygosity has to be determined.

B. In case of positivity of the partner, screening of maternal antibody should be performed at 28th week—if it is negative, anti-D immunoglobulin has to be administered. Though the mode of action of Rh immunoglobulin is not known, but Rh immunoglobulin will coat the fetal RBC, this coated RBC when enters the maternal circulation will block the immune recognition thus, preventing hemolysis. This antibody is prepared from pooled plasma of donor with high level of antibodies. To prevent hemolytic disease of the newborn, it has to be administered in the following ways:

- **a.** After delivery: In case of Rh-negative woman who delivers Rh-positive infant, Rh immunoglobulin should be administered at a dose of 300 μg as intramuscular injection. It can neutralize 15 mL of fetal blood cells, which is equivalent to 30 mL of whole blood. In case of increased fetomaternal leak after 1–2 hours of delivery, maternal blood sample has to be tested to determine the amount of fetal RBC by acid elution test.
- **b.** During antenatal period in case of Rh-negative women, 300 μg Rh immunoglobulin have to be given intramuscularly at 28–34 weeks of gestation. If infant is Rh positive, Rh immunoglobulin has to be administered following delivery.
- **c.** Any sensitizing events during pregnancy: If any sensitizing event such as amniocentesis, abortion, cordocentesis, ectopic pregnancy, and multiple pregnancy will occur in Rh-negative woman:
  1. Rh immunoglobulin can be given at a dose of 50 μg intramuscularly before 20 weeks' gestation
  2. 100 μg Rh immunoglobulin can be given after 20 weeks' gestation

C. In case of Rh-negative woman with positive antibody screen: In Rh-sensitized gravida, maternal antibody titer should be measured and has to be evaluated at 16–18 weeks' gestation followed by every 2–4 weeks. If the antibody titer is <1:16, the risk of hydrops increases and risk will also increase of mortality.

Treatment of the Fetus

If the optical density is 450, it indicates severely affected fetus. In this case, treatment is governed by lecithin: sphingomyelin ratio, i.e., 2:1.

A. If the ratio is >2:1—prompt delivery is indicated.

B. If the ratio is <2:1—intrauterine fetal transfusion of Rh-negative packed RBCs of <5 days old has to be given by intravascular or intraperitoneal route. Leukocyte-irradiated poor blood should be given to prevent following:

- **a.** Development of alloantibodies against platelets and leukocytes
- **b.** Cytomegalovirus infection
- **c.** Graft-versus-host disease

Transfusion should be given at every 2–4 weeks. Then, prompt delivery is done at 36 weeks.

Treatment of the Neonates

Exchange transfusion: If the unconjugated bilirubin is increased, it cannot be metabolized in the liver due to immaturity of the enzyme. The result is the development of kernicterus and it is more likely in following conditions:

A. Acidosis
B. Hypoxia
C. Sepsis
D. Hypoproteinemia
E. Hypoglycemia

Exchange transfusion can remove:

A. IgG anti-D antibodies
B. Antibody-coated RBCs
C. Correct anemia

In this method, small amount of blood is withdrawn from patient's blood and it will be replaced by equal amount of donor blood of <5 days old at a rate of 2–3 mL/kg/min. Here, donor RBC should be cross-matched with mother's serum because alloantibodies present in the serum of neonates are usually derived from mother's serum.

A. If ABO blood group of both baby and mother are equal, then Rh negative same group of blood has to be given.
B. If ABO blood group of both baby and mother are different, then group O Rh-negative blood is used.

Indications of exchange transfusion:

A. If cord blood hemoglobin concentration is <12 g%
B. If the cord blood bilirubin concentration is >5 mg/dL
C. Rate of rise of unconjugated bilirubin is >0.5 mg/dL/h

Adjunctive Therapy

A. Phototherapy by fluorescent light in the 420–475 nm converts unconjugated bilirubin to soluble form followed by excretion through urine and bile.
B. Albumin infusion as it binds bilirubin in the plasma, thus reducing the risk of kernicterus.

Q54. Current strategies of platelet transfusion.

GMC/2016/MDII (15)

ANSWER

There is recent revolution in the platelet transfusion to treat thrombocytopenia in hematological or nonhematological malignancies receiving chemotherapy. There are three modalities of platelet transfusion.

Role of ABO Incompatibility and Platelet Transfusion: ABO Incompatible Platelet Transfusion

A. Affects the efficacy of transfusion
B. Produces adverse consequences to the recipients

Platelet expresses ABO antigen, but not Rh antigen on cell surface. ABH antigen on the cell surface is the combination of endogenously synthesized intrinsic molecules and adsorbed soluble antigen present in plasma and extrinsic molecules. These A and B determinants are present on platelet glycoproteins and additional ABH antigen is expressed on platelet membrane glycolipids. ABH expression varies from individual to individual as it depends upon serum glycosyltransferase activity and population of platelets. The effectiveness of platelet transfusion depends upon the type of ABO incompatibility of donor and recipient:

a. When donor platelets expressing ABO system are transfused in the recipients containing anti-A and anti-B antibodies in their plasma, major ABO incompatibility occurs. For example, platelet from group A donor is transfused into the recipient containing group O.
b. When donor plasma containing anti-A and anti-B antibodies is transfused into the recipient containing A and B antigen on the RBCs and platelets, minor ABO incompatibility occurs. For example, group O platelets are transfused into the group A or group B recipients.

A. Transfusion of ABO identical platelet concentrates: Indications of ABO identical platelet transfusion—

a. Higher posttransfusion increment
b. Reduction of RBC transfusion requirements
c. Improved outcome in case of any surgical patient

Problems of ABO identical platelet transfusion:

a. Limited availability of ABO identical platelet during urgent need
b. Limited life span of these ABO identical platelets of only 5 days

B. Transfusion of platelets with major ABO incompatibility:

Disadvantages:

a. Lower rate of increment of posttransfusion corrected count at 4 and 24 hours when compared with ABO identical platelet concentrates.

b. Frequent transfusion as compared to ABO identical platelets.

c. There is accelerated destruction of platelets in recipients.

d. Development of alloantibodies such as anti-HLA and antibodies to antihuman platelet antigen.

Outcomes:

a. It is equally effective in controlling major bleeding as compared to ABO identical and minor ABO incompatible recipients.

b. It has no impact on the time of onset of bleeding, i.e., the WHO grade 2 bleeding post-transfusion.

C. Transfusion of platelets with minor ABO incompatibility:

Adverse effects:

a. Development of hemolytic transfusion reaction in the recipients. This is slightly higher with the use of single donor's platelets containing four to eight times plasma as compared to random donor platelets.

b. Poorer platelet increments.

Now "high titer" anti-A and anti-B plasma containing platelets is transfused to "group O" recipients and "nonhigh titer" anti-A and anti-B plasma containing platelets is transfused to "nongroup O" patients.

In this method of transfusion, ABH antigen and ABH glycosylated complexes of recipients combine and inactivate the transfused anti-A and anti-B antibodies and these are harmful to the recipient.

Nowadays, to overcome the ABO barrier during platelet transfusion, following practices are considered:

a. To detect high titer of antibodies screening of platelet donor

b. Washing and resuspension of platelets in the saline

c. Manufacture of instruments, which can validate automated anti-A and anti-B screening

d. Plasma volume of group O apheresis platelet concentrates is to be reduced to 50 mL

e. Replacement of plasma by additive solution or AB plasma after washing

So, following approaches are practiced in case of platelet transfusion:

a. ABO identical platelet is to be transfused, whenever possible

b. Transfusion of these platelets to high-risk patients after proper evaluation

c. Alternatively, random donor platelet concentrates in minor ABO incompatibility cases containing less volume of plasma than single donor platelets

d. Single donor platelet from A2 donor—it is considered as universal platelet donor

Role of Rh D Incompatibility in Case of Platelet Transfusion

Platelet concentrate contains contaminating RBC having Rh D that may produce alloimmunization when transfused into Rh D-negative patient. Though the risk is low, but its clinical impact in women in childbearing age is present as it may be responsible for hemolytic disease of the newborn. Following factors play a protective role in preventing anti-D alloimmunization:

A. ABO incompatibility: It occurs due to destruction of RBC prior to recognition of Rh D antigen by the recipient

B. Patient's immunosuppression

C. Leukoreduction

Nowadays, Rh D-positive platelets are transfused to Rh D-negative patients. Rh D-positive platelet concentrates can be given to Rh-positive patient and women in childbearing age with injection of 125–300 mg Rh immunoglobulin intramuscularly to prevent alloimmunization, but it will not affect the transfused platelets.

Role of HLA in Platelet Transfusion

Platelet expresses HLA class I antigen A, B, and C on their surface, but not HLA class II antigen. Expression of HLA-A and -B is stronger than HLA-C. Platelet synthesizes class I antigen endogenously and mostly contains heavy chain. Most of the HLA molecules on platelet surface are denatured and capable to be detached from the surface during storage. HLA antigen of the donor is recognized directly or indirectly by recipient's immune system. Directly, donor's antigen presenting cells that express HLA class II can be recognized by recipient's T cells. Indirectly, HLA class I antigen of donor can be recognized by antigen presenting cells of the recipient, which is followed by phagocytosis and pinocytosis by splenic macrophages and dendritic cells leading to activation of T cells.

Role of HLA Antigen in Refractoriness of Platelet Transfusion

Platelet refractoriness is characterized by following transfusion of platelets failure to achieve the acceptable increase in platelet count at least in two occasions. It should be measured after 1 hour of transfusion. Corrected count increment (CCI) of 5,500–7,000 or above can be accepted as adequate response. Both immunologic and nonimmunologic mechanisms are responsible for refractoriness. Nonimmunologic mechanisms include:

- **A.** Fever
- **B.** Splenomegaly
- **C.** Disseminated intravascular coagulation
- **D.** Drugs such as amphotericin B

Immunologic mechanism includes recipient's antibodies.

- **A.** Most of the patients with platelet transfusion refractoriness are sensitized with HLA antigens
- **B.** HPA antibodies
- **C.** ABO antibodies

Two processes of platelet transfusion can be implemented in case of platelet refractoriness due to HLA alloimmunization:

- **A.** Transfusion of cross-matched platelets
- **B.** Transfusion of HLA-matched platelets
- **C.** Transfusion of ABO compatible platelets in high doses
- **D.** Administration of Rh immunoglobulin
- **E.** Plasmapheresis

Q55. Targeted therapy in cancer.

BF/OCT2011/MDI (9)

ERA/NOV2012(S)/MDIII (15)

MUHS/NOV2010/MDIII (10)

Cancer chemotherapy.

Maharashtra UNI of Health SC, Vijayawada, 2020 (10)

Explain the role of immune check point inhibitors in the treatment of advanced malignancies. Discuss the mechanism, clinical applications, and challenges associated with this therapy.

WBUHS, 2025 (10)

ANSWER

Definition

Targeted therapy can be defined as the group of drugs that prevent the cancer spread by blocking their growth as a result of interfering with the specific molecules that are responsible for the growth as well as multiplication of the cancer cells. Molecules may be made up of one or more atoms. On the other hand, biological molecules such as proteins and DNA are made up of thousands of atoms.

Goal of Targeted Therapy

The aim of this therapy is to get rid of the cancer cells leaving the normal cells behind; from that point of view, targeted therapy is superior to chemotherapy and radiation therapy. Specific action of targeted therapy is less harmful to normal cells.

Targets of Targeted Therapy

Targeted therapies act on biomarkers or several pathways, which are responsible for cell proliferation and growth.

Biomarkers can be defined as anatomic, physiologic, biochemical, and molecular parameters that are associated with state of the specific disease. But, all the biomarkers are not the target of the medical therapy. Some proteins are involved in cancer process where some may be the byproduct, but both the proteins can direct which patient will respond and which patient will not to certain treatment. But, in true sense, the drug which is directed against the byproduct cannot treat the cancer whereas the drug which is directed against the target protein involved in cancer process may treat the cancer. One example is overexpression of HER2 protein (epidermal growth factor) in case of breast cancer. Many breast cancer patients have too many copies of *HER2* gene and that will help to produce large amount of HER2 protein and this will help the cell to proliferate very quickly. This protein can be blocked by trastuzumab and prevent cell growth.

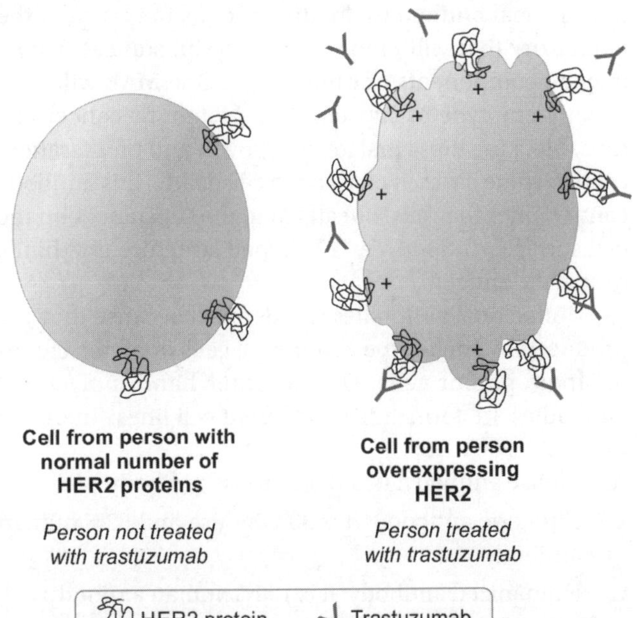

Cell Pathways

It is a chain of events involving many molecules and their interactions, which allow the cells to communicate with one another in their environment. These pathways are sometimes called transduction pathways and sometimes called cell signaling pathways.

A. Cell can release protein-like growth factors and hormones that can alter the behavior of other cells.

B. Some proteins after release bind to the receptor proteins present on the cell surface to make change its shape leading to release of another protein that will react with other cellular components to change them biochemically; as a result, the behavior of the cells will be changed.

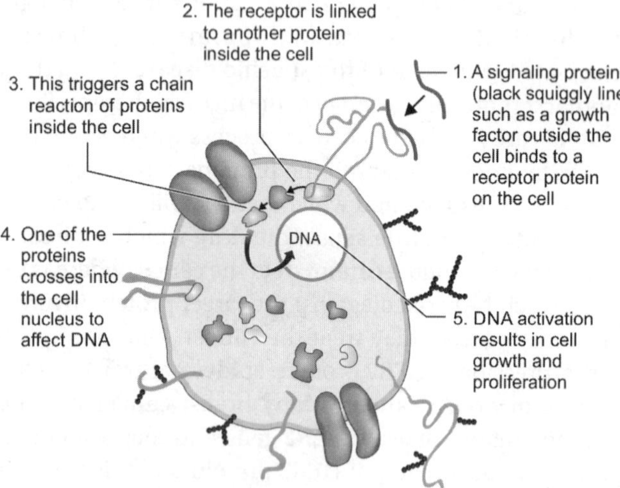

Monoclonal Antibodies

Monoclonal antibodies are the proteins prepared in the laboratory that will bind to the body substances, which may be components of cancer cells. One MAB will bind to only one type of substance or protein or cancer cell thus, blocking the signal for cell growth and proliferation; even in some cases, it can lead to cell death. This antibody cannot enter the cells, but attach to the substances on the cell surface. Antibody is "Y"-shaped structure that binds to specific antigen.

Monoclonal antibodies are identical because they are produced by single type of immune cells or all the clones of single parent cells. On the other hand, polyclonal antibodies are formed from different cell lines. There are three types of MABs:

A. Mouse antibody: It is 100% mouse antibody

B. Chimeric antibody: It is 33% mouse and 67% human antibody

C. Humanized antibody: It is 100% human antibody

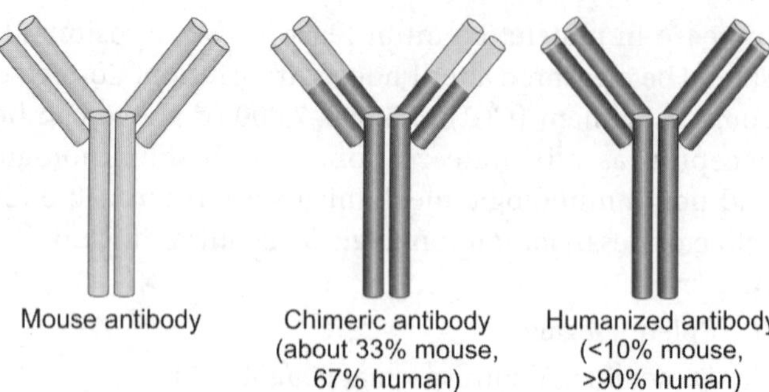

a. All MABs end with—mab

b. Humanized MABs end with—zumab and alemtuzumab

c. Chimeric MAB ends with—ximab and rituximab

d. Mouse MAB ends with—momab

e. Human MAB ends with—mumab

Naked MABs use to work by themselves whereas conjugated MABs act in conjugation with chemotherapeutic drugs or radioactive particles such as:

A. Attached with radioactive particles—ibritumomab

B. Attached with chemotherapeutic drug—brentuximab

Mechanism of Action

A. Direct binding of antibody with antigen on cancer cells: CD20 antibody rituximab and HER2 on breast cancer cells trastuzumab

B. Binding of soluble antigen with antibody prevents growth and survival of tumor cells. For example, siltuximab binds with IL-6 and bevacizumab binds with soluble vascular endothelial growth factor.

C. Toxin delivery into cancer cells: Ado-trastuzumab emtansine carrying microtubule inhibitor DM1 will recognize HER2 and, thus, deliver the inhibitor into HER2-positive cells.

D. Antigen binding with immune cells: After binding, these complexes enhance anticancer immune response. For example, ipilimumab and CTLA4.

E. Bispecific antibodies: These are antibodies type 2 specific. For example, blinatumomab will bind to CD19 receptor present on leukemic cells and CD3 present on T cells directing T cells into the proximity of leukemic cells.

Small Molecule Inhibitors

Kinase is the general term, which is responsible for transfer of phosphate groups from one place to another place within the cell.

Tyrosine kinases are the group of enzymes, which are responsible for transfer of phosphate groups of adenosine triphosphate from important energy molecules within the cell to specific places on the proteins.

Kinase Inhibitors

A. Anaplastic lymphoma kinase (ALK) inhibitors:
- **a.** Alectinib: It inhibits ALK and RET.
- **b.** Ceritinib: It inhibits ALK, insulin like growth factor-1 receptor, insulin receptor (InsR), and ROS1.
- **c.** Crizotinib: It inhibits ALK, hepatocyte growth factor receptor, and RON.

B. BCL2 inhibitors: Overexpression of BCL2 is responsible for CLL. So, drug venetoclax inhibits BCL2, antiapoptotic protein, thus responsible for cellular apoptosis.

C. BCR-ABL inhibitor: It is responsible for CML. Drugs are bosutinib, dasatinib, imatinib, nilotinib, and ponatinib.

D. BRAF and MEK inhibitors: It inhibits reversibly mitogen-activated protein kinase/extracellular signal regulated kinase 1 and 2. Drugs are cobimetinib, dabrafenib, trametinib, and vemurafenib.

E. Bruton's tyrosine kinase inhibitors: It is molecule of B-cell receptor in the signaling pathways. In the BTK active site, it makes a bond with cysteine residue thus, inhibits BTK enzymatic activity. Drug is ibrutinib.

F. Cyclin-dependent kinase 4/6 inhibitors: It prevents cellular proliferation. Drug is palbociclib.

G. Epidermal growth factor receptor inhibitor: Afatinib, erlotinib, and gefitinib.

H. Histone deacetylase inhibitors: It prevents HDAC to catabolize the removal of acetyl groups from lysine residues of histone and nonhistone proteins. Drugs are belinostat and panobinostat.

I. Human epidermal growth factor receptor 2 inhibitors: Lapatinib

J. Janus-associated kinase inhibitors: Ruxolitinib

K. Vascular endothelial growth factor receptor (VEGFR) inhibitor: Axitinib and levatinib

Advantages of Targeted Therapy

A. Therapy is specific to cancer cells leaving the normal cells.

B. It has reduced toxicity and improved tolerability.

C. It has improved efficacy as it shows significant response to cancers.

D. Targeted therapy is based on the genomics of any individual.

E. Combination of multiple targeted therapy can bypass the pathway of resistance.

F. Many drugs are oral, in that case these are very much convenient and compliant to the patient.

G. Some of the targeted agents are capable of crossing the blood brain barrier, in that case they can target the metastatic tumor.

Challenges of Targeted Therapy

A. Due to presence of genetic diversity in a tumor, targeted therapy can treat the tumor partially leaving the residual disease.

B. There may be development of resistance due to following factors:
- **a.** Secondary mutations
- **b.** Bypass pathways
- **c.** Amplification of the alternative signals.

C. Targeted therapy is expensive, so many patient is unable to continue this therapy.

D. All the cancer may not have well defined target.

E. Targeted therapy requires sophisticated investigation that may not be available in the remote areas, so that the patient is unable to select targeted therapy.

In spite of initial efficacy of the targeted therapy, there may be adaptive resistance to this drug leading to progression of the tumor.

Q56. Clinical use of recombinant factor VII.

PGI/NOV2013/MDIII (10)

ANSWER

Introduction

Recently, there is tremendous increase in the use of recombinant factor VII in almost all types of bleeding situations such as traumatic bleed, postoperative bleed, spontaneous cerebral hemorrhage, postpartum hemorrhage, and anticoagulant overdose.

Mechanism of Action

Hemostasis is developed principally on two types of surfaces: One is tissue factor bearing cells and secondly thrombin-activated platelets.

A. Following injury to vessel wall, released tissue factor in the circulation complexes with activated factor VII on the surface of tissue factor containing cells. Here, this complex activates factor X to produce activated factor X, which, in turn, converts prothrombin to thrombin. As a result, limited amount of thrombin is formed, which further activates factors V, VIII, XI, and platelets. These activated platelets change their shape exposing negatively-charged phospholipid, phosphatidylserine and further activate factor X, which results in generation of full thrombin and further activation of factors V, VIII, and XI through positive feedback. This excess thrombin activates thrombin-activatable fibrinolysis inhibitor, thereby preventing premature lysis of fibrin clot by downregulating the fibrinolysis.

B. In absence of tissue factor, activated factor VII binds to activated platelet surface and activates factor X, which, in turn, generates thrombin at the site of injury.

Effect of Clot

Formed clot is strong and complex leading to risk of thromboembolic complications—it is the risk of activated factor VII, but the risk is low.

Activated factor VII is low in presence of decreased level of other factors as well as other cofactors.

Dosage

A. 90 μg/kg of body weight IV bolus dose is recommended, which can be repeated after 2 hours.

B. If the requirement of dosage is more than two in uncomplicated episode of bleeding, then dose interval should be increased to 4 hours for 1–2 days—but it obviously depends upon the size and severity of bleed.

Uses

A. Hemophilia A and B: Treatment with factor VIII/IX leads to produce inhibitor antibodies to these factors. These inhibitor antibodies react with factor VIII/IX rendering these factors replacement ineffective for treating the bleeding episodes. So, here recombinant factor VII acts as "bypassing agent" to activate clotting process.

B. Glanzmann's thrombasthenia: It is autosomal disorder due to defect in GPIIb/IIIa present on the platelet surface resulting in defective binding with fibrinogen. Treatment is recombinant activated factor VII 90 μg/kg intravenously every 2 hours until homeostasis.

C. Factor VII deficiency: Recommended dose is 15–30 μg/kg every 4–6 hours.

D. Emergency bleeding:
   - **a.** Intracranial hemorrhage
   - **b.** Traumatic bleed
   - **c.** Upper gastrointestinal bleeding

E. Oral anticoagulant-induced hemorrhage:
   - **a.** Neurosurgery
   - **b.** Liver resection
   - **c.** Cardiac surgery
   - **d.** Orthotropic liver transplantation

Q57. Oral Janus kinase inhibitors.

MJPRU/2015/MDIV (10)

Oral JAK inhibitors.

DNB 2021 (5)

Discuss how tyrosine kinase inhibitors work? Write briefly about their current uses in treating the diseases.

WBUHS, 2023 (10)

ANSWER

Janus kinase 2 is a tyrosine kinase protein, which is phosphorylated and activated by the receptors of following proteins:

A. Erythropoietin
B. Thrombopoietin
C. Granulocyte colony-stimulating factor
D. Granulocyte-macrophage colony-stimulating factor
E. Interleukin-3

Activated JAK2 starts signaling cascade and in response to growth factor, it initiates proliferation of cells, but mutation of JAK2 by the replacement of valine in place of phenylalanine in exon 14 at 617 position, it starts uncontrollable proliferation of hematopoietic cells in absence of growth factor. This mutation occurs in 95% of polycythemia vera, 50% of essential thrombocythemia or myelofibrosis, and 20% of unclassified myeloproliferative neoplasms. Due to mitotic recombination, this mutation is homozygous. In rare instances, this mutation also occurs in exon 12. Most signaling pathways require more than one JAK, JAK1, JAK3, and Tyk2, but thrombopoietin and EPO require only JAK2.

JAK2 Inhibitors

INCH018424

It is first evaluated for treating primary myelofibrosis and postpolycythemia and essential thrombocythemia myelofibrosis. It is potent JAK1 and JAK2 inhibitors. Its phase III trial is going on.

CEP-701

It is the derivative of indolocarbazole K252. It is staurosporine analog and it is also a JAK2 inhibitor.

XL019

It is a selective and potent inhibitor of JAK2 kinase.

TG101348

It is a selective and potent JAK2 inhibitor.

NS-018

It is in phase I/II trial.

Type 1 Adenosine Triphosphate

It is competitive JAK inhibitor and stabilizes the active conformation of JAKs.

Type 2 inhibitors

They bind as well as stabilize the inactive conformation thus, prevents cycling to its active conformation. It can reverse the persistence of type 1 JAK2 inhibitor and, thus, reduce the burden of mutant allele in murine model than type 1 inhibitor.

JAK2 Inhibitors (Ruxolitinib)

Indications

A. High-risk myelofibrosis:
   a. Postpolycythemia vera myelofibrosis
   b. Primary myelofibrosis
   c. Postessential thrombocythemia myelofibrosis

Mechanism of Action

It inhibits JAK1 and JAK2 signaling, which involves:

A. Recruitment of STAT to cytokine receptors
B. Activation and localization of STATs to the nucleus

The result is modulation of gene transcription.

Pharmacokinetics

It is metabolized in the liver by CYP3A and mostly excreted in feces and partially through the kidney.

Toxicity

A. Thrombocytopenia—it can be tackled by reducing the dose or temporary withdrawal of this drug
B. Anemia
C. Neutropenia
D. Dizziness
E. Headache
F. Occasional symptoms: Anorexia, herpes zoster, and weight gain
G. Rare symptoms: Hypercholesterolemia and raised liver enzymes

Q58. Hypomethylating agents in hematological malignancies.

GMC/2015/MDIV (10)

ANSWER

Altered methylation of DNA by DNA methyltransferase (DNMT) by addition of methyl group through covalent bond at the C5 position of cytosine to form 5-methyltyrosine through promoter or enhancer of DNA methylation activates oncogenes and inactivates tumor suppressor genes leading to modification of cancer cells. There are three DNMTs: DNMT1 methylates hemimethylated DNA and DNMT3A and DNMT3B methylate unmethylated DNA. So, hypomethylation of DNA in malignancies converts the tumor cells to behave like normal cells through different pathways. The drugs responsible for hypomethylation of DNA are nucleoside analogs such as azacitidine and decitabine. These inhibitors make covalent bonds with DNMTs, which lead to degradation of DNMT and hypomethylation during cell cycling. The difference between these drugs is that decitabine incorporates into DNA whereas azacitidine incorporates into both DNA and RNA at low doses. As in high dose, these drugs prevent DNA synthesis and proliferation of DNA, so incorporation of these drugs is not possible as it requires methylation step.

Chemical names	Drugs	Mechanism of action	Drug status
5-azacytidine	Azacitidine	Analog of cytosine	Treatment of MDS
5-aza-2′-deoxycytidine	Decitabine	Analog of cytosine	Treatment of MDS
SGI-110	Guadecitabine	Analog of cytosine	AML—phase III trial
5-fluro-2′-deoxycytidine	FdCyd	Analog of cytosine	Refractory solid tumor—phase II clinical trial
Zebularine		Analog of cytosine	Preclinical trial
CP-4200		Analog of cytosine	Preclinical trial
RG108		Inhibitor of small molecule	Preclinical trial
Nanaomycin A		Inhibitor of small molecule	Preclinical trial

Indications of Treatment

A. High-risk disease to prevent AML evolution or cytopenias, which is severe enough or nonresponsive to supportive care.

Four cycles of drugs should be given prior to assessment of response. Treatment should be continued as long as the clinical benefit continues or till the transplantation is planned.

Resistance

A. Primary resistance:
   a. There is threefold increased risk in case of high ratio of cytosine deaminase: Deoxycytidine kinase
   b. Instability of DNMT inhibitors as both the drugs are rapidly cleared from the circulation.

B. Secondary resistance: It occurs due to mutation in deoxycytidine.

Toxicity

A. Myelosuppression

B. Increased risk of infection

Dose

A. Azacytidine: 75 mg/m^2 intravenously 1–7 days in 28 days cycle.

B. Decitabine: 20 mg/m^2 intravenously over 1 hour × 5 days in 28 days cycle.

Novel Hypomethylating Agent

A. Zebularine: It incorporates into DNA to form reversible complex with DNMT and, thus, methylation.

B. RG108 will bind to catalytic site of DNMT1, which leads to reactivation of tumor suppressor genes such as P16, SFRP1, and TIMP3.

C. CP-4200: It allows azacytidine to enter into the cell without the help of nucleoside transporters.

D. Nanaomycin A: It is selective for DNMT3B.

E. SG110 (guadecitabine): In this, decitabine is linked to deoxyguanosine making it more stable to degradation.

Q59. Blood component therapy with special emphasis on feature of artificial oxygen carrier.

MUHS/MAY2010/MDIV (25)

MGR/SEP2006/MDIV (5)

Artificial blood.

BF/JUN2016/MDIV (10)

Blood component therapy.

NTR UNI of Health SC, Vijayawada, Andhra, 2022 (10)

ANSWER

Blood has two components: Plasma that carries waste nutrients and hormones and formed elements are cells and cellular parts flowing in the plasma. Cells are platelets responsible for forming clot, WBCs responsible for immunity, and RBCs responsible for carrying oxygen and carbon dioxide. Red cell is biconcave disk without any nucleus, so it has large surface area for accommodating oxygen and can permeate through the minute capillaries. It also accommodates nearly 280 million hemoglobin molecules. In case of severe blood loss, most important part of treatment is to maintain the life by providing oxygen and this can be only possible by RBC through blood transfusion. But, there are some challenges, which make it difficult to get blood in proper time. These are:

A. Human blood has to be kept in cool place and shelf-life is 42 days. So, it is impractical to carry it in ambulances into the battlefield.

B. Gradual increase of recipients as compared to donors.

C. Proper cross-matching of the blood is mandatory prior to transfusion.

D. Different deadly viruses can be transmitted through the blood in spite of minute screening

Artificial component of blood neither replaces the lost blood volume and different components such as WBCs and platelets nor work like blood but can carry oxygen where the patient's own red cells are not able to carry sufficient oxygen and, hence, this artificial blood is also known as oxygen therapeutic. It will deliver sufficient oxygen to the body till bone marrow starts regenerating the red cells. Artificial blood can be generated by:

A. Synthetic production

B. Chemical isolation

C. Recombinant biotechnology

Platelet Transfusion

A. Platelet transfusion threshold in case of bleeding patients:
   a. Less than 50,000/cc with severe bleeding and DIC
   b. Less than 30,000/cc platelet if the bleeding is not life threatening or severe.

 c. Less than 100,000/cc platelet for the bleeding in the context of multiple trauma or intracranial bleeding.

B. Prophylactic transfusion threshold if a specific procedure is undertaken to prevent spontaneous bleeding.

C. Prophylactic administration under specific conditions:

 a. Acute promyelocytic anemia
 b. Cardiac surgery with perioperative bleeding
 c. Inherited or acquired platelet disorders in presence of bleeding

Current blood substitutes are:

A. Hemoglobin-based oxygen carrier (HBOC)—it actually uses hemoglobin, RBC component. Pure hemoglobin separated from the RBC cannot be used as it may produce nephrotoxicity. So, various steps are used to produce hemoglobin more safe and useful and these are:

 a. Cross-linking
 b. Polymerization
 c. Encapsulation

 These processes are necessary because RBC is not simple container of hemoglobin but rather complex entity having many biochemical characteristics.

B. Perfluorocarbons (PFCs)—it is based solely on synthetic chemical processes. It is most common. It is completely man-made, hence:

 a. It has advantage over blood substitute such as HBOC that relies on modified hemoglobin
 b. Unlimited manufacturing capabilities
 c. It has ability to be heat sterilized
 d. It is more efficient in delivery of oxygen and removal of carbon dioxide from the tissues
 e. It acts as intravascular oxygen carrier, so that it augments delivery of oxygen
 f. It can be cleared from the bloodstream within 48 hours. It is 40–50 times smaller than hemoglobin and carries several times more oxygen per cc

Composition of PFCs:

A. Perfluorooctyl bromide—28%
B. FO-9982—12%
C. Yolk lecithin—2.4%
D. DSPE-50H—0.12%
E. Distilled water—57.48%

In Japan, first PEBOC, fluosol-DA, is produced by mixture of perfluorodecalin and perfluorotripropylamine along with egg yolk, phospholipids, and Pluronic® F-68 as emulsifying agents. It is able to deliver only 0.4 mL of oxygen per 100 mL. More recently, PFC is developed, which can carry 1.4 mL of oxygen per 100 mL, but 100 mL of normal blood can deliver 5 mL of oxygen.

Advantages of PFCs emulsion are:

A. It will not react with oxygen
B. It can transport oxygen easily to the body
C. It will increase the solubility of oxygen in the plasma
D. It will minimize the effect of temperature and pH in the circulation

Disadvantages of PFCs are:

A. It can produce flu-like symptoms in the body, which may be caused by phagocytosis of PFCs by body's immune system.
B. It is unable to remain mixed as aqueous phase hence, they are produced as emulsions prior to use.
C. Platelet count will be decreased.
D. This product cannot be used by human body hence, it has to be discarded within 18–24 months.
E. As it will absorb oxygen passively hence, the patient is asked to breathe in a linear rate so that proper oxygenation of the tissues will be ensured.
F. It will support the life temporarily, so that the patient in the meantime will regenerate own RBC or will be transfused with RBC.

Hemoglobin-based oxygen carrier: It uses purified animal, human, or recombinant hemoglobin as oxygen carrier.

Advantages of HBOC:

A. Blood transfusion can be avoided in case of surgical or medical conditions with hemoglobin deficiency
B. It can available in large volume
C. It can be stored for prolonged period
D. It can be rapidly administered without typing and cross-matching
E. It can be sterilized by pasteurization

Disadvantages of HBOC:

A. It has reduced circulation half-life
B. Hemodynamic and gastrointestinal perturbations
C. It induces free radical in the body

Real characteristics of artificial blood:

A. It can be used very safely
B. It is fully compatible in human body
C. In case of requirement, it can transport as well as release oxygen in the human body

D. It can be stored for longer duration

E. It is devoid of toxin and pathogen, which can induce immune response in the body

Uses of artificial blood components:

A. As the medical and surgical conditions are increased annually, the requirement of blood is also increased.

B. In the battlefield, rapid and urgent transfusion can be provided by artificial blood component only without any reaction and it does not require blood grouping and cross-matching.

C. In different countries such as South Africa and Nigeria worldwide, there is increased incidence of HIV infection through blood transfusion, so disease-free source of transfusion, i.e., artificial blood is incredibly beneficial in these regions.

D. Though cost of cross-matched blood is low but as the manufacturing becomes refined, cost of the blood component will fall.

E. It has a shelf-life of 1–3 years as compared to donated blood whose shelf-life is 42 days hence, artificial blood can be stored for longer period.

F. In case of any refusal of patients for cultural or religious regions, synthetic oxygen carrier is the right alternative substitute.

G. This substitute will provide full capacity of oxygen transport immediately as compared to donated blood, which takes 24 hours to reach full oxygen transport capacity due to depletion of 2,3-diphosphoglycerate (2,3-DPG). Again, replenishment of lost blood cells requires months. Hence, until replenishment, oxygen carrying substitute can perform this function.

Q60. Discuss the pathophysiology, hematological clinical manifestations, and management of myelodysplastic syndrome (MDS).

MGR/SEP2007/MDIV (20)

Discuss the pathophysiology, hematological, clinical manifestations, and management of myelodysplastic syndrome.

MGR UNI, Tamil Nadu, 2022 (10)

Discuss etiopathogenesis, clinical features, diagnosis, and current guideline on management of MDS.

Veer Narmad South Gujarat UNI, 2021 (20)

ANSWER

Definition

It is group of premalignant conditions affecting hematopoietic stem cells resulting in dysplastic hematopoietic changes and ineffective erythropoiesis. In absence of inciting agents producing secondary myelodysplasia, MDS can be diagnosed. Following factors are responsible for secondary myelodysplasia:

A. Growth factor therapy

B. Viral infection

C. Exposure to toxins and drugs

D. Congenital disorders

E. Immunologic disorders

F. Vitamin deficiencies

G. Supplementation of excessive zinc

H. Deficiency of copper

Classifications

A. According to the FAB classification of MDS mainly based on morphological and dysplastic changes in at least two lineage of cell lines:

- **a.** Refractory anemia: <5% marrow blast
- **b.** Refractory anemia with ring sideroblast: <5% blast + >15% ring sideroblasts
- **c.** Refractory anemia with excess blasts: 5–20% marrow blasts
- **d.** Refractory anemia with excess blasts in transformation: 21–30% marrow blasts
- **e.** Chronic myelomonocytic leukemia: ≤20% marrow blasts + Peripheral blood monocytosis > 1,000/μL
- **f.** Acute myeloid leukemia: >30% marrow blasts

B. The WHO guideline revised the FAB classification and cytogenetic data is eliminated.

- **a.** In AML, marrow blasts should be lowered from 30 to 20%.
- **b.** The category of refractory anemia with excess blasts in transformation is eliminated.

Clinical Features

A. Age > 65 years and the incidence will be increased along with increasing age.

B. Males are affected more than females.

C. Symptoms are nonspecific according to decreased formation of cell lines.

D. Physical findings are usually normal.

Laboratory Diagnosis

Dyshematopoiesis: It is characterized by cytopenias plus normocellular or hypercellular marrow. Components of features are as follows:

A. Dyserythropoiesis:

- **a.** Peripheral blood: Anemia, reticulocytopenia, poikilocytosis, anisocytosis, basophilic stippling, macrocytosis, and dimorphic anemia, i.e., normocytic normochromic or microcytic hypochromic anemia.
- **b.** Bone marrow: Erythroid hyperplasia or erythroid hypoplasia, ring sideroblast, and megaloblastoid maturation characterized by nuclear fragments, multinucleation, karyorrhexis, or vacuolar cytoplasm.
- **c.** Other assays:
  1. Expression of CD55 and CD59 on granulocytes and erythrocytes is decreased—PNH
  2. Periodic acid-Schiff-positive cytochemistry
  3. Fetal hemoglobin levels are increased

B. Dysgranulocytopoiesis:

- **a.** Peripheral blood: (1) Neutropenia, (2) Neutrophil granules are abnormal or decreased, and (3) Neutrophil hyposegmentation or hypersegmentation or bizarre nuclei.
- **b.** Bone marrow demonstrates: (1) Hyperplasia of granulocytes, (2) Presence of decreased granules in neutrophil precursors, and (3) Increased blast cells.
- **c.** Other assays: (1) Neutrophil ALP is decreased and (2) Myeloperoxidase activity is decreased.

C. Dysmegakaryopoiesis:

- **a.** Peripheral blood demonstrates: (1) Thrombocytopenia and (2) Large platelet with decreased granular cytoplasm.
- **b.** Bone marrow demonstrates decreased: (1) Megakaryocytes and micromegakaryocytes and (2) Megakaryocytes containing large single nuclei or small, multiple separated nuclei.

Genetic Abnormalities

A. In presence of cytopenias with proper clinical presentation of MDS, dysmorphological features in bone marrow following cytogenetic abnormalities confirm MDS:

- **a.** Unbalanced abnormalities: (1) –7 or del(7q), (2) –5 or del(5q), and (3) I(17q) or t(17p).
- **b.** Balanced abnormalities: t(11;16)(q23;p13.3), t(3;21)(q26.2;q22.1), etc.

B. Following cytogenetic abnormalities can diagnose AML with any blood count: t(8;21)(q22;q22).

C. 5q- syndrome: It occurs predominantly in females, low risk of AML transformation, and favorable diagnosis.

Molecular Genetics

Most frequently mutated genes are *SF3B1*, *TET2*, *ASX1*, *SRSF1*, and *RUNX1*. These are involved in epigenesist.

Prognosis

A. Life expectancy: Several months to 10 years. It depends upon:

- **a.** Cytogenetics
- **b.** Age
- **c.** Cytopenias
- **d.** Initial presentation

Revised International Scoring System is following:

Items	0	0.5	1.0	1.5	2	3	4
Karyotype	Very good		Good		Intermediate	Poor	Very poor
Blasts (%)	≥2		>2 to <5		5–10	>10	
Hemoglobin (g/dL)	≥10		8 to <10	<8			
Platelet (K/μL)	≥100	50 to <100	<50				
Absolute neutrophil count (K/μL)	≥0.8	<0.8					

Management

It is based on the following:

A. Patient's age

B. Status of performance

C. Revised International Prognostic Scoring System (IPSS-R) status

Supportive Care

A. Transfusion of RBCs and platelets. In case of low-risk cases, only supportive care may be needed.

B. Erythropoietin: It will increase hemoglobin level in 15% of patients and it occurs within 2–3 months. High dose of EPO up to 40,000–60,000 units can be given. Response is likely in following cases:

- **a.** Presence of ring sideroblasts
- **b.** Serum EPO level <500 mU/mL

C. Combination of EPO plus G-CSF in the dose of 1 mg/kg/dL. It can be given in following conditions:

- **a.** It will increase response rate in case of anemia
- **b.** It increases erythropoietic activity where the patient will fail to respond to EPO alone

Remittive Therapies

A. DNA Hypomethylating agents: Azacitidine—it is given in low and intermediate risk of MDS

- **a.** It will improve blood cell count
- **b.** It will eliminate transfusion requirement
- **c.** It will improve both survival
- **d.** It will improve quality of life

B. Lenalidomide: It will be given in low and intermediate risk of MDS and deletion of 5q. It will result in:

- **a.** Decrease in transfusion requirement
- **b.** Improve anemia
- **c.** Improve cytogenetics
- **d.** Increased survival

C. Immunosuppressive drugs: It is indicated in:

- **a.** Low marrow cellularity
- **b.** Absence of blast cells

Curative Therapy

Complete resolution of MDS can be achieved by: induction chemotherapy plus HSCT. But, it depends upon the risk category of the disease.

Q61. Oncogenes.

MUHS/NOV2010/MDI (10)

Cancer genetics.

MGR/SEP2008/MDI (5)

ANSWER

Cancer is the uncontrollable proliferation of organ-specific cell in the body that ultimately leads to development of cancer, which is responsible for >12% of death worldwide. It is caused by different factors such as environment, diet, lifestyle, and genetic factors, but most important is stress. So, normal cell growth is the resultant of balance growth promoting and balance growth restraining signals.

Tumor is caused by alteration in any one of oncogenes, tumor suppressor genes and microRNA genes. Nearly, among 50,000–100,000 genomes, approximately 100 proto-oncogenes, and number of dozens of tumor suppressor genes have been identified; these genes are responsible for cell proliferation and differentiation, cell growth, apoptosis, genomic integrity, and morphologic reactions.

Tumor Suppressor Genes

These are antioncogene, which control cell proliferation by inhibiting effectively in cell growth cycling and its loss or inactivation will lead to cancer. Following are the tumor suppressor genes:

A. *TP53*: Breast, brain, and colorectal cancer

B. *APC*: Adenomatous polyposis coli

C. *BRCA1 and BRCA2*: Familial breast/ovarian cancer

D. *RB1*: Retinoblastoma

E. *NF1*: Neurofibromatosis 1

F. *WT1*: Wilms tumor

p53 acts by driving the cells containing their damaged DNA along the apoptotic pathway. Apoptotic regulators present in the downstream of p53 genes such as *BAX* and *BCL2* are critically responsible for it. Proto-oncogene BCL2 belongs to a big family some of which such as BCL2, BCLXL, BCLW, and MCL1 suppresse apoptosis whereas BAX, BAK, bad, etc., antagonizes the antiapoptotic properties of others.

MicroRNA

It is noncoding RNAs and it is also known as micro-managers of gene expression. It will not encode the proteins. It can anneal to messenger RNA whose nucleotide sequence complements the sequence of microRNA by blocking transcription and translation of proteins and, thereby, regulating gene expression. For example, microRNA-15a and microRNA-16a are involved in CLL. The region of gene responsible for rearrangement of chromosome in cancer cells harbors microRNA. By microRNA microarrays, a large number of microRNAs have been identified as biomarkers of cancer.

Oncogenes

It is a eukaryotic gene coding for protein that fulfills the essential physiological function of any normal cell in normal environment, but has a potentiality to become oncogenic determinant when triggered by any inciting factor. It was first discovered from avian sarcoma virus known as src and gene is called as v-oncogene or v-onc. Normal nononcogenic allele of such genes is known as proto-oncogenes; these are active in normal cells hence, active genes and mutant alleles as active oncogenes. Active oncogene means activation of oncogenic function. These oncogenes may be viral genes when it is inserted into cell by a virus or cellular genes. Their expression ultimately leads to neoplasm.

Virus after entering the cells starts replication and produces oncogenes, which promote cancer. Following some viruses are associated with tumor:

Viruses	Tumors
Epstein–Barr virus	Nasopharyngeal cancer
Hepatitis B virus	Liver
DNA viruses	Burkitt's lymphoma
Papillomaviruses	Cervical cancer and benign wart
HIV-1 virus	Kaposi's sarcoma
HTLV-1	Adult T-cell leukemia
HTLV-2	Hairy cell leukemia
HTLV-5	Cutaneous T-cell leukemia

Following methods are used for identification of oncogenes:

A. Amplification: MYCN and MYCL
B. Chromosomal translocation: ABL, BCL1, and BCL2
C. Homology to retroviruses: HRAS, and KRAS
D. Insertional mutagenesis: EV1 and INT1
E. Transfection assay: MAS, MET, RAS, and TRK

Following means of proto-oncogene activation to form tumor:

A. RNA virus by: Retroviral transduction, enhancer insertion, and transactivation.
B. DNA virus by: Altering activity and expression of host genes through interaction of protein-to-protein.
C. Nonviral by: Amplification, point mutation, and translocation of chromosomes.

Products of oncogenes: Proto-oncogenes encourage cell division and their growth. Four classes of oncoprotein for cell division are encoded by proto-oncogenes. These are the following:

A. Growth factors: These are:
  - **a.** Platelet-derived growth factor
  - **b.** Epidermal growth factor
  - **c.** Insulin-like growth factor 1 and 2
  - **d.** Transforming growth factor-α and -β
  - **e.** Fibroblast growth factor 1-7

B. Growth factor receptor:
  - **a.** Epidermal growth factor family of receptors such as erbB2, erbB3, and erbB4
  - **b.** Platelet-derived growth factor receptor (PDGFR)
  - **c.** Angiotensin receptors

  These are the examples of second-class oncoproteins.

C. Signal transducers: There are two groups of these proteins:
  - **a.** Nonreceptor protein kinases: These are of two types:
    - **1.** Tyrosine kinases: ABL and SRC
    - **2.** Serine and threonine kinases: AKT, MOS, and RAF1
  - **b.** Guanosine triphosphate-binding proteins:
    - **1.** Guanine nucleotide-binding proteins include: RAS, GAP, and GIP
    - **2.** Membrane associated/cytoplasmic tyrosine kinase: ABL and SRC

  Many of the above receptors utilize common signaling pathways. Though there are many intracellular or transduction pathways, but three important pathways are recognized and these are:
    - **1.** PI3 kinase/AKT pathway
    - **2.** RAS/mitogen-activated protein kinase pathway
    - **3.** JAK/STAT

D. Nuclear transcription factors: Transcription factor, being activated by signaling from cytoplasmic signaling molecules, binds with DNA followed by transcription of downstream gene. These transcription factor oncogenes are mutated and overexpressed in cancer. For example, c-myc, proto-oncogenes from chickenpox virus, is translocated to IgG found in B cells in BL resulting in tremendous overexpression of c-myc leading to tumorigenesis.

Sometimes, transcription factors belong to member of multigene families having common structural domains. For example, Fos transcription protein after dimerizing with Jun transcription protein will form AP1 transcription factor and is responsible for overexpression of several oncogenes controlling cell division. Some transcription factors act in the nucleus such as myc, fos, jun, and myb. These factors sometimes upon activation by phosphorylation bind with DNA and start transcription.

Oncogenes act as target: With the advancement of tumor biology, tumor-related genes are isolated and expressed in nontumor cells in vitro to detect its motility, invasion, anchorage, and independent growth—these are the hallmarks of transformed cells. Few cancer-related oncogenes in human being with mode of activation are following:

ABL	CML	Translocation
BCL-2	Follicular B-cell lymphoma	Translocation
l-myc	Lung cancer	Amplification
Ras H	Thyroid cancer	Point mutation
Ras K	Pancreas, colon, and lung cancer	Point mutation
Ras N	AML and ALL	Point mutation

Cancer Therapeutics Through Oncogenes

Modern screening methods of gene analysis evolved a large number of potential molecular targets in cancer. Due to advancement in this study, newer agents are frequently coming up.

Drugs	Oncogenes	Related cancers
Cetuximab	EGFR	Colorectal
Imatinib	ABL, KIT, and PDGFR	CML and gastrointestinal tumor (GIST)
Gefitinib	EGFR	Nonsmall cell lung cancer
Sorafinib	FLT3, VEGFR, and PDGFR	Renal cell carcinoma
Trastuzumab	HER	Breast

Q62. Acanthocytosis.

MUHS/NOV2014/MDIII (10)

ANSWER

Definition

Acantha, a Greek word, means thorn. Spur cell means dense sphenoidal cell containing varying sizes of spiculations distributed all over the cell surface. Cells are contracted, irregular and dense, and irreversibly changed due to alteration of its cell membrane lipid content. As these cells are destroyed by the spleen hence, in case of splenectomy, few numbers of spur cells are present in the circulation.

Diseases Associated with Acanthocytes

Following conditions are associated with acanthocytosis:

A. Alcoholic liver disease
B. Abetalipoproteinemia
C. Infantile pyknocytosis
D. McLeod syndrome
E. Hypothyroidism
F. Anorexia nervosa
G. Lu(null) Lutheran phenotype
H. Idiopathic neonatal hepatitis
I. Zieve syndrome

Echinocyte or Burr cells have uniformly distributed multiple small projections on the red cell surface.

Pathophysiology

Normal ratio of cholesterol to phospholipid is 1:1 in red cell membrane. But, as the proportion of cholesterol increases, surface area also increases leading to formation of flattened cells known as "target cells" in the peripheral blood smear. In case of advanced cirrhosis, abnormal high-density lipoprotein containing large amount of free cholesterol is produced by the liver, which binds to red cell membrane and acts as lipid trap.

These free cholesterol will accumulate in the RBC outer cell membrane that alters the normal cholesterol to phospholipid ratio. As the amount of membrane increases, excess membrane part will be transformed into tiny projections.

Cholesterol damages Na^+/K^+ pump leading to cellular wall deformity. Spleen starts remodeling of these cells that ultimately produces subpopulation of small acanthocytes. As these cells are not further deformable, hence it will be trapped and destroyed.

Clinical Features

A. Features of etiology
B. Chronic diarrhea with foul-smelling stool
C. Loss of appetite with vomiting
D. Neurological features such as ataxia and visual abnormalities
E. Abdominal pain and pallor
F. Dark urine and recurrent infection
G. Orolingual dyskinesia

Workup

A. Complete blood count:
   - **a.** Normocytic normochromic anemia
   - **b.** Elevated reticulocyte count

B. Plasma lipid:
   - **a.** Cholesterol in abetalipoproteinemia <50 mg/dL
   - **b.** Plasma phospholipid level—low
   - **c.** Very low-density lipoprotein (VLDL), apolipoprotein B, and chylomicron—low

d. Plasma triglyceride level < 10 mg/dL
e. Plasma sphingomyelin—high at the expense of lecithin

Treatment

A. Treatment of underlying condition.
B. Dietary restriction:
   a. Restriction of long-chain fatty acids
   b. Medium-chain triglyceride—judicious supplementation
   c. Supplementation of fat-soluble vitamins

Q63. Transfusion hemosiderosis.

MGR/MAY2011/MDII (7)

ANSWER

Normally, there is balance of absorption of iron from small intestine and loss of iron through sweat, stool, menstruation, and shedding in hair and skin. One unit of transfused blood contains 250 mg of iron.

Pathophysiology

In β-thalassemia intermedia due to increased erythropoietic drive, there is deficiency of hepcidin leading to increased absorption of dietary iron in the body and iron overload. In thalassemia major, blood transfusion decreases erythropoietic drive but increases iron overload, which leads to increased hepcidin level. On the contrary, increased hepcidin level decreases absorption of iron from the intestine, retains iron in the macrophages, and increases iron load in the body due to inability of excreting iron in the transfused RBC. After oversaturation of transferrin in transfusion-induced iron overload, excess iron will be circulated as free nontransferrin bound iron, which is taken up by liver, skin, heart, and endocrine organ. In excess iron states, there will be damage of the tissues.

Clinical Features

In case of transfusion-related iron overload, following information are required:

A. Duration of transfusion dependence
B. Yearly number of transfusion
C. History of chelation

Organ-related symptoms are the following:

A. Cardia:
   a. Breathlessness
   b. Paroxysmal nocturnal dyspnea
   c. Orthopnea
   d. Pedal edema
B. Gastrointestinal:
   a. Abdominal pain
   b. Hematemesis with or without melena
   c. Encephalopathy
C. Endocrine manifestations:
   a. Delayed puberty
   b. Delayed growth
   c. Delayed menarche
   d. Decreased libido
   e. Diabetes mellitus

Organ-related signs:

A. Skin:
   a. Bronzing of the skin
   b. Cachexia
   c. Dwarfism
   d. Bruising
   e. Delayed secondary sexual hair growth
   f. Delayed breast development
B. Cardiac signs:
   a. Pedal edema
   b. S3 gallop
   c. Engorged neck vein
   d. Pleural effusion
C. Pulmonary findings:
   a. Loud pulmonary second sound
   b. Basal crepitations
D. Gastrointestinal signs:
   a. Hepatosplenomegaly
   b. Ascites
   c. Umbilical hernia
   d. Caput medusa
E. Neurological findings:
   a. Encephalopathy
   b. Asterixis

Laboratory Findings

A. Biochemical tests:
   a. Serum iron level is increased
   b. Serum ferritin level is increased
   c. Serum total iron-binding capacity is decreased
   d. Transferrin saturation of >50% suggests iron overload
   e. Hepcidin level in serum and urine may be a feasible marker of iron overload

f. Liver enzymes are increased

g. Glycated hemoglobin (HbA1c) and serum glucose will be increased

B. CT scan:

a. Increased density in liver with raised serum ferritin suggests iron overload

b. Superconducting quantum interference device magnetic liver and spleen iron measurement

c. MRI of the liver, spleen, endocrine organ, and joints to measure the deposition of iron

C. Hepatic iron content:

a. Stage 1: Mild < 7 mg/g of dry weight

b. Stage 2: Moderate 7–15 mg/g of dry weight

c. Stage 3: >15 mg/g of dry weight

Treatment

A. Chelation therapy:

a. It will prevent iron accumulation in the organ

b. It helps in excretion of iron from the organ and also from the body

c. Indications:

1. Serum ferritin level > 1,000–1,500 µg/L
2. Liver iron store level > 3–5 mg/g
3. Recipient having transfusion of >2 years

d. Drugs are:

1. Deferoxamine
2. Deferiprone
3. Deferasirox

Q64. Implication of G6PD in clinical practice.
MGR/APR2012/MDII (7)

ANSWER

Introduction and Classification

It is the most common variant of red cell enzymopathy in human being. There are two types of mutations in this enzymopathy.

A. Polymorphic mutations—it occurs in high malaria-endemic areas. It includes:

a. G6PD A—common in Africa and half-life of RBC is 13 days.

b. G6PD Mediterranean—common in India, Middle East, and Mediterranean countries. Half-life of RBC is only several hours.

B. Sporadic mutations—it may occur in any part of the world.

Glucose-6-phosphate dehydrogenase variants associated with G6PD deficiency are:

A. G6PD A

B. G6PD Mediterranean

Glucose-6-phosphate dehydrogenase variants with normal enzyme activity are G6PD B. Life span of RBC is 60 days.

In India, common G6PD variants are:

A. G6PD Mediterranean

B. G6PD Kerala-Kalyan

C. G6PD Orissa

Enzymatic activity decreases with aging of the red cells, so highest activity is found in young RBC and in older RBC lowest activity is found. Due to instability of the enzyme in older RBC, this is more pronounced.

Pathogenesis

A. Glucose-6-phosphate dehydrogenase catalyzes the oxidation of glucose-6-phosphate to glucose-6-phosphogluconate with the formation of NADPH from NADP, so only source of NADPH is G6PD-dependent hexose monophosphate (HMP) shunt.

B. This HMP shunt also produces ribose, essential component of DNA and RNA.

C. Due to presence of NADPH, reduced glutathione converts hydrogen peroxide to water by glutathione peroxidase enzyme. In G6PD deficiency, sufficient glutathione will not be available.

Accumulated hydrogen peroxide oxidize the free SH groups of hemoglobin leading to denaturation and precipitation of globin chains forming Heinz bodies bound to red cell membrane. RBC membrane becomes rigid and trapped by the reticuloendothelial system in the spleen. Heinz bodies are removed by splenic macrophages with resultant loss of RBC membrane that leads to spherocytes formation. These spherocytes are sequestered in the spleen and subsequently phagocytized by splenic macrophages.

In addition to extravascular hemolysis, intravascular destruction of RBC occurs due to peroxidation of membrane lipids.

Relation of Glucose-6-phosphate Dehydrogenase with Malaria

In certain parts of the world, G6PD deficiency is responsible for protection against *Plasmodium falciparum* malaria limited to female heterozygotes. There are two populations of female heterozygotes: G6PD B with normal enzyme and G6PD A with deficient enzyme—it occurs during embryogenesis due to random inactivation of chromosomes.

Parasite growth is inhibited in this deficient RBC but after four to five cycles, malarial parasite can adapt this deficiency by synthesizing its own G6PD enzyme. Hence, in homozygous male, parasite can grow after few cycles but in heterozygous female, parasites invade G6PD-deficient or -normal cells during successive cycles. So, each time, malarial parasite has to adapt to synthesize its own enzyme and it takes time hence, the result is eventual decrease in parasitemia and, thus, severe form of the disease.

Clinical Features

Due to exposure to oxidant stress or infection, there is sudden development of pallor, jaundice, and dark urine due to hemoglobinuria leading to hypotension and acute renal failure in severe cases.

In class III, variant hemolysis is mild-to-moderate and self-limited in spite of taking the offending drugs.

In class II, variant hemolysis is severe and may require blood transfusion.

In class I, variant chronic hemolysis develops in infancy, hepatosplenomegaly, and jaundice and no relation with oxidant drug or infection.

Laboratory Features

Peripheral smear demonstrates: Polychromasia, fragmented RBC, spherocytes, bite cells, half-ghost cells, and Heinz bodies.

Biochemical features demonstrate: Unconjugated hyperbilirubinemia, hemoglobinemia, hemoglobinuria, and absence of haptoglobin.

Q65. Neuroblastoma.

MGR/SEP2010/MDIV (6)

ANSWER

Epidemiology

It is most common congenital tumor occurring 40% in the first year of life, but rarely occurs above 14 years of age. Family clustering has been reported.

Sites

A. Most common site is adrenal gland in 40% of cases presenting as abdominal mass.
B. Involvement of posterior sympathetic ganglion cells presenting as both intrathoracic and intra-abdominal masses known as Dumbbell tumor producing spinal cord compression.

Spread

This disease can present as widespread metastases. Most common metastatic sites are:

A. Bone
B. Bone marrow
C. Liver
D. Lymph nodes
E. Skin

Histology

This tumor closely resembles embryonic sympathetic ganglia. This tumor differentiates into following types:

A. Rosettes
B. Pseudoresettes
C. Mature ganglion cells
D. Immature chromaffin cells

Most primitive histologic type of neuroblastoma is formed by:

A. Small round cells
B. Scanty cytoplasm

Ganglioneuroma is composed of:

A. More mature and larger ganglion cells
B. Abundant cytoplasm

Poor prognosis in neuroblastoma is suggested by:

A. Homogeneously staining regions
B. Double minute chromosomes

Both represent amplified N-myc segments as amplification of this segment is the intrinsic property of poor prognosis tumor. It can be detected by FISH concordant with Southern Blot analysis.

Clinical Features

A. Distended abdomen with abdominal pain
B. Bone pain
C. Constitutional symptoms: Anorexia, malaise, and fever
D. Diarrhea
E. Raccoon eyes—rare
F. Physical signs:
   1. Hepatomegaly
   2. Orbital mass
   3. Subcutaneous nodule mainly in infancy
   4. Intra-abdominal mas
   5. Features of Horner syndrome
   6. Ecchymosis
   7. Hypertension

Laboratory Diagnosis

A. Complete blood count
B. Serum biochemistry for LFT, renal function test, serum cortisol, ACTH, nd aldosterone
C. Urine for homovanillic acid (HVA), VMA, and total catecholamine
D. Bone scan
E. PET-CT of abdomen
F. Bone marrow trephine biopsy for detection of tumor cells
G. Examination of tumor by FISH method to detect *N-myc* gene
H. ^{131}I-metaiodobenzylguanidine—it is specific for neuroblastoma and pheochromocytoma

Prognostic Factors

A. Age: Congenital tumor has highest favorable prognosis even in presence of widespread metastasis as this tumor will spontaneously regresses without treatment. But, as the age of the patient is >1 year, prognosis will be worse.
B. Stage:
   a. For stage I and II—survival rate is >80%
   b. Stage IV—survival rate is <40%
   c. Stage IVS—>90% survival rate
   d. Stage III and IV with presence of amplification of N-myc gene—prognosis is worse
C. Urinary VMA: HVA ratio of <1.5 is present—it produces doubt for this diagnosis, as it is a reflection of indirect measurement of dopamine hydroxylase.

Management

A. Surgery:
   a. Localized disease can be managed by surgical resection.
   b. Metastatic disease—biopsy of primary tumor for detection of *N-myc* gene. After chemotherapy, complete resection can be performed.
B. Radiotherapy: It is done for debulking combined with chemotherapy.
C. Chemotherapy:
   a. For residual localized or advanced disease—multimodal chemotherapy with cyclophosphamide, etoposide, doxorubicin, vincristine, and topotecan plus surgical resection and bone marrow transplantation—it will improve the survival in case of stage III and IV disease.
   b. Congenital tumor: Chemotherapy is not used in asymptomatic patient.
D. Autologous HSCT: In combination with chemotherapy and radiotherapy, it will improve the advanced disease when treated in conjunction with posttransplant 13-cis-retinoic acid.
E. Dinutuximab: It is chimeric GD2 antibody—approved for high-risk neuroblastoma already got partial response to prior chemotherapy regimen.

Q66. Hamartoma.

MGR/SEP2008/MDIII (6)

ANSWER

Definition

It is a noncancerous tumor-like malformation composed of abnormal mixture of cells and tissues present in the growing areas of body. Examples of hamartoma are:
A. Large bowel polyp
B. Bronchial hamartoma
C. Hemangioma as well as other vascular tumors
D. Melanocytic nevi
E. Neuroepithelial cells in tuberous sclerosis

It usually not causes any problem but in following factors may impose problems in the body:
A. Infection
B. Infarction
C. Obstruction
D. Direct or indirect pressure
E. Hemorrhage within the hamartoma
F. Neoplastic transformation
G. Fracture

Classification

Hamartoma can be classified into following four types:
A. Bone forming tumor:
   a. Osteopoikilosis: It is found in small bone of hands and feet and ends of the long bone of feet.
   b. Melorheostosis: It is progressive in linear fashion and cross open epiphyseal plate or joint.
   c. Bone Island: It occurs in ribs, pelvis, humerus, and femur.
B. Cartilage forming tumor:
   a. Osteochondroma: Sessile or pedunculated large masses, surface smooth, or lobulated.

b. Enchondromatosis: It arises from remnants of epiphyseal cartilage and slowly grows.
c. Multiple osteochondroma: It usually terminates at puberty with the epiphyseal plate fusion.

C. Fiber forming tumor:
a. Fibrous dysplasia
b. Nonossifying fibroma

D. Benign nonmatrix forming tumor:
a. Hemangioma of bone
b. Skeletal hemangiomatosis

Etiology

A. Osteopoikilosis: Autosomal dominant trait
B. Osteochondroma: There is abnormality in long arm of chromosome number 8
C. Multiple osteochondroma: Autosomal pattern of inheritance
D. Fibrous dysplasia: It is monostotic and asymptomatic

Clinical Presentations

A. Dull aching pain and swelling or palpable mass—in case of bony hamartoma.
B. Cartilage-forming tumor—palpable mass, pathological fracture, pain, spinal cord compression, venous thrombosis, pseudoaneurysm formation, sometimes unequal length of limbs, and varus or valgus deformity.
C. Fibrous tumor—patient complaints of pain, tenderness, swelling, and deformity
D. Benign nonmatrix-forming tumor—patients complaint of nerve compression, spinal cord compression, collapse of vertebral body, or completely asymptomatic.

Laboratory Workup

A. Blood tests: CBC, renal function tests, and LFT
B. Radiological investigation of bones
C. Histological investigations of hamartoma

Treatment

Surgical therapy.

Q67. Febrile thrombocytopenia.

GMC/2015/MDIII (10)

Approach to a case of fever and thrombocytopenia.

DNB 2019 (10)

ANSWER

According to recent criteria, fever can be defined as:
A. AM temperature if >98.9°F
B. PM temperature if >99.9°F

Variation in daily temperature is 0.5°F.

Thrombocytopenia can be defined as platelet count <150,000/cc. It occurs due to following causes:
A. Decreased production
B. Accelerated destruction
C. Abnormal distribution
D. Artifactual thrombocytopenia

Grade of Thrombocytopenia

A. Mild thrombocytopenia: When platelet count is between 60,000/cc and 150,000/cc
B. Moderate thrombocytopenia: When platelet count is between 20,000/cc and <60,000/cc
C. Severe thrombocytopenia: When platelet count is <20,000/cc

Common Causes of Thrombocytopenia

A. Infections:
a. Dengue
b. Malaria
c. Rickettsia
d. Enteric fever
e. Sepsis
f. Human immunodeficiency virus
g. Leptospirosis
h. Miliary tuberculosis

B. Inflammatory causes:
a. Collagen vascular diseases

C. Malignancy
D. Undifferentiated febrile thrombocytopenia

Clinical Features

A. Features of thrombocytopenia may be present—it will not depend upon the platelet count. It is characterized by bleeding under the subcutaneous tissue and submucosal area as evidenced by ecchymoses, bruises, and intracranial or gastrointestinal bleeding.
B. Features of different infections:
a. In dengue hypotension, fluid is present in different serosal areas of the body.
b. In case of typhoid fever, specific features are different types of temperature—in first week

remittent fever, second week continuous fever, rose spots in the body, relative bradycardia, splenomegaly, and hepatomegaly.

c. In typhus fever, eschar is present in the lower abdomen and high fever.

d. In malaria, typical pattern of fever, hepatosplenomegaly, tachycardia, and anemia are present.

e. In HIV infection, lymphadenopathy and fungal infection in the different mucosal areas and in case of associated HCV infection, evidence of cirrhosis, splenomegaly, and other opportunistic infections may be present.

f. In case of miliary tuberculosis, features will depend on site or organ involvement.

C. In case of inflammatory causes:

a. History of joint pain, lymphadenopathy, skin rash, hematuria, and cough.

b. Physical signs are deforming arthritis, skin rash, lymphadenopathy, and crackles in lung.

D. In case of malignancy, clinical features depend upon the organ involvement and infections.

Laboratory Investigations

A. Hematological test:

a. Leukopenia—dengue, typhus fever, collagen vascular disease, sepsis, and HIV

b. Leukocytosis—malignant disease and sepsis

c. Lymphocytosis—typhoid fever and miliary tuberculosis

d. Erythrocyte sedimentation rate—raised

B. Serum biochemistry:

a. Urea and creatinine—raised in sepsis and dengue shock syndrome

b. Liver function test—deranged in all infectious diseases and collagen diseases

C. Serology:

a. NS1 antigen, IgM dengue, and leptospira IgM

b. Antinuclear antibody (ANA)-HEp-2 and dsDNA/extended collagen vascular disease panel

c. CD4 count decreased—HIV

d. Blood for cartridge-based nucleic acid amplification test (CBNAAT)—tuberculosis

e. Widal test—typhoid

D. Blood culture—typhoid fever

Treatment

A. Treatment of the cause.

B. Platelet transfusion:

a. If platelet count <20,000/cc—platelet transfusion

b. If platelet count >20,000/cc with bleeding—platelet transfusion

c. Any platelet count of <100,000/cc with evidence of bleeding—transfusion

Q68. Discuss in detail the manifestations and management of oncological emergencies.

MGR/FEB2005/MDIII (15)

MGR/MAR2008/MDIV (20)

Oncological emergencies.

MGR UNI, Tamil Nadu, 2022 (10)

Oncologic emergencies.

NTR UNI of Health SC, Vijayawada, 2021 (10)

Discuss regarding oncologic emergencies management.

WBUHS, 2024 (10)

ANSWER

Introduction

Oncologic emergency is very common but some are so subtle that it is overlooked commonly and ultimately it will lead to morbidity and some are very ominous and will lead to mortality, if not treated timely.

Febrile Neutropenia

Nearly 80% of patients who are receiving chemotherapy for hematologic malignancy will develop fever related to neutropenia. Fever increases with duration and severity of neutropenia. Febrile neutropenia can be defined as single axillary or oral temperature of ≥101.3°F or ≥100.4°F sustained for >60 minutes in patient with absolute neutrophil count of <500/cc. Neutropenia is of four types:

1. *Mild*: Absolute neutrophil count 1,000–1,500/cc
2. *Moderate*: Absolute neutrophil count 500–999/cc
3. *Severe*: Absolute neutrophil count 100–499/cc
4. *Profound*: Absolute neutrophil count <100/cc

About 20–35% of fever is due to documented infections from:

A. Gut (*E. coli* and *Enterobacter*)

B. Skin (*Staphylococcus* and *Streptococcus*)

C. Respiratory tract (*Streptococcus*)

Clinical Features

Clinical features are fever with chills, diarrhea, rash, nausea with or without vomiting, dyspnea, and cough. Thorough physical examination should be done to determine the site of involvement.

Treatment

Prior to provide treatment, one well-known scoring tool (MASCC) can be followed:

Characteristics	Points
Burden of febrile neutropenia with or without mild symptoms	5
No hypotension, i.e., systolic blood pressure of >90 mm Hg	5
No evidence of chronic obstructive pulmonary disease	4
Solid tumor or hematologic malignancy with no previous fungal infection	4
Absence of dehydration, which requires parenteral fluid	3
Burden of febrile neutropenia with moderate symptoms	3
Outpatient status	3
Age > 60 years	2

If score is ≥21—these low-risk patients can be treated and monitored for at least 4 hours in emergency department and prior to discharge, cultures from all the sites should be taken. Drugs are 750 mg ciprofloxacin twice daily along with amoxicillin/clavulanate 500/125 mg 8 hourly. Patient may take fluoroquinolone therapy alternatively.

If score is <21—they should be admitted as high-risk group for IV empiric antibiotic followed by definite antibiotics after getting the culture sensitivity report of any secretion. Common antibiotics for use are meropenem, cefepime, imipenem-cilastatin, zosyn, and ceftazidime. In case of gram-positive infection, additionally vancomycin should be started. Defervescence of fever is expected 2–5 days after treatment and urine output should be maintained to >0.5 mL/kg/h.

If the patient remains febrile but hemodynamically stable, re-evaluation of absolute neutrophil count is essential.

A. If the count rises, antibiotic should be continued.

B. If the count will not rise, CT scan of lung and sinuses is considered. At the same time, antifungal treatment should be considered.

Tumor Lysis Syndrome

It is a syndrome characterized by serious metabolic disturbances resulting from imbalance between accumulations of intracellular contents into the bloodstream as a result of lysis of malignant cells and capacity of the kidney to clear these contents containing uric acid, potassium, and phosphate. So, the resultant accumulation of nucleic acid produces hyperuricemia. This accumulated uric acid will crystallize leading to obstruction of renal tubules. There may be associated hyperphosphatemia and hyperkalemia and secondary hypocalcemia. Constellation of these electrolyte abnormalities will ultimately produce lactic acidosis, acute renal failure, and death.

Clinical Features

Symptoms will be started 12–72 hours after initiation of chemotherapy.

A. In hyperkalemia, weakness, paresthesia, cramps, nausea with or without vomiting, diarrhea are present.

B. Hyperuricemia may lead to renal failure as evidenced by fluid overload and decreased urine output.

C. Hypocalcemia can lead to muscle twitches, carpopedal spasm, changes in mental status, seizures, and paresthesia.

Following Cairo–Bishop criteria are usually preferred for this diagnosis.

Two or more of the following criteria either 3 days prior or 7 days after chemotherapy:

A. Uric acid ≥ 8 mg/dL or 25% increase from the baseline

B. Potassium ≥ 6 mEq/L or >25% increase from the baseline

C. Phosphorus ≥ 6.5 mg/dL for children or ≥4.5 mg/dL for adult or 25% increase from the baseline

D. Calcium ≤ 7 mg/dL or 25% decrease from the baseline

Clinical tumor lysis syndrome: It includes laboratory TLS + one or more of the following:

A. Creatinine > 1.5 times of the upper limit of age-adjusted reference range

B. Cardiac dysrhythmia or sudden death

C. Seizures

Treatment

Hyperkalemia

A. Asymptomatic or mild (5–<6 mmol/L):

- **a.** Limitation intake of potassium
- **b.** Electrocardiogram
- **c.** Sodium polystyrene sulfonate 15–30 g orally

B. Moderate (>6–7 mmol/L):
  a. Above treatment
  b. Regular insulin 10 units IV + 100 mL 50% dextrose IV
C. Severe (>7 mmol/L):
  a. Above treatment
  b. Calcium gluconate 10% 10 mL slowly intravenously
  c. Sodium bicarbonate 45–50 mEq slowly intravenously over 5–10 minutes
  d. Albuterol 10–20 mL in 4 mL of saline nebulized over 20 minutes

Hypocalcemia

A. Asymptomatic patient: No treatment is required.
B. Symptomatic patients:
  a. Correction of hyperphosphatemia
  b. 10% 10 mL calcium gluconate slowly intravenously over 10 minutes

Hyperphosphatemia

A. Moderate cases:
  a. Limitation of intake of phosphate
  b. Administration of phosphate binders such as calcium acetate, calcium carbonate, aluminum hydroxide, sevelamer, and lanthanum carbonate
B. Severe cases: Hemodialysis

Hyperuricemia (>8 mg/dL)

A. In low-risk cases:
  a. Intravenous normal saline 150–200 cc/h ± Allopurinol 100 mg thrice daily orally
B. Intermediate-risk cases:
  a. Intravenous normal saline 150–200 mL/h
  b. Allopurinol 100 mg thrice daily
  c. Rasburicase 0.15 mg/kg intravenously for 5–7 days
C. High-risk cases:
  a. Above treatment
  b. Hemodialysis

Increased Intracranial Pressure

There are three compartments in brain and these are:
A. Brain parenchyma: Volume 1.4 L
B. Spinal fluid: Volume 52–160 mL
C. Blood: Volume 150 mL

Increase in any of the three compartments will occur in expense of other two as per Monro-Kellie hypothesis. But, if there is continuous rise in pressure, it will lead to decrease in intracranial compliance compromising cerebral perfusion. Normal intracranial pressure (ICP) is 5-15 mm Hg. Imbalance between CSF production and CSF reabsorption will lead to raised ICP.

Clinical Features

It depends upon the underlying cause and rapidity of obstruction.
A. Slow progressive increase in ICP is associated with mild or no symptom.
B. Dynamic changes may be associated with rapid progression producing headache, which can be relieved by vomiting.

Cushing response will explain body's response to increased ICP:
A. Rise in systolic pressure, widening of pulse pressure, and bradycardia with irregular breathing
B. Without treatment, there is tachycardia, rapid shallow breathing with period of apnea, and decrease in blood pressure
C. If there is no treatment, there will be herniation of brain leading to cardiac or respiratory arrest.

Fundoscopic examination reveals:
A. Absence of venous pulsation in the optic disk center—early findings
B. Papilledema with blurred disk margin and small hemorrhage—late findings

In case of chronic pressure elevation, patient may present with cognitive decline, ataxic gait, and urinary incontinence.

Treatment

Aim is to reduce the ICP. It can be done in following ways:
A. Elevation of head by 30°
B. Febrile antipyretics
C. Osmotic diuresis:
  a. 20% mannitol 0.75–1 g/kg intravenously in bolus followed by 0.25–0.5 g/kg 6 hourly.
  b. Dexamethasone 6–10 mg every 6 hourly up to 100 mg/day to reduce vasogenic edema. But, it should be avoided in case of CNS lymphoma as steroid induces lymphocytic apoptosis thus, obscuring diagnosis.
  c. Rapid and transient method of decreasing ICP is mechanical ventilation.

Spinal Cord Compression

It occurs in 5–10% of breast, prostate, MM, lung, and lymphoma patients through hematogenous seedling in vertebral bodies or direct extension. Colon and prostate cancer produces lumbosacral vertebral metastasis and lung breast cancer in thoracic spine.

Clinical Features

A. Most common presentation is back pain that worsens in recumbent position with maximal intensity in early morning.

B. Cervical spine—headache, pain in shoulder or neck, breathing difficulties, paresis of upper extremities, and sensory loss.

C. Thoracic spine—pain in chest, sensory loss below the level of tumor, bladder and/or bowel abnormalities, positive Babinski sign, and sexual dysfunction.

Physical examination: Tender percussion on spinal column, detection of sensory and motor deficit, straight leg rising sign, and assessment of sphincter tone.

Diagnosis

A. MRI of the spine

B. CT myelography

Treatment

Aim of treatment:

A. Reduction of pain

B. Recovery from neurological disability

C. Prevention of further complication for further growth of tumor

Loading dose of dexamethasone is 10 mg intravenously followed by 4 mg 6 hourly. It reduces swelling around the spinal cord thus, preventing further damage. Further therapy can be guided by following criteria:

A. Clinical picture

B. Availability of histological diagnosis

C. Instability of spinal cord—it requires surgery even in spite of any symptom

D. Previous treatment

Radiation therapy: It can be given to asymptomatic patient or poor candidate of surgery. In case of radiosensitive tumor such as breast, prostate, myeloma, and lymphoma, dose is 3,000–4,000 cGy in 5–10 fractions. In case of palliative treatment, one fraction of 8 Gy is useful.

Systemic chemotherapy can be given in case of small cell carcinoma, Hodgkin and NHL, and breast and prostate cancer.

Superior Vena Cava Syndrome

It is characterized by impairment of venous drainage from upper extremities, head and neck, and upper thorax as a result of occlusion of blood vessels obstructing the blood flow due to external compression by tumor or internal compression by invasion of tumor or fibrosis or thrombus in the vascular lumen. Secondary effect is decreased due to venous return to heart that leads to decreased cardiac output and increased venous congestion of face, head, neck, and upper extremities.

Clinical Features

Clinical features are dyspnea, swelling of face, head, and neck, upper extremities, cough, and pain in chest, occasionally dysphagia.

Treatment

A. Symptomatic treatments are:

- **a.** Moist oxygen inhalation
- **b.** Administration of diuretics
- **c.** Elevation of head end of the bed by 45°
- **d.** Administration of steroids

B. After completion of histological diagnosis, treatment should be tailored by disease.

- **a.** In case of small cell lung carcinoma, chemotherapy with radiotherapy
- **b.** In case of nonsmall cell lung carcinoma, same treatment but with less improvement
- **c.** No treatment modality is superior in case of NHL

C. In case of palliative and urgent intervention:

- **a.** Direct opening of the occluded vessels by endovascular stenting
- **b.** Angioplasty
- **c.** Thrombolysis

D. If early detection of this complication: Fibrinolytic therapy

Q69. Hematopoietic growth factors.
MGR/FEB2005/MDIII (5)

ANSWER

Cellular component of blood, RBC, WBC, and platelets arises from pluripotent or totipotent germ cells called "germ cells" as they have an ability to differentiate to any number of pathways any time to produce mature blood cells. A number of cytokines are present in the microenvironment of pluripotent germ cells, which are responsible for development and differentiation of stem cells in different pathways and produce required number of matured cells. Growth factors are responsible for this hematopoiesis, as they play important following roles:

A. Immunosuppressive drugs can be administered at higher dose
B. Increases the ability of the body to resist infection
C. It will alleviate anemia that reduces the need for RBC transfusion
D. After stem cell transfusion, it will increase the cell counts
E. It will increase the ability to collect stem cells for transfusion

Following are the hematopoietic factors:

A. Granulocyte colony-stimulating factors:
- **a.** It will act primarily on the neutrophil component of the blood to fight against bacteria.
- **b.** Mechanism of action:
  1. It will stimulate granulocyte colonies
  2. It will differentiate progenitor cells toward lineage of neutrophil
  3. It will help in neutrophil maturation
- **c.** Indications:
  1. Chemotherapy-induced neutropenia
  2. Collection of stem cells for transplantation
  3. Transplantation of bone marrow or peripheral stem cells
  4. Congenital neutropenia
  5. Cyclic neutropenia
  6. Idiopathic neutropenia
- **d.** Routes of administration: It can be administered intravenously or subcutaneously.
- **e.** Dose: 5–10 μg/day.
- **f.** Timing of administration: 24 hours prior or after administration of chemotherapy. It should be continued until the neutrophil count rises to >500/cc.
- **g.** Side effects:
  1. Bone pain due to expansion of cell population in the marrow
  2. Fever
  3. Hyperuricemia
  4. Skin rash
  5. Severe reactions:
     - Anaphylaxis
     - Capillary leak syndrome
     - Diffuse alveolar hemorrhage

B. Granulocyte-monocyte colony-stimulating factors:
- **a.** It will stimulate monocytes, neutrophil, and eosinophil colonies.
- **b.** Mechanism of action:
  1. It will increase the number of neutrophils, eosinophils, and monocytes
  2. It will also improve the function of above cells
- **c.** Dose: It is available in USA as sargramostim. Dose is 250–500 μg/m^2.
- **d.** Indications:
  1. Chemotherapy-induced neutropenia
  2. Collection of stem cells for transplantation
  3. Transplantation of bone marrow or peripheral stem cells
- **e.** Side effects are same as that of G-CSF, but here the side effects are more severe due to its effect on inflammatory cytokines.

C. Erythropoietin:
- **a.** It will stimulate stem cells to produce RBCs.
- **b.** Its onset of action is after 7–14 days after administration.
- **c.** Routes of administration: It can be administered intramuscularly, intravenously, or subcutaneously.
- **d.** Prior to administration, serum iron should be estimated to satisfy that adequate iron is present in the body to cope up with increasing hemoglobin production.
- **e.** Indications are anemia due to following causes:
  1. Chronic renal failure
  2. Anemia in premature neonates
  3. Acquired immunodeficiency syndrome
  4. Chemotherapy
  5. Rheumatoid arthritis
  6. To reduce the need of blood transfusion in patients undergoing surgery
- **f.** Dose is 50–150 U/kg/week subcutaneously, but it can be increased up to 300 U/kg/week. Hematocrit level has to be reached to 33–36% and then its dose can be reduced.
- **g.** Side effects:
  1. Headache
  2. Hypertension
  3. Thrombocytosis with occlusion of venous fistula

D. Oprelvekin:

a. It is a recombinant interleukin-11.

b. Mechanism of action:

1. It stimulates megakaryocyte progenitor cells
2. It also helps in maturation of megakaryocytes

c. Indications of administration:

1. It will prevent severe thrombocytopenia
2. It will reduce the need for platelet transfusion following chemotherapy

d. Dose: To start with 50 µg/kg subcutaneously daily within 6–24 hours of chemotherapy.

e. Duration: For up to 21 days after chemotherapy. But, it should be discontinued 2 days prior to administration of chemotherapeutic drugs.

f. Side effects:

1. Most serious side effects are due to increase in plasma volume.
   - Cardiac arrhythmias
   - Dyspnea
   - Nausea
   - Edema

g. Antibodies to this drug have been demonstrated.

Future Applications of Growth factors

A. Gene therapy

B. Expansion of stem cell products from bone marrow, peripheral blood, and liver

C. Alteration of cytokine response to different immunologic events such as infection and rejection of organs.

Q70. Thrombotic thrombocytopenic purpura.

RGUHS/MDIII (10)

What clinical features will make you suspect that a patient is suffering from thrombotic thrombocytopenic purpura? Briefly outline the pathogenesis.

WBUHS, 2023 (10)

ANSWER

Definition

Thrombotic thrombocytopenic purpura, thrombotic microangiopathies, is characterized by features of hemolytic anemia and thrombocytopenia, fever, neurogenic abnormalities, and renal failure resulting from platelet-rich thrombi formation in the arterial and capillary microvascular compartments.

Classification

A. Congenital TTP

B. Acquired or classical TTP

Epidemiology

Its incidence is 3–4/100,000 population with female preponderance. It may occur at increased rate in case of pregnancy and in postpartum period. In case of pregnancy, mean age of onset is 23.5 weeks.

Pathophysiology

Following factors are responsible for platelet aggregation directly or indirectly with or without endothelial damage, which ultimately leads to formation of platelet-rich thrombi in the microvasculature in different organs producing ischemia of those organs:

A. Drugs: These drugs either produce endothelial injury or procoagulatory effect on platelets.

a. Cyclosporine

b. Mitomycin C

c. Quinine

d. Bleomycin

B. Toxins

C. Cytokines

D. Pregnancy

E. Deficient function of VWF cleaving protease called ADAMTS13. Reduced level is found in uremia, pregnancy, malignancy, acute inflammation, and DIC.

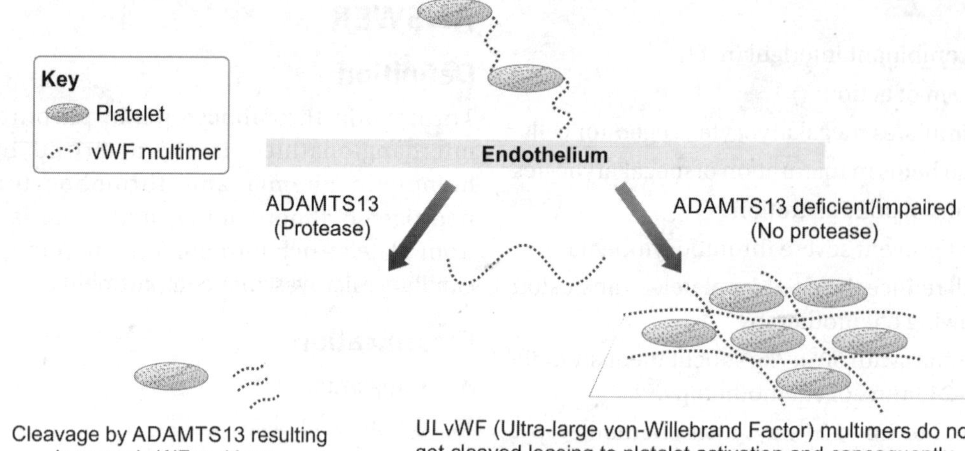

In case of classical TTP: There is formation of autoantibody against ADAMTS13 leading to deficiency of ADAMTS13. Usually, ADAMTS13, a metalloproteinase, will break the newly synthesized ultra-large multimer of VWF into smaller sizes. In absence of ADAMTS13, these ultra-large multimers under shearing stress will bind to platelet more avidly and also activate platelets as compared to short VWF. This will lead to platelet aggregation followed by platelet-rich thrombi formation, which ultimately leads to microangiopathy.

In case of congenital TTP: There is congenital deficiency of ADAMTS13.

In case of pregnancy-associated TTP: In case of congenital deficiency, it occurs in first trimester, otherwise it may be present in second or third trimester.

Clinical Presentation

Pentad of:

A. Fever
B. Microangiopathic hemolytic anemia
C. Purpura
D. Renal involvement—oliguria, anuria, and advanced renal failure
E. Neurological involvement resulting in platelet-rich thrombi in cerebral microvasculature—confusion, seizures, headache, somnolence, confusion, less commonly paresis, and coma

Diagnosis

A. Hematological investigations:
- **a.** Low hemoglobin and haptoglobin
- **b.** High LDH
- **c.** Presence of red cell fragments and FDPs
- **d.** Increased reticulocyte count
- **e.** Thrombocytopenia
- **f.** Raised indirect bilirubin
- **g.** ADAMTS13 activity is low
- **h.** Peripheral blood pictures demonstrate:
  - **1.** Schistocytes
  - **2.** Polychromasia
  - **3.** Occasionally nucleated RBC

Management

A. Plasma exchange is the mainstay of treatment as it will remove the VWF multimer from the circulation. It will be done once daily till normalization of platelet count and LDH level to baseline for at least 2–3 days.

If there is failure, in that case, twice daily exchange can be done. It there is normalization of platelet count and LDH level, then again once daily exchange will be continued. Now, if these parameters are normal for 2–3 days, then this treatment can be discontinued in tapering fashion. But, gradual termination of therapy is better than abrupt termination of therapy.

B. Steroid: It can be given in the initial phase of treatment along with plasma exchange. In case of adult, 1 g methylprednisolone intravenously daily for 3 days or orally prednisolone 1 g/kg/day.

C. Platelet transfusion: It is usually not given as it may produce further platelet-rich thrombi. But, if there is evidence of intracranial bleeding or life-threatening bleeding from any other sites, then platelet can be transfused.

D. Packed RBCs transfusion: It can be given commensurate with the degree of bleeding and hemoglobin level.

E. If there is delay in plasma exchange, in that case, FFP may be administered as a temporary measure. Plasma exchange is better as compared to FFP because:

   a. It will remove the offending agents from the body

   b. It will incur volume overload

F. In refractory and relapsing cases, following second line of treatment should be given:

   a. Addition of steroid

   b. Intravenous immunoglobulin

   c. Vincristine

   d. Cyclophosphamide

   e. Cyclosporine

   f. Splenectomy

   g. Monoclonal antibody rituximab

G. Hemodialysis: More than half of TTP cases may require hemodialysis. 25% of patients will revert back to normal renal function. Some may go into chronic renal failure and will be on maintenance hemodialysis.

Q71. Discuss the mechanism of hemoglobin degradation. Pathogenesis and diagnostic tests for hypercoagulable state.

DNB, 2022 (10)

Hypercoagulable state has been discussed in Page 81.

Heme metabolism.

NTR UNI of Health SC, Vijayawada, Aug, 2021 (10)

ANSWER

A. Macrophages, spleen start degradation by removing old senescent red blood cells from the circulation.

B. Red blood cells are broken down to heme and globin. The globin chain are recycled into the amino acids and these are further catabolized into the intermediates of citric acid cycle and fatty acid oxidation.

C. Heme is broken down to linear tetrapyrrole green pigment biliverdin, ferric iron and carbon monoxide.

D. Biliverdin is further broken down to red-orange pigment bilirubin by biliverdin reductase.

E. Bilirubin is transported into the serum by albumin from the liver where it is conjugated with the help of glucuronyl transferase to bilirubin glucuronide and it is transported into the liver and excreted into the bile.

F. In the intestine bilirubin is carried with bile and here bilirubin is deconjugated to urobilinogen then to stercobilin

G. Some urobilinogen is absorbed and excreted into the urinary tract and excreted in urine as urobilin.

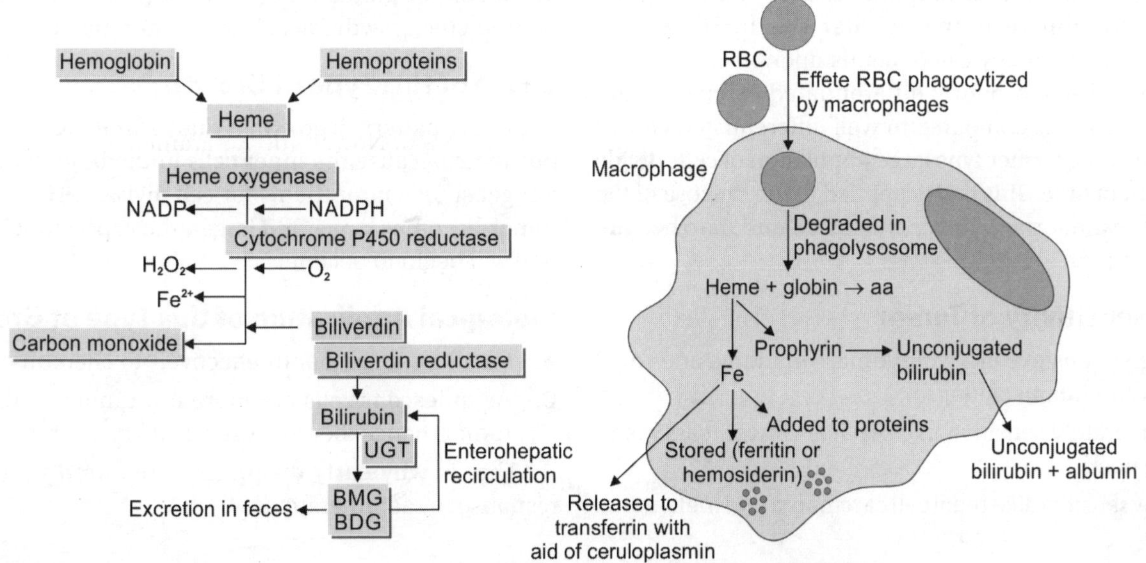

Q72. Principles of radiotherapy in malignancy.

DNB 2020 (5)

ANSWER

Definition

Radiation therapy is the use of directed X-ray either externally or internally or subatomic particles in the management of cancers as curative or palliative therapy.

Types of Radiation

- **A.** External beam radiation
- **B.** Brachytherapy, i.e., internal radiation like photon, protons, etc.
- **C.** Systemic radiation like administration of radio-isotopes I-131c in case of thyroid cancer.

Principles

Most common form of ionizing radiation is photons but electrons are also commonly used for increasing the dose of radiation to the skin.

But exotic particles like neutron, proton carbon ion are also used for certain diagnoses and location of the tumor.

Each type of radiation possess the unique characteristic that can dictate the type of interaction occurring during travelling through the body of the patient.

Therapeutic window of the radiation depends upon the differences in the interactions of DNA between normal versus cancer cells. As a result of break in the DNA there will be mitotic catastrophe leading to interruption of cell division resulting cellular death. Hence the radiosensitivity of any cell depends upon its division. As the cancer cells in poorly differentiated carcinoma are more sensitive as compared to well differentiated cancer because in the former type large population of cells divide at a point of time. This is also applied to the mucosa of the gastrointestinal tract, hence mucositis and diarrhea are more common

Radiosensitivity of Tumor

- **A.** Highly sensitive like lymphoma, seminoma and small cell carcinoma of lung.
- **B.** Moderately sensitive like cervical cancer, cancers in the neck.
- **C.** Low sensitive like renal cell carcinoma and melanoma.

Intent of Radiation Therapy

- **A.** Curative therapy - it should be done along with the surgery or chemotherapy.
- **B.** Adjuvant therapy or neoadjuvant therapy - It should be done after or before surgery to control locally.
- **C.** Palliative therapy - it should be done in case of distant metastases.

Side Effects of Radiation Therapy

- **A.** Acute complications - mucositis, diarrhea, dermatitis
- **B.** Chronic complication - Retroperitoneal fibrosis, secondary malignancy and stricture of the gastrointestinal tract during radiation for cervical cancer or intestine.

Following factors improve the efficacy of the radiation:

- **A.** Rate of the dose
- **B.** Total dose
- **C.** Oxygenation of tumor
- **D.** Phase of the cell cycle.

Q73. Gompertzian growth of the tumor.

DNB 2020 (4)

ANSWER

Definition

This growth is the growth in nonlinear pattern where in the 1st stage there is exponential growth of the tumor followed by the 2nd phase of deceleration phase and lastly in the 3rd phase of plateau. So, there is inverse relationship between the growth fraction and tumor masses.

Cause of this Type of Growth

The above pattern of growth is due to limitation of oxygen, nutrients because the inner cells in the large tumor may not get sufficient nutrients for cell division. Hence as the tumor becomes larger and larger, the exponential growth rate will begin to decline.

Biological Application of this Type of Growth

- **A.** Small tumor responds effectively to chemotherapy.
- **B.** As quiescent cells are more in number in the large tumor, hence they are less sensitive.

That is why early diagnosis is required to get high response to radiotherapy.

Q74. Approach to refractory anemia.

Kerala UNI 2022 (10)

ANSWER

Causes of Refractory Anemia

A. Bone marrow failure:
- **a.** Myelodysplastic syndrome
- **b.** Aplastic anemia

B. Endocrine diseases:
- **a.** Hypothyroidism
- **b.** Hypogonadism

C. Chronic inflammation:
- **a.** Chronic kidney disease
- **b.** Chronic infection
- **c.** Autoimmune diseases

D. Nutritional deficiency:
- **a.** Vitamin B12 deficiency
- **b.** Folate deficiency

E. Malignancy:
- **a.** Leukemia
- **b.** Lymphoma
- **c.** Multiple myeloma

F. Drug induced:
- **a.** Alcohol abuse
- **b.** Lead poisoning
- **c.** Chemotherapy

G. Inherited diseases:
- **a.** Fanconi syndrome
- **b.** Diamond-Blackfan syndrome

Approach to Refractory Anemia

A. History:
- **a.** Bleeding
- **b.** Suffering from long term infection
- **c.** Patient is on chemotherapy
- **d.** Joint pain or swelling
- **e.** Alcohol abuse
- **f.** Severe abdominal pain detect suspected lead poisoning.
- **g.** Vegetarian or non-vegetarian
- **h.** Family history of anemia
- **i.** Presence of blue line in the gum
- **j.** Presence of hepatosplenomegaly and peripheral signs of hepatocellular failure – chronic liver disease.

B. Initial laboratory investigation:
- **a.** Complete blood count to detect the type of anemia.
- **b.** Peripheral blood picture demonstrating types of anemia whether hemolytic or macrocytic, presence of rightward shift of white blood shift toward immature cells, basophilic stippling to detect lead poisoning.
- **c.** Low leukocyte count – Suggests aplastic anemia.
- **d.** Serum vitamin B12 and folic acid or RBC folate to detect the megaloblastic anemia.
- **e.** Serum ferritin increased in anemia of chronic disease, chronic kidney disease, and autoimmune disorders.
- **f.** Serum creatinine and urea to detect chronic kidney disease.
- **g.** Serum thyroid profile to detect the hypothyroidism.
- **h.** Serum alcohol level to detect alcohol abuse.
- **i.** Liver function test to detect chronic liver disease.
- **j.** Serum lactate dehydrogenase to detect the breakdown of red blood cells.
- **k.** Serum haptoglobin to detect hemolytic anemia.
- **l.** Serum ANA and extractable profile of nuclear antigen to detect autoimmune disorder.
- **m.** Ring sideroblast in case of myelodysplastic syndrome.

C. Bone marrow biopsy to detect:
- **a.** Aplastic anemia – hypocellular marrow along with pancytopenia.
- **b.** Fanconi anemia
- **c.** Hematological malignancies
- **d.** Flow cytometry and immunohistochemistry in case of presence of blast cells.
- **e.** Cytogenetics to detect myelodysplastic syndrome.

D. Additional tests:
- **a.** Erythropoietin level – to detect chronic kidney disease.
- **b.** JAK 2 mutation – to detect chronic myeloid leukemia
- **c.** Parvovirus B19 PCR or antibody in case of aplastic anemia.
- **d.** In case of suspected thalassemia – target cells and hemoglobin electrophoresis.

Q75. Cancer chemoprevention.

Kerala UNI, 2022, (10)

Maharashtra UNI of Health SC, Vijayawada, 2022 (10)

ANSWER

Following are the types of chemoprevention:

A. Primary chemoprevention - In case of healthy individual at high risk to prevent cancer. Example is Tamoxifen.

B. Secondary prevention - It means prevention of recurrence or progression of the premalignant lesion. Example is in case of colonic adenoma aspirin can be administered to prevent its progression toward frank malignancy.

C. Tertiary chemoprevention - It is characterized by prevention of the secondary tumor to prevent its recurrence in case of survivors. Administration of retinol in case of tumor of head and neck.

Mechanism of Chemoprotective Agents

A. Prevention of damage of DNA - vitamin C or vitamin E.

B. Blocking of hormone related pathways like Tamoxifen.

C. To prevent progression of chronic inflammation - by aspirin and NSAIDs.

D. Modulation of enzyme by detoxifying enzymes.

E. Drugs used in the modulation of cell cycle and apoptosis.

Examples are the following:

A. To reduce the incidence of breast cancer (ER+) - Tamoxifen or raloxifene.

B. To inhibit 5α reductase and reduce the incidence of prostate cancer -finasteride or Dutasteride.

C. Inhibition of COX and to reduce the formation of polyp in colon, stomach and esophagus by aspirin or NSAIDs.

D. To promote differentiation as well recurrence of the premalignant lesion in the head, neck and lung retinoid is administered.

Risk of Chemoprevention

A. There is chance of thromboembolism and endometrial cancer by administration of Tamoxifen.

B. In some cases, the drug should be administered for long duration.

C. It should be administered in case of high-risk groups like mutated carriers of BCRA.

Q76. Hemoglobin electrophoresis.

MGM UNI, Tamil Nadu, 2022 (5)

ANSWER

This is a procedure commonly done to detect the types of abnormal hemoglobin and separate them based on their movement in the electrical field which occurs due to their different electrical charges and structural variants of hemoglobin. Hemoglobin, a complex protein is composed of hem and globin and is responsible for carrying the oxygen from the pulmonary vascular bed to the peripheral tissues.

Following are the indications of hemoglobinopathies:

A. If the patient is diagnosed as a case of hemolytic anemia.

B. If there is family history of hemolytic anemia if the patient is suspected as a case of hemoglobinopathies.

C. Screening of hemolytic anemia in neonates.

D. If it is unexplained anemia resistant to iron therapy

E. In case of family history of hemolytic anemia or in few countries there routine screening of parents regarding the detection of the hemolytic anemia.

Procedures

A. In the EDTA vial patient's blood has to be collected.

B. From the red blood cells hemolysate should be prepared.

C. If the acetate agar the above sample should be applied.

D. Then on the field electrical current is applied to watch the migration of hemoglobin according to their charges to produce distinct bands.

E. Then the concentration of the band is measured by densitometry or with the comparison bands.

Advantages of this Procedure

A. It is low cost and easily measurable.

B. It is sensitive

C. It is reliable

D. It is used for both adult male and female and neonates.

Disadvantages

A. In case of compound heterogenicity, interpretation may not be possible.

B. Accuracy in terms of quantity may be difficult.

C. In case of low concentration of the abnormal hemoglobin may not be detected.

D. In case of abnormal globin chain, DNA analysis should be required.

Q77. Evaluation and treatment of megaloblastic anemia.

NTR UNI of Health SC, Vijayawada, 2022 (10)

ANSWER

Definition

Megaloblastic anemia is a heterogenous group of anemia which is characterized by presence of megaloblast in the bone marrow resulting from inhibition of nuclear division due to defective synthesis of DNA.

Etiology

A. Deficiencies of folic acid and vitamin B12 in the blood.

B. Inherited causes:

   a. Thiamine responsive megaloblastic anemia syndrome

   b. Inherited deficiency of intrinsic factor or receptors present in the ileum

   c. Congenital folate malabsorption syndrome

Folic acid: It is present in the green vegetables, fruit, meat and liver. Daily requirement is 50 to 100 mcg. Recommended daily allowances in adult is 400 mcg and in pregnant woman 600 μg. It is mainly absorbed from the mucosa in the jejunum. Body stores about 5 mg in the liver which is sufficiently meet the daily demand for 3 to 4 months. Deficiency of folate occurs in:
Following circumstances:

A. Decreased intake:

   a. Alcohol abuse

   b. Poor nutrition

      1. Elderly

      2. Poverty

      3. Special diet

      4. Institutionalized patient

B. Increased demand:

   1. Pregnancy

   2. Hemolysis

   3. Hemodialysis

   4. Malabsorption:

      - Tropical sprue
      - Celiac disease
      - Jejunal resection
      - Crohn's disease

C. Drugs:

   1. Chemotherapeutic agents

   2. Anticonvulsant

Vitamin B12: It is found in meat, fish and eggs and dairy products. It is bound with intrinsic factor produced by the gastric parietal cells in the stomach and absorbed from the ileum. The body stores 2 to 3 mg of vitamin B12 in the liver. The causes of vitamin B12 deficiency are:

A. Autoimmune gastric mucosal atrophy leading to decreased production of intrinsic factor.

B. Gastrectomy

C. Ileal resection

D. Ileitis

E. Zollinger Ellison syndrome

F. Blind loop syndrome

G. Fish tape worm infestation

H. Pancreatic insufficiency

Pathophysiology

Folate donate methyl group in the synthesis of DNA. Vitamin B12 acts as a cofactor in this reaction and recycles 5-methyl tetrahydrofolate to tetrahydrofolate again, this generation of tetrahydrofolate is associated with conversion of homocysteine to methionine.

Lack of vitamin B12 leads to trapping of folate in the 5-methyl tetrahydrofolate resulting deficiency of methionine. So, donation of methyl group acts a crucial role in the DNA synthesis. As hematopoietic precursor cells are rapidly dividing cells, altered DNA synthesis leads to disruption of hematopoiesis. There is arrest in the division of nucleus without any significant alteration in the maturation cycle of cytoplasm. Nucleated precursor cells in the bone marrow develops immature cells and giant metamyelocytes and there are presence of macrocytic red blood cells and hypersegmented neutrophils.

Prolonged deficiency of vitamin B12 leads to intramedullary hemolysis of the erythropoietic precursors.

Pathophysiology of the pernicious anemia involves presence of anti-intrinsic antibodies or parietal cell antibodies in the stomach.

History and Physical Examinations

A. Most common presentation is incidental findings during routine laboratory testing.

B. Common symptoms are:

   a. Shortness of breath

   b. Lightheadedness

   c. Palpitation

   d. Weakness

C. Physical findings include:

   a. Tachycardia

   b. Pallor

   c. Functional systolic murmur

d. Hunter glossitis
e. Splenomegaly
f. In case of intramedullary hematopoiesis jaundice

D. Following are the difference between folate and vitamin B12 deficiency:
  a. In vitamin B12 deficiency
    1. Neurological manifestation will be present characterized by paresthesia and disorder of balance, lancinating pain involving lower extremities.
    2. Visual disturbances due to optic atrophy.
    3. Clinical examination demonstrates:
      - Positive Romberg test
      - Babinski reflex
      - Hyporeflexia
      - Less frequently clonus
    4. Psychological disturbances in the form of dementia.

Evaluation of Anemia

A. MCV more than 100 fL or hypersegmented neutrophil in the peripheral smear.

B. MCV more than 115 fL is specific for vitamin B12 or folate deficiency.

C. Vitamin B12: Normal level is more than 300 pg/mL. Level between 200 and 300 pg/mL is suggestive of borderline deficiency. The level below 200 pg/mL suggests deficiency of vitamin B12.

D. Spurious low level of vitamin B12 are seen in:
  a. Multiple myeloma
  b. Pregnancy
  c. HIV infection
  d. Use of contraceptives
  e. Administration of diphenylhydantoin.

E. Falsely high-level vitamin B12 is seen in:
  a. Myeloproliferative neoplasm
  b. Alcoholic liver disease
  c. Renal disease

F. Folate level in the blood is: 4 ng/mL is normal, 2 to 4 ng/mL is borderline and below 2 ng/mL suggests deficiency of folate deficiency.

G. Methylmalonic acid can differentiate between vitamin B12 and folate deficiency because it is elevated in vitamin B12 deficiency but normal in folate deficiency.

H. Homocysteine level will be increased both in vitamin B12and folate deficiency.

I. Presence of autoantibodies against intrinsic factor is diagnostic of pernicious anemia.

Treatment

A. In absence of any malabsorption, vitamin B12 and folate can be supplemented orally, it takes time to restore the blood level, and hence in case of urgency parenteral supplementation is required.

B. The parenteral administration is required in following circumstances:
  a. Presence of neurological symptoms
  b. Pregnancy
  c. Infancy

C. In case of severe anemia blood transfusion is required as the supplementation cannot correct anemia rapidly.

D. In case adult the recommended dose is 1,000 mcg parenterally once weekly till the correction of the deficiency which is followed by the monthly or alternate monthly supplemental doses.

E. In absence of malabsorption, 1,000 mcg vitamin B12 is equally effective.

F. If the root cause is correctable, in that case the supplementation can be stopped after correction of the deficiency.

G. In case of pernicious anemia, gastric bypass surgery where there is lifelong vitamin B12 deficiency, indefinite supplementation is require.

H. Folate deficiency can be corrected by administration of folate is required at a dose of 1 mg daily. After correction of deficiency, the supplementation can be stopped if the etiology is correctable.

Process of Recovery of Hematopoiesis

A. With adequate supplementation, intramedullary hemolysis will be corrected will improve within 1 week and blood hematocrit and serum hemoglobin levels will normalize within 2 months.

B. Neuropsychiatric symptoms will recover within 12 months.

Q78. Reticular activating system.

MGR University, 2021, (5)

ANSWER

It is mononuclear phagocytic system playing as a central role in the immune response to clear pathogens.

Sites of Re System

A. Liver: Kupffer cells

B. Spleen: Macrophages

C. Lymph nodes: Macrophages
D. Lung: Alveolar macrophages
E. Serosal cavities: Peritoneal macrophages
F. Blood: Monocytes
G. Bone marrow

Functions of Re System

A. Phagocytosis: The cells will engulf bacteria, foreign bodies

B. The cells will present the antigen to the circulating T lymphocytes via MHC II molecules thereby developing adaptive immunity.

C. These cells will release proinflammatory cytokines tumor necrosis factor-alfa, interleukin-1, 6, and others.

D. These cells will breakdown the senescent cells to release iron which will be reused for future red blood cell production.

E. These cells will remove immune complexes, lipoproteins.

F. These cells will help in the tissue repair and fibrosis.

Hyperactivity of these cells:
It occurs in the following circumstances:
A. Infections leading to sepsis
B. Malignancy
C. Hemolytic anemia
D. Hemophagocytic lymphohistiocytosis
E. Autoimmune disorders

Complications in case of hyperactivation of this system:
A. Macrophage activation syndrome
B. Systemic inflammation leading to cytokine storm resulting massive release of proinflammatory cytokines and chemokines.
C. In case of hemolytic anemia and other hematological disorders, there is moderate to massive hepato-splenomegaly.
D. In case of disseminated intravascular coagulation there is damage of the vascular endothelial system leading to release of inflammatory cytokines.
E. Hemophagocytosis resulting phagocytosis of the all the cell lineages.

Q79. Hepcidin.

NTR UNI of Health SC, Vijayawada, 2021, (10)

ANSWER

Hepcidin is a peptide hormone playing a critical role in the iron homeostasis. Iron is essential for carrying oxygen into different tissues in the body and present in hemoglobin, myoglobin and in different electron transport chain.

Synthesis

Hepcidin is synthesized in the liver as preprohormone which is cleaved into prohormone and then to active hormone Hepcidin containing 25 amino acids after further cleavage.

Upregulation of Hepcidin occurs in the following conditions:
A. In the inflammatory states mediated by proinflammatory cytokine IL-6
B. Transferrin, iron binding transport molecules in the blood

Downregulation of Hepcidin production occurs in the following conditions by downregulation of *Hepcidin* genes to construct the new hemoglobin molecules:
A. Erythroferrone, a hormone produced by the erythroblast at the time of erythropoiesis.
B. Hypoxic condition.

Organ system involved: Hepcidin critically regulates the serum iron level by modulating the release of iron from the intracellular storage sites.
A. When the serum level of Hepcidin will be elevated, iron remains bound to ferritin molecule in the intracellular storage form.
B. There is inverse relationship between serum iron and serum Hepcidin level in the inflammatory states, i.e., as the Hepcidin level increases serum iron level decreases which prevent the invaded pathogen to utilize serum iron for their growth, hence Hepcidin is an important mediation of immune defense.

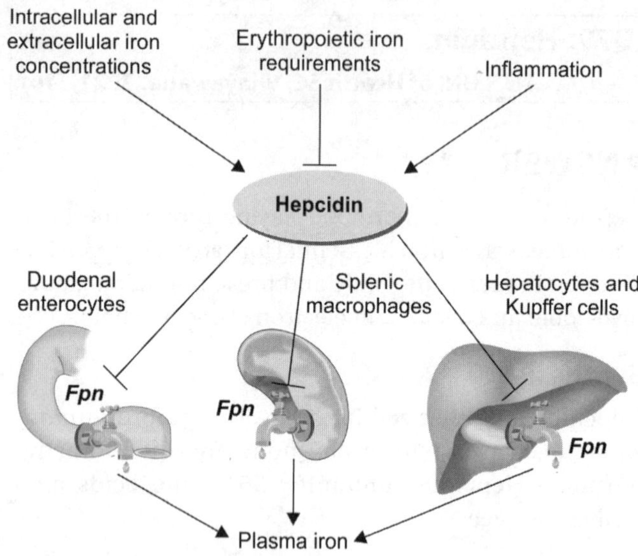

Functions of Hepcidin

Hepcidin controls serum iron through the interaction with the ferroportin-1, which is transmembrane iron exporter present in the macrophages and the enterocytes. As Hepcidin binds to ferroprotin-1, it will cause the cells like macrophages and enterocyte to target hepcidin-ferroportin complex leading to lysosomal degradation. Iron is absorbed from duodenal enterocytes and recovered iron is stored in the reticuloendothelial macrophages. The degradation of the ferroportin will block the absorption of iron from enterocytes and mobilization of iron from the macrophages.

Q80. Trinucleotide repeat disorders.

NTR UNI of Health SC, Vijayawada, 2021, (10)

ANSWER

Definition

Trinucleotide is a specific group of genetic disorders where there is abnormal expansion of the 3 nucleotide sequences leading to disruption of the function of the genes resulting various types of muscle and neurological disorders.

Following are the key features in this disorder:

A. Following are the repeat unit – CAG, CGG, GAA.
B. If the repeat is small in number, it is normal, but if the repeat is excessive, it may produce disease.
C. It is often caused by slippage of replication of DNA and poor mismatch in the repair.
D. It may be autosomal dominant, or autosomal recessive or sex linked.
E. In the successive generation, severity of the disease increases.

Following are the trinucleotide repeat disorders:

Disease	Gene affected	Repeat sequences	Inheritance	Clinical features
Huntington's disease	HTT	CAG	Autosomal dominant	• Chorea • Psychiatric changes • Dementia
Myotonic dystrophy type 1	DMPK	CTG	Autosomal dominant	• Cataract • Myotonia • Cardiac conduction defect • Wasting of muscles
Fragile X syndrome	FMR1	CGG	X-linked dominant	• Large ears • Intellectual disability • Macroorchidism
Spinocerebellar ataxia	Various	CAG	Autosomal dominant	• Dysarthria • Ataxia of gait • Tremor
Kennedy disease	Androgen receptor	CAG	X-linked recessive	• Gynecomastia • Infertility • Weakness of the bulbar muscles

Q81. Causes and management of thrombocytopenia in ICU
NTR UNI of Health SC, Vijayawada, 2021, (10)

ANSWER

Mechanism and Causes of Thrombocytopenia in ICU Settings

Differential diagnoses of thrombocytopenia	Diagnostic clue
Pseudothrombocytopenia	
• EDTA anticoagulated blood • GPIIb/IIIa receptor antagonist therapy	• Platelet count normal • No symptoms related to low platelet count • Preceding therapy with GPIIb/IIIa receptor antagonist
Hemodilution	
Infusion of fluid or plasma	Massive transfusion or infusion due to bleeding
Consumption of platelet	
Loss of blood	• Bleeding • Anemia • Prolonged clotting time
Sepsis	• Fever • Further sepsis criteria • Positive blood cultures
DIC	• Shock • Infection • Obstetric complications • Typical underlying causes · • Prolonged clotting times • Increased fibrin degradation product • Nucleated red cells in the differential count
Massive blunt plasma	• History • Physical examination • Radiological examination
Extracorporeal circuit	Organ failure requiring extracorporeal circuit
Sequestration of platelets	
Hepatosplenomegaly	• History • Cirrhosis of liver • Osteomyelofibrosis • USG • Other radiological examinations

Continued

Continued

Differential diagnoses of thrombocytopenia	Diagnostic clue
Decreased production of platelets	
Intoxication due to alcohol or drugs	• History of abuse or dependence on alcohol • History of intake of drugs
Viral infection like CMV, HCV, HIV, EBV viruses	Different diagnostic method for diagnosis of the viruses
Radiation	History
Infiltration of the bone marrow by leukemia or lymphoma	Complete blood count, bone marrow examination
Chemotherapy	History
Destruction of platelets	
Immune thrombocytopenia	• Antiplatelet antibodies • Increased megakaryocytes in the bone marrow • Response of platelet count to intravenous immunoglobulin or corticosteroids • Comorbidities for secondary ITP like SLE, hepatitis C
Drug induced thrombocytopenia	• History of medication intake – whether new drug started within 7 to 14 days with platelet count of less than 20,000/cc which have been corrected after cessation of suspected drugs • Presence of drug dependent antibodies.
Heparin induced thrombocytopenia	• Platelet count between 20,000 and 80,000/cc between 7 to 14 days of heparin administration in absence of thromboembolic events with ongoing therapy with heparin • Heparin dependent, platelet activating anti-heparin antibodies
Thrombotic microangiopathy	• Hemolysis with negative direct comb test • Fragment red blood cells in the smear • Typical platelet count 10,000–30,000/cc. Elevated LDH • Thrombotic events leading to renal and neurological features • HELLP syndrome

Continued

Continued

Differential diagnoses of thrombocytopenia	Diagnostic clue
Post-transfusion purpura	• History of transfusion • History of pregnancy • Platelet count is less than 10,000/cc • High anti-human platelet antigen antibodies titer
Passive alloimmune thrombocytopenia	After administration of platelet rich product rapid and abrupt and transient fall of platelet count which may be due to presence of platelet alloantibody

Q82. Approach to a patient with purpura.

NTR UNI of Health SC, Vijayawada, 2021, (10)

ANSWER

Classification of Thrombocytopenia

According to the count there three types of thrombocytopenia:

A. Mild thrombocytopenia: ≥100,000–150,000/cc
B. Moderate thrombocytopenia: ≥50,000–<100,000/cc
C. Severe thrombocytopenia: <50,000/cc.

Pathophysiological Classification

Decreased production in the bone marrow:

A. *Congenital*:
- **a.** Fanconi syndrome
- **b.** May–Hegglin anomaly
- **c.** Bernard–Soulier syndrome
- **d.** Wiskott–Aldrich syndrome
- **e.** Thrombocytopenia with absent radius syndrome
- **f.** X-linked thrombocytopenia with thalassemia.
- **g.** Congenital amegakaryocytic thrombocytopenia

B. *Acquired*:
- **a.** Reduced number of megakaryocytic precursor:
  - **1.** Aplastic anemia
  - **2.** Drugs—Chlorothiazide
  - **3.** Toxin
  - **4.** Radiation
  - **5.** Infection:
    - Hepatitis C virus
    - Hepatitis B virus
    - HIV
    - Cytomegalovirus
    - Malaria
    - Babesia
  - **6.** Malignancies:
    - Leukemia
    - Myelodysplastic syndrome
  - **7.** Hemophagocytosis
- **b.** Ineffective erythropoiesis:
  - **1.** Vitamin B12 deficiency
  - **2.** Folic acid deficiency

Increased destruction:

A. Immune thrombocytopenia
B. Thrombotic thrombocytopenic purpura
C. Hemolytic uremic syndrome
D. *Collagen vascular disease*: Systemic lupus erythematosus
E. Antiphospholipid syndrome
F. Post-transfusion purpura
G. Paroxysmal nocturnal hemoglobinuria
H. Neonatal allogenic thrombocytopenia

Increased sequestration:

A. Hypersplenism
B. HIV-associated thrombocytopenia
C. Gestational thrombocytopenia
D. Sepsis:
- **a.** Typhus
- **b.** Dengue

Approach to a Case of Thrombocytopenia

From the clinical presentations:

A. History of jaundice - Hepatitis B or C virus infection
B. History of diarrhea followed by oliguria, hematuria–Hemolytic uremic syndrome
C. History of retro-orbital pain, high fever, nausea with vomiting - Dengue fever
D. History high fever, vomiting, endemic area of Rickettsial disease - Typhus fever
E. History of viral fever in female with chronic course - Immune thrombocytopenia.
F. History of bleeding after 5–10 of platelet transfusion in multiparous female—Post-transfusion thrombocytopenia
G. History of rash, joint pain in females—Systemic lupus erythematosus
H. History of weakness, repeated abortion, recurrent thrombophlebitis—Antiphospholipid syndrome.

I. History of recurrent episodes of thrombocytopenia every 3-4 weeks in female—Cyclic thrombocytopenia

J. History of intake of immunosuppressive drugs in a case of HIV patient—JIV related thrombocytopenia.

K. History of suffering from leukemia—Malignancy

L. Child or young adult suffering from eczema, recurrent bacterial sinopulmonary infection, bloody diarrhea—Wiskott-Aldrich syndrome

M. History of recurrent common cold, respiratory infection, recurrent bleeding from any sites, short stature, poor growth—Fanconi syndrome

N. History of easy fatigability, recurrent bleeding from different sites mainly from mouth, positive family history of bleeding, recurrent blood transfusion—May-Hegglin anomaly.

O. History of shortness of breath, abdominal and back pain, recurrent dark colored urine—Paroxysmal nocturnal hemoglobinuria.

P. Purpura occurs in 2nd and 3rd trimester of pregnancy—TTP

Q. History of neurological symptoms, seizures—TTP.

Classic pentad of thrombotic thrombocytopenic purpura:

- **a.** Microangiopathic hemolytic anemia
- **b.** Fever
- **c.** Thrombocytopenia
- **d.** Renal insufficiency
- **e.** Neurological manifestations.

R. History of following drug ingestion may produce thrombocytopenia—TTP

- **a.** Quinine
- **b.** Mitomycin C
- **c.** Clopidogrel
- **d.** Bleomycin
- **e.** Chlorothiazide

Family history:

A. Autosomal dominant:

- **a.** May-Hegglin anomaly

B. Autosomal recessive disorder:

- **a.** Fanconi anemia
- **b.** Gray platelet syndrome
- **c.** Thrombocytopenia with absent radii.

C. Sex-linked recessive:

- **a.** Wiskott-Aldrich syndrome
- **b.** X-linked thrombocytopenia

Physical Examination

A. Common for all the diseases are:

- **a.** Anemia depending upon the amount of bleeding.
- **b.** Petechiae
- **c.** Ecchymosis
- **d.** Hemorrhagic spot in the retina or subconjunctival area.

B. To identify the etiology of bleeding:

- **a.** Jaundice—Thrombocytopenia with thalassemia, scrub typhus, and dengue fever.
- **b.** Congenital absence of radius bilaterally—Thrombocytopenia with absent radii.
- **c.** Presence of eczema—Wiskott-Aldrich syndrome
- **d.** Short stature/poor growth—Fanconi anemia
- **e.** Splenomegaly—Thrombocytopenia with thalassemia
- **f.** Sternal tenderness—Myelodysplastic syndrome, hyperactive marrow in iron, vitamin B12 and folate deficiency.
- **g.** Butter-fly skin rash, arthritis—Systemic lupus erythematosus.
- **h.** Tender calf region with positive Homan's sign—Antiphospholipid syndrome.
- **i.** Necrosis in different areas of skin after taking heparin mostly due to hypercoagulable state after 5-10 days after 1st exposure or ≤ 1 day after 2nd exposure—Heparin induced thrombocytopenia.

Laboratory Investigations

A. Common to all diseases:

- **a.** Hemoglobin - low.
- **b.** ESR - High
- **c.** Platelet - Low according to the severity, mild, moderate and severe.
    1. Platelet count—<100,000/cc: Immune thrombocytopenic purpura
    2. Severe thrombocytopenia of <20,000/cc immediate or within 5-10 days after taking the causative drugs.
    3. Platelet count may be 10,000/cc: Post platelet transfusion.
    4. Platelet count >70,000/cc in 2nd and 3rd trimester of pregnancy and normal after delivery.

B. For diagnosing the etiology:

- **a.** Serum creatinine—raised in hemolytic uremic syndrome.

b. Leukocyte count—low in Fanconi anemia, aplastic anemia
c. Dengue NS1 antigen dengue IgM antibody—Dengue
d. Scrub typhus IgM antibody—Typhus fever.
e. ANF test—SLE
f. Absence of alfa granules in the platelet—Gray platelet syndrome.
g. Heparin antigen assay or functional assay if pre-test 4T probability score is moderately high.
h. Presence of PIA-1 antibody—Post-transfusion thrombocytopenia.
i. D-dimer will be high—Sepsis, post-transfusion, obstetric complication, malignancy
j. Stool culture—Enteroinvasive *E. coli* or *Shigella* Shiga
k. Toxin demonstration of *Shigella* Shiga
l. Coomb test positive—Thalassemia
m. Raised bilirubin with raised liver enzymes—Dengue, and typhus fever.
n. Estimation of vitamin B12 and folic acid—Nutritional cause.
o. Peripheral smear demonstration:
   1. Giant platelet and large, basophilic well-defined inclusion bodies in granulocytes resembling Dohle bodies - Wiskott-Aldrich syndrome
   2. Fragmented red blood cells, deranged coagulation factors—Microangiopathic hemolytic anemia.
   3. Microcytic normochromic anemia with tear drop cell and positive osmotic fragility test-Thalassemia
   4. Macrothrombocytopenia—Constitutional thrombocytopenia
   5. Platelet anisocytosis—Congenital thrombocytopenia
   6. Clumping of platelet—Pseudo-thrombocytopenia
   7. Atypical cells, immature cells—Leukemia, myelodysplastic syndrome
p. Bone marrow biopsy:
   1. Leukemia
   2. Myelodysplastic syndrome
   3. Aplastic anemia
   4. Fibrosis—Gray platelet syndrome, myelofibrosis, marrow infiltration in case of infection and neoplasia.

Q83. Fever with hepatosplenomegaly.
NTR UNI of Health SC, Vijayawada, 2021 (10)

ANSWER

Causes of Fever with Hepatosplenomegaly

A. Infectious causes:
   a. Viral causes:
      1. Infectious mononucleosis
      2. Hepatitis B and C virus
      3. Cytomegalovirus
      4. Dengue fever
   b. Bacterial causes:
      1. Brucellosis
      2. Leptospirosis
      3. Typhoid fever
      4. Disseminated tuberculosis
      5. Sepsis
   c. Parasitic infestation:
      1. Malaria
      2. Kala-azar
      3. Toxoplasmosis
      4. Schistosomiasis
   d. Fungal infection:
      1. Candidiasis
      2. Histoplasmosis
B. Hematological causes:
   a. Acute and chronic leukemia
   b. Lymphoma
   c. Hemolytic anemia
C. Autoimmune disorders:
   a. Systemic lupus erythematosus
   b. Still's disease
   c. Rheumatoid arthritis
   d. Sarcoidosis
D. Infiltrative diseases:
   a. Amyloidosis
   b. Gaucher disease
E. Other causes:
   a. Metastatic cancer
   b. Hepatocellular carcinoma
   c. Post-transplant lymphoproliferative disorders
   d. Hemophagocytic lymphohistiocytosis

From History

A. Fever:
   a. Sudden onset—Malaria, dengue
   b. Insidious onset—tuberculosis, lymphoma, leukemia, collagen vascular disease
   c. Pattern fever:
      1. 48 hours duration—*Plasmodium vivax, ovale*
      2. 72 hours duration—*Plasmodium malariae*
      3. Undulant fever—brucellosis
      4. Remittent fever—typhoid
      5. Continuous fever—2nd week of typhoid fever, dengue fever.
      6. Intermittent fever—tuberculosis
      7. Pel-Ebstein fever—Infectious mononucleosis
      8. Relapsing fever—Leptospirosis
   d. Associated symptoms:
      1. Associated with chill and rigor - malaria
      2. Night sweat, weight loss—Tuberculosis, leukemia, lymphoma
      3. Associated with nausea, vomiting—Leptospirosis, hepatitis, dengue, hepatocellular carcinoma, hematological disorders

B. Pain abdomen: Leukemia, lymphoma, dengue, malaria, leptospirosis, Kala-azar

C. Yellow urine—Leptospirosis

D. Associated skin rash—Dengue, SLE, drug,

E. Joint involvement—Rheumatoid arthritis, SLE, Still's disease

F. Arthralgia, severe backache—Dengue, malaria,

G. Chest infection, sore throat—Dengue, leukemia, lymphoma

H. Purpura—Dengue, leukemia, disseminated tuberculosis

I. Exposure history:
   a. Travel to endemic areas—Malaria, leishmaniasis
   b. Exposure to contact: Viral hepatitis
   c. Exposure to contaminated water or food: Typhoid, viral hepatitis
   d. Exposure to animals—brucellosis, leptospirosis

J. Drug history:
   a. Reactions—DRESS syndrome
   b. Intake of immunosuppressive therapy—Collagen vascular disease, malignancies, leukemia, lymphoma, post-transplant.

K. Past history:
   a. Bleeding—hematological disorder
   b. Chest infection—tuberculosis
   c. Joint pain—collagen vascular disease
   d. HIV infection

L. Social and family history:
   a. Jaundice—Hepatitis, hepatocellular carcinoma, leptospirosis
   b. Mosquito bite—Malaria, dengue
   c. Sand fly—Kala-azar
   d. Contact with tuberculosis

M. History of blood transfusion—hepatitis B, C, hepatocellular carcinoma

From Systemic Examination

A. Pattern of temperature from recording

B. Hypotension—sepsis, complicated dengue, malarial complications,

C. Anemia—Hematologic malignancy, malaria, dengue, hemolytic anemia

D. Jaundice—Leptospirosis, hepatitis, hemolytic anemia, dengue fever, drug reaction

E. Lymphadenopathy—Leukemia, lymphoma, disseminated tuberculosis, viral hepatitis, infectious mononucleosis

F. Rash - SLE, leukemia, rheumatoid arthritis, dengue, disseminated tuberculosis,

G. Deformity of joints—Rheumatoid arthritis

H. Purpuric spot—Complicated dengue, leukemia, sepsis, hepatitis, any viral infection

I. Abdominal examination:
   a. Liver:
      1. Enlarged tender liver—Malaria, dengue, viral hepatitis, hepatocellular carcinoma
      2. Hard non-tender liver—Leukemia, lymphoma, kala-azar, collagen vascular disease
   b. Spleen:
      1. Tender spleen—Leukemia, lymphoma, acute malaria,
      2. Nontender massive splenomegaly—Kala-azar, chronic myeloid leukemia, myelofibrosis
      3. Moderate splenomegaly—Still's disease, hemolytic anemia, collagen vascular disease.

J. Other systemic examination:
   a. Chest—pleural effusion, cavitary lesion—disseminated tuberculosis, fungal infection in HIV infection.

b. Neurological examination—Malaria, fulminant hepatic failure from viral hepatitis, complicated dengue. Metastasis from malignant leukemia, lymphoma leptospirosis, HIV infection.

From Laboratory Examination

A. Baseline investigation:
   a. Anemia—malaria, complicated dengue, collagen vascular disease, sepsis, hemolytic anemia, leukemia, lymphoma, kala-azar.
   b. Different dots in the red blood cells—different species of malaria.
   c. Peripheral blood picture:
      1. Different types of red blood cell—hemolytic anemia
      2. Different types of abnormal immature white blood cells—leukemia
   d. Liver function test: Transaminitis—Malaria, complicated dengue, hepatitis, hepatocellular carcinoma, leptospirosis, brucellosis, drug reaction, disseminated tuberculosis
   e. Raised urea and creatinine - Leptospirosis, sepsis, HIV infection
   f. Blood culture—Typhoid, sepsis

B. Specific investigations:
   a. Dual antigen—malaria
   b. rK39—Kala-azar
   c. Typhi-dot M—Typhoid infection
   d. Widal test after 7 days—Typhoid
   e. Mantoux test/IGRA/line probe assay—Tuberculosis
   f. Ana, DsDNA—SLE
   g. Rheumatoid factor, anti-CCP antibody—Rheumatoid arthritis
   h. Extractable NA—Different types of collagen vascular disease.
   i. Serological tests—hepatitis, cytomegalovirus, HIV, Epstein-Barr virus, *Brucella*, *Leptospira*.
   j. NS1 antigen, Dengue IgM antibody—Dengue infection
   k. Bone marrow:
      1. Abnormal white blood cells—Leukemia
      2. Reed-Sternberg giant cell—Lymphoma
      3. LD bodies —Kala-azar
      4. Excessive collagen and fibrosis—primary myelofibrosis
   l. Lymph node—lymphoma, infiltrative disease, metastasis, tuberculosis
   m. Liver biopsy—Hepatoma, infiltrative disease, hepatitis, granuloma

C. Imaging:
   a. Ultrasound of the abdomen—hepatosplenomegaly, abdominal lymphadenopathy
   b. Chest X-ray—tuberculosis, different types of infections.

Q84. Myelophthisic anemia.

NTR UNI of Health SC, Vijayawada, AUG 2022 (10)

ANSWER

Definition

Myelophthisic anemia is characterized by immature erythrocytes in the peripheral circulation due to infiltration of the bone marrow with abnormal tissue resulting inadequate production of red blood cells in the bone marrow.

Etiology:

A. Bone marrow infiltration by the following tissue:
   a. Metastatic cancers - from Breast, prostate
   b. Hematologic malignancy
   c. Granulomatous lesions
   d. Lipid storage disorder
   e. Primary myelofibrosis

B. Fibrosis of the bone marrow from:
   a. Disseminated microbial infection
   b. Autoimmune diseases
   c. Renal osteodystrophy
   d. Hypoparathyroidism
   e. Hyperparathyroidism

Histopathology

A. Peripheral blood picture demonstrates:
   a. Leukoerythroblastic reaction
   b. Immature myeloid and nucleated erythrocytes
      1. Schistocytes
      2. Dacrocytes (tear drop cells)
      3. Anisocytosis
      4. Poikilocytosis

History and Physical Examination

A. History of malignancy of prostate, breast and lung cancer
B. History of chronic inflammatory diseases
C. Features related to anemia
D. Features of thrombocytopenia
E. Physical examination demonstrates:
   a. Pallor
   b. Delayed capillary refilling
   c. Tachycardia
   d. Splenomegaly
   e. Hepatomegaly

Evaluation

A. Complete blood count:
   a. Hemoglobin
   b. White blood cells
   c. Platelet count
   d. Hematocrit
   e. MCV
   f. MCH
   g. MCHC
   h. PCV
   i. Red blood cell width
B. Peripheral blood picture as described above
C. Bone marrow picture

Treatment

A. Treatment of the cause of infiltration in the bone marrow.
B. Myelophthisis can respond to check point inhibitors like Pembrolizumab favorably
C. Infusion of packed red blood cells

Q85. Transfusion threshold for various blood components.

NTR UNI of Health SC, Vijayawada, 2021 (10)

ANSWER

A. Packed red blood cells transfusion:
   a. Medically non-bleeder patient—hemoglobin <7 g/dL
   b. Postoperative patients having cardiovascular disease—hemoglobin <8 g/dL
   c. Acute coronary syndrome or moderately severe anemia - hemoglobin <8 to 9 g/dL.
   d. Anemia of chronic kidney disease or myelodysplastic syndrome—It varies according to individual patient.
B. Platelet transfusion:
   a. Prophylactic transfusion—platelet less than 10.000/cc to prevent spontaneous bleeding.
   b. A patient suffering from fever or sepsis—less than 20,000/cc as this patient has risk of bleeding.
   c. Prior to different procedure like central line insertion—less than 20,000 to 50,000/cc, though it varies according to procedure of choice.
   d. Prior to major surgery—less than 100,000/cc as there is high risk of post-procedural bleeding.
   e. Massive transfusion of platelet toward the target of more than 50,000 to 100,000/cc.
C. Fresh frozen plasma transfusion:
   a. In case of bleeding with coagulopathy—INR more than 1.5 PT and APTT is high.
   b. In patient with coagulopathy—INR is more than 1.5 to 1.8 in case of invasive procedure.
   c. Massive transfusion is given which varies according to the patient only to maintain hemostasis.
D. Cryoprecipitate transfusion:
   a. In case of invasive procedure or replacement of fibrinogen if the serum fibrinogen level is less than 150 to 150 mg/dL—if the patient suffers from liver disease, disseminated intravascular coagulation.
   b. In case of patient suffering from congenital fibrinogen deficiency with fibrinogen level is less than 100 mg/dL and fibrinogen concentrate is not available.
   c. In case of von Willebrand disease or if the factor VIII is deficient.
E. *Granulocyte transfusion*:
   a. If absolute neutrophil count is less than 500/cc with sepsis, patient with aplastic anemia or patient is receiving chemotherapy.

Q86. Hemoglobin E.

Maharashtra UNI of Health SC, Vijayawada, 2021 (10)

ANSWER

Hemoglobin E is an extremely common β-hemoglobin variant in Asian population produced at a reduced rate, hence known as mild form of β-thalassemia. It is a genetic condition where person contains one normal gene for normal hemoglobin and the other from abnormal hemoglobin E.

Hemoglobin E can be classified as:

A. Hemoglobin E heterozygote – α globin gene
   a. $\alpha\alpha/\alpha\alpha$ – clinically normal
   b. $-\alpha/\alpha\alpha$ – clinically normal
   c. $--/\alpha\alpha$ – clinically normal
   d. $--/-\alpha$ – Thalassemia intermedia (AE Bart disease)
B. Hemoglobin E homozygote:
   a. $\alpha\alpha/\alpha\alpha$ – clinically normal
   b. $-\alpha/\alpha\alpha$ – clinically normal
   c. $--/\alpha\alpha$ – clinically normal
   d. $--/-\alpha$ – Thalassemia intermedia (AE Bart disease)
C. Hemoglobin E β thalassemia:
   a. $\alpha\alpha/\alpha\alpha$ – Clinically mild to moderately severe disease
   b. $-\alpha/\alpha\alpha$ – Mild disease
   c. $--/\alpha\alpha$ – Mild disease
   d. $--/-\alpha$ – Thalassemia intermedia (EF Bart's disease)

Pathophysiology

Hemoglobin E develops from the point mutation in the codon 26 present in the gene of β globin leading to formation of abnormal hemoglobin and reduced synthesis of β globin.

Hemoglobin E Trait

A. Here one normal β gene and the other hemoglobin E gene.
B. Clinically patient may be asymptomatic or mildly anemic.
C. Laboratory investigations demonstrate:
   a. Mild microcytosis
   b. Hemoglobin electrophoresis demonstrates 30% hemoglobin E. Rest is hemoglobin A.

Hemoglobin E Disease

A. Here both β globin chain are mutated.
B. Clinical features:
   a. Mild hypochromic microcytic anemia
   b. May be splenomegaly
   c. Mild symptoms
C. Laboratory investigation demonstrates:
   a. Microcytosis
   b. Evidence of target cells
   c. Hemoglobin electrophoresis demonstrates 90% is hemoglobin E and rest is hemoglobin A.

Hemoglobin E/β-thalassemia

A. Genetically compound heterozygote where one gene is hemoglobin E gene and the other β-thalassemia gene.
B. Clinical picture:
   a. Retardation of growth
   b. Presence of enlarged spleen
   c. Deformities of the bone
C. Laboratory investigation:
   a. Patient is severely anemic
   b. Peripheral blood picture demonstrates hypochromic microcytosis.
   c. Hemoglobin electrophoresis demonstrates increased level of hemoglobin F and E.

Treatment

A. First two types of thalassemia do not require treatment.
B. Last one variant requires:
   a. If severe anemia – regular blood transfusion
   b. In case massive blood transfusion – chelation of iron is required.
   c. In selected case requiring massive blood transfusion – splenectomy should be done.
   d. In refractory cases – bone marrow transplantation is required.

Q87. Immunohistochemistry in cancerous diseases.

Kerala University, 2020 (10)

ANSWER

Indications of Immunohistochemistry in Cancerous Diseases

A. Classification and typing of the tumor: It can distinguish between adenocarcinoma (CK7+, CK20+) and squamous cell carcinoma (p63+n and p40+)
B. It can help in the detection and prognosis of the cancers: Overexpression of HER2 in the breast cancer, proliferation index can be diagnosed by Ki-67
C. In case of metastasis or poorly differentiated cancer it can help in determining the tissue of origin. In case of lung cancer TTF-1 is used, in case of prostate cancer PSA should be assayed.
D. Target should be detected for treatment – In lung cancer PD-L1 should be detected for administering immunotherapy.

E. It can differentiate between neoplastic and reactive lesion – To differentiate melanoma from melanocytic nevi, HMB-45 and MELAN-A should be used.

Contraindication for Immunohistochemistry in Case of Cancerous Diseases

A. Poor preservation or fixation of tissue because antigenicity may be lost during the process of autolysis or the fixation is suboptimal.

B. If the tissue is poorly stained or cross-reactive, there is chance of misdiagnosis and cannot be properly interpreted.

C. If the antibody is not properly selected, in that case there is chance of false positivity or false negativity.

D. Sample tissue must be adequate for proper processing.

Advantages of Immunohistochemistry

A. It is highly specific and highly sensitive.

B. It can localize, preserves morphology and can identify the cell types in the tissue architecture.

C. There is wide range of diagnostic as well as prognostic applications for guiding the targeted therapy.

D. This process is rapid, fast and cost effective.

Disadvantages of Immunohistochemistry

A. It is very subject specific as this diagnosis is very much observer-dependent.

B. There is every chance of false positivity or false negativity because of the cross positivity.

C. There may be variability from batch to batch because of limited quality of antibodies.

D. It cannot replace the genetic testing.

Q88. Congenital Methemoglobinemia.

Kerala University, 2020 (8)

ANSWER

Methemoglobinemia is a life-threatening condition which is characterized by decreased oxygen carrying capacity of the circulating hemoglobin due to conversion of one or all iron from reduced ferrous form to oxidized ferric form.

Etiology

Congenital methemoglobinemia due to:

A. Autosomal recessive defect in the enzyme cytochrome b5 reductase (CYB5R) or,

B. Autosomal dominant mutation in the gene encoding protein globin which is known collectively as hemoglobin M. There are multiple variants of hemoglobin M like Boston, Hyde Park, Fort Ripley, Osaka, etc.

There are different types of methemoglobinemia:

A. Congenital methemoglobinemia type I: Here there is defect in the CYB5R which is expressed only in erythrocytes.

B. Congenital methemoglobinemia type II: Here all the cells express the defect.

Due to possible multiple mutations occurring in the alfa and beta chains of hemoglobin near to heme iron leading to oxidation of ferrous iron to ferric state. As a result, there is allosteric change in the molecule and thereby oxygen dissociation curve will be shifted to the left. The hemoglobin fails to release the oxygen to the tissue leading to tissue hypoxia.

There is also a genetic mutation encoding the one globin protein leading to substitution of one amino acid with tyrosine that allows the ferric form to become stabilized. So, this patient with hemoglobin M has level of methemoglobin is 15% to 30%.

Normally cytochrome b-5 reductase utilizes NADH which is formed during glycolysis to reduce the methemoglobin back into the functional type of hemoglobin.

There is another pathway for reduction of the methemoglobin is nicotinamide adenine dinucleotide phosphate hydrogen methemoglobin (NADPH-MetHb) that utilizes the NADPH formed during the action of glucose 6 phosphate dehydrogenase in the hexose monophosphate shunt, but its contribution in the reduction of methemoglobin is little normally, but in methemoglobinemia this pathway will very much enhanced by the presence of exogenous electron donor, as for example, methylene blue.

History and Physical Examination

A. Symptoms are:

- **a.** Cyanosis
- **b.** Pallor
- **c.** Fatigue
- **d.** Weakness
- **e.** Headache
- **f.** Depression
- **g.** Metabolic acidosis
- **h.** Seizures
- **i.** Dysrhythmias

j. Coma
k. Death

Degree of symptoms depends upon the following factors:
A. Percentage of the methemoglobin in the patient
B. Rate of accumulation of methemoglobin
C. Ability of the patient to clear the methemoglobin
D. Underlying health status of the patient

Percentage of methemoglobin can be calculated as (the concentration of the methemoglobin)/(concentration of total hemoglobin). Percentage of methemoglobin is better indicator as compared to overall hemoglobin concentration, as for example, concentration of methemoglobin of 1.5 g/dL is only 10% in normal subject with baseline hemoglobin concentration 15 g/dL, but in case of anemic person with hemoglobin of 8 g/dL methemoglobin 1.5 g/dL is amount to 18.75%.

EVALUATION

A. Pulse oxymetry: It may be falsely low and the diagnostic clue is refractory hypoxemia.
B. Arterial blood gases—PaO_2 normal and it will rule out hypoxemia.
C. C-oximetry: It is the definitive test measures total hemoglobin can differentiate oxyhemoglobin, oxyhemoglobin, and carboxyhemoglobin.

   If methemoglobin more than 1 to 2%—abnormal, if it is more than 10% to 15%—patient is symptomatic and if it is more than 70%—very severe.
D. NADPH methemoglobin reductase activity - should be measured.
E. Hemoglobin electrophoresis demonstrates hemoglobin M.

Treatment

Methylene blue reacts rapidly with the secondary pathway of reduction of methemoglobin where NADPH-MetHb reductase will reduce the methylene blue to leukomethylene blue which acts an electron donor thereby reducing the methemoglobin to hemoglobin. Dose of methylene blue is 1 to 2 mg/Kg intravenously over 5 minutes and can be repeated within 1 hour.

Q89. Unstable hemoglobin

NTR UNI of Health SC, Vijayawada, Andhra, 2022 (10)

ANSWER

Definition

Unstable hemoglobin is a group of inherited blood disorders characterized by formation of unstable hemoglobin molecules leading to its precipitation within the inner membrane of the red blood cells as a consequence of mutation in the genetic coding.

Genetic Basis of Unstable Hemoglobin

Beta globin gene (HBB) or alfa globin genes (HBA1 and HBA2) are present in the chromosome number 11 and 16 respectively. Following types of genetic mutation are seen:
A. Missense mutation where there is substitution of single nucleotide leading to changes in the amino acid sequences
B. Deletion of the nucleotide od addition of one nucleotide leads to abnormal length of the protein.
C. Stop codon mutation leads to truncated or elongated chains of nucleotide.

Effect of this mutation:
A. There is alteration of the quaternary or tertiary structure of the hemoglobin.
B. Interaction between the heme and globin chains will be destabilized.
C. There is precipitation of the unstable hemoglobin in the red blood cells leading to formation of Heinz bodies, as a result RBC becomes fragile and there is intravascular or extravascular hemolysis.

Examples of unstable hemoglobin:
A. Hb Koln—Mutation in β28 valine to methionine
B. Hb Zurich—Mutation of β63 histidine to arginine
C. Hb Gun Hill—Deletion of β121

Clinical Features

A. Hemolytic anemia
B. Jaundice
C. Splenomegaly
D. Severity depends unstable hemoglobinopathies depends upon specific types of mutations and the stability of the hemoglobin variant.

Diagnosis

A. Microcytic normochromic anemia
B. Heinz bodies—precipitation of hemoglobin

Treatment

A. Supportive therapy
B. Blood transfusion in moderate to severe cases
C. Supplementation of folic acids

Q90. Tumor markers in clinical practice.

NTR UNI of Health SC, Vijayawada, 2020 (10)

Discuss the role of tumor markers in clinical practice.

WBUHS, 2023 (10)

ANSWER

It has been discussed in question number 124 in updated general metabolism, poisoning chapter.

Q91. Functions of neutrophils.

MGR University, Tamil Nadu, 2020 (5)

ANSWER

Following are the functions of the neutrophils:

A. Phagocytosis: Neutrophils engulf bacteria, fungi and cellular debris producing phagosome which fuses with lysozymes to form phagolysozymes and digest them.
B. Neutrophils contains primary antimicrobial granules containing various enzymes like myeloperoxidase, defensins and lysozymes, and secondary granules like lactoferrin and collagenase and tertiary granules like gelatinase, antimicrobial peptides which are released to kill the pathogenic bacteria.
C. Neutrophils produce superoxide, hydrogen peroxide and hypochlorous acids which are toxic to microbes thereby kill the bacteria.
D. Neutrophils release their proteins and DNA leading to formation of neutrophil extracellular traps which trap the pathogens and kill them.
E. Neutrophils release signaling molecules which recruit the other inflammatory cells and proinflammatory cytokines like interleukin 1β and tumor necrosis factor and chemokines like interleukin-8 at the site of injury.
F. Neutrophils clear the damaged cellular debris and release growth factors leading to repairing of the tissues.
G. Neutrophils react and thereby modulates the function of the dendritic cells, T cells and macrophages leading to development of adaptive and innate immunity.
H. Prolonged activation of neutrophils leads to tissue damage as seen in case of autoimmune diseases and sepsis.

Section 3 Pancreatology

Q1. Autoimmune pancreatitis.

PGI/APR2014 (10)

Describe the pathophysiology and clinical features of autoimmune hepatitis. Discuss the management of autoimmune hepatitis.

DNB (JUN2022) (10)

Diagnostic approach to acute pancreatitis in a 57-year-old lady.

ALLMS, BHU 2020 (10)

ANSWER

Definition

It can be defined as autoimmune disorder involving pancreas with its characteristic histologic, chemical, and morphological manifestation with or without autoimmune involvement of other organs, like bile duct, lymph node, and retroperitoneum. It is also known as nonalcoholic duct destructive pancreatitis, sclerosing pancreatitis, and tumefactive pancreatitis.

Histological Findings

Characteristic findings are:

A. Extensive inflammatory infiltrates extending transmurally and around small veins and nerves containing lymphocytes, plasma cells, polymorphonuclear leukocytes, and sparing of epithelial cells.
B. Dense fibrosis
C. Obliterative phlebitis
D. Varying parenchymal atrophy
E. Pancreatic duct becomes slit-like or star-shaped

Histological Classification of Autoimmune Pancreatitis

Two types:

A. Type 1 autoimmune pancreatitis: It is characterized by:
   a. More than 10 immunoglobulin G_4 (IgG_4) plasma cells
   b. Lymphoplasmacytic sclerosing pancreatitis
   c. Periductal lymphoplasmacytic infiltrate
   d. Obliterative phlebitis
   e. Dense fibrosis
   f. Relapse rate is very high
B. Type 2 autoimmune pancreatitis:
   a. Minimal IgG_4 plasma cells
   b. Granulocytic epithelial cell infiltration
   c. Relapse rate is low as compared to type 1

Clinical Features

A. Males:female (2:1)
B. Abdominal pain may be mild
C. Features of obstructive jaundice
D. Weight loss
E. Associated feature other extrapancreatic autoimmune diseases, like:
   a. Rheumatoid arthritis
   b. Sjögren syndrome
   c. Ulcerative colitis
   d. Autoimmune thyroiditis
   e. Retroperitoneal fibrosis
   f. Mediastinal adenopathy

Laboratory Findings

A. Features of obstructive jaundice, like minimal increase in aminotransferases level with marked elevated alkaline phosphatase

B. Elevated level of IgG_4—but:
- **a.** Its amount can differentiate type 1 and 2 autoimmune pancreatitis
- **b.** Its level will decrease during treatment with corticosteroid

C. Interleukin-10 producing CD4+ and CD25 high Tregs is positively correlated with IgG4 autoimmune pancreatitis

D. Antibodies to plasminogen binding protein peptide in 19–20% of patients

Imaging Studies

A. Computed tomography (CT):
- **a.** Diffuse or focal enlargement or normal
- **b.** Lack of vascular encasement
- **c.** Calcification and peripancreatic fluid
- **d.** Stranding in the pancreas
- **e.** Enlarged peripancreatic lymph node

B. Endoscopic retrograde cholangiopancreatography (ERCP):
- **a.** Stricture of common bile duct (CBD) or proximal bile duct or intrahepatic duct or in combination
- **b.** Stricture of pancreatic duct
- **c.** Sclerosing pancreatitis

C. Magnetic resonance imaging (MRI): Rim-like encasement of pancreatic head

D. Endoscopic ultrasound: Irregular focal or diffuse hypoechoic pancreatic enlargement

Treatment

A. Corticosteroid therapy:

Following are the clinical parameters:
- **a.** Symptoms relief
- **b.** Serial changes in abdominal imaging of bile duct and pancreas
- **c.** Decreased IgG_4
- **d.** Improvement in liver test

Dosage: 40 mg/day for 4 weeks with gradual tapering of dosage by 5 mg/week based on the above clinical parameters.

Response: 50–70% patients will respond to this drug but 20% patients require second dose.

B. Immunomodulatory drugs:
- **a.** Drugs studied in patients relapsed after withdrawal of steroids are mycophenolate mofetil, azathioprine, and cyclophosphamide but with varying response.
- **b.** Monoclonal antibody rituximab was tried in patient's refractory to steroid and 6 mercaptopurine.

Q2. Causes, diagnostic evaluation, and complication of acute severe pancreatitis.

DNBIIIB/DEC2015 (10)

Discuss the etiopathogenesis, clinical manifestation, lab diagnosis, management and complications of acute pancreatitis.

MGR/APR2015/MDIV (15)

Adverse factors in acute pancreatitis. Discuss autoimmune pancreatitis.

MGR/OCT2012 MDIV (7)

Discuss the etiology, pathogenesis, course of the disease, laboratory data, diagnosis, treatment and complications of acute pancreatitis.

MGR/SEP2008/MDIV (20)

Discuss the clinical features, complications, diagnosis and management of acute pancreatitis.

MGR/OCT2003/MDI (15)

Indicating the severity of acute pancreatitis.

PGI/APR2014/MDII (10)

Assessment of severity in acute pancreatitis.

PGI/APR2013/MDIII (10)

Discuss the etiopathogenesis, complications and management of a case of acute pancreatitis.

BF/OCT2010/MDII (30)

Medical causes. Diagnosis and treatment of drug induced acute pancreatitis.

KUHS/MAY2013/MDIII (10)

Describe functions of pancreas and complications and management of acute pancreatitis.

ERA/MAY2012/MDII (10)

Acute pancreatitis.

MUZ/MAY/2016/MDIV (6)

Classify acute pancreatitis. Write down the causes, severity markers, and complications.

DNB (DEC2021)(10)

Causes and complications of acute pancreatitis.

DNB (DEC2019) (4)

Acute pancreatitis – pathophysiology, clinical, diagnosis, management, and complication.

SCBMCH, 2009 (20)

Enlist the causes of acute pancreatitis. Discuss the complications and management of acute pancreatitis.

DNB 2024, MAY(10)

Describe etiology, pathophysiology, clinical features, and management of acute pancreatitis.

NTR UNI of Health SC, Vijayawada, 2020 (10)

Ranson criteria for prediction of pancreatitis mortality.

Sarada Patel University, 2019 (5)

Write clinical features, complications, and management of acute pancreatitis. Write in short about recent advantages in treatment modalities.

Bharati Vidyapeeth Deemed UNI, Jhelum, 2019 (15)

Management of acute pancreatitis.

Teerthanker Mahaveer University, 2018 (10)

Risk factors and management of acute pancreatitis.

Manipur University, 2018 (10)

Describe the clinical pathophysiology of acute pancreatitis. How will you manage a case of acute pancreatitis.

Manipur University, 2021 (10)

Describe the physiology of pancreatic exocrine function. Enumerate the acute complications and management of acute pancreatitis.

Manipur University, 2021 (10)

Write assessment and management of acute pancreatitis in first 72 hours.

WBUHS, 2020 (10)

ANSWER

Pancreatic exocrine functions have been described in question number 4.

Introduction

Acute pancreatitis can be defined as an inflammatory condition of functionally and morphologically normal pancreas. According to Atlanta classification system it can be defined as "an acute inflammatory process of the pancreas with variable involvement of regional tissues or remote organ systems."

Etiopathogenesis

A. Common causes:
- **a.** Gallstones of <5 cm in diameter
- **b.** Acute or chronic alcoholism
- **c.** Hypertriglyceridemia: When serum triglyceride level is >1,000 mg/dL. It may be associated with disordered lipid metabolism
- **d.** ERCP induced, it can be reduced by use of rectal nonsteroidal anti-inflammatory drugs (NSAIDs) and indomethacin
- **e.** Deficiency of apolipoprotein CII: This will activate lipoprotein lipase and it is important for clearing of chylomicron from the blood
- **f.** Trauma
- **g.** Drugs:
  1. Azathioprine
  2. Estrogen
  3. 6-mercaptopurine
  4. Valproic acid

B. Uncommon causes:
- **a.** Hypercalcemia
- **b.** Pancreatic carcinoma
- **c.** Pancreatic divisum

- **d.** Hereditary pancreatitis
- **e.** Cystic fibrosis
- **f.** Infections:
  - **1.** Measles
  - **2.** Mumps
  - **3.** Echovirus
  - **4.** Coxsackievirus
- **g.** Type 1 and 2 autoimmune pancreatitis

C. Causes producing recurrent acute pancreatitis without any obvious etiology:
- **a.** Alcoholism
- **b.** Hereditary pancreatitis
- **c.** Intraductal papillary mucinous neoplasm
- **d.** Drugs
- **e.** Autoimmune causes
- **f.** Metabolic causes:
  - **1.** Hypertriglyceridemia
  - **2.** Hypercalcemia
- **g.** Idiopathic

In case of ERCP-induced pancreatitis following are the risk factors:

- **A.** Sphincterotomy of minor papilla
- **B.** Dysfunction of sphincter of Oddi
- **C.** Previous history of ERCP-induced pancreatitis
- **D.** Age is <60 years
- **E.** More than 2 injection of contrast into pancreatic duct
- **F.** Involvement of endoscopic trainee

There are three theories regarding the development of acute pancreatitis:

A. Common channel theory: According to this theory as the ampulla of vater is obstructed with gallstone the accumulated bile beyond the stone enters into the pancreatic duct producing inflammation of pancreatic tissue leading to acute pancreatitis.

B. Second theory: As the stone passes through the ampulla of vater the valve becomes incompetent, so the duodenal reflux will enter through the incompetent valve into the pancreatic duct producing pancreatic inflammation leading to acute pancreatitis.

C. Third theory or autodigestion theory: According to this theory if pancreatic stone obstruct the pancreatic duct accumulated proteolytic enzymes, like trypsinogen, chymotrypsinogen, proelastase, and lipolytic enzymes like phospholipase A_2 will be activated in the acinar cells of pancreas not in the interstitial lumen. Following factors enhance this mechanism:
- **a.** Oxidative stress
- **b.** Lysosomal calcium
- **c.** Direct trauma
- **d.** Exotoxins
- **e.** Endotoxins
- **f.** Ischemia
- **g.** Viral infections

Activated enzymes mainly trypsin will digest both pancreatic and peripancreatic tissues and also further activate other enzyme.

Effects of pancreatic enzymes in the development of acute pancreatitis:

Acute pancreatitis occurs in three phases:

A. In the initial phase lysosomal hydrolases like cathepsin B will be colocalized in the pancreatic organelles and activate pancreatic proteolytic enzyme trypsin leading to injury to acinar cells.

B. In the second phase there is activation, chemoattraction followed by sequestration of neutrophils and macrophages in the pancreatic tissues leading to pancreatic inflammation. Neutrophils also activate trypsin. So, there are two steps in the activation of trypsin, first one is neutrophil-independent process and second one is neutrophil-dependent process.

C. In the third phase due to released cytokines and activated enzymes digest cellular membrane leading to proteolysis, interstitial hemorrhage, edema, coagulation and fat necrosis, and vascular damages which ultimately produce pancreatic necrosis. As a result of cellular death following substances are released:
- **a.** Bradykinins
- **b.** Vasoactive substances
- **c.** Histamine

These substances are responsible for:
- **a.** Vasodilatation
- **b.** Increased vascular permeability
- **c.** Effect on different vital organs in the body:
  - **1.** Acute lung injury
  - **2.** Systemic inflammatory response syndrome (SIRS)
  - **3.** Multiorgan failure

Clinical Features

Symptoms:

A. Abdominal pain:
- **a.** Site: It will start in in both upper quadrants but may start in lower abdomen
- **b.** Onset is acute

c. Referred pain will go to mid-central back, chest, flanks, and lower abdomen
d. Character: It is boring knife-like. It is gradually progressive and ultimately becomes constant.
e. Relieving factors: Pain will be diminished in upright position, leaning forward and on lateral side with knee drawing forward.

B. Nausea and vomiting:
a. Vomitus: It contains food particles and bilious fluid.
b. There is associated retching which may lead to tear in the lower end of esophagus producing Mallory-Weiss tear.
c. It can be relieved by introduction of nasogastric tube into stomach cavity which can decompress the stomach and at the same time reduces abdominal pain.

C. Low-grade fever

Signs:
A. Raised temperature
B. Tachycardia
C. Hypotension
D. Shock: It is unusual but may result from:
a. Exudation of blood and plasma proteins into retroperitoneal space resulting hypovolemia
b. Large amount of Kinin peptides released produce increased vascular permeability as well as vasodilatation.
c. Systemic effect of lipolytic and proteolytic enzymes released into circulation.

E. Jaundice: It occurs in case of:
a. Pancreatic head involvement as it will compress the intrapancreatic portion of CBD
b. Stone in the CBD as a cause of obstruction.

F. Erythematous nodules in the skin due to subcutaneous fat necrosis.
G. Pulmonary features:
a. Crepitations
b. Left-sided pleural effusion
c. Atelectasis

H. Abdominal features:
a. Upper abdomen is tender with or without a swelling with muscle guard and rigidity in variable degree.
b. Bowel sound is absent or diminished.
c. Grey Turner sign: It is due to ecchymoses in the flank due to retroperitoneal bleeding.
d. Cullen sign: It is due to periumbilical ecchymoses due to retroperitoneal bleeding.

I. Carpopedal spasm due to hypocalcemia
J. Drowsiness due to:
a. Drug
b. Hypoxemia
c. Alcohol abuse
d. Release of cytokines from pancreas
e. Hypotension

Laboratory Investigations

A. Hematological investigations:
a. Leukocytosis (15,000–20,000/cc)
b. In severe cases hemoconcentration with hematocrit value of >44%.

B. Biochemical investigations:
a. Amylase: In pancreatitis serum isoamylase is specific and sensitive. However, threefold rise in amylase level in serum in absence of perforation, ischemia, or gut infarction is diagnostic of acute pancreatitis. It will be elevated within few hours of the onset and in uncomplicated cases it will be elevated up to 5 days.
b. Lipase: In this disease sensitivity and specificity of elevated serum lipase is 85% and 100%. Three times of the normal level is diagnostic of acute pancreatitis and it will be elevated for 7–14 days after onset. Its elevation can differentiate from other causes of hyperamylasemia.
c. Other pancreatic enzymes like phospholipase A, carboxypeptidase A, colipase elastase, and phospholipase A2 can be measured but cannot be available.
d. Hyperglycemia: It may occur due to:
1. Decreased release of insulin
2. Increased glucagon release
3. Increased release of catecholamine and corticosteroids
e. Hypocalcemia: It may occur due to:
1. Decreased response of parathyroid gland to low calcium level.
2. In the areas of fat necrosis intraperitoneal saponification of calcium by fatty acids
f. Serum bilirubin >4 g/dL in 10% of patient with involvement of pancreatic head.
g. If associated elevation occurs in serum alkaline phosphatase and aspartate aminotransferase—it indicates gallbladder related or pancreatic head-related disease.

h. Hypertriglyceridemia: It occurs in 5–10% patients.
i. Hypoxemia with PO_2 level ≤ 60% suggests onset of acute respiratory distress syndrome (ARDS).
j. Serum markers of acute pancreatitis:
   1. Trypsinogen activation peptide measurement in urine is useful as it activates trypsinogen to trypsin in the early event in acute pancreatitis.
   2. Polymorphonuclear elastase
   3. Procalcitonin
   4. Pancreatic-associated protein
   5. Interleukin-1, -6, and -8—sensitivity is about 74–90%.
   6. Other nonspecific markers are C-reactive protein (CRP), complement levels, and tumor necrosis factor.

C. Radiological investigations:
   a. Chest X-ray:
      1. Left-sided pleural effusion
      2. Pulmonary infiltrates

      Both indicate pancreatic necrosis and organ failure.
   b. CT scan of abdomen: It is done for severity of pancreatitis and necrosis. CT severity index of pancreatitis:

Point (A)	Grade
A. Normal pancreas	0
B. Pancreatic enlargement	1
C. Pancreatic or peripancreatic fat inflammation	2
D. Single peripancreatic fluid collection	3
E. More than 2 fluid collection and/or retroperitoneal air	4
Degree of pancreatic necrosis based on contrast CT findings (Point B)	
A. No pancreatic necrosis	0
B. Up to 30% of the gland	2
C. 30–50% of the gland	4
D. >50% of the gland	6

CT severity index (A + B):

Mild pancreatitis: 0–2

Moderate pancreatitis: 3–6

Severity pancreatitis: 7–10

   c. MRI in case pancreatitis: Features are:
      1. Fluid collection
      2. Necrotic pancreatic parenchyma
      3. Hemorrhagic foci
      4. Disruption of pancreatic duct

According to revised Atlanta criteria morphologic variation of acute pancreatitis by CT scan:

A. Interstitial edematous pancreatitis:
   a. Definition: Acute inflammation of pancreatic parenchyma as well as peripancreatic tissues but without recognizable necrosis of the tissue.
   b. CT criteria:
      1. Enhancement of pancreatic parenchyma by intravenous contrast agent.
      2. No findings of peripancreatic necrosis

B. Necrotizing pancreatitis:
   a. Definition: Inflammation associated with pancreatic and/or peripancreatic necrosis.
   b. CT scan criteria: Lack of pancreatic parenchymal enhancement by intravenous contrast agent and/or presence of findings of peripancreatic necrosis (see below—acute necrotic collection and walled off necrosis).

C. Acute pancreatic fluid collection:
   a. Peripancreatic fluid-associated interstitial edematous pancreatitis with no associated peripancreatic necrosis. This term is applied to only areas of peripancreatic fluid seen within first 4 weeks after the onset of interstitial edematous pancreatitis and without the features of a pseudocyst.
   b. CT scan criteria:
      1. It occurs in the setting of interstitial edematous pancreatitis.
      2. Homogeneous collection with fluid density
      3. It is confined by normal peripancreatic fascial planes.
      4. No definable wall encapsulating the collection
      5. Adjacent to pancreas but no intrapancreatic extension

D. Pancreatic pseudocyst:
   a. Definition: It is characterized by encapsulated collection of fluid having well-defined inflammatory wall usually outside the pancreas with minimal or no necrosis which occurs >4 weeks after the onset of interstitial edematous pancreatitis.
   b. CT scan criteria:
      1. Fluid density is homogeneous.
      2. Absence of nonliquid component
      3. Wall is well-defined and completely encapsulated.
      4. It requires >4 weeks to become mature after the onset of acute pancreatitis.

E. Acute necrotic collection:

a. Definition: A collection containing variable amounts of fluid as well as necrotic tissue associated with necrotizing pancreatitis. This necrosis can involve pancreatic parenchyma and/or peripancreatic tissue.

b. CT scan criteria:

1. It occurs in the setting of acute necrotizing pancreatitis.
2. Heterogenous and nonliquid density of varying degrees in different locations
3. No definable wall for encapsulating the collection
4. Collection may be intrapancreatic or extrapancreatic.

F. Walled-off necrosis:

a. Definition: It can be defined as a mature encapsulated collection of pancreatic and peripancreatic necrotic tissue that has developed a well-defined inflammatory wall occurring in >4 weeks after onset of necrotizing pancreatitis.

b. CT scan criteria:

1. Heterogenous collection with liquid and nonliquid density of varying degrees of loculations but some may appear homogenous.
2. Well-defined wall, i.e., completely encapsulated
3. This collection is extrapancreatic or intrapancreatic.
4. It will mature 4 weeks after the onset of acute necrotizing pancreatitis.

Clinical Course and Complications of Acute Pancreatitis

Revised Atlanta criteria defines acute pancreatitis into two phases:

A. Early phases of acute pancreatitis:

a. It lasts for 1–2 weeks.

b. Severity can be detected by following clinical parameters:

1. SIRS: It can be defined by presence of ≥ 2 criteria:
   - Core temperature <36°C or >38°C
   - Heart rate >90 beats/min
   - Respiratory rate >20 breaths/min or PCO_2 < 32 mm Hg.
   - White blood cell count <4,000/cc or >12,000/cc or 10% bands
2. APACHE (Acute Physiology and Chronic Health Evaluation) score II.
3. Bedside index of severity in acute pancreatitis (BISAP) score:
   - (B) Blood urea nitrogen > 25 mg/dL
   - (I) Impaired mental status
   - (S) SIRS ≥ 2 or 4 present
   - (A) Age > 60 years
   - (P) Pleural effusion
4. Organ failure (Modified Marshal Score):
   - Cardiovascular:
     - Systolic blood pressure <90 mm Hg
     - Heart rate >130 beats/min
   - Pulmonary: PaO_2 < 60 mm Hg
   - Renal: Serum creatinine > 2 mg/dL

Marker of severity of acute pancreatitis is persistent organ failure of >48 hours.

B. Late phase of acute pancreatitis:

a. It lasts for >2 weeks.

b. Important clinical parameters are:

1. Persistent organ failure
2. There may be requirement of:
   - Renal dialysis
   - Ventilatory support
   - Supplemental nutrition via parenteral or nasojejunal tube

According to revised Atlanta criteria severity of acute pancreatitis:

A. Mild acute pancreatitis:

a. No local complication
b. No organ failure
c. Patients develop acute interstitial pancreatitis.
d. It is self-limited and spontaneously subsided within 3–27 days after starting treatment.
e. Oral intake can be started if the patient becomes hungry or bowel functions normal.

B. Moderately severe pancreatitis:

a. Presence of transient organ failure which resolves within 48 hours.
b. Lack of local or systemic complications in absence of persistent organ failure.
c. Local complication may be fluid collection for which requires >1 week hospital stay.

C. Severe acute pancreatitis:

a. Persistent organ failure for >48 hours

b. There may be single or multiorgan failure.
c. In presence of local complication its management can be dictated by clinical symptoms, like infection, maturity of fluid collection.
d. Antibiotic is not recommended prophylactically.

Ranson criteria for predicting severity of acute pancreatitis:

At the time of admission	
Age	>55 years
White blood cell count	>16,000/cc
Blood glucose	>200 mg/dL
Lactate dehydrogenase	>350 U/L
Aspartate aminotransferases	>250 U/L
48 hours after admission	
Hematocrit	Fall by >10%
Blood urea antigen (1.8 mmol/L despite)	Increase by >5 mg/dL fluids
Serum calcium	<8 mg/dL
pO_2	<60 mm Hg
Base deficit	>4 mEq/L
Fluid sequestration	>6,000/mL

Treatment of Acute Pancreatitis

A. Careful monitoring of the patients:
   a. Full hemodynamic monitoring including:
      1. Heart rate
      2. Arterial blood pressure
      3. ECG
      4. Central venous pressure
      5. Hourly urine output
   b. Central line should be done in cases of:
      1. Sepsis
      2. Pulmonary complications
      3. Hemodynamically unstable patients
      4. Large volume deficit
   c. To detect complications:
      1. Complete blood count
      2. Blood biochemistry
      3. Serum electrolytes
   d. Arterial blood gases in case of any respiratory complication
   e. Serial ultrasound to evaluate any retroperitoneal complication

B. To provide relief from pain:
   a. Tramadol 100 mg intravenously 8 hourly
   b. Buprenorphine 150 µg dissolving in 10–20 mL of normal saline and to be given slowly intravenously 8 hourly via epidural catheter; it will reduce respiratory complications.

C. Correction of hemodynamic defects:
   a. Volume replacement has to be done to replenish fluid lost in the retroperitoneal space, peritoneal cavity, and intestine. In case of severe pancreatitis >8–10 Liters of fluid in the form of crystalloids or colloids have to be given with constant monitoring of central venous pressure to maintain at 12–15 mm Hg.
   b. In case of retroperitoneal hemorrhage due to extravasation of proteolytic enzymes.
   c. In case of hypoalbuminemia transfusion of 100 mL of 20% albumin can be given.
   d. In spite of adequate fluid replacement if the patient is hypotensive, ionotropic support in the form of dopamine at a rate of 10–15 µg/kg/min or dobutamine (if there is already vasoconstriction) or both the drugs can be administered to maximize oxygen delivery or transport. Sometimes in spite of normal arterial blood pressure adequate oxygen perfusion cannot be done. The other indicators of hypoperfusion are:
      1. Presence of lactic acidosis
      2. Low mixed venous oxygen difference <35 mm Hg.

   The results of proper fluid replacement are:
   a. Normal pulse rate and volume
   b. Normal arterial blood pressure
   c. Good urine output
   d. Improved mixed venous oxygen difference

D. Correction of metabolic abnormalities:
   a. Hypokalemia
   b. Hypoglycemia
   c. Hypocalcemia
   d. Hypomagnesemia

E. Control of secretion of pancreatic enzymes: There is no definite way of reduction of secretion of pancreatic enzymes. But there are some methods of reduction of enzyme secretion:
   a. Nasogastric suction can be done to:
      1. Reduce paralytic ileus
      2. Decrease continuous vomiting
      3. Reduce pancreatic secretion
   b. Proton pump inhibitor intravenously:
      1. It will reduce gastric acid secretion

2. It will reduce bleeding from gastric erosions
3. Reduce the pancreatic enzyme secretion

c. Somatostatin 500 μg bolus intravenously followed by continuous infusion of 250 μg over 4 hours to suppress pancreatic enzyme secretion.

F. Support of other organs:

a. Respiratory support: Ventilatory support in patients with respiratory rate >30 breaths/min or PaO_2 <60 mm Hg.

b. Renal support:

1. In patients with low urine output low-dose dopamine should be given.
2. In patients with increasing level of urea and creatinine temporary hemodialysis or hemofiltration should be done.

G. Nutritional support: In case of acute pancreatitis all oral feeds have to be stopped as intragastric and intradudenal contents will stimulate pancreas. So, first priority is:

a. Restitution of fluid and electrolyte loss
b. Stability of hemodynamic conditions

Recently two types of nutrition are offered to these patients:

a. Total enteral nutrition through nasojejunal tube to early use of gut will help in the following:

1. Maintaining the integrity of the small intestine
2. It will prevent translocation of intestinal bacteria into pancreatic tissue as it will prevent infection and mortality and morbidity.

b. Total parenteral nutrition through central line in case of fulminating pancreatitis where early oral nutrition is not possible at all because it is associated with:

1. Paralytic ileus
2. Vomiting
3. Peritonitis
4. Severe sepsis
5. Abdominal distension

But there is grave danger of catheter-induced infection in these patients on parenteral nutrition.

Criteria of starting oral feedings are:

1. Absence of abdominal pain
2. Normalization of pancreatic amylase and lipase
3. Absence of complications like pancreatic fistulas
4. Returning of bowel sounds

H. Administration of antibiotics: Gram-negative infections are present in retroperitoneal necrotic area and occur in case of fulminating pancreatitis. The antibiotics of choice are:

a. Third-generation cephalosporins
b. Metronidazole
c. Ciprofloxacin
d. Aminoglycosides
e. Imipenem and meropenem

Complications of Pancreatitis

A. Pancreatic necrosis: In case of acute pancreatitis devitalization of pancreatic tissue leading to necrosis within few days to few weeks of onset of the disease.

Pathophysiology:

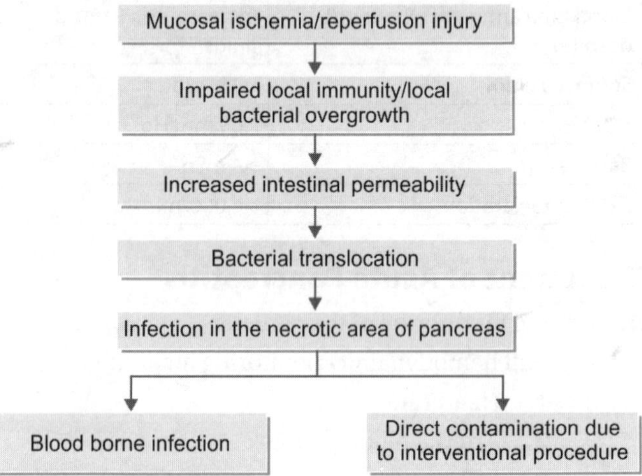

Clinical features: Persistent low-grade fever, abdominal pain, and leukocytosis

Fate:

a. <1 cm: It will resolve spontaneously.
b. 2–4 cm: It is demarcated by macrophages which gradually phagocytose necrotic material and inner content becomes liquefied.
c. >5 cm: Here macrophages are rich in hemosiderin and other immune cells forming a layer of granulation tissue within 20 days from onset which becomes thickened producing fibrotic capsule. Necrotic area is gradually resolved and replaced by fibrotic tissue.

Diagnosis: It can be diagnosed by contrast-enhanced CT (CECT) scan, MRI, and endoscopic ultrasound.

Prognostic markers are CRP, IL-6, polymorphonuclear elastase, phospholipase A2, procalcitonin, and urinary trypsinogen-activating peptide.

B. Pancreatic pseudocyst: It is characterized by collection of fluid within well-defined capsule presenting after 4 weeks of onset containing no capsule.

Location: It is close proximity to pancreas but it can extend to paracolic gutter, pelvis, scrotum, mediastinum, and thorax.

Composition: Wall is thick fibrotic capsule but no epithelial lining. Fluid concentration is similar to that of plasma with high concentration of amylase, lipase, and enterokinase. In case of hemorrhage fluid may contain blood clot, becomes xanthochromic.

Pathophysiology:

Acute pancreatitis: Necrosis

Chronic pancreatitis: Elevated intraductal pressure from stricture and calculi.

Trauma:

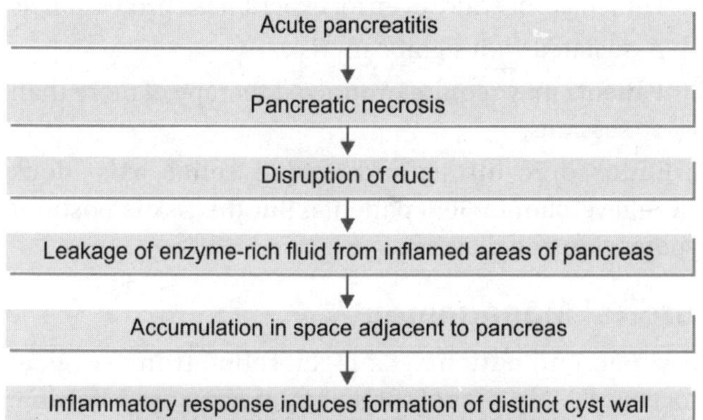

D'edigo classification of pancreatic pseudocyst:

Type	Context	Pancreatic duct	Duct—pseudocyst communication
I	Acute postnecrotic pancreatitis	Normal	No
II	Acute on chronic pancreatitis	Abnormal (no stricture)	50:50
III	Chronic pancreatitis	Abnormal (stricture)	Yes

Presentation:

Persistent abdominal pain, early satiety, nausea, vomiting, bloating, anorexia, weight loss, and abdominal mass.

Signs are tenderness and abdominal fullness.

Complications:

Infections—abscess

Rupture—into gut producing gastrointestinal bleeding, into peritoneum producing peritonitis

Enlargement producing pressure—obstructive jaundice, bowel obstruction

Erosion to vessel—hemorrhage into the cyst, hemoperitoneum

Diagnosis:

75–90% by ultrasound

100% by CECT

Triphasic CT scan can delineate arteries and veins.

MRI can delineate solid component of the lesion.

ERCP

MRCP

C. Pancreatic fat necrosis

D. Systemic complications:

- **a.** Acute liver failure
- **b.** Acute renal failure
- **c.** Adult respiratory distress syndrome
- **d.** Disseminated intravascular coagulation (DIC)
- **e.** Encephalopathy
- **f.** Gut ischemia
- **g.** Paralytic ileus
- **h.** Hypocalcemia
- **i.** Shock

Q3. Management of chronic pancreatitis and its complications.

BF/NOV2013/MDII (10)

Chronic pancreatitis.

MGR/MAR2010/MDII (6)

Discuss tests of exocrine pancreatic function. Describe the complications of chronic pancreatitis.

DNB (JUN2022) (10)

ANSWER

Exocrine functions are discussed in question number 4.

Management of Pain in Chronic Pancreatitis

A. Acid-suppressing agents:

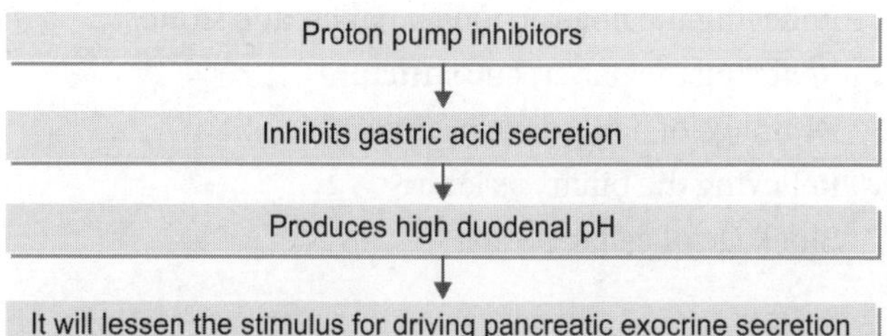

B. Analgesic and pain modulators: It is like three step ladder of WHO for relief of cancer pain:

  a. Step 1: In case of mild-to-moderate pain: Nonopioid analgesic

  b. Step 2: In case of moderate-to-severe pain opioid like analgesic like dextromethorphan, tramadol.

  c. Step 3: Morphine

C. Octreotide: It is somatostatin analog; it will reduce cholecystokinin level.

D. Supplementation of pancreatic enzymes:

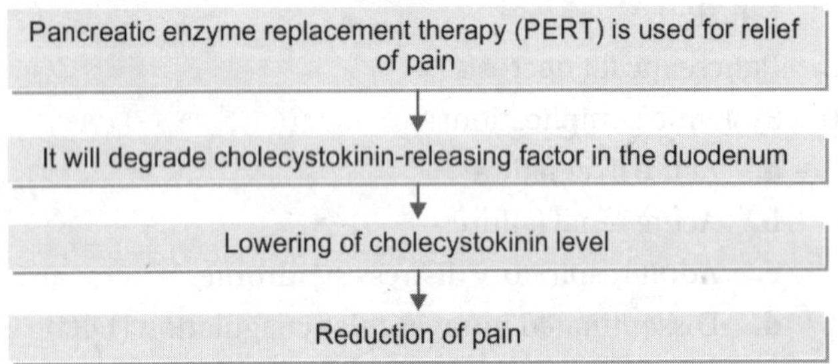

E. Antioxidants:

  a. It will reduce the oxidative stress thus improves pain

  b. It will supply micronutrients thus improves the quality-of-life.

  c. Supplied micronutrients may halt the progress of chronic pancreatitis.

F. Blockage of nerve plexus: Visceral afferent from celiac ganglia present adjacent to aorta at the level of celiac trunk below the diaphragm, then it courses along the sympathetic nerve, crosses the midline to follow the path of splanchnic nerves and synapses in the dorsal root ganglia and sends in the dorsal horn of spinal cord. So, celiac plexus or splanchnic nerves can be blocked by:

  a. Injection of anesthetics or corticosteroids for temporary block—celiac axis block

  b. Injection of absolute alcohol for destroying celiac plexus permanently—celiac axis neurolysis. This effect will last for 24 months. Risks of blockage are diarrhea and postural hypotension.

Endoscopic Management

Goal of endotherapy:

A. Relieving the obstruction by pancreatic stones

B. Relieving the pancreatic structure

C. Drainage of pancreatic pseudocyst

D. Relieving the biliary stricture

E. Blockage of celiac plexus

Endotherapy is:

A. Biliary sphincterotomy

B. Dilatation of stricture and stenting

C. Extraction of stones

D. Lithotripsy

Pain may be relieved after stenting but this procedure is associated with following complications:

A. Blockage of stent

B. Migration of stones

C. Development of new strictures

According to European Society of Gastroenterology in asymptomatic as well as uncomplicated patients with chronic pancreatitis endotherapy is not useful.

Extracorporeal shock wave lithotripsy: It is a difficult procedure for pancreatic stones but it is:

A. Difficult procedure even for experienced professionals

B. Associated with significant risk

C. Patients may require protracted therapy of more than 10 sessions.

Endoscopic ultrasound-guided celiac axis block will relieve pain in 50% patients. But the risk is postural hypotension and diarrhea.

Surgical Management

Fifty percent patients can get relief from surgical procedure. Main aims of surgical treatments are following:

A. To ameliorate intractable pain

B. To treat local complications

C. To preserve exocrine and endocrine functions

D. To improve exocrine and endocrine functions

In case of dilated and obstructed pancreatic duct—drainage and decompression of the duct.

In case of dominant inflammatory mass resection of the mass is recommended.

In absence of above two features no definite option is present.

A. Drainage procedure:

  a. Procedure is lateral pancreatico-jejunostomy (modified Puestow-Gillesby procedure): In this procedure pancreatic duct is drained in presence of multiple pancreatic strictures or multiple stones without performing distal pancreatectomy and splenectomy.

  b. Aim is to decompress intrapancreatic ductal and parenchymal pressure.

  c. But following conditions have to be fulfilled:

    1. Pancreatic ductal diameter will be at least 7 mm in diameter.

2. There is absence of inflammatory mass in the pancreas.

d. It is associated with low mortality.

B. Resection procedure: Pancreatic head is recognized as pacemaker of the disease process, so resection of pancreatic head in patient with nondilated pancreatic duct is option of surgical management. Procedures are:

a. Duodenum-preserving pancreatic head resection (Beger procedure): It will remove the inflammatory areas but preserves upper gastrointestinal tract because duodenum is very essential for regulation of glucose metabolism. Indications are:

1. CBD obstruction
2. Pancreatic duct stenosis
3. Obstruction of retroperitoneal vessels by inflammatory mass removal

Procedure-related mortality is 0–2%.

b. Total pancreatectomy with islet cell autotransplantation is of future choice in case of diffuse inflammatory process.

C. Resection and drainage procedure:

a. Frey procedure: It is modified duodenum-preserving pancreatic head resection procedure where longitudinal pancreatico-jejunostomy with local resection of head of pancreas being performed. It will reduce pain in 90% patients.

b. Izbicki procedure: Here "V"-shaped excision of ventral part of pancreas along with drainage of secondary and tertiary duct into Roux loop of jejunum is performed.

Management of Pancreatic Insufficiency

In case of pancreatic exocrine insufficiency there is decreased secretion of bicarbonate and digestive enzymes which affect >50% patients with chronic pancreatitis and it will develop when more than 90% of pancreatic exocrine function will be lost. This exocrine function insufficiency is characterized by:

A. Steatorrhea
B. Weight loss
C. Vitamin and mineral deficiency
D. Metabolic bone disease
E. Signs of malnutrition

This can be diagnosed by:

A. Fecal elastase—<200 μg/g of stool is specific
B. Serum trypsin—<20 μg/mL

Treatment is enteric-coated capsule containing lipase 10,000–25,000 IU. Normally with each main meal 90,000 USP units of lipase is excreted from pancreas. So, starting dose is 40,000–50,000 USP units of lipase with each meal and half of that dose is for snacks time. Along with this proton pump inhibitors has to be given to suppress the gastric acid as pancreatic lipase is irreversibly inactivated at pH below 4.

So, in this case low-fat diet is not recommended to reduce steatorrhea as it may produce deficiencies of fat-soluble vitamin.

Management of Diabetes Mellitus

Diabetes due to chronic pancreatitis is also known as type 3c diabetes mellitus or pancreatogenic diabetes mellitus which occurs due to total loss of islet cell mass and this type of diabetes is resistant to ketosis. Another characteristic in these patients that they are more susceptable to hypoglycemia as counter-regulatory hormones like glucagon and pancreatic polypeptide will be lost. These patients are at risk of secondary pancreatic carcinoma and this can be reduced by insulin-sensitizing agent like metformin. Again in patients with exocrine insufficiency higher level of gut hormones like GLP-1 reduces the efficacy of insulin secretagogues and incretin drugs. So, in this case administration of enzymes can improve this condition.

Q4. Exocrine function of pancreas.

MGR/OCT2014/MDI (5)

Write physiology of secretion of pancreatic enzymes and their functions in normal metabolism.

Manipur University, 2019 (10)

ANSWER

Daily secretion is 1,200–1,500 mL. It is colorless fluid.

pH is 7.8–8.4 due to high bicarbonate concentration. It is 4–5 times that of plasma concentration.

Electrolytes:

Cations: Sodium, potassium, calcium, magnesium, and zinc.

Anions: Bicarbonate, chloride, and sulfate

Enzymes:

A. Pancreatic α-amylase: It will break α-1-4 glycosidic bonds in the starch and digest boiled and unboiled starch to maltose.

B. Pancreatic lipase: In the pH between 7 and 9 hydrolyses neutral fats to glycerol esters and fatty acids.

   Another pancreatic lipase which is known as bile salt-activated lipase will catalyze the hydrolysis of cholesterol esters, triglyceride, and phospholipids.

C. Pancreatic esterase: It will convert cholesterol esters to cholesterol.

D. Pancreatic pro-phospholipase A2: It will be activated to phospholipase A2 by trypsin and this phospholipase A2 splits a fatty acid off from the lecithin to form lysolecithin and it will damage the cell membrane.

E. Pancreatic proteolytic enzymes:
   - **a.** Trypsinogen: It will be activated to trypsin with the help of enterokinase released from duodenal mucosa and also activated by trypsin itself as autocatalyst to form active trypsin. It will hydrolyze proteins by splitting the bonds containing L-lysine and L-arginine to form small peptides and some amino acids by hydrolyzing dipeptides also.
   - **b.** Chymotrypsinogen: It will be activated to chymotrypsin catalyzed by trypsin and digests protein to small peptides.
   - **c.** Procarboxypeptidase A and B: These will be activated to carboxypeptidase A and B by enterokinase along with trypsin and split removes amino acids stepwise from carboxyl group which is present at the end of peptide chain.
   - **d.** Ribonuclease
   - **e.** Deoxyribonuclease: It will split nucleic acids of ribose and deoxyribose.
   - **f.** Proelastase: It will be broken down to elastase by trypsin and it will convert elastin into simplified substances.

Regulation of pancreatic juice is done by two mechanisms:

A. Nervous regulation: Stimulation of vagus nerve produces:
   - **a.** Secretion of enzyme-rich pancreatic juice
   - **b.** Causes disappearance of zymogen granules from the glandular cells.

B. Humoral regulation: It can be done by two gastrointestinal hormones:
   - **a.** Secretin:
     1. Will act on the ductal cells in the pancreatic gland to produce the flow of alkaline enzyme-poor pancreatic juice.
     2. It will also stimulate secretion of bile.
     3. It will potentiate the effect of cholecystokinin-pancreozymin.
     4. It will constrict pyloric sphincter and delay the gastric emptying.
   - **b.** Cholecystokinin-pancreozymin:
     1. It causes contraction of gallbladder and release bile.
     2. It will secrete enzyme-rich pancreatic juice by discharging zymogen granules from acinar cells of pancreas.
     3. It produces trophic effect on the pancreas.

Q5. Development of pancreas.

MGR/MAY2011/MDI (5)

A. Formation: At approximately 5 weeks of gestation pancreas first appears as two outpouchings of endodermal lining of the duodenum distal to newly forming stomach, one is dorsal bud and the other is ventral bud; dorsal bud grows rapidly as compared to ventral bud.

B. Rotation: Again ventral bud rotates toward dorsal bud and is carried by CBD.

C. Ultimately dorsal and ventral buds fuse along with ductal system so that secretion from ventral bud enters the shared ductal system of ventral pancreas as well as CBD. At last pancreatic head forms from ventral and dorsal pancreatic bud, ventral portion is called uncinated process and body and tail will be originated from dorsal pancreas.

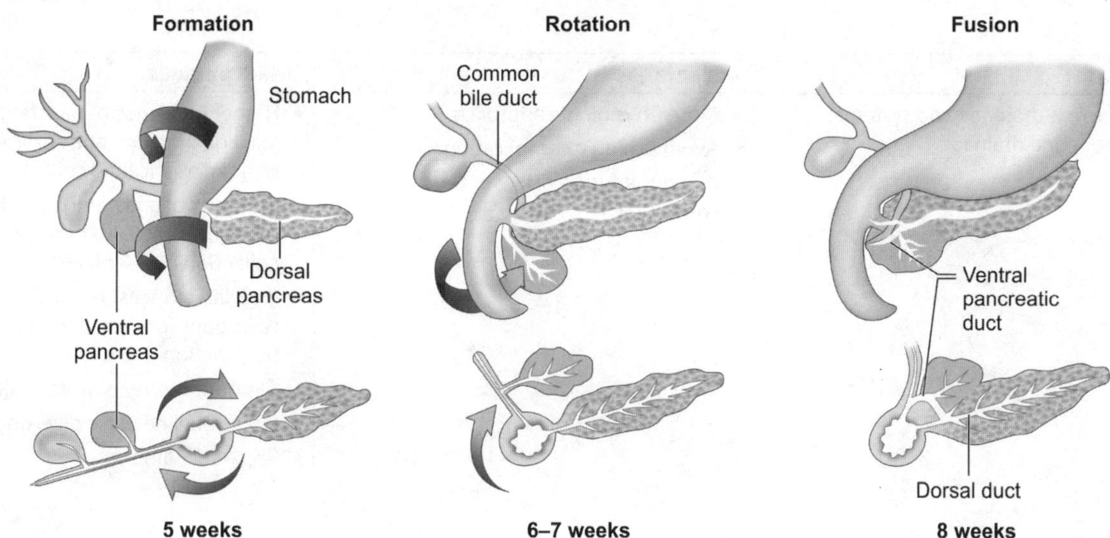

Signaling pathways for pancreatic development are:

A. Hedgehog system: Inhibition of this system will lead to ectopic budding of pancreas into the stomach and duodenum.

B. Homeobox gene Pdx1 pathways: Its expression in the duodenum will mark the location of development of pancreatic bud.

C. Notch signaling pathways: It will inhibit differentiation of endocrine cells and promotes differentiation of exocrine cells. Its blocking will do the reverse.

Q6. Pancreatic transplantation.

MGR/MAR2010/MDII (7)

ANSWER

Pancreas transplantation was first done in 1966 in University by William Kelly and Richard Lilleheiat. There are three modes of pancreas transplantation:

A. In case type 2 diabetes mellitus with end-stage kidney disease there is simultaneous kidney and pancreas transplantation.

B. In case type 1 diabetes mellitus with successful transplantation of kidney allograft pancreas can be transplanted after kidney transplantation. Here the patient has to face surgical risk twice but it is highly recommended.

C. Pancreas transplantation alone and here only pancreas transplantation will show good result.

Procedure	Advantages	Disadvantages
Bladder exocrine drainage and systemic venous endocrine drainage	• Pancreatic dysfunction can be detected early by changes of urinary amylase • Easley accessible for biopsy • Reduced rate of infection due to the relative sterility of the lower urinary tract • Technical considerations (bladder vasculature promote healing, bladder mobilization permits tension-free, multi-layer anastomosis, control of anastomotic leakage can be achieved by bladder catheter)	• Fluid and electrolyte imbalance • Metabolic acidosis • Urologic complications (cystitis, hematuria, urethritis, balanitis and urethral stricture) • Lower urinary tract infection and stone formation • Reflux pancreatitis • Enteric conversion if indicated will expose the patient to another major surgery

Contined

Contined

Procedure	Advantages	Disadvantages
Enteric exocrine drainage and systemic venous endocrine drainage 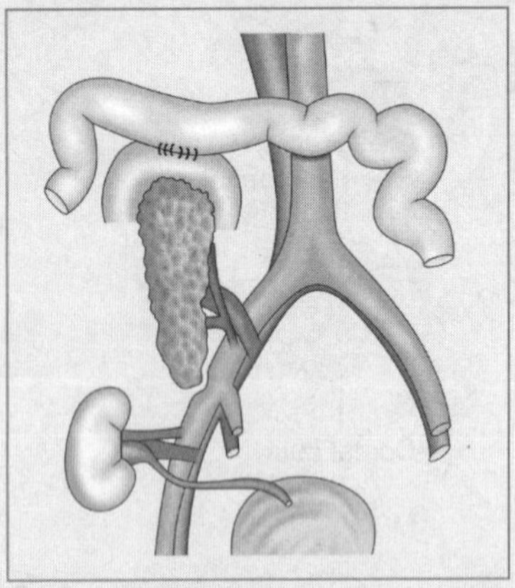	• More physiologic approach • Avoid urologic complications • Avoid the future risk of enteric conversion	• Higher incidence of pancreatitis, leakage of pancreatic enzymes, and peripancreatic fluid collections • More risk of anastomotic leakage, peritonitis, intra-abdominal collection and sepsis • Inability to measure exocrine secretions for early detection of graft dysfunction • Allograft biopsy is more challenging • Occasional need for diverting • Roux-en-Y limb
Enteric exocrine drainage and portal venous endocrine drainage 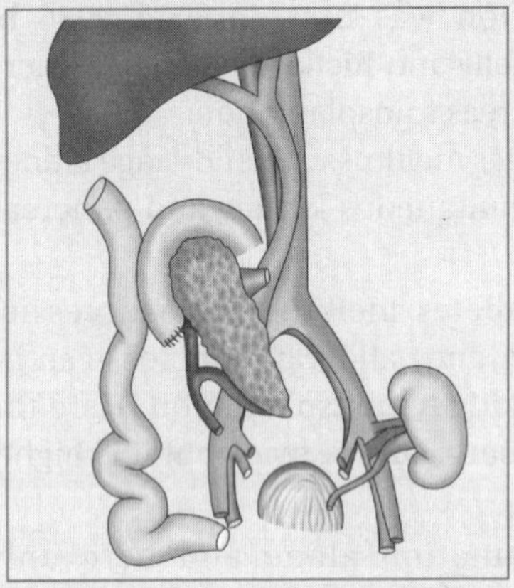	Same advantages mentioned above in addition to: • Avoid the risk of postprandial hypoglycemia • Better lipoprotein metabolism	Same points as mentioned above in addition to: Higher risk of vascular thrombosis
Duodenal exocrine drainage and systemic venous endocrine drainage 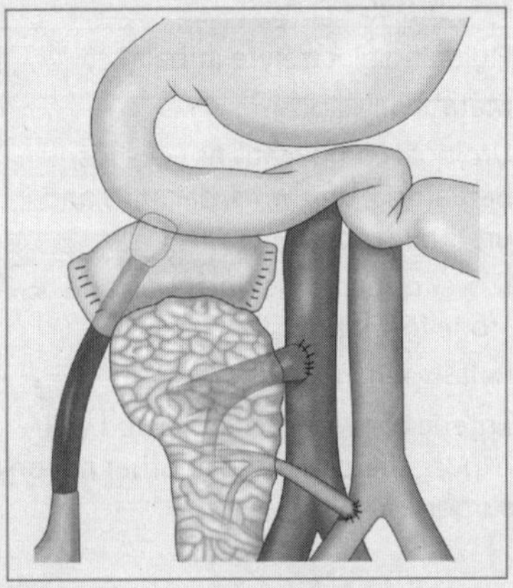	A modification of enteric exocrine drainage with systemic venous endocrine drainage with additional benefits in the form of: • Improved accessibility for biopsy via endoscopy • It expands the options for exocrine drainage sites, especially in cases of pancreas retransplantation	Same disadvantages mentioned above with enteric exocrine drainage and systemic venous endocrine drainage except for relatively easily accessible allograft

Complications of pancreas transplantation:

Post-transplant early complication	
Allograft parenchymal complications	Acute pancreatitis
	Necrotizing pancreatitis
	Fistulous tracts
Infections with or without abscesses	
Enteric complications	Ileus colonic infection
	Anastomotic leakage at duodenoenterostomy
Vascular complications	Acute bleeding
	Venous and arterial graft thrombosis
Post-transplant late complications	
Allograft parenchymal complications	Pseudocyst formation
	Rejection
	Post-transplant lymphoproliferative disease
Enteric complications	Obstruction in small bowel
	Colonic infection
Vascular complications	Arterial and venous thromboembolism

Post-transplant immunosuppression: Induction and maintenance immunosuppression has to be given recently:

A. For induction therapy: Antilymphocyte serum like daclizumab (anti-CD25 antibody like interleukin-2 receptor) plus basiliximab. Now this therapy has been shifted toward T-lymphocyte depleting agents like alemtuzumab and thymoglobulin.

B. For maintenance therapy: Prednisolone, mycophenolate mofetil, and tacrolimus (calcineurin inhibitor). Nowadays sirolimus and everolimus are found to be effective in case of simultaneous pancreas and kidney transplantation to avoid kidney-related complications.

Islet cell transplantation is the emerging technique for management of type 1 diabetes.
In this method:

A. First collection of islet cells from the donor's whole pancreas

B. Next is the infusion of these isolated cells into the portal vein of the recipient through percutaneous catheter.

Since endocrine cells are a small scattered part of cells as compared to large number of exocrine cells hence this requires only minimal invasive technique thus avoid vascular and allograft duodenal anastomoses.

Q7. Artificial pancreas.

Baba Farid UNI of Health SC, 2018 (10)

ANSWER

Definition

Artificial pancreas is a closed-loop insulin delivery system that automatically adjust and monitor the serum blood glucose levels in patients suffering from type 1 diabetes mellitus.

Types of Artificial Pancreas

A. Hybrid closed loop system that automatically adjust basal insulin but the patient can adjust insulin doses during meal time. The examples are Medtronic MiniMed™, Tandem t:slim X2.

B. Fully closed loop system where it is fully automated without any type of intervention of the patients. But it bihormonal is under research.

C. Bihormonal systems which can monitor and inject both glucagon as well as insulin thereby functions like living pancreatic tissue.

D. Dual hormone with adjuncts where amylin analog is used with insulin with or without glucagon.

Evolution of Artificial Pancreas

A. Phase 1: Sensor augmented pump therapy which consists of CGM + insulin pump but absence of automated communication.

B. Phase 2: Here pump suspends before development of hypoglycemia

C. Phase 3: Hybrid closed loop monitoring

D. Phase 4: It is fully automated where insulin pump delivers both basal and bolus insulin.

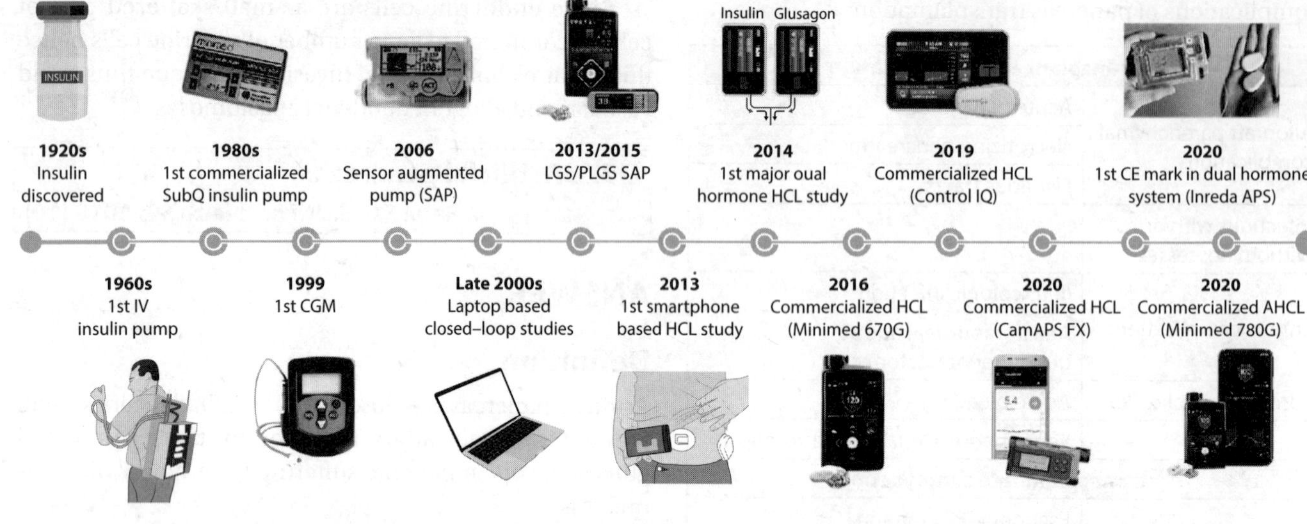

Following are the key features of sensor augmented pump and artificial pancreas system:

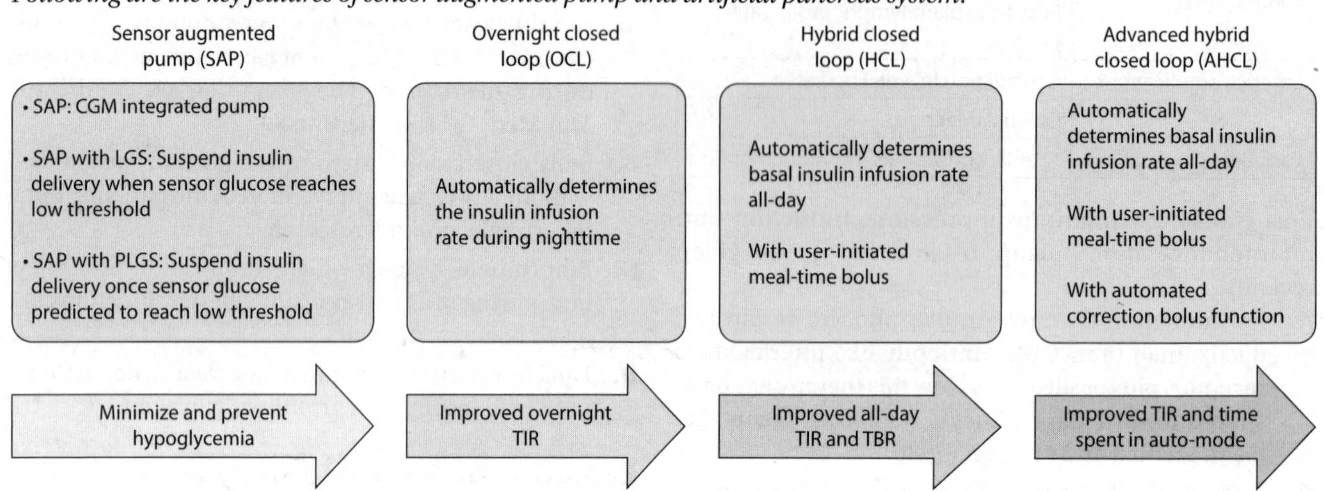

Indications of Use of Artificial Pancreas

A. Type 1 diabetes mellitus who is unaware regarding hypoglycemia but has wide glycemic variability.

B. Type 2 diabetes mellitus on intensive insulin therapy and high blood glucose variability.

C. Type 1 pregnant diabetic woman to prevent fetal complication.

D. Adolescent type 1 diabetic mellitus.

Advantages of Artificial Pancreas

A. It will improve the glycemic control

B. Decreased incidence of glycemic variability

C. It will reduce the episodes of hypoglycemia

D. Patient develops better quality of life.

E. It will prevent long term diabetic complication.

Section 4 Gastroenterology

Q1. Causes and diagnostic evaluation of a patient with acute diarrhea.

DNBI/DEC2010 (10)

Discuss etiology, pathophysiology, clinical features, and management of viral gastroenteritis.

MGR/OCT2015/MDIII (15)

Viral gastroenteritis in pediatrics.

MGR/APR2015/MDIV (7)
MGR/OCT2013/MDIV (7)

ANSWER

Normally 10 L of fluid enters into the jejunum of which 9 L will be absorbed and 1 L will enter into colon. Normal stool output is 100–200 g/day.

Diarrhea is a constellation of the following symptoms:

A. Increase in stool frequency more than 3 times per day

B. Increase in stool volume

C. Decrease in stool consistency

Acute Diarrhea

It is an adverse reaction of many inciting events, such as infection, drug reaction, ischemia, and inflammatory bowel disease (IBD). It can be defined as the presence of diarrhea for <4 weeks.

Causes of acute infective diarrhea are:

Viruses	Bacteria	Protozoa
Rotavirus	*Salmonella*	*Entamoeba histolytica*
Norwalk virus	*Shigella*	*Giardia lamblia*
Corona virus	*Campylobacter*	*Cryptosporidium*
Cytomegalovirus	*Yersinia*	*Cyclospora*
Enteric adenovirus	Enteropathogenic *Escherichia coli*	
Herpes simplex virus	Enteroinvasive *E. coli*	
	Enterohemorrhagic *E. coli*	
	Enterotoxigenic *E. coli*	
	Vibrio cholerae	
	Clostridium perfringens	
	Staphylococcus aureus	

Causes of acute diarrhea due to drugs:

A. Clindamycin

B. Amoxycillin

C. Ampicillin

D. Cephalosporin

Evaluation of a Patient with Acute Diarrhea

Classification of infective organisms according to clinical presentation:

Clinical types of presentation	Likely organisms
Watery diarrhea or noninflammatory diarrhea	Rotavirus, Enterotoxigenic *E. coli*, *Campylobacter jejuni*, Enteropathogenic *E. coli*
Dysentery	*Shigella*, Enteroinvasive *E. coli*, *Entamoeba histolytica*, *Campylobacter jejuni*
Protracted diarrhea	*Giardia*, Enteropathogenic *E. coli*, *Yersinia enterocolitica*
Rice water-like stool	*Vibrio cholerae*, Enteropathogenic *E. coli*
Hemorrhagic colitis	Enterohemorrhagic *E. coli*

Infectious diarrhea:

Onset	Characteristics	Duration	Etiology	Source	Lab tests
1–6 hours	Abdominal pain, nausea, vomiting	1–2 days	*Staphylococcus aureus*	Poorly freezed meat, egg, cream pastries	Stool and vomitus for toxins
10–48 hours	Fever, muscle ache, spontaneous abortion, still birth	Varies	*Listeria monocytogenes*	Hot dogs, unpasteurized milk, soft cheese	Not specified
10–72 hours	• Blurred vision • Diplopia • Vomiting	Varies	*Clostridium botulinum*	Poorly canned food, low acid, honey	Stool for toxin, organism
24–48 hours	• Blood and mucus in stool • Cramping abdominal pain	4–7 days	*Shigella* Shiga	Fecal contamination of water and food	Stool for culture and sensitivity
	• Vomiting, diarrhea • Cramping abdominal pain, fever	1–3 weeks	*Yersinia enterocolitica*	Unpasteurized milk, undercooked food	Stool culture
	Watery diarrhea, nausea, vomiting	1–3 days	Norwalk virus	Undercooked salads, fruits and shellfish	Serum antibody titer
1–3 days	Bloody diarrhea, abdominal cramp, fever	2–10 days	*Campylobacter jejuni*	• Unpasteurized milk, contaminated water • Undercooked poultry food	Stool culture
	Rice water diarrhea, vomiting	3–7 days	*Vibrio cholerae*	Shellfish, contaminated water	Stool culture
	Low-grade fever, watery stool, vomiting	4–7 days	Rotavirus	Fecal contaminated foods	Stool for rotaviral antigen
	Cramp, fever with chills, vomiting	4–8 days	*Salmonella paratyphi*	Contaminated egg, water, unpasteurized food	Blood and stool for culture
	Abdominal cramp, vomiting, watery stool	3–7 days	Enterotoxigenic *E. coli*	Fecal contaminated water, food, contact with farm animal	Stool culture
1–8 days	• Bloody diarrhea • Abdominal cramp	5–10 days	Enterohemorrhagic *E. coli*	Unpasteurized milk and juice, undercooked beef	Stool culture
1–12 days	Relapsing diarrhea, weight loss, fatigue	Several weeks to months	*Cyclospora cayetanensis*	Contaminated berries, water and lettuce	Stool culture; During examination under ultraviolet epifluorescence microscopy, evidence of autofluorescence
1–4 weeks	Abdominal bloating, flatulence	Several weeks	Giardia	Contaminated water and foods	Stool for parasites and ova
1–10 weeks	Bloody watery with mucus involving colon, abdominal cramps, fever (pseudomembranous enterocolitis)	Varies	*Clostridium difficile*	Overuse of clindamycin, cephalosporin; inadequate hand hygiene	Stool for toxins by ELISA test
1–10 days	Abdominal cramping, alternate constipation and diarrhea, may be asymptomatic	Several weeks with varying features	*Entamoeba histolytica*	Contaminated food	Stool for trophozoites; serological test for antibody in the serum detected by immunoagglutination or hemagglutination test

Continued

Continued

Onset	Characteristics	Duration	Etiology	Source	Lab tests
1–5 days	Profuse and prolonged diarrhea	2 weeks	*Cryptosporidium parvum*	Immunocompromised host	Immunofluorescence of stool sample demonstrates acid fast stain, PCR testing
7 days	Acute profuse diarrhea	1–2 weeks but may vary	*Isospora belli*	Immunocompromised host, but may be self-limited in case of immunocompetent person	• Small bowel biopsy • Stool for microscopy
5–7 days	Malabsorption, watery stool, nausea and vomiting	1–2 weeks	Microsporidia	Opportunistic infection	Modified Trichome staining of stool sample
1–7 days	Abdominal cramping, mucoid stool	15 days	*Entamoeba histolytica*, Giardia	Ingestion of contaminated water, history of travel, stress, consumption of contaminated food	Microscopy of stool, stool culture

Noninflammatory diarrhea is characterized by:

A. Defect is in the water and electrolyte transport.
B. Pathogens will adhere to the mucosal surface of the small intestine without invasion of the epithelium and produce enterotoxins; thus there is minimal or less mucosal inflammation.
C. Large volume of >1 L/day stool
D. Presence of nausea and vomiting
E. Presence of cramping abdominal pain
F. Absence of fever and systemic signs of illness
G. Absence of blood and pus in the stool
H. Patient will be dehydrated with loss of large amount of electrolytes
I. Presence of right lower quadrant pain with diarrhea suggestive of *Yersinia enterocolitica*

Inflammatory diarrhea is characterized by the following:

A. Direct invasion of intestinal mucosa by the pathogens or inflammatory response resulting from cytotoxins produced by the pathogens. As a result of inflammation, there is formation of ulcers in the colon leading to loss of protein, mucus, and blood into the lumen.
B. Frequent small volume bloody stool
C. Presence of periumbilical cramping abdominal pain in case of small intestinal diarrhea and hypogastric cramping in case of colonic diarrhea.
D. Presence of tenesmus in case of rectal involvement
E. Less watery but more mucoid with or without blood in case of colonic involvement
F. Presence of spiking fever, systemic inflammatory response
G. Patient is less likely dehydrated.

Q2. Discuss irritable bowel syndrome with respect to pathophysiology, clinical presentation, and management.

DNBIII/DEC2010 (10)

What is irritable bowel syndrome? What are the warning signs in a patient with irritable bowel syndrome? Management of irritable bowel syndrome.

DNBII/2016 (10)

Irritable bowel syndrome.

MGR/OCT2013/MDIV (7)

MUHS/MAY2011/MDIII (10)

Describe the definition, clinical features, etiopathogenesis, diagnosis, and management of irritable bowel syndrome.

MGR/MAR2002/MDI (25)

Enumerate functional bowel disorders. Describe the diagnostic criteria, pathophysiology, and recent advances in the therapy of irritable bowel syndrome.

MGR/MAR2007/MDI (15)

What is ROME-IV diagnostic criteria for diagnosing irritable bowel syndrome? Discuss the newer agents introduced for treating IBS.

DNB (DEC2020) (10)

Describe the diagnostic criteria for irritable bowel syndrome. Discuss its pathophysiology and its treatment.

DNB (JUN2022) (10)

Write down the ROME-4 diagnostic criteria for IBS. Discuss the management of IBS.

AIIMS, BBS, 2023 (10)

What are the somatization syndromes? List the diagnostic criteria and management of irritable bowel syndrome.

AIIMS, BBS, 2022 (10)

Recent advances in management of irritable bowel syndrome.

DELHI UNI, 2024 (10)

Irritable bowel syndrome.

SCBMCH, 2020 (10); MAHARASHTRA UNI OF HEALTH SC, VIJAYAWADA, 2021 (10)

ANSWER

Definition

Irritable bowel syndrome (IBS) is a functional disorder characterized by abdominal cramping with changes in bowel habit due to alteration in visceral hypersensitivity, motility, altered processing of peripheral stimuli by the central nervous system, and psychological factors.

Clinical features will follow Rome diagnostic criteria IV.

Diagnostic Criteria (Rome IV)

Presence of abdominal pain for at least 1 day/week in last 3 months associated with any two of the following features:

A. Change in frequency of stool
B. Change in form of the stool
C. Related to defecation

Above criteria should be fulfilled for last 3 months with symptoms onset and at least 6 months prior to diagnosis.

Bristol Stool Forming Scale

A. Type 1: Stool is separated hard lumps like nut, and it is very hard to pass.
B. Type 2: Stool shape is sausage-like, but it is lumpy.
C. Type 3: Stool is sausage-shaped, but there are cracks on the surface of stool.
D. Type 4: Stool is snake-like and soft.
E. Type 5: Stool is soft, blobs having clear-cut edges, and it is passed easily.
F. Type 6: Stool is fluffy pieces having ragged edges; it is mushy stool.
G. Type 7: Stool is watery, entirely liquid.

Types of irritable bowel symptoms on the basis of predominant stool form:

A. IBS-C: It can be diagnosed by:
   a. Bristol stool scale of 1 or 2 in more the 25% of bowel movements or
   b. Bristol stool scale of 6 or 7 in less than 25% of bowel movements.
B. IBS-D: It can be diagnosed by:
   a. Bristol stool scale of 6 or 7 in more than 25% of bowel movements or
   b. Bristol stool scale of 1 or 2 in less than 25% of bowel movements.
C. Mixed IBS or IBS-M: It can be diagnosed by:
   a. Bristol stool scale of 1 or 2 in more than 25% of bowel movements or
   b. Bristol stool scale of 6 or 7 in more than 25% of bowel movements.
D. Unsubtyped IBS: When the criteria will meet any one of the above criteria.

Alarming features of IBS:

A. Male sex
B. Age > 50 years
C. Short history of symptoms
D. Nocturnal symptoms
E. Rectal bleeding
F. Anemia
G. Family history of colonic cancer
H. Recent antibiotic use
I. Unexplained weight loss
J. Family history of IBD

Associated nongastrointestinal symptoms:

A. Lethargy
B. Backache

C. Headache

D. Urinary symptoms:

- **a.** Frequency of micturition
- **b.** Nocturia
- **c.** Urgency of micturition
- **d.** Incomplete emptying of bladder

E. Dyspareunia in women

Other associated diseases:

A. Fibromyalgia

B. Chronic fatigue syndrome

C. Disorders in the temporomandibular joint

D. Chronic pelvic pain

E. Somatic disorders:

- **a.** Mood disorder
- **b.** Anxiety
- **c.** Neuroticism

F. Adverse life event

G. Increased health care seeking

Pathophysiology

A. Hereditary and genetics:

- **a.** Up to 33% of the patients with IBS have a family history of IBS.
- **b.** There is a high rate of IBS in case of monozygotic twins as compared to dizygotic twins.
- **c.** There is an association of functional polymorphism of *SERT* gene and IBS-D.

B. Abnormalities in the motility of gastrointestinal tract:

- **a.** If the motility is increased, it produces diarrhea; if it is decreased, it is constipation. Ileum, colon, and rectum are more responsive to stress and meals.
- **b.** If the amplitude is high, it produces diarrhea associated with abdominal pain; if low and infrequent, it produces constipation.
- **c.** Reduced gas retention from pharmacologic therapy will improve symptoms.

C. Visceral hypersensitivity: Gastrointestinal tract has hypersensitivity to the following:

- **a.** Gas
- **b.** Fluid
- **c.** Regular contraction of the tract
- **d.** Balloon distension of rectum—it will lower pain threshold

As a result, patient will complain of bloating in spite of low volume of gas due to visceral hypersensitivity.

Combination of both peripheral and central nervous systems is responsible for IBS.

- **a.** Peripheral nervous system: As a result of inflammation, a mixture of inflammatory mediators, leukotrienes, prostaglandins, cytokines, etc., acts on nociceptor terminals, which leads to intracellular signaling activation resulting in hypersensitivity and excitability.
- **b.** Increased excitability of spinal neurons both recruits and amplifies nociceptive and non-nociceptive stimuli to gut.

D. Brain–gut axis: This axis is based on neural, endocrine, and neuroimmune pathways and constitutes:

- **a.** Enteric nervous system and gut wall in the periphery
- **b.** Central nervous system
- **c.** Hypothalamic–pituitary–adrenal axis

Neuronal pathways involve:

- **a.** Afferent pathways, which originate from the dorsal root ganglia of T1–T10 of spinal cord and project to cerebral cortex, cingulate, insular, and amygdala areas.
- **b.** Efferent fibers originating from nuclei of brainstem and S2–S4 level of spinal cord carrying parasympathetic sensation and lateral horn cells of T1–L3 carrying sympathetic sensation to smooth muscles and gland

Main pain signaling pathways are:

- **a.** Spinothalamic tract
- **b.** Dorsal columns with descending supraspinal afferents, which originate from the rostral part of ventral medulla

In physiological condition, signals from food intake, digestion, and sensation from gut will go to the brain, which in turn send efferent signal to control motility, immune function, and secretion. Structural and functional disruption of brain–gut axis will change perceptual and reflexive responses of the central nervous system leading to IBS, which can be aggravated in presence of comorbid conditions and psychiatric disorders.

E. Inflammation: Microscopic inflammation in the colon and small intestine increases the level of proinflammatory cytokines, interleukins, and tumor necrosis factors (TNFs) that will change in the wall of the small intestine like:

- **a.** Lymphocytic infiltration in myenteric plexus
- **b.** Neuronal degeneration

c. Colonic mucosal lymphocytes

d. Increased expression of nitric oxide synthetase in the gut wall

F. Postinfectious IBS: Recurrent bacterial gastroenteritis will ultimately lead to six-fold increased risk of developing IBS; the organisms responsible are *E. coli* and *C. jejuni*. Risk factors are:

a. Female sex

b. Prolonged episodes of infectious diarrhea

c. Use of antibiotics

In case of IBS patients, there are fewer *Lactobacillus* and *Bifidobacterium* as compared to healthy controls. These will bind to epithelial cells and prevent the pathological organisms to bind and penetrate the intestinal barrier. These bacteria will not ferment carbohydrate to form gas that will inhibit *Clostridia* species. Probiotics stabilize the colonic bacteria by colonic fermentation leading to reduction of IBS.

G. Bacterial overgrowth: There is conflicting data regarding the bacterial overgrowth in IBS because there is an abnormal breath hydrogen test after giving a test dose of carbohydrate in case of IBS—it suggests bacterial overgrowth that will respond to antibiotics in IBS-D.

H. Sensitivity to foods: Following foods are responsible for diarrhea-predominant IBS:

a. Fermentable food

b. Oligosaccharides

c. Monosaccharides

d. Polyols

These foods get fermented in the distal bowel and colon to increase gas formation, which produce symptoms, such as flatulence, flatus, belching, and pain. So low fructose, low carbohydrate diet can benefit the patients with IBS-D.

Again, patients positive for gluten antibodies without evidence of villus atrophy may get benefited from gluten exclusion, but evaluation for celiac disease has to be done.

I. Psychosocial factors: Stress and psychosocial factors are strongly associated with IBS-D. At least half of the patients are hypochondriacal, anxious, or depressed.

J. Involvement of 5-HT_3 receptors: It has been shown that 5-hydroxytryptamine receptor (5-HT_3) plays an important role in development of diarrhea and perception of pain as anti-5HT_3 antagonist has an important role in the treatment of IBS-D.

Differential Diagnosis

A. Tropical sprue

B. Colonic carcinoma

C. Microscopic colitis

D. Giardiasis

E. Small bowel bacterial overgrowth

F. Bile salt malabsorption

G. Lactose malabsorption

H. Chronic pancreatitis

Diagnostic Evaluation

A. A detailed physical as well as rectal examination to exclude a pre-existing condition

B. Hematological examination: Complete blood count (CBC), erythrocyte sedimentation rate (ESR), and C-reactive protein (CRP) in case of IBS-D

C. Blood biochemistries: Antitissue transglutaminase antibody IgA, antiendomysial antibody IgG to exclude celiac disease

D. Special tests:

a. Lactose breath intolerance test and "milk challenge test" containing 25 g of lactose to exclude malabsorption. Milk challenge test lacks in specificity.

b. In case of suspected small intestinal bacterial overgrowth, hydrogen breath test should be performed.

c. Giardia can be excluded by:

1. Stool test to detect *Giardia lamblia*
2. Duodenal biopsy

d. Sudden onset of large volume diarrhea, mainly nocturnal disturbance, suggests bile salt malabsorption—it can be diagnosed by the SeHCAT (23-seleno-25-homotaurocholic acid, selenium homocholic acid taurine, or taurodeoxycholic acid) test.

e. Continuous upper abdominal pain radiating to back suggests pancreatic disease; it can be diagnosed by:

1. 24-hour stool fat
2. Pancreatic lipase
3. Abdominal spiral computerized tomography

f. In case of microscopic colitis, small intestinal biopsies should be done.

g. Right upper quadrant pain radiating to right shoulder with jaundice—deranged liver function test (LFT), amylase test, and ultrasound to detect sphincter of Oddi dysfunction.

h. History of rectal bleeding and passage of mucus per rectum in the elderly suggest colonic cancer and can be diagnosed by colonoscopy.

i. History of passage of mucus with stool and abdominal pain suggests IBD; it can be diagnosed by CBC, perinuclear antineutrophil cytoplasmic antibody (p-ANCA), cytoplasmic antineutrophil cytoplasmic antibody (c-ANCA), and colonoscopy.

j. In case of IBS-C:

1. Colonic transit time has to be studied.
2. In case of digital history of evacuation of stool at the time of defecation, anorectal manometry with balloon expulsion study should be done.

k. Other tests to be performed are CT scan of abdomen, small bowel enema, and abdominal X-rays.

Treatment

Constipation predominant symptoms:

Methylcellulose	2 g twice daily after meals
Psyllium	3.4 g twice daily after meals
Lactulose	10–20 mL twice daily
Polyethylene glycol	17 g in one glass of water to be taken. It cannot improve abdominal pain
Tegaserod	6 mg twice daily
Lubiprostone	8 µg twice daily after meals
Linaclotide	290 µg once daily. It will improve bowel movement as well as abdominal pain
Plecanatide	3 mg once daily. It will improve bowel movement as well as abdominal pain
Magnesium hydroxide	2–4 tsp once to twice daily

Diarrhea-predominant symptoms:

Loperamide	2–4 mg once daily
Diphenoxylate	1 tablet 3–4 times daily
Alosetron	1 mg twice daily (not used in USA now)
Cholestyramine	4 g with each main meal
Eluxadoline	100 mg twice daily
Colesevelam	1.875 g twice daily

Where abdominal pain is the predominant symptom:

Smooth muscle relaxants: • Mebeverine • Dicyclomine • Hyoscine • Otilonium bromide	1–3 times daily
Tricyclic antidepressants: • Amitriptyline • Clomipramine	1–50 mg at night
Serotonin reuptake inhibitors: • Fluoxetine • Citalopram • Escitalopram • Paroxetine	10–15 once daily

Somatization syndromes in the question number 60.

Q3. Lower gastrointestinal bleeding causes and management.

DNBII/JUN2011 (10)

ANSWER

Definition

Lower gastrointestinal bleeding (LGIB) can be defined as bleeding from the sites in the intestine distal to the ligament of Treitz. Clinical presentation of LGIB presents in the following forms:

A. Maroon-colored stool in case of bleeding from the right side of colon

B. Bright-red colored stool in case of bleeding from the left side of colon

C. Melena in case of bleeding from cecum

D. In case of brisk bleeding from the upper gastrointestinal tract.

Etiology

Causes of LGIB

A. Internal hemorrhoids

B. IBD

C. Colonic neoplasm

D. Diverticular disease

E. Radiation of enterocolitis

F. Vascular ectasia

G. Colonic ulceration

H. Solitary rectal ulcer syndrome
I. Post polypectomy bleeding
J. Aortoenteric fistula
K. Anastomotic bleed

Causes of Obscure LGIB Where Upper and Lower Endoscopy are Negative

A. Small intestinal vascular ectasia
B. Small intestinal adenocarcinoma
C. Small bowel stromal tumor
D. Meckel's diverticulum
E. Ectopic varices
F. Aortoenteric fistula

Causes of Occult Gastrointestinal Bleeding Where Stool for Occult Blood Test is Negative

A. Intestinal or colonic vascular ectasia
B. Colonic carcinoma
C. Hookworm infection
D. Portal gastropathy

Clinical Presentation

A. Hematochezia: It can be defined as presence of gross blood—
- **a.** Present in the toilet paper after defecation
- **b.** Mixed with blood
- **c.** Prior to defecation mixed with blood

B. Rectorrhagia: It can be defined as passage of bright red blood per rectum without stool.

C. Occult bleeding: It can be defined as type of bleeding that is not obvious to the patient but can be diagnosed by occult blood test in the stool. Positive test in stool indicates 2 mL of blood is lost per day.

D. Obscure gastrointestinal bleeding: It can be defined as type of bleeding whose source remains unidentified in spite of detailed endoscopic procedures.

Evaluation of patients with lower gastrointestinal bleeding from history:

A. Presence of abdominal pain:
- **a.** Ischemic colitis
- **b.** IBD

B. Change of stool caliber, weight loss, and anorexia: Clonic neoplasm

C. Painless bleeding suggests bleeding from:
- **a.** Vascular ectasia
- **b.** Internal hemorrhoids
- **c.** Diverticulosis
- **d.** Polyps
- **e.** Angiodysplasia

D. Bloody diarrhea is suggestive of:
- **a.** IBD
- **b.** Infectious colitis

E. Painful rectal bleeding suggests:
- **a.** Anal fissures
- **b.** Rectal ulcers
- **c.** Internal hemorrhoids

F. History of chronic constipation suggests: Internal hemorrhoids

G. Sudden and new onset of constipation with change in bowel habit is suggestive of: Colonic carcinoma

H. Presence of blood on toilet paper or dripping on toilet water is suggestive of:
- **a.** Anal fissure
- **b.** Hemorrhoids
- **c.** Perianal carcinoma
- **d.** Solitary rectal ulcer syndrome

I. Presence of blood coating on the surface of stool:
- **a.** Blood from anal source
- **b.** Colonic polyp

J. Presence of streak of blood on the stool or blood mixed stool:
- **a.** Left-sided colonic polyp
- **b.** Left-sided colonic malignancy

K. Presence of maroon-colored stool suggests:
- **a.** Bleeding from right side of colon
- **b.** Meckel's diverticulum
- **c.** Massive upper gastrointestinal bleeding

L. Massive upper gastrointestinal bleeding suggests:
- **a.** History of intake of nonsteroidal anti-inflammatory drugs (NSAIDs)
- **b.** Diverticular bleeding
- **c.** Small intestinal ulcer

M. Previous history of bloody diarrhea with abdominal pain in an young adult suggests IBD.

N. Presence of bloody diarrhea in elderly with evidence of hypertension and IHD suggests ischemic colitis.

O. Recent history of colonic polypectomy suggests post polypectomy bleeding.

P. Recent history of resection anastomosis of bowel suggests anastomotic bleed.

Q. Recent history of vascular surgery suggests bleeding from aortoenteric fistula.

Evaluation of lower gastrointestinal bleeding from physical examination:

A. Severe anemia suggests severe LGIB.

B. Orthostatic hypertension (fall of blood pressure of >15 mm Hg) suggests loss of 1,000 mL blood.

C. Examination of pulse: Tachycardia suggests—
  - **a.** Severe anemia
  - **b.** Severe bleeding
  - **c.** Continued bleeding

D. Examination of abdomen:
  - **a.** Tenderness suggests:
    1. IBD
    2. Ischemic colitis
    3. Infectious colitis
    4. Radiation colitis
  - **b.** Mass lesion suggests colonic neoplasm
  - **c.** Liver:
    1. Evidence of metastasis
    2. Shrunken in case of cirrhosis suggests:
       - Rectal varices
       - Portal colopathy
  - **d.** Splenomegaly suggests:
    1. Bleeding disorder
    2. Cirrhosis

E. Rectal examination:
  - **a.** Anal fissure
  - **b.** Mass lesion
  - **c.** Rectal carcinoma
  - **d.** Hemorrhoids
  - **e.** Presence of indurated area in the anal region suggests solitary rectal ulcer syndrome.

Management of Lower Gastrointestinal Bleeding

Initial management of these bleeders depend upon the severity of bleeding.

A. If the bleeding is minimal or intermittent and there is no hemodynamic compromise, in that case they can be managed as outpatients.

B. If the bleeding is severe with severe hemodynamic compromise, they should be admitted. Blood should be sent for:
  - **a.** CBC
  - **b.** Blood grouping and cross matching
  - **c.** LFT
  - **d.** Prothrombin time
  - **e.** Activated partial thromboplastin time
  - **f.** Renal profile
  - **g.** Electrolytes

Blood or blood product transfusion:
  - **a.** If thrombocytopenia (platelet count <50,000/cc)—platelet transfusion
  - **b.** If coagulopathy [international normalized ratio (INR) > 1.5]—fresh frozen plasma (FFP) as it will reverse the coagulopathy within 24 hours.
  - **c.** If it will persist >3-5 hours—large volume of FFP is required to reverse coagulopathy completely.
  - **d.** Injection vitamin K to reverse coagulopathy, but it takes at least 24 hours to reverse it.
  - **e.** In case of liver disease, injection of recombinant activated factor VII

Diagnostic procedures:

A. Upper gastrointestinal endoscopy: In 15–17% of cases of LGIB, upper gastrointestinal bleed is responsible; hence, in this case, this procedure is required to exclude this bleeding.

B. Anoscopy: It should be done prior to colonoscopy. It can diagnose:
  - **a.** Anal fissure
  - **b.** Internal hemorrhoids
  - **c.** Anal carcinoma
  - **d.** Rectal carcinoma in the lower part
  - **e.** Solitary rectal ulcer syndrome

C. Sigmoidoscopy: It can be done with minimal preparation. It can diagnose:
  - **a.** IBD
  - **b.** Anal fissure
  - **c.** Internal hemorrhoids
  - **d.** Anal carcinoma
  - **e.** Rectal carcinoma in the lower part
  - **f.** Solitary rectal ulcer syndrome

D. Long colonoscopy: It can diagnose:
  - **a.** IBD—presence of friable ulcerated mucosa with pseudopolyps formation
  - **b.** Diverticulosis
  - **c.** Vascular ectasia
  - **d.** Ischemic colitis—segmental distribution with varying degrees of damage ranging from pale mucosa with petechial bleeding to cyanotic necrotic mucosa.
  - **e.** Colonic carcinoma—ulceroproliferative growth

f. Evidence of dilated submucosal vessels in the anus:
   1. Above the dentate line—internal hemorrhoid
   2. Below the dentate line—external hemorrhoid
g. Presence of stalk with evidence of bleeding or the raw area at the polypectomy site post-polypectomy bleeding
h. Evidence of bleeding with areas of fibrosis and wall narrowing due to chronic mucosal ischemia—radiation colitis

E. Radionuclide scintigraphy: This noninvasive test can detect bleeding at a rate as low as 0.05–0.1 mL/min. There are two methods:
   a. Technetium-99m sulfur colloid—preparation is simple and rapidly cleared from circulation so repeat scan is not possible.
   b. Tecnetium-99m tagged RBC—it has a longer half-life; hence repeat scan is possible.
      These procedures are helpful in the following conditions:
      1. As a guide to surgical resection
      2. As a screening test prior to angiography

F. Angiography: It can diagnose the bleeding when the rate of bleeding is >0.5 mL/min. It is helpful for:
   a. Pharmacologic vasoconstriction
   b. Selective microembolization

   Complications of this procedure are:
   a. Development of hematoma at the site of catheterization
   b. Arterial detection
   c. Contrast reaction
   d. Catheter site infection
   e. Localized ischemia of bowel in case of micro-embolization

G. Radiological investigations:
   a. Multi-detector CT (MDCT):
      1. It is a noninvasive and quickly diagnostic tool.
      2. In case of active bleeding in the arterial phase, the contrast will be extravasated in the focal area in the intestine.

      Portal phase scan:
      1. It will help to detect the venous hemorrhage.
      2. Venous bleeding associated with tumor

   In case of active contrast extravasation, attention values in Hounsfield units can be measured to differentiate active bleeding from the clot.

   Advantages:
   1. It can delineate mesenteric vessels.
   2. It has a faster scanning time.
   3. It allows more accurate acquisition of images in both arterial and venous phases.
   4. There is improved three-dimensional display.

   Single-detector CT scan can detect bleeding rate of 0.3 mL/min.

   Multidetector CT scan can detect bleeding rate of 0.1–0.5 mL/min.

Treatment

A. Endotherapy:
   a. *Injection adrenaline 1: 10,000*:
      Advantages:
      1. Precise localization of bleeding points is not required.
      2. Several injections can be given around the bleeding points.

      Mechanism of action:
      1. Tamponade around the bleeding vessels
      2. Vasoconstriction of bleeding vessels
   b. *Bipolar or multipolar electrocoagulation (Gold probe)*:
      Advantages:
      1. Current is delivered in small area between the two electrodes at the tip of the probe.
      2. Pulse of short duration
      3. Physical pressure will produce tamponade effect.

      Disadvantages: It can stick to underlying tissue so during removal it can produce further bleeding.
   c. Argon plasma coagulation: It is a noncontact monopolar technique.
      Advantages:
      1. Due to its limited penetration, it is safe.
      2. Due to its forward and side-firing catheter, it can progress to awkward positioned lesion.
      3. It has replaced ND:YAG laser.

      Uses:
      1. Radiation-induced proctopathy
      2. Angiodysplasia
   d. Endoclips: Small vessels and mucosal vessels are ideal vessels for clipping.
      Advantages: It will stop bleeding if the vessel is closed.
   e. Banding: It can band bleeding colonic diverticula.
      Disadvantages: There is risk of perforation.

B. *Angiography*:
   a. Intra-arterial infusion of vasopressin
   b. Superselective embolization with:
      1. Gelatin sponge
      2. Microcoils
      3. Polyvinyl alcohol

   Rebleeding rate is 15–40%.

C. Surgery: It is indicated in case of massive and recurrent bleeding. But localization of site of bleeding is necessary for segmental resection.

Q4. Define chronic diarrhea. Discuss its etiology and the diagnostic approach to a case of chronic diarrhea.

DNBI/DEC2012 (10)

Describe diagnostic evaluation, clinical feature, and management of a patient with malabsorption syndrome.

DNB/DEC2011 (10)

Assessment of malabsorption.

RGUHS/MDIII (10)

Investigation for chronic diarrhea.

MGR/SEP2010/MDII (6)

Differential diagnosis, investigations, and treatment of an individual aged about 30 years coming with chronic diarrhea.

MGR/SEP2006/MDIII (20)

Write and discuss the approach to a patient of chronic diarrhea.

MUHS/MAY2013/MDIII (25)

What is malabsorption syndrome? Discuss the clinical approach to its diagnosis and principles of management.

BF/NOV2013/MDIII (10)

Write details regarding the diagnosis and management of malabsorption.

BF/OCT2011/MDII (20)

Define chronic diarrhea. Discuss its causes and management in adult patients.

BF/MAY2013/MDIII (10)

Discuss the etiology and diagnosis of malabsorption syndrome.

ERA/MAY2012/MDII (15)

Etiopathogenesis of malabsorption syndrome.

KUHS/MAY2013/MDI (10)

Malabsorption syndrome.

MGR/APR2016/MD (5)

Secretary diarrhea.

DNB (DEC2020) (5)

Etiology, workup, and treatment of malabsorption syndrome.

DNB (DEC 2019) (6)

What is stool osmotic gap? Write the classification of malabsorption syndrome. Discuss the various diagnostic tests for fat absorption.

DNB, 2024 MAY (10)

Chronic diarrhea.

NTR UNI OF HEALTH SC, VIJAYAWADA, 2021 (10)

What are the diagnostic studies in the different causes of steatorrhea?

NTR UNI OF HEALTH SC, VIJAYAWADA, 2020 (10)

Describe etiopathogenesis, clinical features, diagnosis, and management of malabsorption syndrome.

VEER NARMAD SOUTH GUJARAT UNI, 2019 (12)

Approach to chronic diarrhea.

TEERTHANKER MAHAVEER UNI, 2019 (10)

How will you approach and manage a patient with chronic diarrhea in immune-competent patient?

MANIPUR UNIVERSITY, 2019 (10)

Discuss the approach to a patient of chronic diarrhea.

WBUHS, 2023 (10)

How will you handle a case of chronic diarrhea? Write a brief management of ulcerative colitis.

WBUHS, 2020 (10)

Treatment of IBD has been discussed in question number 8.

ANSWER

Definition

Normally, 10 L of fluid enters into the jejunum, of which 9 L is absorbed and 1 L enters into colon. Normal stool output is 100–200 g/day.

Diarrhea is a constellation of symptoms:

A. Increase in stool frequency more than 3 times per day
B. Increase in stool volume
C. Decrease in stool consistency

Chronic diarrhea can be defined as passage of loose stool for more than 4 weeks.

Causes of Chronic Diarrhea

A. Inflammatory diarrhea:
- **a.** IBD
- **b.** Ischemic colitis
- **c.** Microscopic colitis
- **d.** Infectious causes:
  1. *Giardia lamblia*
  2. *Aeromonas* species
  3. Pseudomembranous enterocolitis
  4. Tuberculosis
  5. Cytomegalovirus infection
- **e.** Radiation enteritis

B. Osmotic diarrhea:
- **a.** Carbohydrate malabsorption:
  1. Lactase deficiency
  2. Pancreatic insufficiency
- **b.** Ingestion of poorly absorbed sugars, such as sorbitol and lactulose
- **c.** Use of osmotic laxatives, such as magnesium phosphate and magnesium sulfate

C. Secretary diarrhea:
- **a.** Endocrine causes:
  1. Hyperthyroidism
  2. Addison's disease
  3. Gastrinoma
  4. Pheochromocytoma
  5. Somatostatinoma
  6. Vasoactive intestinal peptide tumors (VIPoma)
  7. Drugs and poisons
- **b.** Bile salt malabsorption:
  1. Postcholecystectomy
  2. Surgical resection of terminal ileum
- **c.** Bacterial toxins
- **d.** Tumor:
  1. Villous adenoma
  2. Colonic carcinoma
- **e.** Medications: Stimulant laxatives

D. Dysmotility:
- **a.** Diabetic autonomic neuropathy
- **b.** Post-vagotomy
- **c.** IBS
- **d.** Postsympathectomy

E. Fatty acid diarrhea:
- **a.** Maldigestion:
  1. Pancreatic exocrine insufficiency
  2. Atrophic gastritis
  3. Deficiency of bile acids:
     - Resection of terminal ileum
     - Primary biliary cholangitis
     - Primary sclerosing cholangitis (PSC)
- **b.** Celiac disease
- **c.** Chronic mesenteric ischemia
- **d.** Constrictive pericarditis
- **e.** Giardia infection
- **f.** Lymphangiectasia
- **g.** Small bowel bacterial overgrowth

According to epidemiological characteristics, the following are the causes of diarrhea:

A. Traveler's diarrhea:
- **a.** Bacterial infection
- **b.** Protozoal infections, such as amebiasis and giardiasis
- **c.** Tropical sprue

B. Epidemic outbreak:
- **a.** Protozoal infections, such as cryptosporidiosis
- **b.** Epidemic idiopathic secretary diarrhea
- **c.** Viral infections, such as rotaviral diarrhea
- **d.** Bacterial infection

C. Patients with AIDS:
- **a.** Side effects of the drugs
- **b.** Lymphoma

c. Opportunistic infections, such as cryptosporidiosis, herpes simplex, cytomegalovirus, and *Mycobacterium avium* complex

D. Institutionalized patients:

a. Food poisoning

b. Tube feeding

c. *Clostridium difficile* toxin-mediated enterocolitis

d. Side effects of drugs

Diagnostic Approach in Case of Chronic Diarrhea

A. From history:

a. Age:

1. Young age:
   - Lactase deficiency
   - IBD
   - IBS
2. Adult age:
   - IBD
   - IBS
   - Colonic carcinoma

b. Duration of diarrhea:

1. <2 weeks: Acute diarrhea
2. 2–4 weeks: Persistent diarrhea
3. >4 weeks: Chronic diarrhea

c. Stool frequency:

1. More: Colonic diarrhea
2. Less: Ileal pathology

d. Volume of stool:

1. Large volume in case of small intestinal diarrhea
2. Small volume in case of large intestinal diarrhea

e. Consistency of stool:

1. Watery or soupy or greasy stool in case of small intestine
2. Presence of oily particles in the stool in maldigestion
3. Quantity of stool is small but mixed with blood and mucus:
   - IBD
   - Colonic carcinoma

f. Relation with meals:

1. Relationship with meals:
   - After prolonged fasting, diarrhea will stop—osmotic or secretary diarrhea due to fatty acid or bile acid malabsorption
   - In spite of prolonged fasting, diarrhea will continue—secretary or osmotic diarrhea

g. Diurnal variation: Nocturnal diarrhea is associated with organic disease.

h. Production of excessive flatus:

1. Bacterial overgrowth
2. Carbohydrate malabsorption
3. Poorly absorbed carbohydrate

i. Postprandial cramping abdominal pain occurs in partial intestinal obstruction in:

1. Crohn's disease (CD)
2. IBS
3. Radiation enterocolitis

j. Presence of fever:

1. HIV
2. IBD
3. Lymphoma
4. CD

k. Gradual loss of weight occurs in:

1. Intestinal malabsorption
2. IBD
3. Intestinal malignancy
4. Hyperthyroidism

l. Dietary history:

1. Intake of large quantity of carbohydrate occurs in osmotic diarrhea
2. Consumption of excessive amount of coffee
3. Excessive intake of gluten—gluten enteropathy
4. Milk absorption producing diarrhea in case of lactose intolerance

m. Drug history like following:

1. Diuretics
2. Alcohol
3. Abuse of lactose
4. Chemotherapeutic agents
5. Intake of antibiotics of more than 2 weeks

n. Sexual history: History of contact suggests HIV-associated diarrhea

o. History of travel to developing countries suggests:

1. Postinfection IBS
2. Gastrointestinal infection

p. Presence of systemic disease:

1. Hypertension
2. Diabetes
3. Collagen vascular disease

4. Systemic scleroderma
5. Amyloidosis

q. Personal history:
1. Exposure to radiation for the treatment of malignancy (total body exposure is more than 6 and pelvic radiation 3–4 Gy) suggests radiation enterocolitis.
2. Exposure to biological agents: Anti-interleukin-2 therapy
3. Exposure to chemotherapeutic agents: Daunorubicin, cytosine arabinoside therapy, 6-mercaptopurine, 5-fluorouracil, and methotrexate
4. Exposure to contaminated water and minerals—tuberculosis, giardiasis, and amebiasis
5. Intake of tobacco

r. History of previous surgery:
1. Extensive resection of ileum and right colon
2. Short resection of terminal ileum: Bile salt-induced secretory diarrhea
3. Perineal trauma with damage to sphincter: Fecal incontinence
4. Gastric or jejunoileal bypass operation suggests bacterial overgrowth.

s. Family history of:
1. IBD
2. Colonic carcinoma
3. Collagen vascular disease

B. Physical examination:

a. Anemia:
1. Iron deficiency anemia:
   - Pallor
   - Cheilosis
   - Koilonychia
2. Vitamin B12 deficiency:
   - Peripheral neuropathy
   - Glossitis
3. Protein-energy malnutrition:
   - White nails
   - Peripheral edema

b. Important physical examination:
1. Dermatitis herpetiformis: Celiac disease
2. Urticaria pigmentosa: Mastocytosis
3. Facial flushing: Carcinoid tumor
4. Macroglossia, waxy papule and pinch purpura: Amyloidosis
5. Erythema nodosum or Pyoderma gangrenosum: IBD
6. Conjunctivitis and scleritis: CD
7. Koilonychia: Iron deficiency
8. Bitot's spot and follicular hyperkeratosis: Vitamin A deficiency
9. Hyperpigmented dermatitis: Niacin deficiency
10. Acrodermatitis and scaly dermatitis: Essential fatty acid deficiency
11. Increased pigmentation in the skin, crease, inner surface of the lip and in the pressure points:
    - Addison disease
    - Whipple disease
12. Fine tremor, increased sweating, proptosis, and lid retraction: Hyperthyroidism
13. Edema: Protein-losing enteropathy
14. Angular cheilitis and malabsorption: IBD
15. Presence of oral ulcers: IBD
16. Fistulas or perineal disease: CD
17. Decreased tone of sphincter: Fecal incontinence
18. Arthralgia or arthritis, sacroiliitis:
    - *C. jejuni*
    - Common variable immunodeficiency
    - IBD
19. Lymphadenopathy and hepatosplenomegaly:
    - Lymphoma
    - HIV-induced diarrhea
20. Right-sided heart failure and enlarged hard liver: Carcinoid syndrome

c. Systemic examination:
1. Localized or generalized tenderness:
   - IBD
   - Crohn's colitis
   - Pseudomembranous enterocolitis
2. Presence of masses:
   - Lymphoma
   - Diverticulitis
   - CD
   - Intestinal tuberculosis
3. Neurological examination:
   - Cerebellar signs
   - Peripheral neuropathy
   - Posterior column signs—vitamin B12 deficiency

C. Laboratory tests:

a. CBC:

1. Macrocytic anemia suggests gastrointestinal blood loss as a result of:
   - Celiac disease or
   - IBD
2. Leukocytosis indicates:
   - Presence of infection
   - Ischemia
3. Microcytic anemia due to blood loss resulting in iron deficiency anemia:
   - IBD
   - Ischemic colitis
   - Diffuse lesion in the intestine: Whipple disease or celiac disease
4. Macrocytic anemia due to:
   - Ileal disease
   - Ileal resection
   - Intraluminal bacterial overgrowth
5. Normocytic anemia:
   - CD
   - Whipple disease
   - Intestinal lymphoma
6. Raised ESR:
   - IBD
   - Inflammatory diarrhea

b. Complete biochemical examinations:

1. Serum iron and ferritin low in case of microcytic anemia
2. Serum vitamin B12 and folic acid in macrocytic anemia
3. Low serum calcium, albumin, and vitamin D3 suggests mucosal involvement.
4. Thyroid function test—raised T4 and low TSH suggest primary hyperthyroidism.
5. Raised glucose and glycosylated hemoglobin suggests diabetes mellitus.
6. Low triglyceride level—abetalipoproteinemia
7. Low calcium and low phosphorus—vitamin D deficiency
8. Low cholesterol—severe fat malabsorption
9. Prolonged prothrombin time—vitamin K deficiency
10. Low albumin—protein-losing enteropathy
11. Low corticosteroids and raised adrenocorticotropic hormone (ACTH) suggest Addison disease
12. Abnormal LFT and prothrombin time in primary biliary cirrhosis or CLD suggests:
    - IBD
    - Celiac disease
13. Increased serum level of vasoactive intestinal polypeptide in VIPoma
14. Electrolyte abnormalities in the form of hypokalemia, hypomagnesemia, and hyponatremia suggest chronic diarrhea.
15. Serum gastrin level:
    - Raised serum gastrin >1,000 pg/mL (in absence of achlorhydria) suggests gastrinoma.
    - In equivocal cases after secretin injection, serum gastrin level >200 pg/mL is diagnostic.
16. Gastric pH <2 along with volume of gastric fluid of >140 mL in 1 hour will confirm hypersecretion suggesting gastrinoma.

c. Serological tests:

1. CRP—raised in:
   - IBD
   - Infective etiology
2. Antinuclear factor is increased in case of collagen vascular disease.
3. Anti-tissue transglutaminase antibody IgA and IgG, antiendomysial antibody positive in celiac disease
4. Anti-Saccharomyces cerevisiae antibody (ASCA) positive in CD
5. p-ANCA positive in ulcerative colitis (UC)

d. Serum protein electrophoresis:

1. IgA deficiency: Giardiasis
2. Immunoproliferative disease of intestine and intestinal lymphoma
3. Combined immunodeficiency disease associated with variable puzzled intestinal findings suggestive of HIV disease.

e. Stool test:

1. Stool volume:
   - Large volume with less mucus suggests small intestinal pathology.
   - Small volume with increased amount of mucus suggests large intestinal pathology.
2. Presence of frank or occult blood in stool suggests:
   - IBD

- Ischemic colitis
- Amebic colitis
- Colonic carcinoma

3. Stool microscopy:
   - Presence of leukocytes in stool may be suggestive of infective or inflammatory diarrhea.
   - Absence of leukocytes in stool suggests:
     - Osmotic diarrhea
     - Drug induced
     - Giardiasis
   - Stool for ova, parasite, and cyst:
     - Giardiasis
     - Amebiasis
     - Helminth infection
4. Fecal fat estimation:
   - Qualitative method: Visualization of fat globules under microscope after staining with Sudan III; presence of fat globules suggests maldigestion or malabsorption.
   - Quantitative method:
     - *Method*: Patient is asked to consume 100 g of fat per day for 3 days and stool will be collected for 3 days also.
     - Stool fat concentration of >7 g/day suggests malabsorption or maldigestion.
     - If stool fat content is 7–10 g/day, it is suggestive of malabsorption.
     - If stool fat content is >14 g/day, it indicates maldigestion due to either bile sat deficiency or chronic pancreatitis.
5. Fecal osmolar gap: It can differentiate osmotic and secretary diarrhea. Here, three data have to be measured:
   - Stool sodium
   - Stool potassium
   - Stool osmolarity

   Fecal osmotic gap can be measured as:

   $290 - 2\,[(Na^+) + (K^+)]$ mOsm/kg

   - Stool is usually isotonic to plasma. If its osmolarity is low, it suggests factitious diarrhea due to mixing of stool with water or urine.
   - In case of secretary diarrhea, osmotic gap will be <50 mOsm/kg due to presence of unabsorbed electrolytes in the intestinal lumen.
   - In case of osmotic diarrhea, osmotic gap will be >125 mOsm/kg due to retention of water in the intestine.
6. Stool pH:
   - pH of <5.3 indicates carbohydrate malabsorption.
   - pH of >6–7.5 indicates fecal loss of amino acids and fatty acids.
7. Stool for RT-PCR can detect tuberculosis, microsporidia, and coccidia.
8. Stool for ELISA can detect giardia or cryptosporidium antigen.
9. *C. difficile* toxins A and B indicate pseudomembranous enterocolitis.
10. Fecal elastase level of <200 μg/g suggests pancreatic insufficiency, but it may be falsely positive in large volume diarrhea.
11. Fecal calprotectin level will be increased in case of inflammatory diarrhea, and it will differentiate it from noninflammatory diarrhea.
12. Protein malabsorption:
    - Fecal nitrogen content estimation
    - 14C octanoic acid or 13C egg white breath test
13. Fecal alpha-1 antitrypsin is increased in case of protein-losing encephalopathy
14. Serial CD4 count in stool: If CD4 count is >200/μL, stool culture will be positive for:
    - Bacteria: Bacterial overgrowth, tuberculosis
    - Fungal: *Histoplasma*, *Cryptococcus*, *Candida*
    - Protozoal: *Entamoeba histolytica*, microsporidium, cryptosporidium
    - Viral: Cytomegalovirus, herpes virus

    If CD4 count is <200/μL, stool culture will be negative for:
    - AIDS enteropathy
    - Lymphoma
    - Kaposi sarcoma
    - Drugs—protease inhibitor

f. Urine test:

1. 5-hydroxy indole acetic acid and histamine, if increased, suggest carcinoid syndrome.

2. Vanillylmandelic acid (VMA), if increased, suggests pheochromocytoma.

g. Special tests:
   1. Lactose hydrogen breath test: Patient is asked to ingest 20–25 g of lactose. Blood is collected at 15, 30, 60, 120, and 180 minutes:
      - If the breath of hydrogen is raised by 20 ppm at 120 or 180 minutes as compared to previous values, it is indicative of lactose malabsorption.
      - If the breath of hydrogen is raised by 20 ppm at 30 or 60 minutes over the previous values, it indicates small bowel bacterial overgrowth.
   2. D-Xylose absorption test:
      - After overnight, the patient is asked to take 5–25 g of xylose in 240 mL of water and blood sample is collected at 1st and 3rd hour and urine samples in the next 5 hours. It is not metabolized and usually 25% of the dose is excreted in urine.
      - Normal values are ≥1 and ≥5 g, respectively.
      - Low excretion is seen in case of intestinal bacterial overgrowth and mucosal disease of intestine.
      - It can differentiate malabsorption from maldigestion.
      - Limitation is defective gastric emptying and disordered renal function test.
   3. Bile salts malabsorption:
      - Fecal bile acid output
      - ^{14}C taurocholate bile acid absorption
      - Selenium-75 labeled homotaurocholic acid test
   4. Schilling test: Three-stage test—
      - In case of extensive ileal disease, it will be abnormal with or without intrinsic factor because its absorption will be hampered.
      - In case of pernicious anemia, it will be abnormal without intrinsic factor, but with the addition of intrinsic factor, this test will be normal.
      - In case of small bowel bacterial overgrowth, a course of antibiotic will correct the absorption and the test will be normal.
   5. Other tests are:
      - Quantitative culture of small intestinal aspirates for bacterial overgrowth
      - ^{14}C D-xylose breath test for bacterial overgrowth
      - Glucose hydrogen breath test for bacterial overgrowth

h. Imaging studies:
   1. Straight X-ray of abdomen: Calcification is seen in case of—
      - Chronic calcific pancreatitis
      - Alcoholic pancreatitis
   2. Small intestinal follow through:
      - Dilatation of small intestine with coarsening of the mucosal pattern, fragmentation, and flocculation of barium suggests celiac disease.
      - Segmentation, narrowing, fistula formation, and string sign are suggestive of CD.
      - Small intestinal diverticulosis is suggestive of bacterial overgrowth.
      - Entero-enteric or entero-colonic fistula is suggestive of CD.
   3. Barium enema:
      - Lead-pipe, stove-pipe appearance: UC
      - Rectal sparing, skip-lesion: CD
   4. Contrast-enhanced CT (CECT) abdomen: Pancreatic calcification, distortion of parenchymal and ductal architecture, pseudocyst, and venous thrombosis suggest chronic pancreatitis.
   5. CT scan: Tumor of > 1 cm in gastrinoma triangle suggests gastrinoma.
   6. Endosonography: Presence of 5 out of 10 below criteria is suggestive of pancreatitis:
      - Parenchymal features: Atrophy, hyperechoic foci, stranding cysts, lobularity
      - Ductal features: Narrowing, dilatation, cysts, irregularity, dilatation of side branches, hyperechoic walls

i. Upper gastrointestinal endoscopy:
   1. Aspiration of small bowel aspirate for culture is the gold standard for the diagnosis of small bowel bacterial overgrowth.
   2. For biopsy:
      - Inflammation in celiac disease, CD, eosinophilic gastroenteritis, abetalipoproteinemia, amyloidosis, and mastocytosis

- Neoplasm in case of intestinal lymphoma
- Infection in case of *G. lamblia*, mycobacteria, and Whipple disease

j. Histological features of different causes of malabsorption:

1. Presence of collagenous band below the atrophic mucosa: Collagenous sprue
2. Presence of lipid accumulation in the enterocytes: Abetalipoproteinemia
3. Presence of foam cells and acid-fast bacilli: *M. avium* complex
4. Presence of PAS-positive inclusion bodies in the foamy macrophages: Whipple disease
5. Presence of infiltration of mast cells: Mastocytosis
6. Presence of ectatic lymphatic vessels: Lymphangiectasis
7. Presence of epithelioid granuloma: Tuberculosis, CD
8. Presence of parasites in the specimen: Giardiasis, strongyloidiasis

k. Double-balloon enteroscopy: It can demonstrate the following features—

1. Ulcers, stricture—CD
2. Carcinoid tumor
3. Intestinal tuberculosis
4. Biopsy from ulcers from different part of the mucosa

l. Long colonoscopy:

1. Presence of ulceration, erythema, exudates, granularity, and pseudopolyps suggests UC.
2. Presence of ileal or colonic ulceration, skip lesions with intervening normal mucosa, strictures with rectal sparing, and fistula formation suggests CD.
3. Presence of raised yellowish white 2–10 mm plaques overlying edematous rectal and sigmoid mucosa suggests pseudomembranous enterocolitis.
4. Presence of brown-black discoloration more in proximal colon with rectal and sigmoid sparing suggests prolonged use of anthraquinone-containing laxative.
5. Presence of ulcerations, thickening, and stricture at the ileocecal junction suggests tuberculosis, which can be confirmed by biopsy.

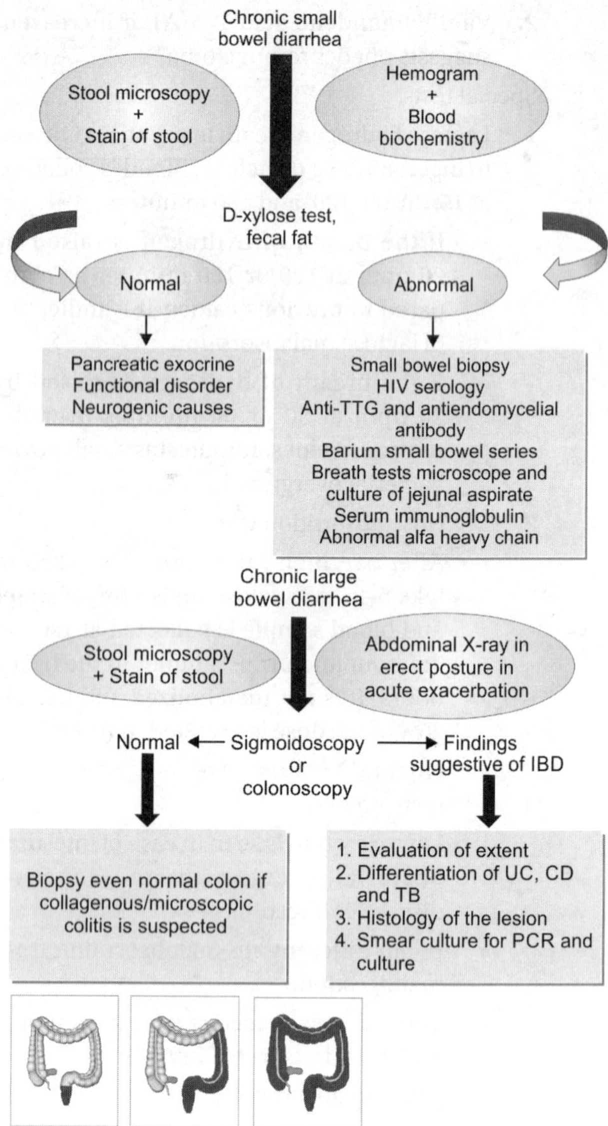

(CD: Crohn's disease; IBD: inflammatory bowel disease; PCR: polymerase chain reaction; UC: ulcerative colitis; TB: tuberculosis)

Treatment

Treatment of celiac disease is described in Question 28.

Treatment of Tropical Sprue

A. Broad-spectrum antibiotic: Tetracycline 500 mg twice daily for 6 months, but signs of improvement can be seen within 1–2 weeks.

B. Folic acid: It will improve appetite, weight, and hematological remission; it also improves small intestinal mucosa.

Treatment of Short Bowel Syndrome

Treatment depends upon:

A. Severity of symptoms

B. Whether the individual can maintain caloric and electrolyte balance

Initial treatment:

A. Initial treatment is administration of opiates to decrease the output of stool.

B. Effective diet:

- **a.** In case of colon in situ:
  1. Low-fat high-carbohydrate diet to minimize diarrhea from stimulation of fatty acids
  2. Medium-chain triglyceride
  3. Low-lactose diet
  4. Soluble fiber-containing diet
- **b.** In absence of ileocecal valve, treatment should be given for possible bacterial overgrowth.
- **c.** In case of gastric acid hypersecretion, a proton pump inhibitor (PPI) has to be given.
- **d.** In case of extensive intestinal resection, home parenteral nutrition is advised. If the patient is parenteral nutrition-dependent, in that case glucagon-like peptide 2 is given:
  1. To improve absorption
  2. To increase intestinal overgrowth
  3. To reduce the requirement of parenteral nutrition

C. Monitoring electrolytes, such as zinc, calcium, iron, and magnesium, and fat-soluble vitamins

Treatment of Bacterial Overgrowth

The first aim is to know whether the stasis or bacterial overgrowth due to the defect is surgically correctable or not.

Surgically correctable anatomical defects are:

A. Stricture

B. Diverticula

C. Proximal afferent loop

Not surgically correctable anatomical defects are:

A. Scleroderma

B. Multiple jejunal diverticulum: In this case, a broad-spectrum antibiotic, tetracycline, should be given. Other antibiotics, such as metronidazole, cephalosporin, amoxicillin-clavulanic acid, and rifaximin can be administered. Duration of treatment is 3 weeks or until the symptoms remit. It should not be repeated until recurrence of symptoms.

Treatment of Whipple disease has been discussed in Question number 32.

Treatment of Protein-losing Enteropathy

Treatment should be directed against the cause rather than to correct hypoproteinemia.

In case of lymphatic obstruction, the nature of obstruction should be searched for.

Q5. Discuss the clinical manifestation of *Helicobacter pylori* infestation, its diagnosis, and recommended treatment regimen.

DNBI/JUN2013 (10)

Role of *H. pylori* in acid peptic disease.

MGR/OCT2012/MDII (7)

Regimens for eradication of *H. pylori*.

MGR/FEB2005/MDIII (5)

***H. pylori* in acid peptic disease.**

MGR/SEP2007/MDIV (5)

Mention the risk factors for *H. pylori* infection. Outline the bacterial and host factors important in determining *H. pylori*-induced gastrointestinal disease. Summarize the potential mechanisms by which *H. pylori* may lead to gastric secretary abnormalities. Describe the recent concepts in management of *H. pylori* infection.

MGR/SEP2002/MDIII (25)

Gut hormones. Diagnostic tests for *H. pylori* infection.

DNB (DEC 2022) (10)

***Helicobacter pylori* infections.**

DR YSR UNI OF HEALTH SC, VIJAYAWADA, ANDHRA, 2022 (10)

***Helicobacter pylori* infection.**

NTR UNI OF HEALTH SC, VIJAYAWADA, 2019 (10)

***Helicobacter pylori* infection management.**

RAJIV GANDHI UNI OF HEALTH SC, KARNATAKA, 2018 (10)

Discuss refractory *H. pylori* infection.

MANIPUR UNIVERSITY, 2024 (10)

Gut hormone has been described in the question number 14.

ANSWER

Helicobacter Pylori

Helicobacter pylori is a spiral microaerophilic short-sheathed gram-negative bacterium containing flagella at one end. There are three metabolically active enzymes that characterize *H. pylori;* these are urease, catalase, and oxidase. These are important for their laboratory identification.

Prevalence of *Helicobacter Pylori*

Prevalence of this organism varies according to geographical areas, age and sex, sanitary condition, and patient's socioeconomic status. It resides in the gastric mucosa, mainly in the antrum and occasionally in the corpus, leading to inflammation, and affects gastric physiology, which may be responsible for gastric ulcers (30–60%), duodenal ulcers (70–90%), chronic gastritis, gastric cancer, and gastric mucosa associated lymphoid tissue (MALT) lymphoma.

Transmission of *Helicobacter Pylori*

Direct contact:

A. Person to person

B. Gastro-oral

C. Feco-oral

D. Oral to oral

E. Salivary route

Pathogenesis

Interactions between host and bacterial genetic factors will direct the differential involvement of the gastroduodenal tract by this bacterium, leading to specific alteration of gastric or duodenal physiology, resulting in the formation of gastric and duodenal ulcers. In the gastric mucosa, it will never invade the gastric mucosal cells but is capable of producing some molecules, such as urea (it converts urea to ammonia and bicarbonate), motility, and chemotactic agent that help it:

A. To survive in the acidic environment though this environment is bactericidal

B. To adhere to gastric mucosal cells

C. To escape host's defense mechanism

Virulence factor of *H. pylori*-associated peptic ulcer disease:

A. Urease molecular complex: It will produce ammonia and bicarbonate that will damage the gastric mucosa:

- **a.** Directly
- **b.** Indirectly derived toxic compound from chemical processing of ammonia
- **c.** As an antigen produce local inflammatory response

B. *H. pylori VacA* gene: It corresponds to anion-channel forming cytotoxin and responsible for formation of intracellular vacuole in epithelial cells. It has three polymorphic regions, signal (s), intermediate (i), and middle (m) and are of two subtypes—type 1 and type 2. Again, s type allele has been subdivided into s1 and s2; s1 again is divided into s1a, s1b, and s3c; these are responsible for transport of toxin to the bacterial membrane and s2 is defective.

Again, i1 is associated with stronger vacuolar activity than i2 type. Cell tropism is broader in case of m1 as compared to m2. So severe peptic ulcer disease is always associated with s1, i1, and m1. In the Eastern region of the World, in case of gastric cancer, m1 is more prevalent suggesting that m1 is more pathogenic; where in Brazil, it is associated mostly with duodenal ulcer disease.

C. *CagA* gene of *H. pylori*: In the type 4 secretion system, *CagA* gene is encoded. Host's complement system is responsible for introducing the gene into the host epithelial cells. In its C-terminal end, EPIYA tyrosine residue is phosphorylated by SFK family kinases, which in turn triggers the following:

- **a.** Abnormal cell proliferation
- **b.** Rearrangement of cytoskeleton
- **c.** Modification of cell signaling pathways

In Western and Southeast Asian countries, *CagA* gene is associated with acid peptic disease.

D. Adhesion molecule BabA: It will adhere to blood group antigen ABO/Lewis B located in the human gastric mucosa leading to increased expression of inflammatory cytokines. There are two genes for BabA—*BabA1* and *BabA2*. BabA encoded by *BabA1* gene is associated with an increased risk of peptic ulcer disease and it will be enhanced by the presence of *CagA*.

E. OipA adhesion molecule: It alters the host cellular signaling pathways induced by tyrosine phosphorylation and actin cytoskeleton. It is associated with:

- **a.** Increased mucosal inflammation by inducing interleukin 8
- **b.** Duodenal ulcer disease

F. Modification of lipopolysaccharide A (LPA) mimicking Lewis blood group antigen results in very low pyrogenic activity as compared to lipopolysaccharide or other enteric bacteria. Genes associated with biosynthetic pathway responsible for LPA production are specific for gastric disease.

G. DupA virulence factor in half strains of bacteria is associated with increased risk of duodenal ulcer disease by the following mechanisms:

- **a.** Increase infiltration of neutrophils
- **b.** Protection against alterations in physiology in case of corpus gastritis

There is regional influence in case of DupA-associated peptic ulcer disease.

H. *IceA* coding gene has two allelic forms—IceA1 and IceA2. IceA1 expression is associated with acute inflammation of antral mucosa by increased interleukin-8 expression in different populations.

I. *H. pylori* will induce reactive oxygen species (ROS) synthesis in gastric mucosa; hence there is a positive correlation between ROS and extent of gastric injury and it can be estimated by measuring the serum level of marker for free radicle-induced DNA damage, 9-hydroxydeoxyguanosine; it will be increased in case of *H. pylori*-infected patients.

Host risk factors associated with *H. pylori*-related peptic ulcer disease:

A. Smoking
B. Alcohol intake
C. Intake of NSAIDs

Pathology of *H. pylori*-related acid peptic disease: Inflammatory infiltrate containing neutrophils in the lamina propria will cross the basement membrane to enter epithelial cells, which recruit neutrophils in the intraepithelial area and plasma cells in the subepithelial region; it is pathognomonic of *H. pylori* infection.

In case of longstanding infection, there is gradual depletion of scattered patches of native gastric mucosal structures throughout the stomach; this is multifocal atrophic gastritis, which may be antrum-predominant or whole stomach.

Later on, this normal mucosa will be replaced by intestinal mucosal cells known as intestinal metaplasia in the antrum or body of stomach.

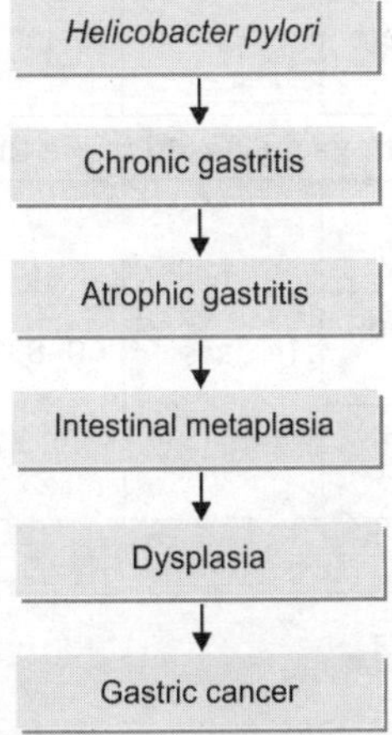

Clinical manifestation of peptic disease related to *H. pylori* infection

A. Symptoms:

- **a.** Patient may be completely asymptomatic; in that case, the patient may present with complications of acid peptic disease, such as perforation, bleeding, obstruction, or penetration of ulcers.
- **b.** Epigastric pain: It is a classical symptom, having gnawing, dull, empty hunger-like character:
  1. In case of duodenal ulcer, pain is relieved by ingestion of food, milk, or antacids and again recurs at night and awakens the patient.
  2. In case of gastric ulcer, eating increases the pain sensitivity, but there is relief in empty stomach. Hence, these patients experience weight loss and anorexia.
  3. Sudden worsening of pain or change of pain characteristic or the pain may be generalized in case of penetration of ulcer or ulcer perforation.
- **c.** Presence of hematemesis, melena, guaiac positive stool, or unexplained anemia suggests bleeding from ulcers.
- **d.** Persistent vomiting or postprandial vomiting suggests pyloric obstruction or duodenal deformity or edema of the ulcer wall.
- **e.** Anorexia, unexplained weight loss, and early satiety suggest gastric cancer.
- **f.** Upper abdominal pain radiating to back suggests penetrating ulcer.

B. Signs:

- **a.** In case of blood loss from ulcer:
  1. Orthostatic hypertension
  2. Tachycardia
  3. Anemia in case of chronic blood loss
- **b.** In case of duodenal ulcer: Duodenal point will be tender
- **c.** In case of perforation of ulcer:
  1. Rebound tenderness in the abdomen
  2. Cardboard rigidity
  3. Generalized tenderness in case of peritonitis
- **d.** In case of pyloric obstruction:
  1. Distended abdomen
  2. Succession splash
- **e.** Age of onset:
  1. Younger age of onset or between 30 and 55 years in case of duodenal ulcer
  2. Between 55 and 70 years with peak at sixth decade in gastric ulcer

Diagnostic Tests

Indications for *H. pylori* test for detection of infection in the patients:

A. Active peptic ulcer disease—gastric and duodenal ulcer
B. Presence of confirmed history of peptic ulcer disease but not previously treated
C. Patients with gastric MALT lymphoma
D. Those who have had a history of resection of gastric cancer
E. Those who have uninvestigated dyspepsia

Indications of endoscopy with biopsy:

A. Upper gastrointestinal bleeding
B. Unexplained weight loss
C. Early satiety
D. Patient is elderly
E. Patients have multiple ulcers
F. Refractory ulcers
G. Ulcers present in unusual locations, such as postbulbar area and jejunum
H. Patients with diarrhea and weight loss as in case of Zollinger–Ellison syndrome
I. Ulcer size greater than 3 cm in diameter
J. Presence of mass in the stomach mucosa

Diagnostic tests for *H. pylori*:

A. Noninvasive testing:
- **a.** Serologic ELISA: Serum immunoassay for immunoglobulin IgG to *H. pylori*:
  1. Sensitivity is 85% and specificity is 79%.
  2. It is not used to detect treatment success as it will remain positive for time post-treatment.
- **b.** Urease test: It can detect the urease activity in the stomach and used for initial diagnosis.
- **c.** Stool for *H. pylori* antigen: It is used for initial diagnosis. It uses polyclonal anti-*H. pylori* capture antibody to detect the *H. pylori* antigen. In case of an antigen-positive patient, one should wait for at least 4 weeks prior to repeat antigen test and provided:
  1. PPI should be stopped for 1–2 weeks.
  2. Antibiotics should be stopped for 4 weeks.
  3. Bismuth compounds should be stopped for 4 weeks.

B. Invasive testing:
- **a.** Urease test: Sensitivity is 89–100% and specificity 92–100%.
- **b.** Histological examination:
  1. Presence of polymorphonuclear leukocytes in the inflamed gastric mucosa
  2. By modified Giemsa, Warthin–Starry or Genta staining to identify *H. pylori*
- **c.** Culture of *H. pylori*—100% specific, but usually not recommended because:
  1. It is very difficult to perform.
  2. It is expensive.

  It can be done in patients who fail to respond to second-line eradication therapy.

Therapy for *H. pylori*-related acid peptic disease:

Drugs	Duration	Eradication rate	Comments
Triple therapy			
Proton-pump inhibitor twice daily Clarithromycin 500 mg twice daily Metronidazole 400 mg twice daily	14 days	70–85%	1st of therapy
Proton-pump inhibitor twice daily Amoxycillin 1,000 mg twice daily Metronidazole 400 mg	14 days	70–85%	1st line of therapy
Quadruple therapy			
Proton-pump inhibitor twice daily Tetracycline 500 mg twice daily Metronidazole 400 mg twice daily Bismuth subsalicylate 525 mg twice daily	14 days	75–90%	2nd line of therapy
Levofloxacin-based triple therapy			
Proton-pump inhibitor twice daily Levofloxacin 500 mg twice daily Amoxycillin 500 mg twice daily	14 days	60–85%	2nd line therapy or rescue therapy

Continued

Continued

Drugs	Duration	Eradication rate	Comments
Clarithromycin-based sequential therapy			
Proton-pump inhibitor twice daily	14 days	75–95%	2nd line therapy or rescue therapy
Amoxycillin 1,000 mg twice daily	First 7 days		
Clarithromycin 500 mg twice daily	Second 7 days		
Levofloxacin-based sequential therapy			
Proton-pump inhibitor twice daily	14 days	65–85%	2nd line therapy or rescue therapy
Amoxycillin 1,000 mg twice daily	First 7 days		
Levofloxacin 500 mg twice daily	Second 7 days		

Q6. Antibiotic-associated diarrhea.

DNBI/JUNE2011 (10)

Fecal microbiota transplant for recurrent *Clostridium difficile* infection.

DELHI UNI, 2024 (10)

Describe the diagnostic procedures for *C. difficile* infection. Enumerate the treatment options for primary *C. difficile* infection.

ODISHA UNI, 2022 (10)

Pseudomembranous colitis.

MGR UNI, TAMIL NADU, 2021 (10)

ANSWER

Introduction

It can be defined as diarrhea that has no known cause other than antibiotic therapy, which is continued concurrently or discontinued 4 weeks prior to incidence of diarrhea. In most of the cases, diarrhea is mild, but it can be mild and can be resolved without treatment or may be severe requiring intensive treatment.

When the ecology of intestinal microbiota is disrupted by antibiotics, diarrhea will ensue, which is antibiotic-associated diarrhea. In some cases, there may be formation of pseudomembranes; in that case, it is called pseudomembranous colitis.

Risk Factors Related to Antibiotic-associated Diarrhea

A. Use of antibiotics:
- **a.** High-risk antibiotics:
  1. Clindamycin
  2. Lincomycin
  3. Amoxycillin
  4. Ampicillin
  5. Cephalosporin
  6. Macrolide groups: Azithromycin
- **b.** Low-risk antibiotics:
  1. Cotrimoxazole
  2. Ciprofloxacin
  3. Penicillin
  4. Ureidopenicillin
- **c.** Rarely:
  1. Metronidazole
  2. Vancomycin

B. Serum level of toxin A antibody IgG

C. Prolonged hospitalization

Following three events are essential for the development of *C. difficile*-induced diarrhea:

A. First event is exposure to antimicrobial agents that produce disruption of normal gastrointestinal microbiota.

B. Second event is exposure to *C. difficile* toxin.

C. Third event is anamnestic response of host to *C. difficile* toxin A and C through the production of IgG.

Following pathogens are responsible for antibiotic-associated diarrhea:

A. *Clostridium difficile*

B. *Clostridium perfringens*

C. *Candida* groups

D. *Staphylococcus aureus*

Pathogenesis

Following postulations will explain pathophysiology of pseudomembranous colitis:

A. Alteration of intestinal microbiota

B. Effects of antibiotics and their metabolites

C. Hypersensitivity reaction

D. Intravenous coagulopathy

E. Localized Schwartzman reaction

F. Toxin elaboration by intestinal flora, production of enzymes, and beta lactamase

Clostridium difficile, gram-positive, spore-forming anaerobic bacillus having usual habitus in the soil is responsible for pseudomembranous colitis. It is normally present in 3% of the adults. This organism is invasive and produces two types of toxins, which will lead to the production of the following adverse effects:

Type A and C toxins are secreted by *C. difficile*, which are enterotoxin and cytotoxin, respectively.

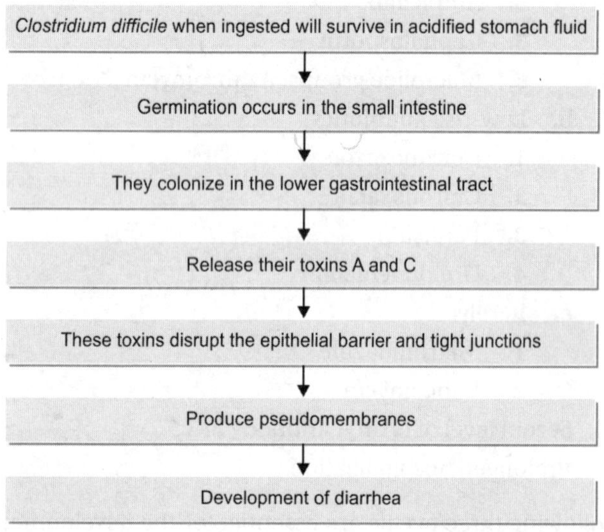

Toxin A also acts as neutrophil chemoattractant.

Both the toxins will glycosylate GTP-binding protein of Rho subfamily, which regulates actin cells of the cytoskeleton. Disruption of cytoskeleton results in loss of adherence and tight junction leading to leakage of fluid into the colonic cavity.

The third type of toxin is CDT, found in 6% of the strains, but is present in all isolates of NAP1/B1/027 strain. It is related to the iota toxin of *Clostridium perfringens*.

Pseudomembranes appear as 1–2 mm plaques with intervening unremarkable mucosa. But with progression of the disease, all the plaques coalesce to form large plaques. The whole colon without rectum is involved.

Microscopically, pseudomembranes consist of fibrin, necrotic leukocytes, cellular debris, and mucus with neutrophilic infiltration.

Stage 1: Normal appearance
Stage 2: Edema with mild erythema
Stage 3: Granular, friable, and hemorrhagic mucosa
Stage 4: Formation of pseudomembranes

Clinical Features

A. Diarrhea—it may be mild-to-severe form and in some cases, there is presence of blood and mucus.
B. A characteristic smell is present.
C. In 22% cases, abdominal pain is present.
D. Features of toxemia characterized by fever, cramps, abdominal pain, nausea with or without vomiting, dyselectrolytemia, severe dehydration, and protein-losing enteropathy are present.
E. Infrequently:
  - **a.** Toxic megacolon
  - **b.** Colonic perforation
  - **c.** Peritonitis
  - **d.** Sepsis
  - **e.** Shock
  - **f.** Death

Fulminant infection can be defined by:

A. Leukocyte count ≥ 15,000/cc
B. Creatinine in serum ≥ 1.5 times of premorbid value
C. Hypotension
D. Shock
E. Ileus
F. Toxic megacolon

Diagnosis

A. Unexpected *C. difficile* infection can be diagnosed by unexplained leukocyte count of >15,000/cc.
B. Diagnosis can be done by fulfilling the following criteria:
  - **a.** ≥3 times passage of unformed stool per day for ≥2 days
  - **b.** Detection of toxin A or B in stool
  - **c.** Detection of *C. difficile* in the stool sample by:
    1. PCR
    2. Culture
    3. Visualization of pseudomembranes in colon by colonoscopy in 50% of the patients having positive *C. difficile* toxin in stool.
    4. According to European guidelines, positive glutamate dehydrogenase along with positive toxins in stool or PCR demonstration of the organism is diagnostic for *C. difficile* infection.

Indicators of severe disease:

A. Leukocyte count ≥ 15,000/cc
B. Creatinine in serum ≥ 1.5 times of premorbid value

Treatment

Clinical conditions	Drugs
Mild-to-moderate initial episodes	Vancomycin 125 mg 6 hourly orally × 10 days Or Fidaxomicin 200 mg twice daily orally × 10 days Or Metronidazole 500 mg thrice daily orally × 10–14 days
Severe initial episode	Vancomycin 125 mg 6 hourly orally × 10 days Or Fidaxomicin 200 mg twice daily orally × 10 days
Initial fulminant episode	Vancomycin 500 mg orally or through nasogastric tube Plus Metronidazole 500 mg 8 hourly intravenously Plus consider Rectal instillation of 500 mg vancomycin in 100 mL of normal saline 6–8 hourly For 2 weeks or till the response
First recurrence	Vancomycin 125 mg orally 4 times daily × 10 days Or Vancomycin orally followed by taper-and-pulse regimen Or Fidaxomicin 200 mg twice daily × 10 days
Multiple recurrences	Vancomycin orally for 10 days followed by taper-and-pulse regimen in the form of: 125 mg orally twice daily × 7 days, then 125 mg orally daily × 7 days, then 125 mg alternate day × 2–8 weeks Or Oral vancomycin 125 mg 4 times daily × 10 days Rifaximin 400 mg twice daily × 2 weeks Or Fidaxomicin 200 mg twice daily × 10 days Or Transplantation of fecal microbiota by enema after antibiotic treatment for ≥2 weeks of *C. difficile* infection
	Other options include: Nitazoxanide 500 mg twice daily × 10 days Or Vancomycin 125 mg 4 times orally daily × 10 days Then Fidaxomicin 200 mg daily orally × 7 doses Then Fidaxomicin 200 mg orally alternate day × 13 doses

Fecal Microbiota Transplant for Recurrent Clostridia Infection

If the standard treatment fails, fecal microbiota transplant comes into action in case of recurrent clostridia infection which can be defined as ≥3 episodes of clostridia infection despite use of antibiotics resulting from inability to restore the microbiome which is protective.

The name of the product of fecal microbiota are:

A. RBX2660

B. SER-109

Rationale for Fecal Microbiota Transplant

A. As a result of prolonged use of antibiotic patients are predisposed to clostridia infection.

B. The gut will be repopularized with healthy bacteria thereby competitively inhibiting the growth of the clostridia difficile.

Indications of Fecal Microbiota in Clostridia Difficile Infection

A. Recurrent infection

B. Fulminant infection

C. Antibiotic dependent clostridia difficile infection

D. High risk group like patient on immunosuppressive therapy, elderly, and inflammatory bowel disease.

Procedure of Application of Fecal Microbiota

A. Through the colonoscopy procedure, fecal microbiota can be delivered directly into the colon.

B. Through the nasogastric tube also fecal microbiota can be administered.

C. By giving enema, it can be administered.
D. Freeze dried fecal material preparation can be administered by giving oral capsule.

Efficacy of the Treatment

A. Treatment is 90% effective.
B. Recurrence rate is low as compared to antibiotic therapy.
C. Response to fecal microbiota transplant is sustained.

Risks of Microbiota Transplantation

A. Risk of transmission of other infectious diseases
B. There is ongoing research regarding development of autoimmunity post fecal microbiota transplant.
C. There may be gut microbiota dysbiosis.

Q7. What is gastroesophageal reflux disorder? Risk factors and management strategies for GERD.
DNBII/APR2016 (10)

Gastroesophageal reflux disease.
MGR/SEP2006/MDI (5) BF/OCT2011/MDII (13)

Describe the recent advantages in the diagnosis and treatment of GERD.
MAHARASHTRA UNI OF HEALTH SC, VIJAYAWADA, 2021 (25)

ANSWER

Definition

Gastroesophageal reflux disorder (GERD) is a chronic disorder characterized by a constellation of symptoms of heart burn, acid regurgitation, and extraesophageal manifestations, such as cough and hoarseness of voice as a result of the retrograde flow of gastric content into the esophagus and adjacent organs with or without tissue damage.

Pathophysiology

Normally antireflux barrier at the lower end of esophagus is divided into the following categories:

A. Anatomical factors extrinsic to lower esophageal sphincter (LES) that prevent reflux:
   a. Distal esophageal mucosal flap
   b. Acute esophago-gastric angle
   c. Compression of gastroesophageal junction by gastric sling fibers
   d. Crus of diaphragm acts as a pinchcock
   e. Sling action of right crus of diaphragm
   f. Intra-abdominal junction of esophagus

   In case of hiatus hernia, gastroesophageal junction moves upward; as a result, there are:
   a. Loss of angulation of gastroesophageal junction
   b. Loss of abdominal esophageal segment supported by diaphragm
   c. Direct transmission of intra-abdominal pressure into intrathoracic LES
B. Efficiency of LES pressure:
   a. 2–4-cm zone of thickened smooth muscle at the gastroesophageal junction
   b. LES maintains high-pressure zone of thickened smooth muscle at the gastroesophageal junction.
   c. LES is controlled by:
      1. Vagus nerve
      2. Myogenic factors
      3. Hormones
   d. Minimum LES pressure required to prevent gastroesophageal reflux is 6–10 mm Hg.

   Diurnal variation of LES pressure:
   a. During swallowing
   b. In increased intragastric pressure
   c. In esophageal distension
C. Gastric factors: It depends upon the following factors—
   a. Gastric volume: It is controlled by:
      1. Volume and composition of gastric content
      2. Rate of increase of gastric secretion
      3. Rate and efficiency of gastric emptying: It depends upon—
         - Duodenal ulcers with duodenal bulbar deformity
         - Pyloric channel ulcer

         Delayed emptying of stomach is due to:
         - Diabetes mellitus
         - Hypothyroidism
         - Collagen vascular disorders
   b. Composition of refluxate:
      1. Gastric acid produces injury to esophageal mucosa by:
         - Protein denaturation
         - Back diffusion of hydrogen ion into the deeper layer of esophageal mucosa

2. Pepsin: It digests esophageal intraepithelial cellular substances.
3. Duodenogastric reflux: It contains bile and pancreatic juice, which reflex into stomach and then to esophagus.
    - It increases permeability of esophageal mucosa to hydrogen ion by back-diffusion.
    - Pancreatic enzymes produce lipolytic injury.

D. Esophageal clearance:

a. Volume clearance: Emptying of esophagus of gastric reflux volume; it can be cleared by the following:

1. Normal esophageal peristalsis
2. Primary esophageal peristalsis initiated by swallowing progressing throughout the entire length of esophagus
   In case of an awakened patient, this peristalsis will occur. But in case of a patient who is sleeping, normal and primary peristalsis will not occur.
3. Secondary peristalsis: It is produced by distension of esophageal food bolus and reflux fluid, but it has limited effect.

b. Acid clearance: This means neutralization of refluxed acid by swallowed saliva.

c. Saliva: It helps in esophageal clearing by the following mechanisms:

1. It will stimulate swallowing.
2. It is secreted at a rate of 0.5 mL/min increased by sucking, eating, or intubation. During stimulation, bicarbonate secretion increases.

E. True resistance of esophageal mucosa:

a. Pre-epithelial resistance:

1. Mucous layer: It is present on the epithelial surface.
   Functions:
    - It acts as an acid lubricant.
    - It acts as a protective barrier against noxious irritants.
    - It prevents back-diffusion of hydrogen ion.
    - It prevents the proteolytic enzyme to act.
2. Unstirred water layer: It produces an alkaline environment as it is rich in bicarbonate.
3. Mucus and bicarbonate ion: It is present just above the lower gastroesophageal junction and just below the upper esophageal sphincter.

b. Postepithelial defense: It is maintained by adequate blood flow and normal tissue acid–base status.

Functions:

1. It removes the waste products.
2. It will supply oxygen, nutrients, and bicarbonate.

F. Epithelial generation:

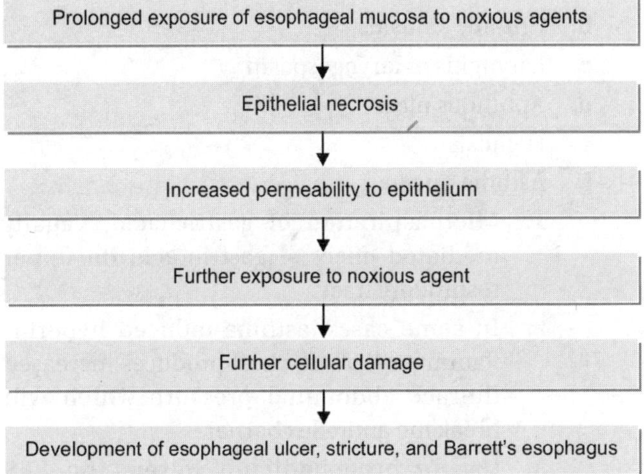

Risk Factors Associated with GERD

A. Obesity
B. Hiatus hernia
C. Tobacco chewing and smoking
D. Eating prior to recumbency
E. Pregnancy—relaxation of LES
F. Diet:

a. High-fat diet
b. Coffee
c. Chocolate
d. Citrus food
e. Alcohol
f. Tomato-based products
g. Vinegar

Clinical Features

A. Esophageal symptoms:

a. Heart burn—burning in the substernal area radiating to neck and back

b. Regurgitation—sensation feeling of contents of stomach flowing in retrograde fashion into the chest and occasionally into the mouth.

c. Dysphagia—difficulty in swallowing in the absence of esophageal inflammation or narrowing.
d. Water brush—sudden appearance of salty water in the mouth due to secretion of saliva in response to acid reflux.
e. Hiccup
f. Painful deglutition known as odynophagia due to severe esophagitis

B. Extra-esophageal symptoms:
a. Dental erosion
b. Chronic sinusitis
c. Laryngitis or laryngospasm
d. Aphthous ulcer
e. Halitosis
f. Asthma due to:
1. Microaspiration of gastric acid, vagally mediated effect of gastric acid on upper respiratory tract
2. In some cases, asthma-induced hyperinflammation of the chest produces increased thoraco-abdominal pressure which will break the antireflex barrier.
3. Use of bronchodilator lowers the LES pressure.
g. Globus hystericus
h. Chronic cough
i. Tracheobronchitis
j. Frequent throat clearing
k. Noncardiac chest pain
l. Aspiration pneumonitis

C. Alarming signs in GERD:
a. Anemia
b. Dysphagia
c. Odynophagia
d. Age > 50 years
e. Family history of esophageal cancer
f. Sudden weight loss
g. Gastrointestinal bleeding

Diagnosis

A. Trial therapy PPI: During a 30-day trial of PPIs, such as omeprazole, rabeprazole, lansoprazole or dexlansoprazole, 1 hour prior to breakfast if the symptom improves within 1–2 weeks, sensitivity being 78% and specificity 54%.

B. Barium swallow:
a. It can detect reflux of barium contrast into esophagus after ingestion of contrast solution.
b. It can detect stricture and neoplasm.

C. Upper gastrointestinal endoscopy: It can detect:
a. Different grades of esophagitis
b. Esophageal stricture
c. Esophageal cancer

Los Angeles classification of grades of esophagitis:

Grade	Mucosal break
A	One or more mucosal breaks ≤5 mm long, none of which extends in between the tops of the mucosal folds
B	One or more mucosal breaks >5 mm long, none of which extends in between the tops of the mucosal folds
C	Greater than one mucosal break that extends between the tops of two mucosal folds, but it involves <75% of esophageal circumference
D	Greater than one mucosal break that extends between the tops of two mucosal folds, but it involves ≥75% of esophageal circumference

D. Ambulatory reflux monitoring: In case of patients with typical esophageal symptoms but normal endoscopy:
Main outcome is acid exposure time (AET) and to be done in "on" and "off" therapy with PPI. AET also has to be done with double-dose PPI therapy to detect refractoriness to PPI.
a. AET of <4% suggests normal or physiological response.
b. AET of >6% suggests abnormal response.

E. Ambulatory esophageal pH monitoring: It can detect only reflux episode. It is acidic in nature. But in case of duodeno-gastric-esophageal reflux, the reflux will be alkaline.

F. Intraluminal multichannel impedance monitoring: It can measure the change in resistance to current flow in between the pairs of impedance electrodes by giving boluses of gases, which increase impedance and giving boluses of liquid, which decrease the impedance. Impedance and pH monitoring can be done in combination. Now distinction is made between acidic (pH <4), weakly acidic (pH 4–7), and alkaline (pH >7) pH.

Advantages:
a. It can detect reflux irrespective of pH.

b. It can detect number of episodes per day and whether they are alkaline or acidic.
c. If the patient is on PPI, then it is the gold standard method.

Results:

a. Number of episodes < 40/day suggests normal or physiological.
b. Number of episodes > 80/day suggests GERD.

G. High-resolution manometry: It is used to assess:
   a. Assess alternate major motor defect
   b. Place pH or pH impedance catheter
   c. Assess function of gastroesophageal junction barrier
   d. Evaluate obstruction at esophagogastric junction

H. Narrow-band imaging: It uses spectral narrow-band filters (415 ± 15 nm, 540 ± 15 nm) as it will visualize superficial 170–210 µm of mucosa. It can detect the following:
   a. Intrapapillary capillary loops
   b. Microerosion
   c. Columnar islands
   d. Ridge/villous pattern
   e. Increased vascularity at the squamocolumnar junction

Management

A. Lifestyle modifications:
   a. It will decrease frequency as well as severity of symptoms.
   b. Process of lifestyle modification includes:
      1. Weight loss
      2. Avoidance of late-night meals
      3. Elevation of head end of the bed by 30° to minimize the acid reflux
      4. Avoidance of spicy and greasy food, acidic foods, such as tomato-based product, and citrus food
      5. Cessation of smoking
      6. Reduction of alcohol intake
      7. Reduction of caffeinated products, such as chocolates and carbonated products

B. Antacid administration:
   a. It will neutralize gastric acids to raise the pH above 4.
   b. It will decrease the reflux symptoms.
   c. Onset of action will start in 5 minutes after ingestion and the effect will last for 90 minutes.
   d. Side-effects include:
      1. Diarrhea in case of magnesium-containing antacids
      2. Constipation in case of aluminum-containing antacids

C. Histamine-2 receptor antagonists:
   a. It will inhibit acid secretion by competitively blocking H_2 receptors present on the gastric parietal cells.
   b. It will prevent heart burn if taken before meals and also ameliorate meal-induced symptoms of heart burn within 15–40 minutes if taken after meals.
   c. It should be given twice daily in patients with GERD to be most effective.
   d. In case of mild-to-moderate esophagitis, the response rate is 75% and in case of severe esophagitis, it is 50%.

D. PPI:
   a. It will block the hydrogen–potassium ATPase irreversibly present on the apical surface of the parietal cells, and thus act on the final common pathway of acid secretion.
   b. Once-a-day dose therapy is the mainstay in this treatment. But in case of severe esophagitis, in order to maintain the intragastric pH above 4 for 15–21 hours, a twice-daily dose has to be introduced.
   c. This drug is most effective if it is administered 15–30 minutes before meals.
   d. Reasons for failure to respond to PPI are:
      1. Poor adherence
      2. Inadequate suppression of acid
      3. Breakthrough of acid secretion
      4. Weakly acid reflux as the cause of symptoms
      5. Delayed emptying of stomach
      6. Functional heart burn
      7. Duodeno-gastric-esophageal reflux
   e. Side effects:
      1. Diarrhea
      2. Headache
      3. Abdominal pain
      4. Increased susceptibility to infection with *C. difficile* enterocolitis
      5. Vitamin B12 deficiency in case of long-term PPI use at least for 5 years may be due to decrease in protein-bound vitamin B12

6. Small intestinal bacterial overgrowth in case of chronic use if there is an underlying intestinal motility disorder
7. Interstitial nephritis
8. Hepatitis
9. It requires dose adjustment of warfarin, diazepam, and phenytoin as it induces cytochrome P450 system.

E. Prokinetic agents: Metoclopramide, a dopamine antagonist, is effective in patients with delayed gastric emptying. Side effects are:

a. Tardive dyskinesia
b. Parkinson-like symptoms

F. GABA-B agonists: Drugs are baclofen and lesogaberan. These are given in those patients who do not respond to PPI. These drugs inhibit transient lower esophageal sphincter relaxations (TLESRs) and prevent reflux episode. Side effects are:

a. Drowsiness
b. Increased risk of seizures
c. Nausea

These drugs are not approved by the Food and Drug Administration (FDA) for the treatment for GERD.

G. Endoscopic therapy:

The goal is:

a. To reduce the reflux
b. To alter the response to acid
c. To improve symptoms

Approaches are:

a. Delivery of radiofrequency energy to gastroesophageal junction
b. Injection of bulking agents in the LES
c. Implantation of a prosthetic device into the LES
d. Endoscopic gastroplication

Complications are:

a. Bleeding
b. Aspiration pneumonitis
c. Mediastinitis
d. Rarely death

H. Surgical therapy: Procedures are—

a. The procedure is Nissen fundoplication; it includes a 360° wrap involving the upper portion of the stomach as it will prevent the retrograde motion of the gastric contents into the stomach and thus allow the mucosa of the esophagus to get healed.
b. Toupet fundoplication—it is a partial wrap in case of poor esophageal motility.
c. New surgical therapy is the placement of bracelet with magnetic beads at the gastroesophageal junction as it will create a barrier at this junction to prevent reflux.

Both the above procedures are done laparoscopically. But these will not reduce the development of Barrett esophagus or adenocarcinoma.

Common adverse effects are:

a. Dysphagia due to tight wrap around LES
b. "Gas-bloat syndrome"—it occurs when it is difficult to expel the air from the stomach.

Surgical therapy is required in the patients:

a. Who respond to therapy but do not tolerate PPIs and require permanent therapy
b. Where PPI decreases heart burn, but regurgitation continues
c. With recurrent complications of GERD, such as stricture or respiratory features

Q8. Describe etiopathogenesis of inflammatory bowel disease. Discuss diagnosis and treatment of ulcerative colitis.

DNBIIIA/DEC2013 (10)

Pathology of ulcerative colitis. Enumerate its extraintestinal manifestations. Medical management of ulcerative colitis.

DNBIIIB/JUN2015 (10) MJPRU/2016/MDIII (15) BF/MAY2010/MDIII (15)

Diagnosis and management of ulcerative colitis.

DNBIIIB/JUN2016 (10)

Ulcerative colitis.

MGR/OCT2014/MDI (5)

Discuss the etiopathogenesis, clinical features, investigations, and management of ulcerative colitis.

MGR/OCT2011/MDII (15)

Extraintestinal manifestation of inflammatory bowel disease.

MGR/FEB2005/MDI (5)

Medical management of inflammatory bowel disease.

MGR/SEP2006/MDIV (5)

Describe the etiology, clinical features, diagnosis, and management of ulcerative colitis.

RGUHS/MAR2008/MDII (20)

Describe pathology, clinical features, and management of inflammatory bowel disease.

MUHS/MAY2012/MDIII (25)

Treatment of ulcerative colitis.

MUHS/MAY2010/MDIII (10)

Diagnosis and management of Crohn's disease.

PGI/APR2013/MDIII (10)

Management of refractory cases of inflammatory bowel disease.

BF/MAY2013/MDII (10)

Discuss recent advances in diagnosis and management of inflammatory bowel disease.

BF/OCT2010/MDIV (8)

Discuss etiopathogenesis, clinical manifestation, and treatment of a case of inflammatory bowel disease.

BF/MAY2010/MDII (30)

Extra-intestinal manifestation of ulcerative colitis.

DNB DEC 2019) (5)

Describe the extraintestinal manifestations of inflammatory bowel disease. Discuss the role of biologic therapies in treatment of inflammatory bowel disease.

DNB (JUN2022) (10)

Discuss the evaluation and treatment of inflammatory bowel disease.

AIIMS, BHU, 2020 (10)

A 46-year-old male presented with intermittent history of diarrhea, rectal bleeding, tenesmus, passage of mucus and cramping abdominal pain. On further investigation there was tenderness on palpation over abdomen and increase in acute phase reactant in the blood.

What is the most probable diagnosis? What are the differential diagnoses? Discuss the diagnostic approach to this condition. How will you manage the condition?

AIIMS, BBS, 2022 (10)

Crohn's disease—pathophysiology, clinical, diagnosis, and treatment.

SCBMCH, 2020 (20)

Enumerate the complications of inflammatory bowel disease. Discuss the treatment of severe ulcerative colitis. Enumerate the novel drugs for the management of IBD.

DNB, OCT2024 (10)

Biologicals and biosimilars in IBD. Enumerate, describe the mechanism of action and their uses.

WBUHS, 2022 (10)

Clinical presentation and management of ulcerative colitis.

NTR UNI OF HEALTH SC, ANDHRA, 2022 (10)

Treatment of inflammatory bowel disease.

MAHARASHTRA UNI OF HEALTH SC, VIJAYAWADA, 2021 (10)

Describe etiology, clinical features, diagnosis, and management of IBD. Discuss the differentiating features between ulcerative colitis and Crohn's disease.

VEER NARMAD SOUTH GUJARAT UNI, 2021 (20)

Extraintestinal manifestations of Crohn's disease.

MAHARASHTRA UNI OF HEALTH SC, VIJAYAWADA, 2020 (10)

Discuss the etiology, pathophysiology, clinical features, investigations, and management of inflammatory bowel disease.

TEERTHANKER MAHAVEER UNI, 2020 (20)

Ulcerative colitis—etiology, clinical features, investigation, and management.

MGR UNIVERSITY, TAMIL NADU, 2020 (15)

Discuss inflammatory bowel disease.

WBUHS, 2020 (10)

Describe etiology, pathophysiology, clinical features, and management of inflammatory bowel disease.

NTR UNI OF HEALTH SC, VIJAYAWADA, 2020 (10)

Extraintestinal manifestations and management of inflammatory bowel disease.

NTR UNI OF HEALTH SC, VIJAYAWADA, 2020 (10)

Differentiating ulcerative colitis from Crohn's disease.

KERALA UNIVERSITY, 2019 (10)

Diagnosis and medical management of Crohn's disease.

BABA FARID UNI OF HEALTH SC, 2019 (10)

Inflammatory bowel disease.

BHARATI VIDYAPEETH DEEMED UNI, JHELUM, 2019 (10)

Management of ulcerative colitis.

RAJIV GANDHI UNI OF HEALTH SC, KARNATAKA, 2018 (10)

Pathology of ulcerative colitis and Crohn's disease.

KERALA UNI, 2018 (10)

A 40-year-old man presented with chronic diarrhea for 6 months. 3–4 episodes per day, mostly mucoid, sometimes bloody. Abdominal pain on and off. Gradually he lost his appetite and 4 kilos of weight. There was no fever. What is your diagnosis? Discuss the etiopathogenesis, clinical features, and management of the disease. List out its complications.

KERALA UNI, 2018 (20)

Clinical features, investigations, and management of ulcerative colitis.

BHARATI VIDYAPEETH DEEMED UNI, 20218 (10)

Management of ulcerative colitis.

MANIPUR UNIVERSITY, 2018 (10)

Diagnosis and treatment of ulcerative colitis.

RAJASTHAN UNIVERSITY, 2018 (8)

Discuss role of biologics in inflammatory bowel disease.

MAHATMA UNIVERSITY, 2022 (10)

Current management of inflammatory bowel disease.

MAHATMA UNIVERSITY, 2019 (10)

Discuss the etiology and management of Crohn's disease.

WBUHS, 2024 (10)

ANSWER

For the last question, the differential diagnoses are:

A. Ulcerative colitis
B. Bacillary dysentery
C. Amebic dysentery
D. Antibiotic-associated colitis

Introduction

Inflammatory bowel disease is a chronic, recurrent, and relapsing immune-mediated intestinal disease consisting of UC and CD.

Etiopathogenesis

In a physiological condition, homeostasis is maintained by following host compartments functioning together in an integrated manner as "supraorganism":

A. Commensal microbiota
B. Intestinal epithelial cells
C. Immune cells within the tissues

The above integrated process will be hampered by the following factors:

A. Environmental factors: These are—
   a. Smoking
   b. Use of antibiotics
   c. Appendectomy
   d. NSAIDs
   e. Oral contraceptive pills (OCPs)
   f. Dietary factors
   g. Childhood hygiene
B. Genetic factors:
   a. Several genetic syndromes are associated with acute, severe, and refractory IBD due to a single genetic defect affecting the immune system. These genetic mutations may occur in IL-10, IL-10 receptor, neutrophil cytosolic factor 2 protein, cytotoxic T-lymphocyte associated protein-4, etc.
   b. In 10% of the affected patients, there are evidences of familial origin. There is an increased concordance rate for monozygotic twins as compared to dizygotic twins.
   c. IBD is a polygenic disorder as evidenced by different subgroups within UC and CD.
   d. Nearly 200 loci have been identified amongst which two thirds are associated with both disease phenotypes whereas others are specific for either CD or UC.
   e. There are associations of other immune-mediated diseases with IBD suggesting common immunogenic pathways of different diseases which account for:
      1. Common responsiveness to similar types of biologic therapies
      2. Simultaneous occurrences of these disorders

      The associated diseases are rheumatoid arthritis (TNFAIP3), type 1 diabetes mellitus (IL-10, PTPN2), asthma (ORMDL3), and psoriasis (IL23R, IL12B).
   f. Genetic factors involving in the fundamental cell biologic processes, such as:
      1. Endoplasmic reticulum and metabolic stress (XBP1, OCTN) regulate the secretory activity of Paneth and goblet cells in response to commensal microbiota.
      2. Innate immunity involving parenchymal and hematopoietic immune cells effectively clears the bacteria, mycobacteria, and viruses.
      3. Adaptive immunity (IL23R, IL12B) will balance between inflammatory and anti-inflammatory cytokines.
      4. Factors (PTGER4, CCR6) that are involved in the process of resolution of inflammation by recruitment of leukocytes and inflammatory mediator production.
C. Commensal microbiota: Human beings are sterile during birth but acquire commensal bacteria during egress from the birth canal and later on from environmental resources and achieve biomass of 10^{12} colony forming units per gram of feces from 3 years of age till adult life. The intestine contains other microbiota, such as protists, archaea, and viruses. The composition and function of intestinal microbiota are under control of environmental and genetic factors and intestinal immune cell responses. Structural component and metabolic activity of microbiota influence the host's epithelial and immune functions through epigenetic effects. Commensal microbacteria present in IBD are different from noninfected individuals, such as:
   a. Proteobacteria, i.e., enteroinvasive and adherent *E. coli* that drive the disease
   b. Loss of micro-organisms, such as *Faecalibacterium prausnitzii*, that hinders inflammation

   Few drugs, such as metronidazole, elemental diet, and fecal diversion alter the intestinal microbiota and thus improve the CD.
D. Defective immune regulation: Mucosal tolerance to luminal contents or intramuscular soluble antigen involves multiple mechanisms:
   a. Deletion or anergy of antigen-reactive T cells
   b. Induction of CD4+ cells that will suppress inflammation in the gut preventing anti-inflammatory cytokines, such as IL-10, IL-35, and transforming growth factor-β (TGF-β).

In case of IBD, this suppression will be altered, which leads to uncontrolled inflammation by an unknown mechanism.

In case of a transgenic mouse model, it has been seen that the following factors will lead to spontaneous colitis:

a. Deletion of cytokines IL-2 and IL-10
b. Deletion of cytokine receptors
c. Deletion of molecules that are associated with recognition of T-cell antigen
d. Interference with function of intestinal epithelial cell (IEC) barrier
e. Interfering the regulation of response to commensal bacteria

Again, absence of some bacteria will activate certain elements of the immune system in the intestine suggesting the protective properties present in some bacteria.

Therefore, specific changes in the host or intestinal microbiota will lead to activation of the immune system, thus initiating intestinal inflammation.

E. Inflammatory cascade in IBD: Genetic and environmental factors initiate inflammation in the intestine by parenchymal and hematopoietic cells, which will be perpetuated by T-cell activation coupled with inadequate regulatory pathways.

Cytokines from innate immune cells, such as IL-1, IL-6, and TNF:

a. Will promote fibrogenesis
b. Will promote production of collagen
c. Will produce other inflammatory mediators
d. Will activate tissue metalloproteinase
e. Will activate coagulation cascade in local blood vessels through increased production of Von Willebrand factor

In case of any infection, this coagulation cascade will be activated but will be turned off at an appropriate time to prevent further tissue damage. But in case of IBD, it will not be inhibited and not regulated, leading to imbalance between proinflammatory and anti-inflammatory cytokines:

a. Some cytokines activate macrophages and B cells.
b. Some cytokines indirectly recruit from blood stream inflammatory leukocytes and mononuclear cells into intestine and it is done through interactions between:
   1. Homing receptors present on the lymphocytes
   2. Addressins present on vascular endothelium
c. Three types of CD4+ T helper cells promote inflammation. These are:
   1. T_H1 cells secrete interferon γ and induce granulomatous inflammation, such as CD.
   2. T_H2 cells secrete IL-4, IL-5, and IL-13 and produce superficial mucosal inflammation like UC.
   3. T_H17 cells secrete IL-17 and IL-21, these will recruit neutrophils.

   These T cells cross regulate each other as follows:
   1. IL-4 together with IL-6 induces T_H2.
   2. IL-23 together with TGF induces T_H17.
   3. Activated macrophages secrete IL-6 and TNF.
d. Innate immune cells lacking T-cell receptors also participate in IBD.

Clinical Features

Symptoms

Features	UC	CD
Abdominal pain	Cramping in the left lower quadrant, but in severe cases pain will be worse due to inflamed wall of the colon during muscular contraction	Frequent in the right lower quadrant: As the food bolus will pass through the narrow segment, receptors in the bowel wall will be stretched
Rectal bleeding	• Always present in active cases; in severe cases, intensity increased • In rectal involvement, blood streak with mucus on the surface of hard stool • With proximal involvement, liquid stool with pus and blood • Presence of blood clot suggests cancer or hemorrhoids	Rare but may occur in distal colon involvement
Diarrhea	• Frequent in adult due to increased mucosal permeability • Reduced activity of Na^+/K^+ ATPase pump • Altered membrane phospholipids	Present in active disease due to: • Increased mucosal permeability • Mucosal inflammation

Continued

Continued

Features	UC	CD
	• Sometimes, it is nocturnal or postprandial	• Imbalanced concentration of luminal bile acids • Bacterial overgrowth syndrome
Weight loss	Occurs due to: • Hypercatabolism • Loss of protein through the inflamed mucosa • Downregulation of synthesis of albumin	Increased due to: • Diseased bowel • Resection of the intestine
Fever	Occurs in severe attack	Occurs due to: Release of IL-1, IL-6, TNF-α
Anorexia	Present in severe attack	Present due to: • Release of TNF-α • Delayed gastric emptying
Smoking	Protective effect	It is associated with early onset due to: • Altered smooth muscle tone • More frequent use of immunosuppressant • Increased oxidative stress • Endothelial dysfunction • Altered gut mucosal integrity
Diet	Low-fiber diet is required	• Increased risk is with low-fiber diet • High-fiber diet is beneficial as it inhibits proinflammatory mediators
Appen-dectomy	No relation	Accepted as risk factor
Stress	Present	Present

On physical examination in case of CD:

A. Anemia:

  a. Iron deficiency due to:

    1. Bleeding

    2. Decreased erythropoietin production due to inhibition by INF-α, INF-λ, and IL-1

  b. Vitamin B12 deficiency due to extensive ileal involvement

  c. Folic acid deficiency due to sulfasalazine

B. Edema due to hypoproteinemia

C. In the mouth aphthous ulcer

D. Extraintestinal involvement of different organs in the body

E. Abdominal examination:

  a. Abdominal distension with signs of intestinal obstruction due to stricture

  b. Hepatomegaly in 10% patients

F. Digital rectal examination:

  a. Anal fissure

  b. Anal stenosis

  c. Fistula

  d. Abscess

  e. On palpation:

    1. Perianal tenderness

    2. Blood at the fingertip

On physical examination in case of UC:

A. In case of mild disease, there may not be any physical sign.

B. Anemia due to: Blood loss

C. Jaundice due to PSC

D. Edema due to hypoalbuminemia in case of extensive colitis

E. Tachycardia

F. Aphthous ulcer in the mouth

G. Extraintestinal involvement of other organs of the body

H. Abdominal examination:

  a. Abdominal tenderness in the affected part of the colon

  b. Hepatic tympany in case of toxic megacolon

  c. In case of perforation signs of peritonitis

I. Digital rectal examination:

  a. Feeling of velvety and edematous mucosa

  b. Presence of blood with or without mucus at the fingertip

Complications of UC:

A. Severe hemorrhage

B. Toxic megacolon: It is characterized by >6 cm diameter involving right or transverse colon with loss of haustration in case of severe UC. It is triggered by use of narcotics or electrolyte abnormalities.

C. Perforation

D. Colorectal cancer

E. Stricture in 5–10% patients with UC because of presence of neoplasia or inflammation followed by fibrosis.

Truelove and Witt's criteria of disease severity assessment:

Characteristics	Mild UC	Moderate UC	Severe UC
Stool pass	<4 times/day	>4 times/day	>6 times/day
Systemic disturbances	Nil	Minimal	Moderate-to-severe
ESR	Normal	Normal	>30 mm in 1st hour

Mayo score of activity of UC:

Parameter	Sub score (0–3)
Stool frequency	0 = Normal number of stools
	1 = 1–2 stools more than normal
	2 = 3–4 stools more than normal
	3 = 5 or more stools more than normal
Bleeding per rectum	0 = No blood is seen
	1 = Streak of blood with stool less one half of the time
	2 = Obvious blood with stool most of the time
	3 = Blood alone passed without stool
Endoscopic findings	0 = Normal or inactive disease
	1 = Mild disease characterized by erythema, decreased vascular pattern, and mild friability
	2 = Moderate disease characterized by lack of vascular pattern, marked erythema, friability, and erosions
	3 = Severe disease characterized by spontaneous bleeding and ulceration
Global assessment by physician	0 = Normal
	1 = Mild disease
	2 = Moderate disease
	3 = Severe disease

Extraintestinal Complications of UC

A. Dermatological manifestation:

- **a.** Erythema nodosum: It is characterized by red or violet, tender subcutaneous nodules 1–5 cm in diameter, present on the anterior extensor surface of lower extremities in 10% of UC and 15% CD.
- **b.** Pyoderma gangrenosum: It is characterized by erythematous nodules or pustule spreading to adjacent skin, which will be converted into deep burrowing ulcer having violaceous edges with surrounding erythema, present on the dorsum of the legs and feet, but may develop on the arm, chest, and even on the face. It may occur during or prior to occurrence of UC and may occur years postcolectomy.
- **c.** Pyoderma vegetans occurring in the intertriginous areas
- **d.** Pyostomatitis vegetans involving the mucous membrane
- **e.** Sweet's syndrome: It is characterized by tender papulosquamous exanthema or nodules present on the arms, legs, trunks, or face.
- **f.** Psoriasis occurs in 5–10% UC patients suggesting the immunological basis of the disease.
- **g.** Perianal tag present in 75–80% patients of CD and rarely in UC.

B. Mouth:

- **a.** Sore tongue
- **b.** Aphthous ulcer
- **c.** Stomatitis

C. Eye:

- **a.** Conjunctivitis
- **b.** Iritis
- **c.** Episcleritis: It is characterized by painless hyperemia of the sclera and conjunctiva.
- **d.** Anterior uveitis occurs in UC during disease process, during remission, or after medical or surgical treatment.

D. Joint:

- **a.** Sacroiliitis. It is symmetrical, more common in UC, may be asymptomatic, no correlation with bowel disease, and may not progress to ankylosing spondylitis.
- **b.** Ankylosing spondylitis in 10% of IBD. It is more common in CD as compared to UC. Two thirds of the patients are HLA-B27 positive. Presenting complaints are low back pain, pain in buttock, and morning stiffness. Course is progressive and may develop permanent skeletal damage.
- **c.** Anterior arthropathy:
  1. *Type 1*: Pauciarticular, asymmetrical, migratory, and self-limiting, involving <5 large joints, mainly knee joints
  2. *Type 2*: Polyarticular, symmetrical, nonmigratory, involving >5 joints, mainly metacarpophalangeal joints

E. Liver:

- **a.** PSC due to inflammation of intrahepatic and extrahepatic bile ducts followed by fibrosis leading to cirrhosis and hepatocellular failure. It occurs more commonly in UC and may occur postcolectomy.

b. Hepatic steatosis present in half of IBD patients.
c. Fatty liver occurs due to:
    1. Chronic debilitating illness
    2. Malnutrition
    3. Glucocorticoid therapy
d. Gallbladder polyps: There is a chance of gallbladder malignancy.
e. Small PSC involves small caliber duct; it is a variant of PSC.
f. Cholelithiasis occurs in CD with:
    1. Ileitis
    2. Ileal resection
    3. Malabsorption of bile acids due to:
        - Bile salt depletion
        - Secretion of lithogenic bile

F. Urologic:
a. Ureteric calculi, mainly oxalate stones, result from increased absorption of oxalate. In a physiological condition, calcium combines with oxalate in the intestinal lumen to form insoluble calcium oxalate. But in case of CD, nonabsorbable fatty acid combines with calcium, leaving oxalate free for absorption from the large intestine in the presence of inflammation.
b. Ureteral obstruction

G. Metabolic bone disorders:
a. Low bone mass in 14–42% of the IBD patients in the following conditions:
    1. Glucocorticoids
    2. Cyclosporine A (CSA)
    3. Methotrexate
    4. Total parenteral nutrition (TPN)
    5. Malabsorption due to release of IL-1, IL-6, and TNF

Therefore, there is a chance of fractures in the rib, spine, hip, and wrist, which is more common in the elderly.

b. Osteonecrosis: It is characterized by osteocytes and adipocytes, leading to collapse of bone, mainly affecting the hip, shoulders, and knees.

H. Thromboembolism involving small, medium, and large vessels:
a. Arterial thromboembolism
b. Venous thromboembolism

The causes of hypercoagulable states are:
    1. Platelet–endothelial dysfunction
    2. Hyperhomocysteinemia
    3. Impaired fibrinolysis
    4. Coagulation cascade alteration
    5. Involvement of tissue factor bearing microvesicles
    6. Coagulation system alteration by developed autoantibodies
    7. Genetic predisposition

I. Cardiac manifestations:
a. Endocarditis
b. Myocarditis
c. Pericarditis

J. Lung:
a. Pleuritis
b. Interstitial lung disease (ILD)

K. Others:
a. Amyloidosis: Here systemic deposition of amyloid material produces:
    1. Constipation
    2. Diarrhea
    3. Renal failure
b. Pancreatitis resulting from:
    1. Duodenal fistula
    2. Ampullary CD
    3. Gallstones
    4. Primary sclerosing cholangitis
    5. 6-mercaptopurine and azathioprine
    6. Autoimmune phenomenon
    7. Primary CD in the pancreas

Diagnosis

A. Hematological:
a. Raised ESR
b. Leukocytosis
c. Raised platelet count

B. Biochemical:
a. Liver function test: Hypoalbuminemia
b. Altered in case of PSC
c. Abnormal coagulation factors by factor assay
d. Calcium level
e. Oxalate level

C. Serological:
a. CRP
b. ANCA
c. p-ANCA

D. Stool examination:

a. *Clostridial difficile* examination will be ruled out.

b. *Escherichia coli, Shigella, Salmonella,* and *C. jejuni* have to be excluded.

c. Fecal lactoferrin—it is present in activated neutrophil; it is a highly specific and sensitive marker of interstitial inflammation.

d. Fecal calprotectin present in monocytes and neutrophils. It is elevated in:

1. Inflammatory colitis
2. Infectious colitis

But it is normal in case of IBS.

It can assess in case of UC:

1. Disease activity, more in endoscopically severe disease
2. Response
3. Relapse of the disease
4. Histological inflammation

E. Colonoscopic appearances:

a. It usually involves from rectum up to cecum

b. No intervening normal mucosa

c. In early cases, there is:

1. Superficial erosion
2. Mucosal hyperemia
3. Decreased vascular pattern
4. Mild friability

d. In moderate cases:

1. Mucosa is granular and friable. Granular mucosa means presence of tissue like rough grain-sized mass consisting of fibroblast and blood vessels
2. Complete loss of vascular pattern
3. Extensive erosions
4. Marked erythema

e. In severe cases:

1. Diffuse ulcerations
2. Spontaneous bleeding
3. Presence of pseudopolyps

f. In 10–20% cases, 5 cm of ileum may be involved, called backward ileitis.

Endoscopy can diagnose and assess therapeutic progression or the frequency of relapse.

F. Straight X-ray of abdomen:

It can demonstrate the following features:

a. Normal

b. Edematous wall

c. Irregular margin of the colon

d. Thickening of the colonic wall

e. Dilated colonic segments of >6 cm with loss of haustration involving right or transverse colon

G. Barium enema:

a. It is rarely used in IBD.

b. Double-contrast barium enema can be done in mild-to-moderate disease.

c. It can diagnose stricture of bowel.

d. In case of severe disease, it is contraindicated as it may produce toxic megacolon.

e. It can visualize the following features:

1. Irregularly thickened mucosa
2. Granular mucosa
3. Shortening of colon
4. Presence of pseudopolyps
5. Ulcerations—superficial or deep
6. Haustral folds—thickened and edematous.
7. Widening of prerectal space of >1 cm

H. CT colography:

a. Colonoscopy is superior in case of an ulcerated lesion in colon whereas in case of an elevated lesion, CT colonography is superior.

b. But biopsies are required for diagnosis of UC or neoplasm or any infection; hence CT colonography is rarely indicated.

I. MR colonography: It can diagnose:

a. Wall thickening from rectum to proximal colon

b. Increased enhancement of mucosa without any enhancement in submucosa

J. Histopathology:

a. Main differentiating feature is distortion of glandular architecture like distortion of vertical alignment of glands with irregular branching in UC, which is not present in infectious colitis.

b. The earliest finding is acute cryptitis due to leukocytes migration into cryptic epithelium from the basal capillary of the lamina propria, which ultimately leads to cryptic abscess.

Histological assessment of disease severity according to True Love criteria:

Grade	Features
0	Normal
1	Inflammation is not significant
2	• Edema • Vascularity

Continued

Continued

Grade	Features
	• Increased acute and chronic inflammatory cells • Intact epithelium
3	• Large number of inflammatory cells • Cryptic abscess • Ulceration of surface epithelium

Treatment

Aim of Therapy

A. Primary therapy:

a. Induction of remission

b. Maintenance of remission

B. Secondary therapy:

a. Maintenance of nutrition

b. Improvement of quality-of-life

Different types of remission:

A. Symptomatic remission—improvement of patient-related outcomes

B. Endoscopic remission—evidence of restoration to intact mucosa and absence of friability

C. Corticosteroid-free remissions—it is based on symptoms and endoscopic findings in absence of use of corticosteroids

D. Deep remission—it is the combination of symptomatic remission plus endoscopic remission.

Oral 5-aminosalicylic acid (5-ASA) Preparations

Mechanism of action:

A. It will scavenge free radicals.

B. It will downregulate NF-kB activity.

C. It will decrease IL-1 and TNF.

D. T-cell proliferation will be decreased.

E. Adhesion of neutrophil and macrophages will be decreased.

F. Antigen presentation to T cells will be decreased.

Preparation	Formulation	Site of release	Dose per day	Adverse effect
		Azo bond		
Sulfasalazine	Sulfapyridine + ASA	In the colon broken down by Azo reductase of bacteria to release 5 ASA	In mild-to-moderate UC: • In acute case: 3–6 g • In maintenance phase: 2–4 g	Hypersensitivity to sulfa: • Rash, fever, pneumonitis, agranulocytosis, worsening of colitis, pancreatitis • >6 g produces anorexia, nausea, vomiting, headache
Balsalazide	Aminobenzoyl-alanine-5-ASA	It is released into colon,	6.75–9 g	
		Delayed release drug		
Enteric-coated mesalamine like Delzicol, Asacol		• At pH > 7, it will disintegrate from the small intestine to colon up to splenic flexure • If taken with meal, it shows increased gastric resistance	• In acute case: 2.4–4.8 g • In maintenance phase: 1.6–4.8 g	In very high dose, it has adverse effects in the male reproductive system
Mesalamine like Lialda	Mesalamine is incorporated into lipophilic matric and encapsulated in AC polymer, which is resistant to degradation at pH < 7.5	It will be released into ileum to colon	2.4–4.8 g; it is given once daily	• Headache, nausea, abdominal pain, and hair loss • Rare effects: Hematuria, pancreatitis, and paradoxical worsening of colitis

Continued

Continued

Preparation	Formulation	Site of release	Dose per day	Adverse effect
		Delayed and extended-release tablets		
Apriso	It encapsulated mesalamine	It will deliver the granules into ileum and colon as outer coating will be dissolved at pH >6. Its polymer matrix core helps to release the granules throughout the colon		
		Controlled-release tablet		
Pentasa	• Its ethyl cellulose coating helps the small beads of mesalamine to absorb and dissolve 5-ASA in water and that will diffuse from the beads into the lumen • This disintegration occurs in the stomach and will be distributed throughout the small intestine up to the distal colon in fed and fasted conditions	Stomach to colon	• In acute phase: 2–4 g • In maintenance phase: 1.5–4 g	
		Mesalamine enema		
Rowasa	Topical enema	Distal colon	1–4 g	

Glucocorticoids

Oral corticosteroid is used in case of active UC not responding to 5-ASA therapy. Another locally acting steroid, budesonide, has minimal adverse effects due to its first-pass metabolism.

Mechanism of action:

A. Neutrophilic phagocytic activity will be decreased.

B. It has numerous anti-inflammatory and immunosuppressive activities.

C. It downregulates the NF-kB activity.

D. Elastase, collagenase, and nitric oxide synthetase activity will be inhibited.

E. There will be inhibition of expression of proinflammatory cytokines.

F. It inhibits adhesion molecules and leukotrienes.

Doses of the drugs:

A. In case of severe colitis not responding to 5-ASA, intravenous hydrocortisone 100 mg every 6 hourly or methylprednisolone 40–60 mg/day is given.

B. In case of moderately active disease unresponsive to 5-ASA, oral prednisolone 40–60 mg per day is given.

C. For mild disease not responding to 5-ASA, oral prednisolone 20 mg/day is given.

D. In case of budesonide, the dose is 9 mg/day for 8 weeks.

All the systemic steroids have to be tapered within 8–12 weeks.

Adverse effects:

A. Bone loss or osteoporosis

B. Myopathy

C. Glucose intolerance

D. Adrenocortical suppression

E. Neuropsychiatric symptoms, such as insomnia and mood disturbance

F. Posterior subcapsular cataract

Topical corticosteroids: In case of proctosigmoiditis, with or without proximal colon involvement, hydrocortisone enema or foam can be given once or twice daily in addition to oral 5-ASA or oral steroid therapy. But long-term topical steroid preparation should not be continued as it may produce profuse adrenocortical suppression.

Immunosuppressive Agents

Azathioprine and 6-mercaptopurine:

a. Pro-drug azathioprine will be converted in the liver to 6-mercaptopurine and inhibit cellular proliferation by inhibiting purine biosynthesis. It is used in active disease and also in maintenance phase.

b. Dose:
    1. Azathioprine 2–2.5 mg/kg/day
    2. 6-mercaptopurine 1–1.5 mg/kg/day

c. Side effects: Fever, nausea, vomiting, and pancreatitis. Bone marrow suppression, mainly leukopenia, may occur in deficiency of thiopurine methyl transferase.

Cyclosporine:

a. Mechanism of action: It works by interfering with IL-2 production and inhibits proliferation and activation of T-helper cells.
b. Dose: 2–4 mg/kg intravenously. In case of sudden discontinuation, there is relapse to a fulminant variety.
c. Adverse effects: Hypertrichosis, tremor, nephrotoxicity, gingival hyperplasia, nausea, vomiting, seizures, etc.

Tacrolimus:

a. Mechanism of action: By interfering IL-2 production, it will inhibit proliferation and activation of T-helper cells, but its onset of action is rapid and more potent.
b. Adverse effects: Hypertrichosis, tremor, nephrotoxicity, gingival hyperplasia, nausea, vomiting, seizures, etc.

Methotrexate:

a. Mechanism of action:
    1. It inhibits dihydrofolate reductase, thus impairing DNA synthesis.
    2. It decreases the production of IL-2.
b. Dose: 15–25 mg/week intramuscularly or subcutaneously
c. Toxicities: Hepatic fibrosis requiring evaluation of liver enzymes periodically; leukopenia requiring periodical evaluation of CBC

Biological Agents

Infliximab: It is a chimeric monoclonal antibody against TNF-α and binds with both membrane-bound and soluble forms of TNF-α.

Adalimumab: It is a fully humanized monoclonal antibody against TNF-α and is administered subcutaneously.

Golimumab: It is a fully humanized monoclonal antibody against TNF-α and is administered subcutaneously.

Ustekinumab: It is human monoclonal antibody that binds with p40 subunits of interleukin 12 and 23, thereby prevents their interaction with the receptors on the cell surface and reduces the immune response. Adverse effects are headache, upper respiratory infection, risk of malignancies and reversible posterior leukoencephalopathy syndrome.

Certolizumab: It is the first pegylated humanized monoclonal antibody against TNF-α.

Dose: 5 mg/kg infliximab at 0, 2, and 6 weeks followed by maintenance dose every 8th week along with 2.5 mg/kg orally; azathioprine is superior to monotherapy.

Side effects of infliximab: Pruritus, urticarial rash, nausea, chest discomfort, flushing, headache, dizziness, myalgia, etc.

Vedolizumab: It inhibits a-4 beta-7 integrins. It is effective, inducing remission in case of moderate-to-severe UC.

Tofacitinib: It is a nonselective Janus kinase inhibitor, dose is 10 mg twice daily, and can be used in case anti-TNF-alfa non-responsive patients. Complication is herpes zoster.

Filgotinib: It is a nonselective Janus kinase inhibitor, dose being 200 mg orally daily.

Natalizumab: It is humanized monoclonal antibody that inhibits α4 integrin thereby prevents adhesion of leukocytes as well as migration of leukocytes across the endothelium. Adverse effects are PML and reaction at the sites of infusion.

In spite of initial good response, two types of response may occur:

a. Primary nonresponse in 20% of patients
b. Secondary loss of response in 10–15% of patients

This may occur due to:

a. Concurrent intestinal infection
b. Inadequate therapeutic concentration of the drugs
c. Overlapping irritable bowel syndrome

Following are the causes of low drug level:

a. Increased inflammatory burden
b. Loss of protein from the inflamed mucosa
c. Development of neutralizing antidrug antibodies, which can be benefitted from escalation of the dose of that drug

In maintenance therapy, the concentrations of the drugs are:

a. In case of infliximab, 3–7 μg/mL
b. In case of adalimumab, 5–10 μg/mL

These optimum concentrations are associated with:

a. Clinical response
b. Normalization of CRP
c. Mucosal healing

Antibiotics

Antibiotics have no role in the treatment of UC.

Probiotics

Combination of 5-ASA with a probiotic at a daily dose of 3.63×10^{12} colony forming unit/day can improve symptom as compared to no treatment.

Fecal Microbiota Transplant

It shows variable benefits, but it has no steroid-sparing effect because of the variability of donor, system of delivery, and treatment duration. Hence, it is not recommended.

Surgery

Indications:

A. Complication of severe attack
B. Colonic dysplasia or colonic carcinoma
C. Severe attack, which cannot be cured by medical therapy
D. Chronic and continuous disease, which may impair the quality-of-life of the patient
E. Failure to discontinue the steroid therapy in spite of other medical interventions

Method of surgery:

A. Subtotal colectomy with ileostomy
B. Total colectomy with ileoanal anastomosis
C. Proctocolectomy with Brooke ileostomy
D. Proctocolectomy with ileal-pouch anal anastomosis

In case of mild-to-moderate UC:

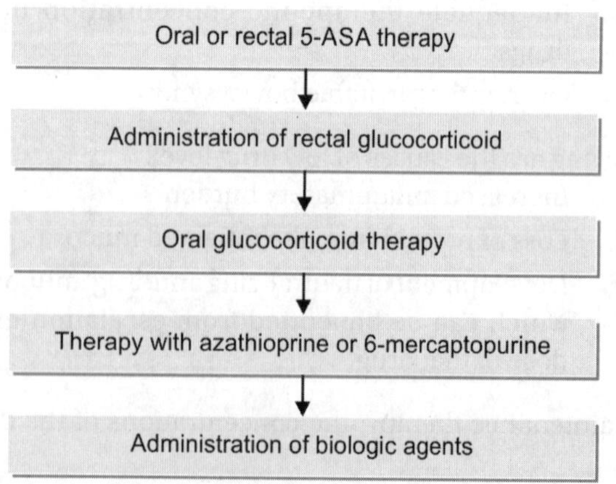

In case of severe UC:

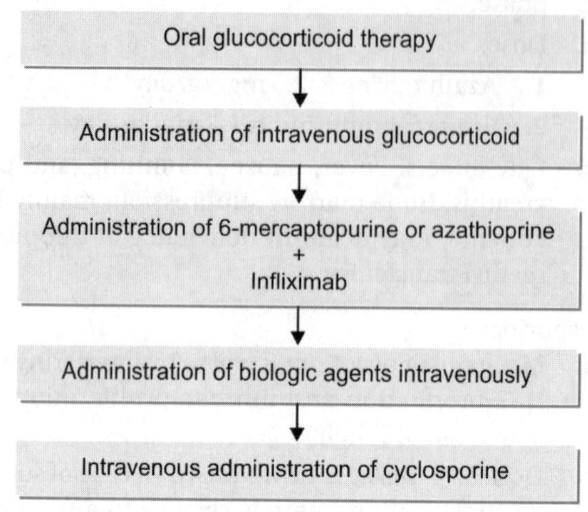

Q9. Meckel's diverticulum.

MGR/OCT2013/MDI (5)

ANSWER

Meckel's diverticulum is the most common (2% of population) congenital abnormality of the gastrointestinal tract, where a blind sac arises from the antimesenteric border of ileum, approximately 40–100 cm away from the ileo-cecal valve; its length is 5 cm and diameter 2 cm. Arterial supply is from a branch of the ileocolic artery, which is a branch of the superior mesenteric artery.

Embryology

In an embryo, mid gut communicates with yolk sac temporarily with omphalomesenteric duct, which will become obliterated progressively in the 5th or 6th week. But if this obliteration is incomplete, it will give rise to various abnormalities, such as ileo-umbilical fistula, fibrous cord between ileum and umbilicus, or Meckel's diverticulum when the intestinal end of that duct fails to close.

Histopathology

It contains all the layers of ileal mucosa along with some heterotopic tissues from:

a. Gastric mucosa
b. Pancreas
c. Jejunum
d. Brunner's gland

e. Combined gastric and duodenal mucosa
f. Hepatobiliary
g. Colonic

Clinical Features

A. Mostly, it is asymptomatic and can be diagnosed during laparotomy or contrast study or during laparoscopic procedures.
B. Other symptomatic features are:
   a. Gastrointestinal hemorrhage
   b. Intestinal obstruction
   c. Inflammation
   d. Intussusception
   e. Umbilical sinus
   f. Umbilical fistula
   g. Lithiasis of diverticulum
   h. Entrapment of ileal loop by a band, which is stretched in between the base of the mesentery and the ileal loop
   i. Gallstone ileus
   j. Phytobezoar formation
   k. Impacted meconium in neonates
   l. Carcinoid, mesenchymal tumors

Diagnosis

A. Radioimaging:
   a. In case of distention in the diverticulum, gas-filled viscus may be seen in the middle of the abdomen or right iliac fossa.
   b. In case of perforation, pneumoperitoneum can be seen in the erect position in case of straight X-ray of abdomen.
   c. Meckel's diverticulum may be seen as a contrast-filled pouch in the ileum at the antimesenteric border.
   d. Inflammation of Meckel's diverticulum may produce gas–fluid levels in the cecal region.
B. Ultrasonography: It will demonstrate—
   a. Tubular diverticulum swollen with fluid in the region away from the cecum
   b. Invagination of Meckel's diverticulum
   c. Segmental thickening of the bowel wall
   d. Pelvic abscess
   e. Presence of anomalous vessels by Doppler study
C. CT scan: It will demonstrate:
   a. Gas-filled structure in continuity with small intestine
   b. Blind end fluid containing structure in continuity with small intestine
   c. Inverted diverticulum shown as interior nucleus of fat attenuation encircled by annulus of soft tissue
D. Angiography: It will demonstrate:
   a. Location of hemorrhage
   b. Reason for hemorrhage
E. Nuclear imaging by Technetium 99m-Pertechnetate: It will concentrate on the ectopic gastric tissue. Pretreatment with pentagastrin will accelerate tissue uptake of technetium.
F. Capsule endoscopy: It can visualize the small intestine and Meckel's diverticulum. It is contraindicated under 10 years of age.
G. Double-balloon small bowel enteroscopy can visualize small bowel and, if required, biopsy can be taken.
H. CT enterography can maximize the visibility of the bowel structure as well as mucosa and peri-enteral abnormalities and detection of bowel wall lesion.
I. MR enterography assesses the functional abnormalities of the small intestine.

Treatment

Treatment of choice is resection of Meckel's diverticulum by laparotomy or laparoscopy. Accordingly, the patients who follow the below criteria should undergo resection of diverticulum:
   a. Patient's age is <55 years
   b. Male sex
   c. >2-cm length of diverticulum
   d. Histopathology of tissue demonstrates presence of abnormal tissue
   e. Broad-based diverticulum in patients who are prone to develop complications
   f. Presence of broad band attached to diverticulum

Methods are:
   a. Resection of diverticulum with end-to-end anastomosis
   b. Resection of associated intestine with end-to-end anastomosis
   c. In case of gastrointestinal bleeding, segmental ileal resection

Q10. Diagnosis and management of tuberculosis of intestine.

DNBIIIB/DEC2015 (10)

Gastrointestinal tuberculosis.

RAJIV GANDHI UNI OF HEALTH SC, KARNATAKA, 2019 (10)

ANSWER

Introduction

Gastrointestinal tuberculosis is 1–3% of all tuberculosis worldwide. It may be the primary disease of intestine or secondary to pulmonary involvement.

Etiology

Mycobacteria can infect the gastrointestinal tract in the following ways:

- **a.** Ingestion of sputum containing *Mycobacterium tuberculosis* in a patient having active pulmonary disease
- **b.** Hematogenous spread from distant tubercular focus
- **c.** From infected lymph nodes through lymphatic spread
- **d.** From direct extension of contagious sites
- **e.** Consumption of raw milk infected with *Mycobacterium tuberculosis*

Gastrointestinal tuberculosis can be classified into two types:

- **a.** Primary tuberculosis due to direct ingestion of infected milk
- **b.** Secondary tuberculosis due to spread of human tuberculous bacteria from patients suffering from tuberculosis

Site of infection: The main site is the terminal ileum with the ileocecal valve due to a combination of the following factors:

- **a.** Narrow lumen
- **b.** Increased physiological stasis
- **c.** Minimal digestive activity
- **d.** Presence of M cells in the lymphatic tissue that are capable of taking tubercle bacilli

Proximal gastrointestinal tract is not usually involved as the fatty capsules of tubercle bacilli are not digested in these sites, thus preventing release of bacilli.

Pathophysiology

A. Esophagus is involved from contagious tissues in the middle third at the level of carina.

B. Gastric lesion is rare due to:

- **a.** Presence of protective fatty acid capsule
- **b.** Rapid transit time
- **c.** High acidic environment
- **d.** Absence of lymphoid tissue

But it may involve secondary to pulmonary involvement. In that case, it may produce gastric outlet obstruction.

C. In case of small and large intestines:

- **a.** Ulcerative form (20%):
  1. Malnourished adults are affected.
  2. Presence of multiple ulcers distributed transverse to long axis of colon, called "girdle ulcer".
  3. Ulcer margins are everted and indented and may penetrate beyond muscularis propria.
  4. Healing of ulcers is followed by stricture formation.
  5. There may be adhesion between the loops.
- **b.** Hypertrophic form (10%):
  1. Well-nourished young patients are affected.
  2. Due to low-grade and low-virulent infection and high immunity of host, there will be formation of mass consisting of mesenteric nodes, adherent bowel, and adherent lymph nodes.
  3. There is a hypertrophic germinal center and hyperplasia of lymphoid follicles, but absence of granuloma.
  4. Presence of exophytic mass arising from mucosa simulating carcinoma.
- **c.** Ulcerohypertrophic form (70%):
  1. It is most common—70%.
  2. Infection is of low virulence with high-grade host immunity.

D. In case of rectum having multiple fistulae and, after a recent anal surgery, the lesion may not heal or there may be a circumferential lesion resembling mass.

E. Gallbladder and liver may be involved as a result of hematogenous spread or direct intra-abdominal spread.

F. Peritoneal involvement: Peritoneum is involved due to rupture of necrotic lymph nodes of retroperitoneum and mesentery or these can caseate and calcify resulting ascitic fluid formation. Tuberculous peritonitis shows in five forms:

- **a.** Ascitic form
- **b.** Fibrous form
- **c.** Plastic form
- **d.** Purulent form
- **e.** Nodular form

Clinical Features

A. Present history:

- **a.** Abdominal pain:
  - **1.** Colicky abdominal pain due to subacute abdominal obstruction due to narrowing
  - **2.** Diffuse abdominal pain due to involvement of peritoneum or mesentery
  - **3.** Pain in right iliac fossa due to presence of tender lump
- **b.** Diarrhea:
  - **1.** Blood in stool due to ulcer in the intestine but rarely massive.
  - **2.** It may be due to multiple factors:
    - Malabsorption
    - Inflammatory response in the intestine leading to effect of leukotrienes, cytokines, and prostaglandins on intestinal fluid, thus increasing intestinal motility.
- **c.** Features of malabsorption due to:
  - **1.** Extensive ulceration
  - **2.** Decrease in absorptive areas
  - **3.** Lymphatic obstruction
  - **4.** Bacterial overgrowth in the small intestine
- **d.** Weight loss
- **e.** Low-grade fever
- **f.** Past history of pulmonary tuberculosis
- **g.** Family history of pulmonary tuberculosis
- **h.** Dysphagia or odynophagia
- **i.** Repeated postprandial vomiting due to gastric outlet obstruction

A. General examination:

- **a.** Signs of malnutrition
- **b.** Pallor
- **c.** Disseminated disease lymphadenopathy
- **d.** Cutaneous markers of tuberculosis

B. Abdominal examination:

- **a.** Doughy abdomen due to abdominal inflammation and fibrous adhesion
- **b.** Hepatomegaly
- **c.** Splenomegaly
- **d.** Ascites
- **e.** Lump in the right iliac fossa
- **f.** Lymphadenopathy
- **g.** Abdominal mass
- **h.** Rectal bleeding

C. Respiratory system examination:

- **a.** Features of parenchymal involvement
- **b.** Features of pleural effusion in case of disseminated tuberculosis

Evaluation or Diagnosis

A. Routine investigations:

- **a.** Hemoglobin—low
- **b.** ESR—high
- **c.** Lymphocytic leukocytosis
- **d.** Serum albumin—low
- **e.** CRP—raised

B. Mantoux test: In patients with ileocecal tuberculosis, this test has many limitations:

- **a.** There is cross reactivity with BCG.
- **b.** There is a high prevalence of environmental mycobacteria.
- **c.** There is presence of widespread latent mycobacterial tuberculosis infection

C. Chest X-ray: In 10—15% patients, there is evidence of active pulmonary tuberculosis.

D. Plain X-ray of abdomen:

- **a.** Presence of calcified granuloma or calcified lymph node
- **b.** Evidence of dilated terminal ileum
- **c.** Presence of multiple dilated loops showing air–fluid levels

E. Barium study:

- **a.** Hypersegmentation and flocculation of barium is the early sign.
- **b.** Circumferential distribution of ulcers, irregular thickened mucosal folds
- **c.** Inverted umbrella sign or Fleischer's sign: There is a triangular appearance of the ileocecal valve with its base present near the cecum.
- **d.** String sign: Presence of a narrowed segment before the ileocecal valve
- **e.** Sterling sign: Rapid transit of barium and lack of retention of barium in the terminal cecum

F. Ultrasonography of abdomen: Following are the features of intestinal tuberculosis:
  - **a.** Presence of ascites
  - **b.** Presence of bowel mass consisting of bowel loops and omentum
  - **c.** Due to interloop ascitic fluid, loops look like club sandwich
  - **d.** Evidence of concentric thickening as compared to eccentric thickening in case of CD
  - **e.** Appearance of matted lymph nodes like heterogenous as compared to homogenous appearance of nodes in case of lymphoma
  - **f.** In some cases, pulling up of the ileocecal region in the subhepatic areas producing a pseudo-kidney sign

G. CT scan of abdomen demonstrates the following features:
  - **a.** Intraluminal or extraluminal pathology
  - **b.** Extent of the disease
  - **c.** Thickening and narrowing of the intestinal wall with or without luminal narrowing
  - **d.** Presence of lymphadenopathy with central necrosis or calcification

H. Colonoscopy will demonstrate the following features:
  - **a.** Concentric ulcers surrounded by inflamed mucosa
  - **b.** Fish mouth opening of the ileocecal valve due to a patulous valve with surrounding heaped-up folds suggestive of tubercular rather than Crohn's etiology
  - **c.** Presence of hyperemic nodules, ulcers, or polyps in the terminal ileum or cecum
  - **d.** Stricture may be present at the ileocecal region

I. TB gold of blood for tuberculosis. Though used previously, according to new guidelines, it is not used nowadays.

J. Measurement of gamma-producing T-cell response to early secreted antigenic targets of *Mycobacterium tuberculosis* is used and shows excellent results.

K. GeneXpert *Mycobacterium tuberculosis* assay— it can simultaneously identify tubercle bacilli and resistance to rifampicin.

L. PCR and ultra-PCR are highly sensitive and highly specific for diagnosis of tuberculosis of intestine accurately and can at the same time differentiate it from CD.

M. Line probe assay: It uses PCR and reverse hybridization:
  - **a.** To detect *Mycobacterium tuberculosis* complex
  - **b.** To detect rapidly mutation in mycobacterial genome associated with drug resistance against rifampicin and isoniazid in case of MTBDRplus and fluoroquinolone resistance in case of MTBDRs1

N. Ascitic fluid test:
  - **a.** Serum-ascites albumin gradient (SAAG) value is <1.1.
  - **b.** Adenosine deaminase (ADA) value is >39.
  - **c.** Ziehl–Neelsen staining of ascitic fluid—sensitivity is 0.6%, culture—sensitivity is 20%.
  - **d.** GeneXpert assay of ascitic fluid—sensitivity is lower than that of culture.

O. Fine needle aspiration cytology from the mass during endoscopic ultrasound or transabdominal ultrasound for definite diagnosis

P. Laparoscopy can help in taking biopsy of peritoneal tubercle.

Q. Histology of tubercle contain:
  - **a.** Band of epithelioid macrophages
  - **b.** Langhans giant cells
  - **c.** Lymphocytes
  - **d.** Cheese-like caseation in the central area
  - **e.** On acid-fast staining, there is presence of acid-fast bacilli

Management of Intestinal Tuberculosis

A. Medical management: 6 months' course of four antituberculous drugs with rifampicin, isoniazid, ethambutol, and pyrazinamide for 2 months followed by two-drug therapy with rifampicin and isoniazid for 4 months. It will heal tubercular ulcers but not the deformity. But in case of disseminated disease, prolonged therapy is needed.

B. Surgery: Indications of surgery:
  - **a.** Obstruction
  - **b.** Free perforation
  - **c.** Fistula
  - **d.** Hemorrhage
  - **e.** Abscess

  Process: It can be classified into three broad groups:
  - **a.** Bypassing the involved segment: It can be done by:
    1. Entero-enterostomy
    2. Ileo-transverse colostomy

    The above procedures are complicated by:
    1. Fistula formation
    2. Blind loop syndrome
    3. Recurrence of the disease

b. Radical resection of involved segments: Procedure is hemicolectomy. This procedure is accompanied by antitubercular treatment. But this procedure can be hindered by low nourishment of the patient.

c. Conservative surgery: Strictureplasty can be done in the patients who are on antithyroid drug (ATD) treatment but have persistent strictures or multiple strictures.

Q11. Define and classify gastrointestinal neuroendocrine tumors. How are they diagnosed and managed?

DNBIIB/DEC2014 (10)

ANSWER

Neuroendocrine tumors are the interface between two main systems, endocrine and endocrine systems. These tumors can be distinguished from other solid tumors by their ability to secrete some molecules having ability to produce systemic syndrome. The tumors are classified as follows:

A. Carcinoid tumor: This tumor arises from enterochromaffin cells of the aerodigestive tract. It will convert dietary tryptophan to serotonin, which will be converted into 5-hydroxyindoleacetic acid. It can be described according to its origin and distribution.

Site	Location	Hormone secreted	Carcinoid features	Associated features
Foregut	• Stomach • Duodenum • Lung • Pancreas	• Elevated gastrin • Histamine • Majority nonfunctional	Rare (associated with bronchial carcinoid and liver metastasis)	• Atrophic gastritis • Pernicious anemia • Multiple endocrine neoplasia 1 • Zollinger–Ellison syndrome
Midgut	• Small intestine • Proximal colon • Appendix	Vasoactive substances, such as: • Histamine • Tachykinin • Kallikrein • Prostaglandin	Classical features with liver metastasis	• Obstruction • Intussusception • Abdominal pain
Hindgut	• Distal colon • Rectum • Genitourinary tract	Nonsecretory	Rare, but associated with testicular or ovarian tumor	Alteration of bowel habit, bleeding obstruction

Typical features are flushing and diarrhea mainly from small intestinal tumors.

Treatment:

a. Since abdominal rectal carcinoid tumor is <2 cm—segmental resection with mesenteric lymphadenectomy

b. If the size of appendicular carcinoid is >2 cm or there is posterior margin invasion—right hemicolectomy

c. Liver metastasis can be treated by:
   1. Local surgical debulking
   2. Embolization of hepatic artery
   3. Chemoembolization
   4. Cryotherapy
   5. Radiofrequency ablation

d. Patient can be medically treated with octreotide having antitumor activity

e. Telotristat ethyl targeting tryptophan hydroxylase can be administered orally in association with the somatostatin analog, octreotide.

f. Other chemotherapeutic active agents are streptozocin, 5-fluorouracil, doxorubicin, and interferon.

B. Pancreatic neuroendocrine tumor: It is an islet cell tumor arising from the beta cells of pancreas; 75% of these are nonfunctioning and 25% are functioning.

Following is the description of pancreatic neuroendocrine tumors:

Name	Secreted hormone	Clinical feature	Diagnosis
Insulinoma	Insulin	Hypoglycemia	• Increased serum insulin • Raised C-peptide • Low glucose level
Zollinger–Ellison syndrome or gastrinoma	Gastrin	• Secretory diarrhea • Peptic ulcer	• Serum gastrin >1,000 pg/mL • If serum gastrin <1,000 pg/mL, secretin stimulation test
Somatostatinoma	Glucagon	• Weight loss • Abdominal pain • Diarrhea • Diabetes mellitus • Stones in gallbladder	Fasting somatostatin level >160 pg/mL
Glucagonoma	Somatostatin	• Cheilitis • Anemia • Weight loss • Diabetes • Necrotizing migrating erythema	Serum level of glucagon >500 pg/mL
VIPoma	VIP	• Profuse watery diarrhea • Hypochlorhydria • Hypokalemia	Serum VIP level >75 pg/mL

Treatment of gastrinoma:

a. In case of sporadic gastrinoma without metastasis—surgical resection of the tumor

b. Gastrin secretion can be controlled by:

1. PPIs
2. Somatostatin analog or octreotide
3. Sunitinib and everolimus are approved by the FDA for treatment of a well-differentiated pancreatic tumor.
4. Active chemotherapeutic agents are streptozocin, doxorubicin, 5-fluorouracil, and dacarbazine.

Treatment of Insulinoma:

a. Surgery is the treatment of choice.

b. In case of recurrence of disease or metastases to liver, surgical resection along with liver-directed therapy, such as chemoembolization or radiofrequency ablation

c. Refractory hypoglycemia can be treated by oral diazoxide, as it inhibits secretion of pancreatic insulin.

d. Sunitinib and everolimus are approved by the FDA for the treatment of a well-differentiated pancreatic tumor

e. Active chemotherapeutic agents are streptozocin, doxorubicin, 5-fluorouracil, and dacarbazine.

Treatment of VIPoma:

a. Diarrhea can be treated by octreotide and correction of water and electrolyte imbalance.

b. In case of recurrence of disease or metastases to liver surgical resection along with liver-directed therapy like chemoembolization or radiofrequency ablation

c. Sunitinib and everolimus are approved by the FDA for the treatment of a well-differentiated pancreatic tumor.

Treatment of glucagonoma:

a. Patients with a dermatological lesion can be treated by amino acid infusion and zinc supplements.

b. Surgery

c. Somatostatin analog

d. Anticoagulant in case of thromboembolism

e. Targeted chemotherapy

Treatment of glucagonoma:

a. Surgery

b. Targeted therapy/chemotherapy

Q12. Splanchnic circulation.

MGR/OCT2013/MDI (5)

ANSWER

This circulation involves the stomach, pancreas, spleen, pancreas, small and large intestines, three branches of the abdominal aorta:

A. Celiac artery: It is a major division at the T12 level: Branches are:

- **a.** Left gastric artery
- **b.** Common hepatic artery
- **c.** Splenic artery

Supplied to the following organs:

- **a.** Stomach
- **b.** Upper duodenum
- **c.** Spleen
- **d.** Pancreas

B. Superior mesenteric artery: It arises at the level of L1 and contains >10% of cardiac output. Branches are:

- **a.** Inferior pancreaticoduodenal artery
- **b.** Intestinal arteries
- **c.** Ileocolic artery
- **d.** Right colic artery
- **e.** Middle colic artery

Supplied to the following organs:

- **a.** Lower part of the duodenum
- **b.** Jejunum
- **c.** Ileum
- **d.** Cecum
- **e.** Appendix
- **f.** Ascending colon
- **g.** Two-thirds of transverse colon

C. Inferior mesenteric artery: It arises anteriorly at the level of L3. Branches are:

- **a.** Left colic artery
- **b.** Sigmoidal branches
- **c.** Superior rectal artery

Supplied organs are:

- **a.** Lateral one-third of transverse colon
- **b.** Descending colon
- **c.** Upper rectum

Physiology

In a resting state, blood flow is 30 mL/min/100 g of tissue. In case of low cardiac output, it will decrease to <10 mL/min/100 g of tissue and after meals, it will peak to 250 mL/min/100 g of tissues. This flow can be controlled by two mechanisms:

A. Intrinsic control: There are two proposed mechanisms—

- **a.** Myogenic control: In this method, the vessel will respond to increased transmural pressure or stretching by constricting and thus maintains blood flow at baseline.
- **b.** Metabolic control: It will depend upon oxygen supply and demand. Metabolites such as adenosine, K^+, H^+, and carbon dioxide during poor oxygen supply and tissue hypoxia will produce vasodilatation, which in turn increases the blood flow.

B. Extrinsic control:

- **a.** Sympathetic stimulation releases noradrenaline leading to α-adrenergic vasoconstriction. In case of sympathetic stimulation, there is a triphasic pattern of alteration of blood flow:
  1. Initial reduction of flow to near normal within minutes of stimulation
  2. Reactionary hyperemia on cessation of all activities
  3. Normalization of blood flow

  During this period, blood will be distributed throughout the body.
- **b.** Parasympathetic stimulation: Its stimulation increases intestinal motility and increases secretions, which in turn increases the blood flow. Activation of muscarinic receptors by acetylcholine nitric oxide will be released, which in turn increases mucosal blood flow through producing smooth muscles relaxation.

C. Humoral control:

- **a.** Vasodilators are:
  1. Increased PCO_2
  2. Decreased O_2
  3. Acetylcholine
  4. Vasoactive intestinal polypeptide (VIP)
  5. Gastric inhibitory polypeptide (GIP)
  6. Nitric oxide
  7. Dopamine
  8. Gastrin
  9. Secretin
- **b.** Vasoconstrictors:
  1. Decreased PCO_2
  2. Increased O_2

3. Increased H^+
4. Vasopressin
5. Peptide YY
6. Angiotensin II

Disorders of Splanchnic Circulation

A. Ischemic reperfusion injury and gut origin hypothesis: In case of critical cases like hypovolemic states, low cardiac output states, and abdominal compartment syndrome, perfusion of vital organ is maintained in expense of splanchnic circulation, which can lead to nonocclusive mesenteric ischemia. Reperfusion develops following the sequence of events:

a. Formation of ROS producing tissue damage

b. Adhesion of polymorphs to the endothelial cells

The result is systemic inflammatory response syndrome due to the following factors:

a. Release of inflammatory cytokines into systemic circulation

b. Vascular permeability

If untreated, it ultimately leads to multiorgan dysfunction syndrome having mortality of 40%.

In case of systemic inflammation, bacterial translocation from the intestinal wall due to disruption of the gut barrier function leads to liberation of proinflammatory cytokines, which ultimately produce multiple organ dysfunction syndrome (MODS), starting acute lung injury.

In gut-lymph hypothesis, proinflammatory cytokines from the ischemic gut via mesenteric lymph nodes in the thoracic duct into the systemic circulation bypassing the liver to the subclavian vein and then to the lung.

B. Splanchnic blood flow (SBF) in systemic inflammatory response syndrome (SIRS): In case of systemic infection, there is compromise in the SBF by the microcirculatory condition which is mediated by:

a. Local metabolic factors

b. Paracrine factors

c. Redistribution of blood flow between mucus and muscularis mucosae

Microcirculatory flow is influenced by systemic vascular resistance and cardiac output.

C. Splanchnic circulation in case of liver disease: The main cause of disruption of splanchnic circulation is portal circulation.

D. In case of anesthetic agents:

a. Volatile anesthetic agents have recognized effects on systemic hemodynamics and also changes in regional distribution of blood flow to splanchnic circulation.

b. In case of intravenous anesthetic agents, there is no relation with SBF.

E. In case of ventilation, there is a direct positive effect of positive-pressure ventilation and SBF due to:

a. Large tidal volume

b. High level of positive end expiratory pressure

c. High inspiratory pressure

These effects are due to:

a. Increased hepatic venous pressure

b. Increased mesenteric vascular resistance along with reduction of portal venous flow

F. Sympathomimetic agents:

a. Effect of norepinephrine in the splanchnic circulation is minimal.

b. Dobutamine, dopamine, and dopexamine have a positive vasodilatory effect on SBF.

c. Vasopressin administration is associated with vasoconstriction in the splanchnic circulation.

Q13. Test of gastric function.

MGR/OCT2011/MDI (5)

ANSWER

Following are the tests for gastric function:

A. Fractional test meal: All the fasting stomach content has to be aspirated; then gastric secretion is stimulated by providing test meals, and acidity of each sample has to be measured.

B. Pentagastrin stimulation test:

a. In the fasting state, gastric juice is aspirated by Ryle's tube—it is residual juice.

b. Then after 1 hour, gastric juice is collected as a single sample.

c. Then, pentagastrin will be injected and gastric secretion is collected every 15 minutes for the next 1 hour.

1. Basal output (BAO): It is the acid output in mmol/h in absence of all avoidable and intentional stimulation.
2. Maximal acid output (MAO): It is the acid output in mmol/h measured by addition of all 15-minute samples after pentagastrin stimulation.
3. Peak acid output (PAO): It is the acid output in mmol/h measured by adding two consecutive peak samples collected at 15-minute interval.

	Acid output in mmol/h			
	Men		Women	
	Lower limit	Upper limit	Lower limit	Upper limit
BAO	–	10	–	5.5
MAO	7	45	5	30
PAO	12	60	8	40

Interpretation of gastric juice analysis:

a. In case of Zollinger–Ellison syndrome:
  1. BAO is >15 mmol/h
  2. BAO/MAO: ≥0.6

b. In case of CDU:
  1. BAO, MAO, and PAO all are elevated.
  2. BAO vary from 4 to 6 mmol/h
  3. BAO/PAO ratio ≥ 0.3 suggests increased basal secretory drive.

Causes of hyperacidity:

a. Duodenal ulcer
b. Carcinoid tumor
c. Zollinger–Ellison syndrome
d. Gastric cell hyperplasia
e. Multiple endocrine neoplasia (MEN)

Causes of hypoacidity:

a. Gastritis
b. Gastric carcinoma
c. Pernicious anemia
d. Chronic iron deficiency anemia

C. Gastric motility function tests:

Tests	Parameters to be measured	Radiation exposure	Clinical importance
Scintigraphic gastric emptying	Emptying of stomach	+	• It will guide the therapy • It will predict the outcome
Stable isotope breath test	Emptying of stomach cavity	Nil	• It will guide the therapy • It will predict the outcome
USG	• Emptying of stomach • Transpyloric flow • Accommodation in the stomach	Nil	Under investigation
Drink test	Not known exactly	Nil	No proved clinical utility
Electrogastrogram	Measurement of myoelectrical activity	Nil	It is under investigation
Antroduodenal manometry	Measures: • Antropyloroduodenal coupling • Contraction of stomach and intestine	+	• It can differentiate normal from gastroparesis or gastric obstruction • It can predict the response to enteral feeding response • It can predict the response to prokinetic therapy
MRI	• Antral contraction • Accommodation in stomach cavity • Gastric emptying	Nil	Under investigation
Single photon emission computerized tomography	Accommodation in stomach cavity	+	Under investigation

Q14. Gut hormones.

MGR/SEP2010/MDI (5) MGR/MAR2009/MDI (5) RGUHS/MDI (10)

Gastric secretion and their hormones.

MGR/SEP2009/MDI (5)

Gut hormones and their physiology.

BF/MAY2010/MDI (8)

Gut hormones in health and diseases.

WBUHS, 2022 (10)

Gut hormones.

RAJIV GANDHI UNI OF HEALTH SC, KARNATAKA, 2018 (10)

Gut hormones in health and diseases.

RAJASTHAN UNIVERSITY, 2017 (10)

ANSWER

Name of hormone	Site of origin	Actions	Stimulant of secretion
Gastrin	• G cell of stomach • TG cells of GI tract • Islets cells of pancreas in fetus • Anterior pituitary • Brain	Stimulates: • Gastrin secretion • Motility • Release and secretion of pancreatic hormones • Secretion of pancreatic juice • Promotes growth of gastric mucosa	• Presence of stomach cavity • Stimulation of nerve plexus of stomach and small intestine • Gastrin-releasing peptide released from vagal nerve endings
Secretin	S cells in the small intestine	• Stimulates watery and alkaline pancreatic juice secretion • Inhibits motility and gastric secretion • Constricts pyloric sphincter • Potentiates action of cholecystokinin	• Presence of active chime in the duodenum from stomach • Product of protein digestion
Cholecystokinin	I cells in the small intestine	• Stimulates pancreatic enzyme secretion • Contracts gallbladder • Increases secretion of enterokinase • Increases gastric and intestinal motility and pyloric sphincter contraction • Accelerates activity of secretin • Induces tolerance to opioids	Presence of chyme containing fat, protein, peptides, and amino acids in the upper small intestine
Gastric inhibitory polypeptide (GIP)	K cells of duodenum, jejunum, antrum of stomach	• Stimulates secretion of insulin • Inhibition of gastric motility and secretion	Chyme containing glucose and fat in duodenum
Vasoactive intestinal polypeptide	• Small and large intestines • Stomach	• Dilatation of splanchnic blood vessels • Inhibition of HCl in gastric juice • Stimulation of succus entericus and insulin secretion • Intestinal smooth muscle relaxation	Presence of acid containing chyme in stomach and intestine
Glucagon	• Alpha cell of pancreas • Alpha cell of stomach • L cells in small intestine	Rise in blood sugar level	Presence of increased fat and protein content in stomach cavity
Glicentin	L cells in duodenum and jejunum	Rise in blood sugar level	Chyme containing fat and protein in small intestine
Glucagon like polypeptide-1 (GLP-1)	• Alpha cell in pancreas • Brain	• Inhibits gastric motility • Stimulation of secretion of insulin	Presence of food containing glucose in small intestine
GLP-2	L cells in ileum and colon	Suppression of appetite	Presence of food containing glucose in small intestine
Somatostatin	• D cells in pancreas, stomach and small intestine • Hypothalamus	Inhibits: GH secretion, gastric secretion, pancreatic juice, and other gastrointestinal hormone secretions	Presence of food containing glucose and protein in small intestine
Pancreatic polypeptide	PP cells in pancreas and small intestine	• Decrease pancreatic secretion • Increase glucagon secretion	Presence of food containing protein in small intestine, hypoglycemia, exercise
Peptide YY	L cells in ileum and colon	• Inhibits gastric and intestinal motility • Suppresses appetite • Reduces pancreatic juice secretion	Presence of food containing fat in small intestine

Continued

Continued

Name of hormone	Site of origin	Actions	Stimulant of secretion
Neuropeptide Y	• Ileum • Colon • Automatic nervous system	Increases the enteric blood flow	Presence of food containing fat in small intestine
Motilin	• Mo cells of stomach and small intestine • Enterochromaffin cells in intestine	Increases gastric motility and intestinal peristalsis	Entry of food from stomach into intestine
Substance P	• Brain • Small intestine	Increases intestinal motility	Presence of food in small intestine
Ghrelin	• Pituitary • Stomach • Kidney • Placenta • Hypothalamus	• Increases GH • Induces food intake • Stimulates gastric emptying	Fasting

Gut Hormones in Diseases

Hormones	Diseases
Gastrin	Its level is increased in Zollinger-Ellison syndrome
Ghrelin	Its level is increased in Prader-Willi syndrome associated with cachexia and obesity
Cholecystokinin	Its level is decreased in pancreatic insufficiency and obesity
Motilin	Its level is decreased in constipation type irritable bowel syndrome and gastroparesis
Secretin	Its level is decreased in the duodenal ulcer
Glucagon like peptide 1	In diabetes and obesity, agonist to GLP-1 is used as treatment
Peptide YY	Its level is decreased in obesity and metabolic disorders
Glucagon like peptide 2	In case of short bowel syndrome it is the therapeutic target
Somatostatin	It is used as treatment in case hormone producing tumor like carcinoid syndrome
Vasoactive intestinal polypeptide	It is produced in large quantity in case of VIPoma
Enteroglucagon	Its production is increased in glucagonoma
Neurotensin	Its level is increased in neuroendocrine tumor

Q15. Etiology, investigation, and treatment of bacillary dysentery.

MGR/APR2013/MDIII (7)

ANSWER

Definition of Case

It is a mild-to-severe intestinal infection characterized by passage of mucus and blood due to infection with four species of gram-negative nonspore-forming bacilli.

Etiology

Four types of bacilli:

A. *Shigella dysenteriae*: Type 1 *Shigella dysenteriae* is responsible for severe infection; in case of untreated infection, disease-related mortality is 20%.

B. *Shigella flexneri*: It produces disease of intermediate severity.

C. *Shigella boydii*

D. *Shigella sonnei*: It is more common in industrialized countries. It produces least severe disease.

Shigella dysenteriae, flexneri, and *boydii* usually occur in developing countries.

Pathogenesis

Incubation period is 1–3 days, but in untreated cases, it will last for ≥5 days.

Reservoir of infection is human beings.

Sources are:

A. Infected stool from symptomatic human being, but asymptomatic patients with normal stool may be the source rarely.

B. Contaminated food

C. Flies serves as a vector for *Shigella* infection.

Route of transmission:

A. Feco-oral route

B. Person-to-person contact—it mainly occurs in children

C. Sexual contact

Infective dose is few like 100 viable organisms.
The sites of affection are distal ileum and whole colon, but the rectosigmoid area is most severely affected and proximal colon involvement is less severe.

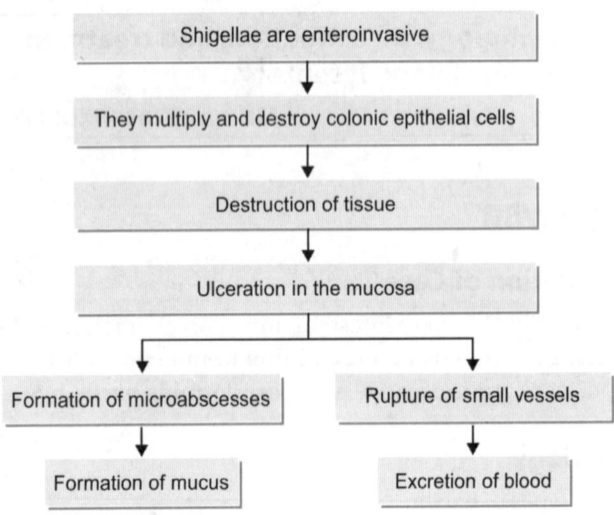

Shigella infection results in local profound inflammatory response leading to release of outpouring of polymorphonuclear leukocytes as well as mucus. Combination of mucus and blood from the colonic epithelium results in production of dysenteric stool. *Shigella* also produces systemic inflammatory response resulting in fever with chill, body ache, malaise, etc.

Virulence of *Shigella* is controlled by 202 kb weighing virulence plasmid containing genes, which aid in adherence and penetration of colonic epithelium and spread in between the cells. This plasmid makes *E. coli* distinct from *Shigella.*

Survival of Shiga is influenced by induction of apoptosis in macrophages, which circumvent an important component of host response.

Exotoxin Shiga produced by *Shigella* Shiga:

A. Inhibits protein synthesis

B. Induces vascular damage resulting in severe colitis

C. Produces severe colitis like hemolytic uremic syndrome and leukemoid reaction

Non-*Shigella* dysenteriae type 1 can produce toxin via lysosomal bacteriophages.

Shigella enterotoxins 1 and 2 produce watery diarrhea.

Clinical Features

Hallmarks of *Shigella* infection are:

A. Cramping abdominal pain with tenesmus

B. Passage of small volume stool containing mucus, blood, and few fecal matters

In case of children, there is presence of rectal prolapse as a result of severe tenesmus.
In case of *Shigella sonnei*, there is watery diarrhea.

Systemic features:

A. Fever (as high as 40°C with chill)

B. In case of children, there may be seizures which may be due to high fever or metabolic complications

C. Lethargy

D. Confusion

E. Obtundation

F. Coma

The above mental changes result from metabolic complications because *Shigella dysenteriae* is responsible for neurologic complications.

Complications of shigellosis:

Complications	Organisms	Pathophysiology	Treatment
Intestinal complications			
Rectal prolapse	• *Shigella dysenteriae* 1 • *Shigella flexneri*	• Increased abdominal pressure • Repeated tenesmus	Compression with magnesium sulfate reduces edema

Continued

Continued

Complications	Organisms	Pathophysiology	Treatment
Toxic megacolon	*Shigella dysenteriae* 1	• Transmural inflammation of colonic mucosa • Increased NO production in the colonic musculature	• Intravenous fluid • Antibiotic to cure sepsis and infection
Intestinal perforation	*Shigella dysenteriae* 1	Transmural colonic ulcer with surrounding inflammation	Surgical repair under cover of broad-spectrum antibiotics
		Extraintestinal complications	
Severe dehydration	*Shigella sonnei*	• Watery diarrhea due to *Shigella* enterotoxins 1 and 2 • Fever • Decreased intake of fluid	Administration of oral or intravenous fluids
Hypoglycemia	*Shigella dysenteriae* 1	• Impaired gluconeogenesis • Depletion of glycogen store	Intravenous administration of 25% dextrose
Hypoproteinemia	• *Shigella dysenteriae* 1 • *Shigella flexneri*	• Loss of protein through stool • Due to inflammation, protein synthesis is decreased	• Treatment of edema • High-protein diet
Hyponatremia	• *Shigella dysenteriae* 1 • *Shigella flexneri*	Inappropriate secretion of antidiuretic hormone	• If Na is <120 mmol/L, administration of 3% NaCl • If Na is 120–130 mmol/L, administration of 0.9% NaCl
		Systemic complications	
• Seizures • Encephalopathy	*Shigella sonnei* and other *Shigella* species	• Fever • Metabolic complications • Sepsis • Shiga toxin type 1	• Correction of metabolic disorders • Treatment of fever • Anticonvulsive treatment
Septicemia	• *Shigella* type 1 • Other *Shigella* species	• Colonic perforation • Transmural inflammation producing leakage • Contamination of intravenous needles	• Administration of intravenous fluid to correct shock • Administration of broad-spectrum antibiotics
Hemolytic uremic syndrome	*Shigella* type 1	*Shigella* shiga toxin	• Restriction of fluid • Dialysis if required • In case of anemia blood transfusion
Leukemoid reaction	*Shigella dysenteriae* 1	• Features of hemolytic uremic syndrome • Related to Shiga toxin	Treatment of primary infection
Reactive arthritis	• *Shigella sonnei* • *Shigella flexneri*	Autoimmune reaction	• Administration of anti-inflammatory drugs • Pain-relieving drugs
• Conjunctivitis • Vaginitis	All species of *Shigella*	Occasional infection	Administration of antibiotics
Malnutrition	• *Shigella dysenteriae* 1 • *Shigella flexneri*	• Anorexia • Increased protein loss • Metabolism is increased due to fever, inflammation • Decreased synthesis of protein	• Adequate feeding ensured • High protein diet

Evaluation of bacillary dysentery:

A. Laboratory diagnosis:
   - **a.** Fresh stool sample to be examined within 2 hours of passing: By Gram stain—large number of polymorphonuclear cells and red blood cells
   - **b.** Blood: Leukocytosis
   - **c.** Stool culture: It should be immediately plated at bedside to detect gram-negative organism. In case of any delay, it should be transported in Cary–Blair transport media. In the culture, *Shigella* produces white or colorless colony, as it is a nonlactose fermenter. Then it is further analyzed by a definite biochemical test.
   - **d.** To detect the complication:
      1. Serum electrolytes, such as sodium, potassium, and magnesium
      2. Serum sugar
      3. Serum urea and creatinine
      4. Serum iron profile
   - **e.** Straight X-ray of abdomen:
      1. Toxic megacolon
      2. Paralytic ileus

Management

Proper Treatment

A. Will shorten the duration of illness

B. Will shorten the excretion of pathogens

C. Will reduce the mortality and complications

Following are the characteristics of shigellosis treatment:

A. It should be systematically absorbed.

B. It is active against *Shigella.*

C. It is inexpensive.

D. The active concentration of the drugs should be more than the minimum inhibitory concentration of the infective strain.

E. It can be administered orally.

F. It has a high therapeutic index.

G. In case of children, it is available in a liquid form.

The antibiotics of choice are:

A. Ciprofloxacin 500 mg 12 hourly for 3–5 days

B. Azithromycin 500 mg daily for 5 days

Alternate therapy of choice: Ceftriaxone 1–1.5 g intravenously twice daily for 5 days

Supportive therapies:

A. Severe dehydration can be treated by intravenous fluids.

B. High-protein diet can treat the nutritional deterioration.

C. Correction of hypoglycemia

D. Zinc supplementation:
   - **a.** Reduces severity of diarrhea
   - **b.** Reduces the incidence of diarrhea

E. Vitamin A supplementation will provide benefit in acute infection.

F. Treatment of complications

G. In case of fever—antipyretics

Q16. Infectious esophagitis.

MGR/APR2014/MDIII (7)

ANSWER

In case of immunosuppressed patients or in patients with AIDS, infections of esophagitis are:

A. *Candida albicans*

B. Herpes simplex

C. Cytomegalovirus

In case of HIV, patients with infectious esophagitis CD4 count should be between 100 and <200. In case of HIV patients, the disease spectrum may be:

A. At the time of seroconversion, self-limited syndrome consists of oral ulcers plus acute esophageal ulcers plus maculopapular rash.

B. In case of advanced disease, deep persistent esophageal ulcers are present, which are treated with steroids and thalidomide

But in case of nonimmunized patients, the infections responsible for esophagitis are:

A. *Candida albicans*

B. Herpes simplex

C. *Candida* esophagitis:
   - **a.** Organism is *Candida albicans*, normal commensals in the throat.
   - **b.** Risk factors are:
      1. Compromised host
      2. Esophageal stasis in case of esophageal motility disorder or esophageal diverticula
      3. Diabetes
      4. Adrenal insufficiency
      5. Alcoholism
      6. Use of antibiotics

c. Clinical features:
   1. Dysphagia
   2. Odynophagia
d. Complications:
   1. Bleeding
   2. Perforation
   3. Stricture
   4. Invasion to systemic circulation
e. Endoscopic findings:
   1. Presence of raised yellowish-white small plaques, which are surrounded by erythema
   2. In case of extensive disease, presence of confluent linear and nodular plaques
f. Confirmation of candida by brush cytology and examination under a microscope, which demonstrates hyphae and masses of budding yeast
g. Treatment:
   1. Initial therapy is 200–400 mg on the 1st day followed by 100–200 mg daily for 14–21 days.
   2. Patient refractory to fluconazole will respond to voriconazole.
   3. If the patient cannot tolerate oral medication, intravenous echinocandin like caspofungin or micafungin or amphotericin B can be given.

Other two viral esophagitis are herpes simplex and cytomegalovirus esophagitis described below:

Viruses	Herpes simplex	Cytomegalovirus
Patients involved	Immunocompromised and nonimmunocompromised	It is primarily in immunocompromised patients
Clinical features	Dysphagia, odynophagia	Dysphagia, odynophagia
Location	Distal third	Lower or middle third
Endoscopy	Multiple punched-out ulcer limited to squamous epithelium	Serpiginous ulcers mainly to distal part
Biopsy taken from	Edge of the ulcer	Center of the ulcer
Histology	• Eosinophilic Cowdry type A inclusion bodies • Ground glass nuclei multinucleated giant cells	• Perinuclear halo • Intranuclear inclusions • Cytoplasmic inclusions
PCR	Acyclovir-resistant strain can be identified	Can be identified
Treatment	• In case of nonimmunocompromised patients, orally acyclovir 200 mg 5 times daily for 7–10 days though it is self-limited after 1–2 weeks • In case of an immunocompromised host, acyclovir 400 mg orally 5 times daily, famciclovir 500 mg 3 times, or valacyclovir 1 g 3 times daily for 14–21 days • In severe odynophagia, 5 mg/kg intravenous acyclovir 3 times daily for 7–14 days	Ganciclovir 5 mg/kg 12 hourly intravenously or valganciclovir 500 mg orally 12 hourly for 3–6 weeks

Q17. Achlorhydria.

MGR/OCT2011/MDIV (7)

ANSWER

Etiopathogenesis

Gastric fluid is composed of hydrochloric acid, potassium chloride, and sodium chloride. Parietal cells are responsible for secretion of hydrochloric acid. Achlorhydria is a condition where the secretion of hydrochloric acid is negligible or absent due to the varieties of medical and surgical conditions.

There are variations of secretory cells lining the invagination, consisting of exocrine glands, endocrine glands, and paracrine glands. There are three types of exocrine cells present on the wall of gastric sac and oxyntic gastric mucosal glands:

A. Mucous cells secrete watery mucus.
B. Chief cells secrete precursor of pepsinogen enzyme.
C. Parietal cells produce hydrochloric acid and intrinsic factor.

Gastric pH is maintained between 1 and 2.
Following factors will affect the acidity of stomach:

A. Type of food intake
B. Integrity of nervous system
C. Level of micronutrients in the blood
D. Individual emotional atmosphere
E. Protein intake
F. Unstable emotional state

Functions of hydrochloric acid are as follows:

A. It will activate pepsinogen enzyme precursor to pepsin and acid produces optimal environment for activity of pepsin.

B. It helps in breakdown of connective tissue and muscle fibers present in the food resulting in formation of more absorbable tiny particles.

C. It with eliminate microbacteria present in the food along with salivary lysozyme.

So, gastric acid secretion can be affected by the following medical and surgical conditions:

A. *Pernicious anemia*: Here antiparietal cell or anti-intrinsic factor antibodies are responsible for autoimmune destruction of parietal cells leading to the development of atrophic gastritis.

B. Long-term use of PPIs

C. In case of acute infection of gastric epithelial cells with *H. pylori*, the alpha subunit of H-K-ATPase gene expression is repressed, resulting in transient achlorhydria, and *H. pylori* proliferation is suppressed.

D. Gastritis may occur due to ingestion of different dietary ingredients interfering with gastric mucosal and tight junctions. If this process is chronic and ongoing, it will lead to gastric atrophy producing achlorhydria.

E. Food in the small intestine will retard the gastric acid secretion.

F. If gastric pH will fall below 3, released somatostatin will decrease gastrin secretion and this will lead to acid suppression.

G. Gastric bypass surgery in the treatment of obesity results in lowering of gastrin secretion leading to achlorhydria.

H. VIPoma: VIP is secreted from beta pancreatic cells; if it is associated with MEN1, it produces massive watery diarrhea, achlorhydria, hypokalemia, hypercalcemia, hyperglycemia, and vasodilatation.

I. Thyroid hormone plays a role in acid secretion from the stomach. Hence, hypothyroidism can produce achlorhydria.

J. Gastric cancer

K. Radiation of stomach

Clinical Features

Most common symptoms are:

A. Abdominal pain

B. Fatigue

C. Diarrhea

D. Belching or bloating

E. Frequent exhaustion

F. Chest burning

G. Malaise

H. Pruritus ani

I. Nausea with or without vomiting

J. Abdominal fullness

K. Dry mouth

Most common features are:

A. Chronic candidiasis

B. Chronic anemia

C. Glossitis

D. Acne

E. Fragile nails

F. Presence of undigested food in the feces

Evaluation of achlorhydria:

A. Presence of antiparietal cells and anti-intrinsic factor antibodies

B. Gastric pH monitoring

C. Serum gastrin level between 500 and 1,000 pg/mL indicates achlorhydria.

D. If serum pepsinogen level is low, it indicates achlorhydria.

E. Biopsy from stomach

F. *H. pylori* detection:

- **a.** *H. pylori* antigen in the stool
- **b.** Urea breath test
- **c.** Polymerase chain reaction for *H. pylori*
- **d.** Fluorescence in situ hybridization (FISH)

G. Serum hemoglobin and vitamin B12 levels

Treatment for achlorhydria: There is no specific treatment for achlorhydria. Usually, the treatment is:

A. Eradication of *H. pylori*

B. Replacement of:

- **a.** Calcium
- **b.** Vitamin B12
- **c.** Iron

Q18. Classify chronic gastritis. Note the treatment of *H. pylori* infection.

MGR/APR2012/MDIV (7)

ANSWER

Inflammation of gastric epithelium can be classified into two types:

A. Gastropathy when there is epithelial injury along with regeneration without much inflammation

B. Gastritis when there is much inflammation of the gastric mucosa with inflammatory infiltrate

Following are the types of chronic gastritis:

Pathologic diagnosis	Histologic diagnosis	Etiology	Endoscopic findings	Clinical associations
Chronic and chronic active gastritis	Inflammatory cells like neutrophils, plasma cells + Foveolar hyperplasia + lymphoid aggregates + erosions + ulcers + intestinal metaplasia + atrophy	*H. pylori*	• Normal or erythema, nodularity, friability • In some areas, ulceration or erosion	Asymptomatic or duodenal ulcer, gastric ulcer, gastric adenocarcinoma, or functional dyspepsia
Granulomatous gastritis	Multifocal active chronic containing epithelioid granuloma	• Crohn's disease • Fungal, spirochete, and tubercular infections Idiopathic isolated granulomatous gastritis, vasculitis, drugs related, and sarcoidosis	Thickened folds and ulcerations	It depends on underlying cause
Lymphocytic gastritis	Presence of chronic active inflammation with intraepithelial lymphocytes but absence of foveolar hyperplasia, erosion, or ulcer	Hypersensitivity of gliadin, unknown agents, may be autoimmune	Varioliform or chronic active gastritis (presence of nodules or central ulcer), Ménétrier's disease	Ménétrier's disease Celiac sprue
Eosinophilic gastritis	Presence of sheets of eosinophils	Allergy to food, drug, and parasitic disease	Normal or presence of hyperemia, nodularity or ulcers	• Nausea with vomiting • Abdominal pain, weight loss, anorexia, anemia
Hypertrophic lymphocytic gastritis	Presence of chronic active inflammation with intraepithelial lymphocytes and foveolar hyperplasia, but no erosion or ulcer	Etiological agent not known	Hypertrophic gastropathy	Hypertrophic gastropathy

Treatment of *H. pylori*-related acid peptic disease is discussed in question number 6.

Q19. Causes and mechanism due to disorders of gut mucosal function and structure.

DNBIIIA/DEC2014 (10)

ANSWER

Anatomy of Mucosal Barriers

A. Extracellular components of mucosal barrier: Mucin secreted by gastric foveolar mucous cells and intestinal goblet cells provides mucosal barrier and thus prevents large particles and bacteria from contacting with the epithelial layer. Hydration of mucus is very important as hyperviscous mucus leads to pancreatic, interstitial, and pulmonary diseases.

Small molecules pass through the heavily glycosylated mucus layer, but bulk flow is not possible due to an unstirred mucus layer on the epithelial surface, which is protected from convective mixing forces. In the stomach, this property of unstirred layer along with bicarbonate secretion by the epithelial cells will maintain the zone of alkalinity on the mucosal surface.

In the small intestine, this layer:

a. Reduces the movement of nutrients to transporting protein-rich microvilli of brush border
b. Also limits the extent of loss of nutrients released by the activities of digestive enzymes present in the brush border into the intestinal limen. The thickness of the unstirred layer is increased in case of celiac disease to create malabsorption of the nutrients.

B. Cellular component of mucosal barrier: Normally, epithelial cells in absence of specific transporters are impermeable to hydrophilic solutes. But cytotoxic agents, chemotherapeutic agents, and mucosal irritants directly damage the epithelial cells leading to loss of barrier function.

At the same time, paracellular pathways in between the cells must be sealed by tight junction and subjacent adherens junction. These junctions are supported by a dense peri-junctional ring of actin and myosin regulating the barrier function. This adherens junction along with desmosomes maintains the close proximity between cells. Loss of adherens junction is responsible for:

a. Disruption of cell-to-cell and cell-to-matrix contact
b. Polarization and differentiation of epithelial cells
c. Premature of apoptosis

Adherens junctions are composed of family of cadherins, amongst which E-cadherin interacts with δ1-catenin and β-catenin directly. β-catenin in turn will bind with α-catenin 1 and regulate assembly of local actin, which ultimately forms a perijunctional actomyosin ring.

Tight junctions are composed of multiprotein complexes, such as:

a. Transmembrane proteins:
   1. Most important is claudin family, which regulates several aspects of tight junction permeability. Mutation of deletion of claudin family can produce profound effect on organ function.
   2. Occludin interacts directly with claudin and actin.
b. Peripheral zonal membrane proteins—Zonula occludens 1 and 2 help in assembly and maintenance of tight junctions. These proteins have multiple domains for interaction of actin, claudin, and occludin.
c. Regulatory molecules like kinases

The paracellular pathway is more permeable to solute flux as compared to the transcellular pathway, and tight junctions control this flux and act as a rate-limiting step in the transepithelial transport of the solute. The barrier function of tight junction is based on its charge and size selectivity.

There are two routes through which the solutes are transported across the tight junction:

a. One is leak pathway, which allows paracellular transport of large solutes, large protein and bacterial polysaccharides, but whole bacteria cannot pass through. This pathway is not charge-selective. Transport across this leak pathway is increased by cytokines, such as interferon and TNF.
b. The second pathway is the small pores having a radius larger than 4 A. These are associated with claudin proteins and are charge selective. Specificity of the claudin varies in different organs and different regions of a single organ and can be modified by cytokines.

Interdependence of Transport Routes

Transepithelial transport requires a selective permeable barrier: Transcellular secretion and absorption require generation of a transepithelial concentration gradient. Diffusion will equalize the concentration on both sides of the epithelium; hence, a tight junctional barrier is required for transepithelial transport. An intact tight junctional barrier controls the active transcellular transport. Selective permeability of the tight junctional barrier allows paracellular transport of water and ions.

Example: In a normal condition, there is paracellular absorption of magnesium and calcium ions in the thick ascending limb of loop of Henle through the cation-selective claudin-16 protein at the tight junctional barrier. But in familial hypomagnesemia with hypercalciuria and nephrocalcinosis, there is mutation of claudin-16 protein necessary for cation selectivity in the tight junction.

Example: Apical Na^+-H^+-exchange protein 3 is responsible for transcellular absorption of Na in the renal tubule and intestine and creates a transepithelial gradient, which drives water and small solutes like glucose paracellularly, but efflux of Na is prevented by tight junction and thus dissipation of gradient produced by the exchange protein. This is seen when oral rehydration solution containing sodium and glucose is consumed in case of infectious diarrhea or after exercise. On the contrary, TNF activates both protein kinase Ca and myosin light chain kinase to produce diarrhea. Inhibition of apical Na^+-H^+-exchange protein 3 mediated by protein kinase Ca will reduce the transcellular Na gradient leading to decreased absorption of water. This is associated with myosin light-chain kinase-mediated increased permeability of tight junction, thus allowing large volume of water to flow into the lumen producing large volume diarrhea.

Tight junction barrier modifies absorption: Intracellular signaling being stimulated by transcellular transport controls tight junction barrier.

Example: Apical Na^+-nutrient co-transporter increases the paracellular absorption of water and nutrients amplifying total transcellular absorption of nutrients when intraluminal water and nutrient content exceed the capacity of these cotransporters. Later on, it was found that myosin light-chain kinase (Ca^{++}-calmodulin dependent serine-threonine protein kinase) controls this tight junction induced by cotransporters and increases its permeability.

Immunogenic Regulation of Tight Junction

Following are the cytokine-mediated loss-of-barrier functions:

A. Increased transcription of tight junction protein
B. Vesicular removal of protein from tight junction
C. Degradation of protein of tight junction
D. Activation of kinases
E. Modulation of cytoskeleton
F. Extensive apoptosis of the epithelial cells leading to barrier loss

Cytoskeleton regulates the tight junction: Tumor necrosis factor-α and interferon-γ control and modify the tight junction barrier function of intestinal, pulmonary, and renal salivary epithelial cells and in between epithelial cells. In case of intestines, cytokine is responsible for many diseases, such as inflammatory bowel disease, graft-versus-host disease, and intestinal ischemia. Increased production of TNF in the epithelial cells will contribute to increased permeability in the intestine in case of colitis, which can be corrected by TNF antibodies leading to reduction of inflammation. TNF activates myosin light-chain kinase protein to increase the permeability of the paracellular pathway due to activation and transcription and translation and increased activity of this protein. It occurs in case of IBD, and the degree of activity correlates with disease activity. Myosin light-chain kinase activity-induced barrier dysfunction is caused by TNFSF14, IL-1β, enteropathogenic *E. coli* infection, *H. pylori* infection, giardiasis, acetaldehyde, and lipopolysaccharide.

Barrier defect with intestinal diseases:

Disease	Cause of barrier defect	Timing of barrier defect	Effect on cytoskeleton	Role of microorganism
Crohn's disease	Associated with frameshift insertion at 3020 of NOD2 nucleotide	Before clinical onset and clinical relapse	• Claudin-2 upregulation • Occludin downregulation • Myosin light chain kinase activation	Antibiotic maintain remission
Ulcerative colitis	Unknown		• Claudin-2 upregulation • Occludin downregulation • Myosin light-chain kinase activation	Not known
Celiac disease	Not studied	Not studied	Not defined	No role
Systemic T-cell activation	Activation of myosin light-chain kinase	With acute diarrhea	• Activation of myosin light-chain kinase • Occludin endocytosis	Not defined
Dextran sulfate sodium-induced colitis	Damage of epithelial cells	After dextran sulfate sodium treatment but before clinical onset	Not known	Exacerbation by eradication of microorganisms
C. difficile-induced colitis	• Disruption of actinomycin • Glycosylation of Rho protein	With toxin release and disease onset	Loss of zonula occludens 1 and 2	Antibiotic predispose to this disease

Continued

Continued

Enteropathogenic *E. coli* infection	Secretion of type III bacterial protein	Following infection	• Activation of myosin light-chain kinase • Occludin endocytosis	Not defined
Graft-versus-host disease	Increased TNF production	After clinical onset	Not known	Limitation of the disease by eradication of microorganism
Trinitrobenzene-induced colitis	Immunogenic signaling	Not studied	Upregulation of claudin-18	Use of probiotic reduces severity

Epithelium and tight junctional barrier act as an integrator of homeostasis: Bacterial product or dietary antigens enter the lamina propria through a minor defect in the barrier, which either leads to homeostasis or disease.

If foreign materials are taken up by antigen presenting cells (APCs), such as dendritic cells, they will differentiate T helper 1 and T helper 2 cells:

A. APCs and T helper 1 cells release TNF and interferon-γ, which in turn direct epithelial cells to increase the flux through the leak pathway; in this process, bacterial products and dietary antigens also enter the lamina propria from the lumen and thus further amplify the cycle of inflammation; this ultimately culminates in the disease.

B. T helper 2 cells release IL-13, which increases the flux through the small cation-selective pores and potentiates the ongoing disease process.

C. If APCs promote differentiation of regulatory T cells, it is enhanced by TGF-β and retinoic acid. The regulatory T cells possess latency-associated peptide on their surface and release IL-10 and TGF-β to prevent the disease.

Q20. Explain the pathogenesis of peptic ulcer. How would you diagnose, treat, and prevent peptic ulcer?

MGR/APR2013/MDII (15)

Cytoprotective agents in peptic ulcer disease.

KERALA UNIVERSITY, 2020 (10)

Enumerate the causes of peptic ulcers not caused by *H. pylori* and NSAIDs. Write short note on gastroduodenal mucosal defense.

WBUHS, 2024 (10)

ANSWER

Definition

A. Gastroduodenal ulcer results from breakdown of the mucosal defense against hydrochloric acid and proteolytic enzymes secondary to *H. pylori* infection of use of NSAIDs.

B. Gastritis is the inflammatory response of the mucosa due to variety of agents and mechanisms, such as infections, drugs, and autoimmune reaction.

C. Gastropathy is gastric mucosal damage without inflammation resulting from drugs, from infections, and also from vascular congestion in portal hypertension.

D. Ménétrier's disease: It is a type of gastropathy, which results from hypertrophy of gastric mucosa or loss of protein or increased secretion.

Etiopathogenesis

A. *H. pylori* infection: It is responsible for gastritis, peptic ulcer disease, gastric MALT lymphoma, and gastric cancer as a result of an interplay between bacterial and host factors:

Bacterial factors: *H. pylori* induces gastric mucosal injury, able to avoid host defense, and facilitates gastric residence. This bacterium produces different virulence factors:

a. Gamma-glutamyl transpeptidase

b. Cytotoxin-associated gene A (cag A) product

c. Virulence components vacuolating toxin

d. Pathogen-associated molecular patterns:

1. Flagella
2. Lipopolysaccharide

There is one region in the bacterial genome encoding virulence factors cag A and pic B. Vac A is not encoded within the pathogenicity islands.

Functions of these virulence factors:

a. Vac A inhibits proliferation of CD4 T cells and disrupts function of B cells, mast cells, macrophages, and CD8 T cells, thus producing mucosal damage.

b. cag-PAI positive *H. pylori* strains are associated with a high risk of peptic ulcer disease, premalignant gastric ulcer, and gastric cancer.

c. In case of acute infection, *H. pylori* inhibits the activity of H^+K^+-ATPase through cag A-dependent mechanism leading to decreased acid production.

d. Urease by generating ammonia helps the bacteria to reside in the stomach and damages epithelial cells.

e. These bacteria produce chemotactic factors for neutrophils and monocytes leading to epithelial cell injury.

f. Proteases and phospholipases released from these bacteria break down the glycoprotein lipid complexes, the first line of defense in the mucus gel, and thus break down the mucosal defense.

g. These bacteria expresses adhesins they enhance bacterial attachment to the gastric epithelial cells.

h. Lipopolysaccharide of these bacteria has some role in the infection.

Host factors:

A. There may be genetic predisposition in case of *H. pylori* infection.

B. *H. pylori* binds to major histocompatibility complex molecules present on gastric epithelial cells leading to death of the cells, i.e., apoptosis.

C. In case of cag-PIA strains, *H. pylori* cag-A enters and later on damages host cells by the following processes:

  a. Cellular pathways activation leading to production of several cytokines, such as IL-2, IL-6, IL-8, and IL-1α/β that are present in the gastric epithelium, TNF-α, and interferon-γ.

  b. Repression of tumor suppressor genes

D. *H. pylori* also induces both mucosal and humoral immune responses, which prevent eradication of these bacteria, leading to further cellular injury indirectly.

E. The following mechanisms also produce cellular injury:

  a. Activated production of ROS mediated by neutrophils leading to enhanced epithelial cell turnover.

  b. Interaction between T cells and interferon-γ leading to apoptosis

  c. Gastric microbiota is altered by *H. pylori* in the stomach.

  d. Urease secreted by these bacteria will stimulate nitric oxide synthetase expressed on the macrophages present in the gastric epithelial cells, which leads to release of nitric oxide, and it is responsible for the cytopathic effect on the surrounding epithelial cells.

Effect on duodenal ulcer: *H. pylori*-associated duodenal ulcer is more virulent due to the following factors:

A. Duodenal ulcer-promoting gene A present in the bacteria is associated with duodenal ulcer development.

B. Presence of gastric metaplasia in the duodenal mucosa due to high acid exposure will help *H. pylori* to bind the epithelial cells leading to cellular injury.

C. Antral infection due to *H. pylori* leads to increased acid production, thus increasing the concentration of acid in the duodenum. This will further injure the duodenal mucosa.

D. In case of *H. pylori* infection, basal and stimulated gastrin will be increased and on the other hand, somatostatin secreting D cells will be decreased.

E. Proinflammatory cytokines also increase acid secretion through action on D, G, and parietal cells of stomach.

F. There is also decreased bicarbonate production from duodenal mucosa in *H. pylori* infection.

Effect on gastric ulcer: In *H. pylori* infection, there will be pangastritis associated with normal or low acid production.

A. **NSAIDs-induced peptic disease**:

  a. Prostaglandin is responsible for maintaining the integrity of gastric mucosa and its repair. So, any cause that produces interruption of prostaglandin synthesis can produce gastric mucosa injury. As a result, the following things will happen:

    1. Increased secretion of hydrochloric acid
    2. Decreased bicarbonate secretion
    3. Decreased secretion of mucin
    4. Decreased secretion of surface-active phospholipid
    5. Decreased proliferation of epithelial cells

  b. Direct toxic effect of NSAIDs: Direct injury to the gastric mucosa increases permeability of epithelial surface. Aspirin being weak acid will remain in a nonionized lipophilic form. It will cross the lipid membranes and trapped intracellularly as ionized form and damage the cells.

c. NSAIDs damage the surface mucus layer, which leads to back-diffusion of hydrogen ion and pepsin and further cellular damage.

d. Activation of lipoxygenase pathway via production of proinflammatory cytokines, TNF, and leukotrienes; NSAIDs also produce mucosal injury.

Smoking:

Cigarette smoking is responsible for peptic disease through the following mechanisms:

A. Altered gastric emptying

B. Decreased production of proximal duodenal bicarbonate

C. Increase risk of infection with *H. pylori*

D. Induction of noxious mucosal-free radicals

Ulcer is frequent in smokers as compared to nonsmokers due to the following reasons:

A. Decreased rate of healing

B. Impaired response to therapy

C. Increased rate of ulcer-related complications, such as perforation

Genetic causes:

A. First-degree relatives of duodenal ulcer are three times likely to develop an ulcer.

B. Blood group O and nonsecretory status have been associated with duodenal ulcer.

C. NSAID-metabolizing enzymes, i.e., cytochrome P450 *2C9* and *2C8* are the two genes responsible for NSAID-induced peptic ulcer disease.

Specific chronic disorders are associated with peptic ulcer disease:

A. Advanced age

B. Chronic renal failure

C. Chronic pulmonary disease

D. Nephrolithiasis

E. Cirrhosis

F. Alpha-1 antitrypsin deficiency

G. Systemic mastocytosis

Following disorders are associated with acid peptic disease:

A. Coronary artery disease

B. Polycythemia vera

C. Hyperparathyroidism

D. Chronic pancreatitis

E. African-American race

F. Former alcohol use

G. Three or more visits to doctor in a year

Investigations

Investigations are discussed in Question number 5 for *H. pylori* disease.

Barium study: It is rarely used today; sensitivity of duodenal ulcer is 80%. It is decreased in the following cases:

A. In case ulcer of >0.5 cm

B. Presence of previous scarring

C. In case of postoperative patients

In case of gastric ulcers, there is presence of an ulcer crater along with radiating folds that originate from the crater. But if the ulcer size is >3 cm along with presence of mass. It suggests a malignant ulcer.

Upper gastrointestinal endoscopy:

In case of gastric ulcer:

A. Discrete mucosal lesion having a punched-out smooth ulcer base often filled up with fibrinoid exudate

B. Ulcer is solitary, well circumscribed, and sized 0.5–2.5 cm in diameter. The site is at the junction of fundus and antrum along the lesser curvature:

a. In case of benign ulcer: Smooth, regular, round edge, flat base, and smooth with surrounding radiating mucosal folds

b. In case of malignant ulcer: Margin is everted or heaped up; sometimes, mass will protrude into the lumen. Mucosal folds surrounding the ulcer are irregular and often nodular. Endoscopic biopsy from gastric ulcer will confirm the diagnosis.

Serum gastrin level: It should be measured after stopping the PPI for 5 days. The following conditions require serum gastrin estimation:

A. Multiple ulcers

B. Strong family history of acid peptic diseases

C. Post-bulbar ulcer

D. Peptic ulcer associated with diarrhea, weight loss, and/or steatorrhea

E. Peptic ulcer not associated with NSAIDs use or *H. pylori* infection

F. Recurrence of ulcer after surgery

G. Refractory to medical therapy

H. Ulcer associated with renal stones or hypercalcemia

I. Screen for Zollinger–Ellison syndrome

Treatment

Antacids	Aluminum hydroxide with magnesium hydroxide		• Aluminum causes constipation and depletion of phosphate and magnesium causes diarrhea • Contraindication: Chronic renal failure
	Calcium carbonate		Long-term use produces Milk-alkali syndrome
	Sodium bicarbonate		Systemic alkalosis
H2 receptor antagonist	Cimetidine	400 mg twice daily	Reversible gynecomastia, impotence in high dose, elevation of transaminases, creatinine, prolactin
	Ranitidine	300 mg before dinner	These are more potent than cimetidine
	Famotidine	40 mg before dinner	
	Nizatidine	300 mg before dinner	
Proton-pump inhibitor	Omeprazole	20 mg before breakfast	
	Esomeprazole	20 mg before breakfast	S-isomer of omeprazole
	Lansoprazole	30 mg before breakfast	
	Dexlansoprazole	30 mg before breakfast	R-isomer of lansoprazole
	Pantoprazole	40 mg before breakfast	
	Rabeprazole	20 mg before breakfast	
Cytoprotective drug	Sucralfate	1 g 4 times daily	
Bismuth-containing preparation	• Colloidal bismuth subcitrate • Bismuth subsalicylate		Constipation, black stool, darkening of tongue
Prostaglandin analog	Misoprostol	200 µg 4 times daily	• It will enhance the mucosal defense and repair • Toxicity: Diarrhea, uterine bleeding, and contraction • It is contraindicated in pregnant woman and woman of child-bearing age

Some points:

A. S and R isomers are dual delayed-release system and improve gastroesophageal reflux disease.

B. Lansoprazole and omeprazole are administered in enteric-coated granules and dissolved in the small intestines at pH 6 as they are heat labile.

C. Lansoprazole can be given as a disintegrating tablet with or without water and can be given in patients with dysphagia.

D. In case of NSAID-induced gastric injury, lansoprazole–naproxen combination can be given.

E. Omeprazole can be given with sodium bicarbonate in the powder form through the nasogastric tube because:

- **a.** It protects omeprazole from degradation by acids.
- **b.** It promotes rapid gastric alkalization.
- **c.** Subsequent proton-pump activation.

F. Pantoprazole and rabeprazole are lipophilic compounds. After their entry into parietal cells, they are protonated and subsequently trapped in the canalicular tubulovesicular system, thus inhibiting all phases of gastric secretion. The onset of actions is 2–6 hours and the duration of inhibition is 72–96 hours.

G. There is evidence of mild-to-moderate hypergastrinemia in the patients who are on these drugs, but it returns to normal 1–2 weeks after cessation of drugs.

H. There is evidence of gastric acid hypersecretion within 1–2 months after cessation of PPI in *H. pylori*-negative patients and may last for 2 months. Possible mechanisms involve gastrin-induced hyperplasia and hypertrophy of histamine-secreting enterochromaffin-like cells. So, gradual tapering of PPI followed by switching to H2 receptor blocker is done to prevent acid rebound.

I. But acid rebound does not occur in case of *H. pylori*-induced inflammation, which leads to decrease in acid production.

J. Due to large stores of vitamin B12 in the body, vitamin B12-related anemia does not occur in spite of inhibition of intrinsic factor production by PPI.

K. PPI interferes with absorption of ketoconazole, iron, digoxin, and ampicillin. Omeprazole and lansoprazole inhibit the P450 cytochrome system.

L. Long-term suppression of acid by PPI leads to changes in the host microbiota and is responsible for:
   a. Community-acquired pneumonia
   b. Hospital-acquired *C. difficile*-associated disease
   c. Risk of spontaneous bacterial peritonitis

M. Long-term use of PPI is associated with:
   a. Development of hip fractures in older women
   b. Iron, vitamin B12, and magnesium deficiency. Hence CBC, magnesium, and vitamin B12 level should be estimated at a regular interval after 1–2 years of PPI use.
   c. Negative effect on the antiplatelet effect of clopidogrel because of competitive inhibition of the same cytochrome 450 enzyme by PPI. Hence, 12 hours' separation is required between clopidogrel and PPI so that it will minimize this competition. So, PPI should be given before breakfast and clopidogrel should be given before bed time.
   d. Acute and chronic kidney injury
   e. Dementia
   f. Increased cardiac risk

   Patients of ≥65 years of age are at a high risk of developing long-term side effects.

Cytoprotective Agents

Sucralfate: Here hydroxyl group has been substituted by aluminum hydroxide and sulfate. It will bind to ulcer sites in the stomach and duodenum as viscus paste and protect the ulcer by following mechanisms:

A. Acts as physicochemical barrier
B. Produces trophic action by binding with endothelial growth factor.
C. Enhances synthesis of prostaglandin
D. Stimulates bicarbonate as well as mucus secretion
E. Enhancement of mucosal defense and repair.

It has to be avoided in case of chronic renal insufficiency to prevent aluminum related neurotoxicity.

Adverse effects:

A. Constipation
B. Hyperphosphatemia
C. Gastric bezoar formation.

Misoprostol

It is prostaglandin analogue. It acts by the following mechanism:

A. Increases the secretion of bicarbonate and mucus.
B. It will increase the blood flow
C. It will inhibit the acid secretion.

Adverse effects:

A. Diarrhea
B. Abdominal cramps

Contraindication: It is contraindicated in case of pregnancy as it will increase the uterine contraction.

Bismuth Subsalicylate

It acts in the following mechanism:

A. It will form a protective barrier on the ulcer base
B. It will stimulate secretion of prostaglandin and mucus.
C. It has antimicrobial activity against the *H. pylori*.

Adverse effects:

A. Darkened tongue
B. Black stool
C. In high dose encephalopathy

***H. pylori* treatment has been discussed in question number 5.**

Q21. Traveler's diarrhea.

MGR/OCT2011/MDIII (7)
MGR/MAR2008/MDIII (6)
MGR/FEB2005/MDIII (5)
DNB (DEC 2022) (4);
MGR UNI, TAMIL NADU, 2022 (10);
MAHARASHTRA UNI OF HEALTH SC, VIJAYAWADA, 2022 (10)

Enumerate the strains of *E. coli*. Add a note on travelers' diarrhea.

NTR UNI OF HEALTH SC, ANDHRA, 2022 (10)

Travelers' diarrhea.

KERALA UNIVERSITY, 2020 (10)

ANSWER

Definition

Classical traveler's diarrhea can be defined as at least loose to watery stools per day with or without abdominal cramps, nausea, vomiting, fever, or presence of blood in the stool developed in the traveler after arrival in a resource-limited destination.

Method of Transmission

Feco-oral route—Incubation period: The time of onset of symptoms depends upon the incubation period of the pathogen, which may be 2 weeks after returning from that country, but it may be longer in case of infection with protozoa or helminth.

Causes

A. Bacteria:
- **a.** Enterotoxigenic *E. coli*
- **b.** Enteroinvasive *E. coli*
- **c.** Enteropathogenic *E. coli*
- **d.** *Campylobacter jejuni*
- **e.** *Shigella*
- **f.** *Salmonella*
- **g.** *Vibrio cholerae*
- **h.** *Aeromonas*

B. Virus:
- **a.** Rotavirus
- **b.** Norovirus
- **c.** Astrovirus
- **d.** Adenovirus 40/41

C. Protozoa:
- **a.** *Cryptosporidium parvum*
- **b.** *Giardia lamblia*
- **c.** *Entamoeba histolytica*
- **d.** *Cyclospora cayetanensis*

D. Unknown etiology

Risk Factors

A. Host-related:
- **a.** Country of origin: If the traveler comes from a highly industrialized country, the incidence is high.
- **b.** Age: Incidence is increased between 15 and 30 years of age.

B. Travel-related factors:
- **a.** Destination: High incidence in case of travel to Africa, West, Central and South Asia
- **b.** Duration of stay: Incidence will be increased until the day 12 or 14.

Clinical Features and Consequence of Diarrhea

Clinical spectrum varies from:

A. Typically watery stool with cramping abdominal pain in case of Enterotoxigenic *E. coli*

B. Bloody stool in case of *Shigella*

C. Short-lived nausea, vomiting with watery or semi-loose motion in case of food poisoning or norovirus infection

D. Illness is more severe in infants and children.

E. Most of the cases will be resolved within a few days, 10% cases within a week, and 2% cases take about a month to resolve completely.

Complications

A. Hemolytic uremic syndrome from Shiga toxin

B. Guillain-Barré syndrome from *C. jejuni*

C. Postinfectious arthropathy from any invasive bacteria

D. Prolonged illness of >10 days or relapse after return from the outside country associated with weight loss due to *G. lamblia*

E. Development of IBS

Prevention of Traveler's Diarrhea

A. Following food and beverages have to be avoided:
- **a.** Raw undercooked meat, seafood, and fish
- **b.** Unpasteurized milk, ice cream, cheese, and other dairy products
- **c.** Cold sauces and toppings
- **d.** Tap water
- **e.** Ground leafy green vegetables
- **f.** Fruits
- **g.** Cooked food but has been kept at room temperature for long time
- **h.** Foods from street vendor at all unless freshly prepared

B. Hygiene measures:
- **a.** Washing of hand before food intake
- **b.** Intake of water unless it is boiled or treated with chlorine or filtered with filter of ≤1 μm

C. Vaccines: No vaccine can prevent traveler's diarrhea:
- **a.** Enteric vaccine can prevent rotavirus diarrhea.
- **b.** Cholera and typhoid vaccine can be given if indicated but after careful assessment of risk.
- **c.** Some *E. coli* strains produce a heat-labile enterotoxin, which is similar to toxin produced by *V. cholerae.* So killed cholera vaccine containing nontoxic portion of cholerae protein will provide cross-immunity against Enterotoxigenic *E. coli.*

Chemoprophylaxis of Traveler's Diarrhea

A. Bismuth subsalicylate: 525 mg four times per day for 3 weeks

B. Antibiotics:

- **a.** Norfloxacin 400 mg daily orally
- **b.** Ciprofloxacin 500 mg orally daily
- **c.** Rifaximin 400 mg twice daily; since it is poorly absorbed from the gastrointestinal tract, systemic side effects are rare. It is not attractive for enteroinvasive pathogens.

Risks of long-term fluoroquinolone therapy are QT prolongation, tendon rupture, and *C. difficile* infection.

Treatment of Traveler's Diarrhea

A. Hydration: Oral fluid has to be taken to prevent and to treat dehydration:

- **a.** In case of mild dehydration, increased amount of oral fluid or clean water
- **b.** In case of moderate-to-severe dehydration, mainly in children and elderly suffering from chronic morbid illness, oral rehydration fluid as advised by the World Health Organization (WHO)

B. Antidiarrheal medication: In case of mild cases, loperamide alone or in case of moderate-to-severe disease, loperamide with proper antibiotic

C. Antibiotics:

- **a.** Norfloxacin 400 mg twice daily for 3–5 days
- **b.** Ciprofloxacin 500 mg twice daily for 3–5 days
- **c.** Ofloxacin 200 mg twice daily for 3–5 days
- **d.** Levofloxacin 500 once daily for 3–5 days
- **e.** Azithromycin 500 mg daily for 3 days
- **f.** Rifaximin 200 mg thrice daily for 3–5 days

In case of pregnant woman, pre-travel advice has to be followed strictly. In case of diarrhea, azithromycin is the drug of choice, but loperamide and rifaximin are class C drugs of choice.

In case of children: Traveler's diarrhea is more severe and more prolonged, sometimes bloody. In this disease, oral hydration fluid is of choice. Bismuth and loperamide are not recommended. Cefixime or other third-generation cephalosporins may be effective as second line, but azithromycin is the first choice.

Q22. Oral hairy leukoplakia.

MGR/APR2014/MDIII (7)
MGR/SEP2008/MDIII (6)

ANSWER

Clinical Features

Oral hairy leukoplakia is characterized by unilateral or bilateral white or gray adherent patches present on the lingual margin and dorsum or ventral part of the tongue to a lesser extent. The surface of the patches is irregular, with prominent folds or projections resembling hair, but sometimes corrugated in appearances. It may be flat on the ventral part of the tongue. It may occur on:

A. Floor of the mouth
B. Buccal mucosa
C. Oropharyngeal mucosa
D. Soft palate

The patient may be asymptomatic or present with soreness of throat.

Histological Features

A. Hyperparakeratosis
B. Acanthosis
C. Intranuclear inclusions
D. Koilocytosis containing pyknotic nuclei with perinuclear halo in the prickle cell layer
E. Keratinized hair-like projection
F. Few or no Langerhans cell
G. Limited or no inflammatory cellular infiltration in the lamina propria

Causes

A. Immunocompetent individual
B. Immunocompromised individual like HIV infection
C. Epstein–Barr virus (EBV) infection
D. *Candida* infection

Features for Diagnosis of Oral Hairy Leukoplakia

A. Provisional diagnosis: Characteristic gross appearance, which is responsive or nonresponsive to therapy

B. Presumptive diagnosis: Histological features described above

C. Definitive diagnosis: In situ hybridization of histological specimen demonstrates positive staining for EBV DNA or electron microscopy of histological specimen demonstrates herpes virus-like particles.

Treatment

A. In case of an asymptomatic individual, it may resolve spontaneously and has no premalignant potential.

B. 0.1% topical retinoic acid can improve the appearance in spite of its dekeratinizing and immunomodulating effect. However, it can produce a burning sensation over the applied surface.

C. Topical podophyllin can resolute the lesion.

D. Surgical excision or cryotherapy can be applied, but it can recur.

E. Antifungal drug can reduce the extent of the lesion but cannot eradicate infection.

F. Following antiviral drugs can ameliorate the lesion:

- **a.** Acyclovir
- **b.** Zidovudine
- **c.** Ganciclovir
- **d.** Foscarnet

The strains of *E. coli* are the following:

A. *Enterotoxigenic E. coli*: It produces heat stable and heat labile toxins responsible for childhood as well as travelers' diarrhea.

B. *Enteropathogenic E. coli*: It adheres to the intestinal epithelium and responsible for infantile diarrhea.

C. *Enterohemorrhagic E. coli*: It produces Stx-1 and Stx-2 toxins, i.e., Shiga like toxins and responsible for HUS and hemorrhagic colitis.

D. *Enteroaggregative E. coli*: It produces cytotoxins and produces biofilm in the intestinal mucosa leading to production of persistent childhood diarrhea and also in immunocompromised individuals.

E. *Enteroinvasive E. coli*: It invades the intestinal wall mucosa leading to production of hemorrhagic colitis like *Shigella* infection.

F. *Uropathogenic E. coli*: It is responsible for urinary tract infection. Through the adhesion with the uroepithelium by its P-fimbriae.

G. *Neonatal meningitis associated E. coli*: It expresses K1 capsular antigen that helps to evade the immunity leading to sepsis and neonatal meningitis.

Q23. Plummer–Vinson syndrome.

MGR/SEP2008/MDIII (6)

ANSWER

Definition

Plummer–Vinson syndrome or Peterson–Brown Kelly syndrome is characterized by a triad of:

A. Iron deficiency anemia

B. Esophageal web

C. Dysphagia

There is an increased tendency to develop esophageal or pharyngeal cancer.

Epidemiology

It was common in the middle-aged Caucasian women of northern countries, but now-a-days, this disease is extremely rare due to improvement of nutritional status as well as disappearance of iron deficiency.

Etiopathogenesis

A. Iron deficiency with iron supplementation can improve the symptoms.

B. High cell turnover loses iron-dependent enzymes, which in turn causes mucosal degeneration leading to web formation.

C. Malnutrition

D. Genetic predisposition

E. Autoimmune process as there is association with other autoimmune diseases, such as celiac disease, thyroid disease, and rheumatoid arthritis.

Clinical Features

A. White middle-aged woman in the 4th to 7th decade of life

B. Intermittent and progressive dysphagia limited to solids over years

C. Weight loss

D. Iron deficiency anemia as evidenced by:

- **a.** Weakness
- **b.** Tachycardia
- **c.** Fatigue
- **d.** Koilonychia
- **e.** Glossitis
- **f.** Angular cheilitis

E. Splenomegaly may be present.

F. Thyromegaly may be present.

Complications

A. Esophageal cancer

B. Pharyngeal cancer

Diagnosis

A. Hematological:

- **a.** Low hemoglobin, low hematocrit, and mean corpuscular volume
- **b.** Iron profile: Serum iron and ferritin are low, and serum iron-binding capacity is increased.

B. Barium swallow: Presence of esophageal web. It can be best demonstrated in video fluoroscopy—smooth, thin, and gray central or eccentric lumen.

C. Upper gastrointestinal endoscopy: It can be demonstrated. But as it is present in the upper esophagus, it can be ruptured unless it is introduced under direct vision. Web can be described as one or more thin membranes placed horizontally protruding from the anterior wall and progressing laterally.

D. Biopsy of this membrane is composed of squamous epithelium and submucosa.

Management

A. Search for the cause of iron deficiency, such as hemorrhage, malignancy, or celiac disease
B. Administration of iron supplement as it can resolve dysphagia
C. Mechanical dilatation of esophagus

Q24. MALToma.

MGR/MAR2008/MDIV (6)

ANSWER

Definition of MALT

Mucosa-associated lymphoid tissue is the most extensive component of lymphoid tissue and scattered along the mucosal linings throughout the human body like:

A. Gut-associated lymphoid tissue
B. Nose-associated lymphoid tissue
C. Bronchial and tracheal-associated lymphoid tissue
D. Vulvovaginal-associated lymphoid tissue
E. Parotid gland-associated lymphoid tissue

Definition of MALToma

Chronic inflammation due to infection or autoimmune disorder of this MALT will lead to the development of B-cell lymphoma of the marginal type or MALToma. The sites of MALToma are as follows:

A. Stomach
B. Other gastrointestinal sites
C. Skin
D. Salivary gland
E. Thyroid gland
F. Upper respiratory tract
G. Lung
H. Liver

Pathophysiology

MALT consists of small solitary lymph nodes or collection of lymphatic cells having a lightly staining germinal center and dark-staining peripheral region. Presence of MALT in a specific site is key to its function. In the intestinal wall, B cells will be stimulated by an infection to form IgM and IgA, which in turn prevent adherence of virus as well as bacteria to the intestinal epithelium, thus blocking their entry into the subepithelium of intestine.

M cells having microfolds on the luminal side present on the mucosal epithelial surface are responsible for absorption, transport, processing, and presentation of various antigens to subepithelial lymphoid cells, which include IgD/IgM$^+$ B cells and CD4+type 1 helper cells; the former is APCs which react with the latter type 1 cells. These cells and B cells are known as "pocket" of M cells. Follicle-associated epithelium having a true germinal center is observed in this pocket.

Majority of lymphoid tissue is accumulated in the Peyer patches in the lamina propria of intestinal epithelium, which allows the antigen to enter into the lymphoid tissue beneath it.

Dendritic follicular cells stimulate T1 helper cells. B7 costimulatory molecule stimulates CD28 of T1 helper cells resulting in secretion of IL-2 and IFN-γ; in turn IFN-γ suppresses type 2 helper cells which are involved in humoral immunity and IL-10 production by type 2 cells.

The main immune response occurs in the germinal center because a large number of cells congregated here are responsible for immune response. Early, in case of T-cell dependent immune response, B cells are accumulated and rapidly divided in the germinal center and form a dark zone. On the basis of interaction between antigen and antibody on the surface of dendritic follicular cells, B cells will be selected, the process of antigen involves several steps that express type II major histocompatibility complex (MHC). It will begin somatic hypermutation in the dark zone followed by immunoglobulin class-switching and plasma cell precursor and memory cells generation in the apical light zone.

Now efficiency of MALT depends upon adequate function of IgA. It again depends on acquisition of joining chain. In case of selective IgA deficiency, gastrointestinal and genitourinary tracts are prone to infection. In case lymphoma malignancy occurs in MALT, it is called MALToma, extranodal manifestation of marginal zone lymphoma. It is a low-grade lesion; most MALTomas occur in stomach and may be associated with *H. pylori* infection.

Clinical Features

A. Medial age of onset is 65 years.
B. It is more common in females and whites.
C. Nonspecific symptoms of gastric lymphoma:
  a. Low-grade fever
  b. Fatigue
  c. Constipation
  d. Weight loss
  e. Constipation
  f. Anemia

D. Respiratory distress

E. In case of conjunctival MALToma:

- **a.** Blurred vision
- **b.** Defects in visual field

Investigations

A. Laboratory studies:

- **a.** CBC
- **b.** Immunophenotyping of bone marrow lymphocytes, circulating lymphocytes, or biopsy specimen of MALToma
- **c.** MALToma is negative for CD10, CD23, and CD5 but positive for CD20. It is also positive for single type of light chain of CD21 and CD35.
- **d.** Low-grade type is positive for BCL2 whereas intermediate-grade type is negative for BCL2.

B. Imaging studies:

- **a.** Barium contrast studies demonstrate masses and infiltration in stomach and small and large intestines.
- **b.** CT and MRI can demonstrate:
  - **1.** Extent of primary lesion
  - **2.** Spread to distant site
- **c.** PET-CT

C. Endoscopy may demonstrate mucosal rigidity and mucosal hyperplasia.

D. Endoscopic ultrasonography can demonstrate the lesion.

E. Histology

Staging of MALToma

Staging of MALToma is similar to that of non-Hodgkin's lymphoma, but it is extranodal in origin:

A. Stage IE: Lymphoma involves only one area or organ outside the nodes.

B. Stage IIE: Lymphoma involves only one area or organ outside the nodes and lymph nodes around it, other lymph nodes on the same side of diaphragm may be involved.

C. Stage IIIE: Lymphoma is present on both sides of the diaphragm; may spread to area or organ near the spleen or lymph nodes.

D. Stage IV: Lymphoma spreads to other organs in the body with or without involvement of lymph nodes.

Treatment

Treatment depends on whether it is gastric or nongastric.

Conservative treatment is preferable for gastric lymphoma as it is mainly associated with *H. pylori*. Nongastric lymphoma is present in the lung, orbit, head, and neck. Since it is not associated with *H. pylori*, it is treated with radiotherapy, chemotherapy, and monoclonal antibodies administration. Stage IIE can be treated with surgery or radiation. Stage III/IV disease can be treated with the regimen used for follicular lymphoma, such as rituximab, chlorambucil, prednisolone, vincristine, fludarabine, dexamethasone, and mitoxantrone.

If the nongastric lymphoma is transformed to large B-cell lymphoma, it can be treated with R-CHOP.

In case of gastric MALToma, eradication of *H. pylori* with triple therapy (clarithromycin, amoxycillin, PPI or clarithromycin, metronidazole, and PPI in case the patient is allergic to penicillin) can regress low-grade lymphoma by 75%.

Presence of translocation at t(11;18)(q21,q21) indicates poor prognosis. Chemotherapy, radiotherapy, and surgery combination is superior to treatment with antibiotic; hence, endoscopic surveillance is required.

Stage IEII *H. pylori*-negative patient can accept radiation therapy or rituximab therapy.

Q25. Management of obscure gastrointestinal bleeding.

MJPRU/2014/MDIII (10)

How will you approach and manage a case of obscured GI bleeding in a 50-year-old male?

WBUHS 2022 (10)

ANSWER

Definition

Obscure gastrointestinal bleeding can be defined as bleeding from an unknown source, which may recur or persist in spite of negative evaluation by upper and lower gastrointestinal endoscopy, small bowel follow through or enteroclysis. Obscure bleeding can be subcategorized into two types:

A. Obscured-occult bleeding: It can be defined as in absence of gross gastrointestinal hemorrhage; there is a persistent positive occult blood test or presence of iron deficiency anemia or both.

B. Obscured-overt bleeding: It can be defined as persistent or recurrent visible bleeding in the form of hematemesis, melena, or hematochezia without any source of bleeding by endoscopic or radiologic evaluation.

Etiology of Obscured Gastrointestinal Bleeding

A. Upper gastrointestinal tract lesions:
  a. Cameron lesion
  b. Fundal varices
  c. Angiodysplasia
  d. Peptic ulcer
  e. Dieulafoy's lesion
  f. Gastric antral vascular ectasia

B. Lower gastrointestinal tract lesion:
  a. Angioectasia
  b. Neoplasm

C. Mid-gastrointestinal tract lesion:
  a. Below 40 years of age:
    1. Dieulafoy's lesion
    2. Celiac disease
    3. Meckel's diverticulum
    4. CD
  b. More than 40 years of age:
    1. Angioectasia
    2. Enteropathy due to NSAIDs
    3. Celiac disease
    4. Hemobilia
    5. Aortoenteric fistula
    6. Hemosuccus pancreaticus
  c. Rare causes:
    1. Blue rubber bleb nevus syndrome
    2. Osler-Weber-Rendu disease
    3. Plummer-Vinson syndrome
    4. Ehlers-Danlos syndrome
    5. Kaposi's sarcoma in AIDS

Investigations Given in Upper and Lower Gastrointestinal Bleeding

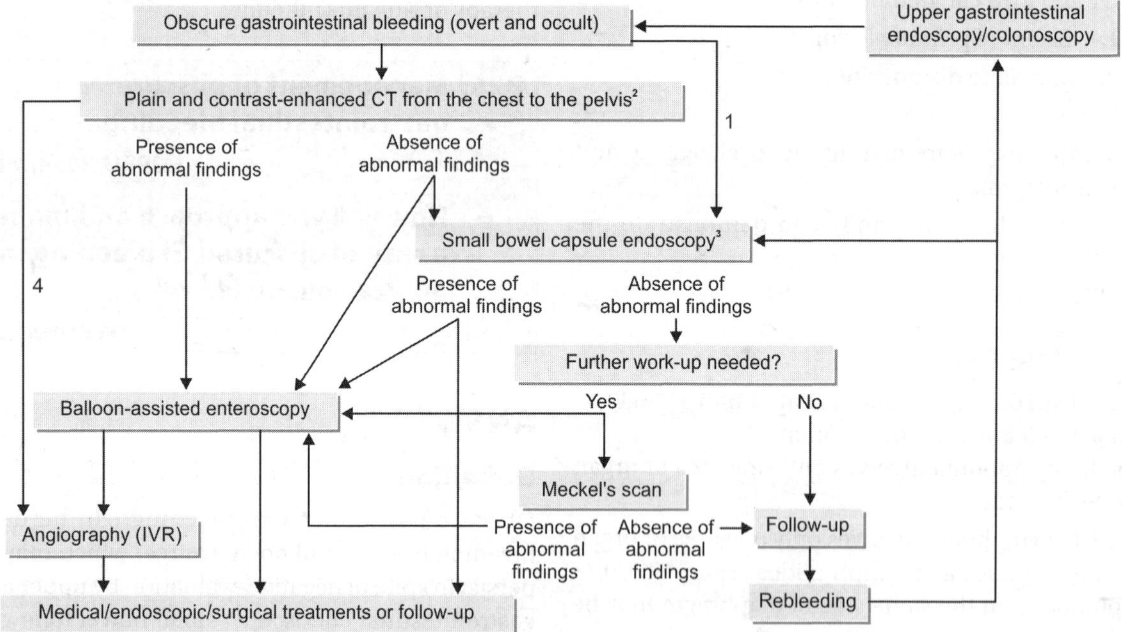

1. In the institutions without CT, capsule endoscopy may be performed at first. In this instance, however, CT should be performed later in another hospital.
2. Dynamic CT is preferable because some lesions can be visualized only by dynamic CT.
3. In cases of suspicious Crohn's disease, presence of abdominal symptoms (pain, distension, etc.), long-term NSAID use, and those with a medical history of abdominal irradiation and surgery, a patency capsule test should be performed first, and then small bowel capsule endoscopy can be undertaken only after confirmation of gastrointestinal patency.
   Note that patients with bowel obstruction (including suspicious obstruction) should not undergo the gastrointestinal patency test using a patency capsule or capsule endoscopy.
4. In the case when endoscopy is difficult to perform or unavailable.

Meckel's scan: ^{99m}Pertechnate is used to identify occult Meckel's bleeding, sensitivity being 75–100% due to presence of ectopic gastric mucosa.

Recommended Management

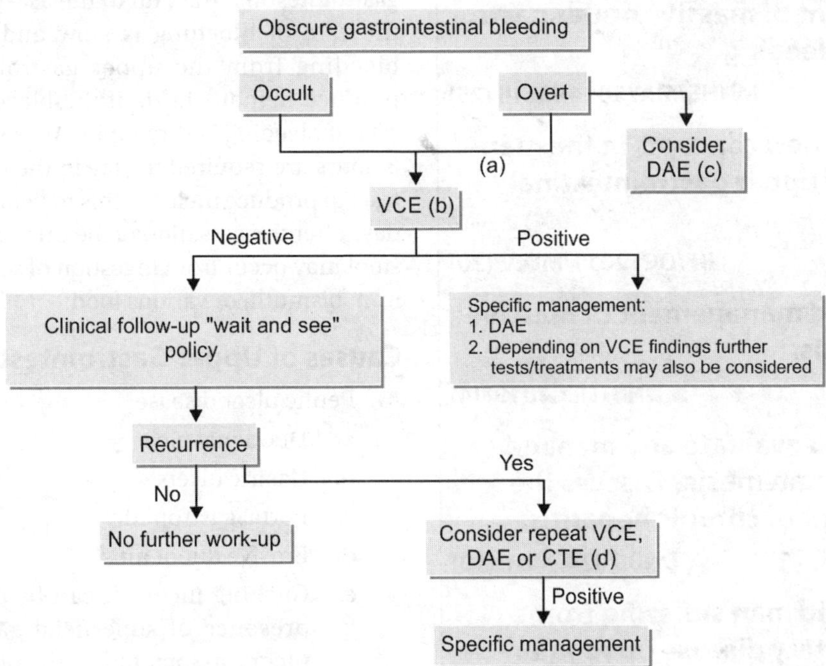

(CTE: computed tomography enterography/enteroclysis; DAE: device-assisted enteroscopy; VCE: video capsule endoscopy)

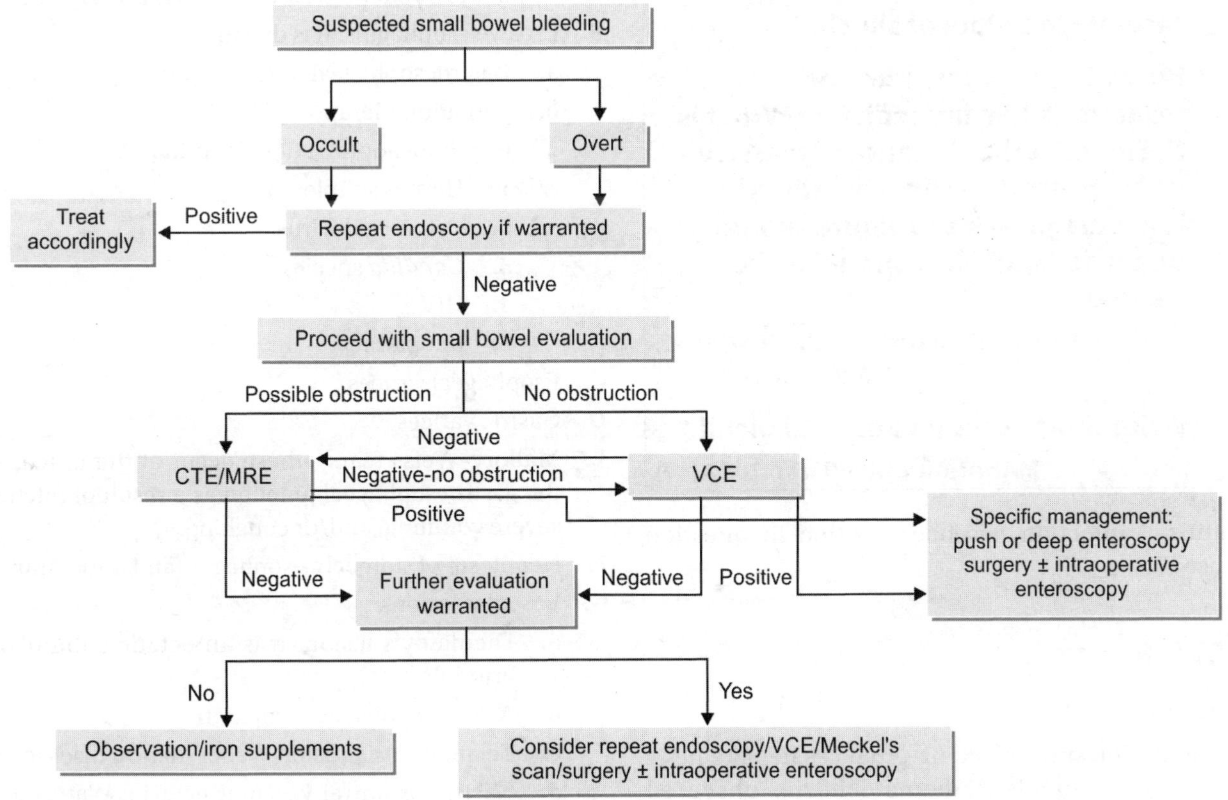

Q26. Describe causes, clinical features, and management of massive upper gastrointestinal bleeding.

MUHS/MAY2014/MDIII (25)

Discuss the new concepts in the management of upper gastrointestinal bleeding.

BF/OCT2011/MDIV (20)

Etiology and management of massive hematemesis.

DNB (DEC2019) (4)

How will you evaluate and manage massive hematemesis? Discuss the management of chronic hepatitis.

DNB 2024, MAY (10)

A 70-year-old man suffering from coronary artery disease on regular follow-up after PCI, suddenly has developed massive bout of hematemesis and is brought to casualty in a state of shock.

How will you assess him and resuscitate him immediately? What is the most probable cause of massive upper gastrointestinal bleeding? What diagnostic procedure should be carried out? How should he be treated?

SRI GURU RAM DAS UNI OF HEALTH SC, AMRITSAR, 2022 (10)

Write short notes on upper GI bleed.

MAHATMA UNIVERSITY, 2022 (10)

Hepatitis B infection has been written in question number 10.

ANSWER

Introduction

Upper gastrointestinal bleeding produces hematemesis with or without melena, hematochezia, obscured bleeding or occult bleeding.

Usually, upper gastrointestinal bleeding from the tract above the ligament of Treitz produces hematemesis and melena, but it may occur from anywhere in the gastrointestinal tract up to the ascending colon provided the rate of bleeding is slow and not brisk, whereas bleeding from the upper gastrointestinal tract may produce hematochezia if the bleeding is brisk and the rate of bleeding is very rapid. At least 60 mL of blood and 8 hours are required to stay in the upper gastrointestinal tract to produce melena. This melena is present for several days after the cessation of the original bleeding site. Black stool may occur from ingestion of some products, such as iron, bismuth, or various food.

Causes of Upper Gastrointestinal Bleeding

A. Peptic ulcer disease:
- **a.** Duodenal ulcer
- **b.** Gastric ulcers
- **c.** Portal gastropathy
- **d.** Erosive duodenitis
- **e.** Cushing ulcer—it can be characterized by the presence of superficial gastric and duodenal ulcers associated with increased intracranial pressure.
- **f.** Curling ulcers—these are acute superficial ulcers in the duodenum associated with severe burns.

B. Erosive esophagitis: It is due to:
- **a.** Gastroesophageal reflux disease
- **b.** Radiation therapy
- **c.** Immunosuppressed patients due to:
  1. Herpes simplex virus
  2. Cytomegalovirus
  3. *Candida* species
  4. HIV
  5. Idiopathic

C. Esophageal varices

D. Gastric varices

E. Mallory-Weiss tears—these occur at the mucosa of the gastroesophageal junction as a result of retching, severe vomiting, and/or coughing.

F. Neoplasm of stomach, esophagus, and duodenum

G. Vascular lesions:
- **a.** Dieulafoy's lesion: It is an ectatic submucosal arteriole.
- **b.** Arteriovenous malformation
- **c.** Telangiectasia: Osler–Weber–Rendu disease
- **d.** Gastric or antral vascular ectasia: Watermelon stomach; it may be associated with portal hypertension, chronic renal failure, or collagen vascular disease.

H. Uncommon causes:

a. Hemobilia: It is characterized by bleeding into the biliary tract in patients who have undergone hepatobiliary manipulation and liver biopsy or experienced liver trauma.

b. Aortoenteric fistula: Here there is communication between aortic aneurysm and aortic graft with the third part of the duodenum. The type of bleeding here is a brief "herald" bleed followed by massive acute bleeding. It is associated with a high mortality rate.

c. Hemosuccus pancreaticus: It is characterized by bleeding into the pancreatic duct in case of:

1. Acute pancreatitis
2. Chronic pancreatitis
3. Pancreatic cancer
4. Manipulation of pancreatic duct.

Causes	Presentation
Peptic ulcer disease	• Hematemesis • Melena • Coffee ground vomiting • Hematochezia
Esophageal and gastric varices	• Splenic vein thrombosis • Chronic liver disease
Erosive esophagitis	• Hematemesis • Melena • Coffee ground vomiting
Mallory–Weiss tear	• Hematemesis • Coffee ground vomiting
Neoplasm	• Occult bleeding • Weight loss • Flatulent dyspepsia • Iron deficiency anemia
Vascular malformation	• Hematemesis • Coffee ground vomiting • Melena • Iron deficiency anemia

Clinical Presentation

Present history:

A. Hematemesis—fresh blood or coffee ground vomiting, frequency, and amount of vomiting. If the amount of blood is >500 mL in vomit, it is called massive hematemesis.

B. Melena—it is black, tarry, foul-smelling stool.

C. Hematochezia—it may occur in case of brisk bleeding.

D. Upper abdominal pain suggests:

a. Peptic ulcer disease

b. Mesenteric ischemia

c. Subacute bacterial peritonitis in case of decompensated liver disease

E. Symptoms of liver decompensation, such as ascites, jaundice, and hepatic encephalopathy, favoring variceal bleeding disorders.

F. Recent ingestion of NSAIDs, corrosive agents, and alcohols

G. History of severe retching followed by vomiting

H. Symptoms of volume contraction, such as postural hypotension, oliguria, dry mouth, and headache

Past history:

A. Variceal bleeding

B. Nonhealing peptic ulcer disease

C. Bleeding from arteriovenous malformation

Personal history:

A. Chronic alcohol consumption

B. Chronic alcoholic liver disease

C. Smoking as it impairs wound healing

General examination:

A. Features of shock:

a. Hypotension

b. Cold clammy extremity

c. Pallor

d. Postural tachycardia—heart rate increases by 10 beats/min; form change of posture from lying down position to standing position

e. Postural hypotension: Drop of systolic blood pressure by 10 mm Hg following posture change from lying down position to sitting up position

f. Low volume pulse: Resting hypotension indicates 20–25% blood loss, whereas postural hypotension as well as postural tachycardia suggest 10–20% blood loss (700-mL blood loss).

B. Acanthosis nigricans—gastrointestinal malignancy

C. Koilonychia—iron deficiency anemia

D. Pigmented lips, soles, and palms—Peutz-Jeghers syndrome

E. Purpura, bruise—vascular disease

F. Stigmata of alcoholic liver disease, such as Dupuytren's contracture, palmar erythema, and parotid enlargement

Abdominal examination:

A. Tenderness in the abdomen—ischemic bowel disease, pancreatitis.

B. Gray turner sign—acute pancreatitis
C. Ascites, splenomegaly, and caput medusae—portal hypertension
D. Abdominal mass—malignancy
E. Umbilical nodule—abdominal malignancy

Risk factors for bleeding:
A. Age > 60 years
B. Onset in the hospital
C. Comorbid diseases
D. Features of shock
E. Recurrent bleeding
F. Severe coagulopathy
G. Active bleeding

Variable	0	1	2	3
Age	*<60 years*	*60–79 years*	*>80 years*	
Shock	• No shock • SBP >l00 • Pulse <100/min	• Tachycardia • SBP >100 • Pulse <100/min	• Hypotension • SBP <100 mm Hg	
Comorbidity	No major comorbidity	• SBP >100 • Pulse <100/min	CF, IHD, etc.	RF, LF, Disse. malignancy
Diagnosis	• M-W tear • No SRH no lesion identified	All other diagnoses	Malignancy of UGI tract	
Major stigmata of RH	None or dark spot only		Blood in UGI tract, adherent clot, visible or spurting	

(DBP: diastolic blood pressure; IHD: ischemic heart disease; LF: liver failure; RF: renal failure; RH: recent hemorrhage; SBP: systolic blood pressure; UGI: upper gastrointestinal tract)

Rockall score:
Score ≤ 2: Low risk of bleeding; chance of rebleeding is 4.3%
Score 3–5: Intermediate chance of bleeding; mortality is 2–7.9%
Score ≥ 6: High incidence of bleeding; mortality is 15.1–39.1%

Management of Upper Gastrointestinal Bleeding

Hemodynamically unstable patients have to be admitted in the intensive care unit.
A. Oxygen supplementation through nasal catheter
B. Close monitoring of vital signs
C. Close monitoring of urine output

Blood transfusion depends upon the following factors:
A. Rate of bleeding
B. Amount of bleeding
C. Underlying condition
D. Vital signs

Blood should be given if the blood hemoglobin level is <7 g/dL, but in case of significant comorbidities, such as ischemic cardiovascular disease, the hemoglobin level should be set at a higher level or at least 8 g/dL. The following measurements should be taken:
A. Two large-bore needles should be introduced intravenously or the central venous line should be made.
B. Intravenous fluid should be administered to expand the intravenous volume.
C. Packed red blood cells should be administered to raise the hemoglobin level to 7–8 g/dL.
D. If the platelet count is <50,000/cc, platelets have to be transfused.
E. In case INR is >2.5, fresh frozen plasma or prothrombin complex should be transfused, but it should be individualized.
F. All types of anticoagulants should be stopped.
G. Antihypertensive drugs can be started with caution.
H. Blood should be drawn for CBC, urea, creatinine, LFT, calcium, prothrombin time, activated partial thromboplastin time, and platelet count.
I. Cardiac enzymes to assess cardiac condition
J. Arterial blood gases
K. Leukocyte count—if it is >15,000/cc, it indicates infection.

Immediately after bleeding, the hematocrit level will not reflect accurately the amount of blood loss. But the hematocrit level will fall only when extravascular fluid enters into the intravascular space with an aim to restore the intravascular volume and it takes 24–72 hours to complete. 2–3% decrease in hematocrit value means loss of 500 mL of blood. So, the aim is to increase the hematocrit level by 30% in elderly, but 20–25% in young individuals.

Again, in case of upper gastrointestinal bleeding, blood urea nitrogen to creatinine ratio of >36 in the absence of underlying renal insufficiency suggests either prerenal azotemia or digested blood absorption during intestinal transit.

Management of Nonvariceal Bleeding

A. Pharmacotherapy: Intravenous infusion of a PPI 80 mg bolus followed by 8 mg/h for 72 hours to raise pH > 6 as it stabilizes clot at the ulcer site by the following mechanisms:

a. Optimization of platelet aggregation
b. Inhibition of fibrinolysis

B. Endoscopic injection therapy:

The goal of endoscopic therapy is:

a. Persistent bleeding
b. Recurrent bleeding

Ability to achieve sustained hemostasis depends on:

a. Controlled access to bleeding vessels
b. Relatively small size of the vessels
c. Absence of significant coagulation defects

The following methods are used:

a. Injection of vasoconstrictor agent 1:10,000 adrenalin at the periphery of the ulcer site reduces blood flow by the following mechanisms:
   1. Creation of local tamponade
   2. Vasoconstriction of the affected blood vessels
   3. If the amount of epinephrine is >13 mL, it will prevent recurrent bleeding in a high-risk patient.
b. Mixture of thrombin and fibrinogen (fibrin-sealant glue) can block the bleeding vessels.
c. Hemostatic powder spray can control bleeding by the following mechanisms:
   1. Adhesive properties of the materials
   2. It will absorb water molecules and dehydrate the tissues.
   3. It acts as a barrier upon contact with moisture.
   4. It has no local or systemic side effects.
d. Endo clot: Hemostatic powder can be injected through endoscopy into the ulcer without coming in direct contact with mucosa.

C. Endoscopic thermal therapy:

a. Compressing and coagulating the bleeding vessels, hemostasis can be achieved.
b. Contact thermal technique: This method will compress bleeding vessels to achieve hemostasis by the following methods:
   1. Heat probe thermal coagulation
   2. Bipolar electrocoagulation

   In some cases, an irrigator channel is used to inject adrenaline to irrigate culprit vessels.
c. Noncontact thermal technique: In this technique, through the beam of ionized argon gas, high-frequency electrical current will produce coagulation and damage the tissue. The methods are laser and argon plasma coagulation.

D. Mechanical technique: The techniques are Endoclips and Hemoclips. In case of bleeding from the posterior wall of the duodenum and lesser curvature of the stomach over the scope clip can only reach and significantly stop bleeding, and it is superior to epinephrine injection.

E. Endoscopic suturing: This method is an attractive aspect in a patient with upper GI bleeding.

F. Cryotherapy:

a. Contact thermal technique: This method has the following drawbacks:
   1. Definite contact is required.
   2. It is expensive.
   3. There is lack of control of depth of injury.
   4. Targeting multiple lesions is difficult.
b. Methods involving freezing tissue by delivering liquid nitrogen or nitrous oxide in case of bleeding lesions

G. Video capsule endoscopy:

a. It can stratify high- and low-risk patients in patients with upper gastrointestinal bleed.
b. It helps to determine needs for intervention.
c. It will reduce the time significantly for doing emergent endoscopic therapy.

Management of Acute Variceal Bleeding

A. Pharmacotherapy:

a. Vasoactive agents are octreotide, terlipressin, vasopressin, and somatostatin. All these drugs produce splanchnic vasoconstriction. But vasopressin produces systemic vasoconstriction. Somatostatin has no cardiovascular adverse effects and octreotide has a longer biological half-life:
   1. Vasopressin: 250 μg bolus intravenously followed by 0.3–1.0 μg/min for 48 hours. Cardiovascular side effects can be treated by intravenous nitroglycerin drip.
   2. Octreotide: 25–100 μg intravenously as a bolus dose followed by 25–50 μg hourly for 72 hours.
   3. Terlipressin: 2 mg intravenously as bolus dose followed by 1 mg 8 hourly for further 72 hours.

B. Endoscopic therapy:

a. Emergency intravariceal or paravariceal sclerotherapy by the following sclerosants:
   1. Ethanolamine oleate
   2. Sodium polydecanol

3. Sodium tetradecyl sulfate
4. Sodium morrhuate

Side effects are:

1. Ulceration
2. Perforation
3. Stricture
4. Fever
5. Sepsis

b. Endoscopic band ligation: It involves banding at the base of the varices.

Complications are:

1. Ulceration
2. Stricture
3. Hastening of portal systemic gastropathy

C. Insertion of a triple-lumen tube "Sengstaken-Blakemore tube":

a. One lumen for evacuating stomach
b. One lumen leads to gastric balloon
c. One lumen leads to esophageal balloon

But it should not be kept for >48 hours.

Complications:

a. Occlusion of airway by esophageal balloon
b. Aspiration of blood and secretion into lung
c. Ischemic necrosis of esophageal mucosa by prolonged compression of the balloon.

D. Transjugular intrahepatic portosystemic shunt (TIPS):

a. Pre-emptive TIPS is helpful in the following cases:
   1. Where there is a high risk of failure of endotherapy
   2. Where there is a chance of rebleeding in Child-Turcotte-Pugh (CTP) class C cirrhosis
   3. Class B with active bleeding on endoscopy
b. Where early TIPS cannot be performed, vasoactive drugs have to be continued intravenously for 2–3 days; then after discontinuation of these drugs, nonselective beta-blockers should be started. Rescue TIPS should be done in the following cases:
   1. Hemorrhage cannot be controlled.
   2. In spite of administration of vasoactive drugs along with AVL, bleeding recurs.

   After successful TIPS, vasoactive drugs can be discontinued. The efficacy of TIPS is 95%.

E. Surgery:

Indications: Endotherapy fails, but TIPS is not available.

Methods:

a. Devascularization procedures
b. Selective portosystemic shunting
c. Calibrated H grafts

Q27. Physiology of gastric acid secretion.

MUHS/NOV2010/MDI (10)

ANSWER

Typical oxyntic gland of stomach consists of three types of cells:

A. Mucus neck cells secreting mucus
B. Chief cells secreting pepsinogens
C. Parietal cells secreting hydrochloric acid and intrinsic factors

After stimulation, parietal cells secrete 160 mmol/L of hydrochloric acid; it is nearly isotonic to body fluid, but the pH of this acidic fluid is 0.8, i.e., extremely acidic.

Parietal cell contains a large number of branched intracellular canaliculi. Hydrochloric acid is produced in the villus-like projected structure inside the canaliculi and then projected toward the secretory end of the cell. The main driving force for secretion of hydrochloric acid from the parietal cell is the hydrogen-potassium pump. Formation of hydrochloric acid in the parietal cell consists of the following steps:

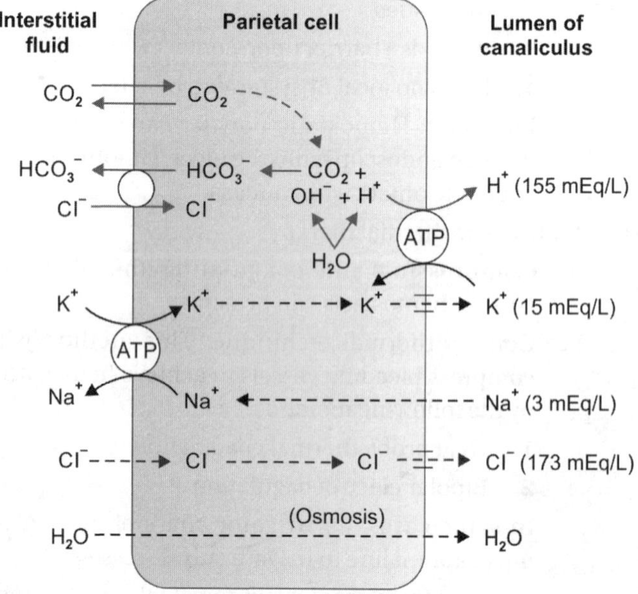

A. In the parietal cellular cytoplasm, water is dissociated to form H^+ and OH^- ions. H^+ ion is actively secreted into canaliculi in exchange of K^+ ion with the help

Na^+-K^+ ATPase. Again, K^+ ion is transported into parietal cellular cytoplasm actively by H^+-K^+-ATPase in exchange of Na^+ from the extracellular fluid on its basolateral membrane, which tends to leak into canaliculi but is reverted into cell by H^+-K^+ ATPase. As a result, intracellular concentration of Na^+ will be decreased, which leads to reabsorption of Na^+ from canaliculi. So, the net result is that most of the Na^+ and K^+ ions are absorbed into the parietal cellular cytoplasm in exchange of H^+ ion, which is secreted into the canaliculi.

B. Accumulated OH^- combines with CO_2 developed to form HCO_3^- catalyzed by carbonic anhydrase. This HCO_3 is transported into extracellular fluid across the basolateral membrane in exchange of Cl^- ion. CO_2 is produced due to cellular metabolism and entered from the extracellular fluid. Cl^- ion is also secreted from the extracellular fluid. Now this Cl^- ion is secreted into canaliculi; as a result, there is production of strong solution of hydrochloric acid. This hydrochloric acid is then secreted into the glandular lumen through the open end of canaliculi.

C. Water is secreted into the canaliculi by osmosis. So, final secretion contains:

a. Water

b. Hydrochloric acid: 150–160 mEq/L

c. Potassium chloride: 15 mEq/L

d. Sodium chloride: Small amount

Now to prevent the back leak of this, hydrochloric acid is attributed to the gastric barrier which is formed by the following:

a. Alkaline mucus

b. Tight junction in between the epithelial cells. If toxic substances, such as alcohol and excessive aspirin use, damage the barrier, acid will be leaked down the electrochemical gradient into the mucosa leading to the mucosal damage.

Stimulation gastric acid secretion:

a. As a result of stimulation of parasympathetic nerve, released acetylcholine excites:

1. Secretion of hydrochloric acid by parietal cells
2. Secretion of pepsinogen by peptic cells
3. Mucus by mucous cells

b. Gastrin and histamine stimulate parietal cells to release hydrochloric acid but not the other cells.

Q28. Diagnosis and treatment of celiac disease.

MUHS/NOV2010/MDIII (10)

Write down clinical features, pathogenesis, diagnosis, and management of celiac disease.

DNB (DEC 2021) (10)

Diagnosis and treatment of celiac disease.

ODISHA UNI, 2020 (10)

Celiac disease.

NTR UNI OF HEALTH SC, VIJAYAWADA, 2021 (10); TEERTHANKER MAHAVEER UNI, 2020 (10); RAJIV GANDHI UNI OF HEALTH SC, KARNATAKA, 2019 (10)

ANSWER

Definition

Celiac disease is an immune-mediated disorder and triggered by gluten-containing diet characterized by the spectrum of presentation from absence or subtle symptoms to severe symptoms including features of malabsorption of nutrients and abdominal discomfort, and, if untreated, results in different gastrointestinal complications.

Incidence

It is worldwide in distribution, occurs 1 in 113 people, and common in the United States and Europe.

Etiopathogenesis

A combination of the following factors will interact to produce this disease:

A. Environmental factor: Important component factor of gluten, gliadin, is present in wheat, rye, and barley, which will trigger innate and adaptive immunity in the small intestinal mucosa.

B. Immunogenic response: It can be suggested by the presence of antigliadin, antiendomysial, and antitissue transaminase antibodies (tTG) IgA in the serum. Endomysial antibodies recognize tTG; it deaminates gliadin. Gliadin is presented to gliadin-specific T cells bound to two human leukocyte antigens, HLA-DQ2 and HLA-DQ8, on the surface of APCs. Activation of gliadin-specific T4+ lymphocytes results in release of more and more cytokines leading to amplification of immune response; as a result there is epithelial damage, villus atrophy, and hyperplasia of crypt. A 4-week course of prednisolone will produce remission in patients who continued gluten-containing diet by improving the small intestinal mucosa.

C. Genetic factors: Its incidence varies widely in different groups of population, high among whites and low in blacks. It is present in 10% of first-degree relatives. All the celiac disease patients have HLA-DQ2 and HLA-DQ8 alleles, but very minority of patients with these alleles have this disease. On the other hand, patients having characteristic symptoms but absence of these alleles will exclude this disease.

Predisposing Factors

A. Northern European ancestry
B. First-degree relatives of celiac disease
C. Type 1 diabetes mellitus
D. Female sex
E. Iron deficiency anemia
F. Autoimmune thyroid disease
G. Osteoporosis
H. IgA deficiency
I. Dermatitis herpetiformis
J. Turner syndrome
K. Down syndrome

Presentation

Symptoms:

A. Gastrointestinal symptoms: Diarrhea associated with abdominal discomfort, abdominal bloating, nausea, and flatulence. Mechanism of diarrhea:
   a. As a result of changes in the jejunal mucosal function, steatorrhea will occur.
   b. As a result of changes in the jejunal brush border enzymatic function, there will be lactate deficiency.
   c. In case of extensive disease involving colon, bile acid induced fluid secretion result in bile acid malabsorption.
   d. As a result of cryptic hyperplasia, there is endogenous fluid secretion.

B. Constitutional symptoms: Anorexia, weight loss, malaise, and decreased energy
C. Some patients present with only constitutional symptoms.
D. In few cases, features are only related to malabsorption of nutrients, such as iron-producing anemia, folate-producing macrocytic anemia, vitamin D-producing osteomalacia, or loss of protein-producing edema.
E. Family history of gastrointestinal disorders
F. Dietary habits, such as intake of wheat, barley, and rye and common irritants, such as artificial sweeteners, alcohol, and caffeine
G. Coexistence of relevant diseases, such as diabetes mellitus type 1, thyroid disease, and osteoporosis

Signs:

A. Pale due to iron and folate deficiency anemia
B. Cardiovascular manifestations, such as tachycardia, due to anemia
C. Mental features, such as lethargy and depression
D. Neurological features, such as tremor and neuropathy
E. Dermatological examination, such as dermatitis herpetiformis, dry mucosa of thyroid disease, and easy bruising

Diagnosis

A. General tests:
   a. CBC to demonstrate anemia
   b. Thyroid function test
   c. Immunoglobulin level like IgA
   d. Vitamin level like vitamin B12 and folic acid
   e. Iron profile

B. Specific to celiac disease:
   a. Anti-tTG antibody IgA—highly sensitive and highly specific. The height of this antibody titer will correlate with the degree of injury of the small intestinal mucosa.
   b. Antigliadin antibodies IgA and IgG
   c. Antiendomysial antibody IgA

   But IgA in serum must be assessed.

   d. Duodenal or jejunal mucosal biopsy demonstrates (at least 4 or more samples should be taken) the following:
      1. Number of intraepithelial lymphocytes are increased.
      2. Height of villi of small intestinal mucosa is decreased toward flattening.

3. Increased proliferation of cryptic mucosa leading to hyperplasia of crypt
4. Loss of villus architecture but there is no mucosal atrophy
5. Lining mucosal cells are cuboidal with presence of nuclei near the apex.
6. In the lamina propria, there is an increased number of lymphocytes and plasma cells.

According to Marsh criteria, the following grades of histological changes are suggestive of celiac disease:

a. Type I celiac disease: Usually >30–40 lymphocytes per 100 lymphocytes—increased intraepithelial lymphocytes
b. Type II celiac disease: Cryptic hyperplasia along with increased intraepithelial lymphocytes
c. Type III celiac disease: Villus atrophy like blunting of epithelial projection in the wall of the intestine along with cryptic hyperplasia and increased intraepithelial lymphocytes

Serial biopsy is required to estimate the response to gluten-free diet.

C. HLA typing: Screening of family members or the patients suffering from the suspected symptoms—HLA-DQ2 and HLA-DQ8
D. Imaging technique:
   a. Upper gastrointestinal endoscopy to detect the characteristic mucosal changes in the small intestine
   b. Wireless capsule endoscopy can detect the following changes:
      1. Extent of small bowel involvement
      2. Presence of this disease which spares the duodenum
      3. The cause of bleeding in case of celiac disease
      4. Presence or absence of intestinal malignancy
   c. Bone densitometry to detect the presence of osteoporosis

Treatment of Celiac Disease

A. Strict adherence to gluten-free diet, such as diets free of Horlicks, rye, and barley
B. Supplementation of nutrients, such as iron, vitamins, proteins, and calcium
C. Use of rice flour in place of wheat flour is helpful.

Complications

A. Development of gastrointestinal or nongastrointestinal cancer and lymphoma—incidence is higher in UK and Ireland. Lymphoma can be suspected when:
   a. Patients previously completely responsive to gluten-free diet suddenly become nonresponsive to gluten-free diet
   b. Patients present with clinical and histological features, which are consistent with celiac disease
B. Collagenous sprue: Here collagen material is deposited beneath the basement membrane. Patients will not respond to gluten-free diet. Prognosis is poor.
C. Intestinal ulceration
D. Refractory sprue: 10% of the patients fail to respond to gluten-free diet because:
   a. They respond to restriction of other dietary proteins, such as soy
   b. They respond to treatment with steroids
   c. Their clinical and morphologic findings will disappear after several months to years
   d. They fail to respond to all the measures or/and will face fatal outcome with or without complications.

   In this case, the therapeutic approach includes:

   a. Use of peptidase to inactivate toxic gliadin peptides
   b. Use of small molecules to block the uptake of toxic peptides across the tight junctions in between the intestinal epithelial cells

Prevention and Management of Complications

A. Successful adherence to gluten-free diet
B. Serological tests should be performed every 3–6 months to see the improvement, and then every 1–2 years to detect any recurrence of symptom.
C. In case of appearance of unexplained symptoms, such as anemia and weight loss, a small intestinal malignancy has to be suspected.
D. Baseline bone densitometry followed by regular calcium and vitamin D supplementation, which is followed by regular monitoring with densitometry, should be done.
E. In case of autoimmune diseases, such as thyroid disease or type 1 diabetes mellitus, serological tests for celiac disease should be done.

Q29. IgG4-related disorders.

PGI/APR2013/MDIV (10)
MJPRU/2015/MDIV (10)

Four IgG related disorders.

NTR UNI OF HEALTH SC, VIJAYAWADA, 2021 (10)

IgG4 related disorders.

BABA FARID UNI OF HEALTH SC, 2019 (10)
NTR UNI OF HEALTH SC, VIJAYAWADA, 2018 (10)

ANSWER

Definition

IgG4-related disorders (IgG-RD) are T helper 2 cells with or without combinations of regulatory T (Treg) cells mediated fibroinflammatory process, having a tendency to produce a tumefactive lesion in a synchronous fashion in different organs in the body.

The following conditions and affected organs in the body in IgG4-RD:

Affected organs	Conditions
Orbits and upper respiratory tract	Eosinophilic angiocentric fibrosis
Dura mater	Hypertrophic pachymeningitis
Mediastinum	Fibrosing mediastinitis
Kidney	Idiopathic hypocomplementemic tubulointerstitial nephritis with extensive tubulointerstitial deposits
Orbit, lung, kidney	Inflammatory pseudotumor
Aorta	Inflammatory aortic aneurysm
Salivary and lacrimal glands	Mikulicz's syndrome
Submandibular gland	Kutner's tumor
Aorta and large vessels	Periaortitis, periarteritis
Thyroid	Riedel's thyroiditis
Retroperitoneum	Retroperitoneal fibrosis
Pancreas	Sclerosing pancreatitis
Mesentery	Sclerosing mesenteritis
Mediastinum, retroperitoneum, orbit, thyroid gland, and other organs	Multifocal fibrosclerosis

Clinical Characteristics

A. Middle-aged to elderly males are affected.
B. Male to female ratio is 3.5:1, but in case of sialadenitis, females are more frequently affected.
C. Nonspecific symptoms, such as fever and malaise
D. Organ-specific symptoms, such as pulmonary and renal symptoms
E. Features of pancreatitis include abdominal pain, jaundice, and weight loss

Pathophysiology

IgG4 antibodies: Only 5% of subclasses of IgG is IgG4. Half of this IgG4 will split randomly owing to variance of amino acid in the hinge region and join with other half molecules to produce FAB-arm exchange. As a result, asymmetric bispecific antibodies are produced having two different binding sites, which hardly bind to Fc receptors and complements to form immune complexes, so their innate immune response will be limited. So IgG4 is regarded as an anti-inflammatory and antiallergic molecule. But on repeated antigenic exposure, IgG4 will be produced in large numbers and represent as a bystander phenomenon rather than a causative factor. But in some cases of thrombotic thrombocytopenic purpura (TTP) or vasculitides, these antibodies may play a role.

B cells: The following features are suggestive of a role of B lymphocytes in IgG4-RD:

A. Extensive presence of B lymphocytes or plasma cells in the affected tissues
B. Rituximab is the effective treatment.
C. CD19+CD20-CD27+CD38+ plasmoblasts are present in increased numbers in the circulation and responsible for displaying oligoclonal expansion and somatic hypermutation. This antigenic-driven response is present in IgG4-RD.

T cells and cytokines: Type 2 helper cells are the key to the pathogenesis in this disease as they will release the following cytokines:

A. IL-4
B. IL-5
C. IL-13
D. IL-10
E. TGF-β

IL-13 and TGF-beta are responsible for activation of fibroblasts leading to fibrosis.

IL-4 and IL-10 cause IgG4-specific class switch recombination with B-lymphocytes.

It has been shown that CD4+ cells initiate IgG4-RD by activating B cells. Other cytokines, such as IL-21 and IL-27 produced by macrophages, play a role in differentiation of T helper cells, thus leading to IL-10 production.

Innate immunity and complement:

A. IgE has been shown to be an important factor in IgG4-RD because mast cells produce IL-4, IL-10, TGF-beta and mast cells are highly positive for IgE.

B. Again, M2 macrophages being activated by Th2 and T-regulatory cytokines, such as IL-10 and IL-13, will be responsible for the fibrosing process.

C. Nucleotide-binding oligomerization domain-like receptor present on the macrophages will class-switch recombination via B cells and will further activate as well as proliferate IgG4 positive B cells.

D. Unknown microbial antigen may trigger immune response and it may be a causative factor in IgG4-RD.

E. A low complement level is found in case of renal involvement, but it may be attributable to concomitant IgG subclass elevation other than IgG4.

Laboratory Testing

A. Organ-specific parameters including renal, pulmonary, hepatic, and pancreatic parameters

B. CRP will be elevated.

C. Low complement level in IgG4-related renal disease

D. Positive rheumatoid factor

E. Elevated ANA in IgG4-RD

F. Serum IgG4: It will be increased but in some cases it may be normal.

Histopathological hallmark of IgG4-RD:

A. Major features:

- **a.** Lymphoplasmacytic infiltrate
- **b.** Storiform fibrosis
- **c.** Obliterative phlebitis
- **d.** High percentage of IgG4-positive plasma cells
- **e.** Mild-to-moderate tissue eosinophilia

B. Minor features:

- **a.** Germinal centers
- **b.** Lymphoid follicles
- **c.** Obliterative arteritis (usually present in the lung)
- **d.** Nonobliterative phlebitis

Flow Cytometry

CD19+, CD20-, and CD27+ plasmoblasts are not present in peripheral circulation normally, but are present in high numbers in IgG4-RD as compared to other inflammatory diseases.

Fluorodeoxyglucose (FDG) PET:

A. It will highlight the inflammatory lesion; thus, it can estimate the extent of the disease.

B. It can stage the disease.

C. It can assess the disease activity.

D. It can assess the response to treatment.

E. It can guide the biopsies.

Comprehensive Diagnostic Criteria for IgG4-RD

A. Clinical examination (clinical history, physical examination, imaging)

B. Immunological examination: IgG4 in the serum >135 mg/dL or elevated IgG4/IgG ratio; optionally accompanied by other laboratory alterations, such as immunoglobulin E, γ-globulin, or complement.

C. Histopathologic examination: Lymphocytic infiltration with Storiform fibrosis and obliterative phlebitis, infiltration by IgG4+ plasma cells (IgG4+/IgG+ >40%)

1 + 2 = Possible IgG4-RD
1 + 3 = Probable IgG4-RD
1 + 2 + 3 = Definite IgG4-RD

Therapy

Indication of Therapy

A. Untreated IgG4-RD involving pancreas or kidney disease though asymptomatic should be treated without delay.

B. Close follow-up is required in the following cases:

- **a.** With no or only mild symptoms
- **b.** Without signs of organ dysfunction
- **c.** Location of IgG4-RD will not produce major complications

C. If treatment not initiated, it will:

- **a.** Worsen the organ function
- **b.** Reduce the chance of remission
- **c.** Increase the chance of complications

Initiation and Maintenance Therapy

A. Glucocorticoids: These are used as first line of therapy. The dose is 30–40 mg/day or 0.6 mg/kg/day, but it can be varied according to urgency or disease activity. Response to corticoids will be started within days or weeks and within few weeks, remission can be achieved.

Slow tapering of the dose of the steroid has to be started within 2–4 weeks after induction therapy and it will last for 3–6 months.

B. Low dose of 2.5–5 mg/day of steroid should be continued for up to 3 years. It will decrease the relapse of pancreatitis.

C. If steroid-sparing drugs, such as azathioprine, methotrexate, and mycophenolate mofetil, can be used as induction and maintenance therapy, the choice depends upon the organ involved or medical specialist.

D. Rituximab will deplete the B cells, which leads to reduction of IgG4 and very effective disease control in case of steroid refractory cases.

Disease activity: This disease is a chronic, relapsing disease; hence, it requires maintenance therapy. Therefore, this patient has to be evaluated regularly to judge disease activity and flaring during remission.

Recently, plasmablast has been emerged as a good indicator of activity of the disease, but application of this parameter will require further research.

Future prospect: Relapse frequently happens in this disease. Glucocorticoid is still regarded as first line of therapy both in induction and in maintenance phases, and steroid-sparing drugs and rituximab are considered in case of relapse or refractory to steroid or if the patient is intolerant to steroid.

Q30. Discuss fat malabsorption. Also discuss investigations and management of fat malabsorption.

BF/NOV2013/MDI (10)

ANSWER

Fat malabsorption arises from either digestion or absorption of fat. Lipid processing is called emulsification which starts in the mouth through mastication, mixing with lingual lipase which will be continued up to stomach cavity where continuous mixing occurs. 15% fat will be digested when it will enter the duodenum and to jejunum. In proximal two thirds of jejunum, the rest of the fat will be digested by gastric and pancreatic lipase. Majority of fat absorption occurs in this part of the jejunum. In the jejunum, the rest of the fat is solubilized by raising the intraluminal pH to 6.5 and forms micelles by mixing with bile salts released from gallbladder. Micelles are formed by aggregation of product of fat digestion and mixture of lipolytic product which will be absorbed. Bile salt will be absorbed in the terminal ileum and recycled through enterohepatic circulation.

Causes of fat malabsorption:

A. Decreasing duodenal pH (normal pH is 6.5): Zollinger–Ellison syndrome: Increased secretion of gastric acid will lower the pH and destroy the pancreatic enzymes.

B. Loss of intestinal absorptive mucosal area: As a result, the intestinal transit time will be decreased and thus decreased exposure time to intestinal enzymes. The causes are:

- **a.** Diffuse mucosal disease:
  1. UC
  2. CD
  3. Celiac disease
- **b.** Small intestinal resection—result of barrier surgery

C. Impaired processing of lipids by bile acids: It usually happens when the amount of bile acids is inadequate for fat absorption, secretion of bile acids is impaired, or bile acids being unabsorbed are present in the intestinal lumen. These unabsorbed bile acids are unavailable for reuse for fat digestion but stimulate colon to secrete electrolytes and water. So the causes are:

- **a.** Liver disease:
  1. Cirrhosis of liver impairs bile acid synthesis.
  2. In case of amyloidosis, amyloid deposition in the hepatic stellate cells prevents synthesis of bile acids.
- **b.** Cholestasis: Intrahepatic or extrahepatic cholestasis will prevent flow of bile into the intestine.

D. Small intestinal bacterial overgrowth: It will disrupt the harmony of bacteria in the small intestine; as a result, few bacteria deconjugate bile acids making it ineffective for fat digestion. It may be associated with atrophic gastritis. It can result from:

- **a.** Prolonged lactase deficiency
- **b.** Blind loop syndrome developed as a result of the inflammatory process in IBD
- **c.** Any type of gastric stasis
- **d.** Medical conditions responsible for dumping of gastric food having basic pH

E. Pancreatic exocrine efficiency:

- **a.** Chronic pancreatitis due to alcohol or chronic biliary obstruction
- **b.** Resection of pancreas—loss of pancreatic tissue
- **c.** Cystic fibrosis

d. Pancreatic cancer—loss of functional pancreatic tissue
e. Celiac disease
f. Zollinger–Ellison syndrome
g. Gastric surgery

F. Defect in chylomicron/lipoprotein secretion—abetalipoproteinemia due to mutation of *MTP* gene

G. Lymphatic disorders:
a. Intestinal lymphangiectasia
b. Whipple disease

Diagnosis

A. Hematological tests:
a. CBC for evaluation of anemia
b. Metabolic panel for evaluation of:
1. Liver function
2. Renal function
3. Electrolyte imbalance
c. Iron panel
d. Vitamins to evaluate:
1. Vitamin B12
2. Folic acid
3. Vitamin D3

B. Fecal test for evaluation of fat malabsorption:
a. Measurement of fecal fat in single specimen: If it is positive, then 72-hour stool fat estimation will be necessary.
b. 72-hour fecal fat estimation: It is the gold standard for the diagnosis of steatorrhea.
c. Sudan III—in one stool sample
d. Acid steatocrit
e. Near-infrared reflectance analysis—it measures accurately 72-hour fecal fat excretion. It also measures carbohydrate and nitrogen during the measurement of fat.

C. Specific evaluation of malabsorption syndrome:
a. Jejunal aspirate culture for evaluation of bacterial overgrowth
b. Computerized tomography or MRI: Pancreatitis
c. Magnetic resonance cholangiopancreatography (MRCP) for chronic pancreatic insufficiency
d. Endoscopic retrograde cholangiopancreatography (ERCP) to evaluate chronic pancreatitis if history is suggestive of alcohol intake and high fecal elastase.
e. Endoscopy with biopsy to detect:
1. CD: Cobble-stoning of duodenal mucosa
2. Jejunoileitis
3. Celiac disease—blunted duodenal folds or scalloping of the duodenal mucosa
4. Acid fast stain for differentiating *Tropheryma whipplei* from *M. avium*

Treatment

A. Treatment should follow the cause.

B. To decrease the peristalsis—loperamide, it acts on mu-receptor on the gut epithelium

C. Dietary modification:
a. Avoidance of fat
b. Avoidance of alcohol
c. Intake of low fiber diet

D. Administration of bile acid binding resin, cholestyramine

E. In case of depression, tricyclic antidepressant

F. In case of diarrhea due to opioid withdrawal, clonidine as alpha-2 adrenergic blocker can slow the intestinal transit.

Q31. Describe the clinical features and management of carcinoid tumor.
BF/MAY2013/MDI (10)

ANSWER

Definition

It is a slowly growing neuroendocrine tumor arising from enterochromaffin cells distributed throughout the gastrointestinal tract and bronchopulmonary system in the body. But it can arise from thymus, hepatobiliary system, mediastinum, ovaries, kidney, and prostate.

Tumor Biology

The term "enterochromaffin cells" refers to its ability to be stained with chromium salts. Biologically active substance secreted by these cells in the tumor is vasoactive peptide 5-HT synthesized from the amino acid tryptophan and released into systemic circulation producing classical symptoms, such as episodic flushing, diarrhea, and bronchopulmonary constriction. Other products of this tumor are acid phosphatase, amylin, dopamine, catecholamines, alpha-1 antitrypsin, gastrin, fibroblastic growth factor, bombesin, glucagon, histamine, insulin, kinin, motilin, etc.

Classification

It can be classified according to the location in the primitive gut:

A. Foregut carcinoid tumor: It is divided into—
  a. Sporadic primary tumor: Stomach, proximal duodenum, pancreas, bronchus, thymus, and lung
  b. Tumor secondary achlorhydria

B. Midgut carcinoid tumor: It is derived from:
  a. Second portion of duodenum
  b. Jejunum
  c. Ileum
  d. Appendix
  e. Right colon

C. Hindgut carcinoid tumor: It arises from:
  a. Transverse colon
  b. Left colon
  c. Rectum

According to the WHO, the carcinoid tumor has been classified into the following types based on its malignant potential:

A. Well-differentiated endocrine tumor (proliferative index is <2%)

B. Well-differentiated endocrine carcinoma (proliferative index is >2% but <15%)

C. Poorly differentiated endocrine carcinoma (proliferative index is >15%)

D. Mixed exocrine–endocrine tumor

E. Tumor-like lesions

Pathophysiology

This tumor originates from primitive stem cells giving rise to multiple cell lineages. In the GI tract, it is developed deep in the mucosa and then grows and extends slowly toward the mucosal surface, resulting in the formation of nodules bulging into the lumen. The color of the tumor is yellow due to accumulation of cholesterol and lipid in the tumor. Microscopically, this tumor has five different patterns:

A. Solid, nodular, and insular cord

B. Trabecular pattern with anastomosing features

C. Rosette patterns of glands and tubules

D. Poorly differentiated

E. Mixed patterns

In case of midgut carcinoids, the cells are round, regular, and closely packed monomorphous masses.

Clinical Presentations

A. In case of intestinal carcinoids producing periodic abdominal pain due to:
  a. Fibrosis of the mesentery
  b. Kinking of the intestine
  c. Intestinal obstruction

B. VIP produces symptoms like those of neuroblastoma, especially in the children.

C. In foregut carcinoid tumor, features of Cushing syndrome or ectopic ACTH

D. Carcinoid crisis occurs in response to stress, chemotherapy, or anesthesia. Features are intense flushing, abdominal pain, diarrhea, hypertension or hypotension, tachycardia, alteration in mental status, and coma.

E. In case of midgut tumor, cutaneous flushing affecting the head and neck, itching, upper body erythema, lacrimation, diaphoresis, salivation, and diarrhea. These are triggered by stress, exercise, and cheese.

F. Wheeze due to bronchoconstriction, shortness of breath, and cough

G. Other features are:
  a. Cardiac valvular lesion involving the right side of the heart due to fibrosis of endocardium on its ventricular aspect
  b. Lacrimation, arthritis, joint pain, and ophthalmologic features with flushing
  c. Skin hyperkeratosis and hyperpigmentation

Laboratory Investigations

A. Urinary 5-HIAA—increased in this tumor

B. Fasting plasma 5-HIAA is more stable than whole blood assay of serotonin and more stable than 24-hour urinary 5-HIAA.

C. Imaging studies:
  a. CT and scintigraphy can diagnose chest tumor.
  b. Liver metastasis and mesenteric invasion can be diagnosed by CT scan.
  c. PET scanning is used for follow-up of the tumor.
  d. Scintigraphy with MIBG can detect carcinoid tumor.
  e. Octreotide scanning is more sensitive in detection of tumor as compared to MIBG scanning.
  f. Radionuclide imaging attached to radioactive tracer with somatostatin analog is used. The

radiotracer used is yttrium or ^{111}In-DTPA which has affinity for somatostatin receptor subtypes SSTR-1 to SSTR-5; amongst them, SSTR-2 has the highest affinity and SSTR-1 and SSTR-4 have the lowest affinity. It can identify primary and metastatic diseases.

g. Colonoscopy and upper gastrointestinal endoscopy

h. CECT of thorax to see primary or metastasis in lung

Treatment

A. The following chemotherapeutic agents are used for metastatic carcinoid disease:

- **a.** Alkylating agents
- **b.** 5-fluorouracil
- **c.** Doxorubicin
- **d.** Cisplatin
- **e.** Etoposide
- **f.** Streptozocin
- **g.** Interferon-alpha
- **h.** Somatostatin analogs

B. In case of metastatic liver disease, chemoembolization of hepatic artery can be given in adult.

C. The somatostatin analog, octreotide, can be used to reduce symptoms, but by reducing the growth factor it can impair growth in children. Intermittent administration of octreotide can normalize insulin-like growth factor 1 in blood and suppress plasma growth hormone-releasing hormone.

D. In case of a nonresectable tumor, octreotide attached to radioactive load using yttrium-90 can be given.

E. Surgical treatment:

a. In case of appendicular carcinoid with a small lesion, appendectomy can be given. If the lesion is >2 cm, or a perforated appendix or base of the appendix is involved, block dissection of the tumor should be done. More extensive surgery (hemicolectomy) is indicated if:

1. The tumor size is >2 cm along with lymphatic involvement
2. Infiltration of mesoappendix
3. Positive resection margin
4. Cellular pleomorphism along with a high mitotic index

b. In case of a rectal tumor, endoscopic resection of the tumor is of choice if:

1. Tumor size is <1 cm
2. Tumor is limited to mucosa
3. Adequate margin at presentation

c. If the tumor is of large size, debulking may give symptomatic relief

d. In case of a hepatic tumor, ligation of the hepatic artery can produce necrosis of the tumor cells and at the same time preserve the normal liver cells.

e. In case of endoluminal bronchial carcinoid, bronchoscopic cryotherapy can be given successfully.

Q32. Whipple disease.

KUHS/NOV2013(S)/MDIII (10)

ANSWER

Definition

Whipple disease is a multisystem disease caused by gram-positive bacteria, *T. whipplei,* identified by polymerase chain reaction, and characterized by steatorrhea, loss of weight, arthralgia, central nervous system, and cardiac manifestations.

Etiology

Gram-positive actinobacteria *T. whipplei* it is of low virulence but highly infective, which leads to production of minimal symptoms as compared to burden of bacteria.

Pathophysiology

These bacteria infiltrate different body tissues. Now the body's immune system will incorporate these organisms into tissue macrophages which are PAS positive. These organism-laden macrophages will infiltrate the lamina propria of the intestinal wall disrupting normal villus function. It will also infiltrate the heart valves, synovial tissues, central nervous system, and rarely in the lungs.

The route of exposure is from soil and animals.

Clinical Presentation

A. Males are commonly affected with a ratio of 8:1.

B. Middle-aged males are affected.

C. Migratory large joint arthropathy

D. Fever

E. Diarrhea and steatorrhea due to intestinal mucosal injury and lymphatic obstruction

F. Lymphadenopathy

G. Occult gastrointestinal bleeding

Physical manifestations:

A. Cachexia

B. Distended abdomen

C. Lymphadenopathy

D. Vitamin deficiency in the form of glossitis, angular stomatitis, and night blindness

E. Chvostek sign and Trousseau sign—features of calcium deficiency

F. Hyperpigmentation around the orbital and malar areas

G. CNS signs, such as tremor, ataxia, and clonus

Diagnosis

A. Basic studies:

  a. Serum albumin

  b. Serum carotene

  c. Prothrombin time

  d. Sudan stain of stool

  e. 72-hour fecal fat estimation

B. Radiological features:

  a. Small bowel series demonstrate the presence of malabsorption.

  b. Brain MRI

C. Definite diagnosis is done by tissue biopsy from different involved organs including intestinal wall. It will demonstrate PAS-positive macrophages containing *T. whipplei* within the lamina propria. It may be present in other cases like in case of *M. avium* complex, which is also responsible for diarrhea in HIV patients. But presence of *T. whipplei* outside the macrophages is more diagnostic of this active disease.

D. RT-PCR targeting segment of *rpoB* gene as it is specific for *T. whipplei*—it is highly specific.

Treatment

A. Antibiotic administration: Antibiotic of choice is intravenous administration of ceftriaxone or meropenem twice daily for 2 weeks followed by trimethoprim/cotrimoxazole (160/800) orally twice daily for 1 year.

Biopsy containing PAS-positive macrophages may persist indefinitely after treatment, but presence of bacilli outside the macrophages is the sign of:

  a. Persistence of infection

  b. Early sign of relapse

B. A case of a patient with dementia along with recurrence of disease is prognostically poor and requires antibiotics that can cross the blood–brain barrier.

C. In case of intolerance to trimethoprim/cotrimoxazole, chloramphenicol can be administered.

Q33. Venous drainage of rectum and anal canal.

MGR/APR2016/MDI (5)

ANSWER

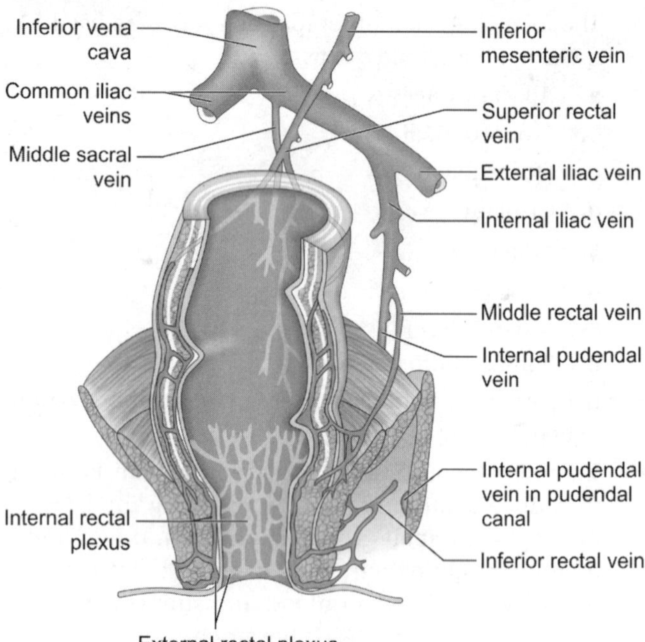

A. Venous drainage of rectum and anal canal is the mirror image of arterial supply to these orgAnswer Venous blood will enter into valveless perirectal venous plexus from valveless intramural venous plexus; from there, the blood will be carried by the superior rectal vein. This vein runs along the side of the superior rectal artery, crosses the pelvic brim from below upward, and ultimately becomes the inferior mesenteric vein, which on its way takes the blood from the sigmoid colon, descending colon, and splenic flexure and ultimately drains into the splenic vein.

B. Some amount of venous blood from perirectal as well as intramural venous plexus runs bilaterally in the middle rectal veins, which ultimately drain into the internal iliac vein.

C. Some amount of venous blood from rectal plexuses runs through the anal wall and drain into inferior rectal veins, which in turn drain via internal pudendal veins into the internal iliac vein.

D. Venous drainage of anal canal:

   a. Above the pectinate line, venous blood will drain into the venous plexus, which in turn drains into the superior rectal vein and ultimately drains into the systemic vein through the inferior mesenteric vein (portal circulation).

   b. Below the pectinate line, venous blood drains into the internal pudendal vein, which ultimately drains into the portal venous system through the internal iliac vein (systemic circulation).

   In between the two systems of drainage, there is presence of portosystemic anastomoses to maintain connection between two systems.

   As a result, if there is much more pressure in one system as compared to the other, it will lead to formation of anorectal varices.

Q34. Nerve supply of tongue.

MGR/APR2016/MDI (5)

ANSWER

Tongue is supplied by motor and sensory nerves. Motor supply of the tongue is as follows:

A. All the intrinsic muscles and all the extrinsic muscles except the palatoglossus are supplied by the 12th cranial nerve, i.e., hypoglossal nerve. This nerve originates from the hypoglossal nucleus in the medulla, exits from the skull through the hypoglossal canal, and passes straight up to a point below the angle of mandible; from here, it runs forward, crosses the external carotid artery first and then the loop of lingual artery, and follows the hyoglossus muscle to reach the tongue through the oropharyngeal triangle.

B. The vagus nerve supplies the palatoglossus muscle via branches of pharyngeal plexus placed on the middle pharyngeal constrictor muscle.

Tongue is supplied by the following sensory nerves:

A. Glossopharyngeal nerve carries:

   a. General sensory information from the posterior one-third part of the tongue

   b. Special sensory information from the vallate papillae

   This 9th cranial nerve leaves the skull through the jugular foramen, descends along the lateral surface of the stylopharyngeus muscle, and reaches the oropharynx; from here it enters the tongue inferiorly to hyoglossus and styloglossus muscles.

B. General sensation from the anterior two-thirds of tongue is carried by the mandibular branch of the trigeminal nerve. It will pass through the oropharyngeal triangle to reach the floor of the oral cavity.

C. Special sensation from the anterior two-thirds of tongue is carried by the facial nerve. The fibers carrying the sensation leave the tongue as a part of lingual nerve and join with the chorda tympani branch of the facial nerve at the infratemporal fossa.

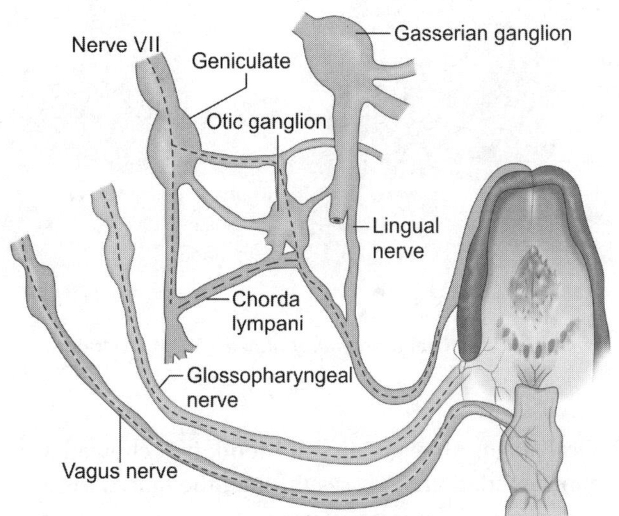

Q35. Mechanism of deglutition.

MGR/APR2016/MDI (5)

ANSWER

Swallowing process has been subdivided according to the position of the bolus into oral, pharyngeal, and esophageal phases. The oral phase is again subdivided into two—preparatory phase and propulsive phase:

A. Oral preparatory phase: After taking the liquid, this liquid bolus is placed on the floor of the mouth or on the anterior upper surface of the tongue against the hard palate and surrounded by upper dental arch. Posteriorly, the oral cavity is closed by the close contact between the soft palate and tongue, thus preventing the liquid from leaking into the oropharynx. But in the elderly, due to laxity of the muscles, there may be some leaking of the fluid.

B. Oral propulsive phase: In this phase:

a. Tip of the tongue rises to touch the alveolar edges of the hard palate behind the upper teeth and at the same the posterior part of the tongue drops to open the back of oral cavity.

b. Upper surface of the tongue will be moved upward and gradually expanded to increase the contact between the upper surface of the tongue and the hard palate from anterior to posterior and thus squeezing the liquid bolus posteriorly toward the pharynx along the palate.

c. During this stage, the pharyngeal stage usually begins.

In case of eating solid food, the following are the stages of deglutition:

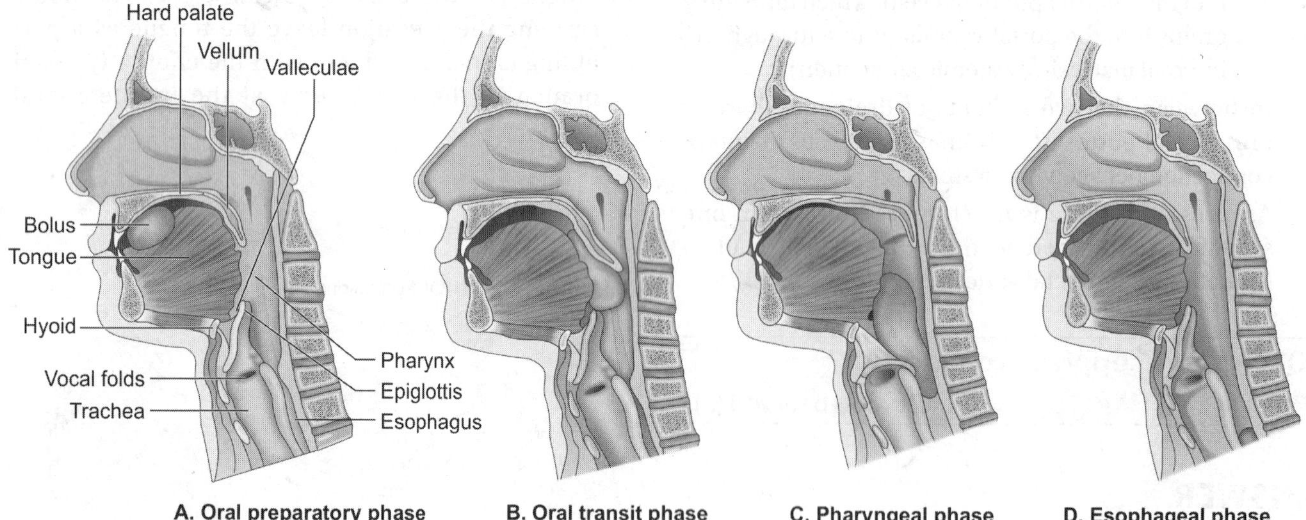

A. Oral stage: After taking solid food, it is chewed and moistened; then it passes through the fauces to form bolus in the oropharynx prior to commencement of the swallowing phase. So the oral stage is subdivided into the following stages:

a. Stage I transport: After ingestion, the food is carried to the postcanine region by the tongue where it will be rotated laterally to place the food onto the occlusal surface of the lower teeth for processing the food.

b. Food processing: By the process of continuous chewing, mastication, and salivation for moistening the food particles, softened food bolus is formed and it will be ready for swallowing. The cyclic movement of the jaw is associated with tightly coordinated movement of muscles of the tongue, cheek, soft palate, and hyoid bone. As compared to the process of drinking, the tongue and soft palate move cyclically associated with coordinated movement of the jaw, which will permit open communication between the pharynx and oral cavity.

c. Stage II transport: It is similar to the oral propulsive phase of drinking the liquid bolus, but this phase here is driven by the tongue as it does not require gravity. Transported food will be accumulated on the pharyngeal surface of tongue as well as valleculae. If any food remains in the oral cavity, the continued process of chewing will push the bolus into the oropharynx to increase the size of the bolus already present in the oropharynx.

Duration of aggregation of bolus in the oropharynx is fraction of seconds to 10 seconds in case of a normal individual.

B. Pharyngeal stage: Pharyngeal process of swallowing consists of two biological features:

a. Propelling the food bolus through pharynx and upper esophageal sphincter to the upper esophagus. In this process, the soft palate will be elevated to come in contact with the posterior and lateral walls of the pharynx and close the nasopharynx to prevent regurgitation of food into it, so that bolus enters into the pharynx. The base of the tongue will be retracted to push the food bolus against the pharyngeal wall. Now pharyngeal constrictor muscles contract from above downward to squeeze the bolus downward and at the same time the vertical length of the pharynx will be shortened to reduce the pharyngeal volume.

b. Insulation of larynx and trachea from pharynx to prevent the food from entering the airway by different protecting mechanisms:

1. Closing or apposition of vocal folds will seal the glottis.
2. Tilting forward of arytenoid to contact epiglottic base before opening of the upper esophageal sphincter
3. Pulling of hyoid bone and larynx upward and forward by the contraction of suprahyoid as well as thyrohyoid muscles. This displacement of larynx will tuck it under the base of the tongue.
4. Epiglottis will be tilted backward to seal the vestibule of larynx.

c. Upper esophageal sphincter (UES) consists of three parts:

1. Inferior pharyngeal constrictor muscles
2. Cricopharyngeus muscle
3. Proximal part of esophagus

It is closed in resting position by tonic contraction of muscles. The following factors are responsible for opening the UES:

1. Cricopharyngeus muscle relaxes prior to arrival of food bolus.
2. Suprahyoid and thyrohyoid muscles contract to pull the hyolaryngeal complex forward and open the sphincter.
3. Pressure of the food bolus will distend the UES and thus open it.

C. Esophageal stage: It is a tubular structure; its lower sphincter is also closed during rest to prevent regurgitation of food from the stomach cavity. Cervical esophagus is formed by striated muscles, but the thoracic part (lower two-thirds) is composed of smooth muscles. As the food bolus passes the UES and enters the esophagus, peristaltic waves carry the bolus down toward the stomach cavity. The peristaltic wave consists of two parts:

1. Initial wave is wave of relaxation for accommodation of bolus into the cavity.
2. Wave of contraction will propel the bolus and gravity will assist this downward propelling of food toward the stomach cavity.

Coordination between breathing, swallowing, and eating: The above three processes are strongly coordinated. In a normal individual, swallowing is dominant to respiration. Breathing stops transiently during swallowing because:

1. Elevation of soft palate and tilting of epiglottis physically close the airway.
2. Suppression of respiration in the brain stem

Swallowing of liquid bolus will start during the expiratory phase of breathing there is pause in respiration for 0.5–1.5 seconds during swallowing; lastly, respiration resumes with expiration. This is one of the mechanisms to prevent food inhalation remaining in the pharyngeal cavity during swallowing. But if the drinking is continued, respiration will resume with inspiration.

Q36. What are the causes of constipation in adults? How will you manage a patient with chronic constipation?

BF/MAY2011/MDIII (20)

ANSWER

Constipation can be defined as bowel symptoms, such as difficult to pass stool or infrequent passage of stool, hardness of stool or feeling of incomplete evacuation, straining during defecation, and digital evacuation of stool.

Classification of Constipation

A. Based on duration of constipation:

a. Acute constipation: It may occur due to adynamic ileus or intra-abdominal disease or trauma.

b. Chronic constipation: According to the American College of Physicians, if the symptoms persist for >3 months and fewer than three bowel movements per week

B. Based on etiology:

a. Functional constipation—it may be due to slow colonic transit or disturbances in the pelvic floor

b. Secondary constipation medical conditions

C. Based on pathophysiology:

a. Slow colonic transit—it may be due to myopathy, i.e., due to colonic smooth muscle dysfunction or neuropathy, i.e., dysfunction of neural innervation. It occurs mainly in females.

b. Dyssynergic defecation: It is due to pelvic floor, abdominal, and anorectal muscles dyssynergia leading to difficulty or inability to expel stool from the rectum.

c. Constipation is predominant in IBS.

Causes of Constipation

A. Surgical conditions:
- **a.** Colorectal tumor
- **b.** External compression from extrinsic tumor
- **c.** Anal fissure
- **d.** Anal stricture
- **e.** Diverticulosis
- **f.** Postsurgical abnormalities

B. Metabolic diseases:
- **a.** Diabetes mellitus
- **b.** Hyper- and hypothyroidism
- **c.** Hyper- and hypomagnesemia
- **d.** Chronic kidney disease
- **e.** Heavy metal poisoning
- **f.** Multiple endocrine neoplasia
- **g.** Porphyria

C. Gastrointestinal conditions:
- **a.** Anal fistula
- **b.** Anal abscess
- **c.** Proctalgia fugax
- **d.** Levator ani syndrome
- **e.** Irritable colon syndrome

D. Musculoskeletal disorders:
- **a.** Scleroderma
- **b.** Dermatomyositis
- **c.** Amyloidosis

E. Dietary:
- **a.** Eating disorders
- **b.** Low-fiber diet
- **c.** Dehydration

F. Depression

G. Medication: Calcium channel blocker, use of senna, cascara

H. Other causes:
- **a.** Cardiac disease
- **b.** Degenerative joint disease
- **c.** Pregnancy

Approach to a Patient with Constipation

A. From history:
- **a.** Absence of urge to pass the stool
- **b.** History of ineffective straining
- **c.** History of ≤3 bowel movements per week
- **d.** Sense of incomplete evacuation
- **e.** Digital evacuation of stool
- **f.** Proper history of consistency, size, shape of the stool, and its mapping with the Bristol stool form chart
- **g.** History of requirement of change of posture to pass the stool effectively and completely
- **h.** History of bleeding per rectum and fecal incontinence
- **i.** History of burning pain during passage of stool
- **j.** History of abdominal bloating or discomfort
- **k.** Repeated enema to evacuate stool
- **l.** Requirement of vaginal or perianal pressure to evacuate stool

B. On physical examination:
- **a.** Pallor indicates presence of neoplasm, internal piles, and anal fissure
- **b.** Abdominal examination:
  1. Presence of abdominal distension
  2. Presence of mass
- **c.** Anorectal inspection:
  1. Anal fissure
  2. Hemorrhoids
  3. Skin tag
  4. Excoriation of skin
- **d.** Perianal sensation may be lost in case of neuropathy. Absence of lower extremity neurologic features suggests damage of puborectalis muscles from pelvic injury or excessive stretching from longstanding chronic constipation.
- **e.** Anocutaneous reflex: By gentle stroking of all four quadrants of perianal skin by cotton bud, if reflex is lost, it suggests neuropathy:
  1. Digital rectal examination demonstrates posterior motion of puborectalis muscles during straining; it denotes proper coordination of pelvic muscles.
  2. Rectal or anal stricture
  3. Rectal or anal cancer
  4. Impaction of stool in the rectum
  5. Dyssynergia: The patient is asked to bear down and at the same time digit will perceive following things:
     - Anterior motion of puborectalis muscles
     - Paradoxical contraction of puborectalis muscles
     - Perineal descent of <1.5 cm during stimulated evacuation of the bowel
     - Relaxation of external anal sphincter

C. Investigations:

a. CBC: Low hemoglobin, raised ESR

b. Thyroid profile: Hypo- or hyperthyroidism

c. Blood sugar: Diabetes mellitus

d. Blood urea and creatinine, potassium, and sodium: Chronic renal insufficiency

e. Serum magnesium: Hypo- or hypermagnesemia

f. Stool test for occult blood

g. Plain X-ray of abdomen can detect dilated loops and abundant gas in colon

h. Barium enema: It can identify:

1. Megacolon
2. Redundant sigmoid colon
3. Megarectum
4. Presence of intraluminal masses
5. Extrinsic compression on the wall of colon

i. Measurement of colonic transit: Transit of radio-marker is easy, safe, repeatable, inexpensive, and reliable. There are several validated methods of test:

1. After ingestion of radio-opaque markers, an abdominal film has to be taken after 5 days of ingestion. In absence of any laxative or enema, it will indicate passage of 80% of markers out of the colon but it will not provide any information regarding the transit profile of stomach and small intestine.
2. After ingestion of 24 radio-opaque markers on 3 consecutive days followed by intake of an abdominal film on the 4th day. The presence of number of markers in the abdominal radiograph can estimate the colonic transit in hours.
3. Estimation of bowel gas in between the lower border of sacroiliac joints and the level of ischial spines can detect the presence of disorder of rectal evacuation.
4. Radioscintigraphy: After administration of delayed released capsule containing radio-particles, delayed colonic transit as well as gastric and small bowel transit can be estimated over 24–48 hours, because it is very important in 20% cases of delayed colonic transit where it may be due to generalized gastrointestinal motility. Its disadvantages are:
   - Expensive
   - Requirement of specific markers prepared in the laboratory of nuclear medicine.

j. Anorectal and pelvic floor tests: Pelvic floor dyssynergia is suggested by the following:

- Feeling of persistent fullness in the rectum
- Failure to evacuate rectum
- Rectal pain during defecation
- Digital evacuation of rectum
- Application of pressure on the posterior wall of vagina during defecation
- During straining support of perineum
- Excessive straining during defecation

Measurement of perineal descent can be measured by placing the patient in the left decubitus position and watching the perineum:

- Inadequate descent of <1.5 cm—pelvic flood dysfunction
- Ballooning of the perineum of >4 cm during straining in relation to bony landmark suggests excessive perineal descent.
- Balloon expulsion test: In this test, a balloon-tipped catheter is placed in the rectum and balloon is filled up with 50 mL of water. A normal patient can expel during sitting in the toilet or in left lateral decubitus position. Expulsion can be facilitated by adding extra weight to facilitate expulsion. Normal expulsion occurs with or without aid within 1 minute.

Anorectal manometry: It can detect:

- High resting pressure of >80 mm Hg
- Squeeze anal sphincter tone suggests spasm of anal sphincter.
- Absence of rectoanal inhibitory reflex suggests Hirschsprung's disease.

Defecography: During expulsion of barium or MR defecogram, the lateral view of dynamic barium enema reveals:

- Changes in rectoanal angle
- Anatomic defect in rectum like prolapse of internal mucosa
- Enterocele
- Rectocele

- Whole thickness intussusception along with complete outlet obstruction due to:
  - Extremely large rectocele which fills during attempts of defecation
  - Funnel-shaped plugging at the anal canal

Electromyography: It is helpful in case of fecal incontinence or obstructed defecation.
Spinal evoked response during electrical stimulation of rectum and/or stimulation of external anal sphincter contraction by stimulating lumbosacral cord can identify neuropathies of the lumbosacral region.

Treatment of Constipation

A. Bowel training: Following meal and walking, colonic activity is greatest. Hence, the patient is advised to defecate in the morning as during this time bowel is most active and also 30 minutes after meals. This is known as gastrocolic reflex.

B. High-fiber diet: Daily recommended fiber intake is 20–30 g/day. Fiber-containing diet is to take fruit, nuts, bran, vegetables, psyllium, and methylcellulose. Increased fiber intake will lead to bulky stool and improve colonic transit.

C. Fluid intake: Patient is advised to take 2–3 L of water per day and decrease the intake of alcohol or tea or coffee.

D. Exercise: Prolonged bed rest decreases the colonic motility whereas regular exercise increases colonic transit.

E. Bulk laxative: Psyllium, calcium polycarbophil, and methylcellulose absorb water and thus increase bulk and colonic motility. These may produce bloating.

F. Osmotic laxatives:

a. Polyethylene glycol in low dose, i.e., 17 g/day, is well tolerated in the elderly, but in high dose, i.e., 34 g/day, it produces abdominal bloating and flatulence.

b. Lactulose:

1. Increases the bulk
2. Increases the colonic motility
3. Decreases the severity of symptoms of constipation

c. Sorbitol:

1. It is less expensive than lactulose.
2. It is better tolerated in elderly.

d. Magnesium-containing laxatives, such as milk of magnesia or magnesium citrate, are less indicated in elderly and in case of chronic renal failure, there is a chance of developing hypermagnesemia.

G. Stimulant laxatives, such as bisacodyl and Dulcolax, increase transport of electrolytes across the intestinal mucosa, thus increasing colonic transit. Side effects of long-term use are hyponatremia, hypokalemia, and abdominal cramps leading to dehydration.

H. Stool softeners, enema: Glycerin suppositories will soften the stool not affecting the colonic motility. It is given in patients with dyssynergia.

I. Prokinetics: The 5-HT4 receptor agonist prucalopride stimulates the gastrointestinal tract. Adverse effects are nausea, diarrhea, and headache, but there are no cardiac side effects. Other 5-HT4 agonists, such as naronapride and velusetrag, will improve the motility of the gastrointestinal tract.

J. Secretagogues:

a. Linaclotide, a selective guanylate cyclase agonist, has secretory and visceral antinociceptive properties:

1. It will bind to GC receptors present on the surface of epithelial cells of the intestine leading to increased cyclic guanosine monophosphate (GMP) levels intracellularly.
2. It will activate cystic fibrosis transmembrane conductance regulator, which leads to stimulation of water, electrolytes, and bicarbonate increasing the stool bulk and colonic transit.

b. Plecanatide: It is also guanylate cyclase-C agonist.

c. Lubiprostone: It is a selective chloride channel activator present in the apical membrane of the GI tract that increases chloride secretion in the intestinal lumen, which leads to increase in the fluid content in the intestinal lumen and increases colonic transit.

d. Colchicine: It may be effective in chronic constipation in the dose of 0.6 mg thrice daily.

K. Mu-opioid receptor antagonist: It will activate central and peripheral μ-opioid receptor, thus regulating intestinal motility and secretion.

L. Treatment of colonic inertia: Combination of diet, exercise, and medication in the form of osmotic and stimulant laxatives is the first line of therapy. If this inertia is refractory to medication, ileorectostomy is the treatment of choice.

M. Treatment of pelvic floor dysfunction:

a. Surgical therapy of rectocele or rectal prolapse can resolute constipation. But prior to this surgery, one has to place a pressure on the posterior of vagina during the process of defecation to see any improvement in defecation.

b. Biofeedback training: It is useful in the paradoxical contraction of puborectalis muscle. In this process, the patient has to receive auditory and visual feedback regarding the function of pelvic floor and anal canal muscles. According to those cues, the patient will relax the pelvic floor muscles during straining during defecation and thus facilitate the rectal evacuation.

Q37. How will you approach and manage a case of chronic diarrhea in a HIV-infected patient?

DNB 2020

ANSWER

Etiology

A. *Infective causes*:
- a. *Bacteria*: *Salmonella, Shigella, Campylobacter, Mycobacterium avium* complex, and *Clostridium difficile*.
- b. *Viral*: Cytomegalovirus and human herpes virus-8
- c. *Protozoa*: *Isospora belli, Cryptosporidium, Microsporidia, Cyclospora cayetanensis, Giardia*

B. *Non-infectious causes*:
- a. HIV enteropathy
- b. ART
- c. Other causes—celiac diseases
- d. Neoplasm-Kaposi's sarcoma, lymphoma.

Clinical Features

As per chronic diarrhea described in question number 4.

Laboratory Investigations

As per chronic diarrhea described in question number 4.

A. *Stool microscopy for*:
- a. Cryptosporidium
- b. Microsporidia
- c. Giardia

B. Stool culture foe above bacteria, *Campylobacter*.

C. Stool antigen for *Clostridium difficile, Entamoeba histolytica*

D. Polymerase chain reaction for virus

E. Acid fast staining for cryptosporidium and isospora

F. Fecal leukocytes to differentiate inflammatory from non-inflammatory diarrhea.

G. *Blood test*:
- a. CD4 count—if it is <200/cc, it denotes chance of opportunistic infection.
- b. Viral load for HIV
- c. Blood culture for *Salmonella, Mycobacterium avium* complex
- d. Serum sodium, potassium, chloride, magnesium,

H. *Endoscopy with biopsy*:
- a. In case of HIV villus atrophy
- b. In cytomegalovirus infection basophilic cytoplasmic inclusions
- c. In case of *Mycobacterium avium* complex – presence of granuloma.

Treatment

A. ART treatment should be continued along with the adjustment of doses according to CD4 count.

B. Symptomatic treatment according to status of dehydration, nutrition in case of high protein loss, vitamin administration in case of clinical suspicion of vitamin loss.

C. Pathogen-specific therapy:
- a. In case of *Cryptosporidium* infection—nitazoxanide
- b. In *Isospora* infection—trimethoprim + cotrimoxazole
- c. In microsporidia infection—albendazole
- d. *Clostridium difficile* infection—vancomycin
- e. In case of cytomegalovirus infection—ganciclovir or valacyclovir
- f. In case *Giardia* infection—metronidazole or tinidazole
- g. In *Mycobacterium avium* complex infection—rifampin + clarithromycin ± ethambutol

Q38. Classify malabsorption syndrome and add a note on tropical sprue.

DR YSR UNI OF HEALTH SC, VIJAYAWADA, ANDHRA, 2022 (10)

Tropical sprue.

BABA FARID UNI OF HEALTH SC, 2019 (10)

MANIPUR UNIVERSITY, 2024 (10)

NTR UNI OF HEALTH SC, VIJAYAWADA, 2019 (10)

ANSWER

Classification of chronic diarrhea described in question number 4.

Tropical Sprue

Etiology

It is a type of malabsorption syndrome seen in the tropical areas characterized by malabsorption, deficiencies of multiple nutritional elements, vitamin B12 and folic acid.

Following factors enhance the pathogens to damage the intestinal mucosa due to following agents:

- **A.** Toxins: Rancid fats may be the possible cause.
- **B.** Deficiency: Vitamin or mineral deficiency
- **C.** Infections: The factors favor the long latent period between the exposure to infection and onset of the disease.

Epidemiology

This disease occurs in the tropical countries in between the latitudes 30° North and 30° South, mainly prevalent in Puerto Rico, Haiti and Cuba in the Western Hemisphere and India and Pakistan in the Eastern Hemisphere.

Histopathology

In the early cases there is no change in the intestinal mucosa. But as the disease progresses,

- **A.** The villi become atrophied,
- **B.** Increased depth of the villus crypt.
- **C.** Nuclear immaturity
- **D.** Enlarged epithelial cells
- **E.** Intraepithelial infiltration of lymphocytes
- **F.** Increased number of inflammatory cells in the lamina propria
- **G.** Accumulation of lipids underneath of the basement membrane.

Clinical Features

- **A.** Residence of tropical or subtropical area
- **B.** Watery and foul-smelling chronic diarrhea
- **C.** Cramping abdominal pain, loud borborygmi, anorexia
- **D.** Steatorrhea
- **E.** Features of anemia secondary to vitamin B12 and folic acid due to malabsorption.
- **F.** Physical examination demonstrates: Cheilitis, glossitis, pedal edema, and distended abdomen
- **G.** Propensity to frequent infection, poor wound healing, irritability.

Laboratory Evaluation

- **A.** Complete blood picture demonstrates: Megaloblastic anemia, low vitamin B12, and folic acid
- **B.** Elevated homocysteine level
- **C.** Elevated methyl malonic acid level is found in case of vitamin B12 deficiency.
- **D.** Low electrolyte level such as sodium, potassium, chloride levels
- **E.** D-xylose test—positive test indicates serum level <20 mg/dL and urine level is <4 g
- **F.** Upper gastrointestinal endoscopy demonstrates absent mucosal folds and presence of scalloped folds and mucosal fissures in the duodenum.
- **G.** Histology—as per above description
- **H.** Barium studies demonstrate increased caliber and thickening of the mucosal folds.

Treatment

It includes

- **A.** Antibiotics mainly 250 mg of tetracycline 4 times daily for 6 months
- **B.** Administration of vitamin B12 and folic acids
- **C.** Electrolyte replacement.
- **D.** Following patient needs hospital-based treatment:
  - **a.** Severe dehydration
  - **b.** Electrolyte imbalance
- **c.** Symptomatic anemia
- **E.** Inadequate treatment may lead to relapse if this disease.

Complications

- **A.** Worsening of anemia
- **B.** Severe vitamin deficiencies
- **C.** Severe malnutrition

All the above will lead to tissue destruction resulting organ dysfunction.

Q39. Zollinger–Ellison syndrome.

RAJIV GANDHI UNI OF HEALTH SC, KARNATAKA, 2020 (10)

ANSWER

Definition

This disease is characterized by features of severe peptic ulcer disease along with diarrhea due to excessive secretion of gastrin from the neuroendocrine tumor in the intestine.

Etiology

These tumor cells arise from the pluripotent cells. Gastrinoma is either sporadic or associated with multiple endocrine metaplasia 1 or MEN-1. It is autosomal dominant disorder due to germline mutation of *MEN-1* gene.

Epidemiology

About 80% to 90% tumor arises from "Gastrinoma triangle" which is bounded by superiorly by confluence of cystic duct and common bile duct, 2nd and 3rd portion of duodenum inferiorly, medially by the neck of the pancreas. This tumor also rarely arises from:

- **a.** Stomach
- **b.** Liver
- **c.** Common bile duct
- **d.** Ovary
- **e.** Heart
- **f.** Associated with small cell cancer of lung.

It is commonly diagnosed in the subject between 20 to 50 years with higher incidence in men.

Pathophysiology

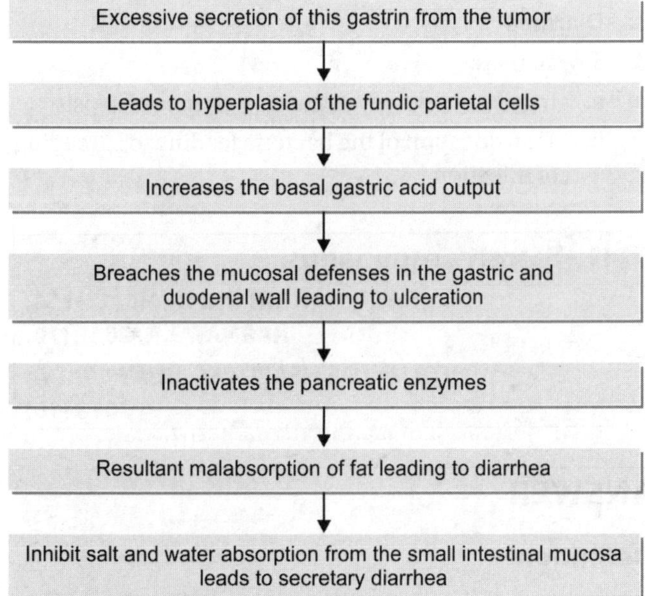

Clinical Features

- **A.** Abdominal pain
- **B.** Chronic diarrhea
- **C.** Gastroesophageal reflux
- **D.** Dyspepsia
- **E.** Gastrointestinal bleeding
- **F.** If the duodenal and gastric ulcer is multiple, gastrinoma should be considered.

Diagnosis

- **A.** Serum gastrin is >1,000 pg/mL
- **B.** Secretin stimulation test demonstrates paradoxical rise in the serum gastrin to >200 pg/mL.
- **C.** Gastric pH is <2.
- **D.** *Imaging*:
  - **a.** Somatostatin receptor scintigraphy with SPECT/CT, gallium somatostatin analog PET-CT localizes the tumor, and it can evaluate the extent of the metastatic spread.
  - **b.** Presence of peri-pancreatic lymph nodes or metastasis in the liver suggests malignancy.
- **E.** All these patients have to be evaluated for serum calcium level and ultrasonography to detect MEN-1.
- **F.** Endoscopic ultrasound can detect the small duodenal tumor.

Treatment

- **A.** High dose of proton pump inhibitors to suppress the acid secretion.
- **B.** Surgery is the only treatment in case of gastrinoma. But prior to operation any evidence of metastasis should be sought.
- **C.** In case of MEN-1, surgery can be done if the tumor size is >2 cm.
- **D.** Surgery in MEN-1 should not be recommended in case of:
  - **a.** Multiplicity of the tumors
  - **b.** Extra-pancreatic location
  - **c.** Co-existent metastatic disease
- **E.** Chemotherapy: It should be done in case of widespread metastasis 1st line of treatment is streptozotocin and 5-fluorouracil or doxorubicin. But these treatments have considerable toxicity.
- **F.** Hormonal therapy by octreotide or lanreotide, human somatostatin analog can reduce the gastric acid secretion also has anti-tumor activity.

Complications

- **A.** During surgery, the surgeon fails to locate the tumor
- **B.** Metastases
- **C.** Severe diarrhea leading to gross loss of weight

D. Failure to remove the whole cancer tissue
E. Intestinal bleeding
F. Perforation from the gastric or duodenal ulcers.

Q40. Probiotics.

MAHARASHTRA UNI OF HEALTH SC. VIJAYAWADA, 2022 (5)

ANSWER

Definition

Probiotics are the living organisms which when administered in sufficient amount can restore the gut microbial flora.

Name of the Probiotics

A. Lactic acid bacteria:
   a. *Lactobacillus* species
   b. *Streptococcus thermophilus*
B. *Bifidobacterium*:
   a. *Bifidobacterium bifidum*
   b. *Bifidobacterium longum*
   c. *Bifidobacterium infantis*
C. Yeast: *Saccharomyces boulardii*
D. Non-lactic acid bacteria:
   a. *Escherichia coli* Nissle 1917
   b. *Bacillus subtilis*
E. Emerging probiotics:
   a. *Faecalibacterium prausnitzii*
   b. *Akkermansia muciniphila*

Uses of Probiotic

A. Gastrointestinal causes:
   a. In case of irritable bowel syndrome diarrheal type: *Bifidobacterium infantis, Lactobacillus*
   b. Inflammatory bowel disease: *Lactobacillus plantarum, Bifidobacterium infantis*
   c. Antibiotic associated diarrhea: *Saccharomyces boulardii, Lactobacillus*
   d. Constipation associated irritable bowel syndrome: *Bifidobacterium lactis*
B. Blood sugar level should be modulated in case of diabetes.
C. In case of dyslipidemia cholesterol level can be improved by administration of *Lactobacillus reuteri.*
D. Dental carries can be prevented by *Lactobacillus reuteri.*
E. Dermatological diseases can be prevented by *Lactobacillus rhamnosus* GG. The diseases are:
   a. Eczema
   b. Atopic dermatitis
F. Modulation of immune function by *Bifidobacterium bifidum.*
G. Mental health like depression and anxiety can be prevented by *Lactobacillus* species and *Bifidobacterium longum.*

Advantages of probiotic

A. It will improve the immune function, inflammation and reduce the oxidative stress.
B. It will reduce the incidence of infection by improving the immune function.
C. It will improve the mental health like anxiety and depression.
D. It will restore the gut microflora.
E. It will reduce the hypertension by improving the dyslipidemia.

Disadvantages of Probiotic

A. Abdominal flatulence and bloating
B. Diarrhea
C. Severe risks:
   a. In case of severely ill patient, chance of sepsis
   b. Translocation of the bacteria leading to spreading of infection.

Q41. Barrett's esophagus.

RAJIV GANDHI UNI OF HEALTH SC, KARNATAKA, 2019 (10)

NTR UNI OF HEALTH SC, VIJAYAWADA, 2018 (10)

ANSWER

Definition

It is a pre-malignant condition characterized by salmon colored mucosa extending up to 1 cm above the lower gastroesophageal junction which on biopsy demonstrates evidences of intestinal metaplasia.

Etiopathogenesis

Long standing acid and bile regurgitation into the esophageal cavity through the lax gastroesophageal junction. Lining mucosa of the stomach is columnar which can withstand the acidic environment whereas, esophageal mucosa is squamous which will be irritated by the environment, so the mucosa becomes inflamed upon exposure to gastric acid. But persistent acidic exposure leads to metaplastic reaction in the esophageal mucosa with eventual development of intestinal metaplastic cells characterized by presence of goblet cells. Bile acids upregulate intestinal differentiation factor *CDX2, MUC2* genes, goblet cells specific genes within the intestinal columnar and esophageal cancer cell lines.

Additional risk factors enhancing the development of Barrett esophagus are:

A. Non-Hispanic white race
B. Male sex
C. More than 50 years old
D. Central obesity
E. History of smoking
F. History of Barrett esophagus or esophageal adenocarcinoma in the 1st degree relatives
G. Sometimes genetic mutation may be responsible

Histopathology

Following specific histopathological pictures are demonstrated:

A. Indefinite dysplasia where types of neoplasia cannot be described but mucosal atypia may be seen overlapping low grade dysplasia.
B. Low grade intestinal dysplasia where there is evidence of goblet cells with elongation and enlargement of nuclei, lymphocytosis with increased nuclear cytoplasmic ratio and nuclear stratification that involves basal half of cellular cytoplasm.
C. High grade intestinal dysplasia characterized by increased number of lymphocytes, greater degree of nuclear enlargement, stratification nucleus involving full thickness of the mucosa and nuclear polymorphism like loss of nuclear polarity, irregular shape of the nucleus.
D. Intramucosal carcinoma characterized by invasion of the lamina propria by the individual cancer cells having no cryptic connection, sheets of malignant cells, irregular glands in the lamina propria or muscularis mucosae.

Clinical Features

A. Retrosternal burning after taking food
B. Acid regurgitation
C. Sore throat
D. Chronic cough
E. Hoarseness of voice
F. Weight loos

Evaluation

According to American College of Gastroenterology Screening of Barrett esophagus should be recommended who have additional risk factors like age more than 50 years, male genotype, past or present history of smoking, white race, presence of Barrett esophagus or esophageal adenocarcinoma in the 1st degree relatives. Biopsy should be taken from 2 cm from each quadrant, at an interval of 2 cm for the shorter segments of Barrett mucosa.

A. Upper gastrointestinal endoscopy with four quadrant biopsy
B. High-definition white light and chemoendoscopy using topical acetic acid will increase the sensitivity and specificity in the identification of high-grade dysplasia or adenocarcinoma

Diagnosis of Barrett esophagus demonstrates at least 1 cm long salmon pink colored columnar metaplasia proximal to the gastroesophageal junction confirmed by biopsy showing intestinal metaplasia with goblet cells.

Surveillance Protocol of the Barrett Esophagus

A. If no dysplasia, endoscopy is recommended every 3 years in Barrett segment is >3 cm long and every 5 years if the Barrett segment is at least 3 cm in length.
B. Indefinite dysplasia: Endoscopy should be recommended after 6 months on PPI therapy twice daily and it should be taken 30 to 45 minutes prior to meal. If there is no change as compared to prior findings in endoscopy, then it should be recommended annually,
C. Low-grade dysplasia: If endoscopic eradiation therapy is not done or cannot be performed due to some reasons, in that case then endoscopy should be performed after 6 months, then again after 6 months and then annually if the endoscopic feature is unchanged.
D. High-grade dysplasia: If the mucosa is flat, in that case endoscopic eradication therapy should be performed to eliminate the whole area of intestinal metaplasia.

Following are the methods of eradication technique:

A. Radiofrequency ablation: The complications are—
  a. Chest pain for 14 days
  b. Aspiration

c. Bleeding
d. Surface laceration
e. Deeper perforation
f. Strictures

B. Cryotherapy with liquid nitrogen cryospray
C. Hybrid argon plasma coagulation—it should be used for small islands of metaplasia.
D. Endoscopic mucosal resection.

Q42. The role of microbiota in maintaining gastrointestinal health.

AIIMS (BHU), 2024 (10)

Gut microbiota.

MANIPUR UNIVERSITY, 2018 (10)

SRI GURU RAM DAS UNI OF HEALTH SC, AMRITSAR, 2022 (10)

ANSWER

Composition of Microbiota

A. Dominant group of bacteria:
   a. Firmicutes:
      1. *Clostridium, Enterococcus, Lactobacillus Ruminococcus*
      2. Functions:
         - These bacteria produce short chain fatty acids,
         - These bacteria modulate immunity.
   b. Bacteroides:
      1. *Prevotella*, Bacteroides
      2. *Functions*:
         - They will break down complex carbohydrates.
         - They will tolerate immunity.

B. Minor group of bacteria:
   a. Actinobacteria:
      1. *Bifidobacterium*
      2. Functions:
         - They will colonize the gastrointestinal tract in children.
         - They will ferment carbohydrate in the intestine.
   b. Proteobacteria:
      1. *Salmonella* species
      2. *Escherichia* species
      3. Function:
         - These bacteria will overgrow in in the intestine during disease and inflammation, but normally low during good health.
   c. Verrucomicrobia:
      1. *Akkermansia*
      2. *Muciniphila*
      3. *Function*:
         - These bacteria degrade mucus.
         - These bacteria link to the metabolic health.

C. Non-bacterial groups of microbiota:
   a. Bacteriophage that infects bacteria.
   b. Fungi - *Candida* species
   c. Protozoa that will colonize the gut but not producing the disease.
   d. Archaea: Methane producing organism—*Methanobrevibacter*.

Following factors have influence on the composition of the bacteria:

A. Age: There is different composition of microbiota in children and adults.
B. Use of different antibiotics
C. Dietary composition like carbohydrate, protein, or fat.
D. Mode of birth like whether the child born vaginally or by cesarean section
E. Geographical location
F. Lifestyle of an individual

Role of microbiota in the gastrointestinal health:

A. Metabolism of nutrition: They will nourish the colonic epithelial cells by breaking down the dietary fibers into short chain fatty acids like acetate, butyrate, propionate resulting energy metabolism. They will also help in synthesizing the vitamin B and K.
B. Function as barrier: They will tighten the transcellular junction and increase the mucus production thereby form a barrier against the invasion by the bacteria.
C. Immunomodulation: They will promote the production of harmless pathogen at the same time retard the production of defensive barrier against the pathogenic bacteria.
D. They will maintain the balance between the pro-inflammatory and anti-inflammatory response.

E. These bacteria competitively block the intake of nutrients and attachment sites the pathogenic bacteria in the colonic mucosa.

F. They will produce antimicrobial substances that will either kill of inhibit the pathogenic bacteria.

G. These bacteria develop tolerance to the pathogenic bacteria to the antigen produced by these bacteria and thereby prevent allergic reaction against them.

H. They will produce gut associated lymphoid tissue.

Dysbiosis of the gut microbiota that is associated with the diseases:

A. Inflammatory bowel disease:
   - a. Reduction of Firmicutes
   - b. Increased production of Proteobacteria
   - c. Diversity of the bacteria will be reduced.

   The result is the triggering of the immune cells production in the colonic mucosa leading to development of chronic inflammation.

B. Irritable bowel syndrome:
   - a. This is the result of gross imbalance between the gut-brain axis and imbalance of the microbiota.
   - b. Overgrowth of gas producing bacteria along with decreased production of *Bifidobacterium* and *Lactobacillus*.

   The result is visceral hypersensitivity, increased permeability to the mucosa and alteration of the gut motility.

C. Colonic cancer:
   - a. It is result of chronic activity of the pathogenic bacteria.
   - b. Increased production of proinflammatory bacteria
   - c. Decreased production of Firmicutes leading to decreased production of short chain fatty acids.
   - d. The metabolites of the bacteria promote chronic inflammatory response leading to alteration of DNA resulting tumorigenesis.

D. Celiac disease:
   - a. This disease is the result of altered sensitivity to the gluten producing foods.
   - b. Decreased production of Firmicutes and increased production of Proteobacteria.
   - c. Alteration in the microbiota results altered permeability in the colonic mucosa along with signaling of the immune mechanism.

E. Small intestinal bacterial overgrowth:
   - a. There is abnormally high count of the pathogenic bacteria.
   - b. Result is increased sensation of bloating, malabsorption of food, diarrhea.

F. Pseudomembranous enterocolitis:
   - a. The causative organism is overproduction of *Clostridium difficile* leading to increased production of toxin.
   - b. Result is bloody diarrhea.

Q43. Protein losing enteropathy.

MAHATMA UNIVERSITY, 2021 (10)

ANSWER

Definition

It can be defined as a clinical condition where there is massive loss of protein from the gastrointestinal tract leading development of edema, ascites, or bilateral pleural effusion.

Etiology

A. Primary erosive or ulcerative gastrointestinal diseases:
   - a. Inflammatory bowel disease
   - b. Stomach ulcers
   - c. Duodenal ulcers
   - d. Gastrointestinal malignancies

B. Non-erosive or non-ulcerative gastrointestinal disorders:
   - a. Tropical sprue
   - b. Celiac disease
   - c. Ménétrier disease
   - d. Amyloidosis
   - e. Eosinophilic gastroenteritis
   - f. Bacterial overgrowth
   - g. Whipple's disease
   - h. Collagenous colitis
   - i. AIDS
   - j. Mixed connective tissue disorders

C. Increased intestinal pressure or lymphatic obstruction:
   - a. Primary intestinal lymphangiectasia
   - b. Constrictive pericarditis
   - c. Right sided heart failure
   - d. Cirrhosis with portal hypertension

Pathophysiology

Here the protein loss through the intestine exceeds the amount of synthesis of protein in the body leading to development of hypoproteinemia due to increased mucosal permeability in the intestine and poor reabsorption.

In case of increased lymphatic pressure and lymphatic obstruction there is leak of lymph into the gastrointestinal tract and decreased reabsorption of the chylomicron leading to loss of fat-soluble vitamins.

Clinical Features

- **A.** Peripheral edema
- **B.** Ascites
- **C.** Bilateral pleural effusion
- **D.** Gastrointestinal features:
  - **a.** Abdominal bloating
  - **b.** Abdominal pain
  - **c.** Diarrhea
- **E.** Immunocompromised state leading to frequent infection.
- **F.** Features of heart failure.

Evaluation

- **A.** Intestinal clearance of alfa-1 antitrypsin—most commonly performed test. It can be calculated by 24 hours collection of stool and measuring of this anti-trypsin in the stool.

  Alfa-1 antitrypsin clearance = [(Stool volume) × (Stool content of alfa-1 antitrypsin)] / serum alfa-1 antitrypsin. Normal clearance is 13 mL/day. Clearance if greater than 27 mL/day—it indicates increased protein loss. As the clearance will be increased in case of diarrhea, so in case diarrhea the loss greater than 56 mL/day should be used as diagnostic.
- **B.** 51 chromium labeled albumin clearance is the gold standard.
- **C.** Technetium 99 labeled albumin can be done in case of negative intestinal clearance of alfa-1 antitrypsin test.
- **D.** Investigations to detect the etiology.

Treatment

- **A.** Treatment of the underlying pathology.
- **B.** Diet rich in medium chain triglyceride and low in fat should be considered.
- **C.** Replacement of micronutrients, fat soluble vitamins, electrolytes
- **D.** Diuretics in case of heart failure.
- **E.** Pericardiotomy in case of constrictive pericarditis.
- **F.** Immunosuppressive medication in case of inflammatory bowel disease, SLE or rheumatoid arthritis.
- **G.** Octreotide can be considered in case of primary lymphangiectasia.
- **H.** Budesonide and corticosteroids can be administered in case of eosinophilic gastroenteritis.

Q44. Outline the schematic representation of enterohepatic circulation of bile acids and highlight the pathophysiological defect causing disease with examples.

AIIMS, BHU, 2024 (10)

ANSWER

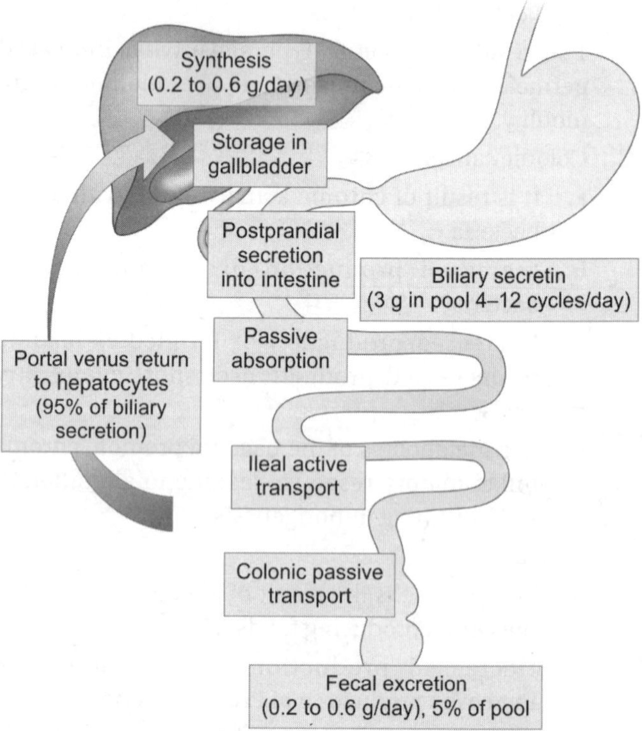

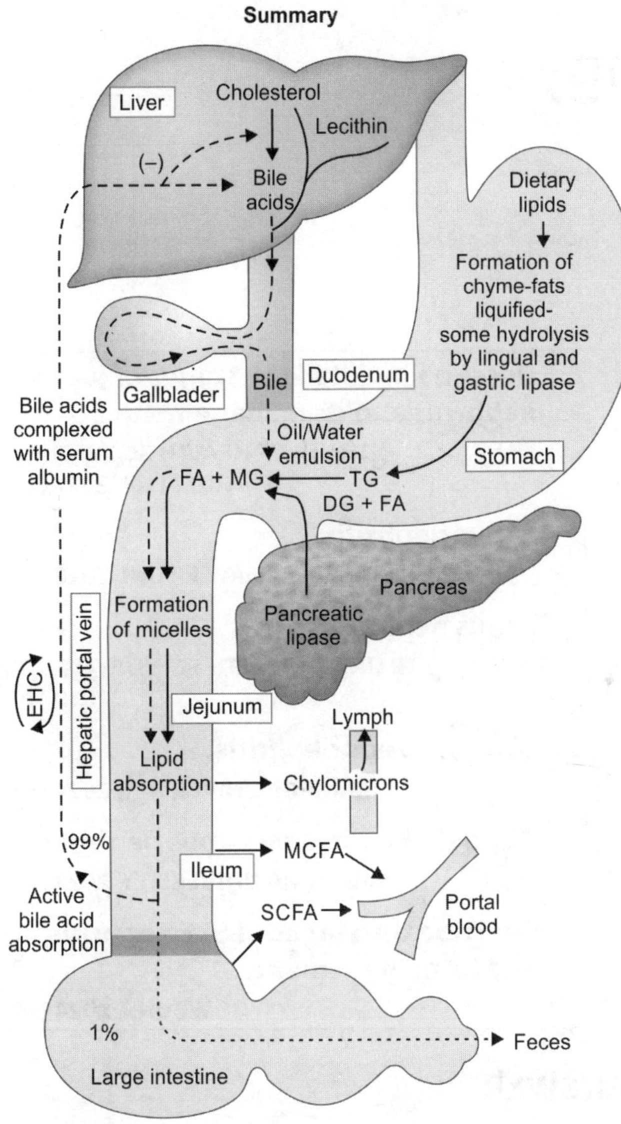

Pathophysiology of Bile Acid Absorption

A. In the terminal ileum as a result of Crohn's disease or tuberculosis or resection of the terminal ileum bile salt will be reabsorbed in little amount due to malabsorption of bile salts results:

- **a.** Bile acid diarrhea
- **b.** Reduced bile acid pool leading to decreased absorption of fat resulting steatorrhea
- **c.** Reduced absorption of fat-soluble vitamins.

B. Due to mutation of apical sodium dependent bile acid transporter gene, there is primary bile acid resorption leading to

- **a.** Poor bile acid pool
- **b.** Poor absorption of fat
- **c.** Chronic diarrhea

C. As a result of excessive deconjugation and dihydroxylation of bile salts there is excessive growth of bacteria in the small bowel resulting malabsorption of fat leading to steatorrhea

D. Due to impaired flow of bile through the biliary canaliculi in primary biliary cholangitis or primary sclerosing cholangitis extrahepatic or intrahepatic bile duct obstruction leads to development the features of cholestatic jaundice and damage of hepatocytes.

E. Due to stimulation of colonic secretion and motility, excess amount of bile acids will enter into the colon leading to bile acid diarrhea.

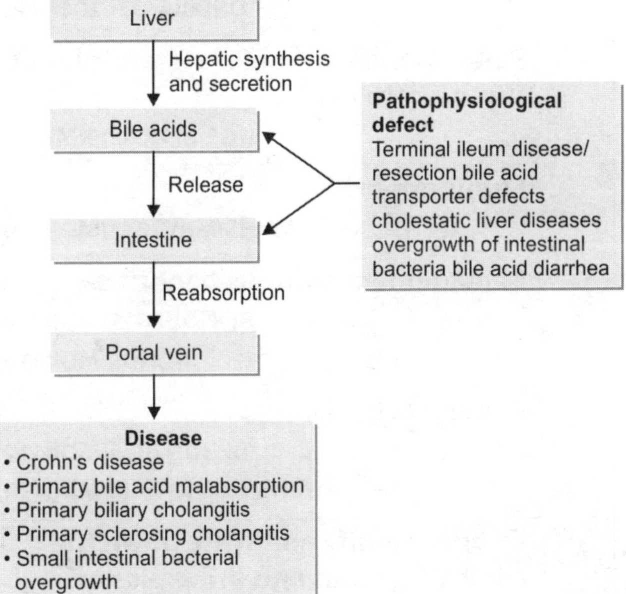

Section 5 Nephrology

Q1. Classify lupus nephritis and outline its management.

DNBI/JUN2010 (10)

Classify lupus nephritis. Describe its clinical features, diagnosis, and management.

DNBIII/DEC2012 (10)

World Health Organization classification of lupus nephritis and its management.

DNBIIIA/DEC2014 (10)

Renal manifestation of systemic lupus erythematosus.

MGR/MAR2009/MDI (5)

Lupus nephritis.

MUHS/MAY2013/MDII (10)

Management of lupus nephritis.

BF/NOV2013/MDII (10)
RGHUS/MDII (10)

Lupus nephritis.

BF/JUN2016/MDII (10)
KUHS/NOV2013(S)/MDII (10)

Define, classify and write down the clinical features and principles of therapy in Lupus nephritis.

DNB (DEC 2021) (10)

Lupus nephritis.

MGR UNI, TAMIL NADU, 2022 (5), 2022 (10)

Describe in detail the stages of lupus nephritis and its management.

DR YSR UNI HEALTH SC. VIJAYAWADA, ANDHRA, 2022 (10)

Describe in detail the stages of lupus nephritis and its management.

NTR UNI OF HEALTH SC, ANDHRA, 2022 (10), 2021 (10)

Lupus nephritis.

TEERTHANKER MAHAVEER UNI, 2020 (10)

Lupus nephritis.

NTR UNI OF HEALTH SC, VIJAYAWADA, 2019 (10)

Discuss Lupus nephritis.

MANIPUR UNIVERSITY, 2024 (10)

Write short notes on Lupus nephritis.

MAHATMA UNIVERSITY, 2022 (10)

Describe the stages of SLE nephritis and its management.

WBUHS, 2024 (10)

ANSWER

Introduction

Lupus nephritis (LN) occurs in 50% patients with systemic lupus erythematosus (SLE), but in case of male LN is more aggressive and more likely develop renal failure as compared to women. It occurs at younger age in the early course of SLE within 6–36 months, sometimes it may be the initial diagnosis.

Risk Factors

A. Younger age
B. Male sex
C. Non-European ancestry: Black and Hispanic people are more likely progress to renal failure.

International Society of Nephrology and the Renal Pathology Society classification of lupus nephritis:

Class	Histology	Modification in histology	Clinical findings
1	• *Light microscopy*: Normal • *Immunofluorescence microscopy*: Mesangial immune complexes	Nil	None relevant to kidney
2	Mesangial cell proliferation/ mesangial immune complexes	Nil	Hematuria, low-grade proteinuria, renal insufficiency, nephrotic syndrome is not expected
3	Mesangial and subendothelial immune complexes/ <50% glomeruli showed segmental endocapillary proliferation	Lesions can be active, chronic or both	Proteinuria, hematuria seen in most of the patients, renal insufficiency, and nephrotic syndrome is not unusual
4	Mesangial and subendothelial immune complexes/≥50% glomeruli showed segmental or global endocapillary proliferation	Lesions can be active, chronic or both	Proteinuria, hematuria seen in most of the patients, renal insufficiency, and nephrotic syndrome is not unusual
5	Numerous subepithelial immune complexes involving >50% glomerular capillaries	Nil	Possible hematuria, proteinuria often in nephrotic range, usually no renal insufficiency
6	Glomerulosclerosis involving >90% glomeruli	Nil	Renal insufficiency, often hematuria and proteinuria may be present

Classification of lupus nephritis according to World Health Organization (WHO):

Class 1	• Minimal mesangial glomerulonephritis • Histologically normal in light microscopy but on electron microscopy there is mesangial deposits
Class 2	• Mesangial proliferative lupus nephritis • Typically responds completely to corticosteroids
Class 3	• Focal proliferative nephritis • Often responds successfully to treatment with high dose of corticosteroids
Class 4	• Diffuse proliferative nephritis • Mainly treated with corticosteroids and immunosuppressive drugs
Class 5	• Membranous nephritis • Characterized by extreme edema and protein loss
Class 6	Glomerulosclerosis

Classifications with Clinical Features

Classification category	Features
Class I: Minimal mesangial	• Normal/minimal proteinuria, normal creatinine • Earliest and mildest form of glomerular involvement
Class II: Mesangial proliferative	• Microscopic hematuria +/– proteinuria • Hypertension uncommon and nephrotic syndrome plus renal insufficiency rarely seen
Class III: Focal lupus nephritis	Hematuria, proteinuria, hypertension, reduced eGFR +/– nephrotic syndrome
Class IV: Diffuse lupus nephritis	• Most common and severe form of lupus nephritis • Clinical features as for class III but also significantly low C3 and high dsDNA, especially in active disease
Class V: Membranous nephropathy	• Nephrotic syndrome, microscopic hematuria, hypertension, normal/high creatinine • Can present without other clinical or serological manifestations of SLE but electron microscopy features will distinguish it from the idiopathic form
Class VI: Advanced sclerosing lupus	Slowly progressive renal failure with proteinuria and bland urine sediment

(dsDNA: double-stranded deoxyribonucleic acid; SLE: systemic lupus erythematosus)

Treatment of Lupus Nephritis

In case of class 1 and 2 lupus nephritis:

A. No clinical manifestation
B. Normal renal function
C. Excellent prognosis
D. Patient usually does not require any treatment.

In case of class 3, 4, and 5 lupus nephritis:

A. Induction of remission:
   a. Pulse methyl prednisolone 0.25–1 g/day infusion in 100 mL of normal saline for 3 days followed by oral prednisolone 0.5–1 mg/kg of body weight (maximum 80 mg/day) to be tapered over several months to 7.5 mg/day over months as maintenance therapy.
   b. If no response or in case of severe disease:
      1. If glomerular filtration rate (GFR) >60 mL/min, intravenous 750 mg cyclophosphamide in 250 mL of normal saline to be given in 30 minutes monthly for 6 months. White blood cell count has to be screened 10–14 days after this injection.
      2. If GFR <60 mL/min dose of cyclophosphamide has to be reduced to 500 mg.
      3. Oral cyclophosphamide 1.5–2 mg/kg/day (maximum 150 mg/day) for 4–8 weeks followed by maintenance therapy
      4. Mycophenolate mofetil 0.5–1 g twice daily can be given as an alternative to cyclophosphamide.

Response

A. If the patient shows worsening of the disease, alternate induction therapy should be chosen:
   a. Multitarget therapy—mycophenolate mofetil
   b. Rituximab
   c. Intravenous immunoglobulin
   d. Leflunomide

   But the patient is refractory to this alternate treatment regimen, in that case:
   a. Diagnosis has to be confirmed.
   b. Determination of histologic activity whether active or chronic
   c. Evaluation of any complicating factor, such as thrombotic microangiopathy
B. If the patient is stable, partial or in complete remission to first induction regimen then maintenance therapy by:
   a. Mycophenolate mofetil 1–2 g/day or
   b. Azathioprine 1.5–2 mg/kg/day
   c. Steroid to its minimal dose of 7.5 mg/day
C. After 12–18 months of maintenance dose:
   a. If the patient is in partial remission:
      1. Diagnosis has to be confirmed.
      2. Determination of histologic activity whether active or chronic
      3. Evaluation of any complicating factor, such as thrombotic microangiopathy
   b. If the patient is in complete remission, the maintenance therapy has to be continued to further 18 months then the drugs should be tapered with close monitoring of lupus flare.

Response Criteria

A. According to (Kidney Disease: Improving Global Outcomes) KDIGO:
   a. Complete response: Urine protein creatinine ratio decline to ≤5 g/g and return of serum creatinine to baseline
   b. Partial response: >50% reduction of urine protein creatinine ratio; in case of nephrotic range of proteinuria reduction should be <3,000 mg/g, stabilization or improvement of serum creatinine but not to normal range.
   c. No response: Failure to achieve partial or complete remission
B. According to American College of Rheumatology (ACR):
   a. Complete response: Urine protein creatinine ratio <0.2 g/g, normal serum creatinine, or 25% improvement in estimated glomerular filtration rate (eGFR) if it is abnormal during lupus nephritis flare, inactive urinary sediment.
   b. Partial response: Urine protein creatinine ratio 0.2–2 g/g, eGFR is in the baseline or 25% improvement if it is abnormal in LN flare, inactive urinary sediment.
   c. No response: No worsening or no change of proteinuria, eGFR declines by ≥25%, active urinary sediment.

Q2. Describe the nerve supply of urinary bladder and discuss the physiologic basis of automatic bladder.

DNBIV/DEC2011 (10)

Urinary bladder control.

MGR/OCT2012/MDI (5)

Physiology of micturition.
MGR/OCT2011/MDI (5) MGR/MAR2010/MDI (5)

Micturition reflex.
MGR/SEP2010/MDI (5)

Nerve supply to urinary bladder.
MGR/MAR2010/MDI (5) MGR/SEP2008/MDI (5)
MGR/MAR2007/MDI (5)

Nervous control of urinary bladder.
MGR/MAR2009/MDI (5) RGUHS/SEP2008/MDII (6)

Describe nerve supply of urinary bladder. Discuss neurogenic bladder.
MUHS/MAY2009/MDI (25)

ANSWER

Neuroanatomy of the Bladder

Normally, bladder control is under control of three sets of peripheral nerves:

A. Sympathetic nerve
B. Parasympathetic nerve
C. Somatic nerve

All the above sets of nerve are under control of two areas of brain, i.e., (1) brainstem and (2) cortex. A number of brain structures send their signal to periaqueductal gray matter which in turn send the signals to pontine micturition center (PMC) which ultimately exert the stimulatory or inhibitory effect on the bladder function. So higher cortical center will determine the voiding place is acceptable or not—in case of unacceptable place, it will exert inhibitory effect on PMC or in case socially acceptable place for voiding, it will exert the opposite effect on PMC. Cortical micturition center is composed of the following areas:

A. Superior frontal gyrus
B. Anterior aspect of cingulate gyrus

Subcortical micturition center is composed of the following areas:

A. Red nucleus
B. Hypothalamus
C. Limbic system
D. Substantia nigra

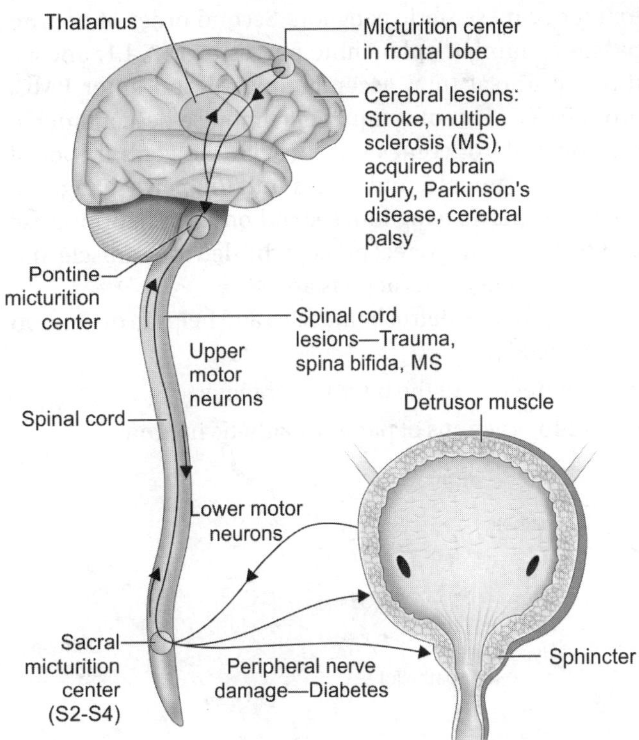

Brainstem

In the brainstem, pons contains a micturition center (PMC) which receives the afferent signals from the urinary bladder and sends it to cortical center through periaqueductal gray matter. Cortical center sends efferent inhibitory or excitatory signal to PMC through periaqueductal gray matter. This cortical control over PMC develops when infant starts social training during growth and development and gets toilet training.

If the bladder becomes full, the stretch receptors present in the detrusor muscles of the bladder and send their afferent signal to PMC which send this impulse to cortical cognitive centers. In case of acceptable place for micturition, cortex sends excitatory signals to PMC through periaqueductal gray matter to contract the bladder muscles to void.

Spinal Cord

In the vertebral column, spinal canal contains the spinal cord floating in cerebrospinal fluid—it acts as a conduit between lumbosacral segment and pons.

Sympathetic afferent neuron from the detrusor muscles of bladder and internal sphincter muscles passes through the hypogastric nerve through hypogastric plexus to inferior mesenteric ganglion. Second order of neuron passes as lumbar splanchnic nerves to T12, L1, and L2 through dorsal root, ascends upward and enter PMC. From PMC, efferent sympathetic impulse descend down the spinal cord, comes out through the ventral root of the same segments, and enters into the pelvic ganglion. From this pelvic ganglion, second order of neuron arise and relay into the β_2 receptors in the detrusor muscle and external sphincter. Its actions are:

A. Inhibition of detrusor muscles and helps in distention of bladder
B. Contraction of the internal sphincter
C. Inhibits actions of parasympathetic neuron

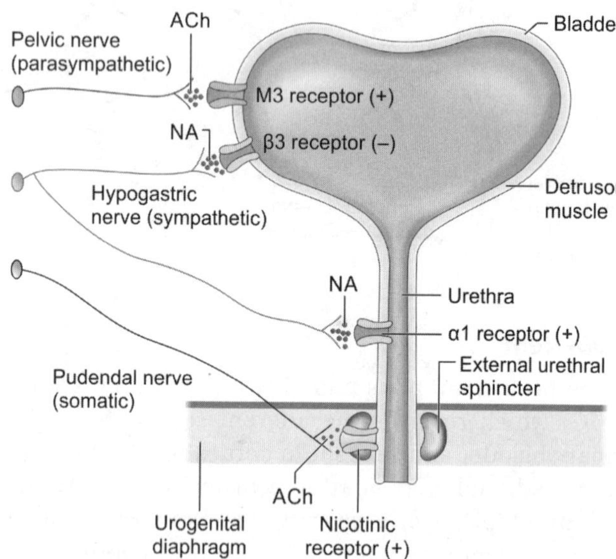

Parasympathetic afferent neuron from the stretch receptors on the detrusor muscles in the bladder and internal sphincter muscle passes through the pelvic nerve and enters through dorsal horn of S2, S3, and S4 and relays in the dorsal root ganglia. From there, second order of neuron ascends upward along the spinal cord and relays into the PMC. From PMC, efferent excitatory signal descend along the spinal cord into intermediolateral cell in the S2, S3, and S4 segments. From there, second order of neuron releases through the anterior horn of spinal cord and relays into the pelvic ganglion cells, here it releases acetylcholine which stimulates third order of parasympathetic neuron and relays on the parasympathetic receptors on the detrusor muscles and internal sphincter and releases acetylcholine which serves following functions:

A. Contraction of detrusor muscles of bladder and helps in complete evacuation of the bladder.
B. Relaxation of internal sphincter muscle

Somatic nerve: Afferent neuron from external sphincter containing α fibers reach the sacral segments and activate the Onuf nucleus of S2, S3, and S3 segments of spinal cord. This α fiber also travels to periaqueductal gray matter and from there to PMC. PMC will send signals to reticulospinal tract, from there efferent signals reach the Onuf nucleus. Efferent pudendal nerve originates from the Onuf nucleus situated in the ventral gray horn of S2, S3, and S4 and reaches to external sphincter muscle and levator ani muscles in the pelvic diaphragm. This pathway is responsible for guarding reflex. This reflex is very essential during coughing, sneezing reflexes, and during weight bearing, because during this act increased abdominal pressure will exert pressure of the bladder wall which helps in voiding in any place. But this guarding reflex helps in contraction of external sphincter muscle and pelvic floor muscles thus inhibit voiding. During voluntary micturition this reflex will be abolished.

Physiology of Micturition

Normal human being voids 6–8 times per day. There are two phases in voiding:

A. Filling phase: In this phase urine starts accumulating in the urinary bladder which acts as a low-pressure receptacle, so the pressure in the bladder will be low. At the same time, pressure of the internal sphincter will be high so that pressure within the bladder remains low as compared to pressure in the sphincter. This filling phase occurs due to the following mechanisms:
   a. Sympathetic nerve-induced relaxation of detrusor muscle
   b. Sympathetic nerve-induced constriction of internal sphincter
   c. Sympathetic nerve-induced inhibition of parasympathetic nerve as the latter helps in contraction of detrusor muscles

Continence reflex and stress incontinence: As the bladder fills, pudendal nerve will also be stimulated. As a result of stimulation, there is contraction of external sphincter muscle. So combined pressure of internal and external sphincter muscle will be more than that in urinary bladder. This will prevent dribbling of urine. This is continence reflex. Reverse in the pressure of urinary bladder as well as internal and external sphincter results urinary incontinence.

Stress incontinence: Again, in response to stress, coughing, laughing or sneezing increased abdominal pressure will transmit the pressure in the urinary bladder, if this pressure is more than combined pressure of both the sphincters, incontinence occurs—it is stress incontinence.

B. Phase of emptying: This phase may be of two types:

a. Involuntary reflex: It occurs in infant when there is no cortical control over the bladder. So, when the bladder fills, the stretch receptor will be stimulated, signal will enter the sacral segments, which in turn send signal to contract the detrusor muscles and the voidance occurs. But as the infant grows and starts habit formation to go to proper place for voiding, cortex will also starts taking control over the bladder.

b. Voluntary reflex: When the bladder fills up, stretch receptor will be stimulated, this stimulation will pass along the both afferent sympathetic and parasympathetic and somatic afferent pathways. The result will be:

1. Inhibition of sympathetic pathway, thus there will be relaxation of internal sphincter.
2. Stimulation of parasympathetic pathway resulting contraction of bladder and relaxation of internal sphincter.
3. Stimulation of pudendal nerve produces relaxation of external sphincter and relaxation of pelvic floor muscles.

Resultant effect is emptying of bladder.

Delay in voiding: Instinct of any individual is his or her ability to control micturition on command despite full bladder because this will be governed by cortex that makes the final decision whether to or not to void. When the sympathetic and parasympathetic afferent signals enter the PMC, it will send these signals to cognitive cortex through the periaqueductal gray matter, efferent signals from cortex will depend upon the proper place of voiding. If the place is not suitable cortex will send inhibitory signal to PMC and it will stimulate sympathetic pathway and inhibit parasympathetic pathway, but if the pace is suitable for voiding, reverse stimulation occurs, i.e., sympathetic inhibition and parasympathetic stimulation, patient will perceive the sensation of fullness of the bladder and will void in proper place.

Neurogenic Bladder

Neurogenic bladder has been classified based on site of neurologic lesion as it can help in taking decision regarding pharmacological or surgical therapies:

A. In stroke or brain tumor, where the lesion is above the pontine micturition center there is uninhibited bladder, which is characterized by the following:

a. Reduced awareness of bladder fullness

b. Due to subcortical and cortical structural damage reduced inhibition of pontine micturition center the bladder capacity will be low.

c. Normal opposition of detrusor muscle and internal/external sphincteric tone will be maintained thus there will be no increase in pressure in the bladder which may be responsible of urinary tract damage in future.

B. Any lesion between pontine micturition center and sacral spinal cord due to multiple sclerosis or trauma or syringomyelia produces upper motor neuron bladder, which is characterized by:

a. Detrusor-sphincter dyssynergia, as a result high pressure will be developed in the bladder (up to 80–90 cmH_2O) leading to vesicoureteral reflux due to compromise of the oblique course of the ureter through hypertrophic detrusor muscle.

b. If the lesion is above T10 level, i.e., above the sympathetic innervation of bladder, the bladder will be spastic.

c. Bladder capacity will be reduced due to highly tonus detrusor muscle.

d. But, if the pressure of detrusor muscle exceeds that of sphincter tone incontinence develops.

C. Any sacral lesion that damage the detrusor nucleus but spares pudendal nucleus will produce mixed type A bladder which is characterized by the following:

a. Detrusor muscle will be flaccid (detrusor reflexia) due to damage of detrusor nucleus but external urinary sphincter is hypertonic due to intact pudendal nucleus. So bladder will be large but with low pressure, as a result there is urinary retention.

b. Due to low tone of detrusor, there is no evidence of vesicoureteral reflux.

c. No incontinence

D. Any sacral lesion that spare the detrusor nucleus but damages pudendal nucleus will produce mixed type B bladder which is characterized by the following:

a. External sphincter will be flaccid due to damage of pudendal nucleus but urinary bladder will be spastic due to disinhibited detrusor muscle.

b. Bladder capacity will be low and vesicle pressure will not be elevated because urine will be expelled due to little resistance to outflow.

E. Due to sacral nerve root injury lower motor neuron bladder develops. This is characterized by the following:

a. Bladder capacity is high due to decreased detrusor muscle tone.

b. Innervation of internal sphincter is intact.
c. There is overflow incontinence which may occasionally produce urinary tract infection.

Q3. Define cardiorenal syndrome. Discuss its etiopathology and management.
DNBIII/JUN2012 (10)

Cardiorenal syndrome.
DNBIIA/DEC2014 (10) MLB/MAY2009/MDII (20)

Discuss cardiorenal syndrome—types and management.
BF/MAY2011/MDIV (20)

Biomarkers in cardiorenal syndrome.
DNB (DEC 2022) (4)

Cardiorenal syndrome.
DNB (DEC 2020) (5)

Pathophysiology, diagnostic evaluation and management OF CARDIO-RENAL syndrome.
DNB (DEC2018) (10)

Cardiorenal syndrome.
SCB MED COL, (10)
MGR UNI, TAMIL NADU, 2021 (10)
MAHARASHTRA UNI OF HEALTH SC, VIJAYAWADA, 2020 (10)

Pathophysiology of cardiorenal syndrome and its implications in the management.
WBUHS, 2025 (10)

ANSWER

Definition

Cardiorenal syndrome can be defined as direct and indirect effect of heart or kidney which is dysfunctional and can initiate as well as perpetuate the combined disorder already present in these organs through a complex neurohormonal feedback process. There are five types of cardiorenal syndrome.

Pathophysiology

Type 1 Cardiorenal Syndrome

Acute heart failure (hypertensive pulmonary edema with preserved left ventricular systolic function), acute severe decompensated heart failure, predominantly right ventricular failure, and cardiogenic shock produces acute renal injury in the following mechanisms:

A. Decreased cardiac output leading to acute hypoperfusion on kidney thus reduced oxygen delivery in kidney which will be responsible for renal necrosis.
B. Administration of angiotensin-converting enzyme (ACE) inhibitors, diuretics, contrast media other exogenous factors produce toxic vasoconstriction leading to necrosis or apoptosis
C. Increased secretion of brain natriuretic peptide (BNP) from heart producing natriuresis
D. Humoral signaling from the heart will produce immune-mediated damage through cytokine release due to activation of monocytes and endothelial cells, apoptosis of cardiac and kidney tissue through caspase activation.

On the other hand, cardiac injury can occur due to acute kidney injury, due to hypoperfusion, reduced delivery of oxygen, acute renal necrosis, and resistance to atrial natriuretic peptide (ANP) or BNP through the following mechanisms:

a. Activation of sympathetic nervous system produces vasoconstriction leading to hypertension, cardiac ischemia, and myocardial infarction.
b. Activation of renin–angiotensin–aldosterone system (RAAS) leading to sodium and water retention as well as vasoconstriction produce cardiac afterload and cardiac ischemia.

Here the biomarkers involved are the following:

A. Classical biomarker is creatinine
B. Neutrophil gelatinase-associated lipocalin—it is one of the earliest marker of acute kidney injury (AKI) in both adult and child.
C. Cystatin-C—it is the better predictor of GFR as its level is not affected by age, sex, race, or muscle mass.
D. N-acetyl-β-(D) glucosaminidase and interleukin-18 (IL-18)—are associated with development of AKI.
E. B type natriuretic peptide, which is elevated in acute heart failure.
F. High sensitivity troponin (hs-cTnT): It indicates injury to the myocardium.
G. ST2 (Suppression of tumorigenicity 2): It indicates cardiac remodeling.
H. Kidney injury molecule 1 (KIM 1): It indicates extent of renal tubular damage.

Type 2 Cardiorenal Syndrome

Chronic heart disease produces chronic progressive renal injury through the following mechanisms:

A. Low cardiac output along with different morbid factors, such as obesity, hypertension, and diabetes mellitus

B. Chronic hypoperfusion, embolism, increased vascular resistance, and increased venous pressure.

Chronic hypoperfusion of kidney along with different types of macrovascular disease produce apoptosis and necrosis of the renal tissue leading to sclerosis as well as fibrosis of kidney. This will affect heart through the following mechanisms:

A. Anemia due to low erythropoietin production

B. Increased activation of RAAS leading to vasoconstriction and sodium and water retention which produce hypertension and left ventricular hypertrophy

C. Abnormalities of calcium and phosphate metabolism

Here the biomarkers involved are:

A. Brain natriuretic peptide/NT-ProBNP—in indicates elevated chronic heart failure.

B. Gelectin-3—it is marker of progressive myocardial fibrosis and progression of heart failure.

C. Serum creatinine and effective glomerular filtration rate—it indicates progression of chronic kidney disease.

D. Urinary albumin-creatinine ratio—it is a marker of renal damage and microalbuminuria.

E. Fibroblastic growth factor 23—it indicates progression of chronic kidney disease as well as cardiovascular incidence.

F. Biomarkers of endothelial dysfunction like asymmetric dimethyl arginine which is linked to vascular dysfunction.

Type 3 CRS (Acute Renocardiac Syndrome)

Here sudden and primary worsening of renal function, such as acute kidney injury, ischemia, or glomerulonephritis produce acute cardiac injury, such as heart failure, arrhythmias, and ischemia through the following mechanisms:

A. Acute fluid overload leads to development of pulmonary edema.

B. Hyperkalemia produces cardiac arrhythmias leading to death.

C. In uremia, uremic toxins will affect through myocardial depressant factors, myocardial contractility, and pericarditis.

D. Metabolic acidosis produces:

- **a.** Pulmonary vasoconstriction leading to right-sided heart failure
- **b.** Negative ionotropic effect through electrolyte imbalances leading to arrhythmias

E. Renal ischemia releases cytokines and other inflammatory mediators which leads to acute cardiac dysfunction.

In this syndrome following biomarkers released are:

- **a.** Cardiac troponins for myocardial injury
- **b.** Biomarker for myocyte stress BNP responsible for acute decompensated cardiac failure. This will not prevent progression of this disease.
- **c.** Marker of myocyte metabolism, inflammation, and oxidative stress. Oxidative stress produces myocyte apoptosis followed by necrosis, arrhythmias, and endothelial dysfunction.
- **d.** Inflammatory mediators, such as IL-1, IL-6, tumor necrosis factor-α produce myocyte apoptosis.
- **e.** NGAL, Cystatin C and KIM-1—these indicates early acute renal injury.
- **f.** Urinary fatty acid fatty acid binding protein—it will indicate renal tubular injury.
- **g.** Raised NT-pro BNP—indicates cardiac overload as a result of renal failure.
- **h.** Troponins—it indicates acute myocardial injury.
- **i.** Oxidative stress biomarkers like myeloperoxidase malondialdehyde may be raised.

Type 4 CRS (Chronic Renocardiac Syndrome)

Here chronic kidney disease (CKD) affects cardiac remodeling, left ventricular hypertrophy with dysfunction, reduced coronary perfusion with increased ischemic risk, and coronary and tissue calcification. There are five stages of CKD:

A. In stage 1–2 CKD: It affects heart in association with morbid factors, such as obesity, hypertension, smoking, dyslipidemia, diabetes, and chronic inflammation in genetically susceptible patient

B. In stage 3–4 CKD, the effect of anemia, uremic toxins, malnutrition, sodium, and water overload along with mediators of chronic inflammation affects heart.

C. In stage 5 CKD: Above all factors derived in stage 3–4 CKD affect cardiac function. Chronic inflammation releases cytokines responsible for:

- **a.** Endothelial dysfunction
- **b.** Bone remodeling
- **c.** Increased catabolism in muscles
- **d.** Decreased appetite
- **e.** Release of acute phase reactants in the liver
- **f.** Increased production of adipocytokine in fat cells
- **g.** Increased insulin resistance

The biomarkers involved are the following:

- **a.** Cardiac troponin
- **b.** Natriuretic peptides
- **c.** Acute phase reactant
- **d.** C-reactive protein
- **e.** Asymmetric dimethylarginine
- **f.** Serum amyloid protein A
- **g.** Ischemia-modified albumin
- **h.** Troponins: It indicates chronic myocardial stress in patients with chronic kidney disease.
- **i.** Parathormone, vitamin D and phosphate—these are raised in cardiovascular disease in a case of CKD.
- **j.** Osteoprotegerin—it indicates vascular calcification.

Type 5 Cardiorenal Syndrome (Secondary Cardiorenal Syndrome)

Cardiorenal syndrome due to systemic diseases resulting both cardiac and renal dysfunctions. Examples are diabetes, sepsis, amyloidosis, cirrhosis and vasculitis.

The biomarkers are the following:

- **A.** IL-6, TNF-α, CRP, procalcitonin—indicates chronic inflammation.
- **B.** BNP/NT-Pro BNP—indicates inflammation related heart failure.
- **C.** Troponins—indicate involvement of myocardium in case of systemic diseases.
- **D.** NGAL, Cystatin C and KIM-1—these indicates early acute renal injury.

Management of Cardiorenal Syndrome

Diuretic use is used as surrogate marker for poor prognosis in patients with congestive cardiac failure (CCF). The probable mechanisms are the following:

- **A.** Inadequate dose of diuretics
- **B.** Excessive intake of sodium
- **C.** Decreased excretion of diuretics in urine
- **D.** Gut mucosal edema of intestine leading to decreased absorption
- **E.** Increased resorption of sodium from distal convoluted tubule which is not blocked by diuretics
- **F.** Concomitant use of nonsteroidal anti-inflammatory drugs (NSAIDs) diminish synthesis of vasodilators and natriuretic prostaglandins.

So, there are several management options:

A. Loop diuretics:

- **a.** Dose of the loop diuretics should be doubled rather increasing the frequency.
- **b.** Restriction of sodium to achieve net fluid loss
- **c.** Intravenous diuretic therapy should be given to avoid the bioavailability in case of:
  1. Reduced gastrointestinal blood flow
  2. Reduced peristalsis of the intestine
  3. Increased intestinal wall edema

Here continuous furosemide infusion produces better diuresis than bolus dose administration, it will decrease mortality and hospital stay will be reduced.

B. Thiazide diuretic: It blocks the sodium reabsorption in the distal tubule.

C. Potassium sparing diuretics

D. Salt poor albumin: It will enhance the delivery of furosemide to the kidney, if furosemide is added.

E. Angiotensin-converting enzyme (ACE) inhibitor: This drugs should be used cautiously in these patients with close monitoring of renal function but it should not be avoided. If the is deterioration of renal function even after long-term use of these drugs, concomitant reduction of dose of diuretic should be reduced to facilitate safe uptitration of ACE inhibitor. Simultaneous use of NSAIDs should not be started to prevent the deterioration of renal function.

F. Inotropic support: In case of acute decompensated heart failure resulting hypotension and reduced renal perfusion inotropes should be used to increase the cardiac output which can increase the renal blood flow. Dopamine reduces the renovascular resistance. According to European Society of Cardiology (ESC) guideline, dobutamine, dopamine, and milrinone can be used as class IIa level B, class IIa level C, and class IIb level B respectively.

G. Nesiritide: It is analog of BNP, indices vasodilatation, reduces filling pressure, and augment cardiac output. It is under phase III trial.

H. Future novel treatment:

a. Patients who are resistant to diuretic therapy can get benefit from ultrafiltration or aquapheresis. It removes a large amount of fluid without producing severe hypotension.

b. Vaptan: It is vasopressin antagonist, it normalizes the serum sodium and reduces body weight without any adverse effect on blood pressure, heart rate, and renal function. It also reduces pulmonary artery, pulmonary capillary wedge and right atrial pressure and increases the urine output keeping the renal function intact.

c. Adenosine A1 receptor antagonist: Adenosine level is increased in heart failure. So adenosine A1 receptor antagonist prevents the action of serum adenosine, but randomized trial failed to demonstrate any benefit regarding this drug.

d. Hypertonic saline solution (HSS): It may be an useful adjunct with intravenous furosemide in CRS for their few postulated mechanisms:

1. Mobilization of fluid from extracellular to intracellular compartment by osmotic effect.
2. It increases renal blood flow which will help to overcome the diuretic resistance.

But its routine use is rare.

Q4. Renal tubular acidosis, classification, and principles of treatment.

DNBI/JUN2011 (10)

Renal tubular acidosis.

MGR/MAY2011/MDIV (7)
MGR/MAR2002/MDI (10)
MGR/SEP2007/MDIV (5)
KUHS/NOV2013(S)/MDII (10)
DNB (DEC 2022) (5)

Discuss the clinical approach in a patient with renal tubular acidosis.

BF/MAY2013/MDIII (10)

Renal tubular acidosis.

SCBMCH, 2021 (20)

Describe the etiology, diagnosis of renal tubular acidosis. Outline the approach to the treatment of renal tubular acidosis.

DNB, 2024, OCT (10)

What are the types of renal tubular acidosis? Briefly outline the etiology, basic pathophysiology and manifestations of different types of renal tubular acidosis.

WBUHS, 2021 (10)

Describe the types of renal tubular acidosis, diagnosis and management.

NTR UNI OF HEALTH SC, VIJAYAWADA, 2020 (10)

Enumerate the types of renal tubular acidosis. Discuss the evolution and management of renal tubular acidosis.

AIIMS (BHU), 2024 (10)

ANSWER

Renal tubular acidosis is a group of transport defect in bicarbonate reabsorption or excretion of hydrogen ions or both characterized by:

A. Metabolic acidosis
B. Normal GFR
C. Hyperchloremia
D. Normal anion gap

It can be differentiated from uremic acidosis by the following:

A. Normo- or hypochloremia
B. Low GFR
C. Metabolic acidosis
D. Increased anion gap

Renal acid-base homeostasis is maintained by the following two mechanisms:

A. Resorption of bicarbonate by proximal convoluted tubule

B. Excretion of ammonium and titration of urinary buffers through excretion of fixed acids by distal convoluted tubule

Proximal Tubular Bicarbonate Resorption

A. From proximal tubular cell H^+ secreted through luminal membrane in exchange of H^+ by Na^+/H^+ exchanger-3 (NHE-3). This transport depends upon the lumen-to-cell concentration gradient of sodium which is stimulated by intracellular acidosis and inhibited by drug amiloride.

B. In the basolateral membrane HCO_3^- secreted along with Na^+ passively by N^+/H^+ cotransporter (NBC-1).

C. In the lumen, filtered bicarbonate combines with secreted H^+ to form carbonic acid which at once will be broken down to CO_2 and H_2O by carbonic anhydrase IV.

D. CO_2 diffuses freely into the proximal tubular cells where it combines with H_2O to form H_2CO_3 by carbonic anhydrase II. This H_2CO_3 will be dissociated into H^+ and HCO_3^+.

E. Substantial portion of HCO_3 is absorbed by vacuolar ATPase (adenosine triphosphatase).

Distal Renal Tubular Acidification

A. Secretion of ammonia: Ammonia is formed in the proximal tubular cells in the following form:

- **a.** 60% ammonia is formed from deamination of glutamine coming from metabolism of amino acids in the liver.
- **b.** 30% ammonia is formed from deamination of glutamic acid.
- **c.** 10% ammonia is produced from deamination of other amino acids.

B. Formation of ammonium ion: Ammonia is secreted into tubular lumen along its concentration gradient as nonionic diffusion. In the lumen, it combines with ammonia to form ammonium ion and prevents the pH of urine to fall. Ammonium ion is absorbed at loop of Henle in substitution of K^+ by Na^+ K^+ Cl^- system and K^+ H^+ antiport system. But thick ascending limb of loop of Henle is impermeable to ammonium thus increasing the concentration of ammonium in medullary interstitium. It helps in diffusion of ammonium into collecting tubule facilitated by high acidity of tubular fluid.

C. In the collecting tubule, principal cells are responsible for Na reabsorption and K secretion and two types of intercalated cells are responsible for both H^+ and HCO_3^- secretion:

- **a.** α-type intercalated cell secretes H^+ by vacuolar H^+ ATPase controlled by electronegativity of sodium transport by principal cells. Another ATPase, H^+ K^+ ion ATPase also involves in H^+ secretion in exchange of potassium.
- **b.** β-type intercalated cell secretes HCO_3^-

D. Medullary collecting tubule only carry hydrogen ion but neither reabsorbs sodium ion nor secretes potassium ion, so lumen is positive. Here hydrogen ion has to be secreted against electrochemical gradient via vacuolar H^+ ATPase.

E. Terminal inner medullary collecting duct secretes hydrogen ion like α-type intercalated cell. Luminal carbonic anhydrase IV helps in bicarbonate ion absorption.

Classification of Renal Tubular Acidosis

There are four types of Renal Tubular Acidosis (RTA)

A. Proximal renal tubular acidosis or type 2 RTA:

Causes:

- **a.** Primary causes:
  1. Hereditary (persistent): It is autosomal dominant
  2. Sporadic (transient in infancy)
- **b.** Secondary causes:
  1. Fanconi syndrome
  2. Administration of drugs and toxins
  3. Other causes: Vitamin D deficiency, hyperparathyroidism, chronic hypocapnia, Alport syndrome, medullary cystic disease.

Pathophysiology: Here the main defect is impairment of bicarbonate absorption by proximal tubule characterized by decreased renal threshold for bicarbonate ion (normal is 26 mmol/L). As a result large amount of bicarbonate ion will enter into distal tubule but it cannot handle that large amount of ion, as a result it will be excreted in urine making the urine pH alkaline.

Distal acidification system is intact. When the plasma concentration of bicarbonate ion will be sufficiently low, large amount of ammonium ion will excrete through urine and urine pH is below 5.5.

B. Distal renal tubule acidosis or type 1 RTA:

Causes:

- **a.** Primary causes:

  Persistent:
  1. Classic form
  2. Associated sensorineural deafness (autosomal recessive)
  3. Associated with bicarbonate wasting (infants and children)
  4. Incomplete distal RTA

  Transient:
- **b.** Secondary causes:
  1. Genetic diseases
  2. Disorders due to calcium metabolism
  3. Autoimmune disorders
  4. Hypothyroidism

5. Tubulointerstitial disorders:
   - Obstructive uropathy
   - Pyelonephritis
   - Interstitial nephritis
6. Hyponatriuretic state (nephrotic syndrome, cirrhosis)
7. Dysproteinemia syndrome
8. Drugs and toxins

Pathophysiology: This type is characterized by impaired acidification of urine under stimulus of acidemia, so there is inability to lower the pH of urine. There is also inability of distal tubule to secrete NH_4^+ in urine. Here bicarbonate absorption is normal.

C. Combined proximal and distal renal tubular acidosis (type 3 RTA): In this type of RTA there is sharing both the features of both type 1 and type 2 RTA. In this RTA:
   a. There is striking reduction of tubular reclamation of filtered load of HCO_3^-.
   b. Inability to acidify maximally the urine in spite of severe degree of acidemia. It is seen in children and infants, transiently in distal RTA.

D. Type 4 RTA or hyperchloremic RTA: This RTA is caused by impaired ammoniagenesis and is characterized by:
   a. Normal ability to acidify urine in response to high-acid load
   b. Subnormal net excretion due to low excretion of ammonium ion
   c. Renal tubular absorption of bicarbonate ion is reduced in the face of normal concentration of bicarbonate ion in serum.

This type in children is associated with primary pseudohypoaldosteronism type 1 characterized by salt wasting, hyperkalemia, metabolic acidosis, and increased plasma renin activity.

Diagnosis of Different Types of Renal Tubular Acidosis

	Proximal RTA	Classic distal RTA	Type 3 RTA	Type 4 RTA
In metabolic acidosis (spontaneous or in response to acid loading)				
Plasma potassium	Normal or decreased	Normal or decreased	Normal or decreased	Increased
Urine anion gap	Negative	Positive	Positive	Positive
Urine pH	<5.5	>5.5	>5.5	<5.5
Ammonium excretion	Normal	Decreased	Decreased	Decreased
Fractional potassium excretion	Normal or increased	Increased	Increased	Decreased
Calcium excretion	Normal	Increased	Increased	Normal or decreased
Citrate excretion	Normal	Decreased	Decreased	Normal
In case of normal acid base equilibrium (after acid loading)				
Fractional bicarbonate excretion	>10–15%	<5%	>5–15%	>5–10%
Other defect in tubules	Often present	Absent	Absent	Absent
Nephrolithiasis	Absent	Often present	Often present	Absent
Involvement of bone	Often present	Rarely present	Rarely present	Absent

Approach to Case of RTA

A. In a patient with hyperchloremic metabolic acidosis with negative urine anion gap:
   a. Gastrointestinal HCO_3^- loss: Urinary sodium
   b. Hydrochloric acid intake
   c. Proximal RTA: In this case:
      1. Increased acid load urine pH <5.5
      2. Sodium bicarbonate load:
         - Fractional excretion of bicarbonate >10–15%
         - Urine to blood PCO_2 >20 mm Hg

B. In a patient with hyperchloremic metabolic acidosis with positive urine anion gap:

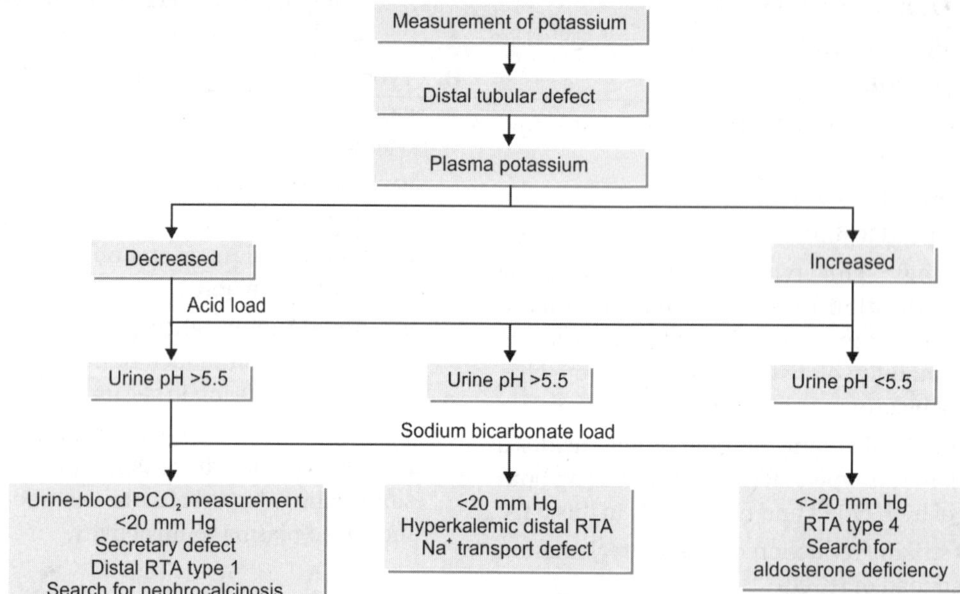

Treatment of Renal Tubular Acidosis

A. For proximal renal tubular acidosis type 2:

a. Potassium or sodium citrate 10–20 mmol/kg/h due to massive urinary loss of HCO_3. This dose should be separated to several divided dosages along the day and night. Since alkali therapy is unpalatable, so long-term compliance is poor.

b. Concurrent thiazide diuretics may be helpful to reduce the base requirement but it may worsen the hypokalemia.

Prognosis depends upon the etiology, especially in the context of Fanconi syndrome. But in case of sporadic isolated proximal RTA, it can be improved over time.

B. For distal renal tubular acidosis type 1:

a. Here the aim of treatment is to balance the hydrogen ion production by adequate base administration. Hydrogen ion production is higher in case of children as compared to adult due to release of this ion during bone growth. Sodium or potassium citrate or bicarbonate salt can be given at a dose of 5–8 mmol/kg of body weight in infant, 1–2 mmol/kg in adult are required.

b. Correction of hyperuricemia is mandatory as because excretion of urinary citrate remains subnormal. So calcium to creatinine ratio or citrate to creatinine ratio monitoring can estimate the exact amount of alkali administration required.

c. Overcorrection of acidosis may be paradoxically harmful as it will increase the extracellular volume as well as increases urinary calcium excretion.

C. Type 4 renal tubular acidosis:

Treatment depends on underlying cause:

a. Potassium sparing diuretic has to be withdrawn.

b. Fludrocortisone can be given in case of hyporeninemic hypoaldosteronism in combination with loop diuretic, furosemide to prevent extracellular volume expansion.

c. Alkali supplementation may be required in few cases at a dose of 2 mmol/kg of body weight.

Q5. Define acute kidney injury. Describe its pathogenesis, clinical presentation, and treatment.

DNBIV/JUN2012 (10)

Define acute kidney injury. Discuss etiology and management of acute tubular necrosis.

DNBI/JUNE2013 (10)

Classify major causes of acute renal failure. Discuss the pathophysiology, clinical features, and management of acute tubular necrosis.

MGR/OCT2013/MDII (15)

Acute renal failure.

MGR/SEP2009/MDII (6)

Discuss the etiopathogenesis, clinical features, and management of acute renal failure.

MGR/APR2012/MDIII (15)

Describe causes, clinical features, and management of acute renal failure in Indian scenario.

MGR/SEP2006/MDIII (15)

Write about the types and causes of acute renal failure.

MUHS/NOV2014/MDIV (10)

Acute kidney injury: Criteria and diagnosis.

PGI/NOV2012/MDI (10)

Discuss etiopathogenesis and management of acute renal failure.

SNMC/MAY2008/MDIII (15)

Enumerate causes of acute renal failure. Describe the management and preventive guidelines in such patients.

DNBIII/DEC2011 (10)

Classify the major causes of acute kidney injury (AKI). Role of urinary sediment findings in AKI. List the indications for dialysis of AKI.

DNBIIIB/JUN2016 (10)

Markers of acute kidney injury.

MGR/APR2014/MDI (5)

Briefly enumerate the new biomarkers in acute kidney injury. Short notes on non-calcium containing phosphate binding drugs.

AIIMS, BHU, 2020 (10)

AKI- diagnosis and management.

SCBMCH, 2019 (20)

Describe the complications and briefly outline their management in patients of acute kidney injury.

ORISA UNI, 2021 (10)

Discuss the pathophysiology of ischemic acute kidney injury. Enumerate the novel biomarkers of acute kidney injury. Discuss the complications of peritoneal dialysis.

DNB, 2024 MAY (10)

Discuss dialysis therapy and biomarkers in acute kidney injury.

KERALA UNI, 2022 (10)

Peritoneal dialysis has been explained in the question number 7.

Phosphate binding drugs has been written in question number 6.

Dialysis part has been discussed in question number 7.

Discuss etiology, clinical features, investigations and treatment of acute renal failure.

VEER NARMAD SOUTH GUJARAT UNI, 2022 (25)

Classify major causes of ARF. Discuss the pathophysiology, clinical features and management of ATN.

MGR UNI, TAMIL NADU, 2021 (15)

Write AKIN criteria for acute kidney injury. Describe etiopathogenesis, clinical features, diagnosis and management of acute kidney injury.

MAHARASHTRA UNI OF HEALTH SC, VIJAYAWADA, 2021 (25)

Describe anatomy of nephron. Discuss etiopathogenesis, clinical features and management of ARF.

VEER NARMAD SOUTH GUJARAT UNI, 2021 (20)

Acute kidney injury.

KERALA UNIVERSITY, 2020 (10)

Acute tubular necrosis.

NTR UNI OF HEALTH SC, VIJAYAWADA, 2020 (10)

Describe the etiology, pathophysiology, clinical features and management of acute kidney injury.

NTR UNI OF HEALTH SC, VIJAYAWADA, 2020 (10)

Classify major causes of acute renal failure – discuss the pathophysiology, clinical feature and management of acute tubular necrosis.

MGR UNI, TAMIL NADU, 2019 (15)

Describe pathogenesis of acute tubular necrosis and metabolic changes related to it. How will you manage a case?

VEER NARMAD SOUTH GUJARAT UNI, 2019 (25)

Markers of acute kidney injury.

BABA FARID UNI OF HEAKTH SC, 2019 (10)

Discuss the causes, clinical features and management of acute renal failure in tropics.

MAHARASHTRA UNI OF HEALTH SC, 2019 (25)

Classify acute kidney failure and outline their etiopathogenesis. How do you investigate and manage a case of acute kidney failure.

BHARATI VIDYAPEETH DEEM UNI, LHELAM, 2019, (15)

Acute kidney injury.

RAJIV GANDHI UNI OF HEALTH SC, KARNATAKA, 2018 (10)

TEERTHANKER MAHAVEER UNIVERSITY, 2018 (10)

Acute renal failure in tropics.

NTR UNI OF HEALTH SC, VIJAYAWADA, 2018 (10)

Briefly review normal kidney physiology and narrate the pathogenesis of acute kidney injury.

WBUHS 2024 (10)

Pathogenesis of acute kidney injury in septic shock.

AIIMS, BHU, 2024 (10)

Pathophysiology of acute kidney injury.

MANIPUR UNIVERSITY, 2018 (10)

Classify the major causes of ARF. Discuss the pathophysiology, clinical features and management of ATN.

WBUHS, 2023 (10)

Narrate the major causes, clinical features and diagnostic modalities for pre-renal acute kidney injury.

WBUHS, 2024 (10)

Briefly review the kidney physiology and narrate the pathogenesis of acute kidney injury.

WBUHS, 2024 (10)

ANSWER

Kidney performs the following functions to do normal homeostasis:

A. Acid base homeostasis
B. Excretion of urea and creatinine
C. Maintenance of fluid and electrolytes balance
D. Activation of vitamin D
E. Secretion of erythropoietin
F. Control of blood pressure

Acute kidney injury: There are two criteria of acute kidney injury (AKI) and based on these criteria acute kidney injury can be defined. These criteria are:

A. Acute kidney injury network (AKIN)
B. Risk, Injury, Failure, Loss, and End-stage renal failure (RIFLE)

Acute kidney injury network criteria:

Stage	Serum creatinine	Urine output
1	≥3 mg/dL increase or ≥1.5 to 2-fold increase from baseline	<0.5 mL/kg/h for >6 hours
2	>2 to 3-fold increase from baseline	<0.5 mL/kg/h for >12 hours
3	>3-fold increase from baseline or baseline of ≥ 4 mg/mL with acute rise of ≥0.5 mg/dL or on renal replacement therapy	<0.5 mL/kg/h for >24 hours or anuria for 12 hours
Time	<48 hours	

RIFLE criteria:

Class	Serum creatinine	GFR
Risk	1.5 times increased	Decreased to >25%
Injury	2 times increased	Decreased to >50%

Continued

Continued

Class	Serum creatinine	GFR
Failure	3 times increased or >4 mg/dL from baseline with acute rise of >0.5 mg/dL	Decreased to >75%
Loss		Persistent AKI = complete loss of kidney function for >4 weeks
ESRD		>3 months
Time	1–7 days	
	Sustained for >24 hours	

(AKI: acute kidney injury; ESRD: end-stage renal disease; GFR: glomerular filtration rate)

Etiopathogenesis of Acute Kidney Injury

Prerenal azotemia: This type of azotemia occurs to hypoperfusion of kidney with minimal cellular damage of the renal tissue. This can be reverted to normal function within 24–72 hours of correction of the hypoperfusion state. The causes of hypoperfusion states are the following:

A. Total intravascular volume depletion:
- **a.** Hemorrhage
- **b.** Gastrointestinal loss of fluid:
  1. Diarrhea
  2. Vomiting
  3. Lavage through the nasogastric tube
- **c.** Fluid loss in third space:
  1. Peritonitis
  2. Necrotizing pancreatitis
  3. Severe hypoproteinemia
  4. Systemic inflammatory syndrome
- **d.** Renal fluid loss:
  1. Excessive use of diuretics
  2. Osmotic diuresis—mannitol administration, glycosuria
  3. Primary adrenal insufficiency
  4. Salt loosing nephropathy
  5. Diabetes insipidus

B. Arterial underfilling due to effective volume depletion: Here total intravascular volume is normal or even increased but decreased cardiac output or arterial vasodilatation in different clinical settings are responsible for arterial underfilling. The causes are the following:
- **a.** Diminished cardiac output:
  1. Cardiogenic shock in myocardial infarction
  2. Pericardial tamponade
  3. Acute decompensated heart failure
  4. Massive pulmonary embolism
- **b.** Peripheral vasodilatation:
  1. Anaphylaxis
  2. Sepsis
  3. Antihypertensive drugs
  4. Chronic liver diseases

C. Intrarenal hemodynamic changes: Either afferent arteriolar vasoconstriction or efferent arteriolar vasodilatation may produce intrarenal changes in perfusion. The causes are:
- **a.** Afferent arteriolar vasoconstriction:
  1. Cyclosporine
  2. Nonsteroidal anti-inflammatory agents
  3. Cyclooxygenase-2 (COX-2) inhibitors
  4. Tacrolimus
  5. Hypercalcemia
  6. Radiocontrast dye
- **b.** Efferent arteriolar vasodilatation (postglomerular effect):
  1. Angiotensin II receptor blocker
  2. Angiotensin-converting enzyme inhibitors

Postrenal acute kidney injury: It occurs due to acute obstruction to the flow of urine, the site may be in the ureter, bladder neck, or urethra. In case of male prostatic hypertrophy or prostatic cancer may produce partial or complete obstruction of urine. On the other hand in case of women pelvic irradiation or pelvic surgery may lead to urinary tract obstruction. The causes are:

A. Bilateral obstruction of ureter or in case single kidney unilateral obstruction:
- **a.** Extraureteral obstruction:
  1. Retroperitoneal fibrosis
  2. Pelvic or abdominal malignancy
  3. During pelvic surgery accidental ureteral ligation
- **b.** Intraureteral ligation:
  1. Stone
  2. Tumor—transitional carcinoma
  3. Blood clot
  4. Intrawall edema
  5. Pyogenic debris

c. Bladder neck obstruction:
  1. Blood clot
  2. Bladder carcinoma
  3. Bladder stone
  4. Prostatic carcinoma
  5. Fungal ball
  6. Benign prostatic hypertrophy
  7. Autonomic neuropathy

d. Urethral obstruction:
  1. Urethral stricture
  2. Blood clot

Intrinsic acute kidney injury: Here azotemia may be due to vascular, glomerular, interstitial or tubular causes—which may be of systemic or vascular origin which cannot be changed by repletion of fluid, improving cardiac function or removal of obstruction:

A. Vascular causes: It can be classified according to involvement of size of the vessels:
  a. Large and medium size vessel involvement:
    1. Polyarteritis nodosa
    2. Renal artery thrombosis
    3. Bilateral renal vein thrombosis
    4. Arterial clamping during operation
  b. Small vessel involvement:
    1. Malignant hypertension
    2. Thrombotic-thrombocytopenic purpura
    3. Hemolytic uremic syndrome
    4. Atheroembolic disease
    5. Scleroderma renal crisis
    6. Postpartum acute kidney injury

B. Glomerular causes:
  a. Nephrotic syndrome: Though it is uncommonly associated with acute kidney injury but following causes are associated with this:
    1. Minimal disease
    2. Focal segmental glomerulonephritis
  b. Nephritic syndrome: Here proteinuria is 1–2 g/day. The causes are:
    1. Glomerulonephritis
    2. Rapidly progressive glomerulonephritis or crescentic nephritis—there is rising creatinine, hematuria, and proteinuria. There is damage in the capillary wall leading to inflammation, fibrosis, and crescent formation thus destruction of glomeruli. The causes are the following:
      - Antiglomerular basement membrane (anti-GBM) antibody deposition in linear fashion along the basement membrane:
        - Goodpasture syndrome
        - Kidney-limited Goodpasture syndrome
      - Granular immune complex deposition:
        - Lupus nephritis
        - Acute postinfectious glomerulonephritis
        - Immunoglobulin A glomerulonephritis
        - Membranoproliferative glomerulonephritis
        - Cryoglobulinemia
        - Infective endocarditis
        - Henoch–Schönlein purpura
      - Pauci-immune glomerulonephritis:
        - Microscopic polyangiitis
        - Idiopathic crescentic glomerulonephritis
        - Churg–Strauss syndrome
        - Wegener granulomatosis

C. Interstitial involvement: The most important cause is interstitial nephritis where there is marked interstitial edema, focal diffuse infiltration with inflammatory cells, such as lymphocytes, eosinophils in the interstitium. It occurs due to the following causes:
  a. Drug-induced interstitial nephritis:
    1. Diuretics—thiazide, chlorthalidone, and furosemide
    2. Antibiotics—methicillin, erythromycin, rifampicin, and ciprofloxacin
    3. Nonsteroidal anti-inflammatory drugs
    4. Allopurinol
    5. Anticonvulsant—phenytoin
  b. Infections:
    1. Tuberculosis
    2. Bacteria—*Streptococcus* and *Staphylococcus*
    3. Viral—Epstein–Barr virus and cytomegalovirus

D. Tubular involvement: Here proximal tubular dysfunction produces abrupt decrease in glomerular dysfunction. Microscopically, there is swelling, loss of brush border, apical blebbing, vacuolization, and loss of basolateral infoldings of tubular cells. In case of ischemic or nephrotoxic injury tubular dysfunction will be reversible in presence of continued presence of renal blood flow. Ischemic injury may be due to decreased blood volume or underfilling of arteries with redistribution of away from the kidney which may be present in the following conditions:

a. Renal ischemia:
   1. Hemorrhage
   2. Shock
   3. Pancreatitis
   4. Trauma
   5. Gram-negative sepsis
   6. Hypotension

b. Nephrotoxic drugs:
   1. Aminoglycoside drugs
   2. Acyclovir
   3. Amphotericin B
   4. Antineoplastic agent
   5. Ethylene glycol

c. Endogenous toxins:
   1. Myoglobin—in rhabdomyolysis
   2. Hemoglobin—acute falciparum malaria, incompatible blood transfusion

E. Sepsis: In sepsis, decline in renal function is due to the following factors:
   a. Intrinsic damage of the tubule
   b. Vascular factors affecting autoregulation leading to decrease in GFR.

Clinical Features

A. In case of prerenal azotemia:

a. In case of reduction of intravascular volume:
   1. Orthostatic hypotension
   2. Loss of axillary sweat
   3. Dry mucous membrane, tachycardia, thready pulse
   4. Weight reduction
   5. Tenting of skin in the upper thorax when it is pinched in between the fingers.
   6. Collapsed jugular vein

b. In case of arterial underfilling with excess extracellular fluid volume:
   1. Engorged pulsatile jugular vein
   2. Dependent edema
   3. Inspiratory crackles in both lung bases
   4. S3 gallop
   5. Anasarca
   6. Ascites
   7. Evidence of liver failure:
      - Jaundice
      - Palmar erythema
      - Shrunken size of liver

B. In case of postrenal azotemia:

a. In case of confused or unconscious patient agitation

b. Abdominal examination:
   1. Distended tender bladder or bilateral hydronephrosis
   2. Catheterization of urinary bladder is not recommended because
      - Diagnostic utility of ultrasound will be lost.
      - It will alter the diagnostic utility of urinalysis.

c. If there is no urine output, catheter is recommended and it is the procedure of choice.

d. Patient is asked to void and urine output after bladder catheterization has to be recorded and it should be <50 mL.

C. In case of intrinsic renal disease:

a. Evidence of cholesterol emboli in the form of:
   1. Livedo reticularis
   2. Blue toe syndrome
   3. Peripheral necrotic areas
   4. Abdominal pain due to presence of emboli in the gut and pancreas

b. In case of thrombotic microangiopathy:
   1. Microangiopathic hemolytic anemia
   2. Thrombocytopenia
   3. Eye findings:
      - Papilledema
      - Retinal hemorrhage
   4. Involvement of lung characterized by:
      - Shortness of breath from pulmonary edema
      - Chest pain
   5. Neurological manifestation producing confusion
   6. Features of scleroderma

c. In case of glomerular disease from nephrotic syndrome:
   1. Hypertension
   2. Pitting edema

3. Periorbital edema
4. Anasarca

d. In case of glomerular disease from nephritic syndrome:
1. Dermatological manifestations:
• Palpable purpura
• Skin rash
2. Joint involvement: Arthralgia, arthritis
3. Lung—hemoptysis
4. Heart—murmur
5. Neurological examination—acute neuropathy
6. Abdominal pain

e. In case of acute interstitial nephritis:
1. Fever
2. Maculopapular rash and petechial skin eruption
3. Abdominal pain in the flank

Diagnosis of Acute Kidney Injury

A. Urinary diagnostic indices:

Indices	Prerenal azotemia	Acute tubular necrosis
Urinary sodium (mEq/L)	<20	>40
Urinary osmolarity (mOsm/kg H_2O)	>500	<350
Urine creatinine to plasma creatinine	>40	<20
BUN/serum creatinine	>20	≤10
Fractional excretion of urea = [(UNa/PNa)/(UCr/PCr)] × 100	<1	>1

(BUN: blood urea nitrogen)

B. Urinary findings in acute kidney injury:

Dipstick	Prerenal azotemia	Postrenal azotemia	Small-vessel vasculitis	Nephrotic glomerular	Nephritic glomerular	AIN	ATN
Leukocyte esterase	Nil	Nil	Nil	Nil	Nil	Present	Nil
Heme	Nil	Nil	Present	Nil or trace	Present	Present	Nil
Protein	Nil	Nil	Present	Present	Present	Present	Nil or trace
Specific gravity	>1.020	1.010	Variable	Variable	Variable	1.010	1.010
Microscopy							
RBCs	Nil	Nil	Present	Nil or few	Present	Present	Nil
WBCs	Nil	Nil	Nil	Nil	Nil	Present	Nil
RBC cast	Nil	Nil	Present	Nil	Present	Nil	Nil
WBC cast	Nil	Nil	Nil	Nil	Nil	Present	Nil
Granular cast	Nil	Nil	Nil	Nil	Nil	Nil	Present
Renal tubular epithelial cells	Nil	Nil	Nil	Nil	Nil	Nil	Present
Tests							
Osmolarity (mOsm/L)	>500	≤350	Variable	Variable	Variable	≤350	≤350
Protein g/dL	Nil	Nil	1–2	>3	1–2	1–2	≤1

(AIN: acute interstitial nephritis; ATN: acute tubular necrosis; RBC: red blood cell; WBC: red blood cell)

C. Diagnostic criteria of hepatorenal syndrome (HRS):

a. Presence of cirrhosis
b. Serum creatinine is >1.5 mg/dL
c. Absence of other cause of AKI
d. Absence of shock
e. No history of use of nephrotoxic drugs
f. Absence of sustained improvement in renal function following 2 days of complete withdrawal of diuretics along with volume expansion with albumin at a dose of 1 g/kg/day to maximum 100 g/day.

D. In case of postrenal azotemia:

a. Renal ultrasonography: Hydronephrosis—but it may not occur in case of early obstruction and in case of compression due to compression by retroperitoneal fibrosis or tumor. Again there may be functional hydronephrosis in pregnancy or anatomical variants of collecting duct system which can be differentiated by furosemide isotope renogram which can decrease hydronephrosis in later cases.

b. Isotope renography: It is performed with intravenous administration of radionucleotide as well as furosemide. If there is rapid washout of the dye with increase urinary flow—it suggests no obstruction. But if there is persistence of isotope in the renal parenchyma—it suggests obstruction.
c. Noncontrast computerized tomography: It can identify the site of obstruction.
d. Cystoscopy and retrograde or anterograde pyelography: It can identify blood clot, tumor, stone, pyogenic debris. Pyelography should be done even in case of negative ultrasonographic findings.

E. In case renal vessel disease:
  a. Raised lactate dehydrogenase
  b. Doppler ultrasonography: It can assess renal vein thrombosis and renal blood flow.
  c. CT and MR angiography: It can detect clot in inferior vena cava or renal vein.
  d. Angiography can be done in case of acute anuria and acute renal embolization.

F. In case of small vessel disease:
  a. Increased erythrocyte sedimentation rate (ESR)
  b. Eosinophilia
  c. Hypocomplementemia where C3 is low but C4 will be normal.
  d. Kidney will reveal intravascular cholesterol crystal.

G. In case of thrombotic microangiopathy:
  a. Peripheral smear demonstrates fragmented red blood cells, thrombocytopenia
  b. Elevated lactate dehydrogenase (LDH) due to hemolysis

H. In case of glomerular disease:
  a. Perinuclear antineutrophil cytoplasmic antibody (p-ANCA) and cytoplasmic antineutrophil cytoplasmic antibody (c-ANCA) is sensitive test for screening but these are elevated in glomerulonephritis or other than vasculitis. So these should be tested against specific antigen targets proteinase 3 and myeloperoxidase, former antibody PR3-ANCA is responsible for c-ANCA staining (positive for Wegener granulomatosis) and myeloperoxidase ANCA (MPO-ANCA) for p-ANCA staining (positive for microscopic polyangiitis). 50% of Churg–Strauss syndrome is positive for both antibody in equal frequency.
  b. Anti-GBM antibody is positive in Goodpasture syndrome.
  c. Hypocomplementemia is present in:
    1. Lupus nephritis
    2. Membranoproliferative glomerulonephritis
    3. Mixed cryoglobulinemia
    4. Atheroembolic renal disease
    5. Sepsis
    6. Acute pancreatitis
    7. Advanced liver disease

I. In case of acute interstitial nephritis: Eosinophilia

Markers of Acute Kidney Injury

A. Serum creatinine: Normal value is 0.6–1.2 mg/dL. But the correlation between serum creatinine and glomerular filtration rate is confounded by several factors:
  a. Certain medicine, such as trimethoprim interfere with secretion of creatinine without interfering GFR.
  b. Creatinine excretion depends upon muscle mass which is again depends on age and illness. So, in a cachectic-aged patient creatinine value of 1.3 reflects severely impaired GFR as compared to weight-lifter aged patient having weight of 100 kg.
  c. Excretion and secretion of creatinine must come to a steady state prior to actual level of creatinine.

B. Blood urea nitrogen: Normal value is 8–18 mg/dL. It is filtered but not secreted. But urea is absorbed from proximal tubule and by arginine vasopressin sensitive urea transporters in the collecting duct in case of volume depletion. Blood level rises without rise in serum creatinine which results the blood urea nitrogen (BUN) to creatinine ratio of >20. Blood urea rises without alteration of GFR are:
  a. Hypercatabolic state
  b. Increased serum protein
  c. Upper gastrointestinal bleeding
  d. Administration of high dose of steroids

  Blood urea will rise in the face of low GFR:
  a. Low protein diet
  b. Severe liver disease
  c. Severely malnourished person

C. Cystatin C: It is produced by all nucleated cells, filtered by glomerulus but completely reabsorbed by proximal tubules and not secreted by the tubule, it is best measured by immunonephelometric assay. In case of AKI serum, cystatin C measurement is more accurate than serum creatinine. It is mainly measured in case of reduced muscle mass or liver cirrhosis.

D. Biomarkers of AKI: It is released into the urine as well as into the blood by injured kidney and is more sensitive and specific. These are usually increased 1–2 days prior to increase in serum creatinine after AKI. These are:

- **a.** Urinary interleukin-18
- **b.** Neutrophil gelatinase-associated lipocalin or NGAL: It is also known as siderocalin or lipocalin-2. It will bind to iron siderophore complexes and responsible for many tissue protective effects in the proximal tubule. It will be upregulated very quickly inflammatory kidney injury and in case of cardiopulmonary bypass associated kidney injury it can be detected within 2 hours in blood and urine.
- **c.** Kidney injury molecule-1 (KIM-1): Normally it is expressed in small amount in absence of injury to kidney, but it will be expressed in large amount very shortly in response to kidney injury by nephrotoxic drugs like cisplatin so that it can be estimated in urine. Its role is:
    1. To provide phagocytic properties to the tubular cells so that the cells will engulf and clear the debris from the tubular lumen.
    2. To reduce the inflammatory response to injury
- **d.** Tubular enzymes
- **e.** Insulin-like growth factor binding protein 7 and metalloproteinase-2 are predictive biomarkers in case of moderate to severe renal injury in case of critically ill patients.
- **f.** Liver fatty acid binding protein

Kidney Biopsy

It will provide definite diagnostic and prognostic information regarding AKI. It can diagnose different types of glomerulonephritis, interstitial nephritis, vasculitis, myeloma kidney, hemolytic-uremic syndrome, thrombotic thrombocytopenic purpura, and dysfunction of allograft. It is required when prerenal azotemia, acute interstitial nephritis, and ischemic injury have been excluded. In presence of coagulopathy or thrombocytopenia, this procedure may produce severe bleeding.

Management of Acute Kidney Injury

In Case of Prerenal Azotemia

A. In case of volume depletion:

- **a.** If the volume depletion is due to hemorrhage, blood group matched packed RBC should be given. In some cases, intravenous normal saline or Ringer lactate can be given for the time being till the availability of blood.
- **b.** If the volume depletion is due to loss of fluid, 0.9% saline or Ringer lactate can be given. In case of administration of 1 L of normal saline only 250 mL will remain in intravascular space and rest 750 mL will enter into interstitial compartment. Again, one study demonstrates that albumin is no more effective than normal saline in fluid resuscitation.

    Again, in normal saline 154 mEq/L sodium and chloride are present whereas, in plasma sodium concentration is 135 mEq/L and chloride is 109 mEq/L. So, administration of normal saline may produce hyperchloremic metabolic acidosis and aggravates AKI. On the other hand, Ringer lactate may produce or aggravate hyperkalemia and increases the serum concentration of lactate.

    Clinical situation dictates the amount of fluid to be administrated and rapidity of fluid administration:

    1. In young stable patient one time bolus of 500–1,000 mL of fluid has to be administered over 1 hour.
    2. In case of elderly or in patient with unknown cardiac status 250 mL of fluid has to be given over 1 hour.
    3. Then clinical evaluation of sustained hypovolemia or volume overload should be done by the following:
        - Measurement of blood pressure in lying down and sitting position
        - Pulse
        - Jugular venous pressure: In lying down position usually it can be seen. But in severe hypovolemia, it will disappear. So post fluid administration, the reappearance of jugular pulse suggests normalization of central venous pressure.
        - Presence of third heart sound—it indicates fluid overload
        - Inspiratory basal crackles suggests fluid overload.

B. In case arterial underfilling with extracellular volume excess:

a. In case of heart failure, to increase the cardiac output and to improve renal blood flow diuretics, beta-blockers, ACE inhibitors, angiotensin receptor blockers (ARBs), hydralazine, and nitrates are used. Furosemide is given as bolus dose of 200 mg followed by 10–40 mg/h as slow intravenous infusion. Dopamine can be administered at low dose to increase the salt and water excretion through kidney but in case of intrinsic AKI different trials failed to demonstrate any benefit. In case of advanced heart failure, refractory or partially responsive to the above agents following procedures can be done:

1. Continuous venovenous hemofiltration (CVVH)
2. Continuous ultrafiltration
3. Intermittent ultrafiltration without dialysis

b. In case of cirrhosis, it can be treated with sodium restriction, loop diuretics, and aldosterone antagonists. In case of diuretic-resistant patient, large volume paracentesis, transjugular intrahepatic portosystemic shunt, or transplantation of liver may be of choice.

c. In case of type I HRS, vasopressin analog with albumin or transjugular intrahepatic portosystemic shunt (TIPS) are given to improve the renal blood flow

d. In case of type II HRS, liver transplantation is the method of choice.

C. In case of postrenal AKI:

a. In case of bladder-neck obstruction, Foley's catheter drainage followed by removal of prostate are of choice. But in some cases α-blocker can be given.

b. In case of ureteral obstruction, cystoscopy followed by ureteral stent with removal of stones should be done which allows the passage of stones, sludge, and pus. In case of tumor infiltration, prograde stent followed by nephrostomies under radiological supervision are of choices.

D. In case of primary glomerular diseases:

a. Therapeutic options are steroids with or without immunosuppressive drugs, and in case of Goodpasture syndrome—plasmapheresis.

b. In case of scleroderma renal crisis drug of choice is ACE inhibitor.

c. Hemolytic-uremic syndrome (HUS) or thrombotic thrombocytopenic purpura (TTP) should be treated with plasmapheresis. Pharmacologic blockade of complement activation may be given in atypical HUS.

E. In case of acute interstitial nephritis:

a. Removal of offending drugs or radiocontrast material

b. Prednisolone 1 mg/kg for 2–4 weeks followed by slow taper within 2–4 months

F. In case of rhabdomyolysis, there is no specific therapy. Initial fluid requirement is 10 L/day. Alkaline fluid produced by 75 mmol/L sodium bicarbonate in 0.45% saline prevents formation of cast and tubular injury but there is chance of worsening of hypocalcemia. Diuretics cannot achieve urinary flow to 200–300 mL/h, hence not recommended.

G. Malnutrition: AKI is a catabolic disease, nitrogen balance is negative for the following causes:

a. Sepsis with or without multiorgan dysfunction

b. Postsurgery

c. Renal factors:

1. Uremia
2. Metabolic acidosis
3. Abnormalities of parathyroid hormone (PTH)
4. Inadequate intake of protein
5. Protein losses

So according to Kidney Disease Improving Global Outcomes (KDIGO) guidelines:

a. Total intake of energy: 20–30 kcal/kg

b. Protein intake—it depends upon the severity of AKI:

1. In noncatabolic AKI without the requirement of dialysis—0.8–1.0 g/kg/day
2. In case of patient under dialysis 1.0–1.5 g/kg/day, maximum to 1.7 g/kg/day in hypercatabolic patient on continuous renal replacement therapy (CRRT)

H. Anemia: In AKI, it is multifactorial origin. It is not improved by erythropoietin because of its delayed action, presence of bone marrow resistance. Bleeding in uremia will respond to desmopressin or estrogen and in long-standing case dialysis.

I. Gastrointestinal prophylaxis can be provided by proton pump inhibitors or histamine receptor blockers.

J. In case of venous thromboembolism low molecular heparin and factor Xa inhibitors.

K. Electrolyte and acid-bases abnormalities:

a. Hyponatremia:

1. Restriction intake of free water and minimization of administration of hypotonic solutions and dextrose solutions
2. Hypertonic saline is rarely required.

b. Hyperkalemia:

1. Potassium intake should be restricted.
2. Avoidance of potassium sparing diuretics
3. If the potassium level is >5.5–6.5 mEq/L—potassium-binding resin (sodium polystyrene sulfonate) orally.
4. If potassium level is >6.5–7.5 mEq/L—10 units of insulin in 50 mL of 50% dextrose has to be given to promote potassium intracellularly in addition to potassium-binding resin.
5. If potassium level is >7.5 mEq/L—10% 10 mL calcium gluconate or 10% 10 mL calcium chloride should be given to stabilize the cardiac muscle cell against potassium.

c. Hypocalcemia: In case of symptomatic patient calcium gluconate or calcium carbonate.

d. Hyperphosphatemia:

1. Restriction of dietary phosphate intake
2. Phosphate-binding agents, such as calcium acetate, sevelamer hydrochloride, aluminum hydroxide with meals.

e. Hyperuricemia: Treatment is not required usually except in case of tumor lysis syndrome.

Dialysis

A. Indications:

a. Severe hyperkalemia
b. Volume overload
c. Metabolic acidosis
d. Toxin ingestion
e. Complications of uremia

B. Timing of dialysis: There is debate regarding that:

a. If dialysis is done in late, there is chance of volume overload, metabolic complications, and electrolyte abnormalities.

b. If dialysis starts early:

1. There is chance of unnecessary exposure to intravenous lines.
2. Infection
3. Bleeding
4. Hypotension
5. Procedural complications

C. Mechanism of actions in dialysis: Removal of small solutes across the semipermeable membrane along the concentration gradient by the method of diffusion and movement of plasma water in convection method.

D. Choice of the modality of dialysis depends upon:

a. Technical skill
b. Immediate availability of the procedure

E. Procedure:

a. Access to peritoneal cavity by peritoneal dialysis: It is uncommonly used in AKI. It is used in patients with minimal catabolism who has no life-threatening indications of dialysis. Exchange of 1.5–2 L of fluid has to be introduced into the peritoneal cavity. Major risks are peritonitis and infection.

b. Access to large blood vessels by hemodialysis

F. Hemodialysis:

a. It can be done continuously or intermittently
b. By either convection and diffusion method or both
c. Vascular access: Femoral, subclavian or internal jugular vein
d. This procedure is performed thrice to 4 times weekly
e. Duration of each session is 3–4 hours per day, but first session must be 2 hours.
f. Major complication is hypotension in critically ill patients

G. Types of hemodialysis:

a. Intermittent hemodialysis: It is done in otherwise stable patients who can tolerate the removal of fluid at a rate of 1 L/h. Duration is 4 hours per session, it can be done daily or alternate day. Target level of clearance of urea ranges from 1.2 to 1.4 (Kt/V).

b. Continuous renal replacement therapy: There are four types of CRRT:

1. Continuous venovenous hemofiltration (CVVH): By this method large amount of plasma accompanied by solute forcibly across the semipermeable membrane which will be replaced by physiological crystalloid solution by convection.

2. Continuous venovenous hemodialysis (CVVHD): This method transports solutes, such as urea across the membrane along the concentration gradient by diffusion. Here dialysate flow rate is 15–40 mL/min.
3. Continuous venovenous hemodiafiltration (CVVHDF): Here both diffusion as well as convection methods are used to replace plasma and solute with physiological solution.
4. Sustained low-efficiency dialysis (SLED): It is hybrid form of RRT and CRRT:
   - Dialysate flow rate 100–200 mL/min similar to blood flow rate
   - Duration is 10–12 hours.
   - Anticoagulation is not required in 75% of cases.
   - It requires modified dialysis machine but not replacement fluids, special filters.
   - Fewer hemodynamic alteration as compared to intermittent hemodialysis
   - It is usually done at night time so various procedures can be done in day time.
   - It is successfully introduced in sepsis.
   - It is recommended to administer drugs after the procedure but with close monitoring of the blood level of the drug.

Q6. Diagnosis and management of renal osteodystrophy.

DNBI/DEC2010 (10)

Pathogenesis of renal osteodystrophy.

MGR/APR2012/MDIII (7)

Metabolic bone diseases in chronic kidney disease.

MUHS/MAY2013/MDI (10)

Renal osteodystrophy.

BF/NOV2012/MDII (11)

Bone involvement in chronic kidney disease.

DNB (DEC 2022) (5)

Classification of chronic kidney disease. Bone manifestations of CKD. Causes of anemia in CKD and its management.

DNB (DEC2019) (10)

Describe different presentation of bone disease in chronic kidney disease and its management.

DR. YSR UNI OF HEALTH SC, VIJAYAWADA, ANDHRA, 2022 (10)

Renal osteodystrophy.

NTR UNI OF HEALTH SCIENCES, VIJAYAWADA, 2018 (10)

BHARATI VIDYAPEETH DEEMED UNI, 2018 (10)

Explain bone disease in CKD.

MGU, 2024 (5)

Chronic kidney disease is described in question 15.

Anemia in CKD is described in question 16.

Discuss the pathogenesis and management of mineral and bone disorder in chronic kidney disease.

WBUHS, 2024 (10)

ANSWER

Bone disease in chronic renal disease is classified into four types:

A. High bone turnover along with high parathormone level (osteitis fibrosa cystica—it is the classical sign of secondary hyperparathyroidism)
B. Osteomalacia due reduced action of active vitamin D3
C. Low bone turnover with low or normal parathormone level—adynamic bone disease
D. Combination of above

Pathophysiology

Dynamic bone disease with secondary hyperparathyroidism relating to abnormal metabolism due to the following factors:

A. Retention of phosphate due to low excretion of phosphate as a consequence of low GFR
B. Retained phosphate in turn stimulates synthesis of fibroblastic growth factor-23 (FGF-23) by osteocytes and also stimulates growth of parathyroid gland mass.
C. Reduced level of ionized calcium as a result of suppression of calcitriol production by kidney failure and FGF-23
D. Retained phosphate stimulate parathormone production

E. Low calcitriol level leads to hypocalcemia by which parathyroid gene transcription directly responsible for the development of hyperparathyroidism.

F. FGF-23 is a risk factor for:
   a. Left ventricular hypertrophy
   b. Mortality in chronic kidney disease (CKD)
   c. Kidney transplant patient

So, increased level of FGF-23 even in presence of normal level of phosphate needs urgent treatment.

When the GFR is below 60 mL/min, the above pathophysiology will start.

Fibroblastic growth factor-23, a member of family of phosphatonins secreted by osteocytes starts increasing in early stage of chronic kidney disease before retention of phosphate leading to hyperphosphatemia. FGF-23 increases the excretion of phosphate through any of the following mechanisms:

A. Increased excretion of phosphate through urine
B. Through stimulation of parathormone increases the excretion of phosphate through urine
C. Diminished absorption of phosphate from the intestine due to suppressed formation of $1,25(OH)_2D_3$.

There is increased turnover of bone in case of hyperparathyroidism which ultimately leads to osteitis fibrosa cystica. Histology of that bone demonstrates the following:

A. Abnormal osteoid
B. Fibrosis of bone and bone marrow
C. In advanced stage, there is formation of cyst in the bone. If this cyst contains blood due to hemorrhage the color of the cyst becomes brown, called brown tumor.

Clinical of severe hyperparathyroidism are:

A. Bone pain
B. Increased fragility of bone
C. Brown tumor
D. Compression syndrome
E. Due to bone marrow fibrosis there is development of resistance to erythropoietin.
F. PTH also behaves like uremic toxin and produces:
   a. Weakness of muscles
   b. Fibrosis of cardiac muscle
   c. Constitutional symptoms

Adynamic bone disease: It occurs in elderly and diabetic patients. It occurs due to:

A. Excessive suppression of parathormone which results from:
   a. Use of vitamin D preparations
   b. Excessive use of calcium-containing phosphate binders
   c. Use of high calcium-containing dialysis solutions
B. Chronic inflammation
C. In combination of both
D. Metabolic acidosis
E. Continuous ambulatory peritoneal dialysis (CAPD)
F. Aluminum deposition

Features are reduced mineralization of bone and reduced bone volume.

Clinical features are musculoskeletal pain due to inability of repair of microfractures that may develop during ordinary physical activity.

Complications of adynamic bone disease is increased incidence of fracture and bone pain which may be associated with soft tissue calcifications in the cardiac muscles and vascular tissue. In the soft tissue, the large concretions of calcium may produce tumoral calcinosis.

Osteomalacia may develop as a result of nonmineralized osteoid due to reduced production of $1,25(OH)_2D_3$. It occurs in case of aluminum deposition, metabolic acidosis, and vitamin D deficiency.

In case of cardiovascular system: There is strong association between cardiovascular mortality and earlier and late stage of chronic kidney disease. Hyperphosphatemia and hypercalcemia are associated with ectopic calcification in coronary arteries and cardiac heart valves. The magnitude of calcification is related to:

A. Age of the patient
B. Hyperphosphatemia
C. Low parathormone level
D. Low bone turnover: In this case calcium will be deposited in the extraosseous sites. There is also association between vascular calcification and osteoporosis. In case of hyperphosphatemia, there is change in expression of gene in the vascular cells to osteoblast-like profile which leads to vascular calcification even to ossification.

Radiological Findings

A. Resorption of subperiosteal bone in the distal and middle phalanges of hands and feet.
B. Osteosclerosis (Rugger-Jersey spine on lateral film)

Calciphylaxis: In advanced chronic kidney disease, there is advanced patches of necrotic areas in legs, thigh, abdomen, and breast, called livedo reticularis—which develops due to occlusion of vessels associated with extensive vascular calcification. Though previously it was thought to develop in case of hyperthyroidism but recently it occurs due to increased use of calcium phosphate binder and oral anticoagulant warfarin therapy. Vitamin K-dependent regeneration of Gla protein prevents vascular calcification. Warfarin decrease the formation of this protein thus leading to development of vascular calcification.

Pathologically, mural calcification with intimal proliferation and fibrosis involving vessels of skin, soft tissue, visceral organ, and skeletal muscles.

Risk factors are:

A. Uremia

B. Caucasian race

C. Raised PTH

D. Malnutrition

E. Diabetes mellitus

F. Protein C and S deficiency

Treatment

A. Dietary restriction of phosphate (cereals, meat, egg, and milk)

B. Phosphate binders:

- **a.** Calcium based binders—calcium acetate, calcium carbonate:
  1. Advantages: Suppression of pH and inexpensive
  2. Disadvantage: Hypercalcemia which leads to ectopic calcification.
- **b.** Aluminum-based binders: Alludrox gel:
  1. Advantages: Inexpensive and very effective
  2. Disadvantage: There is risk of aluminum toxicity.
- **c.** Sevelamer hydrochloride:
  1. Advantage: It avoids aluminum and calcium
  2. Disadvantages: Expensive, gastrointestinal intolerance, need of large dosage, and mild metabolic acidosis
- **d.** Lanthanum carbonate:
  1. Advantage: Avoids calcium and aluminum
  2. Disadvantage: Expensive

C. Vitamin D analog:

- **a.** It directly suppresses PTH secretion
- **b.** It also suppresses PTH secretion by increasing the concentration of ionizing calcium
- **c.** It increases calcium and phosphate absorption from gastrointestinal tract
- **d.** Dose is 0.25 μg/day to start with and gradually increases up to 1 μg/day.

D. Calcimimetic agent:

- **a.** These agents bind to calcium sensing receptors on the parathyroid gland and mimic the effect of increased extracellular calcium.
- **b.** The result is:
  1. PTH level will be decreased
  2. Calcium level will be decreased
  3. Parallel level of phosphate level and the product of calcium and phosphate
- **c.** Side effect: Gastrointestinal intolerance

Q7. Define renal replacement therapy and enumerate the strategies. Discuss the indications and complications of hemodialysis.

DNBII/DEC2012 (10)

Enumerate the problems with hemodialysis. Note on intermittent hemodialysis.

MGR/APR2012/MDIV (7)

Complications of dialysis.

RGUHS/SEP2002/MDII (10)

Dialysis.

MJPRU/2015/MDIII (10) MJPRU/2015/MDI (10)

Continuous renal replacement therapy.

MUHS/MAY2010/MDIV (10)
SNMC/MAY2013/MDIV (10)

Renal replacement therapy.

PGI/APR2013/MDII (10)
SNMC/MAY2013/MDII (10)
MUHS/MAY2011/MDII (10)

Describe principles governing renal replacement therapy.

ERA/MAY2011/MDII (10)

Absolute indications of renal replacement therapy. Different modalities of RRT. Principles of hemodialysis.

AIIMS, BHU, 2020 (10)

Renal replacement therapy—types and indications.

DR. YSR UNIVERSITY OF HEALTH SC, VIJAYAWADA, ANDHRA, 2022 (10)

Dialysis dementia.

MGR UNIVERSITY, TAMIL NADU, 2020 (10)

Renal replacement therapy.

BHARATI VIDYAPEETH DEEMED UNI, JHELUM, 2019 (10)

NTR UNI OF HEALTH SC, VIJAYAWADA, 2018 (10)

Continuous renal replacement therapy.

RAJIV GANDHI UNI OF HEALTH SC, KARNATAKA, 2018 (10)

Enumerate emergency indications of dialysis in chronic kidney disease patients and describe the complications which can occur during hemodialysis and its related managements.

MANIPUR UNIVERSITY, 2019 (10)

Renal replacement therapy.

RAJASTHAN UNIVERSITY, 2018 (25)

ANSWER

Indications of Dialysis

A. Absolute indications:
- **a.** Hyperkalemia >6.5 mmol/L or rapidly rising potassium level regardless the ECG changes
- **b.** Volume overload—pulmonary edema refractory to diuretics

B. Relative indications:
- **a.** Intractable acidosis (pH < 7.1)
- **b.** Uremia:
  1. Uremic pericarditis
  2. Uremic symptoms with blood urea level >40 mmol/L
- **c.** Critically unwell patients present in intensive therapy unit:
  1. Start before toxin accumulation
  2. Allow safe administration of volume, feeding, and transfusion.
- **d.** Hyperthermia
- **e.** Removal of toxins and poisons—lithium, antimicrobials, and ethylene glycol
- **f.** Bleeding diathesis
- **g.** eGFR < 10 mL/min

Complications of Hemodialysis

A. Intradialytic hypotension: It is the most common complication of dialysis procedure characterized by lightheadedness, cramping, dizziness, and nausea as the blood pressure goes down to very low level. This hypotension has been divided into four categories:
- **a.** Volume related issues: It occurs due to:
  1. High ultrafiltration rate
  2. Incorrectly low dry weight
  3. Low level of sodium in dialysate fluid
- **b.** Inadequate vasoconstriction: It occurs due to:
  1. Use of antihypertensive drugs just prior to dialysis
  2. If temperature of dialysate is higher than that of patient's body
  3. Autonomic neuropathy
  4. Eating during the time of dialysis
- **c.** Cardiac factors:
  1. Cardiac failure
  2. Ischemic heart disease—myocardial infarction due to hypotension
  3. Cardiac arrhythmias—preexisting cardiovascular disease, electrolyte imbalance, acidosis, and hypotension
- **d.** Other causes:
  1. Air embolism: It occurs due to inadvertent entry of air into the circuit.
  2. Reaction with dialyzer
  3. Hemolysis: It occurs due to the following:
     - Obstruction or narrowing of blood lines due to kinking, defective manufacturing, use of small-gauge needles
     - Incorrect electrolyte concentration, contaminated with chemicals in dialysate
  4. Myocardial infarction
  5. Septicemia
  6. Pericardial tamponade
  7. Severe anemia

B. Dialysis disequilibrium syndrome: It occurs in acutely uremic subjects with high blood urea level >150 mmol/L and he will be subjected prolonged hemodynamic session.

Pathophysiology: In dialysis, rapid correction of blood urea will reduce the blood urea as compared to brain cell urea level. So, due to intracellular hypertonicity water will enter into the brain cell leading to cerebral edema with or without intracerebral acidosis.

Clinical features are:

a. In mild cases: Nausea, vomiting, restlessness, and headache

b. In severe cases: Seizures, obtundation, stupor, and coma

C. Technical complications:

a. Vascular access:

1. Infectious complications due to gram-positive bacteria, such as *Staphylococcus aureus* and coagulase-negative staphylococci.

2. Stenosis of arteriovenous fistula or arteriovenous graft. It leads to swelling of the arms, difficult cannulation and prolonged postdialysis bleeding.

b. Rupture of the dialyzer

c. Failure of water purification system

d. Dialyzer reaction: There are two types of reactions:

1. Type A reaction or anaphylactic reaction: It occurs within first several minutes of dialysis but it may occurs after >30 minutes of dialysis. It occurs due to contaminated dialysate, allergy to ethylene oxide, AN-069 dialysis membrane, reuse of dialyzer, or heparin:

- Milder symptoms are cough, sneezing, abdominal cramping, diarrhea, and itching.
- Severe symptoms are breathlessness, sense of warmth feeling, sense of impending doom, cardiac arrest leading to death.

2. Type B reaction: It starts after 20–60 minutes after start of treatment. Symptoms are chest pain and back pain.

D. Long-term complications:

a. Infections

b. Cardiovascular disease

c. Bone disease

d. Malnutrition

e. Dermatological manifestations

f. Intracranial bleeding—hypertension and pre-existing vascular disease

Complications of Peritoneal Dialysis

A. Peritonitis: It occurs due to infection of the peritoneal membrane. It occurs from the following:

a. Contamination by touch due to improper technique

b. Extension of infecting organism around the peritoneal catheter

c. Translocation of bacteria across the intestinal wall

d. Blood-borne infection from bacteremia or sepsis from another source

Types of peritonitis:

a. Refractory peritonitis: It is characterized by failure of peritoneal effluent to clear after 5 days of treatment with antibiotics.

b. Relapsing peritonitis: It is characterized by reoccurrence of peritonitis with same organism after an episode of sterile peritonitis developing within 4 weeks after completion of treatment of previous episode.

c. Fungal peritonitis

d. Peritonitis with the growth of multiple enteric organisms

e. Repeat peritonitis: Reoccurrence of peritonitis with same organism 4 weeks after treatment with antibiotic

f. Sclerosing encapsulating peritonitis

B. Tunnel infection: Catheter site infection by *Staphylococcus* or *Pseudomonas* infection. It is characterized by purulent drainage with or without development of erythema around the exit site.

C. Leakage in peritoneum: It is characterized by leakage of dialyzing fluid around the entrance site into the different tissue planes, rectus muscle sheath, or Scarpa's fascia leading to peritoneal wall edema. It may be due to defect in intrinsic peritoneum, abdominal wall, and diaphragm.

D. Electrolyte imbalance: Hypokalemia can develop which affect cardiovascular and other infection.

E. Hypoalbuminemia is frequent and is associated with increased morbidity and mortality.

Renal Replacement Therapy

It can be defined as removal of excess electrolytes, toxins, drugs, and fluid which accumulate in intravascular as well as extravascular spaces in case of acute kidney injury due to different causes. Most of the time it can be done through the venovenous extracorporeal route where blood pump drives the venous blood through artificial membrane.

Absolute indications of renal replacement therapy:

A. Severe metabolic acidosis having pH <7.1 refractory to medical therapy

B. Severe hyperkalemia having potassium level >6.5 mEq/L refractory to medical therapy

C. Severe hypercalcemia
D. Severe hypermagnesemia
E. Drugs intoxication:
  a. Ethylene glycol
  b. Methanol
  c. Lithium
  d. Salicylates
  e. Theophylline
F. Severe pulmonary edema refractory to diuretic therapy and severe respiratory distress and worsening of the cardiac function
G. Symptomatic uremia:
  a. Uremic pericarditis
  b. Uremic encephalopathy
  c. Severe and intractable vomiting

Different Types of Renal Replacement Therapy

Continuous renal replacement therapy (CRRT): Principles of CRRT:

A. Diffusion: Here large particle, such as albumin or cells cannot pass through semipermeable membrane but small molecules, such as potassium and urea pass across the concentration gradient from plasma to dialysate. Dialysate flow rate is 15,040 mL/min in CRRT but in intermittent hemodialysis (IHD) it is 300–450 mL/min. Example is continuous venovenous hemodialysis.
B. Convection: Here plasma water is pushed across the semipermeable membrane by negative filtering pressure in the dialyzer and takes solute with it just like glomerular filtration. So, here large volume of fluid replacement solution is required. Example is continuous venovenous hemofiltration.
C. Diffusion plus convection: Here both dialysate and replacement fluid are utilized. This is the principle of continuous venovenous hemodiafiltration.
D. Ultrafiltration: Here the fluid is taken out without any solute or replacement fluid. This is the principle of SCUF (slow continuous ultrafiltration).

Here assessment of body fluid status is very essential:

A. Hypovolemia: No ultrafiltration is required.
B. Euvolemia: No ultrafiltration is required.
C. Volume overload: Here 2–3 L of fluid has to be removed in first 2 hours.

Sustained Low-efficiency Dialysis

It is hybrid form between intermittent hemodialysis and CRRT:

A. Dialysate flow: 100–200 mL/min, similar to blood flow rate
B. Duration: 10–12 × hours
C. It requires modified dialysis machine but not replacement fluid, special filters.
D. Anticoagulation is not required in 75% of cases.
E. Fewer hemodynamic complication as compared to IHD.
F. It is usually done at night time, so various procedures are done during day time.
G. It is successfully done in sepsis, acute kidney injury with adequate urea clearance.
H. It is recommended to administer drugs after the procedure but with close monitoring of the blood level of the drug.

Intermittent Hemodialysis

This modality of extracorporeal therapy is based on diffusive clearance of solute at a definite period of time. It is usually done as outpatient basis 2–3 times weekly. Clearance depends upon the blood flow rate and dialysate rate. In IHD:

A. First session is 2 hours, second session is 3 hours and subsequent session is 4 hours.
B. Blood flow is slow 100–200 mL/min and subsequent increment per session is 50 mL/min/session.
C. Frequency: Since there is frequent rebound rise in blood urea—hence dialysis should be done against blood urea level or uremic symptoms.
D. Small dialyzer is preferable.
E. Fluid removal by ultrafiltration
F. First session should be heparin free or minimize heparin in critical stage or in sepsis because there is chance of bleeding from various sites.

Dialysis Dementia

It is a rare neurological complication in patient undergoing chronic hemodialysis and it is linked to aluminum toxicity.

Etiopathogenesis:

A. Aluminum containing phosphate binders used previously in case of hyperphosphatemia

B. Aluminum contaminated dialysate used in case of dialysis can lead to its accumulation in the brain.

C. Impaired excretion of aluminum through the kidney in case of end stage renal failure.

Clinical features:

A. Cognitive dysfunction like dementia and memory loss.

B. Slurred speech

C. Myoclonus

D. Seizures

E. Depression

F. Anxiety

G. Gait disturbances

H. Tremor

Diagnosis:

A. Progression of the symptoms along with the progression of the dialysis.

B. Serum level of aluminum

C. Electroencephalography demonstrating slowing of the brain activity

D. MRI brain demonstrating cortical atrophy.

Management:

A. Aluminum containing phosphate binders should be avoided

B. Purified water should be used.

C. Chelating agents like deferoxamine should be used to chelate aluminum from the body.

D. Supportive therapy like anti-seizure drugs,

E. Regular monitoring of the aluminum level.

Q8. Discuss the etiology, clinical features, and diagnostic evaluation of urinary tract infection.

DNBIII/JUN2013 (10)

Etiology, pathogenesis, and treatment of acute uncomplicated urinary tract infection.

DNBIIIB/JUN2015 (10)

Treatment of acute uncomplicated urinary tract infection.

MGR/OCT2012/MDII (7)

Management of recurrent urinary tract infection.

MUHS/MAY2013/MDII (10)

Recurrent urinary tract infection.

BF/MAY2012/MDII (12)

Discuss causes and diagnosis of recurrent urinary tract infection in a 60-year-old male.

ERA/MAY2012/MDIV (10)

Enumerate the causes of recurrent urinary tract infection. Clinical features and management of emphysematous pyelonephritis.

DNB (DEC2018) (10)

Describe the diagnostic approach and outlines of management in urinary tract infection.

ODISHA UNI, 2022 (10)

How can you evaluate recurrent urinary tract infection in a 25 years old female?

DNB, 2024 MAY (10)

Diagnosis of acute pyelonephritis and write a short note on emphysematous pyelonephritis.

NTR UNI OF HEALTH SC, ANDHRA, 2022 (10)

Emphysematous pyelonephritis has been written in the question number 40.

ANSWER

Definition

Urinary tract infection (UTI) can be defined as microbial invasion starting from urethral orifice to renal cortex. So presence of bacteriuria proves that anywhere in urinary tract is at risk of microbial invasion. Upper urinary tract involves kidney but lower urinary tract involves urinary bladder, prostate, and urethra.

Recurrent Urinary Tract Infection

Recurrent urinary tract infection may be of two types: (1) Reinfection and (2) relapse.

Reinfection can be defined as occurrence of two uncomplicated infections within the span of 6 months or three uncomplicated infections within 1 year with different pathogens, but according to recent studies 50% of recurrent infection occurs by identical drug susceptible pathogens. Example is cystourethritis.

Relapse can be defined as infection by same often drug-resistant pathogen requiring longer course of treatment, urologic evaluation, and surgical interventions. Examples are acute pyelonephritis and prostatitis.

Uncomplicated Urinary Tract Infection

This infection is nothing but cystourethritis due to colonization of pathogens in the bladder and urethral mucosa in absence of upper urinary tract disease and the sequelae is rare in absence of morbidity associated with reinfection mainly in women.

Pathogenesis of Urinary Tract Infection

Bacteria involved are:

A. *Escherichia coli*
B. *Klebsiella*
C. *Staphylococcus saprophyticus*
D. *Enterococcus faecalis*
E. *Proteus mirabilis*
F. *Pseudomonas aeruginosa*
G. *Citrobacter*

Risk factors that are associated with UTI are the following:

A. Age
B. Pregnancy
C. Use of diaphragm
D. Sexual intercourse
E. Condom
F. Spermicides especially nonoxynol-9
G. Menopause
H. Delayed postcoital micturition
I. History of recent UTI

Factors that are not associated with increased risk:

A. Use of tampons
B. Use of clothing
C. Personal hygiene, such as cleaning after defecation and during bathing

Enteric flora gain access from the gastrointestinal tract to genitourinary tract due to its close proximity, but how the pathogen migrates is not exactly known. P-fimbriated strain of *E. coli* after entry will colonize in the uroepithelial cell, where glycolipids act as receptors in women who secretes blood group antigen. Escherichia coli encodes for type 1 pilus that contains adhesion FimH, recognizes different cell types associated with meningitis, sepsis, and cystitis. Opsonizing factors are acid pH, normal vaginal flora as well as type-specific cervicovaginal antibodies. This is the stage of persistent asymptomatic bacteriuria. Then the pathogen enters into:

A. Urinary bladder through urethra
B. Kidney through ureter
C. Prostate through ejaculatory duct

Urethra and ureter act as mechanical barrier preventing ascent. But except mechanical obstruction or instrumentation the method of ascent is not known.

In the bladder, normally the growth of uropathogens are prevented by the following though urine supports the bacterial growth:

A. Urinary slime containing mucopolysaccharide layer prevents bacterial colonization
B. Tamm–Horsfall protein, component of uromucoid prevent bacterial colonization by adhering to P-fimbriae.
C. Constant flow of urine
D. Bladder contraction prevents stasis of urine and thus bacterial colonization

In the bladder, bacteria multiply and enter into the bladder mucosa producing bacteriuria. From the bladder pathogen migrates into kidney, here P-fimbriated *E. coli* adheres to the renal tubular cells by Gal-α and Gal-β disaccharide galabiose adhesin producing acute pyelonephritis. Following host factors prevents renal infection:

A. High urine osmolality
B. High ammonium concentration
C. Phagocytic activity
D. Increased rate of urine flow

In case of urethral catheterization defense mechanism against the invasion of pathogen is lost by the following mechanisms:

A. Disruption of glycosaminoglycan layer of bladder
B. Biofilm formation on the introduced catheter—it protects the pathogen against the following:
  a. Flushing by urine
  b. Antibiotics
  c. Host defense

These pathogens including *P. mirabilis*, *Morganella morganii*, and *Providencia stuartii* colonizing the catheter are less virulent because of their lack of P-fimbria thus showing lower incidence of febrile bacteriuria.

In case of spinal cord injuries, catheter may be present for long duration, in that case there may be lower urinary tract obstruction by the following mechanisms:

A. Catheter blockage by:
  a. Encrustations
  b. Urinary tract stones

B. Associated complications:

a. Scrotal abscesses

b. Epididymitis

c. Prostatitis

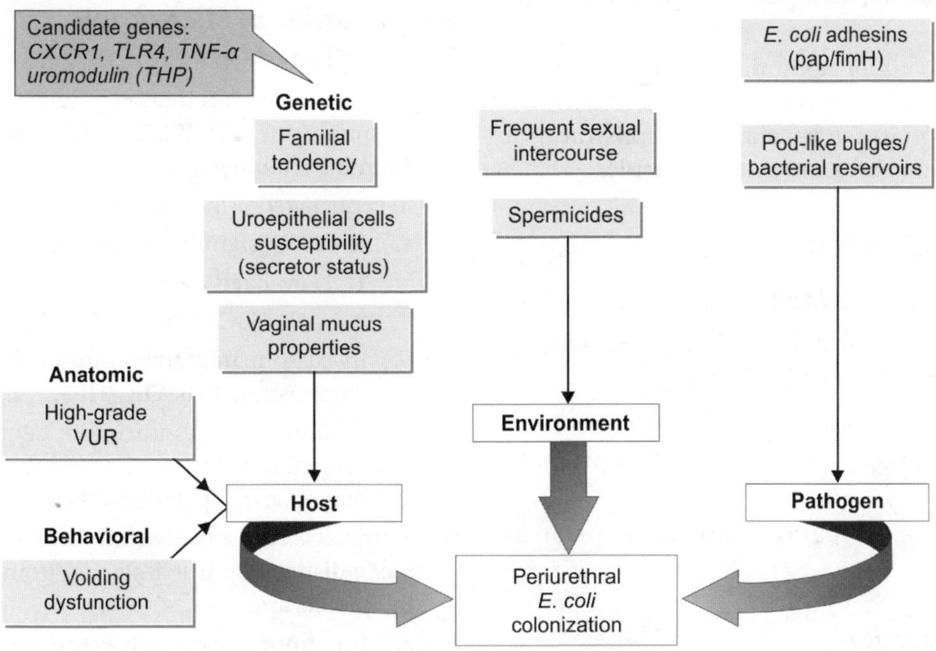

(TLR4: toll-like receptor 4; TNF-α: tumor necrosis factor alpha; UTI: urinary tract infection; VUR: vesicoureteral reflux)

Clinical Features

A. In case of lower urinary tract infection:

a. Dysuria

b. Frequency of micturition

c. Urgency

d. Stranguria

e. Hematuria

f. Suprapubic discomfort

g. In case of recurrent urinary tract infection women can diagnose by herself in nearly 90% of cases.

h. In case of elderly:

1. May present with confusion without incontinence

2. Urinary retention

B. In case of upper urinary tract infection:

a. Fever with chill and rigor

b. Nausea with vomiting

c. Loin pain

d. On examination, there may be costovertebral tenderness.

C. In case of infant, it commonly occurs in boys presenting with fever and failure to thrive.

D. In patients with indwelling catheter present with fever without localizing findings relating to genitourinary tract. But they may present with obstruction of catheter with or without costovertebral tenderness.

E. Prostatitis: It is frequently seen in younger and middle-aged men. 90% of patients with urinary tract infection may present with asymptomatic prostatitis with increased prostate-specific antigen (PSA) which may be elevated for 1 year along with increased volume of prostate. Prostatic syndrome can be divided into four types:

a. Acute bacterial prostatitis: Presenting features are fever with chill and rigor, urgency and frequency of urine, dysuria, perineal pain, low back pain, and other constitutional symptoms. On rectal examination, prostate gland is tender, worm, and swollen.

b. Chronic bacterial prostatitis: Its hallmark is relapsing urinary tract infection presenting with urgency, frequency, nocturia, perineal and low back pain, may be afebrile, prostate examination may be unremarkable. In this case, urine demonstrates positive microscopic examination and uropathogens in culture.

c. Nonbacterial prostatitis: Clinical features are same as that of chronic bacterial prostatitis but urine or prostatic massage sample shows sterile culture.

d. Prostatodynia or noninflammatory prostatitis: Here clinical features are same but urine or prostatic massage specimen demonstrates no inflammatory cells and culture is sterile.

Diagnostic Evaluation

Major Indications of Urine Culture

A. Patients with clinical features of urinary tract infection
B. Removal of indwelling urinary catheter
C. Recently treated urinary tract infection follow-up
D. During pregnancy screening of asymptomatic bacteriuria
E. In obstructive uropathy and stasis prior to instrumentation

Methods of Collection

A. Midstream clean-catch collection of urine after proper washing of external genitalia in a sterile container.
B. Urine collected by single catheterization
C. Suprapubic aspiration of urinary bladder
D. Collection of urine by sterile method from the tube of closed catheter drainage

During collection of urine, introduction of infection into urinary tract at the time of catheterization should be avoided in the following cases:
A. Elderly patients confined in the bed
B. In male with condom catheter
C. Dysfunctional bladder in diabetic patient

Interpretation of Urine Culture

A. In case of properly collected and transported urine specimen 10^5 colony forming unit (CFU)/mL.
B. In case of symptomatic young female with urethritis and pyuria 10^3 CFU/mL.
Poor method of collection, delayed transport of urine is indicated by presence of mixed flora or intermediate colony count.
C. In case of suprapubic needle aspiration of urine ≥ 2 colonies (≤200 CFU/mL) showing same organism suggests growth of specific bacteria.
D. In case of prostatic secretion of patient with UTI shows >10–15 WBC/HPF leukocytes along with lipid laden macrophages suggests prostatic inflammation. Colony count of $\geq 10^5$ CFU/mL of same pathogen suggests acute bacterial prostatitis.

Interpretation of Microscopic Examination of Urine

Microscopic urine examination is done from:
A. Unspun urine: ≥10 WBC/cc/HPF while examined in counting chamber
B. In centrifuged urine sediment:
   a. In case of significant bacteriuria:
      1. Few bacteria/HPF
      2. ≥10 WBC/HPF
   b. In case of negative culture, 25% patients will demonstrate ≥10 WBC/HPF.
C. Gram stain of unspun urine or centrifuged urinary sediment shows specific morphology and stain characteristics of specific pathogen.
D. Pyuria: It is very sensitive indicator of inflammation as it can distinguish true infection from contamination. But pitfalls are:
   a. It cannot distinguish acute urethral syndrome from bacterial UTI
   b. Tuberculosis is cause of pyuria with negative urine culture

Clinical Situations Related to Presence of Bacteriuria

A. Staghorn calculi in kidney harbors urea-splitting organism—proteus
B. Hospital-acquired infections—*Klebsiella*, *Pseudomonas aeruginosa*
C. *Staphylococcus aureus* due to staphylococcal bacteremia
D. *Enterococcus* and coagulase-negative staphylococci in elderly indicates recent catheterization or instrumentation.
E. *Candida* infection in patient with prolonged antibiotic therapy

Localization of Site of Infection

Localization of site is very important because upper urinary tract involvement can denote uropathy, such as:
A. Vesicoureteral reflux
B. Renal stone
C. Congenital abnormalities
D. Occlusion of ureter
E. Prostatic hypertrophy
F. Neurogenic bladder

Findings are: WBC cast, So, duration of treatment is much longer—10–14 days and relapse is common.

Whereas, lower urinary tract infection, such as cystitis is rarely complicated, so duration of treatment is 3–5 days and relapse is rare. Here cast is not present.

Other Diagnostic Procedures

A. Plain X-ray of abdomen: Radio-opaque shadow indicates kidney stones
B. Ultrasonography (USG) of kidneys, ureters, and bladder (KUB):
   a. Kidney size enlarged: Acute pyelonephritis
   b. Small kidney size: Chronic pyelonephritis
   c. Incomplete bladder emptying
   d. Hydronephrosis
C. Intravenous urography:
   a. It will exclude anatomical abnormalities after resolution of infection.
   b. Ureteric stone or pelvic stone
   c. Any stricture in the ureter or urethra
D. Cystourethrography: It will detect vesicoureteral reflux, indicates reflux nephropathy.
E. Cystoscopy: It can detect:
   a. Bladder cancer
   b. Incomplete bladder emptying
   c. Prostatic cancer
   d. Enlarged median lobe of prostate
F. Technetium-99m dimercaptosuccinic acid (99mTc-DMSA) scanning can detect scars (reflux nephropathy)

Treatment of Uncomplicated Urinary Tract Infection

A. Acute uncomplicated cystitis:
   a. First-line drugs:
      1. Nitrofurantoin: 50–100 mg twice daily
      2. Fosfomycin: 3 g single dose
      3. Pivmecillinam: 400 mg twice daily
   b. Second-line drugs:
      1. Ciprofloxacin: 500 mg twice daily
      2. Levofloxacin: 500 mg daily
      3. Cephalexin: 500 mg four times daily
      4. Cefixime: 400 mg four times daily
      5. Doxycycline: 100 mg twice daily

   Duration is 3–5 days.
B. Acute uncomplicated pyelonephritis: In case of urosepsis 2–3 days course of intravenous antibiotics followed by oral antibiotics of same dose as in case acute uncomplicated cystitis. Intravenous drugs are the parenteral form of above drugs including ceftriaxone 2 g intravenously twice daily.

   But here the duration of treatment is 14 days.

Management of Recurrent Urinary Tract Infection

A. Increased fluid intake to >2 L/day
B. Spermicide lubricated condom should be discouraged.
C. Avoid estrogen cream per vagina in postmenopausal women
D. Postcoital single dose of following antibiotics:
   a. Nitrofurantoin 50 mg
   b. Trimethoprim 100 mg
   c. Norfloxacin 200 mg
   d. Cephalexin 250 mg.
E. Long-term low dose of above drugs can be given for 4 weeks.

In all above uncomplicated upper or lower UTI or recurrent UTI antibiotic can be changed according to the culture and sensitivity of urine after 48–72 hours.

Causes of recurrent urinary tract infection in 25 years old female:

A. Anatomical factors:
   a. Short urethra that helps to reach the bacteria in the urinary tract.
   b. Urinary tract obstruction due to stones or stricture
B. Physiological factors:
   a. Vesicoureteral reflux leading to back flow of the urinary flow into the ureter from urinary bladder.
   b. Neurogenic bladder: Incomplete emptying of the bladder due to neurologic condition.
C. Behavioral factors:
   a. Poor genital hygiene
   b. Frequent sexual activity
D. Life style factors:
   a. Spermicide or diaphragm use leading to introduction of bacteria into the urethra.
   b. Incomplete emptying of the bladder leading to increased proliferation of the bacteria.
E. Systemic diseases:
   a. Diabetes mellitus
   b. Immunosuppression due to chemotherapy or HIV infection or estrogen deficiency.

  - c. Increased genetic susceptibility to *E. coli* infection due to increased adhesion of these bacteria to the wall of the wall of the urinary tract.

F. Decreased amount of lactobacilli leading to increased propensity to bacterial proliferation.

G. Chronic urinary tract infection either due to colonization with multidrug resistant bacteria or inadequate treatment which is most common cause.

H. Gynecological causes:

  - a. Prolapse of uterus leading to development of cystocele resulting infection.

I. Sexually transmitted diseases like chlamydia

Approach can be written from the above causes.

Clinical features of emphysematous pyelonephritis:

Q9. Discuss the etiopathogenesis, differential diagnosis, and treatment of rapidly progressive glomerulonephritis.

DNBIIA/DEC2013 (10)

Rapidly progressive glomerulonephritis.

MGR/MAR2010/MDI (5)
MUHS/MAY2010/MDII (10)
MGR/OCT2011/MDI (5)

Discuss approach to a patient of rapidly progressive glomerulonephritis. Discuss treatment of immune glomerulonephritis.

MUHS/NOV2013/MDII (25)

What is rapidly progressive crescentic glomerulonephritis? Discuss its pathology and management.

BF/MAY2013/MDI (10)

Management of patient with rapidly progressive renal failure.

BF/NOV2012/MDIII (20)

Discuss the approach to rapidly progressive glomerulonephritis.

AIIMS, BBS 2020 (10)

Describe the pathophysiology of RPGN.

AIIMS, BBS, 2023 (10)

Discuss the etiopathogenesis, clinical features, investigations and management of rapidly progressive glomerulonephritis.

MAHARASHTRA UNI OF HEALTH SC, VIJAYAWADA, 2022 (25)

Rapidly progressive glomerulonephritis.

MGR UNIVERSITY, TAMIL NADU, 2020 (5)

Rapidly progressive glomerulonephritis.

MAHATMA UNIVERSITY, 2015 (10)

ANSWER

Definition

Rapidly progressive glomerulonephritis (RPGN) is characterized by presence of glomerular disease as evidenced by hematuria, red blood cell casts, and proteinuria along with rapid and progressive loss of kidney function leading to renal failure over days to weeks. Clinical hallmark of this disease is presence of crescents for which it can also be known as crescentic nephritis.

Classification

A. Primary causes:

  - a. Type 1 RPGN: Anti-GBM antibody disease (Goodpasture syndrome)
  - b. Type 2 RPGN: Granular glomerular immune complex disease
  - c. Type 3 RPGN: Pauci-immune RPGN

B. Secondary due to systemic diseases:

  - a. Poststreptococcal glomerulonephritis
  - b. Postviral glomerulonephritis
  - c. Vasculitis:
    1. Small vessel vasculitis (immune complex):
       - Cryoglobulinemia
       - Systemic lupus erythematosus
       - Henoch–Schönlein purpura
    2. Small vessel vasculitis (pauci-immune):
       - Microscopic polyangiitis
       - Eosinophillic granulomatosis
       - Wegener granulomatosis
    3. Median vessel disease:
       - Polyarteritis nodosa
       - Goodpasture syndrome

4. Medication related:
   - Minocycline
   - Hydralazine
   - Propylthiouracil
   - Drug-induced lupus
   - Rifampicin
   - Penicillamine

Pathophysiology

Primary feature is formation of crescent in the following way:

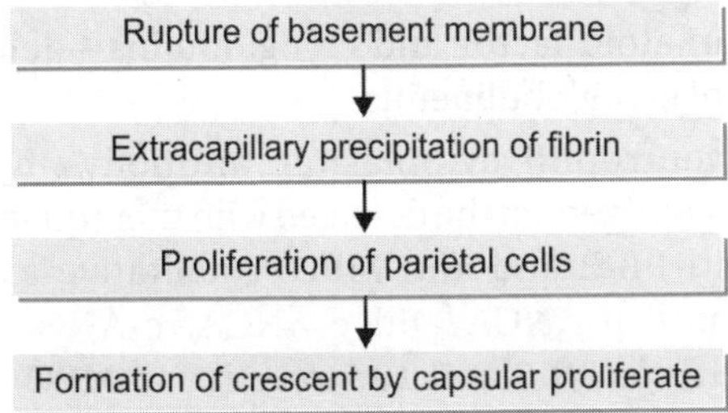

Each above disease will follow the different pathways leading to formation of crescent as follows:

A. In case of anti-GBM disorder: Here immunoglobulin G (IgG) antibodies developed against α-3 chain of type IV collagen in noncollagenous domain of glomerular as well as pulmonary capillary basement membrane will damage the capillary wall by activation of polymorphs and local complement. Triggering factors for development of antibodies are smoking and hydrocarbon. There is also evidence of association with human leukocyte antigen (HLA)-DR15.

B. In 10–15% cases, there is deposition of immune complexes in the tuft of glomerular capillaries in two ways:

a. Immune complexes are formed in the circulation and then deposited in the capillary wall.

b. Immune complexes may be formed in situ.

Triggering antigen may be:

a. Exogenous, such as bacteria or virus

b. Endogenous, such as nuclear or tumor antigen

Immune complex disease may be multisystem disease or may be a complication of another primary glomerular disease.

C. In 50–70% cases, there is involvement of antinuclear cytoplasmic antibody developed against either myeloperoxidase (MPO) or proteinase-3 (PR-3) or both (in case of drug-induced disease). This antibody activates polymorphs and systemic complement in alternate pathway and injures capillary wall conjointly with tumor necrosis factor-α and different cytokines. During this process, anti-plasminogen as well as plasminogen activator antibodies are formed which by inhibiting fibrinolysis produces fibrinoid necrosis and thrombophilia.

D. Ultimately crescent is formed by:

a. Proliferation of both parietal and visceral cells

b. Polymerization of fibrin

c. Monocytes, macrophages and T cells infiltration

d. Myofibroblast cells invasion from interstitium

Following factors play crucial role in the formation of crescent:

a. Tumor necrosis factor-α and β

b. Macrophage inflammatory factor

c. Interleukin-1

d. Macrophage chemotactic protein-1

Histology

A. Primary lesion is rupture of capillary wall along with proliferation of visceral and parietal cells in the Bowmen's space in the form of crescent.

B. Proliferation of podocytes along with infiltration of myofibroblast, lymphocytes, and macrophages.

C. Antineutrophil cytoplasmic antibody (ANCA) is found in different stages of crescent, such as cellular, fibrocellular, and fibrous stages. But in case of anti-GBM disease all lesions are found in the same stage.

D. In the periglomerular region there is evidence of interstitial inflammation.

E. Later on within few days to weeks fibrosis develops in the form of sclerosis and obliteration of glomerulus.

F. Immunofluorescence microscope can demonstrate:

a. Linear deposition of anti-GBM antibodies along the capillary wall and the lesions are in same stage.

b. In case of immune complex disease, there are deposition of IgG, IgA, and IgM along the glomerular capillary wall; here, the lesions are present in different stages.

G. In case of pauci-immune rapidly progressive glomerulonephritis:

a. There may be no deposit.

b. There may be scanty deposit of IgG or IgM or C3 as seen by immunofluorescence microscope.

Clinical Features

In all cases, there is ultimate rapid decline in renal function with nonspecific clinical features, but in some cases, the presentation may be shortness of breath with or without hemoptysis:

A. In case of anti-GBM disease, there may be shortness of breath, hemoptysis due to pulmonary involvement along with hematuria, edema with rapidly progressive renal failure within weeks to months.

B. External manifestations of ANCA vasculitis are:

   a. Skin—palpable purpura, livedo reticularis

   b. Eye—scleritis, episcleritis

   c. Nose—sinusitis, nasal cartilage necrosis, epistaxis

   d. Ear—impairment of hearing, otitis media

   e. Central nervous manifestation—mononeuritis multiplex, numbness of extremities, blurred vision, weakness of extremities

   f. Gastrointestinal—abdominal pain due to ischemia or infarction, nausea, vomiting

   g. Respiratory system—tracheal or bronchial ulceration, hoarseness of voice, cough, shortness of breath

   h. Pulmonary hemorrhage, diffuse pulmonary infiltrate

   i. Oral mucosa—ulcers

   j. Constitutional symptoms—fever, arthralgia, night sweat, weight loss

So, this disease should be assessed as quickly as possible otherwise the patient will enter into rapidly progressive renal failure and at that time patient presents with weight loss, nausea, vomiting, and oliguria.

Evaluation of Rapidly Progressive Glomerulonephritis

A. Urine analysis for microscopic hematuria and proteinuria:

   a. Dysmorphic red blood cells—glomerular hematuria

   b. Protein—it can suggest nephrotic or subnephrotic range proteinuria.

B. Serum electrolytes to see evidence of hyper- or hyponatremia, hyperkalemia, hypocalcemia

C. Serum creatinine to assess the status of renal failure

D. Complete blood count—eosinophilia suggests eosinophilic granulomatosis with microscopic polyangiitis.

E. Serology:

   a. Detection of anti-GBM antibodies by enzyme-linked immunosorbent assay (ELISA) or Western blot test, which are negative for that antibodies but history is suggestive of Goodpasture syndrome, in those patient kidney biopsy should be undertaken to detect that antibody.

   b. Hepatitis B virus (HBV)

   c. Hepatitis C virus (HCV) antibody

   d. Human immunodeficiency virus (HIV)

   e. Antistreptolysin O for poststreptococcal infection

   f. Lupus—antinuclear antibody, anti-ds-DNA antibody, anti-Smith antibody

F. Complement, C3, and C4 level: Low in case of granular immune complex disease due to systemic lupus erythematosus (SLE), cryoglobulinemia, primary membranoproliferative glomerulonephritis

G. Rheumatoid factor and cryoglobulins—detected in case of cryoglobulinemia

H. Antineutrophil cytoplasmic antibody—by ELISA newer antigen can be detected with titer (quantitative) of anti-PR-3 and anti-MPO. Qualitative assay can estimate p-ANCA and c-ANCA. c-ANCA is 90% reactive to PR-3 and 10% reactive to MPO and just opposite in case of p-ANCA where it is 90% reactive to MPO and 10% reactive to PR-3.

I. New two antibodies are recently found in case of ANCA positive patients. These are:

   a. Lysosome-associated membrane protein-2 (LAMP-2)—this antibody directly activates neutrophil thus damaging endothelium directly. It is found in >90% patients with ANCA positive and ANCA negative having pauci-immune crescentic glomerulonephritis.

   b. Anti-plasminogen antibody present in both MPO and PRO-3 positive patients and correlates with venous thromboembolism.

J. Chest X-ray—demonstrate:

   a. Cavitary lesion—vasculitis

   b. Diffuse infiltrate—Goodpasture syndrome

K. Bronchoscopy—diffuse alveolar hemorrhage

L. Skin biopsy—to detect vasculitis

M. Otolaryngologic evaluation—ulcer in nasal septum—Wegener granulomatosis

N. Kidney biopsy is the main stay of diagnosis of RPGN

O. To exclude thrombotic thrombocytopenic purpura serum lactate dehydrogenase, anti-cardiolipin antibody, reticulocyte, and platelet count are required.

Treatment

This patient requires urgent treatment even prior to definite diagnosis. So, empirical treatment has to be started at earliest.

Empiric Treatment

A. Intravenous methylprednisolone 500–1,000 g daily for 3 days

B. Plasmapheresis—it has to be provided if there is associated hemoptysis (suggestive of Goodpasture syndrome).

Antiglomerular basement membrane disease:

A. Pulse methylprednisolone—500–1,000 g intravenously in 100 mL 0.9% saline for 3 days.

This is followed by (oral prednisolone 1 mg/kg/day to maximum 60 g/day plus cyclophosphamide 1–2 mg/kg/day) for 3–6 months.

If the patient is intolerant to cyclophosphamide mycophenolate mofetil or rituximab can be given.

B. Plasma exchange—8–10 treatment in <2 weeks (by two-third volume of 4.5% albumin and one-third fresh frozen plasma).

Serum anti-GBM antibodies titer should be estimated weekly to confirm the treatment efficacy.

Discontinuation of treatment:

a. Treatment should be stopped with the anti-GBM titer will be negative. It takes about 4–6 weeks.

b. In the maintenance phase low dose of prednisolone with azathioprine can be considered.

C. According to recent study immunoadsorption treatment can be of great benefit.

Antineutrophil cytoplasmic antibody positive pauci-immune crescentic glomerulonephritis:

A. Intravenous methylprednisolone for 3 days followed by oral prednisolone.

B. Intravenous or oral cyclophosphamide, in case of intolerance to cyclophosphamide rituximab

C. Plasmapheresis: It is indicated in:

a. Rapid deterioration of renal function

b. Severe renal involvement during presentation

D. Hemodialysis in:

a. Serum creatinine if >4 mg/mL

b. There is pulmonary hemorrhage

c. If the patient has anti-GBM antibodies

Duration of therapy is 12–16 weeks but maintenance therapy must be continued.

In case of immune complex glomerulonephritis:

A. Here treat should be done according to etiology.

B. Poststreptococcal glomerulonephritis can be recovered spontaneously but very rarely glucocorticoid can be administered in crescentic nephritis.

In case of drug-induced glomerulonephritis:

A. Most of the patients recover spontaneously after removal of offending drug

B. But in few cases treatment of pauci-immune disease has to be given.

In case double-positive antibody glomerulonephritis (GN): Here the treatment is similar to pauci-immune GN, plasmapheresis should be added.

Q10. Pathogenesis, natural history, and management of diabetic nephropathy.

DNBIB/JUN2015 (10)

Discuss the clinical features, diagnosis staging, and treatment of diabetic nephropathy.

MGR/MAR2009/MDII (20)

Mention the steps for slowing progression of diabetic nephropathy.

DNBIIIA/DEC2015 (5)

What are the common causes of nephrotic syndrome? How will you diagnose and manage a case of diabetic nephropathy?

MJPRU/2016/MDIII (20)

Pathology of diabetic kidney disease.

KERALA UNI, 2022 (10)

Diabetic nephropathy.

KERALA UNI, 2021 (10)

MGR UNI, TAMIL NADU, 2021 (5)

Diabetic nephropathy.

NTR UNI OF HEALTH SC, VIJAYAWADA (10)

Describe the structure of nephron. Explain the pathological classification of diabetic nephropathy.

AIIMS (BHU), 2024 (10)

Structure of nephron has been described in question 18, 25, 29.

Histopathology in diabetic nephropathy.

RAJASTHAN UNIVERSITY, 2017 (10)

ANSWER

Definition

Diabetic nephropathy is a clinical syndrome characterized by:

A. Persistent albuminuria (>300 mg/day) is confirmed at least two occasions 3–6 months apart.

B. Progressive decline in effective filtration rate

C. Progressive increase in arterial blood pressure

Pathogenesis of Diabetic Nephropathy

Risk Factors for Diabetic Nephropathy

A. Demographic factors:

- **a.** Male sex
- **b.** Elderly age
- **c.** Race: Black, American, Indian, and Hispanic

B. Hereditary factors:

- **a.** Genetic history of kidney disease
- **b.** Family history of diabetic kidney disease

C. Systemic disease:

- **a.** Hypertension: In type 2 diabetes mellitus (DM) patients 10 mm Hg increase in systolic blood pressure over 140 mm Hg is associated with increase in hazard ratio for development of micro- and macroalbuminuria and impaired function of kidney is characterized by doubling of baseline creatinine level and baseline eGFR < 60 mL/min.
- **b.** Obesity
- **c.** Hyperglycemia: In type 1 DM, intense glycemic control targeting HbA1c level ≤ 7% is associated with reduced risk of microalbuminuria.

D. Injury to the kidney:

- **a.** Toxins
- **b.** Acute kidney injury
- **c.** Smoking

E. Diet: High-protein intake

Pathophysiology

Sorbitol-aldose Reductase Pathway

In hyperglycemia high level of intracellular glucose activate polyol pathway, where aldose reductase with the help of nicotinamide adenine dinucleotide phosphate (NADPH) as a cofactor reduces glucose to sorbitol, which is further metabolized into fructose by sorbitol dehydrogenase with the help of nicotinamide adenine dinucleotide (NAD) as a cofactor. As a result, intracellular sorbitol level will be increased and produces potential harmful osmotic consequences. Fructose on the other hand will be converted into fructose-3-phosphate and then into 3-deoxyglucosone—both these substrates participate in the advanced glycation end product.

As a result of excessive use of NADPH, less NADPH will be available for action of glutathione reductase to maintain normal pool of reduced glutathione which leads to less capability of the cells to respond oxidative stress and increased activity of compensatory mechanism, such as glucose monophosphate shunt which supplies NADPH.

As a result of increased usage of NAD by sorbitol dehydrogenase the ration NADH: NAD will be increased leading to alteration of cellular function, such as NADH is a substrate for NADH oxidase leading to generation of intracellular oxidant species.

Protein Kinase C

Various isoforms of protein kinase C phosphorylate different target proteins which are responsible for intracellular transduction that regulates vascular contractility, permeability, vascular function, flow in the vessel, and cell proliferation. Activation of this protein kinase C is responsible for the following harmful effects:

A. Increased angiogenesis

B. Increased vascular permeability

C. Capillary obliteration

D. Fibrosis of the involved organ

E. Increase endothelin-1, prostaglandin E2, induction of vascular endothelial growth factor, and transforming growth factor

F. Reduced nitric oxide production

G. Overexpression of fibrinolytic inhibitor, plasminogen activator inhibitor-1

H. Inflammatory mediators

I. Oxidative stress stimulation

Advanced Glycation End Products

These products through ligation with specific receptors of podocytes, smooth muscle cells, endothelial, mesangial, and tubular epithelial cells produce following consequences:

A. Generation of reactive oxygen species

B. Release of inflammatory cytokines:

- **a.** Interleukin-1
- **b.** Interleukin-6
- **c.** Tumor necrosis factors
- **d.** Activation of transcription factors

C. Increases production of type IV collagen

Oxidative Stress

It is the resultant of imbalance between production of oxidants and the capacity to detoxify reactive intermediates by biological system leading to oxidation of protein, carbohydrates, lipids, and DNA that is responsible for diabetic macro- as well as microvascular complications. Reactive oxygen species include superoxide, hydroxyl, peroxyl, and hydrogen peroxide.

Growth Factors

Extracellular matrix provides mechanical support renal cells, helps in cell to cell and cell to other elements interactions. Growth factor controls the formation and turnover of extracellular matrix:

A. Transforming growth factor-beta: This prothrombotic growth factor plays a critical role in fibrotic and sclerotic manifestations of nephron, such as glomerulosclerosis and interstitial fibrosis.

B. Connective tissue growth factor: It increases the production of extracellular matrix proteins leading to change in structure of cytoskeleton. It also directly mediates prothrombotic activity.

C. Vascular endothelial growth factor: It maintains the integrity and viability of endothelium through the following mechanisms:

- **a.** Promoting endothelial cell proliferation and survival
- **b.** Remodeling of interstitial matrix
- **c.** Mediating endothelium-dependent vasodilatation

It also helps in neovascularization and glomerulosclerosis.

Podocytes also affects glomerular blood flow by altering the synthesis of GBM constituents.

Adipocytokines

These bioactive peptides secreted by adipose tissue act locally or distally through autocrine and paracrine effects:

A. Adiponectin: It acts through receptors AdipoR1 and AdipoR2 and participates in activated protein kinase and cyclic adenosine monophosphate (AMP)-dependent protein kinase. It generates reactive oxygen species (ROS).

B. Leptin: It has following proinflammatory effects:

- **a.** Impairment of endothelial functions
- **b.** Stimulation of inflammatory signaling pathways
- **c.** Increase in oxidative stress
- **d.** Stimulation of aggregation and migration of platelet
- **e.** Stimulation of hypertrophy and proliferation of vascular endothelial cells

C. Visfantin: It is produced by visceral fat and performs in the following functions:

- **a.** Promotes maturation of B cells.
- **b.** It inhibits apoptosis of neutrophils

Chemokines

Monocyte-activated chemokines attract macrophages from the vessels along the endothelial gradient.

Adhesion Molecules

These help in binding between the cells and with extracellular matrix. These are composed of three domains, such as intracellular, transmembrane, and extracellular domains:

A. Intercellular adhesion molecule-1: This endothelial and leukocyte-associated transmembrane protein facilitates leukocyte endothelial transmigration. It produces proinflammatory effects and recruit inflammatory leukocytes.

B. Vascular cell adhesion molecule-1: It helps in adhesion of monocytes, eosinophils, basophils, and lymphocytes with vascular endothelium.

Proinflammatory Cytokines

These act as final regulator of effectors. These are interleukin-1 (IL-1), interleukin-6 (IL-6), interleukin-18 (IL-18), and TNF-α. Interleukins increase endothelial permeability, cellular proliferation of mesangial cells, and synthesis of matrix and intraglomerular hemodynamic abnormalities. IL-6 increases expression of fibronectin, endothelial permeability and affects dynamics of extracellular matrix. IL-18 is the early predictor of renal dysfunction.

Tumor necrosis factor-alpha: The functions are:

A. It inhibits collagenase synthesis

B. It stimulates the metalloproteinase inhibitors thus reducing the degradation of extracellular matrix.

C. It produces abnormal extracellular matrix thus responsible for glomerular sclerosis and tubulointerstitial injury.

D. It increases local release of angiotensin II thus affecting renal hemodynamics.

Stages of Diabetic Nephropathy

Class	Description	Inclusion criteria
1	• Light microscopy—nonspecific • Electron microscopy—thickening of GBM	• Glomerular hyperfiltration • Normoalbuminuria (<30 mg/g)
2a	Mild-mesangial expansion in >25% of the observed mesangium	• Mild thickening of GBM • Albuminuria (<30 mg/g) • Normal GFR
2b	Severe mesangial expansion in >25% of observed mesangium	• Mild-to-moderate thickening of GBM and variable mesangial sclerosis • Albuminuria—30–300 mg/g • Normal or mildly decreased GFR
3	Nodular sclerosis (Kimmelstiel–Wilson lesion—at least one convincing lesion seen)	• Marked thickening of GBM • Diffuse mesangial sclerosis • Albuminuria >300 mg/g • Decreased GFR • Hypertension
4	Advanced diabetic glomerulosclerosis	• Diffuse global glomerulosclerosis • Decreasing albuminuria • GFR <15 mL/min • Hypertension

(GBM: glomerular basement membrane; GFR: glomerular filtration rate)

Natural History of Diabetic Nephropathy

A. Earliest clinical manifestation is microalbuminuria in the range of 30–300 mg/g:

- **a.** In case of type 1 DM: It can appear 5–10 years after the onset of diagnosis, so this test should be started 5 years after the diagnosis and thereafter every year.
- **b.** In case of type 2 DM: Time of onset of diabetes is unknown, so this test should be done at the time of diagnosis and thereafter every year.
- **c.** In type 2 DM, microalbuminuria is a potential risk factor for:
  1. Cardiovascular events, such as myocardial infarction and congestive cardiac failure
  2. Death before the progress of the disease toward proteinuria and renal failure

B. Microalbuminuria progresses to gross and frank proteinuria and nephrotic syndrome—proteinuria being from 500 mg to 3.5 g/day

C. More than 90% of type 1 DM with diabetic nephropathy develop diabetic retinopathy

D. There is strong correlation between K-W nodules and retinopathy

E. After the onset of proteinuria—50% develops renal failure in another 5–10 years.

F. 60% type 2 DM with diabetic nephropathy develop diabetic retinopathy

G. 10–20 years are required from early manifestation of microalbuminuria to frank renal failure.

Diagnosis

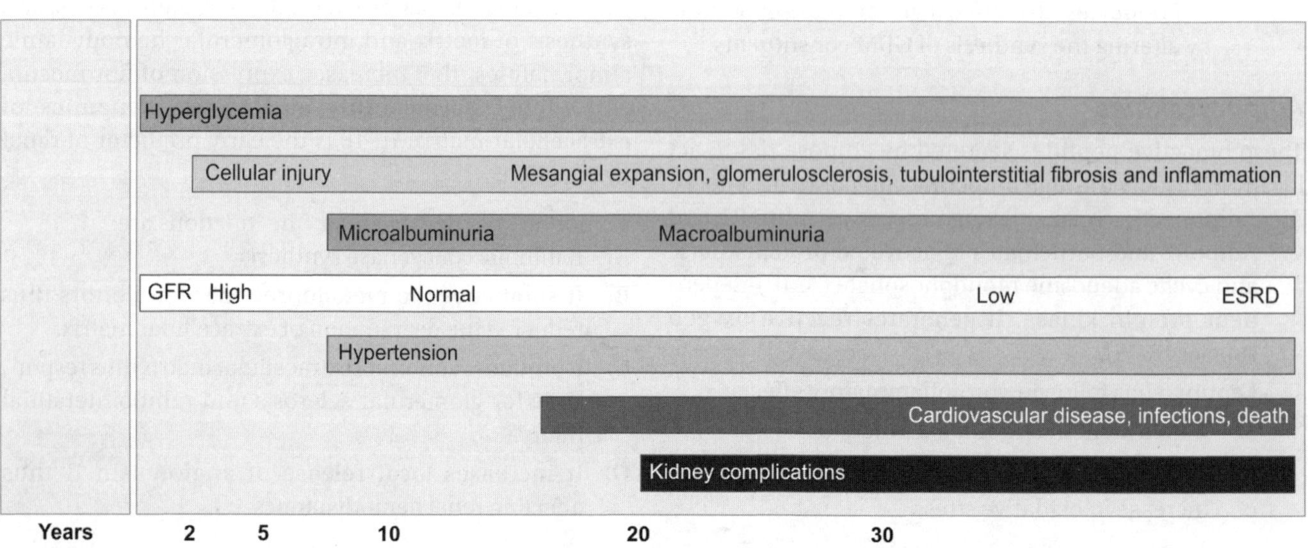

(ESRD: end-stage renal disease; GFR: glomerular filtration rate)

Treatment of Diabetic Nephropathy

Glycemic Control

Intense glycemic control in early course of diabetes is well established in both type 1 and 2. But in long-standing DM, this stringent glycemic control cannot reduce the microvascular or macrovascular complications and reduce the progression of renal disease, on the other hand it increases the incidence of hypoglycemia. So, according to American Diabetes Association, target of hypoglycemia varies according the age, comorbidities, and life expectancy of the patients:

A. HbA1c should be <6.5% in patients with diabetes of short duration, younger age, and in absence of any complication.

B. HbA1c should be maintained at <8% in patients with long-standing DM, elderly patients in presence of micro- or macrovascular complications.

Again, according to KDIGO guideline target of HbA1c should be 7% to prevent or delay micro- or macrovascular complications.

In a diabetic patient with CKD treatment will be complicated because:

A. Increased insulin resistance

B. Kidney is responsible for degradation of one-third exogenous insulin

C. Kidney is responsible for metabolism and excretion of many oral antidiabetic drugs.

Following antidiabetic medications should be continued:

A. Metformin: At GFR ≥ 30–45 mL/min/1.73 m^2, this drug can be given, but ≤30 mL/min there is risk of lactic acidosis.

B. Glucagon-like peptide-1 (GLP-1) receptor agonists, dipeptidyl dipeptidase-4 (DPP-4) inhibitors, and sodium-glucose cotransporter-2 (SGLT-2) inhibitors are contraindicated, if GFR will be <30 mL/min/1.73 m^2.

Management of Hypertension

A. It should be done according to Eighth Joint National Committee (JNC-8) guideline. Pharmacologic treatment should be started when the blood pressure is ≥140/90 mm Hg. Drugs are the following:

- **a.** Thiazide diuretics
- **b.** Calcium channel blocker
- **c.** Angiotensin-converting enzyme inhibitor: In early and late course of type 1 diabetic nephropathy, slower the decline of eGFR toward ESRD.
- **d.** Angiotensin receptor blocker

B. In black diabetic patients:

- **a.** Thiazide diuretics
- **b.** Calcium channel blocker

C. In diabetic patient with high level of albuminuria:

- **a.** ACE inhibitor or ARB
- **b.** Combination with another drug class

D. According to KDIGO guidelines: ARB or ACE inhibitor is recommended to maintain blood pressure at 130/80 mm Hg in any patients with CKD with albuminuria irrespective of DM.

Control of Hyperlipidemia

A. HMG-CoA reductase inhibitor:

- **a.** It reduces cardiac complications
- **b.** It reduces proteinuria
- **c.** It will preserve GFR in overt nephropathy.

Sodium Restriction

High dietary sodium intake produces hypervolemia leading to hypertension with adverse cardiovascular outcome.

On the other hand low sodium intake enhances antiproteinuric effect.

Novel Agents for Therapy

Targets are:

A. Glomerular hyperfiltration

B. Glomerular inflammation and fibrosis prevention

Drugs that are most promising are:

A. Ruboxistaurin: It is protein kinase C-β inhibitor

B. Baricitinib: A selective Janus kinase 1 and Janus kinase 2 inhibitor

C. Pentoxifylline: Anti-inflammatory and antifibrotic agent—it will block inflammatory cytokines and leukotrienes associated with DM.

D. Atrasentan: Selective endothelin A receptor antagonist—it will produce vasodilatation, decreases extracellular matrix accumulation thus prevents interstitial fibrosis.

E. Finerenone: Highly selective nonsteroidal mineralocorticoid receptor antagonist—it reduces proteinuria when used alone but produces additive effect combined with ACE inhibitor or ARB.

F. Selective serotonin receptor antagonists: These drugs prevent mesangial proliferation, platelet aggregation, decrease type IV collagen deposition, and regulate tissue vasculature.

There are no data, regarding phase III trial of above drugs, are available.

Q11. Pathophysiology of hemolytic uremic syndrome.

PGI/APR2013/MDI (10)

Diagnosis and management of atypical hemolytic uremic syndrome.

PGI/APR2013/MDIV (10)

Hemolytic uremic syndrome in clinical practice.

BF/NOV2013/MDIII (10)

Hemolytic uremic syndrome.

BF/MAY2009/MDIV (10)

MUHS/MAY2012/MDII (10)

Hemolytic uremic syndrome.

SCBMCH, 2020 (10)

Describe renal circulation and hemolytic syndrome.

ORISA UNI, 2021 (10)

Renal circulation has been described in question number 18.

ANSWER

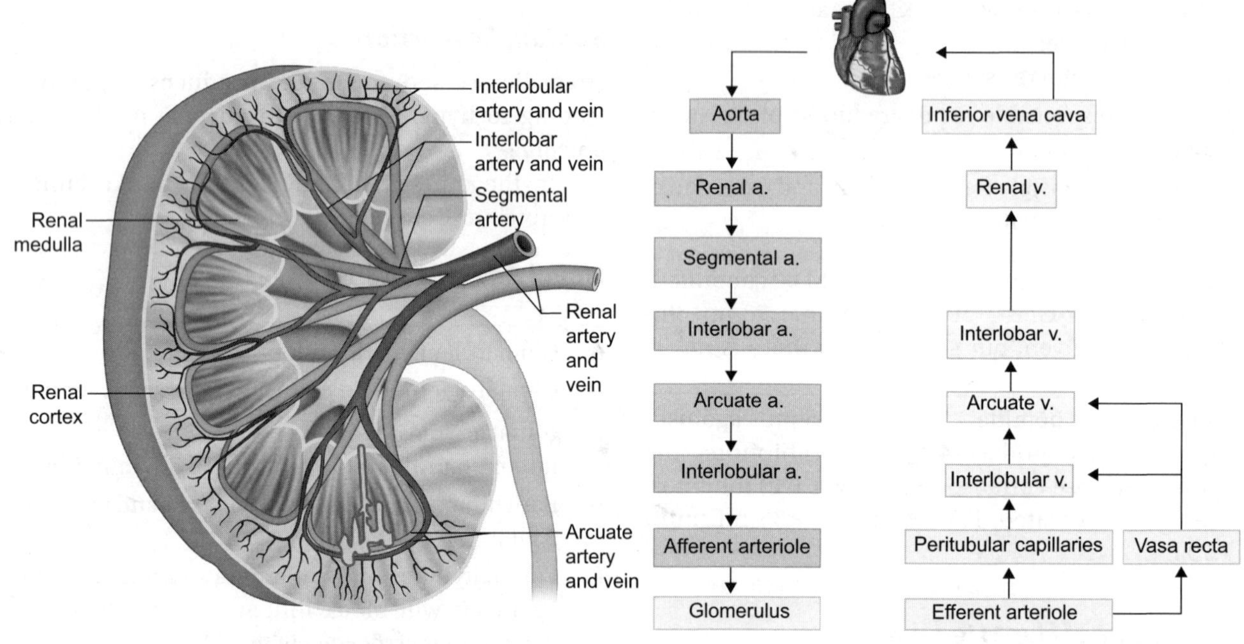

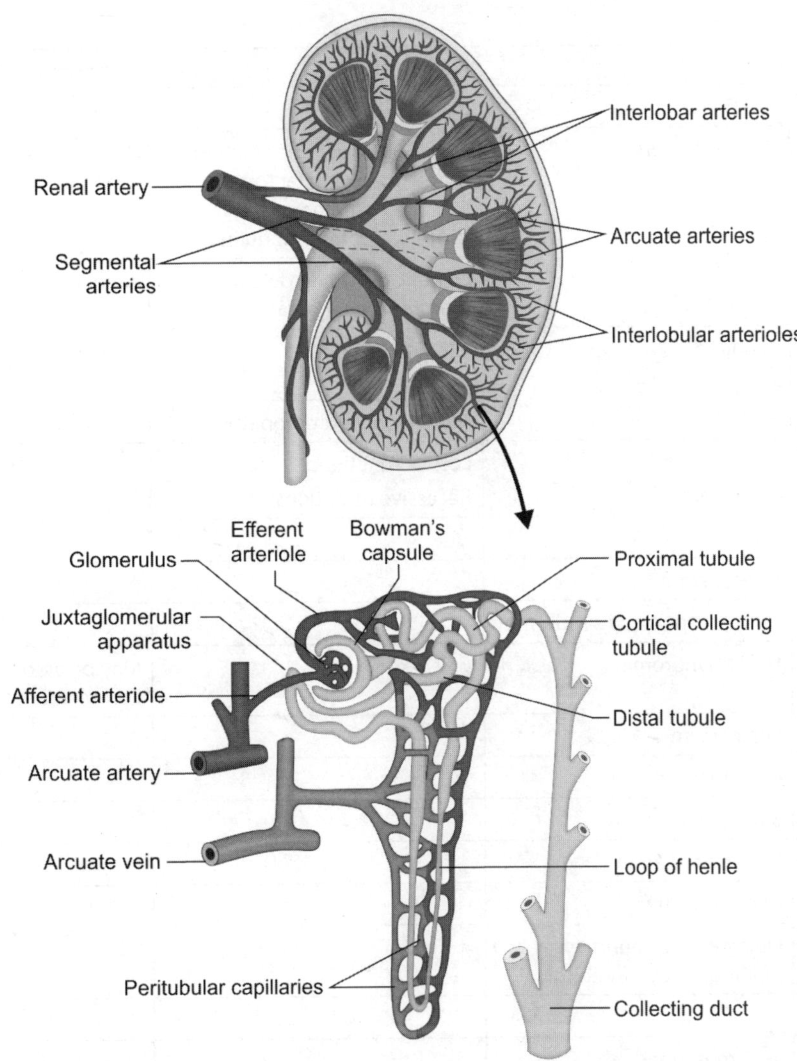

Definition

Hemolytic uremic syndrome is characterized by simultaneous occurrence of the following:

A. Renal failure
B. Immune hemolytic anemia
C. Peripheral thrombocytopenia

Classification According to Etiologies

Etiologies	Causes	Descriptions	Comments
Specific infectious agents	Shiga toxin-producing bacteria	Enteroinvasive *Escherichia coli*	Serotypes are O157, O26, and O104
		Shigella dysenteriae type 1	
		Citrobacter freundii	
	Streptococcus pneumoniae		Neuraminidase production
	Influenza A	H1N1	Neuraminidase production
	Enteroviruses	Coxsackie A and B viruses Echoviruses	
	HIV		
	Pseudomonas aeruginosa		

Continued

Continued

Etiologies	Causes	Descriptions	Comments
		Atypical HUS	
Dysregulation of complement	Genetic factors	Mutation of genetic encoding for the following factors: Factor 1, B and H, membrane cofactor protein, thrombomodulin	Activation of complement via alternate pathway
		Genetic encoding deletion or rearrangement of factor H	Associated antibody to factor H
	Acquired	Factor H antibodies	Associated with genetic encoding deletion or rearrangement of factor H
		Monoclonal gummopathy	
Diacylglycerol-ε mutation		Loss of function, Recessive mutations	
Autoimmune disease	SLE		
	Scleroderma		
	Anti-phospholipid syndrome		
Pregnancy related	HELLP syndrome		May be associated dysregulation of complement
	Postpartum		
Transplantation	Bone marrow		
	Solid organ		
Malignancy	Ionizing radiation		
	Chemotherapy		
Drugs	Quinine, calcineurin inhibitors, VEGF inhibitors		
Malignant hypertension			
Denys–Drash syndrome	WT1 mutations		
Cobalamin metabolism	Cobalamin type C MMACHC mutations. Homocystinuria		
Unknown	May be familial		

(HELLP: hemolysis, elevated liver enzymes, and low platelet; SLE: systemic lupus erythematosus; VEGF: vascular endothelial growth factor; WT1: Wilms tumor 1)

Pathophysiology

The common feature is endothelial cell injury in the kidney or any other organ less frequently. The damage may be due to:

A. Extrinsic and transient due to *Streptococcus*, toxigenic *E. coli*, drugs and cancer, so it will abate if the triggering factors can be removed.

B. Intrinsic or endogenous and sustained factor due to dysregulation of complement alternative pathways or loss or mutation of *DGKE* gene or deficiency of cobalamin. Here hemolytic uremic syndrome (HUS) can relapse and outcome is poor.

In case of type 1 HUS:

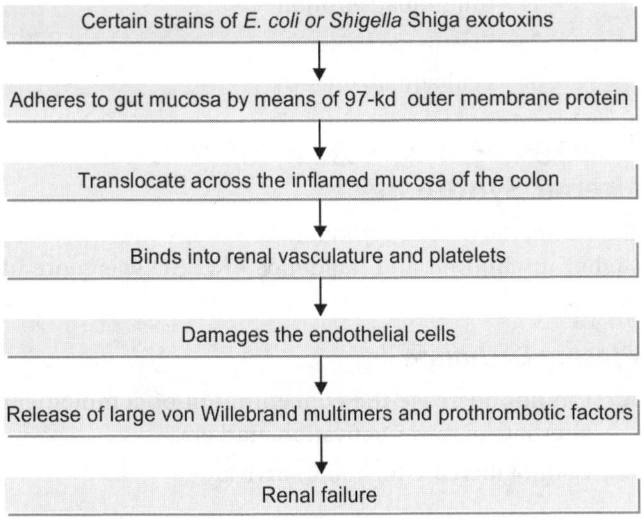

In case of type 2 HUS:

A. Genetic predisposition responsible for deficiency of factor H

↓

Leading to hyperactivation of alternate pathway of complement

B. Drugs responsible for HUS are cyclosporine, quinine, rapamycin, and tacrolimus

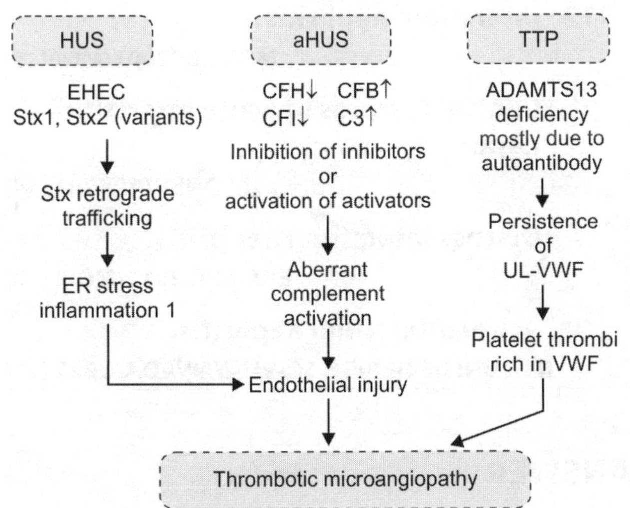

(aHUS: atypical hemolytic uremic syndrome; HUS: hemolytic uremic syndrome; TTP: thrombotic thrombocytopenic purpura)

When shiga toxin is within the blood stream it will bind to Gb3 recepters on the surface of the platelets. Then the toxin is internalized within the cells. Then the activated cells will release these toxins as microvesicles containing toxins. These microvesicle will reach the target organs, here they are taken up by the endothelial cells.

Symptoms

Triad of:

A. Microangiopathic hemolytic anemia
B. Thrombocytopenia
C. Renal failure

In case of D+ HUS:

A. Diarrhea
B. Raised blood pressure
C. Fever
D. Oliguria
E. Fluid overload

Ultimately the patient will go into:

A. Multiorgan dysfunction syndrome
B. Pancreatitis
C. Cardiomyopathy

Laboratory Diagnosis

Department	Features	Assay
Hematological parameters	Hemolysis	Reticulocyte count
		Lactate dehydrogenase
		Unconjugated bilirubin
		Haptoglobin
		Peripheral blood smear
		Direct antiglobulin test
	Thrombocytopenia	Platelet count
	Leukocytosis	Neutrophil count
	Coagulation is normal	Screening of coagulation
Biochemical parameters	Renal failure	Raised serum creatinine, urea
		Hyperkalemia
		Metabolic acidosis
	Pancreatic effects	Hyperglycemia
	Gastrointestinal losses	Hypoalbuminemia
		Hyponatremia
	Hepatic effects	Deranged liver function test
Microbiological parameters	Gastrointestinal infections	Stools for culture, PCR of *EHEC* genes, ELISA for free Shiga toxins
		Serology: EHEC virulence factor by ELISA

Continued

Continued

	Bacteremia	• Blood culture • Spinal fluid culture
	Urinary tract infection	Culture
	Streptococcus pneumoniae infection	T-antigen lectin-binding assay
Urinalysis	Hematuria	• Microscopy • Chemistry
	Proteinuria	Routine urine test 24 hours urine protein estimation
	Injury to glomerulus	

(ELISA: enzyme-linked immunosorbent assay)

Treatment

A. Supportive treatment:
- **a.** Renal replacement therapy—peritoneal dialysis or continuous hemodialysis in unstable patients.
- **b.** Adequate hydration and nutrition
- **c.** Correction of electrolyte imbalance and acidosis
- **d.** Control of hypertension
- **e.** Control of seizures
- **f.** Blood transfusion:
  - **1.** In case of children if hemoglobin is below 6 g/dL
  - **2.** In adult it will depend upon the comorbidities.
- **g.** Platelet transfusion should be done if the platelet level below 10,000/cc.

B. Management of EHEC-related HUS:
- **a.** Administration of intravenous fluid reduces the risk of HUS and also need for dialysis.
- **b.** In pre-HUS phase antibiotic should be avoided as it has an effect on bacteriophage lysogenesis as well as release of toxin thus increasing the risk of developing HUS. But after the development of HUS antibiotic can be administered to eradicate exotoxins. Antibiotics can be recommended in case of hemorrhagic colitis by *Shigella*:
  - **1.** It shortens the duration of diarrhea
  - **2.** It will decrease the duration of diarrhea
  - **3.** It reduces the risk of transmission
  - **4.** It shortens the duration of bacterial shedding.
- **c.** In case of ESRD:
  - **1.** Immunoadsorption
  - **2.** Plasma exchange
  - **3.** Eculizumab therapy

Management of Atypical Hemolytic Uremic Syndrome

Before the advent of eculizumab therapy mortality was higher in children and incidence of ESRD was more in adult.

Plasma Exchange

A. Cannot decrease the concentration of complement alternate pathway activation markers.

B. Cannot increase the renal survival

Eculizumab

It is monoclonal anti-CD5 antibody which blocks the entry of C5 into C5 convertase. Main risk is the development of infection with encapsulated organisms. Hence, prophylaxis against meningococcus, *Haemophilus influenzae*, hence prophylaxis against these organisms has to be given. But discontinuation of this drug is associated with recurrence of HUS. Lesion may be focal or diffuse.

Q12. Interstitial nephritis.

MGR/SEP2007/MDIV (5)

Clinical features of acute interstitial nephritis.

DNBII/APR2016 (4)

Discuss interstitial nephritis.

ERA/MAY2011/MDIII (10)

Acute interstitial nephritis.

NTR UNI OF HEALTH SC, VIJAYAWADA, 2021 (10)

ANSWER

Interstitial Nephritis

Definition

Tubulointerstitial nephritis can be defined as immune-mediated infiltration of inflammatory cells in the interstitium of kidney which can lead to oliguric or nonoliguric renal injury or chronic changes in the interstitium leading to development of chronic kidney injury.

Etiology

A. Drug induced:
- **a.** Nonsteroidal anti-inflammatory drugs (NSAIDs)
- **b.** Antimicrobials
- **c.** Diuretics

B. Infections:
- **a.** Viral:
  - **1.** Hepatitis virus
  - **2.** Cytomegalovirus
  - **3.** Poliovirus
  - **4.** Human immunodeficiency virus
- **b.** Bacterial:
  - **1.** *Salmonella*
  - **2.** *Leptospirosis*
  - **3.** *Streptococcus*
- **c.** Fungal: Histoplasmosis
- **d.** Parasitic: Toxoplasma

C. Immune mediated:
- **a.** SLE
- **b.** Sarcoidosis
- **c.** Inflammatory bowel disease (IBD)
- **d.** Sjögren syndrome

D. Idiopathic

E. Tubulointerstitial nephritis and uveitis syndrome

F. Granulomatous tubulointerstitial nephritis

Chronic Tubulointerstitial Nephritis

A. Vesicoureteral reflux

B. Sickle cell disease

C. Lithium

D. Heavy metals

E. Chronic exposure to toxins and therapeutic agents

F. Calcineurin inhibitors

Pathophysiology

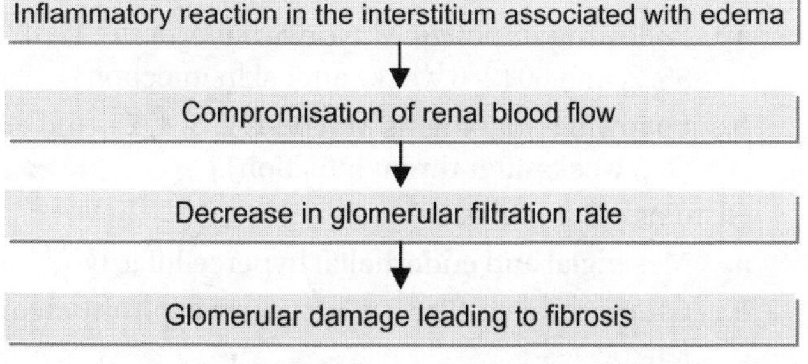

High metabolic demand of the tubular interstitium makes it very much susceptible to injury.

In case of acute tubulointerstitial nephritis (TIN), there is accumulation of lymphocytes and plasma cells along with inflammatory edema leading to decreased glomerular filtration rate. But if prolonged, there is accumulation of extracellular matrix leading to interstitial fibrosis and tubular atrophy and irreversible impairment of renal function. Macrophages though initially help in repair of acute injury but in chronic case it may aggravate inflammation and produce fibrogenic cytokines. Tumor growth factor-beta may also aggravate fibrogenesis. Drug-induced TIN may be immune-mediated or allergic which are supported by the following:

A. No dose dependence

B. Patient can develop systemic manifestation of hypersensitivity reaction.

C. It occurs in small portion of patients only.

D. It can occur after re-exposure to this drug.

E. Presence of eosinophils in renal biopsy

Pathology

Tubulointerstitial infiltrate contains lymphocytes, eosinophils, and interstitial edema. But in case of drug-induced TIN, eosinophil infiltration is extensive.

In case granulomatous TIN, there is presence of granuloma which are nonnecrotic, few granuloma. But necrotic granuloma is found in bacterial and fungal infection.

Clinical Presentation

A. Classical presentation of hypersensitivity reaction are fever, rash, and arthralgia

B. Loin pain due to increased size of kidney, due to accumulation of inflammatory cells, and edema.

C. Oliguric renal failure may occur within 7–10 days of treatment with methicillin or β-lactam antibiotic except in case of rifampin, the presentation will be much faster.

This disease should be suspected when features of hypokalemia, hyperchloremic metabolic acidosis are out of proportion of dysfunction of kidney.

D. Patient may present with the features of Fanconi syndrome as evidenced by hypokalemia, hyperchloremic metabolic acidosis, elevated fractional excretion of sodium, glycosuria, and aminoaciduria.

E. Urine may demonstrate pyuria, hematuria, mild proteinuria, and eosinophiluria.

In case of TIN with uveitis syndrome: Clinical presentations are:

A. Features of TIN

B. Features of uveitis, such as pain in eye, photophobia, redness, eyelid edema, rapid and progressive loss of vision, anterior or posterior synechiae along with systemic manifestations. Ocular changes are bilateral in 80% cases.

Diagnosis: Gold standard for the diagnosis of acute interstitial nephritis (AIN) is renal biopsy. But there are following contraindications to renal biopsy:

Absolute contraindications:

A. End-stage renal disease (ESRD)

B. Uncontrollable bleeding diathesis

C. Severe uncontrolled hypertension

D. Non-cooperative patients

Relative contraindications:

A. Renal, perirenal bilateral multiple renal cysts

B. Pregnancy

C. Hydronephrosis

D. Solitary native kidney

Treatment

A. Drug-induced TIN will be spontaneously cured by cessation of drug administration if identified early.

B. Treatment of the infectious etiology

C. Corticosteroid can be given to accelerate recovery but does not any impact on long-term survival. In granulomatous disease corticosteroid treatment is associated with better prognosis irrespective of tubulointerstitial fibrosis.

D. Mycophenolate mofetil can be used for treatment of TIN.

E. Systemic rheumatologic and inflammatory conditions should be treated with corticosteroids.

F. In case of uveitis, topical corticosteroid and cycloplegic agents are effective in 50% of patients. Systemic steroid is also given to treat TIN. But if the patient does not respond to systemic steroid or develop toxicity to steroid in that case cyclosporin A, azathioprine, and mycophenolate mofetil may be used to treat uveitis.

Q13. Discuss the biochemical and histological changes in acute nephritic syndrome.

BF/JUN2016/MDI (10)

Hematological consequences of nephritic syndrome.

MGR/OCT2011/MDIV (7)

Discuss the pathophysiology and types of glomerular disorders.

BF/NOV2013/MDI (10)

Discuss the etiopathogenesis, clinical features, and management of glomerular disease with nephritis presentation.

MGR/FEB2005/MDII (15)

Membranoproliferative glomerulonephritis.

DNB (DEC2022) (5)

Enumerate the causes of acute nephritic syndrome. Classify Nephritis.

AIIMS, 2020 (10)

Acute nephritic syndrome.

KERALA UNIVERSITY, 2019 (10)

ANSWER

Lupus nephritis has described in question 1.

Acute Nephritic Syndrome

Definition

This syndrome is characterized by hypertension, hematuria, pyuria, mild-to-moderate proteinuria ranges from 200 mg/day to 10 g/day, red blood cell cast in urine with gradual fall in glomerular filtration rate leading to uremic symptoms like retention of salt and water followed by edema and hypertension.

Etiology

A. Infectious causes:

- **a.** Following impetigo M type *Streptococcus* 47, 49, 55, 2, and 60 (2–6 weeks after skin infection)
- **b.** Following pharyngitis M type 1, 2, 3, 4, 25, and 49 (1–3 weeks after throat infection).

Histological findings:

- **a.** Mesangial and endothelial hypercellularity
- **b.** Glomerular infiltrate of polymorphonuclear leukocytes
- **c.** Granular subendothelial deposits of IgG, IgM, C3, C4, and C5-9'

d. Subepithelial deposits like hump

Biochemical changes:

a. In the first week, 90% patients have depressed CH_{50}, decreased C3, and normal C4 level

b. Positive rheumatoid factor

c. Cryoglobulin

d. Circulating immune complexes

e. In 10% cases, positive ANCA against myeloperoxidase (MPO)

f. Antihyaluronidase antibodies

B. Subacute bacterial endocarditis: It occurs in right-sided endocarditis or negative blood culture and untreated for long time.

Histological changes:

a. Focal proliferation around foci of necrosis

b. Subendothelial and subepithelial deposits of IgM, IgM and C3

c. Crescent formation

Biochemical and serological changes:

a. Normocytic anemia

b. Elevated ESR

c. Hypocomplementemia

d. High titer rheumatoid factor

e. Type III cryoglobulinemia

f. Elevated serum creatinine

C. Antiglomerular basement membrane disease: This disease is characterized by deposition of antibasement membrane antibodies leading to development of glomerulonephritis. If this patient develop hemoptysis, it is known as Goodpasture syndrome.

Histological changes:

a. Linear deposits of IgG and C3 along the glomerular basement membrane by immunofluorescent studies—it is particularly against the target of α_3 NC1 domain of collagen IV.

b. 10–15% patients demonstrates MPO-positive ANCA antibodies

c. In advanced cases, diffuse nephritis with segmental and total necrosis with extensive crescent formation

Biochemical and serological findings:

a. Presence of circulating IgG antibodies

b. Low complement C3

D. IgA nephropathy: It is characterized by two most common presentations like recurrent episodes of macroscopic hematuria with proteinuria following or during upper respiratory tract infection and persistent microscopic asymptomatic hematuria.

Histological changes:

a. Diffuse mesangial deposits of IgA along with codeposition of IgG, IgM, and complements with mesangial hypercellularity as evidenced by immunofluorescence microscopy.

b. IgA is polymeric and of IgA1 subclass.

c. In case of rapid deterioration of renal function there may be segmental necrosis, rarely segmental necrosis with cellular crescent formation.

Serological and biochemical findings: Elevated level of serum IgA

E. Small vessel vasculitis: It involves arterioles, capillaries and venules producing small vessels vasculitis, and glomerulonephritis. Three antibodies are involved in it, these are antiproteinase 3 antibodies, anti-myeloperoxidase (anti-MPO) antibodies, and anti-LAMP 2 antibodies. ANCA produced by T cells positive for anti-MPO antibodies damage the small blood vessels. The diseases involved are:

a. Microscopic polyangiitis

b. Churg–Strauss syndrome

Anti-PR3 antibodies positive disease is granulomatosis with polyangiitis.

Histological findings:

a. Necrotizing capillary lesion, immune deposits: It can be divided into four types:

  1. Focal

  2. Segmental

  3. Crescentic

  4. Sclerotic lesions

b. Crescent formation

c. Negative for immunofluorescent and electron microscope hence it is "pauci-immune".

d. In case of C3 glomerulopathy, there is glomerular accumulation of C3 with little or no immunoglobulin deposition.

Biochemical and serological findings: Serum anti-PR3 antibodies or anti-MPO antibodies

F. Membranoproliferative glomerulonephritis (MPGN): Pathologically, it has been subsided into three types:

a. Type I is commonly associated with persistent hepatitis C, autoimmune diseases, and neoplastic diseases.

b. Type II and III MPGN are idiopathic, driven by classical complement pathway.

Histological changes:

- **a.** Type I MPGN: It is characterized by:
  - **1.** Subendothelial deposits, it may be primary or secondary to cryoglobulinemia
  - **2.** Mesangial proliferation and lobular segmentation
  - **3.** Mesangial deposition in between capillary basement membrane and endothelial cells looking like "tram-tracking" appearance.
- **b.** Type II MPGN: It is characterized by subendothelial deposits with occasional intramesangial deposits due to deficiency of compliment factor H—it is dense deposit disease.
- **c.** Type III MPGN: It is subendothelial and subepithelial deposits. Subepithelial deposits may occur along widened segments of glomerular basement membrane.

Biochemical and serological findings:

- **a.** Low level of C3 in type II MPGN
- **b.** Circulating immune complexes

G. Mesangioproliferative glomerulonephritis:

Histological findings:

- **a.** Expansion of mesangium
- **b.** Mesangial hypercellularity
- **c.** Thin single contour capillary walls
- **d.** Deposition of immune complexes containing IgM, C1q and C3.

Biochemical and serological findings:

- **a.** Low C3 level
- **b.** Increased immune complexes

Q14. Discuss donor selection for renal transplant.
ERA/MAY2012/MDIV (10)

Kidney transplant.
BF/MAY2009/MDI (8)

Post-transplant renal replacement therapy.
PGI/APR2014/MDII (10)

Renal transplantation in the Indian set-up.
RGUHS/MDII (10)

Renal transplantation.
MGR/SEP2010/MDIV (6) MGR/MAR2009/MDIV (6)

Donor nephrectomy.
MGR/OCT2011/MDIV (7)

Discuss briefly the postrenal transplant management.
MGR/APR2015/MDIV (7)

Enumerate indications and contraindications of renal transplantation. Immunosuppressive therapy in the recipient of renal transplant.
DNB (DEC2018) (10)

Renal transplantation—complications, post-transplant management.
SCBMCH, 2020 (20)

Discuss the donor selection in renal transplant. Enumerate the potent diseases that occurs in transplanted kidney.
WBUHS, 2022 (10)

Write details about infection in renal transplant recipients and its management.
MGR UNI, TAMIL NADU, 2021 (15)

Renal transplantation.
MGR UNI, TAMIL NADU, 2019 (10)

Post kidney transplant treatment.
NTR UNI OF HEALTH SC, VIJAYAWADA, 2019 (10)

Write down the management of a post-kidney transplant patient.
MANIPUR UNIVERSITY, 2020 (10)

Explain the principles of renal transplantation. Discuss the complications associated with the procedure and their management.
WBUHS, 2025 (10)

ANSWER

Indications of Transplant

- **A.** Chronic kidney disease
- **B.** Renal tumor

Following diseases can recur in transplanted kidney:

- **A.** Oxalosis
- **B.** Reflux nephropathy

C. Diabetes
D. Certain glomerulopathies
E. IgA nephropathy
F. HUS in pediatric transplanted kidney

Following are the contraindications for receiving kidney transplant:
A. Active infection
B. Ongoing active immunologic disease leading to kidney failure
C. Metastatic malignancy
D. Due to medical or psychological regions, patient is unable to follow medical regimens.
E. Age >70 years with comorbid conditions having less demonstrable benefit for survival.
F. Serious cardiac and peripheral vascular diseases
G. Serious conditions that are unlikely to improve after kidney transplantation
H. Demonstrated of repeated episodes of medical non-compatibility to perform rehabilitation adequately after transplantation
I. Active immunologic disease

Human immunodeficiency virus positivity is not a contraindication for kidney transplantation provided patients meet the following criteria:
A. CD4 count has been higher than 200 cells/μL for at least 6 months
B. HIV-RNA is undetectable
C. The patient has been stable on antiretroviral therapy for at least 3 months
D. Patient has no major infectious or neoplastic complication.

Evaluation of Recipients

Advantages of Pretransplant Evaluation

A. Renal transplantation is technically possible
B. Improvement of patient's survival
C. Patient has no risk of premature death owing to other medical problem.
D. Minimal surgery related complications
E. Search of preexisting conditions which do not deteriorate post-transplantation.

Following comorbid conditions which may affect the immunosuppression should be considered:
A. Age: In any age it can be done. But in case of cadaveric renal transplant age is should be <65 years.
B. Diabetes
C. Abnormal electrocardiogram
D. Congestive cardiac failure
E. Angina:
So, following cardiac tests should be done:
- **a.** Stress test to be done in case of:
  - **1.** Age > 50 years
  - **2.** Presence of diabetes mellitus
  - **3.** Presence of abnormal ECG other than left ventricular hypertrophy (LVH)
  - **4.** Presence of history of coronary artery disease
- **b.** Who cannot perform stress test, following tests can be done:
  - **1.** Dipyridamole-thallium imaging
  - **2.** Stress echocardiography
  - **3.** Coronary angiography
- **c.** Other tests to be done:
  - **1.** History of claudication, if there is presence of arterial insufficiency, Doppler studies.
  - **2.** In presence of history of transient ischemic attack (TIA) carotid Doppler study

F. Screening of the patients suffered from malignancy because 2–5 years remissions is required before performing transplantation but it also requires:
- **a.** Type of tumor
- **b.** Tumor invasiveness
- **c.** Any prior treatment

G. Screening of infections:
- **a.** Hepatitis B virus
- **b.** Hepatitis C virus
- **c.** HIV
- **d.** Serological status of cytomegalovirus and varicella virus
- **e.** Epstein–Barr virus

Here assessment should be done by fibroscan or liver biopsy to assess liver damage.

H. Malignancy:
- **a.** In case of malignancy other than nonmelanoma of skin if there is no evidence of malignancy for 2 years post-treatment
- **b.** In malignancy of colorectal, uterus, breast, and malignant melanoma waiting time may be >5 years.
- **c.** In case of low-grade bladder carcinoma, focal cancer, renal carcinoma, in-situ cancer, and basal-cell cancer no waiting time is required.
- **d.** Prior post-transplant lymphoproliferative disorders is not a contraindication.

When the recipient will be accepted as a candidate then initial medical screening should be started. Recipient's blood should be screened for human leukocyte antigen (HLA) antibodies using single antigen beads. If the recipient receives prior transfusion or organ transplantation or accept pregnancy then antibodies against HLA of another individual are produced. This antibodies can be detected and overall degree of HLA sensitization or calculated panel reactive antibody (cPRA) have to be calculated. If the antibodies are declared clinically significant by transplant center then corresponding HLA antigen is listed as "unacceptable" for that recipient, in that case donor kidney containing that antigen will never be offered. So higher the value of cPRA longer will be the time of waiting for kidney transplant. This process is known as "virtual cross-matching".

Evaluation of the Donor

A. Living donor: After the assurance of ABO incompatibility and negative cross-match, donor has to be evaluated as the following diseases which are relatively contraindicated to donation has to be screened:

- **a.** Hypertension
- **b.** Obesity
- **c.** Kidney stones
- **d.** Structural kidney disease
- **e.** Functional kidney disease
- **f.** Proteinuria
- **g.** Diabetes mellitus in patient with family history of diabetes

If the recipient is affected by polycystic kidney disease or hereditary nephritis, these diseases have to be ruled out in the donor clinically or genetic testing prior to selection.

Radiological imaging of the kidneys has to be done by CT scan and angiography.

Postoperative mild hypertension and proteinuria may occur after kidney transplant. In 15% donors after transplant bleeding, infection, and postoperative complications may occur.

In case of patient's family member: As the body can function perfectly well with just one healthy kidney, a family member with two healthy kidney may choose to donate one of them to the patient.

If the tissue and blood of family member of the patient match patient's blood and tissue, he can schedule a planned donation.

Receiving a kidney from the family member is a good option as it reduces the risk that the patient's body will reject the kidney and it enables you to bypass the multiyear waiting list for a deceased donor. Allograft survival time is 12 years.

B. Deceased donor: These are also called cadaveric donor. These are the people who died usually as a result of accident rather than a disease. Either donor or their family has chosen to donate their organ or tissues. Patient's body is more likely to reject a kidney from an unrelated donor.

However, a cadaveric organ is a good alternative if you do not have any family member or friend who is willing or able to donate a kidney.

Allograft survival time is 8 years.

Following conditions preclude donation:

- **a.** Widespread infection
- **b.** HIV
- **c.** Unknown cause of death
- **d.** Presence of metastases
- **e.** Advanced age
- **f.** Elevated serum creatinine
- **g.** Oliguria
- **h.** Hypertension
- **i.** Dependence on pressure support

Hepatitis C donor can donate the kidney to hepatitis C recipient.

Standard criteria donor (SCD): This donor is such who has been died due to primary brain death while cardiac and respiratory function remain intact and also do not follow the expanded donor criteria.

Expanded criteria donor (ECD): This donor can be defined as:

- **a.** Any donor older than 60 years
- **b.** Any donor older than 50 years with at least any two of the following:
  1. Terminal serum creatinine >1.5
  2. Cerebrovascular accident as a cause of death
  3. Preexisting hypertension

Expanded criteria donor has 1.7 relative risk as compared to SCD.

In case of complete HLA mismatch, 5 years survival rate somewhat poorer in both types of donors.

Immunology

A. Major histocompatibility complex (MHC) It has two functions:

- **a.** Identification of self from nonself
- **b.** It will coordinate the T-cell receptor recognition of antigen

These molecules are divided into two groups:

- **a.** MHC I molecule is present on the surface of all nucleated cells and known as HLA-A, HLA-B, and HLA-C.
- **b.** MHC II molecules are present on the antigen-presenting cells (APCs) and are known as HLA-DR, HLA-DP, and HLA-DQ.

In case of renal transplantation, HLA-A, HLA-B, and HLA-DR are determine due to their specific immunogenicity. If there is no mismatch in these HLA-A, B, and DR then it is called "zero-antigen mismatched kidney".

B. Antigen presenting cells: These monocytes, macrophages, dendritic cells, and activated B cells are distributed throughout the body tissues and they will recognize foreign antigen. The captured foreign antigen degrade them and express them on MHC II molecules.

C. T cells: These are processed in thymus and responsible for cellular immunity. There are two classes of cells:

- **a.** T helper cells or CD4+ cells recognize MHC class II molecules on the surface of APCs.
- **b.** Cytotoxic T cells or CD8+ cells are restricted to recognition of MHC class I.

Cellular immunity is mediated by lymphocytes in response to organ specific HLA antigen. In response to HLA class II incompatibility CD4+ cells proliferate followed by release of proinflammatory cytokines leading to proliferation of immune system.

CD8+ cells responds to MHC class I molecule and will mature into cytotoxic effector cells and produce organ damage through direct effect and direct target cell lysis.

T Cells and APCs Interaction

In case of allograft rejection, there are several interactions between T cells and APCs:

- **a.** Signal 1: In this signal through interactions between TCR/CD3 as well as expressed foreign peptide in MHC complex there is initial binding of T cells to APCs. This process is calcium-dependent process resulting activation of calcineurin.
- **b.** Signal 2: It is also known as costimulation. Here
  1. There is signal between CD28 present on resting T cells and B7 on APC surface—it will lead to intracellular signaling, production of interleukin-2 (IL-2) followed by T cell activation.
  2. Cytotoxic T-lymphocyte antigen-4 immunoglobulin (Ig) is expressed on activated T cells, it will bind to B7 on APC surface leading to inactivation of immune response and provide potent negative feedback.
  3. There is another molecule CD40 present on activated B cells and APCs. It will bind to CD40 ligand present on T cells. This CD40/CD40 ligand are responsible for immunoglobulin production through the activation of B cells.

B Cells

These are produced in liver, spleen, lymph nodes, and other areas of the body. In response to interaction between T cells and APCs, B cells are activated to produce antibodies against foreign MHC antigens—these are called donor-specific antibodies which ultimately lead to cellular toxicity and subsequent cellular lysis.

Pharmacotherapies

It can be divided into two main categories:

A. Induction therapy: It is used prior to transplant. The drugs are:

- **a.** Antithymocyte globulin: Polyclonal immunoglobulin will neutralize lymphocytes by multiple antibody-mediated mechanism and has a sustained effect on proliferation. In case of acute rejection, it is more effective than basiliximab. Dose is 1.5 mg/kg intravenously for 3–5 days.
- **b.** Basiliximab: This chimeric/human monoclonal antibody inhibits IL-2-induced T-cell activation as well as its proliferation without T-cell depletion by binding with IL-2 receptor present on the activated T cells. Dose is 20 mg intravenously at the time of transplant and next dose after 4 days.
- **c.** Alemtuzumab: This humanized anti-CD-52 antibody will deplete both T and B cells due to its potent immunosuppressive properties. But there is high susceptibility to infection and autoimmune syndrome. Dose is 30 mg intravenously at the time of transplant.
- **d.** Rituximab: This monoclonal antibody causes rapid and sustained depletion of B lymphocytes. It is used for:
  1. Treatment of acute humoral rejection
  2. Desensitization and ABO-incompatible kidney
  3. Treatment of secondary diseases, such as focal segmental glomerulosclerosis (FSGS) and post-transplant lymphoproliferative disorders.

B. Maintenance therapy: It will prevent allograft rejection and/or treatment for acute rejection. Following drugs are given:

a. Calcineurin inhibitors: The drugs are:

1. Cyclosporin A: Starting dose is 6–8 mg/kg/day in divided doses twice daily followed by gradual tapering of doses.

2. Tacrolimus: Starting dose is 0.15–0.3 mg/kg/day in divided doses twice daily followed by gradual tapering of dose.

Both the above drugs bind to intracellular calcineurin thus inhibits translocation of transcription factor of activated T cells which leads to inhibition of cytokine-induced cell proliferation.

Side effects are hypertension, hirsutism, hyperlipidemia, gingival hyperplasia. Post-transplant diabetes and neurotoxicity is more common with tacrolimus.

b. Mammalian target of rapamycin inhibitors (mTor-Is): The drugs are:

1. Sirolimus

2. Everolimus

Both these drugs inhibit IL-2-mediated signal transduction and proliferation of cells.

Toxicities include hypertriglyceridemia, cytopenia, hypercholesterolemia, pneumonitis, delayed wound healing, and proteinuria. Dose is 2–5 mg/day.

c. Antimetabolites: The drugs are:

1. Mycophenolate mofetil

2. Mycophenolic acid

3. Azathioprine

These drugs can be used with calcineurin inhibitors. They inhibit synthesis of purine which leads to lymphocyte proliferation. Dose is 1 mg for mycophenolate mofetil and 720 mg in case of mycophenolic acid twice daily. Dose of azathioprine is 1.5 mg/kg daily. Toxicities are diarrhea and discomfort in gastrointestinal tract.

d. Corticosteroids: It will inhibit immune response by inhibiting inflammatory mediators. Dose is ≥0.1 mg/kg.

e. Belatacept: This fusion protein:

1. Will bind to B7 on the surface of APCs with high affinity

2. Inhibits CD28-mediated T-cell costimulation (signal 2).

Transplantation

A. Prior to transplantation cross-matching between recipient and the donor will minimize both hyperacute and acute antibody-mediated rejection, can be done by:

a. Complement-mediated cytotoxicity

b. Solid-phase single antigen bead (SAB) assay

c. Cell based flow cytometry

d. Combination of above

If the cross match is positive following decision can be made:

a. Cancellation of the procedure

b. Transplant center experience

c. Desensitization procedure which again depends upon previous risk of rejection. It will reduce rejection risk. The therapy aims at treating the antibody-mediated rejection, such as plasma exchange followed by low dose of intravenous immunoglobulin until the next cross match will be negative and high dose of intravenous immunoglobulin along with or without rituximab.

B. Induction: In most of the cases, high dose of steroid is given at the time of transplantation and it is followed by tapering of the drug. Antibody therapy is given as induction in the following conditions where there is increased risk of rejection:

a. Increased plasma renin activity

b. Previous transplant

c. Africans-Americans

Antibody therapies include:

a. Antithymocyte globulin

b. IL-2 receptor antagonists

c. Alemtuzumab

C. Donor nephrectomy: Living donor nephrectomy can be done by open or laparoscopic surgery.

Choice of kidney is left kidney because it is more accessible and renal vein is longer.

Laparoscopic approach is more acceptable because:

a. Shorter hospital stay

b. Quicker return to work

c. Less pain

Disadvantages of laparoscopic approach:

a. High cost

b. Longer operating time

c. Learning curve to decrease the rate of morbidity

In case of deceased donor kidney is removed with patch of aorta and inferior vena cava as part of multiorgan surgery. Then after separation, separated organ is preserved in hypothalamic preservation solution mainly in expanded criteria donor and donation of kidney after death.

D. Transplant surgery:

  a. Donor kidney is placed in left or right iliac fossa
  b. Donor renal vein is connected end to end with external iliac vein
  c. Donor renal artery is connected end to end with external iliac artery
  d. To prevent lymphocele lymphatics are ligated.
  e. Ureter is implanted into the bladder and to prevent urine leak a tunnel is formed by pulling the bladder mucosa over the ureter.
  f. Sometimes ureteral stent is placed during surgery to confirm patency and to prevent leakage of urine.
  g. Foley's catheter is done during surgery and will be kept for up to 5 days after operation.
  h. In absence of technical complications of kidney transplantation prompt urine will be formed.

Complications of Transplantation

A. Surgical complications:

  a. Urine leak: It may occur due to ureteral necrosis due to distal ureteral blood supply interruption or at the site of ureteral implantation in the bladder.
  b. Ureteric obstruction: It occurs secondary to ureteral ischemia.
  c. Vesicoureteral reflux
  d. Arterial or venous thrombosis
  e. Lymphocele
  f. Wound complication
  g. Infection

B. Renal complications:

  a. Accelerated rejection:
    1. Hyperacute rejection: It occurs within 2 days due to graft thrombosis or loss
    2. Delayed hyperacute rejection: It occurs within first few days of transplant.
    3. Acute cellular rejection: It occurs in first few weeks to months of life.
  b. Chronic allograft failure: In this case, characteristic findings are tubular atrophy and interstitial fibrosis.
  c. Recurrence of disease

Infections in renal transplant recipients:

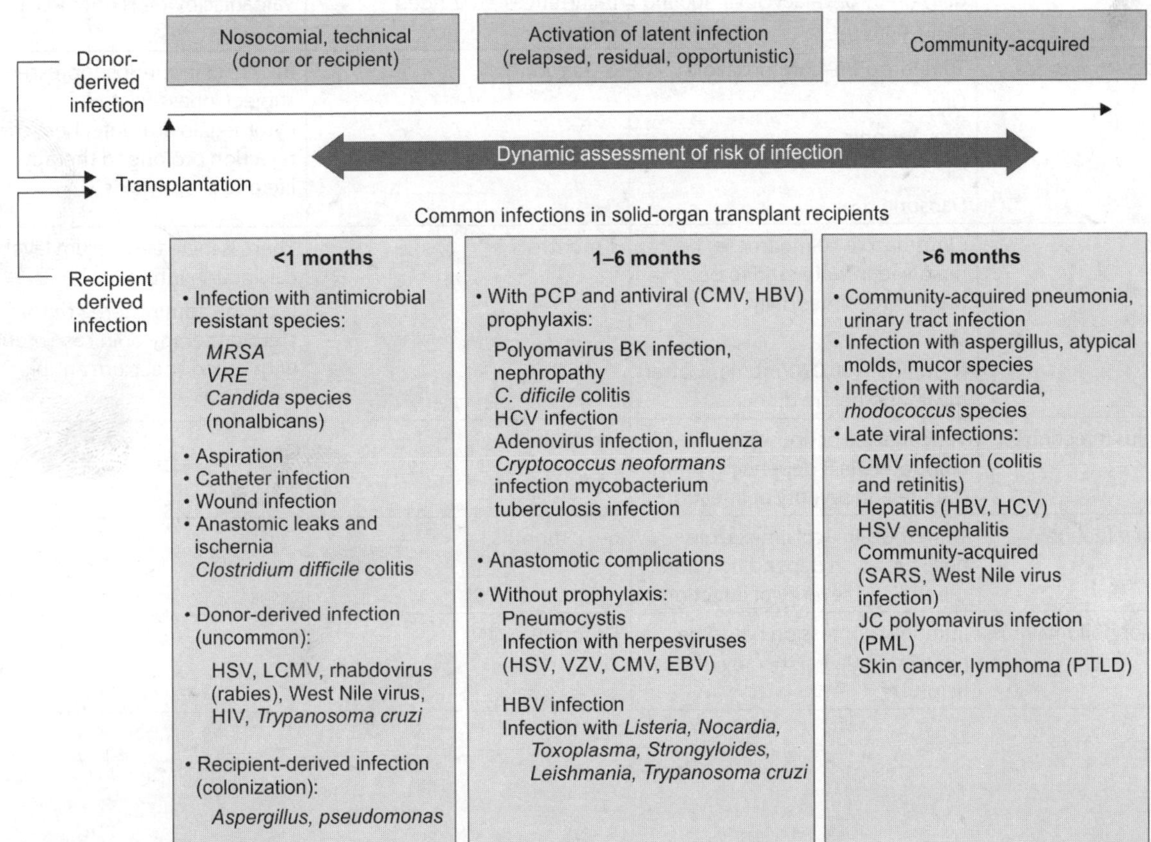

	Days 1–30	Months 1–6	More than 6 months
Bacteria	Hospital acquired, includes surgical site and device related; may involve resistant donor-derived pyogenic organisms	Opportunistic bacteria including listeria, nocardia, tuberculosis, and non-tuberculous mycobacteria Donor-derived bacteria	• Encapsulated organisms, especially sinopulmonary • Urinary tract infections • Pancreaticobiliary and diverticular-associated infections
Viral	• Herpes simplex • Healthcare-associated respiratory viruses • Donor-derived (LCMV, WNV, etc)	• CMV • EBV/PTLD • Varicella zoster/herpes zoster • Polyomaviruses (especially BK) • Donor-derived	• Community-acquired respiratory viruses • CMV (delayed onset due to prophylaxis) • EBV/PTLD (less common after year 1)
Fungal	• *Candida* • Donor derived	• Molds, especially aspergillus • *Cryptococcus* • PJP if no prophylaxis	• Endemic/environmental mycoses • *Cryptococcus*
Parasitical/ Protozoal	Donor derived (e.g., *Balamuthia*)	• *Strongyloides* • *Toxoplasmosis* • *Trypanosoma cruzi*	Variable risk based on exposures

Following prophylactic antibiotics are commonly used following renal transplantation:

Pathogenic organisms	Antibiotics	Duration	Comments
Cytomegalovirus	Valganciclovir 900 mg orally daily and it should be adjusted as per renal function	Based on the risk Donor positive/recipient negative – 6 months Recipient positive—3 months	Valganciclovir for lower risk (donor negative/recipient negative), monitoring (preemptive therapy)
Herpes simplex	Acyclovir 400 mg three times daily orally or valacyclovir 900 mg orally daily	3 months, but in case recurrences prolonged therapy	If the patient is already on Valganciclovir it is not indicated
Pneumocystis Jirovecii	Trimethoprim–cotrimoxazole Or Atovaquone Or Dapsone	6–12 months	In case of immunosuppressed subject, or associated cytomegalovirus infection, chronic rejection prolonged therapy or lifelong prophylaxis
Candida	Clotrimazole 10 mg troche dissolved in water and to be taken three times daily Or Nystatin—100,000/mL, 4 mL after meals and before dinner	1 month	There is increased serum level of calcineurin inhibitors It can be administered during steroid therapy or in case of therapy with broad spectrum antibiotics
Aspergillus infection	Voriconazole or liposomal amphotericin B depending upon the site and severity of infection	6 months	
Nocardia infection	Trimethoprim–cotrimoxazole—dose based on depending upon the site and severity of infection	6–12 months.	
BK virus or poliomavirus	Immunosuppression has to be reduced. Antiviral therapy of least helpful	6 months	

Q15. Discuss the epidemiology, differential diagnosis, laboratory features, and treatment of chronic kidney disease.

MGR/SEP2007/MDI (15)

Causes and diagnosis of chronic renal failure.

MGR/APR2003/MDIII (10)

Action plan of predialysis management of chronic kidney disease.

MJPRU/2014/MDIII (10)

Management of chronic kidney disease.

MUHS/MAY2014/MDII (10)

Discuss the pathophysiology and staging of chronic kidney disease. Write clinical features and managements.

MGR/OCT2011/MDIII (15)

What do you understand by ESRD? Describe the causes and discuss the management.

AIIMS, BBS, 2023 (10)

CKD – etiopathogenesis, clinical diagnosis and management.

SCBMCH, 2020 (20)

Describe the physiology of nephron. Discuss the etiopathogenesis, clinical feature and management of chronic kidney disease.

VEER NARMAD SOUTH GUJARAT UNI, 2022 (25)

Write down the Kidney Disease improving Global Outcome (KDIGO) classification of chronic kidney disease. Discuss the current treatment of CKD.

AIIMS (BHU), 2024 (10)

Management of metabolic acidosis in CKD.

RAJASTHAN UNIVERSITY, 2023 (8)

ANSWER

Dialysis part of treatment has been described in question 7 and transplantation part in 14.

Definition

It can be defined as damage of kidney for 3 months or longer due to structural and functional abnormalities of kidney in presence or absence of decreased glomerular filtration rate which can be manifested by pathological abnormalities or abnormalities in imaging tests or blood or urine.

Chronic kidney disease also can be defined by glomerular filtration rate of <60 mL/min/1.73 m^2 for 3 months or longer in presence or absence of kidney damage.

Epidemiology

A. Gender: Overall incidence of end-stage renal disease is greater in males than in females.

B. Age: Normal annual decline in GFR occurs with age from the age of 30 years.
In normal adult, male GFR is 120 mL/min/1.73 m^2 and in normal adult, female GFR is 188 mL/min/1.73 m^2.
Decline in GFR occurs at 1 mL/min/1.73 m^2.

C. Smoking: It is associated with proteinuria and chronic kidney disease in patients with type 1 or 2 diabetes mellitus or immunoglobulin A deficiency. Polycystic disease of kidney or lupus nephritis. So cessation of smoking may regress the kidney disease in type 1 diabetes mellitus.

D. Ethnicity: As compared to white patients, African-American peoples are 3-fold increased risk of developing end-stage renal failure.

E. Suboptimal control of glucose, blood pressure

F. Low socioeconomic status

G. Consumption of nonnarcotic analgesic, such as phenacetin

H. Previous episodes of acute kidney injury

I. Family history of renal disease

J. Abnormal urinary sediment

Stages of Chronic Renal Failure

There are five stages in chronic failure.

Prognosis of CKD according to GFR and albuminuria	Persistent albuminuria		
	A1	A2	A3
	Normal to mild increase	Moderate increase	Severe increase
	<30 mg/g	30–300 mg/g	>300 mg/g

Continued

Continued

GFR categories description with range	G1	Normal or high	≥90			
	G2	Mild decrease	60–89			
	G3a	Mild-to-moderate decrease	45–59			
	G3b	Moderate-to-severe	30–44			
	G4	Severe decrease	15–29			
	G5	Kidney failure	<15			

(CKD: chronic kidney disease; GFR: glomerular filtration rate)

Causes of ESRD

A. Diabetes mellitus
B. Hypertension
C. Vascular disease
- **a.** Renal artery stenosis
- **b.** ANCA-negative vasculitis
- **c.** Hypertensive nephrosclerosis
- **d.** Atheroemboli
- **e.** Renal vein thrombosis

D. Glomerular disease:
- **a.** Membranous nephropathy
- **b.** Alport syndrome
- **c.** Minimal change disease
- **d.** Focal and segmental glomerulosclerosis
- **e.** Rapidly progressive glomerulonephritis

E. Tubulointerstitial disease:
- **a.** Drugs like sulfonamides
- **b.** Infection
- **c.** Chronic hypokalemia
- **d.** Chronic hypercalcemia
- **e.** Multiple myeloma
- **f.** Heavy metals
- **g.** Radiation
- **h.** Sarcoidosis

F. Recurrent kidney stone
G. Urinary tract obstruction
H. Uncovered acute kidney injury
I. Congenital defect in the kidney and urinary bladder
J. Drugs

Following factors may hasten the renal injury:
A. Systemic hypertension
B. Dehydration
C. Proteinuria
D. Smoking
E. Hyperlipidemia
F. Uncontrolled diabetes
G. Hyperlipoidemia
H. Hyperphosphatemia

In ESRD, severe metabolic acidosis will occur but anion gap should not be >20 mEq/L. In this stage, anion gap will be increased due to accumulation of phosphates, sulfates and other organic ions. Metabolic acidosis has deleterious effect on the protein balance leading to the following:
A. Negative nitrogen balance
B. Increased degradation of protein
C. Reduced synthesis of albumin
D. Increased oxidation of essential amino acids
E. Lack of adaptation to low protein diet

Features in Different Stages of Chronic Kidney Disease

A. In stage 1–2 CKD:
- **a.** Asymptomatic
- **b.** Patient present with following symptoms:
  1. Edema of nephritic syndrome
  2. Hypertension
  3. Features of some types of glomerulonephritis
  4. Features of other parenchymal or vascular disease
  5. Features of collagen vascular disease

B. In stage 3–4 CKD:
- **a.** Clinical and laboratory complications of CKD
- **b.** Symptoms related to involvement of all organs in the body
- **c.** Acid-base imbalance
- **d.** Electrolyte imbalance

C. In stage 5 CKD:
- **a.** This is end-stage renal failure
- **b.** Marked imbalance in electrolyte and water imbalance
- **c.** Patient may develop uremic syndrome

Causes of Chronic Renal Disease

A. Hypertension
B. Diabetes mellitus

C. Glomerulonephritis

D. Primary glomerular disease with associated hypertension

E. Autosomal dominant kidney disease

F. Cystic kidney disease

G. Tubulointerstitial nephropathy

H. Collagen vascular disease

Laboratory Investigations

This should be done to evaluate:

- **a.** Underlying causative agents
- **b.** Degree of renal damage
- **c.** Consequence of renal damage

A. Serum and urine protein electrophoresis in patients with anemia and normal or elevated serum level of calcium in presence of CKD—multiple myeloma should be excluded.

B. In patients with glomerulonephritis—exclude autoimmune disease, such as SLE and infections, such as hepatitis B and C.

C. Serum iron, total iron-binding capacity (TIBC), and ferritin in case of ferritin to assess degree of iron store and severity of anemia.

D. Serum folate and vitamin B12 to assess the type of anemia

E. Serum calcium, phosphorus, and parathormone—to evaluate metabolic bone disease

F. 24-hour urine collection to estimate protein excretion of >300 mg is an indication of therapy with ARB or ACE inhibitors.

G. Specific tests:

- **a.** Serum DsDNA, ANA for SLE
- **b.** Serum complement levels
- **c.** C-ANCA and P-ANCA to diagnose granulomatosis polyangiitis and microscopic polyangiitis
- **d.** Antiglomerular antibody in the serum in case of suspected Goodpasture syndrome
- **e.** Viral serology

Imaging Studies

A. Renal ultrasound: It can detect:

- **a.** Presence or absence of two kidneys
- **b.** Asymmetry in the size of two kidneys
- **c.** Rule out renal masses
- **d.** Any evidence of obstruction

It can be diagnose by:

- **a.** Bilateral small: Scarred small kidneys with increased echogenicity—chronic kidney disease of long duration.
- **b.** If the size is normal the disease may acute or subacute.
- **c.** Large kidney:
  1. Diabetic nephropathy, where it is increased at the onset of diabetic nephropathy before the onset of CKD.
  2. Amyloidosis
  3. HIV nephropathy
- **d.** Enlarged kidney with multiple cysts—polycystic kidneys
- **e.** Discrepancy in the size of >1 cm in both the kidneys suggests:
  1. Unilateral developmental anomalies
  2. Renovascular disease

B. Renovascular disease can be diagnosed by:

- **a.** Doppler ultrasonography
- **b.** Nuclear medicine studies
- **c.** CT scan
- **d.** MRI

C. To detect reflux nephropathy as a cause of CKD in patients with recurrent urinary tract infection or asymmetry in renal size with scarred renal pole voiding cystourethrography to see any evidence of reflux. This reflux is resolved in patient with CKD. If this is present, this cannot be resolved by renal replacement.

D. Radiographic contrast media is not helpful in the investigation of CKD because:

- **a.** In case of diabetic nephropathy, it may precipitate renal failure
- **b.** If this is unavoidable caution must be taken:
  1. To avoid hyperkalemia
  2. Minimization of dye load
  3. Choice of least nephrotoxic radiographic contrast agent
- **c.** To attenuate contrast-induced worsening renal function:
  1. Judicious use of sodium bicarbonate solution
  2. N-acetylcysteine

E. Renal biopsy: It is not advised in case of bilateral small scarred kidneys because:

- **a.** Greater likelihood of causing bleeding and other adverse consequences.

b. Severe scarring may not give the features of underlying renal disease.
c. Specific therapy cannot be applied for specific disease because CKD has already been developed.

Contraindications:

a. Uncontrolled hypertension
b. Severe obesity
c. Bleeding diathesis
d. Active urinary tract infection

Treatment of Chronic Renal Failure

A. Slowing the progression of chronic renal failure: Reduction of intraglomerular hypertension and proteinuria:

a. Blood pressure target in CKD:

Without proteinuria (PCR < 100 mg/mmol):

1. Treat at 140/90 mm Hg
2. Target—130/80 mm Hg

b. With proteinuria (PCR > 100 mg/mmol):

1. Treat at 130/80 mm Hg
2. Target—120/75 mm Hg

c. Diabetes: Target is 120/70 mm Hg
d. The level of HbA1c should be less than 7% to prevent or delay in the microvascular complication. In case of type 2 diabetes mellitus, SGLT-2 inhibitors should be given to reduce the disease burden in these patients.

Increased intraglomerular pressure + hypertrophy of glomerulus produce loss of nephron ultimately lead to decreased function of the kidney in spite of resolution or treatment of the inciting events. Angiotensin-converting enzyme inhibitors and angiotensin receptor blockers can decrease intraglomerular pressure and decrease the proteinuria by dilatation of efferent arteriole and constriction of afferent arteriole.

Adverse effects of the above drugs:

a. Cough and angioedema with ACE inhibitor
b. Anaphylaxis and hyperkalemia—with both of the above drugs
c. Progression of serum creatinine with above agents may suggest renovascular disease involving large and small arteries.

So the second-line drugs should be advised: Calcium channel blockers, such as verapamil and diltiazem—these may exhibit superior renoprotective and antiproteinuric effect as compared to dihydropyridines.

In case where contribution of intraglomerular hypertension in developing CKD but contribution of proteinuria is minimal or absent while taking other antihypertensive drugs.

So order of antihypertensive therapies in case of CKD:

a. Lifestyle changes—salt intake <5 g/day
b. ACE inhibitor—if PCR > 100 g/mmol
c. Loop diuretics (furosemide or metolazone) in case of salt and water overload
d. Addition of ARBs if PCR remains > 100 mg/mmol.
e. Dihydropyridine calcium channel blocker (nifedipine, amlodipine)
f. Potassium lowering gastrointestinal tract binder, such as patiromer improves potassium excretion along with control of blood pressure
g. Beta blockers (bisoprolol, atenolol)
h. Centrally acting agents (moxonidine)
i. Alpha-blockers (doxazosin)
j. Vascular smooth muscle relaxant (minoxidil)

B. Control of blood sugar—excellent blood sugar control in type 1 and 2 diabetes mellitus may retard the progression of the disease:

a. Target is:

1. Fasting blood sugar is 90–130 mg/dL.
2. HbA1c is <7%.

b. Dose of the drugs to be prohibited in CKD:

1. Chlorpropamide—produces prolonged hypoglycemia
2. Metformin produces lactic acidosis
3. Thiazolidinediones (rosiglitazone and pioglitazone)—increase salt and water retention leading to fluid overload states
4. Dose of the insulin should be reduced and adjusted due to decreased degradation as well as renal excretion of insulin

C. Control of hyperlipidemia:

a. Target is <4.0 mmol/L for cholesterol and <2.0 mmol/L for low density lipoprotein (LDL)

D. Metabolic acidosis should be controlled by supplementation of bicarbonate

E. Volume overload should be controlled by loop diuretics and if required by ultrafiltration.

F. Hyperphosphatemia should be corrected by phosphate binders like calcium acetate, sevelamer carbonate and lanthanum carbonate along with dietary phosphate restriction.

G. Hypocalcemia should be corrected by vitamin D3 6k weekly before breakfast for 8–10 weeks.

H. Life style modification in the form of:

a. Low salt 2 g/day

b. Low phosphorus and low potassium diet
c. Daily protein restriction to 0.8 g/kg of body weight.

The drugs are atorvastatin and rosuvastatin.

a. Complications are:
   1. Myalgia
   2. Rhabdomyolysis
   3. Small rise in creatine phosphokinase (CPK)

I. Avoidance of some drugs that are excreted through urine:
   a. Oral antidiabetic drugs
   b. NSAIDs
   c. Meperidine
   d. Nephrotoxic agent, such as gadolinium must be avoided
   e. Many antibiotics require dose reduction or change in the dose of these drugs. Dose reduction of some drugs has to adjusted according to estimated GFR that can be found in the website (http://www.globalrph.com/index_renal.htm)

J. KDOQI guidelines of daily protein intake:
   a. Daily protein intake 0.60–0.75 g/kg/day of which 50% of protein intake of high biological value
   b. In CKD stage 5—spontaneous protein intake tends to decrease, patient may enter a stage of protein energy malnutrition. The protein intake should be increased up to 0.90 g/kg/day.
   c. Energy intake—35 kcal/kg—recommended

K. Control of calcium and phosphate metabolism

L. Control of anemia

Patient suffering from ESRD should be educated in the following:

A. Avoid taking NSAIDs
B. Low phosphorus and low potassium rich diet.
C. Placement and maintenance of vascular access for continuous hemodialysis.
D. Pregnancy should be prohibited in these patients.
E. Avoid intake of too much fluid and salt.
F. Protein restricted diet as will delay the progression of the disease related symptoms

Physiology of Nephrons

Proximal convoluted tubule:

A. Resorption of 60–70% sodium occurs by Na^+/K^+ ATPase through the basolateral membrane of the cells along with the water by osmosis.
B. 65% of water is absorbed will be absorbed through the aquaporin as well as tight junctions.
C. 100% of the glucose and amino acids are reabsorbed sodium dependent transporters.
D. 90% of bicarbonate will be reabsorbed through the carbonic anhydrate inhibitors.
E. Secretion of penicillin, ammonia and creatinine are secreted actively
F. Phosphate absorption is strictly regulated by Parathormone, it will inhibit Parathormone resorption leading to phosphaturia whereas calcium is absorbed passively.

Distal convoluted tubule:

A. 5-10% sodium is reabsorbed in the proximal tubule through the Na^+/K^+ symporters. Here based on the sodium level in the blood, aldosterone is secreted from the macula densa and stimulate reabsorption of sodium form and excretion of potassium into the tubule.
B. Calcium from the tubule will be reabsorbed via Parathormone via TRPV5 channels.
C. Acid base balance should be maintained active secretion of hydrogen ion and Secretion of ammonia buffer the urinary acid.

Loop of Henle: It has been described in question number 41.

Function of collecting duct has been discussed in question number 29.

Q16. Describe the etiology and management of anemia in chronic renal failure.

SNMC/MAY2013/MDIII (10)

Discuss kidney as an endocrine. How would you manage anemia in CKD.

AMU/2011/MDIII (20)

Etiopathogenesis of anemia in chronic kidney disease.

DNBIIIB/JUN2015 (5)

Newer therapies in anemia in CKD.

AIIMS, BHU 2020 (5)

Anemia in CKD.

SCBMCH, 2020 (10)

What is hypoxia inducible factor stabilizers? Discuss the updated management of anemia in CKD.

WBUHS, 2020 (10)

ANSWER

In hematology chapter question number 42—answer given.

Kidney as an Endocrine Organ

A. Renin production: Renin, a rate limiting step in the renin-angiotensin system acts by converting angiotensinogen to angiotensin I. It is produced at the juxtaglomerular apparatus through the following mechanisms:

a. Sensing of baroreceptor in the afferent arteriole to lowering of blood pressure

b. Decreased concentration of sodium chloride in the macula densa

c. Increased level of catecholamines stimulate beta adrenergic receptors on the juxtaglomerular cells

Angiotensin I is converted to angiotensin II by angiotensin-converting enzyme which leads to:

a. Production of antidiuretic hormone

b. Vasoconstriction

c. Aldosterone secretion

d. Sodium resorption

e. Water retention

B. Erythropoietin production: It originates from fibroblast of renal cortex and controls erythropoiesis by increasing erythropoietic precursors and its differentiation. Hypoxia stimulates erythropoietin enhancer and suppresses erythropoietin enhancer GATA-2.

C. Vitamin D production: Vitamin D is produced by interaction of ultraviolet rays of sunlight and 7-dehydrocholesterol present in the skin. Now vitamin D3 is hydroxylated in the liver to 25-hydroxy vitamin D3, which in turn again hydroxylated by 1-α-hydroxylase produced by proximal renal tubular cells in kidney to form 1,25$(OH)_2$ vitamin D3, this will play an active role in calcium-phosphorus homeostasis.

D. Prostaglandin metabolism: Prostaglandin is produced throughout the body and takes part in vasodilatation and inflammation. It regulates vascular tone and salt—water homeostasis in kidney. PGI_2 and PGE_2 increases renal blood flow in spite of decreased effecting circulating volume. Cyclooxygenase acts as rate limiting stem in prostaglandin synthesis. Cyclooxygenase inhibitor decreases the production of PGE_2.

E. Insulin metabolism: Kidney is primary site for insulin clearance from the circulation by two process:

1. Proximal tubular reabsorption: After absorption insulin becomes endocytosed and degrade to different fragment and delivered to lysosomes. This degradation is dramatically reduced in renal failure. Similarly sulfonylurea is at risk of hypoglycemia because of its decreased degradation.

2. Glomerular filtration

F. Gastrin metabolism: Gastrin produced by G cells in the stomach stimulates hydrochloric acid from the stomach. Serum gastrin level is increased in case of chronic kidney disease suggesting its metabolism in kidney.

G. Parathormone metabolism: Parathormone secreted by chief cells in the parathyroid gland is responsible for increased calcium absorption and decreased phosphate resorption from the kidney. In chronic kidney disease decreased ability to excrete phosphate and activation of vitamin D will lead to hypocalcemia and hyperphosphatemia.

H. Glucose metabolism: Medulla of kidney will take part in neoglucogenesis by glucose phosphorylation and glycolytic enzyme activity. Renal cortical cells also contain glucose-6-phosphatase which help in releasing free glucose into the circulation. Renal acidosis also increases neoglucogenesis.

I. Generation of thrombopoietin: Proximal tubular cells of kidney produces small amount of thrombopoietin which is responsible for production and activation of platelets.

J. Urodilatin: It is a specific type of atrial natriuretic peptide secreted by tubular cells and it inhibits sodium reabsorption and renal, coronary, and pulmonary vasodilatation.

Hypoxia Inducible Factor Stabilizers

It is a group of drug that inhibits prolyl hydroxylase thereby stabilize and activates the hypoxia inducible factors which in turn regulate cellular response to hypoxia by:

A. Promoting production of erythropoietin

B. Promoting angiogenesis

C. Promoting iron metabolism

D. Promoting glucose metabolism

Under normal condition this factor (HIF)-alpha subunits are hydroxylated by prolyl hydroxylase through von-Hippel-Lindau ubiquitin pathway. The HIF stabilizer inhibits this pathway thereby preventing degradation of HIF-alpha and allows transcription of the hypoxia-responsive genes.

Applications: This stabilizer is used in case of anemia due to chronic kidney disease.

The approved stabilizers are:

A. Roxadustat: 1st-in-class stabilizers that is approved in this treatment
B. Daprodustat
C. Vadadustat
D. Enarodustat
E. Molidustat

It has following advantages over erythropoietin:

A. It is administered orally.
B. There is least fluctuation of the hemoglobin level thereby reduction of the cardiovascular risk.
C. Metabolism of iron is improved, so the need for intravenous iron administration will be reduced.

This stabilizer has following risks:

A. There is risk of thrombosis leading to cerebral and cardiovascular complications.
B. In case of long term use the angiogenesis may lead to development of tumor.
C. Risk of hypertension will be increased.

Q17. Proteinuria.

ERA/NOV2012(S)/MDIII (10)
KUHS/MAY2014/MDI (10)
MGR/APR2003/MDIII (10)

Causes and diagnostic approach for a patient with proteinuria.

PGI/APR2013/MDI (10)

Approach to proteinuria.

AIIMS, BBS 2020 (10)

Proteinuria—significance and treatment.

SAURASHTRA UNI, RAJKOT, 2022 (20)

Mention with examples of types of proteinuria. How can you approach to a case of proteinuria?

WBUHS, 2025 (10)

ANSWER

Proteinuria

Normally, a person excretes <150 mg of protein per day. Usually <20 mg of albumin is filtered through glomerulus but reabsorbed followed by broken down in the proximal tubule. Nearly 50% proteins Tamm–Horsfall protein called uromodulin, excreted through urine is secreted by tubular cells of distal convoluted tubule and loop of Henle. Rest 50% proteins are plasma proteins, albumin, immunoglobulin, light chain, β-2 microglobulin, and others. But abnormal proteinuria may be due to increased glomerular filtration or tubular reabsorption of both. Abnormal proteinuria can be classified based on physiology:

A. Overflow proteinuria: When abnormally large amount of small molecular weight proteins are filtered through glomerulus which exceeds the capacity of the tubular absorption capacity—it is called overflow proteinuria. The causes are:

a. Intravascular hemolysis-producing hemoglobinuria
b. Rhabdomyolysis-producing myoglobinuria
c. Multiple myeloma excreting light chains

Hemoglobinuria and myoglobinuria cannot be detected by dipstick but can be recognized by:

a. Presence of red urine
b. Presence of heme positive red supernatant after centrifugation

Light chain can be detected by urine immunofixation.

B. Tubular proteinuria: When there failure of the tubulo-interstitium to reabsorb normally filtered protein having small molecular weight, such as light chain, retinol-binding protein, β-2 microglobulin, and breakdown product of albumin.

Due to injury of tubular epithelial cells, brush border and cellular enzymes, such as lysozymes and N-acetylglucosamine and incase of cellular injury involving loop of Henle or distal convoluted tubule uromodulin are excreted in urine.

Tubular proteinuria will never excrete >1–2 g protein per day whereas >3 mg in case of glomerular proteinuria.

These proteins cannot be detected by dipstick but to detect the source of proteinuria, following two methods are used:

a. Urine protein electrophoresis—in case of glomerular proteinuria only albumin is detected but in case tubular variety, small molecular proteins are detected. But it is true the either of these proteinuria is not exclusive as glomerular disease is accompanied by tubulointerstitial injury or inflammation.
b. Immunofixation can detect light chain.

C. Glomerular proteinuria: Glomerular filtration barrier is composed of:

a. Fenestrated endothelial cells—its disruption occurs in preeclampsia.

b. Glomerular basement membrane—its disruption occurs in Alport syndrome

c. Glomerular epithelial cells or podocytes—its disruption occurs in focal-segmental glomerulosclerosis.

Genetic mutations in different proteins responsible for heavy proteinuria:

a. Genetic mutations in the proteins of slit-diaphragm in infants and children.

b. Genetic mutations of podocytes enzymes

c. Genetic mutations of different constituents of glomerular basement membrane.

Following types of charge-selective injury to filtration barrier may produce heavy proteinuria:

a. Due to change in size-selective properties high molecular weight proteins or cells (in crescentic glomerulonephritis)

b. Due to change in charge-selective properties there is ultrafiltration of negatively charged proteins as in case of minimal chain disease.

Mesangial injury interferes with normal mesangial clearance leading to heavy proteinuria.

Gradation of glomerular proteinuria:

a. Mild grade—when albumin excretion is 30–300 mg/day.

b. Moderate grade—when albumin excretion is 1–3 g/day

c. Severe grade—when albumin excretion is >3–20 g/day.

D. Postrenal proteinuria: Small to moderate amount of proteinuria occurs due to inflammation of urinary tract, nephrolithiasis, and tumors.

E. Isolated proteinuria: Less than 2 g/day proteinuria in absence of decreased GFR or hematuria, diabetes mellitus, hypertension, or systemic diseases occurs and it is usually benign but these patients are required constant follow-up.

F. Transient proteinuria: Low grade, i.e., <2 g/day proteinuria occurs in children, young adult, and adolescents. It can occur in the following conditions:

a. Fever

b. Exercise—these patients may show >2 g/day proteinuria and hematuria.

c. Upright position—it is called orthostatic proteinuria. It is diagnosed if first morning urine is negative for protein but day time collection shows positive for protein. These patients do not require follow-up.

d. Uncontrolled diabetes mellitus

e. Hyperglycemia

f. Hypertension

g. Heart failure

Detection and quantification of proteinuria:

A. Dipstick method: It is neither sensitive nor quantitative. Negative dipstick result cannot exclude proteinuria as it can only detect albumin and is concentration gradient.

B. Sulfosalicylic acid test: It can detect all proteins including albumin. So, dipstick negative but positive Sjögren's syndrome A (SSA) test indicate presence of any protein except albumin in urine.

After positive dipstick results quantitative estimation of proteinuria can be done by the following methods:

a. 24-hour urine collection: In this case to ensure adequacy of collection total urinary creatinine has to be measured simultaneously with measurement of 24 hours urinary protein. If the creatinine level is outside the normal range, it suggests the urine collection is inaccurate. Total 24 hours urinary excretion of creatinine levels are:

1. In case normal females under 50 years of age is 15–20 mg/kg

2. In case of normal male under 50 years of age is 18–25 mg/kg

3. In case of adult of >50 years of age creatinine level decreases due to progressive muscle mass reduction.

b. Spot urine protein to creatinine ratio in first voided morning urine: It should be assumed that normal individual excretes 1 g of creatinine per day, normal spot urine protein to creatinine ratio is below 0.2 g protein/g of creatinine. If the value is >0.3—it suggests presence of nephrotic range of proteinuria. It can detect whether the proteinuria is mild or nephrotic range. This distinction is essential because:

1. Nephrotic range is due to glomerular disease but nonnephrotic range is due to tubular disease or glomerular origin.

2. Glomerular disease may have worse prognosis and treatment is different.

c. Urinary albumin-creatinine ratio: In case of healthy adult, it is 5–15 mg albumin/g of creatinine. If it is >30, it suggests incipient diabetic nephropathy.

Causes of proteinuria:

A. Infections:
  a. Hepatitis B and C
  b. HIV
  c. Secondary syphilis
  d. Amyloidosis
  e. Malaria

B. Immunologic:
  a. Systemic lupus erythematosus (SLE)
  b. Sjögren syndrome
  c. Sarcoidosis
  d. Post-bone marrow transplantation
  e. Rheumatoid arthritis

C. Metabolic:
  a. Obesity
  b. Diabetes mellitus

D. Neoplasms:
  a. Multiple myeloma
  b. Breast cancer
  c. Lung cancer
  d. Lymphoma
  e. Leukemia

E. Medications:
  a. Penicillamine
  b. Nonsteroidal anti-inflammatory drugs (NSAIDs)
  c. Tyrosine kinase inhibitors
  d. Vascular endothelial growth factor

F. Genetic:
  a. Alport syndrome
  b. Autosomal dominant polycystic kidney disease (ADPKD)
  c. Congenital nephrotic syndrome
  d. Nail-patella syndrome

G. Miscellaneous:
  a. Reflux nephropathy
  b. Sickle cell disease

Management of proteinuria:

A. General management:
  a. Control of sugar to make the HbA1c less than 7%
  b. Blood should be maintained to maintain 130/80 mm Hg.
  c. Weight reduction to reduce obesity.
  d. Smoking cessation
  e. Dietary factors:
    1. Sodium intake to less than 2 g daily.
    2. Protein intake to 0.8–1 g daily.
  f. vaccination against hepatitis b virus, *Pneumococcus.*

B. Medications:
  a. ACEI in case of chronic kidney disease with proteinuria
  b. ARBs in case of chronic kidney disease with proteinuria
  c. Dapagliflozin and empagliflozin in case to diabetic kidney disease with proteinuria to slow the progression of the kidney disease as well as heart failure.
  d. Aldosterone antagonists in case of resistant cases but there is risk of hyperkalemia.
  e. Endothelial receptor antagonists like Sparsentan and Atrasentan
  f. Statin in case of hyperlipidemia
  g. Immunosuppressantincaseofglomerulonephritis related proteinuria.

C. Disease specific medications:
  a. In case glomerulonephritis steroids, other immunosuppressant and in refractory cases plasma exchange.
  b. In case nephrotic syndrome steroids, immunosuppressant, calcineurin inhibitor
  c. In case of lupus nephritis steroids, cyclophosphamide, mycophenolate mofetil and belimumab.
  d. In case of diabetic nephropathy RAAS, SGLT2 inhibitors

Q18. Histology of kidney.

MGR/APR2016/MDI (10)

Histology of kidney in health.

MGR/SEP2008/MDIII (20)

Microscopic structure of kidney.

MGR/APR2013/MDI (5)

Describe the anatomy and physiology of different segments of the nephron and outline the renal function tests used for the diagnosis of tubule-interstitial renal disease.

DNB (DEC 2020) (10)

Tubular function test described in question number 20

Draw the structure of nephron. Write about the complete urine examination with its significance.

DR YSR UNI OF HEALTH SC, VIJAYAWADA, ANDHRA, 2022 (10)

Describe the ultrastructure of the glomerulus. How do you approach to a patient with proteinuria?

MANIPUR UNIVERSITY, 2019 (10)

Structure of the glomerulus of kidney and its role in the regulation of blood pressure.

MANIPUR UNIVERSITY, 2024 (10)

ANSWER

Role of regulation of blood pressure described in question number 24.

Urine examination has been described in question number 20 and 30.

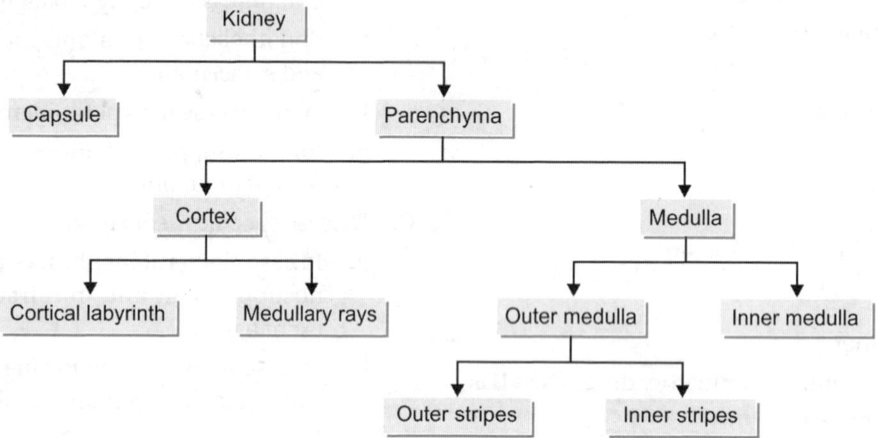

Capsule: It is made up of collagen fibers, smooth muscle cells, and blood capillaries.

Parenchyma is composed of millions of nephrons, renal arteries, and their branches, corresponding veins, lymphatics, and nerves.

Nephrons are functional as well as structural units of kidney.

Depending on the locations of the glomeruli nephrons are classified into two types:

- **A.** Superficial type
- **B.** Juxtamedullary type

On the basis of length of loop of Henle they are classified into two types:

- **A.** Short-looped: It is generally superficial or mid-cortical glomeruli, its tubule extends up to outer medulla from where they will reflect back to cortex.
- **B.** Long-looped: It is juxtamedullary glomeruli, its tubule extends up to inner medulla from where it will reflect back.

Nephron is composed of:

- **A.** Renal corpuscles:
  - **a.** Glomerulus:
    - **1.** Glomerular capillaries
    - **2.** Mesangium
  - **b.** Bowmen's capsule:
    - **1.** Parietal layer
    - **2.** Visceral layer
- **B.** Proximal tubule:
  - **a.** Proximal convoluted tubule
  - **b.** Proximal straight tubule
- **C.** Henle's loop:
  - **a.** Thin descending portion
  - **b.** Thin ascending portion
  - **c.** Thick ascending portion
- **D.** Distal convoluted tubule:
- **E.** Connecting segment

F. Collecting duct:
  a. Arcade: It is initial collecting tubule
  b. Straight portion:
    1. Cortical collecting duct
    2. Outer medullary duct
    3. Inner medullary duct

Histology of Glomerulus

Glomerulus is formed by invagination of a tuft of capillaries into the Bowman's capsule. These capillaries enter into this capsule from afferent arteriole and leaves the capsule through efferent arteriole at vascular pole. This glomerulus is composed of five layers. These are:

A. Layer 1: Foot processes of podocytes. Visceral epithelial cells give series of processes known as podocytes that lay over the second layer. In between the podocytes there are slit-like diaphragm.
B. Layer 2: Lamina rara externa or outer cement layer. Foot processes preset on it.
C. Layer 3: Lamina densa: It is the dense structural part of basement membrane.
D. Layer 4: Lamina rara interna or inner cement layer: It acts as a bed for capillary endothelium.
E. Layer 5: Endothelial cell layer of glomerular capillaries having fenestration of 100 nm in diameter.

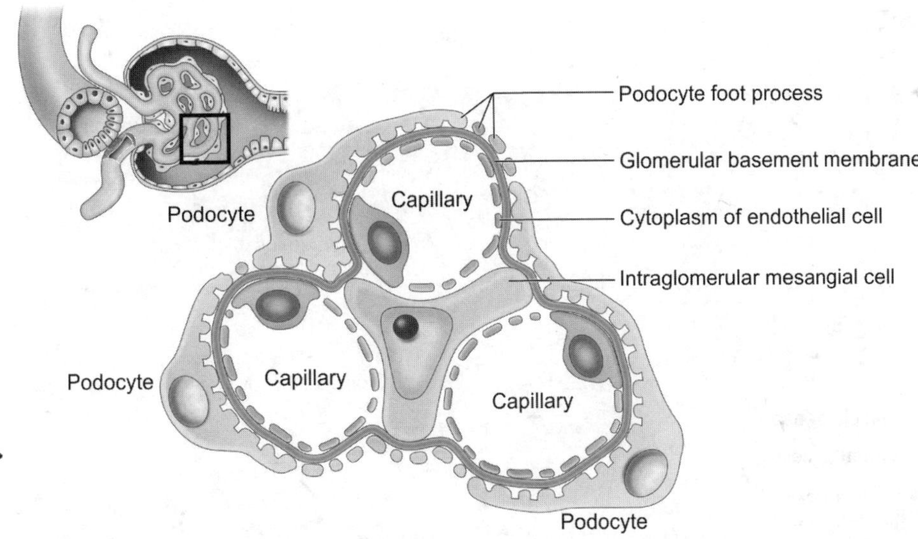

Each glomerulus contains six lobules, each lobule consists of 3–6 capillary loops. There are many anastomoses present between the capillaries in any one lobule.

Urinary pole is opposite to the vascular pole, here Bowmen's space will open into the proximal convoluted tubule.

Visceral layer of Bowmen's capsule is present beneath the glomerular basement membrane.

Mesangium: It is the core of the glomerulus, it is composed of specialized contractile cells which are embedded in acellular matrix.

Mesangial cells contain bundles of microfilaments formed by contractile proteins, these cells have elongated irregular processes. Functions of these cells are:

A. Phagocytosis
B. Production of mesangial matrix
C. Maintenance of capillary loops
D. Maintenance of blood flow

Bowman's capsule is the initial dilated part of nephron having epithelial lining of 5 μm thick. Within it glomerulus is present. Bowman's capsule along with glomerulus is called Malpighian corpuscle. It has two layers:

A. Visceral cell layer: It is very closely applied to capillary loops and it will surround each loop. It is continuous with the parietal cell layer at the site of entrance of afferent and efferent arterioles. It is formed by podocytes having primary, secondary, and tertiary processes, smallest is called foot processes or pedicles. In between the foot processes there is space called slit diaphragm.
B. Parietal cell layer: This layer is applied to proper Bowman's capsule and forms the outer lining of glomerulus. It is continuous with parietal cell layer of proximal convoluted tubule.
C. Additional epithelial cells in the Bowmen's capsule present at the vascular pole in the junction between visceral and parietal cell layer called peripolar cells.

The space present in between the visceral and parietal cell layer is called Bowman's space.

Proximal tubule:

A. It will twist and turn in the cortical labyrinth hence is called proximal convoluted tubule then it will enter into the medullary rays and becomes straight hence called proximal straight tubule.

B. It is lined by simple cuboidal epithelial cells with brush border due to presence of numerous microvilli from the apical cell membrane.

C. Single spherical nucleus is present at the basal part of the cell in eosinophilic cytoplasm.

D. Lumen is uneven and small.

Loop of Henle

A. Thin limb is lined by simple squamous epithelium which gradually changes to cuboidal cells at the end of this segment.

B. Thick ascending limb has simple cuboidal epithelium having apical microprojections with undulated cell borders but no brush borders.

Distal Convoluted Tubule

A. It is lined by tall cuboidal epithelium having brush border.

B. Nucleus is located close to apical cell border.

C. Lumen appears larger as compared to proximal convoluted tubule (PCT).

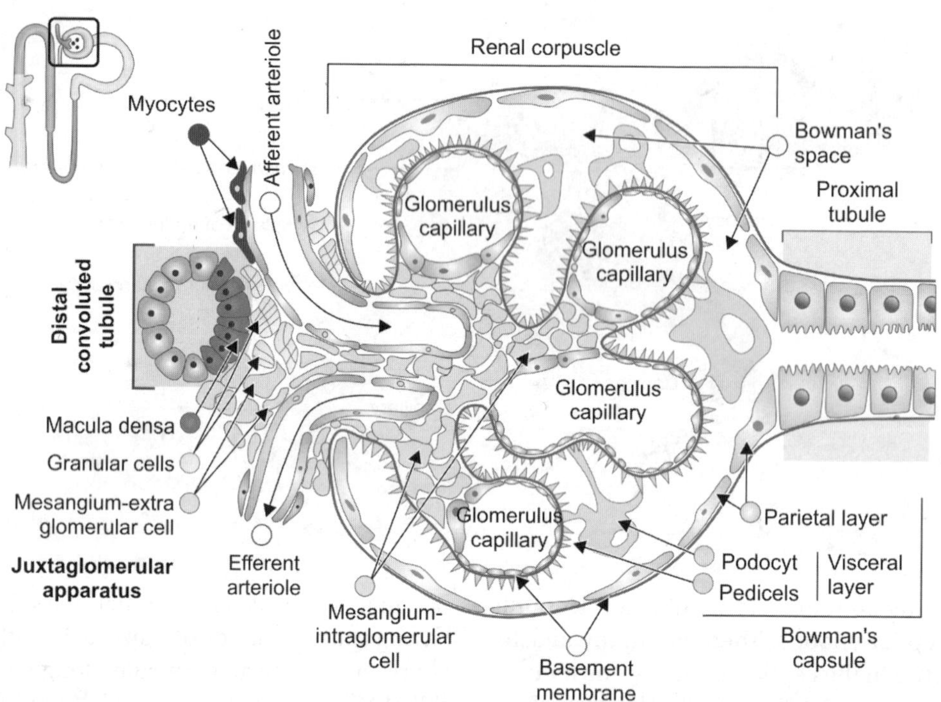

Connecting Segment

A. It contains different types of cells, these are cuboidal cells, connecting segment cells, intercalated cells, and principal cells (low cuboidal cells with short microprojection from its smooth apical surface).

B. Intercalated cells are associated with acid-base homeostasis.

Collecting System of the Kidney

It is formed by joining of distal convoluted tubule of several nephrons. Its length is 20 mm. It is lined by cuboidal epithelium. This tubule will pass through the renal cortex and medulla to drain into the renal pelvis at the apices of medullary pyramid. Collecting ducts at the tip of the pyramid are called duct of Bellini.

The epithelium of the collecting tubule consists of two types of cells:

A. P-cells or principal cells: It contains two types of receptors:

a. Receptors for antidiuretic hormone

b. Receptors for aldosterone

These receptors after being activated increases the permeability to water through aquaporin-2 by increasing the pore size and increasing cyclic adenosine monophosphate (cAMP). Thus 10–12% water is reabsorbed. This cell also is involved in resorption of sodium.

B. I-cells or intercalated cells: It will secrete 5% of the total hydrogen ion and helps to reabsorb bicarbonate ion through Na^+ for K^+ or H^+ which leads to acid urine.

Juxtaglomerular Apparatus

It is located at the vascular pole of glomerulus. It is composed of:

A. Macula densa: It is thick specialized tall and narrow cells in thick ascending limb during its passage in between efferent and afferent arteriole and responsible for renin-angiotensin system.

B. Lacis cells: It is found between macula densa and two arteriole.

C. Juxtaglomerular cells: It is specialized epithelial cells found in afferent arterioles.

Q19. Clinical features, diagnosis, and treatment of immunoglobulin A nephropathy.

KUHS/MAY2014/MDII (10)

Berger's disease and immunoglobulin A nephropathy.

MGR/OCT2013/MDI (5)

IgA nephropathy.

SCBMCH, 2013 (20)

BHARATI VIDYAPEETH DEEMED UNI, JHELUM, 2018 (10)

ANSWER

Introduction

Immunoglobulin A (IgA) nephropathy can be characterized by episodic hematuria along with deposition of IgA in the mesangial area.

Epidemiology

A. It is the most common form of glomerulonephritis throughout the world.

B. Males are predominantly affected.

C. Peak incidence occurs in the second and third decade of life.

D. Geographically 30% occurs in Asian and Pacific rims and 20% in South Europe.

E. Familial forms are more prevalent in northern Italy as well as Eastern Kentucky.

F. There is close similarities are between IgA nephropathy and Henoch–Schönlein purpura but last one can be differentiated by its younger age of incidence, abdominal complaints, and preceding infections.

Pathophysiology

This is a multistep process as there is evidence of therapeutic target in different steps:

A. Immunoglobulin A is produced in the intestinal mucosa by plasma cells through T-cell dependent and T-cell independent process. Cytokines produced by T cells a proliferation-inducing ligand (APRIL) will promote B cells to switch over to IgA1-producing plasma cells.

So first therapeutic target is production of inhibitors of cytokines.

Second therapeutic target is B cell and plasma cell inhibitors to decrease the production of IgA. These are rituximab and bortezomib.

B. Immunoglobulin A1 produced in patient with IgA nephropathy will be under-glycosylated [galactose deficient (Gd)-IgA1] in the hinge region thus exposing N-acetylgalactosamine in truncated hinge region. Susceptible individual will produce autoantibodies IgG against the exposed region.

In this step, antiproliferative agents can prevent this autoantibody production.

C. These Gd-IgA1-autoantibody immune complexes are present in the circulation or in situ activate alternate pathway complement.

So, complement inhibitors will prevent formation of immune complexes.

D. Galactose deficient IgA1 will evade the catabolism by the liver and deposits in the mesangium and produces immune complexes.

E. As the immune complexes are nephritogenic, it will produce local inflammation, cellular proliferation which ultimately leads to fibrosis.

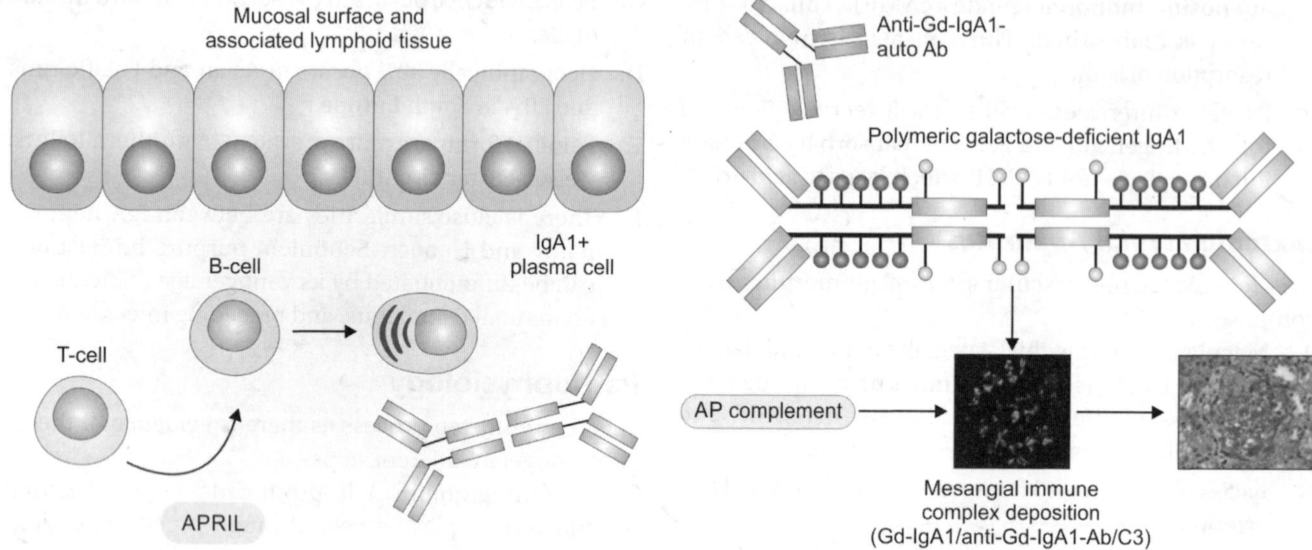

(AP: alternative pathway; APRIL: a proliferation-inducing ligand; auto Ab: autoantibody; Gd-IgA1: galactose deficient immunoglobulin A1)

Pathology

Renal biopsy is the method to confirm diagnosis.

A. Light microscopy findings:
   a. Mesangial cell proliferation and expansion of matrix
   b. In case of rapid deterioration of renal function more diffuse proliferation of both capillary and mesangial cells, segmental necrosis, and crescent formation.
B. On immunofluorescence microscopy: Hallmark is presence of prominent globular mesangial dominant or codominant deposits of IgA1.
C. On electron microscopy: Typical finding is dense deposit.

Etiology

A. Primary IgA nephropathy
B. Secondary IgA nephropathy:
   a. Henoch–Schönlein purpura
   b. Gut disorders:
      1. Alcoholic cirrhosis
      2. Celiac disease
      3. Inflammatory bowel disease (IBD)
   c. Skin and joint disorders:
      1. Spondyloarthropathies
      2. Dermatitis herpetiformis
      3. Psoriasis

Clinical Presentation

A. About 30–50% patients present with:
   a. Recurrent gross hematuria within few days of upper respiratory tract infection
   b. More common in children and young adult
   c. Dull flank pain with fever of low grade
B. About 30–50% patients:
   a. May be asymptomatic detected only during routine examination (positive for microscopic hematuria and mild proteinuria of <500 mg/day)
   b. May present with systemic hypertension
C. Less than 5% patients present with acute oliguric renal failure may be due to:
   a. Tubular damage
   b. Dysfunction due to tubular cast
D. At least 20% patients present with chronic kidney disease due to long-standing underdiagnosed disease presenting with:
   a. Hypertension
   b. Mild-to-moderate proteinuria
   c. Hematuria of undetermined duration

Course of the Disease

A. Immunoglobulin A nephropathy is a benign disease
B. 5–30% will go into remission, rest of the patient may present with hematuria but with well-preserved renal function.

C. Very few patients will enter into renal failure over 20–25 years. Risk factors are:
   a. Hypertension
   b. Proteinuria
   c. Absence of episodes of macroscopic hematuria
   d. Male sex
   e. Older age of onset
   f. Renal biopsy demonstrates extensive glomerulosclerosis or interstitial fibrosis.

Diagnosis

A. Urine analysis: RBC, RBC cast, albumin
B. Blood for liver function test (LFT), lipid level, and serum IgA1 level
C. Renal biopsy
D. 24-hour urine protein determination
E. Skin biopsy to show deposition of IgA in immunofluorescence microscopy
F. Estimated glomerular filtration rate (eGFR) measurement:
   a. Normal: ≥60
   b. <60 to ≥15: Moderate
   c. <15: End-stage renal failure

Prognosis

Poor prognostic features are the following:
A. Impaired renal function
B. Heavy proteinuria > 3 g/day
C. Difficult to treat hypertension
D. Tubulointerstitial fibrosis or glomerulosclerosis on kidney biopsy
E. Rapid progressive crescent IgA nephropathy

Treatment

Treatment varies according to the risk of the patients:
A. In case of low-risk patients:
   a. Normal renal function
   b. Episodic macroscopic hematuria
   c. Proteinuria < 1 g/day
   d. No hypertension

   Here no treatment is required but regular surveillance by:
   a. Measuring blood pressure
   b. Serum creatinine
   c. Dipstick for worsening of proteinuria
B. In case of moderate risk patients:
   a. Older age
   b. Proteinuria >1 g/day
   c. Hypertension

   Treatment should be:
   To maintain target BP to 130/75 mm Hg:
   1. Angiotensin-converting enzyme (ACE) inhibitor
   2. Angiotensin receptor blocker (ARB)

   Increase the dose of above drugs to decrease the proteinuria.

   But regular monitoring of blood pressure, serum creatinine, and potassium are essential for continuation of treatment.
C. In case of high risk patients: It is difficult to treat and these patients will progress to end-stage renal failure despite therapy:
   a. If ACE inhibitor or ARB fails to reduce blood pressure and proteinuria
   b. Start prednisolone 0.5 mg/kg/day for 6 months
   c. If proteinuria is in the nephrotic range—prednisolone 0.5–1 mg/kg/day for 8 weeks.
   d. If crescentic IgA nephropathy:

   Prednisolone 0.5–1 mg/kg/day + cyclophosphamide 2 mg/kg/day for 8 weeks.

Budesonide: It is a novel therapy as it locally acts in lymphoid tissue in the distal ileum and proximal large intestine to modulate IgA function. High first pass metabolism will minimize the side effects.

Q20. Discuss the structure and functions of glomerulus. Describe in detail the various glomerular function tests.
BF/MAY2010/MDI (25)

Determinants of glomerular filtration.
BF/MAY2012/MDII (12)

Renal tubular function test.
MUHS/MAY2011/MDI (10)

Kidney function test.
MGR/SEP2009/MDI (5) MGR/OCT2012/MDI (5)

Estimation of glomerular filtration rate. Pathophysiology of diabetic kidney disease.
DNB (DEC, 2022) (10)

Creatinine clearance.
SCBMCH, 2021 (10)

Diabetic nephropathy answer written in question number 10

Discuss renal tubular function test.
MAHARASHTRA UNI OF HEALTH SC, VIJAYAWADA, 2021 (10)

Glomerular filtration rate.
NTR UNI OF HEALTH SC, VIJAYAWADA, 2020 (10)

Renal tubular function test
MAHARASHTRA UNI OF HEALTH SC, VIJAYAWADA, 2019 (10)

Estimation of glomerular filtration rate.
MGR UNIVERSITY, TAMIL NADU, 2018 (5)

ANSWER

Glomerulus is formed by invagination of a tuft of capillaries into the Bowman's capsule. These capillaries enter into this capsule from afferent arteriole and leaves the capsule through efferent arteriole. This glomerulus is composed of five layers. These are:

F. Layer 1: Foot processes of podocytes. Visceral epithelial cells give series of processes known as podocytes that lay over the second layer. In between the podocytes there are slit-like diaphragm.

G. Layer 2: Lamina rara externa or outer cement layer. Foot processes preset on it.

H. Layer 3: Lamina densa: It is the dense structural part of basement membrane.

I. Layer 4: Lamina rara interna or inner cement layer: It acts as a bed for capillary endothelium.

J. Layer 5: Endothelial cell layer of glomerular capillaries having fenestration of 100 nm in diameter.

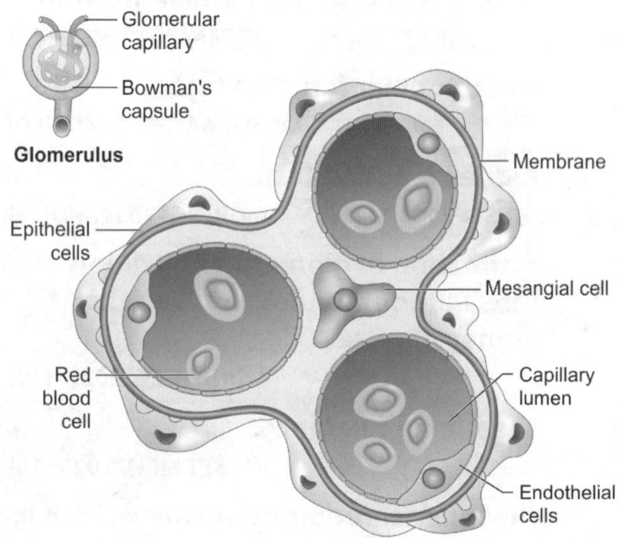

Each glomerulus contains six lobules, each lobule consists of 3–6 capillary loops. There are many anastomoses present between the capillaries in any one lobule.

Physiology of glomerulus: Glomerular capillary pressure is 45 mm Hg as compared to other systemic capillaries which is 25 mm Hg. Glomerular filtration rate is 125 mL/min which is 170–180 L/day.

Mechanism of glomerular filtration: It is governed by the following:

A. Hydrostatic pressure gradient across the capillary wall

B. Osmotic pressure gradient across the capillary wall

C. Capillary wall permeability

D. Size of the capillary bed

Hydrostatic pressure within the capillary = 45 mm Hg

Hydrostatic pressure within the Bowman's capsule = 10 mm Hg

Colloidal osmotic pressure of plasma within the capillaries = 25 mm Hg

Colloidal osmotic pressure of filtrate present within the Bowmen's capsule = 0 as no protein is present.

The Four Basic Functions of the Kidneys

Ultrafiltration by glomerular capillaries:

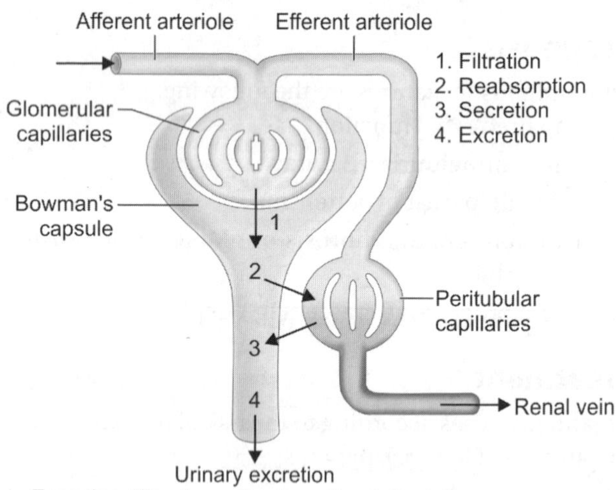

Excretion: Filtration – Reabsorption + Secretion

Glomerular filtration rate = K × effective filtration pressure

K = filtration coefficient of glomerular membrane. Kf = function of surface area of the capillaries and membrane permeability. Its value = 12.5

So, GFR = 12.5 × (45 - 10) - (25 - 0) = 12.5 × 10 = 125 mL/min

Factors affecting the GFR:

A. Advanced age decreases the glomerular filtration rate

B. Glomerular filtration rate (GFR) has a linear relationship with renal blood flow

C. Hydrostatic pressure changes in glomerular capillaries. It depends upon:

- **a.** Changes in the systemic blood pressure
- **b.** Constriction of afferent arteriole reduces renal blood flow and GFR
- **c.** Constriction of efferent arteriole reduces renal blood flow but increases GFR

D. Hydrostatic pressure changes in Bowman's capsule:

- **a.** Ureteral obstruction increases this pressure and decreases the GFR
- **b.** Edema inside the kidney due to tight renal capsule decreases GFR

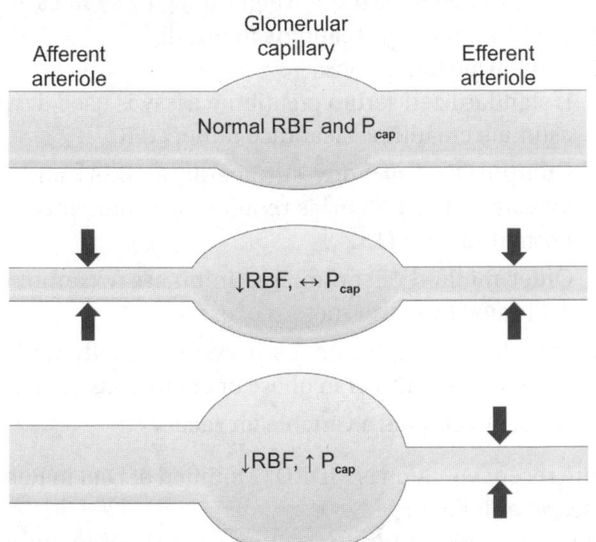

(RBF: renal blood flow)

E. Plasma protein concentration:

- **a.** Hypoproteinemia decreases capillary oncotic pressure thus increases GFR
- **b.** Dehydration increases capillary oncotic pressure thus decreases GFR

F. State of glomerular membrane

G. Size of capillary bed

H. Thickness or permeability of the filtration area

I. Surface area of the filter changes of the value of K

Classification of Renal Function Tests

A. To screen for kidney disease:

- **a.** Full urine analysis
- **b.** Estimation of urea and creatinine
- **c.** Estimation of plasma electrolytes

B. Assess of renal function:

- **a.** Glomerular filtration rate: Clearance test
- **b.** Permeability of glomerulus: Proteinuria

C. Assessment of tubular function:

- **a.** Studies of reabsorption
- **b.** Test for secretion
- **c.** Tests for concentration and dilution
- **d.** Renal acidification

Glomerular Function Tests

Clearance: It can be defined as volume of plasma or blood cleared of a substance per unit volume and expressed as mL of plasma/min.

i.e., Clearance = Mg of plasma excreted per min/mg of substance per mL of plasma and it is expressed as:

$$C = (U \times V)/P$$

Where U = Concentration of substance in urine, V = Volume of urine excreted in mL per minute, and P = Concentration of substance in plasma or blood.

Following are the relationship between clearance and glomerular filtration rate:

Mechanisms	Results	Examples
Substances are secreted but neither absorbed nor secreted	Glomerular filtration rate = Clearance	Uric acid
Substances are filtered but reabsorbed and again excreted	Glomerular filtration rate > Clearance	Urea
Substances are filtered and partially reabsorbed	Glomerular filtration rate < Clearance	PAH, diodrast

(PAH: para-aminohippurate)

A. Following are the methods to assess the clearance (CL) and GFR:

- **a.** Plasma clearance (CL/min): Amount of solute infused into the plasma per unit time (mg/min)/ Average concentration in plasma (mg/mL)

  Plasma clearance (CL_P) = Renal clearance (CL_U) + Extrarenal clearance (CL_E) from gut and and liver.
- **b.** Urinary clearance (U × V in mg/min):

  [Filtered load (GFR × plasma concentration × sieving coefficient)] + Tubular secretion (TS in mg/min) – Tubular resorption (TR in mg/min)

  Or, $U \times V = (GFR \times P) + TS - TR$

  Urinary clearance (CL_U) can be measured as: Amount of markers excreted in urine per unit volume (U × V)/Plasma concentration of marker during the period of collection of urine:

  Or, $CL_U = (U \times V)/P$

  So, $CL_U = [\{(GFR \times P) + TS\} - TR]/P$

c. Estimation of GFR from plasma concentration of endogenous filtration markers: In normal, steady-state constant plasma concentration of filtration marker (P in mg/mL) is constant due to generation (G in mg/mL) is equal to urinary excretion (U × V in mg/mL) plus extrarenal excretion (E in mg/mL).

$U \times V = (GFR \times P) + TS - TR$

$G - E = (GFR \times P) + TS - TR$

Or, $GFR = (TS - TR - G + E)/P$

Glomerular filtration rate = (Tubular secretion – Tubular resorption – Generation of marker + Extrarenal excretion of marker)/Plasma concentration of marker.

Following tests are done to assess function of kidney:

Constituents	Levels in blood	Factors affecting it
Urea	15–40 mg/dL	Catabolism of proteins, dietary protein, renal blood flow
Creatinine	• 0.7–1.4 mg/dL (male) • 0.4–1.3 mg/dL (female)	Glomerular filtration rate, tubular secretion, age, sex, muscle mass
Uric acid	• 3–7 mg/dL (male) • 2–5 mg/dL (female)	Tubular excretion, purine catabolism
Sodium	135–142 mEq/L	Dietary sodium, renal function, hydration state
Potassium	3.5–5 mEq/L	Dietary potassium, renal function, acid-base balance
Calcium	9–11 mg/dL	Calcium in diet, renal function, parathormone

Creatinine Clearance Test

Creatinine level of >1.5 mg/dL indicates impairment of renal function.

Following factors affecting the serum creatinine:

A. Factors reducing the serum creatinine:

- **a.** Sex—female sex
- **b.** Low muscle mass
- **c.** Malnutrition
- **d.** Medicines:
  1. Vancomycin
  2. Thiazide

B. Factors increasing the serum creatinine:

- **a.** Sex—male
- **b.** Old age
- **c.** Renal disease
- **d.** Renal disease
- **e.** Pyelonephritis
- **f.** Glomerulonephritis
- **g.** Renal failure
- **h.** Dehydration
- **i.** Congestive cardiac failure
- **j.** Medicines:
  1. Amphotericin B
  2. Cephalosporins

Estimated GFR can measure the creatinine clearance and thus GFR by creatinine level by following formula:

Ccr = (140—age in years) × weight in kg (0.85 in case of females)/72 × plasma creatinine in mg/dL.

It has following limitations:

A. If standardized serum creatinine assay is used, it will estimate creatinine clearance rather GFR.

B. Computation of body surface area (BSA) and its adjustment to 1.73 m^2 is required for comparison of normal values of CLcr.

C. Older method of serum creatinine assay cannot be calibrated by newer metods of assay.

D. It includes weight, hence it systematically underestimates the mCLcr in obese or edematous patients.

E. It will not contain a variable for race.

More recent equation is MDRD (Modified of Diet in Renal Disease) as follows:

Estimated GFR (mL/min/1.73 m^2) = 186 × (creatinine /88.4) × 1.154 × (age) – 0.203 × 0.742 (if female)

It has following limitations:

A. It will underestimate eGFR at higher GFR

B. Variable "race" includes only coefficients for African-American versus White.

Creatinine Coefficient

Here urinary creatinine is expressed in mg/kg. Normal value 20–28 mg/kg. It is elevated in muscular dystrophy.

Cystatin C as Filtration Marker

Normal level is 0.8–1.2 mg/L, it is present in abundant amount of cysteine protease inhibitors. Its blood level does not depend upon sex, age, muscle mass, and inflamatory process. It is not secreted from the tubule hence is extremely sensitive to very minor changes in GFR.

Urea Clearance Test

It is the number of of mL of blood containing urea excreted in a minute by the kidney. It can be calculated by the following formula:

$$U = V/P$$

Where U = Mg of urea per mL of urine, V = ML of urine excreted per minute, P = Mg of urea per mL of plasma. Normal vale is 54 mL/min.

Interpretation of urea clearance: If the value is below 75% of normal then it is called abnormal, it will gradually decrease with fall in renal function. The value in plasma will gradually rise if the clearance value is <50% of normal.

Serum Urea

Normal value is 15–40 mg/dL. It will be decreased in the following conditions:

A. Late pregnancy
B. Starvation
C. Protein deficient diet
D. Hepatic failure

It is increased in prerenal, renal, and postrenal failure.

Inulin Clearance

It is not metabolized in the body and it is not absorbed and secreted by the renal tubules, hence it can accurately measure GFR. But it always requires continuous infusion during the time of estimation of GFR.

Inulin clearance = 125 mL/min, urea clearance = 75 mL/min

Diodrast Clearance and Para-aminohippurate (PAH) Clearance

Both are filtered and excreted in urine, hence it is excreted through kidney through single passage through the kidney. PAH also measures the renal plasma flow which is 700 mL of plasma or 1,200 mL of blood or one-fourth of cardiac output.

Strength and limitations of glomerular filtration rate measurement and filtration markers:

Methods	Strength	Limitations
Urinary clearance		
Catheterization of bladder and IV infusion of markers	Gold standard method	It is invasive process
Blous marker administration	Short duration	At high GFR rapid plasma level decline
24-hour urine collection		Ver cumbersome so very prone to error
Plasma clearance	Urine collection is not required	Less accurate
Nuclear imaging	• Blood samples required • Urine is not required	Less accurate
Markers		
Inulin	• It is gold standard • Side effect is nil	• Expensive • Supply is limited • It is very difficult to dissolve
Creatinine	• Endogenous marker • No question of administration • Its measurement is widely available	Its secretion will vary among different individual
Iothalamate	• Inexpensive • Longer half-life	• Possibility of tubular secretion which can lead to overestimation of GFR • Very expensive assay in case of use of nonradioactive agent • Low dose is used
Iohexol	• Not radioactive • Very sensitive assay allows at low dose	• Possibility of tubular reabsorption which can lead to underestimation of GFR • Very expensive assay • Low dose is used
EDTA	Widely available in Europe chelated ^{59}Cr as tracert	• Possibility of tubular reabsorption which can lead to underestimation of GFR • Requirement for storage administration as well as disposal of radioactive substances
DTPA	• Widely available in US • New sensitive and easy to use assay of gadolinium	• Requirement for storage administration as well as disposal of radioactive substances when ^{99m}Tc is used as tracer • Due to shorter half-life of ^{99m}Tc, it is not suitable in central laboratory

(DTPA: diethylenetriamine pentaacetate; EDTA: ethylenediaminetetraacetic acid; GFR: glomerular filtration rate)

Proteinuria

It is of two types:

A. Glomerular proteinuria: It occurs when glomeruli is damaged. Albumin will pass through the glomerulus. Overnight urine sample is used to measure the protein by dipstick having range of 200–300 mg/L:

- **a.** Benign proteinuria—300 mg/day
- **b.** Pathological proteinuria—300–1,000 mg/day
- **c.** >1,000 mg/day

Microalbuminuria: It is when 30–300 mg/day of albumin is present in urine. It occurs in early diabetic or hypertensive nephropathy.

Albumin-creatinine ratio:

- **a.** In males <23 mg/g of creatinine
- **b.** In females <32 mg/g of creatinine

Overflow proteinuria:

- **a.** Hemoglobinuria
- **b.** Bence-Jones proteinuria: It is due to excretion of light chain produced in plasmacytoma. It starts when urine is being heated to 45°C, maximally precipitated at 60°C and resolves at 80°C and becomes clear at 100°C.

B. Tubular proteinuria: It occurs when large molecular weight protein appears in urine. These are retinol-binding protein and α-1 microglobulin.

Urogenic proteinuria: It occurs due to inflammation of urinary tract.

Functions of Tubules

Compounds	Handling by tubules	Relative concentration
Uric acid	In proximal tubule 90% is secreted, but small amount secreted in distal tubule	Glomerular filtration = Urine
Creatinine	Not reabsorbed, in small amount it is secreted	Glomerular filtration = Urine
Urea	40% is reabsorbed in proximal tubule	Glomerular filtration > Urine
Sodium	Reabsorbed partially	Glomerular filtration > Urine
Amino acids	Reabsorbed completely	Glomerular filtration >> Urine
Glucose	Reabsorbed completely	Glomerular filtration >> Urine

Threshold of some common substances which are secreted in urine:

Substances	Threshold value
Glucose	180 mg/dL
Lactate	60 mg/dL
Bicarbonate	28 mEq/L
Calcium	10 mg/dL

Functions of Renal Tubules

Nephron segment	Reabsorption	Secretion
Proximal convulated tubule	• 85% of sodium, chloride and bicarbonate • 100% of glucose and amino acid • Obligatory absorption of uric acid and water	Hydrogen ion, acids and bases, ammonium ion, diodrast PAH
Loop of Henle	Sodium, chloride, calcium, and magnesium	
Distal convoluted tubule	• Active absorption of sodium and chloride • Facultative water reabsorption	Hydrogen, potassium ion, ammonium ion, uric acid

(PAH: para-aminohippurate)

Tubular Function Tests

Urine Analysis

A. Volume:

- **a.** 1.5 L/day
- **b.** <400 mL/day—oliguria
- **c.** <100 mL/day—anuria
- **d.** >3,000 mL/day—polyuria

B. Color of urine:

Appearance	Significance
Clear	Urine is normally straw colored
Cloudy	It occurs due to precipitation of phosphates, due to refrigeration, presence of pus
High color	Oxidation of urobilinogen to urobilin, concentration of urine
Yellow	Intake of B-complex, jaundice
Brownish red	Hemoglobinuria
Smoky red	Presence of blood
Red color	Intake of beet, porphyria
Orange color	Intake of rifampicin, high bilirubin level

Continued

Continued

Appearance	Significance
Milky urine	Chyluria
Black color	Formic acid poisoning, alkaptonuria
Green urine	Administration of methylene blue, propofol or amitriptyline
White urine	Pyuria, chyluria, propofol
Purple urine	Due to bacteriuria in patients with urinary catheter (purple urine bag syndrome)

C. Specific gravity:
  a. Normal—1005–1025
  b. Low in:
    1. High water intake
    2. Renal tubular dysfunction
    3. Diabetes insipidus
    4. Polydipsia
  c. High specific gravity in:
    1. Inadequate intake of water
    2. Volume depletion

D. pH:
  a. Normal pH: 5.5–6.5
  b. Low pH:
    1. High protein diet
    2. Acidosis
    3. Recent meal—alkaline tide
  c. High pH: In low protein diet

E. Blood: It is found in:
  a. Menstruation
  b. Glomerulonephritis
  c. Trauma
  d. Stones
  e. Tumor
  f. Hemoglobinuria
  g. Hemolysis

F. Protein <150 mg/day. Proteinuria is found in the following conditions:
  a. Orthostatic proteinuria
  b. Exercise
  c. Fever
  d. Urinary tract infection (UTI)
  e. Glomerulonephritis
  f. Tubular disease

G. Glucose: Gycosuria present in the following conditions:
  a. Diabetes mellitus
  b. Renal glycosuria
  c. Fanconi syndrome

H. Ketone bodies present in:
  a. Diabetes mellitus
  b. Starvation

I. Bilirubinuria present in:
  a. Hepatitis
  b. Obstructive jaundice

J. Bile salt is found in obstructive jaundice

K. Nitrite is found in urinary tract infection

L. Urobilinogen:
  a. Normal is <4 mg/day
  b. It is increased in:
    1. Concentrated urine
    2. Intravascular hemolysis
    3. Concentrated urine
  c. Low in obstructive jaundice.

M. Leukocyte esterase is found in:
  a. Urinary tract infection
  b. Fever

Measurement of Osmolarity

Normally, it is 60–1,200 mOsmol/kg. Normal plasma osmolarity is 285–300 mOsmol/kg.

Concentration Test

A. After 12 hours fasting, if the specific gravity is >1022—it suggests adequate renal function.

B. In case of disease progression specific gravity of urine will be fixed and at around 1010. It is called isosthenuria.

C. Urine has to be collected in the day and at night. If the night volume is half of the day volume. If the night volume is more, it is called nocturia which is indicative of tubular dysfunction.

Dilution Test

The patient is asked to empty the bladder at 7 am and 1,200 mL of water is asked to take followed by collection of urine in next 4 hours separately and each time volume, specific gravity, and osmolarity are measured.

Normal person excretes all the water load within 4 hours and specific gravity of one sample must be 1003.

This test is more sensitive but less harmful.

Urine Acidification Test

The test is acid loading test and has to be done in case of hyperchloremic metabolic acidosis. Here 0.1 g/kg of body weight ammonium chloride has to be administered into the patient. In the body, this will be dissociated into ammonium and chloride ion. In the liver, ammonium is converted into urea. Chloride ion will combine with hydrogen ion to form hydrochloric acid and excreted in the urine to produce acidification.

Patient's urine has to be collected hourly 2–8 hours of ingestion of ammonium chloride and pH of each urine sample has to be measured. At least one urine sample must demonstrate urine pH $\leq$ 5.3. In case of renal tubular acidosis, this pH cannot be achieved.

Fractional Excretion of Sodium

It can differentiate between prerenal azotemia and acute tubular necrosis.

It can be calculated by:

(Urine sodium × plasma creatinine) / (plasma sodium × urinary creatinine)

If it is <1%—it suggests prerenal causes.
If it is >1%—it suggests acute tubular necrosis.

Urinary Level of Enzymes

A. N-acetyl-β-D-glucosaminidase: It is elevated in tubular injury.

B. B_2 microglobulin: It is increased in case of proximal tubular dysfunction.

Concentration and Dilution Test

A. Water deprivation test: It can assess the ability of the kidney to concentrate the urine.

B. Desmopressin challenge test: It can differentiate between nephrogenic and central diabetes insipidus.

Q21. Membranous glomerulopathy.
PGI/NOV2012/MDII (10)

ANSWER

Definition

It is characterized by subepithelial immune deposits along with formation of perpendicular projection of materials called "spikes" looking alike glomerular basement membrane between the podocytes cytoplasm and glomerular basement membrane. These immune complexes consist of IgG4, complement C3, C5-C9 membrane attack complexes. But in case of secondary membranous nephropathy IgA, IgM, IgG1/IgG3 alo may be seen, and may rarely involve mesangium ("full house pattern").

Etiology

A. Primary: Idiopathic

B. Secondary:

- **a.** Infection: Hepatitis B, hepatitis C, syphilis, leprosy
- **b.** Cancer—breast, lung, stomach, colon
- **c.** Autoimmune disease
- **d.** Drugs: Gold, mercury
- **e.** Other systemic diseases:
  1. Fanconi syndrome
  2. Sickle cell anemia
  3. Sarcoidosis
  4. Crohn's disease

Epidemiology

A. It is the most common cause of nephrotic syndrome in Caucasian adult.

B. Male: female ratio is 2:1.

C. Age: Peak incidence occur in the fourth and fifth decades of life.

Pathophysiology

It is an immunologically mediated disease, immune complexes are deposited in the subepithelial space against the following antigens:

A. Neutral endopeptidase, a biologically active peptides acts as podocytes antigen, is recently identified as target antigen against which antibodies are formed and deposit in the subepithelial space.

B. M-type phospholipase A2 receptor is also demonstrated as another target antigen found in case of idiopathic membranous glomerulonephritis but not in secondary causes.

C. Another antigen thrombospondin type 1 domain containing 7A is found in 2.5–5% of idiopathic variety.

D. Recently, there is colocalization of two other antigens, i.e., (1) specific aldolase reductase and (2) manganese superoxide dismutase antibodies IgG4 and C5-C9 found as electron dense deposits.

E. In case of hepatitis B, HBcAg and HBeAg are the two antigens important in the pathogenesis of MGN.

Immune complexes and complement membrane attack complex (C5-C9):

A. Activates podocytes to produce protease, prostanoids, oxidants, extracellular matrix components, cytokines, as well as transforming growth factor beta.

B. Produces abnormal distribution of slit diaphragm protein and detaches viable podocytes to shed into the Bowmen's space by altering its cytoskeleton.

As a result the functional integrity and disruption of glomerular basement membrane and podocytes and its protein filtration barrier are lost which lead to massive proteinuria.

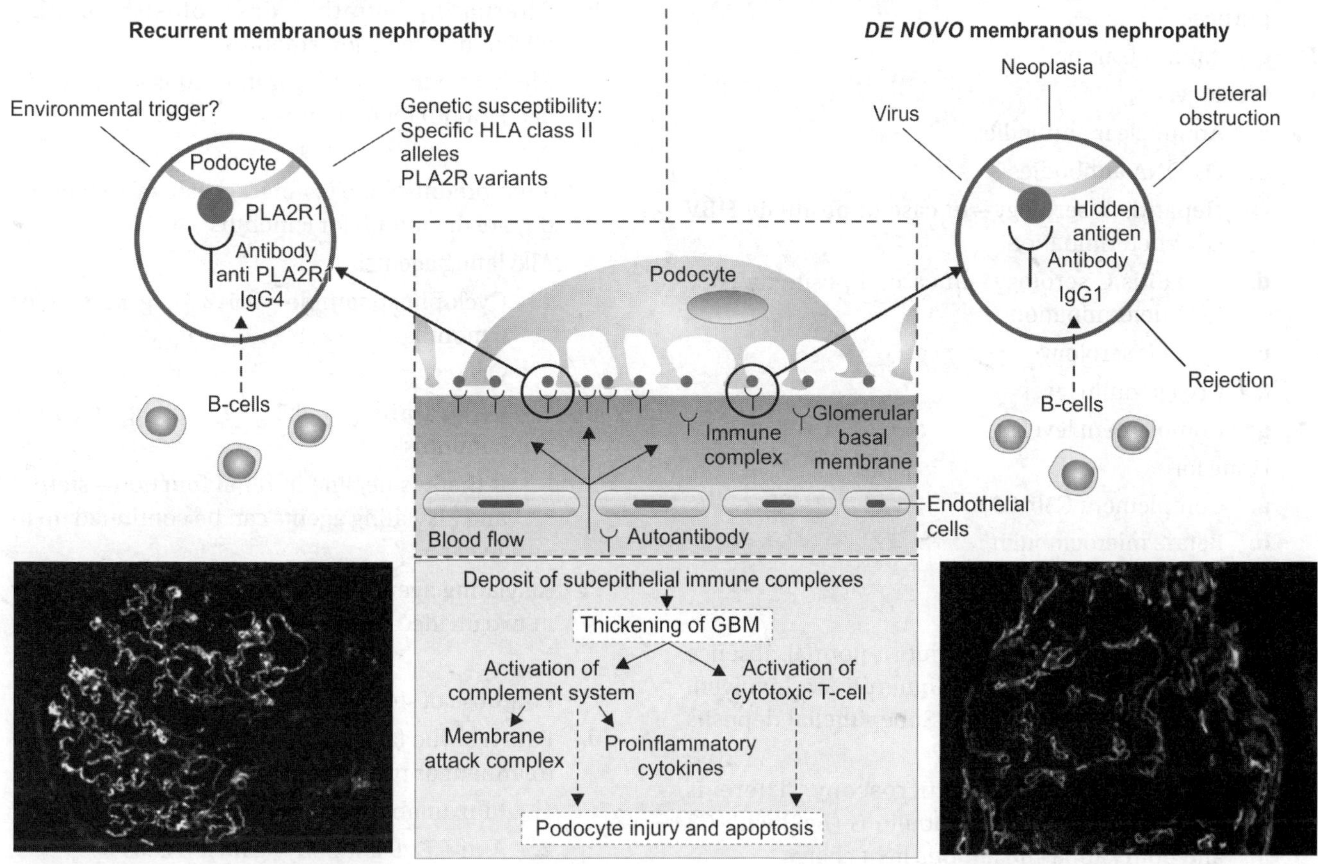

(GBM: glomerular basement membrane; HLA: human leukocyte antigen; IgA1: immunoglobulin A1)

Course

Clinical course may be variable. Patients have been divided into three groups of equal sizes, called "rule of thirds":

A. 25% patients show spontaneous remission: Renal function is normal and there may or may not be any relapse.

B. Variable degree of persistent proteinuria: Here renal function is impaired but is stable.

C. Progressive disease: It leads to end-stage renal disease in small number of patients.

Clinical Presentation

A. The most common presentation is nephrotic range of proteinuria

B. In most patients, there is microscopic hematuria but macroscopic hematuria is rare.

C. In 25% case, there is systemic hypertension.

D. Little alteration of renal function at the time of diagnosis.

E. Edema

F. Flank pain—due to renal vein thrombosis

G. Sudden respiratory distress with proteinuria—pulmonary thromboembolism

H. Features of other deep vein thrombosis

I. Poor appetite

J. Foamy urine

Laboratory Studies

A. Urine analysis: It will demonstrate:

- **a.** Oval fat bodies
- **b.** Fatty cast
- **c.** Proteinuria

B. Blood examinations:

- **a.** Urea
- **b.** Creatinine

- **c.** Albumin
- **d.** Lipid profile
- **e.** Liver function tests

C. Spot urine protein creatinine ratio for screening purpose

D. Creatinine clearance

E. Serology:

- **a.** Antinuclear antibodies
- **b.** Ds-DNA antibodies
- **c.** Hepatitis B serology—in case of positivity HBV DNA determination
- **d.** Hepatitis C serology—in case of positivity HCV RNA determination
- **e.** Syphilis serology
- **f.** Cryoglobulin level
- **g.** Complement levels

F. Urine for:

- **a.** Complement C5b-C9
- **b.** Beta-2 microglobulin

G. Work up of malignancy

H. Histological findings:

- **a.** Light microscopy: Mesangium is normal, absence of hypercellularity. All glomeruli are involved. Thickened capillary wall. Subepithelial deposits are present.
- **b.** Immunofluorescence microscopy: There is deposition of immunoglobulin G (IgG) with C3 and both kappa and lambda light chains.
- **c.** Electron microscopy:
  1. Stage 1: Few electron dense deposits seen in the capillary walls.
  2. Stage 2: Numerous larger deposits with spikes are evidenced.
  3. Stage 3: Evidence of new extracellular material seen surrounding the deposits.
  4. Stage 4: Electron dense deposits become electron lucent and walls of the capillaries are thickened.

Treatment

A. Symptomatic treatment:

- **a.** Low salt diet to reduce anasarca
- **b.** Aggressive treatment of hypertension by angiotensin converting enzyme (ACE) inhibitor and angiotensin receptor blockers (ARBs).
- **c.** Introduction of statins to treat hypercholesterolemia
- **d.** Administration of diuretics to treat edema
- **e.** NSAIDs to reduce proteinuria

B. Specific treatment:

- **a.** Prednisolone 1 mg/kg/day + cyclophosphamide 1.5 mg/kg/day for 6 months followed by slow tapering of the drugs.
- **b.** Alternating monthly dose of steroid plus alkylating agents for 6 months

  Methylprednisolone 1 g intravenously × 3 days in each month for 6 months

  ↓

  Then prednisolone 0.4 mg/kg/day for remaining days of the month for 6 months

  Alkylating agents:

  1. Cyclophosphamide—1.5–2.5 mg/kg/day for 6 months

     Or

     Chlorambucil—0.1–0.2 mg/kg/day for 6 months

     If there is decline in renal function—steroid and alkylating agents can be continued up to 1 year.
- **c.** Alkylating agents—cyclosporine—3.5 mg/kg/day in two divided doses.

  +

  Low dose of steroid for 6–12 months
- **d.** Patients who fail to achieve remission with above treatment or relapse:
  1. Rituximab
  2. Anti-CD20 antibody against B cells
  3. Synthetic adrenocorticotropic hormone

Q22. Diagnostic approach to a patient with hematuria.

PGI/APR2013/MDI (10)

Evaluation of hematuria.

MGR/SEP2010/MDIV (6)

Approach to a patient with hematuria.

NTR UNI OF HEALTH SC, VIJAYAWADA, 2021 (10)

Hematuria.

MAHARASHTRA UNI OF HEALTH SC, VIJAYAWADA, 2021 (10)

ANSWER

Introduction

Hematuria can be defined as presence of blood in urine. If the blood can be detected by naked eye examination it is macroscopic hematuria and if it is detected only by microscopy it is called microscopic hematuria. Microscopic hematuria can be defined as three of more RBCs present in per high power field of urine in 2–3 properly collected urine sample. But the morning midstream urine should be collected. After strenuous exercise, trauma, after intercourse and during menstruation urine sample should be best avoided.

Causes of Hematuria

A. Kidney causes:
- **a.** Inflammation:
  - **1.** Immunoglobulin A (IgA) nephropathy
  - **2.** Hereditary nephritis
  - **3.** Pyelonephritis
  - **4.** Renal tuberculosis
  - **5.** Other glomerulopathies
- **b.** Neoplastic causes:
  - **1.** Renal cell carcinoma
  - **2.** Renal lymphoma
  - **3.** Renal transitional cell carcinoma
- **c.** Stones
- **d.** Anatomic abnormalities:
  - **1.** Autosomal dominant polycystic kidney disease (ADPKD)
  - **2.** Medullary spongy kidney
  - **3.** Hydronephrosis
- **e.** Other causes:
  - **1.** Hypercalciuria
  - **2.** Renal trauma
  - **3.** Papillary necrosis
  - **4.** Renal infarction
  - **5.** Hyperuricosuria

B. Ureter:
- **a.** Ureteral transitional cell carcinoma
- **b.** Stricture
- **c.** Stones

C. Bladder:
- **a.** Malignancy—transitional cell carcinoma
- **b.** Inflammation:
  - **1.** Bacterial cystitis
  - **2.** Radiation cystitis
  - **3.** Tubercular cystitis
  - **4.** *Schistosoma haematobium*
- **c.** Bladder stones
- **d.** Anatomical abnormalities:
  - **1.** Vesicoureteral reflux
  - **2.** Bladder papilloma
  - **3.** Cystocele

D. Prostate:
- **a.** Prostatitis
- **b.** Prostatic cancer
- **c.** Stones
- **d.** Benign prostatic hypertrophy

E. Urethra:
- **a.** Urethritis
- **b.** Malignancy:
  - **1.** Urethral cancer
  - **2.** Penile cancer
- **c.** Anatomic: Stricture

F. Other causes:
- **a.** Abdominal aortic aneurysm
- **b.** Over anticoagulation

Evaluation from History

A. History of fever, sexual intercourse, exercise, infection, trauma

B. History of pain with radiation

C. History of following risk factors, such as male sex, age >35 years, past history of smoking

D. History of urologic disease or disorders

E. History of analgesic abuse

F. History of chronic urinary tract infection

G. History of exposure to chemotherapy, such as alkylating agents

H. History of chronic indwelling into the bladder

According to American Urology Association Symptom Index for assessing the severity of irritative or obstructive features set grades the severity of following symptoms:

A. Incomplete emptying

B. Frequency

C. Intermittency

D. Urgency

E. Weak stream

F. Straining

G. Nocturia

Each symptom has 0–5 grades according to severity. Total maximum score is 35. Now:

A. Mild grade: 0–7

B. Moderate: 8–19

C. Severe: 20–35

Physical Examination

A. Large size palpable kidney—ADPKD, renal cell carcinoma

B. Tender loin—pyelonephritis

C. Suprapubic tenderness—cystitis

D. Palpable tender kidney—Acute pyelonephritis

Laboratory Evaluation

A. Urine analysis: Urine dipstick usually detects peroxidase activity of red blood cells thus:

- **a.** Myoglobin or hemoglobin leading to generation of false positive results
- **b.** Other causes of false positive results:
  1. Exercise
  2. Dehydration
  3. Oxidizing agents
  4. Povidone-iodine
- **c.** Causes of false negative results:
  1. Vitamin C
  2. Air exposure

Urine dipstick can detect 1–2 red blood cells per high power field:

- **a.** In case of glomerular hematuria: Red cells are constantly exposed to urinary pH, osmotic pressure while passing through renal tubules thus making the RBCs dysmorphic:
  1. Presence of 2+ proteinuria or more is suggestive of glomerular hematuria.
  2. There is no blood clot as urokinase and tissue-type plasminogen activator present in glomerular filtrate will dissolve it.
  3. Presence of red blood cell casts is pathognomonic as the main matrix Tamm–Horsfall protein is formed only in distal tubule.
- **b.** In case of nonglomerular hematuria: Red cells are more homogenous and normal in shape.

In case of very dilute urine with specific gravity of 1007, RBCs will be lysed and become false negative.

B. Urine cytology: In three consecutive morning urine samples sensitivity for high-grade tumor is high and for low-grade tumor is low.

C. Urinary tumor markers:

Following tests have to be done:

- **a.** Bladder tumor antigen test
- **b.** Nuclear matrix protein 22
- **c.** Carcinoembryonic antigen
- **d.** Cytokeratin tissue polypeptide-specific antigen
- **e.** Fluorescence in situ hybridization (FISH) assay
- **f.** Lewis X antigen
- **g.** Telomerase activity
- **h.** Urinary bladder cancer tumor marker tests

D. Urine for culture and sensitivity test: It has to be done in case of urinary tract infection.

E. Glomerular filtration rate: In case of glomerular cause of hematuria renal function has to be evaluated by this estimation of GFR. It cannot be measured directly so can be estimated by using urinary clearance of filtration marker.

F. Serum creatinine: This amino acid derivative is freely filtered through glomerulus. It is secreted in the renal tubule and its secretion will decrease with proportionate decrease in renal function and it overestimates GFR. GFR can be calculated from serum creatinine from two different equations. These are Cockcroft–Gault formula and Modification of Diet in Renal Disease (MDRD) formula.

G. Other blood tests:

- **a.** Complete blood count
- **b.** Blood urea nitrogen (BUN)
- **c.** Coagulation studies
- **d.** Serological studies:
  1. Hepatitis B titers
  2. Hepatitis C titers
  3. Antinuclear antibody (ANA)
  4. Antiglomerular basement membrane (anti-GBM) antibody
  5. Complement levels
  6. Antineutrophilic cytoplasmic antibody
  7. Antistreptolysin O titer
  8. Cryoglobulin assay

H. Imaging studies: There are many radiographic methods available for anatomical and functional assessment of full renovascular system. Now three imaging modalities are available for assessment:

- **a.** Ultrasonography: It can detect:
  1. Determination of renal size
  2. Cortical thickness
  3. Renal masses and cysts
- **b.** Color Doppler study can assess:
  1. Renal blood flow
  2. Renal vascular resistance
- **c.** Intravenous urography: It can detect stones in the urinary tract. But it is less reliable in detecting

masses. Its sensitivity 21%, 52%, and 85% in detecting the masses of <2 cm, 2–3 cm, and >3 cm, respectively.

   d. Computerized tomography: It can detect better:
      1. Urinary tract stones
      2. Renal masses

A 30-years-old male with acute onset hematuria with hypertension. Following probable causes are:

A. Primary glomerular diseases:
   a. Post infectious glomerulonephritis
   b. IgA nephropathy
   c. Focal segmental glomerulonephritis
   d. Membranoproliferative glomerulonephritis
   e. Alport syndrome

B. Secondary to systemic diseases:
   a. Lupus nephritis
   b. Goodpasture syndrome
   c. ANCA associated glomerulonephritis

C. Vascular causes:
   a. Renal artery stenosis
   b. Renal vein thrombosis
   c. Thrombotic thrombocytopenic purpura
   d. Hemolytic uremic syndrome

D. Tubulo-interstitial causes:
   a. Acute interstitial nephritis
   b. Pyelonephritis

E. Structural causes:
   a. Adult polycystic kidney diseases
   b. Nephrolithiasis
   c. Urothelial carcinoma

F. Hematological diseases:
   a. Sickle cell disease
   b. Disseminated intravascular coagulation

Clinical features and laboratory investigations have been written in different questions and also in this question.

Q23. Asymptomatic urinary abnormalities.

MJPRU/2015/MDIII (6)

ANSWER

Asymptomatic urinary abnormalities are usually diagnosed by microscopic examination of urine or dipstick examination of urine. The abnormalities are the following:

A. Glycosuria: In absence of hyperglycemia glycosuria suggests either renal glycosuria or proximal tubular disease. It may also occur in pregnancy.

B. Pyuria: More than 3–5 white blood cells per high power field in the face of negative urine culture suggests:
   a. Interstitial nephritis
   b. Renal tuberculosis
   c. Prostatitis

C. Crystalluria: It may be present in the urine as sediment in asymptomatic patients. Most of the crystals are not significant for diagnostic purpose. But hexagonal crystals is indicative of cystinuria.

D. Bacteriuria: It is the frequent contaminent in case of women, But if it is present in pregnant women or children, in that case complete evaluation is required to diagnose urinary tract infection.

E. *Hematuria: It is described in Question number 22.*

F. *Proteinuria: It is described in Question number 17.*

Q24. Diagnosis of renovascular hypertension.

MJPRU/2015/MDII (10)

ANSWER

Introduction

Renovascular hypertension is characterized by progressive occlusive disease of renal artery as evidenced by myriad of symptoms ranges from renovascular hypertension to ischemic kidney damage. Common causes of renovascular hypertension is atherosclerotic renal artery stenosis due to extension of aortic plaque into the renal artery hence, it is usually present at the origin but it may be present anywhere of renal artery and it may be bilateral. Associated risk factors are:

A. Diabetes mellitus
B. Hypertension
C. Smoking
D. Coronary artery disease
E. Peripheral vascular disease

It may be asymptomatic or present with active cardiovascular features, such as refractory hypertension, recurrent flush pulmonary edema ultimately to decline in renal function.

Second most common cause of renovascular hypertension is fibromuscular dysplasia involving intima or fibrous layer in the vascular wall resulting arterial stenosis, formation of aneurysm, occlusion or dissection of medium-sized arteries. There are two subtypes. First one is multifocal fibromuscular dysplasia (FMD) involving midpoint or first bifurcation of renal artery affecting middle-aged women predominantly.

Pathophysiology

Decreased renal perfusion results from fall in pressure of 10–20% in distal to the occlusion which is equivalent to translesional pressure gradient of 20–25 mm Hg with luminal stenosis of 70%. It ultimately leads to increased renin release from juxtaglomerular cells which try to maintain renal perfusion by increasing the systemic as well as distal renal artery pressure.

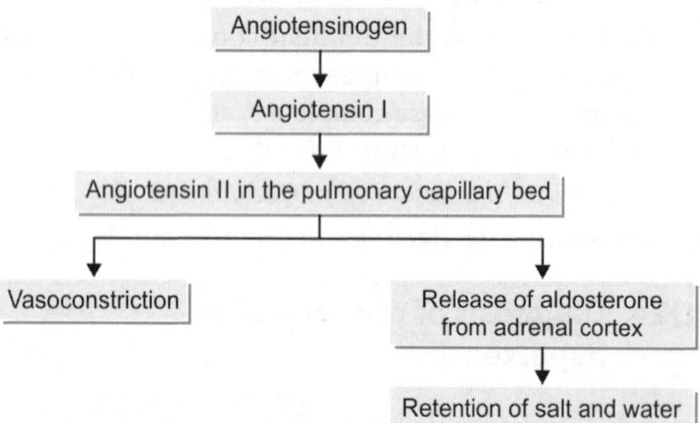

But in presence of normal contralateral nonstenotic kidney, there will be pressure natriuresis thus preventing volume expansion of retention of sodium. On the contrary, if both the kidneys are affected there will be increased retention of sodium and water leading to "volume-dependent hypertension" and the level of renin will also be low in this phase.

Glomerular filtration rate (GFR) is increased in this patient due to constriction of efferent arteriole by angiotensin II. If there is blockade of renin-angiotensin-aldosterone system (RAAS) by angiotensin-converting enzyme (ACE) inhibitor or angiotensin receptor blockers (ARBs) in patient with stenosis of bilateral renal arteries or stenosis of unilateral renal artery; in case of solitary kidney, there will be dramatic fall in GFR.

Clinical Features

A. Multifocal fibromuscular dysplasia occurs in middle-aged women. It rarely produces functional loss of renal tissue.

B. In case of atherosclerotic renal artery stenosis:

- **a.** Features are more widespread due to widespread vascular occlusion.
- **b.** Affects elderly with significant comorbidities.
- **c.** Physical examination reveals bruit over the abdomen or flank area.
- **d.** Sometimes, it can be diagnosed during different imaging procedures, such as coronary angiography and computerized tomography.
- **e.** Sometimes there may be progressive increase in arterial pressure in spite of getting antihypertensive drugs in escalating doses in patients with history of smoking.
- **f.** In presence of activated RAAS additional intake of salt and water will lead to direct damage of target organs as evidenced by left ventricular hypertrophy and renal dysfunction.
- **g.** There may be development of pulmonary edema due to congestive cardiac failure.

So, in following conditions one can suspect of renovascular hypertension:

A. Age < 30 or > 55 years
B. Abrupt onset of hypertension
C. Refractory hypertension
D. Malignant hypertension
E. Accelerated retinopathy of hypertension origin
F. Sudden acceleration of previously controlled hypertension
G. Flash pulmonary edema
H. Abdominal bruit
I. Evidence of generalized atherosclerosis obliterans
J. Asymmetry in the size of kidney on imaging
K. Acute renal failure during treatment with ACE inhibitor or ARBs

Investigations for Renovascular Hypertension

A. Duplex Doppler ultrasonography: It is safe and inexpensive and is regarded as first line of investigation in case of renal artery stenosis:

- **a.** It will directly visualize the renal artery
- **b.** It will also detect some hemodynamic factors:
  1. Comparison of systolic flow velocity between the aorta and renal artery because flow velocity increases with the increasing narrowing by the lesion; so, there is linear relationship between degree of stenosis and increase in flow velocity of blood.
  2. Measurement of end-diastolic flow velocity beyond the lesion

B. Renal arteriography:

- **a.** Lesion usually present concentrically or eccentrically within one-third of renal artery from its origin or at the ostium.
- **b.** In case of fibromuscular dysplasia medial hyperplasia produces string of beads appearance due to involvement of middle to distal portion

of arteries as compared to atherosclerotic renal artery stenosis.

c. It can also measure translesional pressure gradient across the area of stenosis. If this gradient is >20 mm Hg, there is significant chance of improvement of hypertension.

C. Radionucleotide renography with captopril: It can evaluate functional status of each kidney prior to therapeutic nephrectomy. Radionucleotide used in this test is mercaptoacetyltriglycine as it is more reliable in dysfunction.

D. CT angiography:
   a. Specificity and sensitivity are 90% and 94%, respectively.
   b. It can detect small accessory renal artery.
   c. It can be used in implanted service.
   d. It may produce contrast nephropathy in case of renal dysfunction.
   e. In case heavily calcified renal artery, interpretation of images are difficult.
   f. It is contraindicated in case of contrast-induced allergy.

E. MR angiography:
   a. Its sensitivity and specificity are 100%.
   b. Gadolinium is used as contrast but it may lead to nephrogenic systemic fibrosis.
   c. No calcification artifact.

Q25. Bowman's capsule.

MGR/MAR2008/MDI (4)

ANSWER

Anatomy of Bowman's Capsule

Bowman's capsule is the initial dilated part of nephron having epithelial lining of 5 μm thick. Within it glomerulus is present. Bowman's capsule along with glomerulus is called Malpighian corpuscle. It has two layers:

A. Visceral cell layer: It is very closely applied to capillary loops and it will surround each loop. It is continuous with the parietal cell layer at the site of entrance of afferent and efferent arterioles.

B. Parietal cell layer: This layer is applied to proper Bowman's capsule and forms the outer lining of glomerulus. It is continuous with parietal cell layer of proximal convoluted tubule.

The space present in between the visceral and parietal cell layer is called Bowman's space.

Physiology of Bowman's Capsule

A. It helps in the filtration of the blood from the glomerular capillaries. Filtration occurs through the fenestrated capillary endothelium. This fenestration is present in between the endothelium and of 60-80 nm wide. It will also carry negative charges restricting the entry of negatively charged particles into the Bowmen's space. Then these particles and water pass through the three layers of glomerular basement membrane. Mesangial cells present within the glomerulus are responsible for maintaining the integrity of the glomerular basement membrane and capillary loops. Following the glomerular basement membrane filtrate passes through the epithelial layer of Bowmen's capsule which is composed of podocytes. Foot processes of the podocytes interdigitate with each other to create another barrier through which filtrate will run. Parietal cell layer of the Bowmen's capsule will not take part in the filtration. These parietal cells maintains the integrity of the capsule and replace the damaged podocytes.

B. It has a structural function, as it will create an urinary space and through this space urine can enter the nephron and passes to the proximal convoluted tubule. Composition of the filtrate is similar to that of blood except protein and cell content which are being prevented to enter the Bowmen's space normally.

Q26. Discuss the clinical features, diagnosis, staging, and management of renal cell carcinoma.

RGUHS/MAR2008/MDII (20)

Renal cell carcinoma.

MGR/MAR2010/MDII (6)

ANSWER

Introduction

Renal cell carcinoma is a carcinoma of kidney which is comprised of clinically, histologically, and biologically distinct entities.

Etiology and Risk Factors

A. Nonhereditary risk factors:
   a. Hypertension
   b. Intake of tobacco
   c. Obesity
   d. Occupational exposure to cadmium, petroleum, asbestos, and trichloroethylene

e. Chronic kidney disease
f. Acquired cystic disease of kidney

B. Familial syndrome:
a. Von Hippel–Lindau (VHL) disease: Autosomal dominant disease due to deletion of VHL suppressor gene in chromosome 3p25.
b. Hereditary papillary carcinoma: There is multifocal bilateral type 1 papillary renal cell cancer due to mutation of MET proto-oncogene located on long arm of chromosome 7.
c. Birt–Hogg–Dubé (BHD) syndrome: It occurs due to mutation of *BHD* gene or mutation of BHD genetically protein folliculin.
d. Hereditary leiomyomatosis and renal cell carcinoma (HLRCC): It occurs due to mutation of germ line in the gene encoding for Krebs cycle enzyme fumarate hydratase.
e. Succinate dehydrogenase associated with renal cell carcinoma: It occurs due to mutation of SDHA, SDHB, SDHC, and SDHD leading to impaired Krebs cycle function producing metabolic and biochemical alteration.
f. Mutation of LKB1/TSC/mTOR (liver kinase B1/tuberous sclerosis complex/mammalian target of rapamycin) is associated with renal cell carcinoma.

Pathological Classification

A. Clear cell carcinoma: It is composed of cells with clear cytoplasm.

B. Papillary renal cell carcinoma: It is further subdivided into two subtypes:
a. Type 1 papillary renal cell carcinoma
b. Type 2 renal cell carcinoma

C. Chromophobe renal cell carcinoma: It is characterized by sheets of cells containing pale and eosinophilic granular cytoplasm.

D. Renal cell carcinoma associated with HLRCC

E. Collecting duct renal cell carcinoma: Here cancer will develop from collecting duct.

F. Unclassified renal cell carcinoma

G. Renal tumor with sarcomatoid features

Clinical Features

A. It can be detected during routine evaluation during search of other symptoms

B. 10% patients present with classical presentation of:
a. Hematuria
b. Loin pain
c. Flank pain

C. Patient may present with paraneoplastic syndrome, such as:
a. Weight loss
b. Cachexia
c. Anemia
d. Features of polycythemia due to increased erythropoietin level in the blood
e. Hypertension
f. Features of hypercalcemia due to release of parathormone like substance

D. May present with biochemical features: Raised alkaline phosphatase

E. Stauffer syndrome characterized by reversible hepatic dysfunction due to hepatic metastasis.

About 50% patients present with localized disease, 25% with localized advanced disease, and 25% with advanced metastatic disease. Common sites of metastases are the following:
a. Lung
b. Lymph node
c. Bone
d. Liver
e. Central nervous system

Diagnosis

A. History and complete physical examination

B. Complete blood count and differential count

C. Biochemistry: Liver function test, prothrombin time, partial thromboplastin time, and calcium

D. In case of history of hemoptysis, chest pain chest X-ray or CT scan of chest may demonstrate pulmonary or mediastinal involvement.

E. CT scan of abdomen and pelvis with or without contrast agent to evaluate renal mass and regional lymph node or involvement of renal vein and inferior vena cava

F. Bone scan to demonstrate pathologic fracture in case of bone pain

G. In case of neurological feature, brain MRI has to be done to see evidence of metastasis.

H. Isotope renogram has to be done to demonstrate renal function.

Staging

A. Stage 1: Tumor size is not greater than 7 cm in greatest dimension and limited to kidney

B. Stage 2: Tumor size is >7 cm in greatest dimension and limited to kidney.

C. Stage 3: Disease is metastasize to regional lymph node or tumor extends into major veins or perinephric tissues but not involve ipsilateral adrenal gland nor Gerota's fascia.

D. Stage 4: There is evidence of distant metastasis or there is invasion beyond the Gerota's fascia or involvement of ipsilateral adrenal gland.

Treatment of Localized Renal Cell Carcinoma

A. Surgery:

- **a.** In case of early stage of localized renal cell carcinoma total tumor resection can be done in the tumor size is <4 cm.
- **b.** If the tumor size is 4–7 cm radical nephron sparing procedure is the method of choice.
- **c.** If the tumor size is >7 cm radical nephrectomy is the procedure of choice.
- **d.** In case of small renal masses active surveillance of tumor is the alternative option.
- **e.** Following less invasive technique can eradicate smaller renal tumor:
  1. Stereotactic body radiation therapy
  2. Radiofrequency ablation
  3. Cryotherapy

B. Adjuvant therapy:

- **a.** Vascular endothelial growth factor: These tyrosine kinase inhibitors, namely sunitinib and sorafenib
- **b.** Sunitinib has been approved as first line of therapeutic option for metastasis in case of renal cell carcinoma.
- **c.** Pazopanib has been proved as first-line therapy for metastasis of renal cell carcinoma.
- **d.** Adjuvant vascular endothelial growth factor receptor (VEGFR) targeted therapy

Treatment of Metastatic Renal Cell Carcinoma

A. Surgery:

- **a.** In some selected patients with isolated metastases surgical resection of may provide disease-free survival.
- **b.** Cytoreductive nephrectomy can be done in patient with intractable pain or hematuria.

B. Systemic therapy:

- **a.** In case of clear renal cell carcinoma:
  1. Targeted agents directed against vascular endothelial growth factor/platelet-derived growth factor (VEGF/PDGF) as well as rapamycin (mTOR) has been evaluated in case of metastatic cancer.
  2. Novel immunotherapies can be treatment of choice.
- **b.** In case of non-clear cell renal cell carcinomas (RCC) no standard treatment has been demonstrated.

Drugs are:

A. Sunitinib: It will act VEGF receptor 2 and PDGF receptor. It is widely used as first-line agent in metastatic clear cell RCC.

B. Pazopanib: This angiogenesis inhibitor acts on VEGFR-1, 2, and 3, used for advanced RCC.

C. Axitinib: This highly selective tyrosine kinase inhibitor has target on VEGFR-1, 2, and 3, used in advanced RCC.

D. Bevacizumab: It is used in combination with interferon-α.

E. Sorafenib:

F. Cabozantinib

G. mTOR pathway inhibitors:

- **a.** Temsirolimus
- **b.** Everolimus

H. Cytokines:

- **a.** Interleukin-2: Dose is 600,000–720,000 IU/kg 8 hourly, it can be tolerated up to maximum 15 doses.
- **b.** Interferon-α: Dose is 5–18 million IU, 3–5 times/week.

I. Allogeneic stem cell transplantation

J. PD-1/PD-1L inhibitors: Activation of programmed death-1 receptor plays major role in mediating resistance of the tumor to immune surveillance. Inhibitors of PD-1 have demonstrated benefit in case of metastatic RCC. Drugs are:

- **a.** Nivolumab
- **b.** Pembrolizumab

In Case of Non-clear Cell RCC

There is no standard treatment option for non-clear cell RCC. In few trial bevacizumab-based combination (bevacizumab plus erlotinib or bevacizumab plus everolimus) demonstrated efficacy in treating this tumor.

Q27. Renal failure with normal size or enlarged kidney.

MGR/MAR2006/MDI (5)

ANSWER

Renal ultrasound helps in differentiation of kidney size in case of acute and chronic renal failure.

In case of chronic kidney disease both the kidneys are small and scarred but in the following cases kidney size will increased:

A. Diabetic nephropathy
B. HIV-induced nephropathy
C. Infiltrative disease
D. Bilateral adult polycystic kidney diseases

In case of acute renal failure kidney size is usually normal. But in the following cases of acute renal failure kidney size will be increased:

A. Acute interstitial nephritis
B. Acute pyelonephritis
C. Infiltrative disease
D. Urinary tract obstruction due to benign hypertrophy of prostate, retroperitoneal fibrosis, and encasement with tumor.
E. Renal vessel thrombosis

Q28. Indications and contraindications of renal biopsy.

MGR/OCT2012/MDIV (7)

Renal biopsy.

MGU, 2024 (5)

Histology of the kidney has been described in question number 18.

ANSWER

Kidney biopsy is done to establish the diagnosis and thus help in selection of appropriate therapy if the clinical and laboratory tests are inconclusive.

Indications of Renal Biopsy

A. Acute kidney injury, when the cause is unexplained, when it will not cured by supportive therapy.
B. Nephrotic syndrome in case of children with atypical features, steroid resistance or hematuria
C. Systemic diseases:
  - **a.** Vasculitis
  - **b.** Systemic lupus erythematosus
  - **c.** Diabetes mellitus, when the feature is inconsistence with the diabetic nephropathy like persistent hematuria or rapid progression of the disease.
  - **d.** Hypertension
  - **e.** Dysproteinemias

  In these cases biopsy is required for:
  - **a.** Definite diagnosis
  - **b.** Dictating the therapy
  - **c.** Extent of active or chronic changes

D. Infections: Viral, poststreptococcal glomerulonephritis
E. Different types of glomerulonephritis:
  - **a.** Focal glomerulosclerosis
  - **b.** Membranous nephropathy
  - **c.** Membranoproliferative glomerulonephritis
  - **d.** Mesangiocapillary glomerulonephritis

F. Microscopic nonurologic hematuria with proteinuria with or without insufficient kidney function.
G. Microscopic nonurologic hematuria without proteinuria in some unique circumstances, such as insurance, kidney donor, or for employment purpose.
H. Allograft transplant: In case of recipient of kidney transplant, if the recipients develop:
  - **a.** Hematuria
  - **b.** Proteinuria
  - **c.** Dysfunction of kidney transplant

  It is done to differentiate different forms of rejection and other causes of kidney failure.

I. Chronic kidney disease: It is done in case of:
  - **a.** Unexplained chronic kidney disease
  - **b.** Normal-sized kidney in imaging

Contraindications to Kidney Biopsy

A. Absolute contraindications:
  - **a.** Uncooperative patient
  - **b.** Uncontrolled severe hypertension
  - **c.** Uncontrolled bleeding diathesis
  - **d.** Solitary native kidney

B. Relative contraindications:
  - **a.** Perinephric abscess
  - **b.** Active pyelonephritis

c. Hydronephrosis
d. Kidney tumor
e. Hypotension
f. Multiple cyst in kidney
g. Small hyperechoic kidneys
h. Uncontrolled hypertension
i. Skin infection at the site selected for biopsy.

Q29. Collecting system of the kidney.
MGR/SEP2010/MDI (5)

Collecting system of kidney.
MGR UNIVERSITY, TAMIL NADU, 2018 (5)

ANSWER

Collecting system of the kidney is formed by joining of distal convoluted tubule of several nephrons. Its length is 20 mm. It is lined by cuboidal epithelium. This tubule will pass through the renal cortex and medulla to drain into the renal pelvis at the apices of medullary pyramid.

The epithelium of the collecting tubule consists of two types of cells:

A. P-cells or principal cells: It contains two types of receptors:
  a. Receptors for antidiuretic hormone
  b. Receptors for aldosterone

  These receptors after being activated increases the permeability to water through aquaporin-2 by increasing the pore size and increasing cyclic adenosine monophosphate (cAMP). Thus 10–12% water is reabsorbed. This cell also is involved in resorption of sodium.

B. I-cells or intercalated cells: It will secrete 5% of the total hydrogen ion and helps to reabsorb bicarbonate ion through Na^+ for K^+ or H^+ which leads to acid urine.

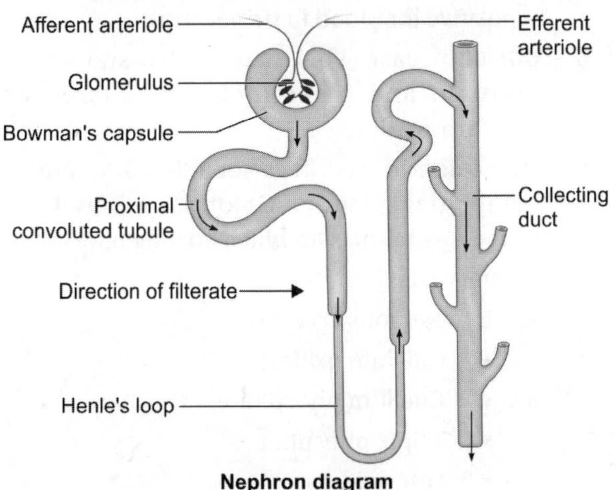

Nephron diagram

Q30. Pathophysiological basis of formation of various renal casts. What is telescoped urinary sediment?
DNBII/APR2016 (7)

Urine microscopy.
MGR UNIVERSITY, TAMIL NADU, 2018 (5)

ANSWER

Cast is the result of solidification of protein in the renal tubular lumen mainly in nephron, and once formed it will be excreted through urine, and it will be in the form of sediment. Presence of casts suggests kidney involvement rather than lower urinary tract involvement. All the casts have basic matrix protein, Tamm–Horsfall mucoprotein to which different cells or materials are added and according to name of added structures. Casts are cylindrical structure taking the shape of tubule with rounded ends. Following are the casts:

A. Hyaline cast: It is least important present in healthy persons and in persons after strenuous exercise. It is formed by solidification of Tamm–Horsfall mucoprotein secreted by tubular cells without significant proteinuria.

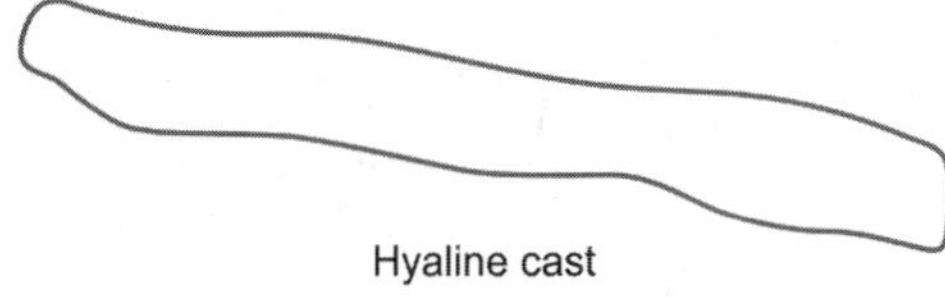
Hyaline cast

B. Cellular casts: In this casts, different types of cells, such as RBC, WBC, and epithelial cell are embedded in protein matrix. In case bacterial cell casts mixture of cell types is present in the protein matrix. Presence of cellular casts indicates the disease:
  a. Red blood cell cast: It is formed due to the following:
    1. Leakage of RBCs through the glomerular membrane
    2. Bleeding into the tubules at any point of nephron

  The causes are:
    1. Poststreptococcal glomerulonephritis
    2. Other acute glomerulonephritis
    3. Immunoglobulin A (IgA) nephropathy
    4. Lupus nephritis
    5. Subacute bacterial endocarditis (SBE)
    6. Renal infarction
    7. Severe acute pyelonephritis (tubulointerstitial disease)

Other form of RBC casts are blood cast and hemoglobin casts which are formed due to degeneration of RBCs present in the cast matrix due to urinary stasis, so cells are no longer visible, but remaining hemoglobin pigment becomes orange-yellow or red-brown color.

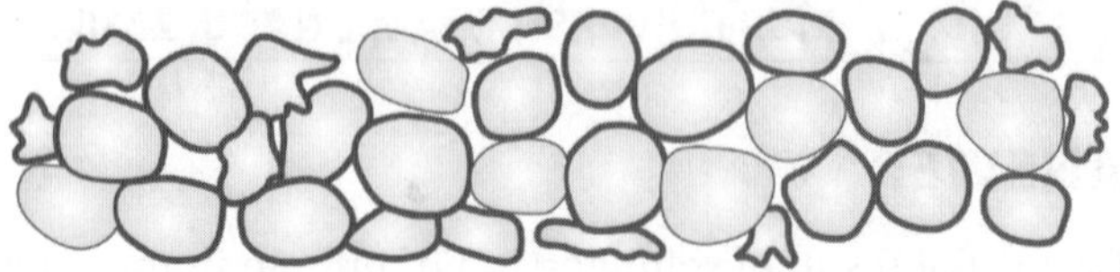

Red blood cells cast

b. White blood cell cast: It is composed of neutrophils:
   1. It is found in acute pyelonephritis, where there is presence of WBCs, and bacteria in the sediment.
   2. In acute glomerulonephritis, presence of RBCs and WBCs in the urinary cast
   3. In acute interstitial nephritis
   4. Acute papillary necrosis
   5. Lupus nephritis

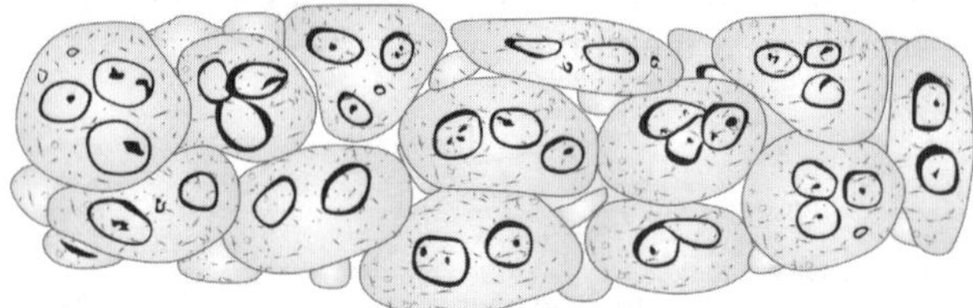

White blood cell cast

c. Bacterial casts: It is composed of bacteria in closely packed or diffusely scattered or concentrated in the protein matrix. Bacteria may be identified in the cytocentrifuged sediment by Gram staining. It is present in:
   1. Acute pyelonephritis
   2. Intrinsic renal infection
d. Epithelial cast: It is composed of epithelial cells and very important findings. These are found in:
   1. Acute tubular necrosis
   2. Viral diseases, such as cytomegalovirus
   3. Exposure to toxins:
      - Mercury
      - Ethylene glycol
      - Various drugs

   These casts are very difficult to distinguish from WBC cast, this can be accomplished by leukocyte esterase test which will be positive in case of WBC cast.
e. Granular cast: These are formed as a result of degeneration of cellular cast. These casts are present in case of tubulointerstitial disease.

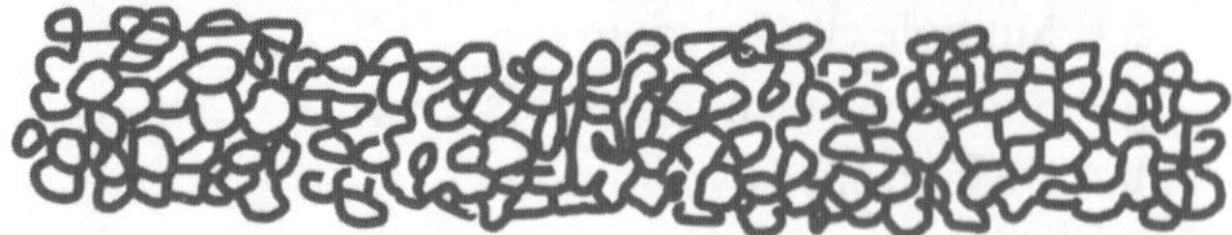

Granular cast

C. Waxy cast: It represents the final stage in the degeneration of cells from cellular to granular and ultimately waxy cast. It is present in case of renal stasis, chronic renal disease, and amyloidosis. Sometimes, they are present as broad cast formed in dilated tubules or collecting tubules due to significant stasis or tubular atrophy hence is called renal failure cast.

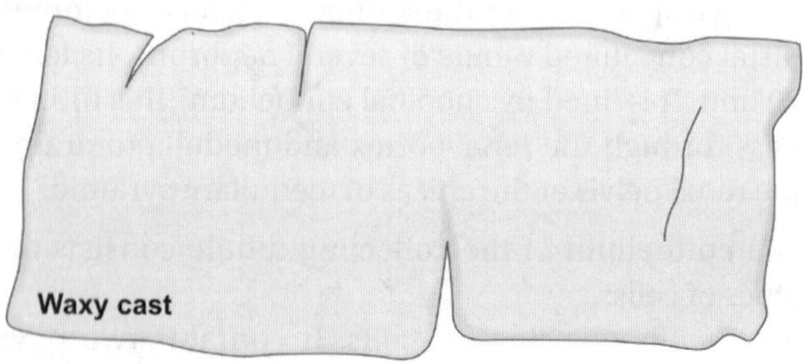

D. Fatty cast: It contains globules of fat as:
   a. Triglyceride or neutral fat: It will stain with Sudan III
   b. Cholesterol: It will polarize as a Maltese cross. It is found in:
      1. Nephrotic syndrome
      2. Diabetic nephropathy
      3. Toxic renal poisoning
E. Other casts:
   a. Myoglobin cast: It is present in myoglobulinuria due to acute muscle damage. Associated finding is positive for blood in urine strip.
   b. Bilirubin cast: This cast is also stained with bilirubin and other intensely colored drug phenazopyridine.
   c. Hemosiderin cast: It is seen 2–3 days after the hemolytic episode. Color is yellow-brown, stained with Prussian blue showing blue color.
   d. Crystal casts:
      1. Endogenous crystals:
         - Calcium oxalate
         - Calcium phosphate
         - Triple phosphate
         - Uric acid

- Bilirubin
- 2,8-dihydroxyadenine
- Cholesterol

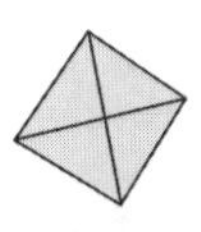
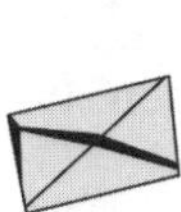

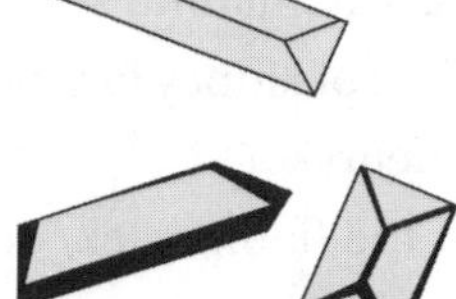

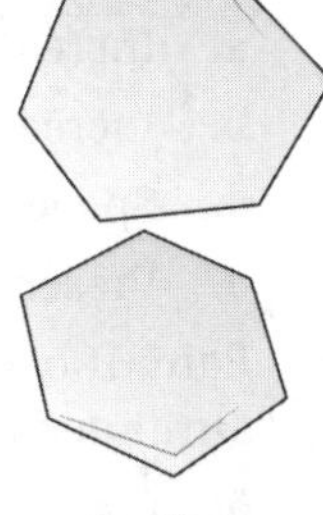

2. Drug related:
   - Acyclovir
   - Methotrexate
   - Acyclovir
   - Amoxicillin

Telescoped Urinary Sediment

It can be defined as urinary sediment, where red blood cells, white blood cells, oval fat bodies, and other types of casts are present in equal proportions. It is found in the following conditions:

A. Lupus nephritis
B. Diabetic glomerulopathy
C. Malignant hypertension
D. Rapidly progressive glomerulonephritis

Q31. Enumerate clinical features of autosomal dominant polycystic kidney disease, methods of diagnosis, and the risk factors that lead to progression of the disease.

DNBIIIB/DEC2013 (10)

Autosomal dominant polycystic kidney disease.

MUHS/NOV2013/MDII (10)

Discuss the etiopathogenesis, clinical manifestations and treatment of autosomal dominant polycystic kidney disease.

DNB (OCT2024) (10)

Polycystic kidney disease.

SAURASHTRA UNI, RAJKOT, 2021 (20)

ANSWER

Polycystic Renal Disease

Etiopathogenesis

It is genetically heterogeneous disease caused by mutation of two different genes:

A. PKD1: It is located in chromosome number 16 and responsible for 85% of cases. It encodes for polycystin-1. PKD1 will develop more cyst starting from very early age and grow faster as compared to PKD2, hence develops more severe disease.

B. PKD2: It is located in chromosome number 4, responsible for 15% of cases, it encodes for polycystin-2.

Polycystin-1 and 2 are membrane-bound glycoprotein present in cilia on the plasma membrane regulating calcium homeostasis. Cyst in the kidney will develop from loss of functional polycystin-1 and 2 along with somatic inactivation of the normal allele, it is consistent with "two hit" mechanism.

C. GANAB: Mutation of this gene is responsible for 3% unresolved autosomal dominant polycystic kidney disease (ADPKD).

Clinical Features

A. May be asymptomatic until fourth or fifth decade

B. Hypertension which may occur from:

  a. Increased activation of renin–angiotensin–aldosterone system
  b. Increased activity of sympathetic nerve
  c. Impaired endothelial cilium function-dependent smooth muscle relaxation of small blood vessels.

C. Flank pain resulting from:

  a. Cyst infection
  b. Gradually increasing size of the cysts
  c. Hemorrhage within the cysts
  d. Nephrolithiasis: Due to uric acid crystals or calcium oxalate crystals. It may occur from:

    1. Defect in distal acidification
    2. Abnormal ammonium transport
    3. Low urine pH
    4. Hypercitrauria

D. Flank pain with recurrent hematuria results from rupture of cyst with hemorrhage into tubule

E. Fever with chill and rigor from infection by gram-negative bacteria in the cyst leading to acute pyelonephritis. It may be the most common cause of death.

Extrarenal Features

A. Cysts in the liver: It is the most common manifestation in ADPKD and prevalence is nearly 90%. Presenting features are:
   a. Asymptomatic with preserved hepatic function
   b. Abdominal pain
   c. Abdominal distention
   d. Liver decompensation

B. Pancreatic cyst: It occurs in 10% of cases. Features are:
   a. Asymptomatic
   b. Features of recurrent pancreatitis due to cystic compression of pancreatic duct
   c. Rarely features of pancreatic carcinoma in case of genetic interaction between ADPKD and pancreatic carcinogenesis.

C. Asymptomatic arachnoid membrane cyst and spinal meningeal cysts:
   a. Asymptomatic
   b. Subdural hematoma
   c. Orthostatic headache due to intracranial hypertension

D. Seminal vesicles cysts

E. Vascular malformation:
   a. Intracranial aneurysm
   b. Dolichoectasia
   c. Thoracic aortic and cervicocephalic artery dissection
   d. Coronary artery aneurysms

F. Cardiac valvular abnormalities:
   a. Mitral valve prolapse is most common.
   b. Aortic regurgitation
   c. Tricuspid prolapse

G. Colonic diverticulosis and diverticulitis

H. Abdominal hernia—paraumbilical, inguinal, and incisional may produce intestinal strangulation or intestinal incarceration.

Complications

A. Hypertension: Prevalence of hypertension is 50% patients of aged 20–30 years in case of end-stage renal disease (ESRD) it will reach to 100%. Pathogenesis of hypertension includes:
   a. Activation of renin–angiotensin–aldosterone axis
   b. Gradual expansion of cyst
   c. Intrarenal ischemia
   d. Decreased expression in the level of polycystin-1 and 2
   e. Availability of nitric oxide

   Uncontrolled hypertension will lead to the following:
   a. Increased risk of proteinuria
   b. Increased risk of hematuria
   c. Speed of decline of kidney function
   d. Presence of aneurysm

B. Pain: It occurs in the flank, back, or abdomen. It is attributed to:
   a. Cystic compression of the kidney capsule
   b. Rupture of cyst
   c. Hemorrhage in cyst: It will resolve within a week. If it is prolonged or if it develops in the patients of >50 years of age, neoplasm has to be excluded.
   d. Infection
   e. Kidney stones

   Acute pain arises from:
   a. Hemorrhage in the cyst
   b. Passage of stones
   c. Urinary tract infection

C. Nephrolithiasis: It occurs in 20–30% of patients, stones being uric acid or calcium oxalate, it occurs due to:
   a. Low citrate in urine
   b. Low urine pH
   c. Decreased excretion of ammonia
   d. Stasis of urine due to distorted anatomy of kidney.

D. Urinary tract infection: It is more frequent in women due to gram-negative bacteria.

E. End-stage renal failure: 45% patients with ADPKD develops ESRD by 60 years of age.

Risk Factors

A. Presence of type of mutated gene
B. Male sex
C. Diagnosis below the age of 30 years
D. First episode of hematuria before the 30 years of age
E. Hyperlipidemia
F. Presence of low density lipoprotein
G. Sickle cell trait
H. Onset of hypertension before 35 years of age.

Diagnosis

A. Positive family history due to autosomal dominant inheritance
B. Presence of bilateral cysts in kidneys

C. In ultrasound:

a. Presence of at least two cysts in each kidney in the age of 30–59 years

b. Presence of at least four cysts in each kidney in the age of >60 years

Sensitivity is 100% and specificity is 100% and false negative rate is 0%.

Due to late onset of ADPKD2 the above criteria is less sensitive.

D. CT scan or T2-MRI can detect smaller size of cyst. But radiation and radiocontrast may produce allergic reaction as well as nephrotoxicity in case of chronic renal insufficiency.

E. T2-MRI with gadolinium can detect cyst of <2–3 mm in diameter, in spite of that many cysts are below the detection level.

F. Genetic testing by:

a. Linkage analyses

b. Mutational analyses

Due to presence of large size *PKD1* gene as well as multiple homologous pseudogenes mutational gene analysis of PKD1 is very costly and difficult.

New technologies for genetic testing will exclude these difficulty, the technologies are:

a. Paired-end next-generation sequencing with multiplexing

b. Matching with bar-coded long range PCR libraries.

Treatment

A. Blood pressure control to 140/90 mm Hg according to Joint National Committee (JNC) guideline. If the systolic blood pressure of 110 mm Hg will be the target in patients with advanced disease, there is compromise in renal blood flow leading to aggravation of renal damage:

a. Low sodium diet < 2 g/day

b. Low cholesterol diet < 200 mg/day

c. Caffeine consumption has to be restricted

d. Protein intake should be restricted to 0.8 g/kg of body weight per day.

e. Drugs:

1. Vasopressin 2 antagonist, such as tolvaptan can be given to reduce the rate of total kidney volume increase as well as decline in kidney function.

2. Somatostatin analog, octreotide like lanreotide reduce the rate of growth of total kidney volume.

B. In case of infection in the cyst lipid soluble antibiotics, such as chloramphenicol, quinolones, and trimethoprim-sulfamethoxazole will cure the gram-negative bacteria as these drugs will penetrate the cyst wall and the cyst is not connected to glomerular filtration.

C. Treatment of kidney stones:

a. Analgesic for relief for pain

b. Proper hydration to maintain adequate flow of urine

D. In case of chronic flank, back, and abdominal pain:

a. Narcotic or nonnarcotic analgesic

b. Nonpharmacologic therapies:

1. Electrical nerve stimulation

2. Acupuncture

3. Biofeed back

4. Surgical decompression of cyst

E. In case of ADPKD with renal failure:

a. Peritoneal dialysis: It is not suitable in the following cases:

1. Massively enlarged polycystic kidneys due to availability of small intraperitoneal space

2. Increased chance of abdominal hernia

3. Back pain

b. Hemodialysis

c. Renal transplantation

In case of massively enlarged polycystic kidney bilateral nephrectomy followed by allograft renal transplantation.

F. Nephrectomy: Indications:

a. Recurrent and severe infection of the cysts

b. Severe renal hemorrhage

c. Intractable pain

d. Renal carcinoma

Pretransplant nephrectomy should be done in the following conditions:

a. Kidney is sufficiently enlarged to interfere the site of implantation of donor kidney.

b. Recurrent infection or hemorrhage in the native kidneys

c. When tumor cannot be ruled out

Q32. Describe clinical presentation and management of HIV-associated nephropathy.

DNBII/DEC2010 (10)

ANSWER

Introduction

Nowadays, due to increased survival in the patients on proper antiretroviral therapy (ART), incidence of chronic renal insufficiency is increased and it is aggravated by following risk factors, such as diabetes mellitus, cardiovascular disease, and infectious diseases, such as hepatitis B and C virus, tuberculosis.

Epidemiology

Measures and incidence of kidney disease in case of HIV varies worldwide and it depends upon:

A. Methods of evaluating renal function
B. Definition of chronic kidney disease
C. Genetic heterogenicity
D. Prevention program
E. Access to healthcare system
F. Initiation of combined ART

Human Immunodeficiency Virus Involvement in Kidney Disease

Human immunodeficiency virus infection damages the kidney through direct and indirect mechanisms:

A. Direct cytopathic effect of virus on the renal parenchymal cells leading to disruption of normal cellular activity.
B. By indirect process pseudopathological process of immune system to HIV virus in the form of:
   a. Deposition of formed immune complexes
   b. Hyperimmune reaction to HIV infection
C. Use of nephrotoxic drugs
D. Superimposed infection

Classification of HIV-induced Kidney Disease

Kidney disease	Directly related to HIV	First-line treatment	Second-line treatment	Adjunct therapies
Predominantly glomerular				
Podocytopathies: • HIV-associated nephropathy • Focal sclerosing glomerulosclerosis	X	Antiretroviral therapy	Steroid, cyclosporin A	ACE inhibitor ARBs
Immune complex-mediated glomerular disease: • Membranoproliferative glomerulonephritis • IgA nephropathy		Antiretroviral therapy	Steroid	ACE inhibitor ARBs
Tubulointerstitial predominant disease				
Tubulointerstitial injury in case of HIV-associated nephropathy	X	Antiretroviral therapy	Steroid	
Drug-induced interstitial nephritis (other than antiretroviral therapy)		Stop the offending drugs	Steroid	
Acute tubular necrosis		Stop the offending drug		
Direct infection of renal parenchyma by pathogens		Treatment of the offending infection		
Immunological dysfunction related inflammation of tubulointerstitium: • Diffuse infiltrative lymphocytosis syndrome • Immune reconstitution inflammatory syndrome		 Antiretroviral therapy Treat opportunistic infection/ART	 Steroid Steroid	 NSAIDs (risk of nephrotoxicity)
Other inflammation of tubulointerstitium in the setting of HIV				
Vascular predominant kidney disease				
Thrombotic microangiopathies: • Thrombotic thrombocytopenic purpura • Hemolytic uremic syndrome	 X X	 ART + plasmapheresis ART + Eculizumab	 Rituximab, bortezomib, cyclosporin A	 Steroid or antiplatelet agents

Continued

Continued

Kidney disease	Directly related to HIV	First-line treatment	Second-line treatment	Adjunct therapies
Arteriosclerosis	X	ART/reduction risk factors for atherosclerosis		
Other causes in the HIV setting				
Diabetic nephropathy		Treatment of diabetes	ACE inhibitor ARBs	
Nephrosclerosis—age related		Antiretroviral therapy	Reduction of factors related to atherosclerosis	

(ACE: angiotensin-converting enzyme; ARBs: angiotensin receptor blockers; HIV: human immunodeficiency virus; IgA: immunoglobulin A; NSAIDs: nonsteroidal anti-inflammatory drugs)

Glomerular-dominant Disease

It is manifested as collapsing glomerulopathy in which collapsed glomerulus with hypertrophy and hyperplasia of glomerular epithelial cells fill the urinary space may be associated with tubulointerstitial disease, such as tubulointerstitial inflammation, tubular atrophy, and interstitial fibrosis. There is presence of immunoglobulin M (IgM), C3, and C1q in the collapsed segments as detected by immunofluorescent microscope.

Human immunodeficiency virus-associated nephropathy is associated with APOL1 allele, low CD4+ count occurs during acute HIV infection.

Q33. Describe pathophysiology, diagnostic evaluation, and treatment of renal amyloidosis.

DNBII/JUN2012 (10)

Amyloid kidney.

MGR UNI, TAMIL NADU, 2021 (5)

Renal amyloidosis.

SRI GURU RAM DAS UNI OF HEALTH SC, AMRITSAR, 2022 (10)

ANSWER

Introduction

Primary fibrillar deposits of immunoglobulin light chain, i.e., amyloid light chain of L in kidney is known as primary amyloidosis or secondary fibrillar deposits of amyloid A protein in kidney is known secondary amyloidosis of kidney.

Types of Renal Amyloidosis

Name of disease	Precursor protein	Amyloid protein	Organ involved
AL amyloidosis	Monoclonal Ig light chain	AL	Kidney, liver, gastrointestinal tract, heart, spleen, nervous system, thyroid gland, adrenal gland
AA amyloidosis	Serum amyloid protein	AA	Kidney, gastrointestinal tract, liver, spleen, thyroid
AH amyloidosis	Monoclonal Ig heavy chain	AH	Very rare, few case of kidney involvement
Hereditary amyloidosis	Transthyretin (TTR)	ATTR	Heart, peripheral nervous system, kidney involvement rare
	Fibrinogen Aα	AFib	Kidney (mainly glomerular involvement), spleen, liver
	Apolipoprotein AI	AApoAI	Kidney (mainly medullary involvement), heart, liver,
	Apolipoprotein AII	AApoAII	Kidney
	Lysozyme	Alys	Kidney, gastrointestinal tract, liver, spleen

(Ig: immunoglobulin)

Pathophysiology

Till date there are 25 structurally unrelated proteins, which are responsible for formation of amyloidosis.

The initial step in fibril formation is misfolding event of "precursor proteins" which can result from any one of the following:

A. Proteolytic cleavage

B. Amino acid substitution, such as transthyretin

C. In presence of specific local factors, such as β_2 microglobulin

D. Intrinsic properties which become significant only at high concentration

Second step is the self-aggregation of these misfolded variants.

Third step is generation of profilaments by self-aggregated misfolded variants.

Final step is interaction of profilaments to form fibrils. These fibrils have characteristic β-pleated sheet which under polarized light produces birefringence after being stained with Congo red dye.

In case of AL amyloidosis:

A. Immunoglobulin light chain produced by clonal plasma cells or its fragment produced by macrophages will be aggregated in acid pH.

B. Here kidney is affected in 50–80% individual. 75% of light chain are of lambda class.

C. 10% of patients suffer from overt myeloma with lytic bone lesion and 30% plasma cells infiltrates bone marrow.

D. 20% patient progress to dialysis.

In case of AA amyloidosis:

A. It occurs due to deposition of β-pleated sheets of amyloid protein, it is acute phage reactant, its physiological functions include:

- **a.** Transport of cholesterol
- **b.** Attraction of immune cells
- **c.** Activation of metalloproteases

B. 40% patients suffer from rheumatoid arthritis

C. 10% suffer from ankylosing spondylitis and psoriatic arthritis.

D. Other disease, such as inflammatory bowel disease, familial Mediterranean fever (FMF), and chronic infection may occur.

E. In FMF and Muckle-Wells syndrome, there are mutations of gene encoding pyrin and cryopyrin proteins:

- **a.** In case of early inflammation, these two proteins are responsible for apoptosis of leukocytes.
- **b.** These proteins are also a part of the pathway called "inflammasome."

F. Mutation of receptor 1 of tumor necrosis factor will also produce chronic inflammation and secondary amyloidosis.

G. Fragment of A amyloid protein increase in number, attach to the receptors for glycation end product and thus self-aggregate in the extracellular environment.

Diagnosis

A. Histological demonstration of amyloid deposits:

- **a.** When stained with Congo red dye, it will show orange-red appearance under light microscopy.
- **b.** It will produce apple-green birefringence under polarized light.
- **c.** Addition of thioflavin T in the amyloid tissue will bind to amyloid fibril and demonstrate yellow-green birefringence under polarized microscope.
- **d.** In case of suspicion of amyloidosis, sensitivities of staining of aspirated abdominal fat are 80–90% and 65–75%, respectively.
- **e.** Salivary gland biopsies and rectal biopsies may demonstrate amyloid tissue.

B. Determination of different types of amyloidogenic proteins:

It can be done in the following ways:

- **a.** Immunohistochemistry of the tissue
- **b.** Immunofluorescence of the extracted tissue

In above cases antibodies to amyloidogenic proteins:

- **c.** Mass spectrometry
- **d.** Sequencing of proteins of amino acids extracted from amyloid deposits

These techniques are not routinely available.

C. In absence of immunoreactivity for λ and k chain for AL amyloidosis:

- **a.** Monoclonal Ig protein in blood clonal plasma cells in the bone marrow or urine. Since monoclonal protein is lower in case of AL amyloidosis as compared to multiple myeloma, hence, immunofixation electrophoresis can detect presence of monoclonal protein.
- **b.** Nephelometric quantification of free light chain present in the serum is done for:
  1. Presence of monoclonal protein
  2. Disease progression
  3. Response to treatment
- **c.** In presence of renal dysfunction, ratio of two light chains isotypes is relevant as light chains are excreted through the kidneys.

D. Bone marrow biopsy to be done for estimation of burden of plasma cells because in absence of multiple myeloma quantity of plasma cells are low in AL amyloidosis.

E. In case of AA amyloidosis, proper history regarding IBD, chronic infections, periodic fever syndrome, and rheumatoid arthritis has to be taken.

F. In case of FMF, proper family history may be absent due to variable penetrance of some diseases.

Features in Kidney Biopsy

A. By light microscopy:

- **a.** Glomerular amyloid presents as amorphous material in the mesangium as well as capillary loops.
- **b.** Sometimes large amount of amyloid tissue in the mesangium may produce small nodules like that of diabetic nephropathy.
- **c.** Deposition of these tissue in tubulointerstitium can produce interstitial fibrosis and tubular atrophy.

B. By immunofluorescence microscopy:

- **a.** Negative for intact Ig, complement and fibrin. But in AL amyloidosis Ig light chain is found.
- **b.** In absence of MM in AL amyloidosis monoclonal protein is of λ and κ type.
- **c.** In case of AA amyloidosis amyloid protein can be identified by using antibodies.

C. By electron microscopy: Randomly distributed nonbranching fibrils of 8–10 mm in diameter with special orientation in the mesangium, interstitium, basement membrane, and vessels.

Treatment of Renal Amyloidosis

Amyloid deposition in kidney is associated with progressive deterioration of renal function which depends upon:

- **a.** Type of amyloid deposition
- **b.** Rapidity of amyloid deposition of amyloidogenic precursor protein.

A. In case of AL amyloidosis: High dose of melphalan intravenously with autologous stem cell transplantation can eliminate clonal plasma cells.

Following factors are responsible for eligibility of above treatment:

- **a.** Cardiac function
- **b.** Function of autonomic nervous system
- **c.** Performance status

In case of toxicity with above treatment following combinations of treatment can be given:

- **a.** Oral melphalan with high dose of dexamethasone
- **b.** Thalidomide or lenalidomide with immunomodulatory drugs or anti-angiogenic drugs effective against plasma cells.

B. In case of AA amyloidosis:

- **a.** Treatment of underlying diseases
- **b.** Long-life treatment with colchicine in case of FMF.
- **c.** Cytotoxic agents or tumor necrosis factor (TNF) antagonists:
  1. It will suppress serum amyloid A (SAA) production which result reduction of AA.
  2. It inhibits expression of receptor for advanced glycation end products (RAGE)
  3. It may reduce interaction between AA fibrils and RAGE.
- **d.** Fibrillogenesis inhibitor with small molecules having structural similarity with glycosaminoglycan (GAG) moieties interferes between GAG and amyloid proteins thus decrease their stability and reduce new amyloid formation.

Regression of amyloid deposits can be detected by scintigraphy using radiolabeled serum amyloid P as it binds to all types of amyloid proteins.

Q34. State the Cockcroft–Gault formula and its use. Describe laboratory findings in prerenal azotemia.

List the modification of diet in renal disease with reasons.

DNBIA/DEC2014 (10)

ANSWER

Cockcroft-Gault Formula

{[(140—age in years) × Lean body weight in kg]/(serum creatinine × 72)} × (0.85 if female)

Q35. Myeloma kidney.

MGR/MAR2007/MDI (5)

ANSWER

Multiple myeloma (MM), 10% of all hematologic malignancies affects mainly in elderly is treated mainly by high dose of chemotherapy and autologous stem cell transplantation. Kidney dysfunction in multiple myeloma may occur in 20% of patients due to acute kidney injury from hypercalcemia or chronic kidney disease due to tubular nephropathy as a result of secretion of immunoglobulin (Ig) or by clone of plasma cell or monoclonal light chain. International Myeloma Working Group definition of multiple myeloma:

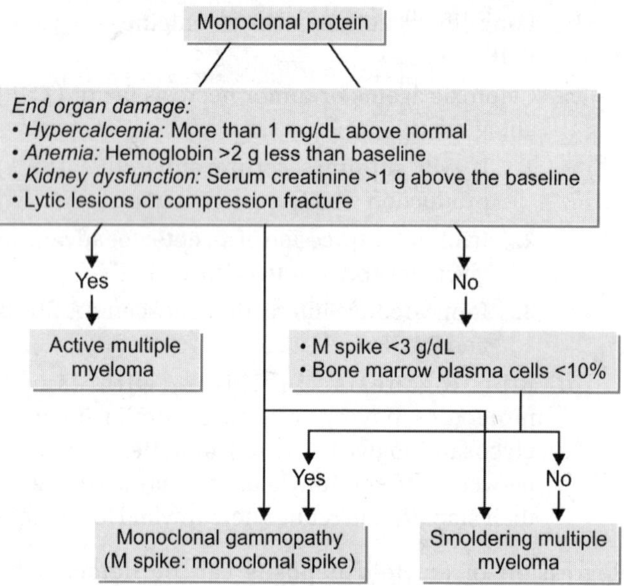

Spectrum of renal disease in case of MM are cast nephropathy, light chain amyloidosis, monoclonal Ig deposition disease, less frequently cryoglobulinemic glomerulonephritis, and proliferative glomerulonephritis.

Following are the association between the clinical manifestation and types of kidney injury:

A. Acute kidney injury:
  - **a.** Myeloma cast nephropathy
  - **b.** Acute kidney necrosis
  - **c.** Direct infiltration of renal parenchyma
  - **d.** Acute tubulointerstitial nephropathy
  - **e.** Iatrogenic effects

B. Nephrotic syndrome:
  - **a.** Monoclonal Ig deposition disease
  - **b.** Rare types of glomerular involvement

C. Chronic kidney disease:
  - **a.** Myeloma cast nephropathy
  - **b.** Amyloidosis
  - **c.** Monoclonal Ig deposition disease

D. Fanconi syndrome: Proximal tubulopathy

Natural Course of Acute Kidney Injury

A. Full recovery
B. To chronic kidney disease
C. Acute on chronic kidney disease
D. End-stage renal failure

In case of acute kidney injury:

Pathology

Normally, light chains after being filtered are endocytosed and metabolized by the tubule but are not deposited in the renal structure, so the light chain produced by neoplastic plasma cells produce dichotomous behavior may be due to mutation in the Ig molecule. Monoclonal free light chains produced by plasma cells are filtered through the glomerulus and are taken up by tubular epithelial cells and mesangial cells and they will activate nuclear factor kappa B (NF-κB) resulting epithelial-mesenchymal transition or apoptosis ultimately leading to transcription of inflammatory cytokines. These cytokines will recruit inflammatory cells into the interstitium leading to development of fibrosis. When the amount of light chain overwhelms the capacity of proximal tubular cells to catabolize the chain. It is triggered by the following factors:

  - **a.** Dehydration
  - **b.** Infection
  - **c.** Hypercalcemia
  - **d.** Contrast medium usage
  - **e.** Use of nephrotoxic medications such as NSAIDs, diuretics, ACE inhibitor, and ARBs
  - **f.** Amount of free light chain >500 mg/L

A. In case of suspected multiple myeloma monoclonal light chain and Bence Jones protein has to be analyzed in concentrated urine by immunofixation.

B. Coincident measurement of serum/urine albumin has to be done in suspected Ig deposition disease.

In case of cast nephropathy: Diagnosis can be confirmed by tubular cast in the distal nephron contains Ig light chain, Ig and other light chain, Tamm–Horsfall glycoprotein, cast is eosinophilic, and brittle because they are fractured and lamellated. Cast may rupture tubules producing interstitial nephritis which ultimately leads to interstitial fibrosis.

In case of chronic kidney disease in multiple myeloma:

A. Triggering factors are:
  - **a.** Dehydration
  - **b.** Hypercalcemia

c. Infection
d. Use of nephrotoxic drugs

Factors associated with progression of chronic kidney disease (CKD) include following causes of CKD, these are:

A. Level of glomerular filtration rate (GFR)
B. Age
C. Level of albuminuria
D. Elevated blood pressure
E. Dyslipidemia
F. Hyperglycemia
G. Smoking
H. Cardiovascular disease
I. Exposure to nephrotoxic agents

Treatment of Kidney Disease in Multiple Myeloma

A. Treatment of cast nephropathy:
   a. Aggressive hydration by 2–3 L/day
   b. Alkalization of urine
   c. Discontinuation of NSAIDs
   d. Avoidance of intravenous contrast media
   e. Administration of bisphosphonates for treatment of hypercalcemia but should be used with caution.
B. Treatment of multiple myeloma:
   a. Apheresis therapy: Induction of remission with chemotherapeutic regimen followed by plasmapheresis. Plasmapheresis involves removal of red blood cells and other substances such as autoreactive antibodies, immune complexes, lipoproteins, paraproteins, and cytokines from the blood by centrifugation with the help of large pore hemofilters thus it maintains normal plasma volume and electrolyte concentrations. Choice of replacement fluid includes crystalloids, human albumin solution, fresh frozen plasma (FFP), liquid stored plasma, and cryoprecipitate.

      If the patient is not suitable for plasmapheresis, melphalan with prednisone is of choice. The preferred approach should be dexamethasone with thalidomide or with cyclophosphamide, vincristine, and doxorubicin followed by autologous stem cell transplantation (ASCT).

      In acute kidney injury (AKI) due to MM can be treated by plasmapheresis with hemodialysis to correct electrolyte concentration along with renal support.
   b. Dialysis therapy in kidney disease in MM: In 65% patient with cast nephropathy may undergo end-stage renal failure within 3 months after diagnosis. These patient has to be treated by hemodialysis.

Pathology of Monoclonal Immunoglobulin Deposition Disease (MIDD)

It can be diagnosed by demonstration of deposition of monoclonal immunoglobulin (Ig) light or heavy or both chains in the basement membrane of kidney and other organs by electron microscope. Extrarenal manifestations of MIDD are:

A. Cardiac disease:
   a. Congestive cardiac failure
   b. Arrhythmias
   c. Cardiomegaly
B. Liver involvement:
   a. Hepatomegaly
   b. Portal hypertension
   c. Hepatic insufficiency
C. Neurological involvement

Pathogenesis in MIDD is interaction of fibrogenic monoclonal Ig with mesangial cells and specific Ig light chain will lead to release of fibrogenic cytokines and production of matrix protein by mesangial cells forming nodules in the glomerulus.

Prognosis of MIDD

Median survival is 4 years. Significant predictors of death are:

A. Age
B. Presence of myeloma
C. Extrarenal manifestation

Therapy of MIDD

A. Melphalan with prednisone or in combination of ASCT. Serum creatinine level of ≤4 mg/dL can be improved with chemotherapy but if creatinine is ≥4 mg/dL will progress to ESRD.
B. High dose of chemotherapy with ASCT can be given to MIDD patients. Renal transplantation should not be tried as it is associated with poor graft and patient survival.

AL Amyloidosis

It is present in 30% patients of MM. Presenting symptoms are proteinuria, nephrotic syndrome, or chronic insufficiency in 50% of cases.

Pathology in AL Amyloidosis in MM

In this case, amyloid fibril is formed by circulating homogeneous and Ig light chains of N-terminal variable portion of light chain fragment.

Prognosis

Median survival is 16 months but patient with λ light chain has poorer prognosis.

Treatment

Inhibition of production of paraprotein by prednisolone, melphalan, and ASCT.

Median time between diagnosis and initiation of hemodialysis is 15 months and median survival on dialysis is 22 months.

Q36. Nephrotic syndrome.

MGR/APR2013/MDI (5)

Discuss clinical evaluation of a case of nephrotic syndrome.

MUHS/NOV2010/MDII (25)

Newer immunosuppressive agents in management of nephrotic syndrome.

AMU/2011/MDIV (20)

Adult nephrotic syndrome.

BABA FARID UNI OF HEALTH SC, 2018 (10)

Discuss etiology, clinical features, investigations and treatment of nephrotic syndrome.

BHARATI VIDYAPEETH DEEMED UNI, JHELUM, 2018 (15)

Enumerate different causes of anasarca. How will you manage a case of nephrotic syndrome?

Causes has been described in question number 208 in general chapter.

MANIPUR UNIVERSITY, 2021 (10)

Nephrotic syndrome.

RAJASTHAN UNIVERSITY, 2023 (9)

ANSWER

Nephrotic syndrome can be defined by presence of physical sign such as pedal edema, biochemical features such as proteinuria of >3.5 g/day, hypoalbuminemia, lipiduria, hyperlipidemia with or without hypertension and in case of adult presence of thrombotic complications.

Thrombotic complication occurs due to:

- **A.** Urinary loss of antithrombin III
- **B.** Increased aggregation of platelets
- **C.** Dysfunction of endothelial cells

Edema occurs due to two distinct mechanisms:

- **A.** According to underfill mechanism hypoalbuminemia leads to the following:
  - **a.** Decreased oncotic pressure
  - **b.** Reduction of effective intravascular compartment size
  - **c.** Renin–angiotensin axis activation
  - **d.** Stimulation of reabsorption of sodium
- **B.** Due to overfill mechanism: Retention of sodium due to corin-mediated activation of sodium channels in the tubular epithelial cells.

In any patient with heavy proteinuria and pedal edema protein: Creatinine ratio > 2 mg/mg indicating nephrotic range of proteinuria.

Causes of Nephrotic Syndrome

- **A.** Primary causes:
  - **a.** Minimal change nephrotic syndrome
  - **b.** Membranous nephropathy
  - **c.** Focal segmental glomerulosclerosis
  - **d.** Membranoproliferative glomerulonephritis
- **B.** Secondary causes:
  - **a.** Metabolic:
    - **1.** Amyloidosis
    - **2.** Diabetic mellitus
  - **b.** Immunological diseases:
    - **1.** Systemic lupus erythematosus (SLE)
    - **2.** Sjögren syndrome
    - **3.** Cryoglobulinemia
    - **4.** Henoch–Schönlein purpura
    - **5.** Microscopic polyangiitis
  - **c.** Neoplastic causes:
    - **1.** Lymphoma
    - **2.** Leukemia
    - **3.** Myeloma
    - **4.** Melanoma
  - **d.** Infections:
    - **1.** Bacterial:
      - Leprosy
      - Syphilis
      - Infective endocarditis

2. Protozoal:
    - Malaria
    - Filariasis
    - Schistosomiasis
3. Viral:
    - Hepatitis B virus (HBV)
    - Hepatitis C virus (HCV)
    - Epstein–Barr virus
    - human immunodeficiency virus (HIV)

e. Drugs:
1. Nonsteroidal anti-inflammatory drugs (NSAIDs)
2. Lithium
3. Heroin

f. Allergic:
1. Poison Ivy
2. Antivenom
3. Stings, venom of snake bites

g. Genetic:
1. Hereditary nephritis (Alport syndrome)
2. Congenital nephrotic syndrome (Finnish type)

Diagnostic Criteria of Nephrotic Syndrome

A. Heavy proteinuria:
  a. Protein to creatinine ratio in spot urine >3–3.5 mg protein/mg of creatinine (300–350 mg/mmol)
  b. 24-hour protein collection of >3–3.5 g/day

B. Hypoalbuminemia: Serum albumin <2.5 g/dL

C. Edema: Clinical sign of pedal edema

D. Hyperlipidemia: Total cholesterol is >350 mg/dL

E. Estimated GFR

F. Creatinine clearance

G. 24-hour urinary protein excretion with selectivity index—it can be calculated as transferrin/immunoglobulin G ratio.

Diagnostic Evaluation in a Patient with Nephrotic Syndrome

A. Step 1: Confirmation of nephrotic syndrome:
  a. Dipstick testing for protein: 2/3/4+
  b. Protein to creatinine ratio >3–3.5 mg protein/mg of creatinine
  c. Measurement of serum albumin

B. Step 2: Assessment of common causes:
  a. Urinalysis: It demonstrate hematuria or different cast—nephritis
  b. Coagulation panel and blood counts abnormal—bleeding disorder
  c. Renal function tests: Elevated level of cystatin C, creatinine suggests acute kidney injury.
  d. Liver function test: Raised transaminases suggest viral hepatitis
  e. Fasting blood glucose level: Raised in diabetes mellitus

C. Step 3: Assessment of underlying conditions:
  a. History:
    1. Fever: Malignancy, infection, collagen disease, and malaria
    2. Rash: SLE
    3. History of different drug ingestion such as NSAIDs, antipsychotic medication
    4. History of addiction to heroin
    5. History of polydipsia, polyphagia, repeated infection: diabetes mellitus
    6. Nasal ulcer: Collagen disease
    7. History of bite by snake, bee sting
    8. History of allergy to snake venom
    9. Family history of nephrotic syndrome: Alport syndrome, congenital nephrotic syndrome.
  b. Systemic examination to search for the causes:
    1. Anemia: Malignancy, malaria
    2. Jaundice: Viral hepatitis, malignancies
    3. Lymphadenopathy: Leukemia, lymphoma, viral hepatitis
    4. Purpura: Henoch–Schönlein purpura, leukemia
    5. Hepatosplenomegaly: Malaria, leukemia, lymphoma, viral hepatitis
    6. Rash: SLE
    7. Leg vein thrombosis: Membranous nephropathy
  c. Special laboratory investigations:
    1. ANA (HEp-2 method), double-stranded DNA antibody
    2. Complement:
        - C3 and C4: Collagen vascular disease for classical and alternate pathways
        - CH50: Screening for red cell lysis—good screening for overall complement activity

3. Antineutrophilic cytoplasmic antibody (ANCA) to diagnose small vessel vasculitis:
    - Cytoplasmic ANCA (cANCA): Antigen is proteinase 3.
    - Perinuclear ANCA: Antigen is myeloperoxidase.
4. Antiglomerular basement antibodies: It is specific for anti-GBM disease.
5. Antistreptolysin O titer: It is diagnostic of streptococcal pharyngitis.
6. Antiphospholipid antibodies: It can diagnose antiphospholipid syndrome.
7. Chest X-Ray: Demonstration of pleural effusion—malignancy, connective tissue disease
8. Echocardiography: Diabetes, collagen vascular disease
9. Presence of cryoglobulinemia: Hepatitis C virus
10. Venous Doppler study: In case history of membranous nephropathy
11. CT scan: Liver disease, lymphoma, leukemia, collagen vascular disease
12. Viral profile: Hepatitis
13. Ultrasonography of kidney: Enlarged in case of acute inflammation

D. Step 4: Assessment of complications: To assess the complication above investigations have to be done to search any aggravation or regression of the parent disease.

E. Step 5: Consideration of renal biopsy:

a. To diagnose the disease and immunological studies

b. To assess the severity of the disease

c. To assess the response to treatment

d. To detect the resistance to treatment

Recent Management of Nephrotic Syndrome

A. Corticosteroid: As an initial treatment corticosteroid can be given as 2 mg/kg/day for 6 weeks orally as a single or divided doses followed by 1.5 mg/kg/day single morning dose at alternate day for next 6 weeks followed by cessation of treatment.

B. Cyclosporine A: It is given at a dose of 4–5 mg/kg daily for 12–24 months. Prednisolone also is administered at a dose of 1.5 mg/kg at alternate day for 2–4 weeks followed by reduction of dose at a rate of 0.15–0.25 mg/kg at every 4th week to a maintenance dose of 0.25–0.5 mg/kg dose and it should be continued for another 6 months. Complication of cyclosporine therapy is hypertension, gum hypertrophy, hirsutism, nephrotoxicity, raised transaminases, hypercholesterolemia. Serum creatinine should be estimated at regular interval of 2–3 months.

Following are the types of remission:

a. Resolution of edema

b. Normalization of serum albumin to ≥3

c. Marked reduction of proteinuria

d. Complete remission:

1. Negative dipstick for protein for three consecutive days
2. <0.3 g/day in adult or urine protein to urine creatinine ratio is 0.3 g/g

e. Partial remission:

1. Urine protein <2 g/day, decreased by 50% and serum albumin will be ≥2.5 mg/dL in children.
2. <3.5 g/day in adult and decreased by 50% in adult.

Following are the three of relapses:

a. Steroid-dependent relapse: Two or more relapses during tapering of steroid or within 2 weeks of steroid discontinuation.

b. Steroid-resistant relapse: Failed to achieve remission with 16 weeks of daily or alternate therapy with steroid.

c. Frequent relapse: There is two or more relapses within 6 months or three or more relapses within any year of achieving remission.

In case of infrequent relapse:

A. Prednisolone—1 mg/kg/day or 2 mg/kg at alternate day (maximum 80 mg/kg or 120 mg/kg at alternate day for 14–16 weeks). Then it should be tapered slowly by 5–10 mg/week but total exposure should not exceed 24 weeks.

In case of steroid-dependent frequent relapse:

Cyclophosphamide—2–2.5 mg/kg/day for 8 weeks.

If relapse in spite of cyclophosphamide or to preserve fertility:

Cyclophosphamide 3–5 mg/kg/day in two divided doses for 1–2 years

Or

Tacrolimus 0.05–0.1 mg/kg/day in two divided doses until 3 months after remission, then will be tapered to minimal effective dose for 1–2 years. Side effects are diarrhea, hyperglycemia and rarely neurotoxicity.

In case of intolerance to steroid, cyclophosphamide, tacrolimus or cyclosporine:

Mycophenolate mofetil 800–1,200 mg/m^2 in divided doses for 1–2 years. Side effects are gastrointestinal disturbances, leukopenia, and diarrhea. Leukocyte count should be monitored every alternate months and treatment should be discontinued if the count will be <4,000/cc.

Q37. Modification of drugs in renal disease.

BF/OCT2010/MDI (8)

Write about drug induced renal toxicity. Discuss complications of hemodialysis.

DNB (JUN2022) (10)

Antibiotic alternatives in hepatic and renal dysfunction.

SAURASHTRA UNI, 2022 (20)

Hemodialysis has been discussed in question number 7.

Drug induced renal toxicity.

WBUHS, 2020 (10)

ANSWER

Pharmacokinetics of drugs is changed in chronic kidney disease (CKD) based on its absorption, distribution, metabolism, and elimination:

A. Absorption of the drugs can be changed in CKD will change the pharmacokinetic behavior of the drugs in the following ways:
   - **a.** In case of CKD saliva becomes more alkaline so the drugs that requires acid milieu for absorption are not absorbed.
   - **b.** Associated nausea and vomiting prevent drug ingestion and absorption
   - **c.** Volume overload state: Absorption of drugs is limited by wall edema
   - **d.** Drug interaction: Some drugs such as phosphate-binding agents used in the management of CKD prevent the absorption of other drugs by binding nonabsorbable complexes.
   - **e.** Gastrointestinal neuropathy: In case of diabetes, uremia may retard the absorption of some drugs by delaying the gastric emptying time.

B. Changes in distribution in coronary heart disease (CHD) can change the pharmacokinetic behavior of the drugs by the following mechanisms:
   - **a.** Volume of distribution (V_0) is the ratio of administered drugs to plasma drug concentration. V_0 represents the size of anatomic space occupied by the drugs if it is present throughout the body. Digoxin with large V_0 is present in small amount in the blood but distributed throughout the tissues.
   - **b.** Malnutrition and proteinuria will reduce the availability of amount of protein available to bind the drugs, as a result free concentration of the drugs will be increased leading to adverse reaction of the drugs.

C. Metabolism of the drugs is changed in CKD in the following mechanisms: CKD will increase or decrease or no change in the pharmacokinetics of the drugs. In some cases active metabolites of the drugs are insignificant in case of normal kidney. In CKD metabolites of morphine, 6- and 3-morphine gluconate is at risk of adverse reactions.

D. Changes in elimination of drugs in CKD in the following mechanisms: Reduction of GFR in CKD will increase the half-life of the drugs that are primarily excreted by kidney. It can be measured by clearance of specific compound.

Following characteristics can determine whether the drug can be removed in dialysis:

A. Molecular weight of the drug: If the molecular weight is <500 Daltons it can be removed by dialysis.

B. Protein binding: If the drug is less protein bound, free drugs can be removed by dialysis.

C. Volume of distribution (V_0): Those drugs with large volume of distribution can be eliminated effectively by dialysis.

D. Water solubility: Drugs which are more water soluble will be eliminated by dialysis as compared to lipid solubility.

E. Dialyzer membrane: Surface area, pore size, and geometry of the membrane will determine the drugs which can be eliminated by membrane.

F. Flow rate of blood and dialysate: Drugs will be eliminated by hemodialysis if the flow rate is increased.

Following drugs produce hyperkalemia in CKD patients:

A. Potassium supplement combination with therapy with diuretics

B. Potassium sparing diuretics inhibiting the potassium elimination through kidney

C. Angiotensin-converting enzyme inhibitor and ARBs alter the RASS

D. Digoxin due to its narrow therapeutic range, overdose can produce and raise the serum potassium.

Following drugs are avoided in CKD patients prior to dialysis:

A. Cephalosporins, carbapenem, monobactam being water soluble small molecules will require supplementation after dialysis.

B. Carbapenem, imipenem lowers the threshold for seizures so have to be avoided in patients on dialysis.

Caution should be required in case of following narcotic drugs in CKD:

A. Following drugs should be avoided:

- **a.** Meperidine
- **b.** Propoxyphene

B. Following drugs should be used with caution:

- **a.** Morphine
- **b.** Codeine

C. Following drugs are used as safe dose:

- **a.** Hydromorphone
- **b.** Fentanyl

Q38. Catheter induced urinary tract infection.

DNB (DEC2022) (5)

Diagnosis and management of catheter associated urinary tract infections.

WBUHS, 2020 (10)

ANSWER

Catheter induced urinary tract infection is very common in hospitalized patients presenting with symptomatic or asymptomatic bacteriuria.

Etiological factors are:

A. *Escherichia coli*

B. *Pseudomonas aeruginosa*

C. *Klebsiella pneumoniae*

D. *Enterococcus species*

E. *Candida*

Pathophysiology

Bacteria while passes through the conduit, it bypass the body's defense mechanism and it will reach the urinary bladder.

Risk Factors

A. Duration of catheterization in the bladder: As the duration of catheterization increases, risk of bacterial colonization will be increased leading to symptomatic or asymptomatic bacteriuria which increases 3–10% per day.

B. Disruption of the natural defense of the body: Body's ability to prevent the natural accent from the periurethral area due to alteration of the flow of urine leading to increased chance of infection.

C. Sex predilection: Women are more prone to develop this type of infection.

D. Improper insertion or improper maintenance leading to this infection.

E. Immunosuppressed patient like patient on immunosuppressive drugs, cancer chemotherapy or transplanted patients.

Clinical Features

A. Patient may be asymptomatic

B. Fever

C. Suprapubic pain

D. In case of elderly, delirium or drowsiness

E. Hematuria

Diagnosis

A. Routine analysis of urine demonstrates:

- **a.** Pus cells in large number
- **b.** Large number of red blood dells
- **c.** Large number of bacteria

B. Urine for culture and sensitivity.

C. Blood: Complete blood count,

Management

A. Removal or change of catheter can cure the infection.

B. Antibiotic therapy: To start with administration of empiric antibiotic therapy after sending the urine for culture and sensitivity, then according to report the antibiotic may be changed.

C. Proper hydration to the patient.

D. Maintenance of close drainage system.

E. Unless required, catheterization should not be done.

Q39. Differential diagnosis of Pulmonary renal syndrome.

DNB (DEC2019) (10)

Pulmonary renal syndrome.

SCBMCH, 2020(20)

Pulmonary renal syndrome.

VEER NARMAD SOUTH GUJARAT UNI, 2021 (10)

ANSWER

Pulmonary renal syndrome is characterized by diffuse pulmonary hemorrhage along with rapidly progressive glomerulonephritis.

The causes of the pulmonary renal syndrome are:

A. Small vessel vasculitis: It is characterized by crescentic glomerulonephritis or pauci-immune necrotizing glomerulonephritis along with pulmonary involvement in the form of:

- **a.** C-ANCA positive Granulomatous polyangiitis: Sinusitis, saddle nose deformity, pulmonary nodules and rapidly proliferative glomerulonephritis.
- **b.** P-ANCA positive microscopic polyangiitis: alveolar hemorrhage, no granuloma, absence of involvement of upper respiratory tract.
- **c.** P-ANCA positive Eosinophilic granulomatosis with polyangiitis: Eosinophilia, neuropathy, asthma.

B. Anti-glomerular basement membrane disease: Risk factors are smoking and exposure to hydrocarbon, presence of anti-GBM antibodies, rapidly proliferative glomerulonephritis, linear deposits of IgG on the glomerular basement membrane and pulmonary capillary basement membrane.

C. Immune complex diseases:

- **a.** Systemic lupus nephritis—ANA and ANTI DS-DNA positive and lupus nephritis.
- **b.** Cryoglobulinemic vasculitis—association with hepatitis C virus and deposition of immune complexes in the basement membranes of kidney and lung.
- **c.** Henoch–Schönlein purpura—pain abdomen, palpable purpuric lesion in the skin, joint pain and renal lesion.
- **d.** Extra-articular manifestations in rheumatoid arthritis.

D. Secondary causes:

- **a.** Drugs: Hydralazine, penicillamine, propylthiouracil, cocaine, levamisole
- **b.** Infections: Tuberculosis, viral, leptospirosis, endocarditis due to bacteria
- **c.** Malignancies: Lymphoma, leukemia, as a part of paraneoplastic syndrome.
- **d.** Thrombotic microangiopathy: Malignant hypertension, antiphospholipid syndrome

Q40. Discuss the risk factors, etiology and management of asymptomatic bacteriuria. Discuss the risk factors and clinical manifestations of emphysematous pyelonephritis.

DNB (JUN2022) (10)

Emphysematous pyelonephritis.

SARDAR PATEL UNIVERSITY, 2019 (5)

MAHATMA UNIVERSITY, 2020 (10)

Discuss the management of asymptomatic bacteriuria.

MAHATMA UNIVERSITY, 2021 (10)

ANSWER

Definition

Asymptomatic bacteriuria can be defined as the presence of bacteria in urine in a patient having no clinical feature of urinary tract infection. It is very common in elderly. Most of this asymptomatic bacteriuria will not turn into symptomatic infection, and has no adverse consequences in future.

Etiology

It is more common in women as compared to men of more than 65 years because of short urethra. It mainly occurs after sexual intercourse and very few of this bacteriuria will turn into symptomatic infection. In aged ale incomplete bladder emptying may lead to asymptomatic bacteriuria.

Following factors increase the likelihood of asymptomatic bacteriuria:

A. Obstructive uropathy due to stones, cystocele or benign prostatic hypertrophy.

B. In women fecal soiling in the perineum.

C. Indwelling urinary catheter

D. Frequent instrumentation in the urinary tract

Diagnostic Criteria

According to Infectious Disease Society of America the criteria is the following:

A. Midstream clean catch urine specimen:

- **a.** In case of women 2 consecutive specimens with isolation of the same bacteria species with at least 100,000 colony forming unit/mL of urine.
- **b.** In case of male, a single specimen with isolation of 1 bacteria species with at least 100,000 colony forming unit/mL of urine.

B. Catheterized specimen:

- **a.** In women or men, a single specimen with isolation of 1 bacteria species with at least 100 colony forming unit/mL of urine.

Urine dipstick to measure the leukocyte esterase can identify pyuria but it is not specific for asymptomatic bacteriuria.

Urine dip stick to measure the nitrate is of limited value because of infection with the non-nitrate producing organism.

Combination of both the above tests are more specific for asymptomatic bacteriuria.

In case of pregnant women, urine should be collected in the 1st trimester to detect asymptomatic bacteriuria. In the 1st few weeks of renal transplantation and resection of prostate urine should be tested to detect asymptomatic bacteriuria.

Treatment

A. In case of patients with spinal cord injuries, children, diabetes mellitus, or in patients with indwelling catheters no treatment should be given as it will not decrease the incidence of symptomatic infections.

B. In case of pregnant women with asymptomatic bacteriuria antibiotic treatment can reduce the incidence of:

- **a.** Pyelonephritis
- **b.** Low birth weight patient
- **c.** Preterm delivery

C. Patients with history of prostatectomy or within 1st three months of renal transplantation should be treated with antibiotics.

D. Drugs safe in pregnancy are:

- **a.** Cephalexin
- **b.** Cefuroxime
- **c.** Amoxicillin
- **d.** Nitrofurantoin

Duration of treatment is 3–7 days. One follow-up culture of the urine should be required.

Emphysematous Pyelonephritis

Definition

Emphysematous pyelonephritis is characterized by the necrotizing infections involving the upper respiratory tract and sometimes the peri-nephric tissues leading to gas formation in the renal parenchyma, collecting systems and sometimes in the perinephric tissues.

The organisms involved are:

A. *E. coli*—most common

B. *Klebsiella pneumoniae*—second most common.

C. *Proteus*

D. *Enterococcus*

E. *Clostridium*

F. *Aspergillus*

G. *Candida*

Risk factors are:

A. Diabetes mellitus

B. Hypertension

C. Obstructive uropathy

D. Immunocompromised conditions:

- **a.** Tuberculosis
- **b.** Alcohol abuse
- **c.** AIDS

E. Adverse risk factors are:

- **a.** Thrombocytopenia
- **b.** Hypoalbuminemia
- **c.** Severe proteinuria
- **d.** Advanced age
- **e.** Altered mentation
- **f.** Acute renal failure
- **g.** Polymicrobial infection

Clinical Features

A. Female to male ration is 4:1

B. Sudden or gradual involvement over 2–3 weeks

C. Fever with chill and rigor

D. Dysuria

E. Nausea with or without vomiting

F. Physical findings are:

- **a.** Abdominal pain
- **b.** Tenderness in the loin

c. Pneumaturia
d. Palpable crepitus

Classifications of Emphysematous Pyelonephritis

A. Micheli classification based on features in the plain abdominal film of kidney and intravenous pyelogram:
   a. Stage 1: Gas in the renal parenchyma or perinephric tissue
   b. Stage 2: Gas in the kidney and its surroundings
   c. Stage 3: Extension of gas through the fascia or bilateral disease.

Treatment

A. Initial treatment:
   a. Oxygen administration
   b. Adequate intravenous fluid administration
   c. Control of blood sugar by administration of insulin
   d. Administration of broad spectrum antibiotics
      1. Preferred single agent is 3rd or 4th generation of cephalosporin or carbapenem
      2. Administration of empirical antibiotic administration will reduce the incidence of mortality and gram negative sepsis.
      3. Administration of combination of therapy are amikacin and 3rd generation cephalosporin decrease the resistance to antibiotics.
   e. Clinical improvement is guided by the following:
      1. Absence of fever
      2. Reduction of leukocytosis
      3. Improvement of patient's well-being.
B. Percutaneous drainage: It is recommended in addition of the antibiotics. But in case of emphysematous pyelitis this drainage can be deferred. Removal of the drainage catheter should be done if there is gradual decrease in the output of secretion.
C. Relief of obstruction in case of hydronephrosis.
D. Nephrectomy or open drainage is not done now-a-days as proper and good antibiotic administration along with advanced drainage technologies by radiological procedure. Nephrectomy should be done if the patient should not respond to conservative therapy. Following types of nephrectomy should be done depending upon the clinical condition of the patient as well as the extent of the disease.

   Management approach according to Huang and Tseng based on the clinical-radiological classification:

A. Class 1 and 2: Medical management ± percutaneous drainage
B. Class 3: It can be subdivided into 2 subtypes:
   a. Type 3A: In patient with ≤ 2 risk factors: Medical management ± percutaneous drainage
   b. Type 3B: In patient with ≥ 2 risk factors: Medical management + percutaneous drainage, if unsuccessful nephrectomy, as 92% cases are unsuccessful with former management.
C. Class 4: Initially medical management + percutaneous drainage.

Q41. Describe the functions of loop of Henle. Enumerate inherited disorders involving the loop of Henle. Add a note on Bartter's syndrome.

DNB (OCT2024) (10)

Bartter syndrome.

MGR UNI, TAMIL NADU, 2022 (10)

ANSWER

Loop of Henle consists of two segments:

A. Descending limb of loop of Henle: This segment is permeable to water and less permeable to solutes. As the surrounding interstitium is hypertonic as compared to descending limb, water is filtered out into the interstitium and the osmolality of the filtrate will be increased.
B. Ascending limb of loop of Henle: This segment is impermeable to water but sodium and chloride ion are reabsorbed into the limb actively. Sodium and chloride ions are reabsorbed actively from the ascending limb into the surrounding interstitium making the interstitium more hypertonic. As a result the urine becomes more dilute and environment in the medulla is hyperosmolar.

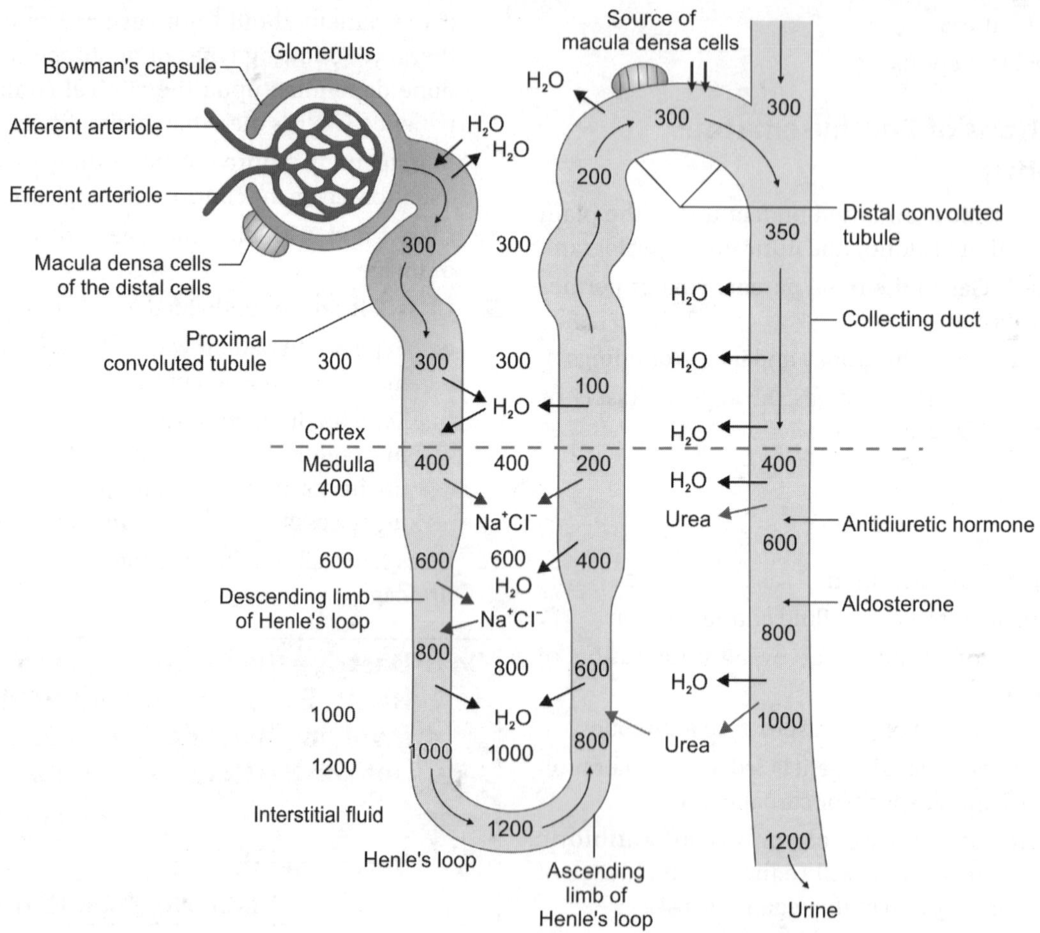

Following are the inherited disorders of the loop of Henle:

A. Bartter syndrome
B. Gitelman syndrome
C. Familial hypercalciuric hypomagnesemia with nephrocalcinosis
D. East syndrome (Epilepsy, ataxia, sensorineural deafness and tubulopathy)
E. Autosomal dominant hypocalcemia type 1.

Bartter Syndrome

It is an autosomal recessive disease involving ascending limb of loop of Henle characterized by defective transport of sodium, chloride and potassium through this limb leasing to development of hypokalemic metabolic alkalosis, hypercalciuria and secondary hyperaldosteronism.

Types and genetic abnormalities in this syndrome:

Types	Genetic mutation	Protein affected	Key features
Type I	SLC12A1	Na-K-2Cl cotransporter	Severe neonatal form of disease
Type II	KCNJ1	Renal outer medullary K^+ channel	Severe neonatal form of disease
Type III	CLCNKB	Chloride channel	Classic form, it is less severe
Type IV	CLCNKB, CLCNCA	Barttin	Associated with sensorineural deafness
Type V	CASR	Calcium-sensing receptor	Excessive loss of calcium

Clinical features:

A. Severe neonatal form (type I and II):
- **a.** Severe dehydration, vomiting
- **b.** Failure to thrive

c. Polyhydramnios
d. Polyuria
e. Nephrocalcinosis
f. Premature death

B. Classic form:
a. Craving for salt
b. Polyuria, polydipsia
c. Hypokalemic metabolic alkalosis
d. Normal or low blood pressure in spite of hyperaldosteronism
e. Retardation of growth

C. In case off type V syndrome there is sensorineural deafness.

Laboratory features:

A. Hypokalemic hypochloremic metabolic alkalosis
B. Hyperreninemia
C. Secondary hyperaldosteronism
D. Hypercalciuria
E. Level of prostaglandin E2 increased in urine.

Treatment:

A. Supplementation of potassium and magnesium to treat hypokalemia
B. Spironolactone to decrease loss of potassium
C. Administration of NSAIDs to decrease the level of prostaglandin in serum
D. Administration of intravenous fluid to replenish body fluids

Prognosis:

A. Type I and II syndrome requires lifelong treatment.
B. Type III syndrome may require treatment
C. Type V syndrome - sensorineural deafness will be permanent but renal features may be treatable.

Q42. Sterile pyuria.

AIIMS, BHU, 2020 (10)

ANSWER

Definition

Sterile pyuria can be defined as when urine contains more than 10 WBC/cc or more than 3 WBC/high power field in the unspun urine or when there is presence of leukocyte esterase or nitrate in dipstick analysis in absence of significant bacteriuria i.e., $\geq 10^5$ colony forming unit/mL.

But advanced testing procedure like next generation sequencing demonstrates that sterile pyuria may not be real absence of bacteriuria.

A distinct form of pyuria is eosinophiluria, which are associated with the following conditions:

A. Allergic interstitial nephritis
B. Urinary tract obstruction
C. Cystitis
D. IgA nephropathy
E. Contrast induced nephropathy
F. Cholesterol emboli

Etiology

A. Infectious diseases:
a. Partially treated or inadequately treated urinary tract infection
b. Difficult to culture organism:
1. *Ureaplasma urealyticum*
2. *Mycobacterium tuberculosis*
3. *Chlamydia trachomatis*
c. Viral infection like adenovirus
d. Fungal infection like candida

B. Noninfectious inflammatory conditions:
a. Glomerulonephritis like lupus nephritis
b. Drug induced or autoimmune interstitial nephritis
c. Sarcoidosis
d. In children Kawasaki disease
e. Rarely sarcoidosis

C. Drug-induced causes:
a. Non-steroidal anti-inflammatory drugs
b. Antibiotics like penicillin, sulfonamides
c. Diuretics like furosemide thiazides
d. Check-point inhibitors like pembrolizumab
e. Proton pump inhibitors
f. Dye
g. Radiation

D. Catheterization

E. Systemic causes:
a. Metabolic disorders:
1. Hyperuricosuria
2. Hypercalciuria
b. Connective tissue disorders like SLE, Sjögren's syndrome

c. Papillary necrosis in
   1. Sickle's disease
   2. Diabetes mellitus

Clinical Features in Sterile Pyuria

A. Dysuria, urgency, and frequency of micturition suggest infection or inflammation.
B. Loin pain indicates renal parenchymal involvement in infection, inflammatory condition, and involvement of papilla
C. Hematuria indicates infection, non-infected inflammatory conditions,
D. Presence of fever, arthralgia, and rash suggest connective or autoimmune diseases.
E. Past history tuberculosis suspects tuberculosis
F. Fatigue, edema, joint pain, and fever suggest systemic pathology.
G. Systemic examination demonstrates:
   a. Suprapubic tenderness—cystitis
   b. Costo-vertebral tenderness—renal parenchymal involvement
   c. Organomegaly—systemic disease

Evaluation of Sterile Pyuria

A. Microscopy of urine detects—WBCs, RBCs, WBC cast, RBC casts
B. Urine culture to rule out common bacterial infection.
C. Special culture to detect mycobacterium tuberculosis, chlamydia etc.
D. PCR of urine to detect rare organisms.

Blood test:

A. Complete blood count—in infection, inflammation,
B. High eosinophil count—in case of allergic conditions.
C. To assess the renal functional abnormality—urea, creatinine
D. In case of suspected electrolyte abnormalities—calcium, magnesium, parathyroid hormone, uric acid, sodium, potassium.
E. ESR or C-reactive protein—to detect systemic inflammation.
F. In case of suspected SLE, ana, DsDNA
G. Interferon gamma release assay in case of suspected tuberculosis.

Imaging studies:

A. Ultrasound of kidney—in case of acute renal parenchymal infection, papillary necrosis, obstructive uropathy.
B. In case of suspected tuberculosis—computerized tomography.

Renal biopsy for histology to detect types of glomerulonephritis.

Treatment in Case of Sterile Pyuria

Disease	Treatment protocol
Genitourinary tuberculosis	Four drugs combination including rifampicin, INH, ethambutol, pyrazinamide for 6 months
Chlamydia trachomatis	100 mg doxycycline orally twice daily Or, Azithromycin 1 gram single dose
Gonorrhea	250 mg ceftriaxone intramuscularly Or, Doxycycline 100 mg twice daily for 7 days
Mycoplasma genitalium	Doxycycline 100 mg twice daily for 7 days followed by azithromycin 1 gram single dose Or, Moxifloxacin 400 mg once daily orally for 7 days
Genital herpes	400 mg acyclovir 3 times daily for 7 to 10 days Or, 1 gram valacyclovir twice daily for 7 to 10 days Or, Famciclovir 250 mg orally thrice daily for 7 to 10 days
Trichomoniasis	500 mg metronidazole orally for 7 days Or, Two gram metronidazole single dose In this case sexual partner should also be treated
Drug-induced nephritis	Discontinuation of the offending drugs Administration of the corticosteroids
Autoimmune inflammatory disease	In lupus nephritis – steroids, immunosuppressive therapies In sarcoidosis steroids
Metabolic causes	Dietary modification Diuretics
Malignancy	Surgery Chemotherapy Immunotherapy

Q43. Oliguria.

SCBMCH, 2020 (10)

ANSWER

Definition

Oliguria can be defined as the volume of urine is less than 400 mL/day or less than 20 mL/hour. It is the earliest sign of renal failure.

Etiopathogenesis

A. Prerenal causes:

- **a.** Hypovolemia due to the following causes:
  1. Gastrointestinal fluid loss
  2. Renal losses
  3. Third space fluid losses
  4. Trauma
  5. Surgery
  6. Burns
  7. Anaphylaxis
  8. Nephrotic syndrome
- **b.** Pump failure due to:
  1. Myocardial infarction
  2. Cardiac tamponade
  3. Congestive cardiac failure
  4. Pulmonary embolism
- **c.** Vascular causes:
  1. Renal artery stenosis
  2. Renal vein thrombosis
  3. Disrupted renal autoregulation secondary ACE inhibitor administration.

B. Renal causes:

- **a.** Acute tubular necrosis
- **b.** Vasculitis
- **c.** Glomerulonephritis
- **d.** Interstitial nephritis
- **e.** Malignant hypertension

C. Post-renal causes:

- **a.** Bilateral upper urinary tract obstruction
- **b.** Lower urinary tract obstruction including bladder neck obstruction due to:
  1. Benign prostatic hypertrophy
  2. Tumor
  3. Drugs

Rest of the pathophysiology, clinical features, evaluation and management have been written in question number 5.

Q44. Metabolic and hormonal functions of the kidney.

SCBMCH, 2020 (10)

ANSWER

Metabolic Functions of the Kidney

A. Gluconeogenesis: During fasting state, renal cortex through the enzyme glucose 6 phosphatase produces glucose.

B. Metabolism of protein and amino acid metabolism:

- **a.** Kidney metabolizes glutamine as a major source of ammonia to maintain the acid base balance.
- **b.** Kidney reabsorbs essential amino acids to conserve them.

C. Lipid synthesis: In the state of energy deficiency oxidizes fatty acids and also participate the synthesis and metabolism of cholesterol.

D. Kidney will detoxify different hormones, toxins and drugs through enzymes in phase I and phase II.

Hormonal Functions of Kidney

A. In response to hypoxia kidney will produce erythropoietin from interstitial fibroblast like cells in the renal cortex thereby stimulate production of red blood cells in the bone marrow.

B. In case of low blood pressure of hyponatremia, autoregulation cells in the renal through the conversion of angiotensinogen to angiotensin I and then to angiotensin II which is a major vasoconstrictor agent.

C. Kidney converts the 25-hydroxy vitamin D to 1,25 dihydroxy vitamin D thereby maintaining the calcium phosphorus homeostasis.

D. Kidney will produce endothelin to maintain the vascular tone as well as handling of sodium.

E. Kidney will release nitric oxide which counteract vasoconstriction and maintain normal renal blood flow.

Q45. Countercurrent mechanism in the kidney.
MGR UNI, TAMIL NADU, 2022 (5)

Counter current multiplier system.
NTR UNI OF HEALTH SCIENCE, VIJAYAWADA, 2020 (10)

ANSWER

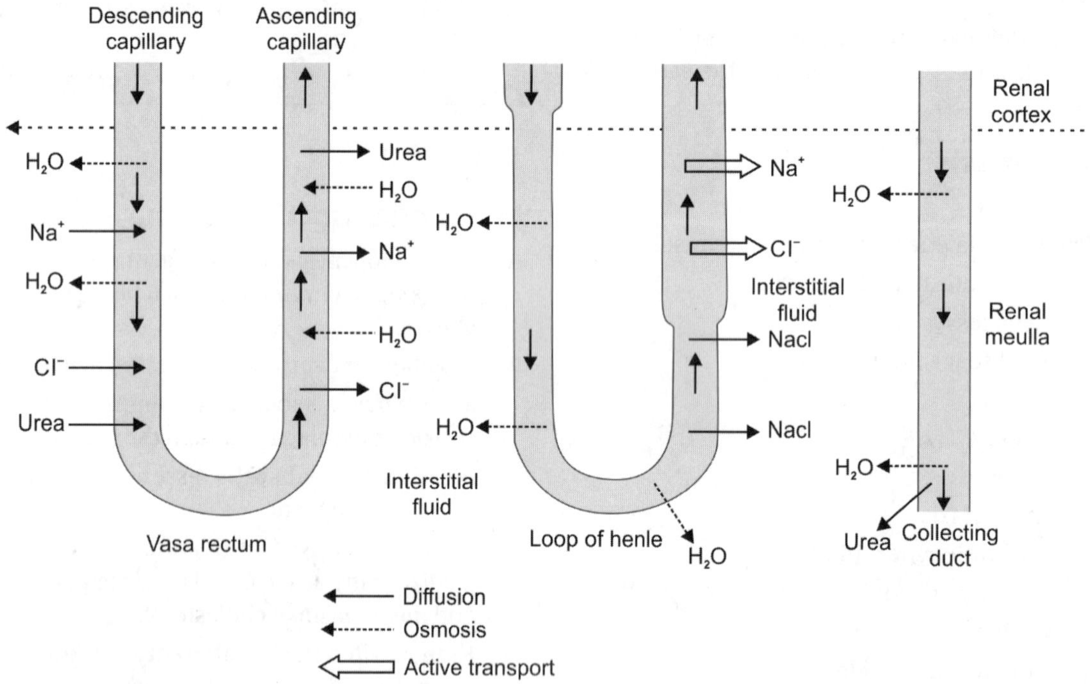

Counter Current Multiplication in the Loop of Henle

A. Descending limb is permeable to water but impermeable to solutes—the result is reabsorption of water from the tubule leading to increased osmolality of the tubular fluid and decreased osmolality of the interstitial fluid

B. Ascending limb of loop of Henle is impermeable to water but there is active transport of solutes—the result is decreased osmolality of the tubular fluid and increased osmolality of the interstitial fluid.

The resultant effect is the increased osmolality of the medullary interstitium which helps in increased reabsorption of the fluid from the collecting duct.

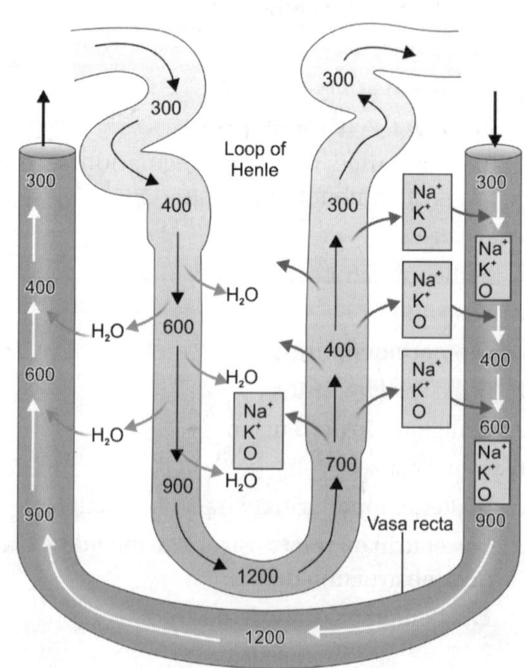

Counter Current Exchanger System

This is performed by vasa recta—it is composed of network of capillaries which maintain the constant gradient in the medullary interstitium which helps in the passive exchange of water and solutes.

A. During its descent into the medulla, it will loss water but gain sodium chloride and the blood hyperosmotic.

B. During ascent of the capillary into the medulla it will gain water but lose sodium chloride making the blood hypoosmolar.

Q46. Juxta glomerular apparatus.

MGR UNI, TAMIL NADU, 2022 (5)

Describe structure and function of juxtaglomerular apparatus.

DR YSR UNI OF HEALTH SC, VIJAYAWADA, ANDHRA, 2022 (10)

ANSWER

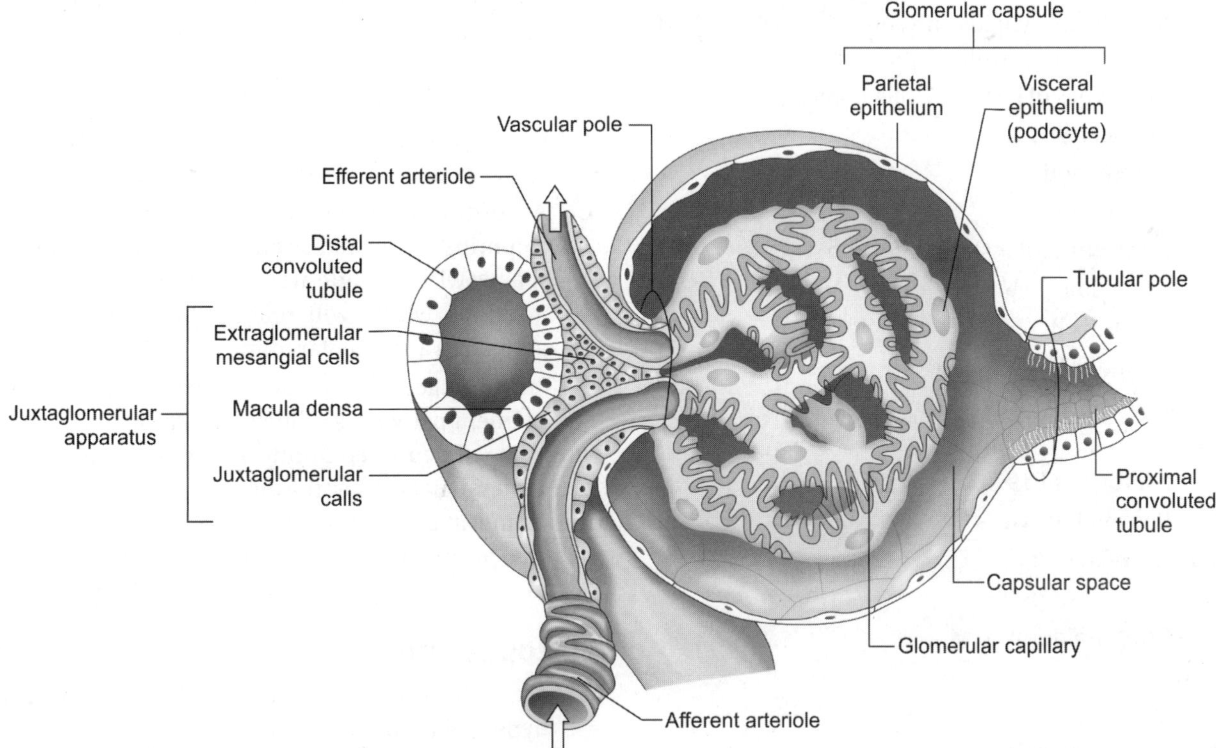

Anatomy and function: Location: This specialized structure is present in the interface between afferent, efferent arterioles and distal convoluted tubule. Its three components are the following:

A. Macula densa: It is composed of densely packed epithelial cells present in the distal convoluted tubule close to afferent arteriole. Its function is to sense the concentration of sodium chloride in the fluid in the distal convoluted tubule.

B. Juxtaglomerular cells: These are modified smooth muscle cells present in the afferent arteriolar wall containing granules containing renin granules. Its function is to sense the changes in the blood pressure.

C. Lacis cells or extraglomerular mesangial cells: These cells are present in the vicinity of afferent, efferent arterioles and macula densa. It will play a role in the secretion of erythropoietin.

Q47. Etiological classification of acute kidney injury. Add a note to post streptococcal glomerulonephritis.

NTR UNI OF HEALTH SC, ANDHRA, 2022 (10)

ANSWER

Classification of acute kidney described in question number 5.

Definition

Post-streptococcal glomerulonephritis is characterized by rapid deterioration of the renal function due to type III hypersensitivity reaction against the A beta hemolytic beta-hemolytic streptococci also known as nephrogenic streptococci.

Etiology

A. Group A hemolytic *Streptococcus*—subtyped based on surface M protein and opacity factor. It causes skin and throat infections. In children 6 weeks after skin infection and 1 to 2 weeks after sore throat kidney will be involved. Serotype M1, M4 and M12 responsible pharyngitis and serotype M49, M50, M57 and M60 are responsible for skin infection.

B. Different types of bacterial infections like:

- **a.** Endocarditis
- **b.** Enterocolitis
- **c.** Pneumonia
- **d.** Intraventricular shunt infection

C. Viral infection:

- **a.** Hepatitis B
- **b.** Hepatitis C
- **c.** Cytomegalovirus
- **d.** HIV
- **e.** Parvovirus B19
- **f.** Epstein Barr virus

D. Fungal infection:

- **a.** Histoplasmosis
- **b.** Coccidioidomycosis

E. Parasitic infections:

- **a.** Malaria
- **b.** Toxoplasmosis
- **c.** Leishmaniasis

Risk Factors

A. Poor hygiene

B. Low socioeconomic status

C. Overcrowding.

D. Genetic factors have role of 40% incidence of PSGN if there is family history of PSGN.

Epidemiology

A. The incidence of the disease has been significantly dropped due to high grade of antibiotic prophylaxis though the incidence of pyoderma is increased.

B. Male to female ratio is 2:1 but it is equal in case of subclinical infection.

C. No racial difference.

D. Frequent affected people are children between the age of 3 years and 12 years and also subject of more than 60 years of age.

Pathophysiology

It is a type III hypersensitivity reaction. The mechanism is not fully known.

A. According some theories, the streptococcal antigen pyrogenic exotoxin B combines with antibody to form immune complexes and will deposit on the kidney glomeruli through the circulation.

B. Again other theory states that there is in-situ formation of immune complexes within the glomeruli due to reaction against streptococcal antigen present in the glomerular basement membrane.

C. According to other theory, streptococcal antigen, Nephritis associated streptococcal plasmin receptor, reacts with the glomerular components to form antibody which will react with the streptococcal antigen as a molecular mimicry.

These antigen-antibody complexes activate alternate complement pathway leading to infiltration of leukocytes at the site of deposited immune complexes, proliferation of the mesangial cells in the glomerulus thereby reducing the glomerular filtration rate. The resultant effects are oliguria, anuria, electrolyte imbalance, volume overload leading to hypertension and generalized edema.

Histopathology

A. Light microscopy demonstrates glomerular hypercellularity by mesangial cells, endothelial cells and inflammatory cells.

B. Electron microscopy demonstrates presence of subepithelial humps characterized by electron dense deposits in the subepithelial space near glomerular basement membrane.

C. Immunofluorescence microscopy demonstrates deposition of IgG, C3 deposits in the 1st to 3rd weeks after commencement of the disease.

Clinical Features

A. Many patients are asymptomatic, can be diagnosed during routine urine analysis.

B. Classical triad are hypertension, edema and hematuria.

C. There may be the preceding history of pharyngitis, impetigo or tonsillitis.
D. Hematuria in the form of cola colored or tea-colored urine,
E. Features of electrolyte imbalance
F. Edema in the form of periorbital puffiness which tends to resolve at the end of the day.
G. There may be the evidence of pulmonary edema leading to respiratory distress.
H. Constitutional symptoms are anorexia, nausea, vomiting.

Laboratory Investigations

A. Evidence of preceding streptococcal infection:
   a. Measurement of antistreptolysin O titer
   b. Increased anti-nicotinamide adenine dinucleotidase following pharyngitis
   c. Elevated level of anti-DNAse B and anti-hyaluronidase in case of both pharyngitis and skin infection.
B. Serum complement C3 level—decreased—it occurs before the elevation of ASO titer.
C. Urine analysis demonstrates:
   a. Microscopic hematuria
   b. RBC casts
   c. Mild proteinuria
   d. WBC casts and other cellular may be present.
D. Renal function test:
   a. Urea and creatinine usually elevated in acute phase which will decline as the patient recovers.
   b. In case of heart failure in PSGN patient increased level of NT-ProBNP
E. Renal biopsy is indicated in the following circumstances:
   a. Anuric renal failure
   b. Progressive decrease in the renal function
   c. If the level of complements are normal.
   d. If there is no rise in streptococcal antibodies
   e. Absence of latent period in between streptococcal infection and acute glomerulonephritis
F. Imaging studies:
   a. Ultrasonography demonstrates enlarged size of the kidney.
   b. Chest X-Ray demonstrates pulmonary congestion which is consistent with the volume overload.

Treatment

A. General measures:
   a. Restriction of salt and water to reduce edema.
   b. In the 1st few days of the disease bed rest and restriction of the daily activities.
   c. Throat culture and sensitivity of the patient and the family members are essential.
B. Pharmacotherapy:
   a. Loop diuretics - it is essential to decrease the volume overload, but effect of this diuretic is minimal if the GFR is less than 30 mL/minute.
   b. Control of blood pressure by salt and water restriction, but in case of uncontrolled blood pressure, calcium channel blocker is recommended. In case of stable glomerular filtration rate ACEI or ARBs may be recommended.
   c. Dialysis it can be recommended to control acid base balance and electrolyte abnormalities.

Complications

A. In acute phase, heart failure or worsening of azotemia.
B. In chronic case nephrotic syndrome or chronic kidney disease may be developed.

Prognosis

A. In case of children, complete recovery is usual and occurs within 6 to 8 weeks.
B. In case of adult, 50% patient will develop proteinuria, reduced renal function and hypertension.
C. Mortality in acute phase is 2–12%

Q48. Contrast induced nephropathy.

NTR UNI OF HEALTH SC, VIJAYAWADA, 2021 (10)

Contrast induced nephropathy.

VEER NARMAD SOUTH GUJARAT UNI, 2019 (12)

Define contrast induced nephropathy. Mention the risk scoring system of contrast induced nephropathy. Discuss about the drugs and procedures for preventing contrast induced nephropathy.

WBUHS, 2020 (10)

ANSWER

Definition

It can be defined as impairment of renal function when the serum creatinine elevates more than 25% above the baseline or increase in the absolute serum creatinine value to more than 0.5 mg% within 48–72 hours after administration of intravenous contrast.

Etiology

This disease occurs in patients with preexisting chronic kidney disease in 8% patients with GFR between 45 and 60 mL/min/m^2 and 13% between 30 and 45 mL/min/m^2 and 27% with GFR less than 30 mL/min/m^2.

Following are the risk factors:

A. Advanced age

B. Diabetes mellitus

C. Peripheral heart failure

D. Female sex

E. Peripheral vascular disease

F. Left ventricular ejection fraction less than 40%

G. Hypertension

Precipitating factors are:

A. Acute coronary syndrome

B. Volume depletion

C. Hypotension

D. Concomitant nephrotoxic medication

E. Anemia

Contrast media affects the distinct anatomical site in the kidney by following mechanisms:

A. Direct toxic effects on the proximal tubules in the kidney

B. Increase the resistance to blood flow in the kidney

C. Increased cellular damage through the reactive oxygen species

D. Increased renal vasoconstriction in the medulla in case of chronic kidney disease.

Pathophysiology of Contrast-induced Nephropathy

The proposed theory is the combination of vasoconstriction, ischemia, direct toxic effect on the renal tubular cells and hypoxia. The risk of injury is higher in case of arterial administration of contrast as compared to intravenous administration. As metformin can produce lactic acidosis, hence this drug should be stopped on the day of the procedure and following 48 hours after administration of drug.

Another cause is catheter induced aeroembolism in the renal vasculature. Renal microcirculation depends upon:

A. Vasodilator—nitric oxide: It is crucial as it has vasodilatory, antiplatelet, antioxidant and anti-inflammatory effects.

B. Vasoconstrictors—adenosine, vasopressin, endothelin and angiotensin 2.

Histopathology

Direct toxic effect of the contrast media in the kidney are the following:

A. Cell vacuolization

B. Cellular necrosis

C. Inflammation of interstitium

The above characteristic changes are known as osmotic nephrosis.

Clinical Presentation

A. Preceding history of administration of the contrast media.

B. Patient develops nom-oliguric renal failure.

C. Features of cholesterol emboli like livedo reticularis and blue toes.

D. Interstitial nephritis secondary to drug as evidenced by rash.

E. Signs of volume depletion.

Laboratory Investigation

A. According KDIGO: Stage 1: Rapid rise in creatinine to more than 0.3 mg/dL within 48 hours or relative rise of more than 50% within 7 days or less Or reduction of urine output 0.5 mL/kg/h for 6–12 hours. Rest of the stage will be governed by rise in the creatinine level.

B. Surrogate marker cystatin C is increased in contrast induced nephropathy.

C. Nonspecific findings in the urine are epithelial casts, granular casts, uric acid crystals.

D. Urine osmolarity is less than 350 mOsmol/Kg.

Treatment

A. In patient with chronic kidney disease pre-procedural administration of intravenous normal saline at a rate of 1 mL/kg/h for 6–12 hours and it should be continued even after the procedure.

B. Administration of bicarbonate as it will alkalinizes the tubular fluid thereby preventing radical injury. Hence sodium bicarbonate can be administered at a rate of 3 mL/kg/h prior to the procedure and it should be continued at a rate of 1 mL/kg/h for another 6 hours.

C. Patient should be treated by high dose of statin prior to the procedure.

D. Administration of ascorbic acid at a dose of 1 g to 3 g for 1–3 days periprocedurally to decrease the incidence of nephropathy.

Complications

A. Acute renal injury

B. Acute on chronic kidney disease

C. Fluid overload leading to pulmonary edema and heart failure

D. Hypersensitivity reaction

E. Contrast induced thyroid dysfunction.

Q49. Analgesic nephropathy.

SARDAR PATEL UNIVERSITY, 2019 (10)

ANSWER

Definition

This analgesic nephropathy is a chronic interstitial nephritis that can occur as a result of chronic use of NSAIDs, acetaminophen and aspirin characterized by the spectrum of manifestations from asymptomatic hematuria, proteinuria or sterile pyuria to symptomatic features of chronic renal disease.

Etiopathogenesis

Analgesics damages the kidney through the following mechanisms:

A. Direct nephrotoxicity where reactive oxygen species developing from the metabolites of phenacetin, paracetamol or NSAIDs produces oxidative damage of the renal tubular cells.

B. Ischemic damage of the kidney occurs due to due to renal vasoconstriction due to decreased synthesis of prostaglandin by NSAIDs leading to decreased blood flow through the renal artery.

C. Coagulative Papillary necrosis results from chronic exposure to analgesic leading to obstruction of the renal tubule resulting progressive renal fibrosis.

D. Persistent inflammation around the renal tubule leading to progressive tubular atrophy and interstitial fibrosis which culminates into chronic renal disease.

Risk Factors

A. Use of combination of analgesics of more than 3 years.

B. Age more than 40 years

C. Female sex

D. Dehydration due to volume depletion

E. Smoking

F. Chronic pain due to arthritis

Histopathologic Pictures of Analgesic Nephropathy

A. Interstitial fibrosis

B. Papillary calcification

C. Metabolic deposits in the medullary interstitium

Clinical Features

A. In early cases:

- **a.** there is decreased concentrating ability resulting polyuria
- **b.** Mild flank pain
- **c.** Nocturia
- **d.** Renal colic with hematuria

B. In established cases:

- **a.** Features of slowly progressive chronic renal disease
- **b.** High blood pressure
- **c.** Sputum
- **d.** Features of urinary tract infection.
- **e.** Features of infection due to papillary necrosis
- **f.** Papillary muscles indicates hematuria

Diagnosis

A. Routine tests:

- **a.** Complete blood count: leukocytosis, normochromic, normocytic anemia.
- **b.** Urinary examination:
  1. Proteinuria
  2. Hematuria
  3. Leukocyturia
  4. Cast – epithelial and granular casts

B. Blood test:

- **a.** Most useful diagnostic test for analgesic nephropathy is urinary protein to urinary creatinine ratio.
- **b.** Electrolyte disturbances:
  1. Hyperkalemia,
  2. Metabolic acidosis

C. Imaging studies:
  a. Ultrasound of KUB demonstrates renal scarring and irregular shape of the kidney.
  b. CT scan of KUB demonstrates:
    1. Decreased renal mass
    2. Renal scarring
    3. Reduction of the renal volume
    4. Irregular surface of the kidney
    5. Papillary calcifications
    6. Parenchymal thinning

Management of Analgesic Nephropathy

A. Discontinuation of the analgesic drugs
B. Supportive treatment:
  a. Proper administration of oral or intravenous fluid to reduce the ischemia of kidney
  b. Control of blood pressure by ACEI or ARBs to slow the progression of the renal disease.
  c. Treatment of anemia by administration of packed red blood cells and if required erythropoietin.
  d. Correction of hyperkalemia
  e. Catheterization of kidney should not be done as there is increased chance of infection.

Q50. Focal segmental glomerulosclerosis.

RAJEEV GANDHI UNI OF HEALTH SC, KARNATAKA, 2019, (10)

ANSWER

Definition

It can be defined as sclerosis of the some part of glomeruli, it is the most prevalent cause of primary glomerulopathy in the adult.

Etiology

A. Primary FSGS:
  a. FSGS with hyalinosis
  b. Progression from IgM nephropathy
  c. Progression from minimal change disease
  d. Progression from mesangial proliferative glomerulonephritis
  e. IgA nephropathy
B. Genetic FSGS:
  a. Mutation of NPHS1 and NPHS2
  b. Polymorphism of APOL1
C. Secondary FSGS secondary to toxins, drugs, inflammation, infection intrarenal and extrarenal hemodynamic alterations.

Proposed Factors Idiopathic Glomerulosclerosis

A. Corticotrophin like cytokine factor 1
B. Apolipoprotein A1-b
C. Anti CD40 antibodies
D. Serum urine type plasminogen activator receptor.

Histologic Variants of FSGS

A. Collapsing variant
B. Tip variant
C. Perihilar variant
D. Cellular variant
E. FSGS with mesangial hypercellularity
F. FSGS with glomerular tip lesion

The glomerulosclerosis occurs due to alteration in the hemodynamics in the kidney—it may be due to decreased renal mass lading to glomerular hypertrophy in the remaining kidney leading glomerular hypertension. Decreased renal mass may be due to:
A. Solitary kidney
B. Kidney allograft
C. Renal agenesis
D. Renal dysplasia
E. Vesicoureteral reflux
F. Segmental hypoplasia

Without decreased renal mass leading to remaining glomerular hypertension resulting sclerosis of the glomeruli:
A. High protein intake
B. Sickle cell nephropathy
C. Obesity
D. Androgen abuse
E. Diabetes
F. Hypertension

Pathophysiology

Injury to the podocytes leads to hypertrophy of the remaining podocytes resulting effacement of the podocytes along with proliferation of the mesangial, endothelial and epithelial cells in the early phase of the disease. In the later phase collapse of the glomerular capillaries, leading to scarring, these may be aided by the different factors.

Proposed mechanisms of injury to podocytes are due to different factors leading to alteration in the intrarenal hemodynamic mechanisms, increased intraglomerular capillary pressure and glomerular hyperperfusion.

Clinical Features

Clinical features are written in the nephrotic syndrome written in question number 36.

Investigations

It is same as that of nephrotic syndrome in question number 36. Rest are the following:

A. In case of idiopathic variety:
- **a.** Vasculitis
- **b.** Gammopathy
- **c.** Hepatitis B and C infections
- **d.** SLE

B. In case of secondary variety:
- **a.** HIV antibody, viral load, CD4 lymphocyte count
- **b.** Test for parvovirus B19
- **c.** Serum level of C3 and C4
- **d.** Antinuclear antibodies
- **e.** DsDNA
- **f.** Urine and serum protein electrophoresis
- **g.** Anti CCP antibodies

Treatment

According to KDIGO 2021 clinical practice guidelines for the management of glomerular disease are as follows:

A. Complete remission:
- **a.** Proteinuria reduces to 300 mg/day
- **b.** Protein creatinine ratio less than 0.3
- **c.** Serum albumin greater than 3.5 mg/dL
- **d.** Stable serum creatinine

B. Partial remission:
- **a.** Proteinuria reduces to 300–3500 mg/day
- **b.** Protein creatinine ratio less than 0.3–3.5
- **c.** Decrease in the proteinuria 50% from the baseline.

C. Relapse:
- **a.** Proteinuria more than 3500 mg/day
- **b.** Protein creatinine ratio greater than 3.5 Or,
- **c.** 50% increase in the proteinuria over the partial remission

D. Steroid resistant G=FSGS:
- **a.** Proteinuria greater than 3500 mg/day Or,
- **b.** Protein creatinine ratio greater than 3.5 after 16 weeks therapy with 1 mg/kg prednisolone

E. Steroid dependent FSGS:
- **a.** Relapse occurs during or within 2 weeks of completion of steroid treatment

F. CNI resistant FSGS:
- **a.** Proteinuria greater than 3500 mg/day or protein creatinine ratio greater than 3.5 after 16 weeks in spite of therapeutic level of the steroids.

G. CNI dependent FSGS:
- **a.** Relapse occurring within or during 2 weeks of completion of CNI therapy for 1 year.

Drugs used:

A. 1 mg/kg/day corticosteroid or 2 mg/kg at alternate day orally for 4 weeks until the remission will be achieved or it should be continued for 16 weeks.
- **a.** If complete remission is achieved, then steroid dose should be tapered after 2 weeks. Prednisolone should be tapered at 5 mg every 2 weeks over total duration of 6 months.
- **b.** If partial remission is achieved, within 8–12 weeks of high dose steroid therapy, it should be continued for 16 weeks to achieve complete remission. Then the steroid dose will be tapered at 5 mg every 1–2 weeks within 6 months.

B. Calcineurin inhibitors:
- **a.** Cyclosporine—3 to 5 mg/kg/day with target trough of 100–175 ng/mL.
- **b.** Tacrolimus—0.05–0.1 mg/kg/day with target trough level of 5–10 ng/mL.

At least 6 months are required to detect their efficacy.

A. If there is no improvement after 6 months - it is known as CNI-resistant FSGS

B. In case of partial remission these drugs should be continued for 12 months, then slow tapering should be started and completed within next 6–12 months.

Q51. Chronic complications in CKD.

BHARATI VIDYAPEETH DEEMED UNI, JHELUM, 2019 (10)

ANSWER

System involved	Complications
Cardiovascular system	• Heart failure • Hypertension • Atherosclerosis • Pericarditis

Continued

Continued

System involved	Complications
Electrolyte imbalance	• Hyperkalemia • Hyponatremia • Hypocalcemia • Hyperphosphatemia
Acid base imbalance	Metabolic acidosis
Hematologic disorders	• Normochromic normocytic anemia • Coagulopathies • Platelet abnormalities
Mineral metabolism	• Osteomalacia • Renal osteodystrophy • Secondary hyperparathyroidism • Vascular calcification
Gastrointestinal complications	• Anorexia • Nausea vomiting • Gastrointestinal bleeding • Constipation
Dermatologic complications	• Pruritus • Uremic frost • Hyperpigmentation
Neurologic complications	• Uremic encephalopathy • Peripheral neuropathy • Sleep disturbances • Restless leg syndrome
Psychiatric complications	• Anxiety • Depression • Cognitive decline
Immunologic complications	Impaired immunity leading to infection

Q52. Explain the use of wearable dialysis devices. What are the potential advantages and challenges associated with these technologies?

WBUHS, 2025 (10)

ANSWER

Wearable dialysis devices are the future of the dialysis of recent technology where sorbitol based dialysis regenerative system known as recirculating dialysis is used where solute waste from spent dialysate will pass through the column containing urease. As a result urea will be hydrolyzed into Carbon dioxide and ammonia, the later one again will be hydrated with water to producing ammonium and bi-carbonate ions. Ammonium as acid remover from the body will bind with nitrogen from the dialysate. This dialysate will pass through the cation and anion exchange columns to remove potassium, calcium and magnesium like cations and anion like toxic organic acids, phosphates and sulphates.

Ultimately this clear dialysate will recharged with potassium and magnesium and will return to dialysate again.

This is a battery operated machine and can be kept in the pocket or attached with the belt.

Uses of this Technologies

A. It is used to replace the center-based dialysis.

B. It is used as continuous procedure mimic like normal kidney.

C. In case of frequent use of dialysis in case of mobile patient this is extremely useful.

D. It can remove the symptoms related uremia, electrolyte imbalance or cardiovascular instability.

Types of Wearable Dialyzer

A. Wearable hemodialysis: It is miniature version of extracorporeal circuit for removal of toxic product and filtration of blood.

B. Wearable peritoneal dialysis: Here peritoneum is used for dialysis for continuous operation as well as regeneration of the dialysate.

C. Sorbent based dialysis system: Here sorbent is used for regenerating dialysate and making the dialyzer for reuse.

Advantages of Wearable Dialyzer

A. It helps in continuous removal of toxins and organic acids maintain the electrolyte balance rather than alternate rise in the cations and anions.

B. Cardiovascular system will be stabilized because of the continuous clearing the toxins and maintain the electrolyte balance in the blood.

C. Increased mobility of the patient as compared to the patients with intermittent dialysis.

D. It will reduce the depression related mentality for the future.

E. It will also decrease the cost of coming to the hospital for regular dialysis.

Challenges of Wearable Dialyzer

A. There is risk of infection for prolonged use of this machine

B. There is limited capacity of clearance of the toxin in this prototype.

C. Technician training is very urgent to introduce of this machine.

Section 6 Cardiovascular Systems

Q1. Clinical presentation, diagnostic evaluation, and management of right ventricular infarction.

DNBI/JUNE2010 (10) DNBIII/DEC2013 (10)

Right ventricular infarction.

MGR UNIVERSITY, TAMIL NADU, 2020 (10)

ANSWER

Definition

Right ventricular infarction, the consequence of inferior wall myocardial infarction, or an isolated event is characterized by increased right ventricular filling pressure in the face of normal left ventricular filling pressure.

Pathophysiology

Normally right ventricle is less susceptible to infarction because of the following reasons:

- **a.** Right ventricle is thin walled chamber having less oxygen demand.
- **b.** It is perfused throughout the both systolic and diastolic phases of cardiac cycle.
- **c.** In case hemodynamic stress its ability to extract oxygen is very high.

Right ventricle is supplied by right coronary artery arising from the right coronary cusp of aorta. Its one division, conus artery supplies the infundibulum of the right ventricle, another division supplies sinoatrial node (SA node). As this right coronary artery passes through the atrioventricular (AV) groove it gives multiple small branches to supply the anterior surface of the right ventricle and ultimately dived into acute marginal branch which runs anteriorly to supply the anterior wall and posterior descending artery runs posteriorly to supply the AV node in 90% patients and in 10% by a branch of left circumflex artery. Posterior descending artery supplies in addition inferior surface of both ventricles.

There is direct correlation between the sites of right coronary artery obstruction and severity of obstruction—more proximal the obstruction more extensive the infarction, but in some cases right ventricle will be infarcted from obstruction of left circumflex artery. If the obstruction in right coronary artery proximal to marginal artery branch and at the same time collateral blood flow from the anterior descending coronary artery is absent, the size of right ventricular infarction will be severe.

In case of impaired contractility and function of right ventricle there is right ventricular diastolic overload and decrease in systolic pressure. In case of concomitant left ventricular dysfunction there is increase in right ventricular afterload leading to decreased right out put which in turn increases right atrial pressure, so here right ventricle acts as poor conduit in between pulmonary artery and right atrium. This elevation of right atrial pressure stimulates to secrete natriuretic factor that worsens further clinical features of right ventricular infarction by virtue of its natriuretic, vasodilating, diuretic, and aldosterone-inhibiting properties. These potential derangements in right ventricular infarction make the patient unusually sensitive to low preloads and loss of AV asynchrony and both these mechanisms results low right and left ventricular output.

Clinical Features

Though 30% patients suffer from right ventricular infarction from inferior wall left ventricular myocardial infarction who present with low cardiac output, but only 10% patients suffer from hemodynamic compromise. Clinical symptoms are:

- **a.** Features of left ventricular infarction
- **b.** Arrhythmias in the form of bradycardia to complete heart block
- **c.** Hypotension
- **d.** Other signs of right ventricular failure including engorged neck vein, clear lung field, and hypotension
- **e.** Peripheral edema

f. Presence of pansystolioc murmur at the lower left sternal border—indicates tricuspid regurgitation increases during inspiration
g. Rarely right ventricular 3rd or 4th heart sound
h. Marked sensitivity to nitrates, diuretics, and morphine suggests the possibility of hemodynamically significant right ventricular infarction.

Evaluation

A. Electrocardiography (ECG) is the first and primary mode of investigation in any patient with chest pain. In case of inferior wall left ventricular infarction ST segment elevation in lead II, III, and aVF. Following are the features of right ventricular infarction:
  a. Disproportionate elevation in lead III more than lead II.
  b. Elevation of ST segment in V_1 is highly suggestive of right ventricular infarction, it is more specific if it is associated with ST depression in V_2.
  c. Usually left-sided ECG is not sensitive for right ventricular infarction because of the position of right side of the heart. Hence in case of right-sided ECG:
    1. ST-segment elevation in V_4R if >1.0 mm—100% sensitive and 87% specific.
    2. Other nonspecific features such as complete conduction block, complete heart block may be present.

B. Cardiac enzymes are elevated both right and left ventricular infarction. Again, in few cases it is not possible to differentiate in hemodynamically significant pulmonary embolism because troponin-I and CPK-MB are elevated in both the cases.

C. Echocardiography has high threshold to detect the right ventricular infarction as it will detect the following:
  a. Right ventricular dilatation
  b. Abnormal right ventricular wall motion
  c. Paradoxical motion of interventricular septum
  d. Tricuspid regurgitation
  e. Pulmonary regurgitation
  f. Measurement of tricuspid annular plane excursion—decreased systolic velocity at the tricuspid annulus—it can indicate poor prognosis.
  g. Myocardial performance index: It can be derived from sum of isovolumic relaxation and contraction time divided by ejection fraction—value greater than ≥ 0.3 suggests presence of right ventricular infarction.

D. Angiography and scintigraphy: Radionuclide angiography and technetium-99m scintigraphy can diagnose right ventricular infarction effectively. Right ventricle will be enlarged, poorly contractile with low or reduced ejection fraction. By technetium-99m "hot spot" can be identified at the site of infarction.

E. Hemodynamic monitoring: Following are the hemodynamic features:
  a. Disproportionally elevated right ventricular filling pressure as compared to left ventricular hemodynamic pressure
  b. Prominent "y" descent in the right atrial pressure
  c. Increase venous or right atrial pressure during inspiration (Kussmaul's sign)
  d. Exaggeration of normal inspiratory decline of systemic arterial pressure known as Pulsus paradoxus
  e. Elevation of right ventricular filling pressure having early diastolic dip as well as plateau

Treatment

These patients should be considered where there is evidence of inferior wall infarction along with hypotension in absence of crepitation.

A. In right ventricular failure left ventricular filling will be limited due to decrease in cardiac output or ventricular interdependence or both. Previously, it was aimed to maintain right ventricular filling pressure adequately to maintain adequate cardiac output. But in case of cardiogenic shock due to right ventricular dysfunction right ventricular end-diastolic pressure will be >20 mm Hg. As a result interventricular septum will be shifted to left ventricular cavity increasing the left atrial pressure but impairing the filling of left ventricle due to bowing of the septum into the left ventricle thereby impairing left ventricular systolic function. In this case noninvasive or invasive assessment of cardiac output along with administration of 500–1,000 L fluid is recommended.

B. Ionotropic support: It should be considered when cardiac output is not maintained in spite of optimization of end-diastolic pressure. Ionotropic drugs used are dobutamine, milrinone, but dopamine should be avoided.
  a. Dobutamine—It acts by:
    1. Improving the right ventricular stroke volume.
    2. Improving the cardiac index.

3. Improving the left ventricular function thus promoting the flow.

b. Combined dobutamine and nitric oxide therapy improve pulmonary vascular resistance thereby reducing the right ventricular afterload and myocardial work.

c. Milrinone, phosphodiesterase III inhibitor, improves right ventricular function through increasing cyclic adenosine monophosphate (AMP) production which will increase right ventricular contractility and decreasing pulmonary vascular resistance.

C. Agent like levosimendan those are calcium sensitizer will improve the right ventricular function. It acts by increasing cardiac myositic activity to intracellular calcium but intracellular calcium remains normal.

D. Afterload can also be reduced by intravenous nitroprusside or intra-aortic balloon pump, but diuretics and vasodilators must be avoided.

E. Like left ventricular myocardial infarction revascularization is the ultimate treatment of choice in right ventricular myocardial infarction. Primary percutaneous coronary intervention (PCI) is the best choice but thrombolytic therapy can also be done.

F. Both surgically or percutaneously implanted ventricular assist devices may also improve survival.

Q2. Clinical features and management of cardiogenic shock.

DNBI/JUN2010 (10)

Pathophysiology and management of cardiogenic shock

MGR/SEP2002/MDIII (10)

Cardiogenic shock.

SNMC/MAY2013/MDIV (10)

MGR UNIVERSITY, 2019 (10)

ANSWER

Definition

Cardiogenic shock can be defined as decreased cardiac output leading to tissue hypoxia in presence of adequate circulating blood volume.

Etiologies

A. Systolic dysfunction resulting decreased myocardial contractility:
   a. Ischemia/Myocardial infarction
   b. Valvular heart disease
   c. Myocardial depressant drugs like beta-blockers and calcium channel blockers (CCBs)
   d. Respiratory acidosis
   e. Myocardial contusion
   f. Severe myocarditis
   g. Metabolic derangements:
      1. Hypocalcemia
      2. Hypophosphatemia
      3. Acidosis
   h. End-stage cardiomyopathy:
   i. Cardiotoxic drugs like doxorubicin

B. Diastolic dysfunction due to stiffness of left ventricle:
   a. Ischemia
   b. Restrictive cardiomyopathy
   c. Prolonged hypovolemic shock
   d. Septic shock
   e. Ventricular interdependence
   f. Extreme condition by pericardial tamponade

C. Valvular or structural abnormalities:
   a. Mitral stenosis
   b. Aortic stenosis
   c. Infective endocarditis
   d. Mitral regurgitation
   e. Aortic regurgitation
   f. Ruptured septum
   g. Cardiac tamponade
   h. Atrial myxoma or tamponade

D. Decreased contractility:
   a. Hypoxia
   b. Ischemia
   c. Acidosis
   d. Right ventricular infarction

Clinical Features

A. From history:
   a. Features of systemic hypoperfusion:
      1. Systolic blood pressure of <90 mm Hg for at least 30 minutes or vasopressor is required to maintain the systolic blood pressure of >90 mm Hg.
      2. Evidence of pulmonary congestion or elevated left ventricular filling pressure
      3. Any one of the following signs of impaired organ perfusion:
         - Altered mental status

- Cold clammy skin
- Oliguria
- Increased serum lactate of >2 mmol/L.

b. Systemic hypotension: It can be defined as:

1. Systolic blood pressure of <90 mm Hg, or
2. Decrease in mean blood pressure of >30 mm Hg

c. History of substernal chest pain radiating to left arm or neck, burning, stabbing in nature. The pain may be atypical in origin like epigastric pain, but it may be absent in diabetic or elderly individual.

d. There may be associated symptoms such as nausea, vomiting, and sweating.

e. History of ingestion of cocaine and previous cardiac diseases

f. Patient should be evaluated for previous cardiac surgery, hyperlipidemia, smoking, and hypertension.

g. Family history of coronary artery disease

h. Other symptoms are:

1. Diaphoresis
2. Exertional dyspnea or at rest
3. Palpitations
4. Presyncope or syncope
5. Anxiety
6. Depression

B. Physical examination:

a. Shock in presence of multiorgan hypoperfusion in presence of hypotension can be defined as:

1. Systolic blood pressure is <90 mm Hg
2. Cardiac index is <2.2 L/min/m^2
3. Presence of normal or elevated pulmonary capillary occlusion pressure of >15 mm Hg
4. Right ventricular end-diastolic pressure of >10 mm Hg

b. Characteristics of the patients are:

1. Patient is ashen or cyanotic.
2. Peripheral cold and clammy extremities
3. Rapid and faint peripheral pulse, pulse may be irregular in presence of arrhythmias
4. Pulsatile engorged jugular vein
5. Crepitation in the lung bases
6. There may be peripheral edema.
7. Heart sound may distant.
8. There may be third or fourth heart sound
9. Pulse pressure will be low.
10. Altered mental status
11. Oliguria

c. Features indicative of specific cardiac cause:

1. Systolic murmur can be heard in—mitral regurgitation or ventricular wall rupture.
2. Parasternal thrill—ventricular septal defect (VSD)
3. Evidence of systolic murmur louder upon prompt standing or Valsalva—suggests hypertrophic obstructive cardiomyopathy (HOCM).

Evaluation of Cardiogenic Shock

A. To assess the proper functioning of the vital organs:

a. Liver function test

b. Renal function test

c. Complete blood count:

1. Anemia—low hemoglobin
2. Leukocytosis—infection or inflammation
3. Thrombocytopenia—coagulopathy or sepsis

d. Serum electrolytes

B. Cardiac enzymes:

a. Myoglobin—foul fold rise in myoglobin level over 2 hours—highly sensitive for myocardial infarction

b. Serum lactate dehydrogenase: It will increase 10 hours after the event, reaches peak by 24–48 hours and then it will come to normal by 6–8 days. Lactate dehydrogenase-1 (LDH1) is primary released by heart but also secreted by kidney, stomach, red blood cells, and pancreas.

c. Troponins: Two types of troponins—troponin I and T. These will be released within few hours of event to reach their peak by 14 hours and after several days again, known as biphasic peak and it will remain abnormal for at least 10 days.

C. Arterial blood gases: It will indicate:

a. Acid-base homeostasis

b. Level of arterial blood oxygenation

Elevation of base deficit correlates with severe shock.

D. Serum lactate level: Elevated level correlates with hypoperfusion and indicators of prognosis.

E. Echocardiography: It can detect:

a. Information regarding regional and global wall function

b. Mechanical causes of shock:

1. Ventricular septal defect
2. Free myocardial wall rupture

3. Pericardial tamponade
4. Rupture of papillary muscles
5. Myocardial regurgitation

c. Other features are:

1. Akinetic or dyskinetic areas of ventricular wall motion
2. Left ventricular ejection fraction

F. Chest X-ray: It demonstrates:

a. Presence of widened mediastinum—indicating aortic dissection

b. Tension pneumothorax

c. Features of left ventricular failure:

1. Pulmonary vascular redistribution
2. Enlarged hilar shadow
3. Presence of Kerley B lines
4. Cardiomegaly
5. Bilateral pleural effusion
6. Bilateral perihilar opacities in butter fly arrangement

G. Coronary angiography: It is indicated in myocardial ischemia or myocardial infarction. It is needed:

1. To identify coronary artery anatomy.
2. It will evaluate the need for urgent revascularization.
3. Evidence of compensatory hyperkinesia in the noninfarcted territory due to severe coronary atherosclerosis

H. Electrocardiography: It will demonstrate:

a. ST segment elevation or depression

b. Presence of Q waves

c. T wave inversion

d. Evidence of right ventricular infarction

Normal ECG cannot rule out the acute myocardial infarction.

I. Invasive hemodynamic monitoring by Swan-Ganz catheterization can exclude other causes of shock like septic shock, volume depletion, or obstructive shock:

a. Cardiac index lower than 2.2 L/min/m^2

b. Pulmonary capillary wedge pressure of >15 mm Hg.

c. Presence of large V wave—severe mitral regurgitation

d. Step up of saturation of oxygen between right atrium and right ventricle—VSD

e. Increased right-sided filling pressure but absence of elevated pulmonary capillary wedge pressure along with ECG criteria—right ventricular infarction

Treatment

According to 2013 American Heart Association (AHA) guidelines of elevated ST segment myocardial infarction if the number of risk factors increase, risk of cardiogenic shock will be increased.

a. Age is >70 years.

b. Systolic blood pressure is <120 mm Hg.

c. Sinus tachycardia = 110 beats/min or heart rate is <60 beats/min

d. Increased time since onset of symptoms of ST-segment elevation myocardial infarction (STEMI)

A. In case of ST segment elevated MI:

a. Immediate transfer to hospital where coronary angiography is done.

b. Primary PCI should be performed irrespective of delay from the onset of MI.

c. If PCI cannot be done, urgent coronary artery bypass graft (CABG) is indicated.

d. Fibrinolytic therapy should be done where PCI or CABG cannot be performed.

e. Beta-blocker is contraindicated.

f. Intra-aortic balloon counter pulsation where pharmacotherapy is contraindicated.

g. Alternative left ventricular assist devices should be used for circulatory support.

Newer recommendations of 2015 AHA guidelines:

a. Rapid transfer to tertiary center with 24 hours cardiac catheterization is performed.

b. Immediate ECG and echocardiography should be done.

c. Continuous ECG and blood pressure monitoring

d. Coronary angiography within 2 hours of admission with the aim of performing revascularization if required.

e. In absence of signs of fluid overload, >200 mL of ringer lactate to be administered in 15–30 minutes as first line of treatment.

f. Intravenous dobutamine should be considered to increase the cardiac output.

In case of non-ST elevated MI:

According to 2014 AHA guideline:

a. Beta-blocker is contraindicated in presence of risk factors for cardiogenic shock.

b. CCB should be administered in patient with cardiogenic shock with risk factors.

c. Early revascularization is required in patients with cardiogenic shock due to pump failure.

d. In case of refractory shock intra-aortic balloon counter pulsation is considered.

Mechanical Circulatory Support

According to 2015 consensus:

- **a.** Percutaneous circulatory assist device which gives superior hemodynamic support as compared to pharmacologic therapy.
- **b.** If the patient fails show the sign of improvement after initial interventions early mechanical support is considered.
- **c.** In case of cardiogenic shock continuous flow pump is better than intra-aortic balloon counter pulsation.
- **d.** In case of patients with impaired gas exchange, extracorporeal membrane oxygenation (ECMO) will provide benefit.

Intra-aortic Balloon Counter Pulsation

Hemodynamic effects:

- **a.** Decrease peak systolic arterial pressure
- **b.** Decrease in heart rate
- **c.** Increase the end-diastolic aortic pressure
- **d.** Normalization of left ventricular end-diastolic pressure and pulmonary capillary wedge pressure
- **e.** Highly increased diastolic aortic pressure
- **f.** Highly increased mean aortic pressure

Q3. Causes, clinical manifestation, and diagnostic approach of superior venacaval obstruction.

DNBII/JUN2010 (10)

What are the causes of superior venacaval obstruction? Describe its clinical presentation and investigational approach.

DNBII/DEC2010 (10)

ANSWER

Introduction

Superior venacaval syndrome is the result of obstruction to blood flow through the superior vena cava as a result of malignant process in the thorax.

Pathophysiology

Venous blood from head, neck, upper thorax, and upper extremities drain into the low pressure thin-walled vascular conduit superior vena cava, present in the middle mediastinum and is surrounded by:

- **a.** Sternum
- **b.** Trachea
- **c.** Right bronchus
- **d.** Aorta
- **e.** Pulmonary artery
- **f.** Lymph nodes—perihilar and paratracheal

Superior vena cava is formed by right and left innominate veins and drains into right atrium, length is 6–8 cm.

Superior vena cava is obstructed by the following:

- **a.** Neoplastic invasion of venous wall with intravascular thrombosis
- **b.** Extrinsic pressure by the tumor within the mediastinum on the thin wall of the vessel
- **c.** Nonmalignant causes are:
    1. Intravascular arterial devices
    2. Vascular diseases like aortic aneurysm
    3. Cardiac causes—pericarditis, atrial myxoma
    4. Thrombosis due to central venous catheter
    5. Mediastinal fibrosis
    6. Infections like histoplasmosis, syphilis, and tuberculosis

This obstructed superior vena cava starts collateral venous return to the heart through the four pathways:

- **a.** Through azygos venous system including:
    1. Azygos vein
    2. Hemiazygos vein
    3. Intercostal veins
- **b.** Internal mammary venous system along with tributaries and secondary communications to inferior and superior epigastric veins
- **c.** Long thoracic venous system with its connection to femoral veins
- **d.** Vertebral veins

In case of superior venacaval obstruction venous pressure is always elevated in upper compartment to as high as 200–500 cm H_2O.

Clinical Features

In early case due partial obstruction patient may be asymptomatic. But as the disease progresses, classical features will arise, these are:

- **a.** Dyspnea—most common
- **b.** Facial swelling
- **c.** Fullness of the head
- **d.** Cough

e. Swelling of the arms
f. Orthopnea
g. Distorted vision
h. Hoarseness of voice
i. Laryngeal stridor
j. Nasal stuffness
k. Pleural effusion

Physical Examination

a. Venous distention in the chest and neck
b. Facial and upper extremity edema
c. Plethora
d. Cyanosis
e. Mental changes
f. Papilledema
g. Stupor
h. Coma

Complications

a. Laryngeal edema
b. Cerebral edema
c. Decreased cardiac output
d. Hypotension
e. Pulmonary embolism

Diagnosis

A. Chest X-ray will demonstrate:
   a. Widened mediastinum
   b. Presence of mass on the right side of the chest
B. Computerized tomography:
   a. It will delineate the lesion from which guided biopsy can be taken by mediastenoscopy or bronchoscopy. Or fine needle aspiration.
   b. It can also diagnose whether the obstruction is due to thrombosis or external compression.
C. MRI: It has following advantages over CT scan:
   a. It can image at different planes.
   b. It will directly visualize the blood flow.
   c. It does not require contrast material hence it is of choice if the patient is allergic to dye or patient has renal failure.
D. Venography: It is the most conclusive diagnostic tool because it precisely defines the cause of obstruction. It is important if surgical management is considered.
E. Radionuclide technetium-99m is minimally invasive alternative method to venography as it will demonstrate flow pattern and patency of the lumen.

Treatment

A. Conservative measures:
   a. Elevation of headend of the bed to decrease the venous pressure
   b. Supplemental oxygen
   c. Corticosteroid and diuretics to reduce cerebral and laryngeal edema.
B. Management of the etiology:
   a. If it is due to indwelling catheter, removal of the device along with anticoagulant therapy and catheter-directed thrombolysis.
   b. In case of acute or subacute thrombus catheter-based thrombolysis or thrombectomy should be done prior to venoplasty or stent placement.
   c. In case of tumor-related obstruction, it is first necessary to diagnose type of tumor and stage of the tumor, then radiotherapy with or without chemotherapy can be given.
   d. Open surgical repair by by-pass grafting with femoral vein, saphenous vein, or polytetrafluoroethylene graft. Dacron graft is universally considered for overcoming superior vena cava (SVC) obstruction. It is usually done in cases where endovascular recanalization is not possible.

Q4. Enumerate acyanotic congenital heart disease and describe in brief the clinical features, diagnostic evaluation and treatment of ventricular septal defect.

DNBIII/JUN2010 (10)

Interventricular septum, Ventricular septal defect.

MANIPUR UNIVERSITY, 2020 (10)

ANSWER

Definition of Acyanotic Congenital Heart Disease

In these diseases blood contains enough oxygen but it is distributed abnormally throughout the body. These defect will not interfere with the amount of blood to be distributed throughout the body.

The acyanotic congenital heart diseases are the following:

A. Aortic stenosis
B. Atrial septal defect

C. Atrioventricular septal defect

D. Bicuspid aortic valve

E. Coarctation of aorta

F. Patent ductus arteriosus

G. Pulmonary stenosis

H. Ventricular septal defect

Heart is developed from the single tubular structure in the third weeks' gestation which undergoes looping to form four chamber heart before birth.

Interventricular septum that divides the ventricle into right and left part develops from four following components:

A. Muscular part which is major portion of the septum develops first from the floor of the 4th ventricle and extends upwards toward the endocardial cushion leaving interventricular foramen.

B. Membranous part which blocks the interventricular foramen in the later part is derived from following three components:

   a. Endocardial cushion

   b. Right and left bulbar ridges forming bulbus cordis region.

   c. Neural crest cells deriving from bulbar ridges.

C. Bulbar septum: It is spiral shaped deriving from conotruncal ridges fuses to form aortopulmonary septum. It also helps to align the aorta with the left ventricle and pulmonary artery with the right ventricle.

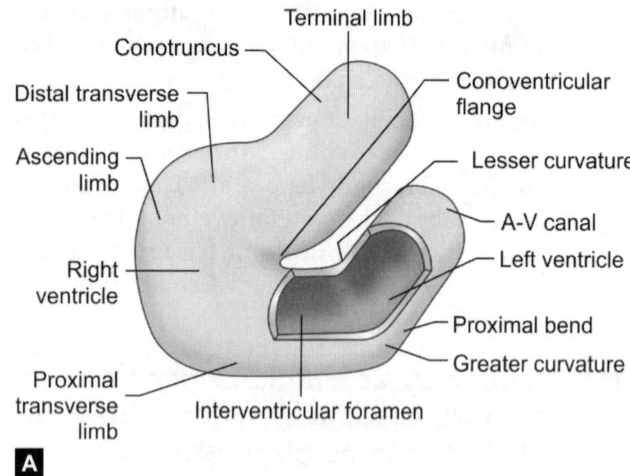

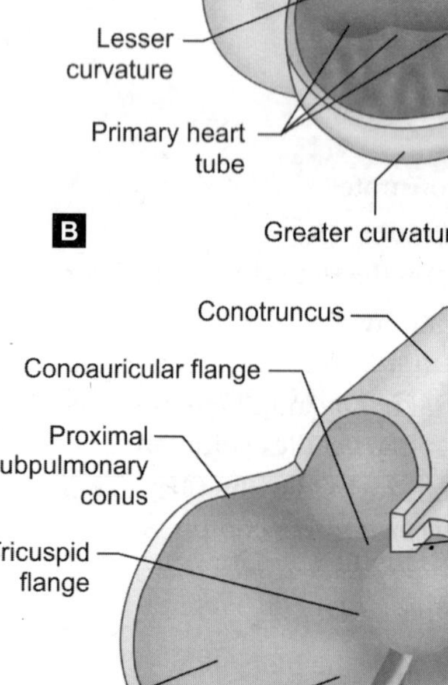

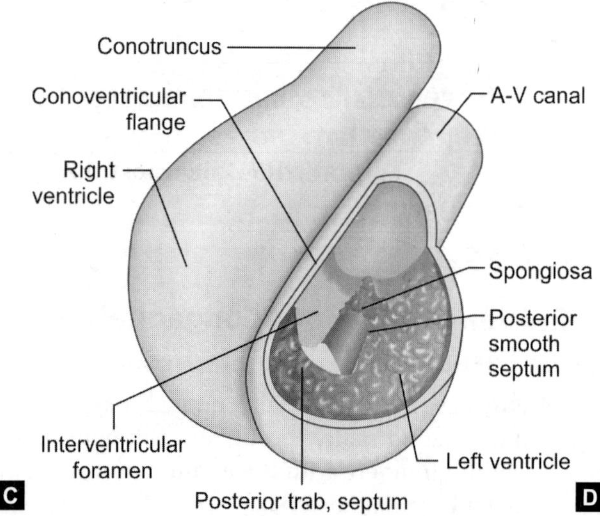

Ventricular Septal Defect

Introduction

It is the most common congenital defect in heart in children and adult. It may be associated with other congenital defects like infundibular stenosis, valvular stenosis, etc. Spontaneous closure of smaller restrictive defect will close before the age of 2 years, 35% of perimembnranous defect will close spontaneously.

Clinical Features

A. Most common symptom in case of hemodynamically significant VSD is exertional dyspnea.

B. Exercise intolerance

Symptoms are related to degree of chronicity of left to right shunt, reversal of shunt from right to left shunt, and pulmonary vascular pressure and pulmonary vascular resistance.

Physical Findings

A. Left parasternal heave due to right ventricular hypertrophy

B. There is associated with palpable systolic thrill in lower left sternum

C. Hollow systolic blowing murmur with varying intensity at the lower left sternum—classical feature

D. There may be early systolic high frequency systolic murmur along with palpable systolic thrill at lower left sternum—due to closure from muscular contraction of septum.

Pitch of the murmur varies according to the size and nature of the defect, hence smaller the size of the defect more and more increase in intensity of the murmur.

E. In the pulmonary area increased intensity of pulmonary component of second heart sound due to increased pulmonary vascular resistance.

F. There may be mid-diastolic rumble due to increased blood flow through the normal mitral valve.

G. There may be presence of early diastolic murmur of aortic insufficiency—it may occur due to subvalvular aortic stenosis.

H. In case of associated lesion like double outlet right ventricle or subvalvular pulmonary stenosis prominent systolic ejection murmur.

I. But if pulmonary hypertension develops with right to left heart shunt patient develops following features:

- **a.** Central cyanosis
- **b.** Exertional dyspnea
- **c.** Clubbing
- **d.** Elevated jugular venous pressure
- **e.** Enlarged pulsatile liver
- **f.** Decrease in the intensity of the previous murmur due to absence of significant pressure gradient across the defect.
- **g.** Systolic blowing murmur of concomitant tricuspid regurgitation may be present.

Diagnostic Evaluation

A. Electrocardiography:

- **a.** In case of small defect unremarkable feature
- **b.** In case of large defect—features of left atrial and left ventricular enlargement
- **c.** In case of AV defect—left axis deviation
- **d.** In case of right ventricular enlargement—right axis deviation
- **e.** After surgical repair—bundle branch block

B. In chest X-ray:

- **a.** Presence of small size or normal size heart and normal pulmonary vascular markings—hemodynamically insignificant defect.
- **b.** Cardiomegaly with left atrial and left ventricular enlargement in left to right shunt.
- **c.** Oligemic lung field in presence of cardiomegaly-associated pulmonary vascular disease.

C. Echocardiography:

- **a.** Color Doppler technique and two-dimensional echocardiography can detect the size and location of the lesion.
- **b.** Presence of pulmonary hypertension is helpful in confirming impending reversal of shunt.
- **c.** Quantification of velocity of shunt: It can estimate the restrictive nature of defect. If velocity is high, it suggests more restrictive nature of defect.
- **d.** In absence of right ventricular outflow tract obstruction pressure gradient across the defect can estimate the right ventricular pressure.
- **e.** Evidence of ventricular septal aneurysm formed by septal leaflet of the tricuspid valve that bows into the defect—it can be associated with perimembnranous VSD.
- **f.** Prolapse of right or left coronary cusp into the VSD producing aortic insufficiency in case of supracrystal VSD.

D. Cardiac catheterization: It can be done in case where there is question of anatomic position in spite of transthoracic or transesophageal echocardiography or in case of suspicion of pulmonary hypertension. Following hemodynamic assessment can be done:

- **a.** Quantification of cardiac index

b. Careful oximetric definition of the shunt level
c. Quantity of shunt
d. Measurement of step-up oxygen saturation that is measured at the pulmonary level confirms left to right shunt across the defect and it should be correlated with pulmonary vascular pressure and resistance.

E. Left ventriculography in left anterior oblique view: It can detect the defect. Right ventriculography cannot opacify the left ventricle adequately except in case of supracrystal defect.
F. Cardiac CT scan and MRI: It can assess the anatomy, location, and shunt fraction of VSD in case of suboptimal image in echocardiography.

Therapy

Indication of Treatment

a. Cardiomegaly in chest X-ray
b. Significant left to right shunt with pulmonary to systemic flow ration > 1.5:1
c. Elevated but responsive pulmonary vascular resistance
d. Symptoms of congestive heart failure
e. Associated lesions like aortic regurgitation
f. Right ventricular or left ventricular outflow tract infection
g. Recurrent infective endocarditis

Medical Management

a. In absence of reversal of shunt with pulmonary hypertension:
   1. Diuretic
   2. Digoxin
b. In case of infective endocarditis:
   1. In case of culture-proven endocarditis 4–5 weeks of antibiotics intravenously before interventions, but it will follow:
      - Patient's clinical status
      - Identification of infecting organisms and its sensitivity
      - Presence of concomitant valvular lesion
      - Use of prosthetic material
c. In case of pulmonary vascular resistance following drugs improve hemodynamics and exercise tolerance:
   1. Use of phosphodiesterase-5 inhibitors
   2. Prostacyclin analog
   3. Endothelin receptor antagonists

Surgical Management

a. Amplatzer muscular VSD occluder: It will close many muscular defects. But perimembnranous defect due to its close proximity of conduction system, AV and semilunar valves may impose problem for transcatheter closure. Complications of this process are:
   1. Late-onset complete heart block
   2. Arrhythmia
   3. Damage of tricuspid valve resulting stenosis or regurgitation
   4. Failure of mechanical device during deployment
b. Surgical closure: Outcome is good in case of children with mortality of 2–3%, in case of adult it is well tolerated with acceptable mortality.

   Contraindications is Eisenmenger complex with pulmonary vascular disease.

   Postoperative sequelae are:
   1. Leak from residual patch
   2. Supraventricular arrhythmias
   3. Ventricular arrhythmias
c. Hybrid patch: It should be done in those patients who cannot tolerate transcatheter approach or surgical repair. In this process through sternotomy device is placed through anterior wall of the right ventricle under the guidance of fluoroscopy or echocardiography.

C. Antibiotic prophylaxis: It is required in the three following situations:
   a. Unrepaired cyanotic defect as in case of VSD with right to left heart shunt
   b. Repaired VSD with prosthetic material or devices within first 6 months
   c. Repaired defect of VSD but residual defect at the prosthetic site.

   In this connection minute oral and dental examination is necessary.

D. Eisenmenger syndrome from irreversible pulmonary hypertension as a result of long-standing left to right shunt as in case of PDA or ASD or VSD—pregnancy should be contraindicated.

Q5. What is perhypertension? Describe the risk factors associated and its management.

DNBI/DEC2010 (10)

ANSWER

Prehypertension: It is in between the normotension and hypertension, associated with subclinical atherosclerosis leading to target organ damage.

Prehypertension can be defined as systolic blood pressure between 120 and 139 mm Hg and diastolic blood pressure between 80 and 89 mm Hg in each of two or more office visits.

Blood pressure category	Systolic mm Hg (upper #)		Diastolic mm Hg (lower #)
Normal	<120	and	<80
Prehypertension	120–139	or	80–89
High blood pressure (Hypertension) Stage 1	140–159	or	90–99
High blood pressure (Hypertension) Stage 2	160 or higher	or	100 or higher
Hypertensive crisis (Emergency care needed)	>180	or	>110

Women of more than 60 years are less likely to develop prehypertension as compared to men.

Following are the predictors of prehypertension:

a. Systolic blood pressure
b. Diastolic blood pressure is significant
c. Age: Older age group are more susceptible.
d. Body mass index: High BMI is associated with prehypertension.

These patients have:

a. High cholesterol and triglyceride
b. High serum glucose
c. Higher homeostasis model assessment-insulin resistance

Pathophysiology

Prehypertension progresses to hypertension at a rate of 19% every 4 year which depends upon blood pressure level and age. In case of high-level prehypertension (130–139 mm Hg and 85–89 mm Hg) progression to hypertension is more rapid as compared to low level prehypertension (120–129 mm Hg and 80–84 mm Hg).

Change in blood pressure will lead to change in the microcirculation and human blood vessels which is more obvious in severe hypertension. In stage 1 hypertension, i.e., prehypertension, few changes are unstable but as the stage increases toward severity, chronic changes in the cardiovascular system will be stable and nonreversible.

Prehypertension is associated with elevation of the following:

a. C-reactive protein (CRP)
b. Tumor necrosis factor-alpha (TNF-α)
c. Oxidized low-density lipoprotein (LDL)
d. Proinflammatory cytokines and chemokines
e. Homocysteine

Clinical Evaluation

A. Proper monitoring of blood pressure:
 a. In case of strong family history of hypertension, i.e., within first degree relatives
 b. Patients with history of smoking and illicit drug use
 c. In case of overweight subject
B. Nocturnal hypertension or nondipping blood pressure: It is early marker of prehypertension or masked hypertension.

Evaluation of Prehypertension

A. Estimation of biomarkers of prehypertension as these levels are increased:
 a. Nitric oxide
 b. Serotonin
 c. Endothelin-1
B. Platelet 5-hydroxytriptamine is lowered in prehypertension.
C. 24 hours ambulatory blood pressuring: It can detect nighttime and 24 hours increase in blood pressure.

Following are the excess risks of prehypertension:

a. Subclinical atherosclerosis
b. Increased coronary atherosclerosis
c. Increased thickness of carotid artery and brachial artery intima-media thickness

Management of Hypertension

Item	Recommendation	Effect of systolic blood pressure in prehypertension	Effect on incidence of prehypertension
DASH dietary pattern Dietary approaches to stop hypertension (limited amount of sweets and meats)	4–5 fruits per day (rich in potassium)	3.5 mm Hg	Decreased by 62%
	4–5 vegetables per day		
	2–3 low-fat dairy product per day (rich in calcium)		
	Less than 25% fat		
Weight loss	Effective blood pressure lowering even without attaining normal basal metabolic rate	1 mm Hg	Decreased by 42%
Physical activity	Moderate exercise ≥30 minutes in most of the days	3–4 mm Hg	N/A
Reduced intake of sodium	Less than 2,400 mg/day	2 mm Hg per decrease in 76 mmol/day	Decreased by 38%
Moderate intake of alcohol	• ≤2 oz per day in men • ≤1 oz per day in women	3.5 mm Hg	N/A

Q6. Describe Duke's criterion for infective endocarditis.

DNBII/DEC2010 (10)

Infective endocarditis.

MGR/SEP2010/MDII (6)

Modified criteria of infective endocarditis.

MGR/OCT2011/MDIV (7)

Duke's criteria for clinical diagnosis of infective endocarditis.

MGR UNIVERSITY, TAMIL NADU, 2021 (10)

ANSWER

Duke criteria for infective endocarditis can be divided into following categories as described here.

Definite Pathological Diagnosis

It is either A or B of the following pathological findings:

A. Microorganisms as demonstrated by culture or histology in vegetation:
   - **a.** Vegetation that has embolized
   - **b.** Intracardiac abscess

B. Pathologic lesions:
   - **a.** Vegetation or intracardiac abscess is present, confirmed by histology showing active endocarditis

Definite Clinical Diagnosis

Two major criteria, or 1 major and 3 minor criteria, or 5 minor criteria are needed.

Possible Clinical Diagnosis

One major and 1 minor criteria, or 3 minor criteria are needed.

For Rejecting the Diagnosis

- **a.** There is firm alternative diagnosis for clinical manifestations
- **b.** Resolution of clinical manifestations with antibiotics within 4 days or less
- **c.** No pathological evidence of infective endocarditis at surgery or autopsy after antibiotic therapy of 4 days or less.

Duke Criteria

Major Clinical Criteria

A. Positive blood culture results for infective endocarditis:
   - **a.** Typical microorganisms (in two or more cultures):
     1. Viridans streptococci
     2. Streptococcus bovis
     3. *HACEK group*
     4. *Streptococcus aureus*
     5. Community-acquired enterococci, in absence of primary foci

b. Persistently positive blood culture:
   1. Recovery of a microorganism consistent with infective endocarditis from two blood cultures drawn more than 12 hours apart.

      Or,

   2. Recovery of a microorganism consistent with infective endocarditis from all of 3 or majority of 4 or more separate blood culture with the first and last drawn at least 1 hour apart.

      Or,

   3. Single positive blood culture for *Coxiella burnetii* or antiphase-1 immunoglobulin G (IgG) antibody titer > 1:800.

B. Evidence of endocardial involvement:

a. Positive echocardiogram:
   1. Oscillating intracardiac mass on valve or supporting structures or in the path of regurgitant jets or on implanted material, in the absence of an alternative anatomic explanation.

      Or,

   2. Abscess

      Or,

   3. New partial dehiscence

      Or,

b. New valvular regurgitation (increase or change in preexisting murmur not sufficient)

Minor Clinical Criteria

A. Predisposition:

a. Predisposing heart condition
b. Injection drug use

B. Fever > 100.4°F

C. Vascular phenomena:

a. Major arterial emboli
b. Septic pulmonary infarct
c. Mycotic aneurysm
d. Intracranial hemorrhage
e. Conjunctival hemorrhage
f. Janeway lesions

D. Immunologic phenomena:

a. Glomerulonephritis
b. Roth's spots
c. Osler's nodes
d. Rheumatoid factor

E. Microbiologic evidence:

a. Positive blood culture but not meeting the major criteria as noted above
b. Serologic evidence of active infection with organism consistent with infective endocarditis

Etiological Agents

A. Underlying cardiac conditions:

a. Mitral valve prolapse with regurgitation
b. Rheumatic heart disease
c. In 10% cases congenital heart disease includes:
   1. VSD
   2. PDA
   3. Bicuspid aortic valve
   4. Tetralogy of Fallot
   5. Coarctation of aorta

B. Source of infection:

a. Dental procedure
b. Infected vascular catheter
c. Infected skin lesion
d. No history of antecedent localized infection

C. Native valve endocarditis:

a. Streptococcal organism
b. Staphylococcal organism
c. *Enterococcus*: It occurs following genitourinary or obstetric procedures.
d. *Streptococcus bovis*: It is associated with colonic cancer or polyp.
e. HACEK
f. Intravenous drug user: *Staphylococcus aureus.* Valve most commonly involved is tricuspid followed by mitral and aortic valves.
g. Enterobacteriaceae—*Escherichia coli, Salmonella, Klebsiella, Proteus, Enterobacter, Serratia, Shigella,* and *Yersinia.*

D. Prosthetic valve: High risk of infection within 6 months of implantation of prosthetic valve.

a. If infection is within 2 months of surgery—intraoperative contamination or nosocomial infection. Organism is most common coagulase negative staphylococci, next is *S. aureus.*
b. If infection is after 2 months of surgery—organisms are similar to that of native valve organisms. Fungi are involved in 15% cases and associated with high mortality.

E. Pace maker or defibrillator:

a. If infective endocarditis develops within 2 months of surgery—it occurs from direct intraoperative seedling of microorganisms.
b. If infective endocarditis occurs after 2 months of surgery—organism are mainly as that of native valve infection.

Q7. Describe clinical manifestation and management of hypertrophic cardiomyopathy.

DNBIII/DEC2010 (10)

Classify cardiomyopathies and discuss the pathophysiology, clinical features, lab diagnosis and management of HOCM.

MGR/MAY2011/MDII (15)

Discuss the types, pathogenesis, clinical features, and management of cardiomyopathies.

TEERTHANKER MAHAVEER UNI, 2020 (20)

(Question 7, 35 and 60)

Mechanism of diastolic dysfunction in hypertrophic and ischemic heart disease.

RAJIV GANDHI UNI OF HEALTH SC, KARNATAKA, 2016 (10)

Describe the etiopathogenesis, clinical features, and management of hypertrophic cardiomyopathy.

BHARATI VIDYAPEETH UNIVERSITY, SUMMER 2017 (10)

Hypertrophic obstructive cardiomyopathy.

BHARATI VIDYAPEETH UNIVERSITY, SUMMER 2018 (10)

RAJIV GANDHI UNI OF HEALTH SC, KARNATAKA, JULY 2020 (10)

Pathophysiology and management of hypertrophic cardiomyopathy.

AIIMS, BBS, 2022 (10)

Explain dynamic auscultatory findings in HOCM.

MGU, 2024 (5)

Discuss the diagnosis and management of hypertrophic cardiomyopathy.

MANIPUR UNIVERSITY, 2021 (10)

Dynamic auscultation in clinical practice.

MANIPUR UNIVERSITY, 2024 (10)

ANSWER

Definition

Hypertrophic cardiomyopathy can be defined as presence of hypertrophy of left ventricle of a nondilated left ventricle in absence of another systemic or cardiac disease which will explain the degree of left ventricular hypertrophy.

Mechanism of Diastolic Dysfunction

A. Increased stiffness of the ventricular wall: Thickened left ventricular myocardium reduces the left ventricular compliance leading to reduced filling of the left ventricle during diastole, as a result the left ventricular filling pressure will be increased.

B. Impaired relaxation of the ventricle during diastole due to myocyte disarray and fibrosis leading to impaired filling of the ventricle during diastole.

C. As a result of the increased stiffness of left ventricular wall and impaired relaxation of the left ventricle left atrial and pulmonary venous pressure will be increased leading to left ventricular failure with preserved ejection fraction.

D. There is non-uniform relaxation of the ventricle due to thickened myocardium and pathchy fibrosis.

Physical Examinations

A. Inspection:
   - a. Prominent a wave in jugular vein: It indicates hypertrophy and lack of compliance of right ventricle.
   - b. Precordial heave: It represents right ventricular strain.

B. Palpation:
   - a. Three components of precordial pulse palpated include:
     1. Presystolic apical impulse
     2. Palpable fourth heart sound
     3. Late systolic bulge of left ventricle
   - b. Pulsus bisferiens—rapid carotid upstroke followed by second peak—is caused by hyperdynamic left ventricle.

C. Auscultation:
   - a. First heart sound is normal; it is preceded by fourth heart sound.
   - b. Second heart sound may paradoxically split due to prolonged ejection time through the pulmonary artery from right ventricle.

c. Harsh crescendo-decrescendo systolic murmur is heard in the left sternal border radiating down the lower left sternum but never to neck and axilla.

d. Intensity of murmur varies according to following maneuvers which can be differentiated from mitral incompetence and aortic stenosis.

Maneuvers	Physiologic effects	Hypertrophic cardiomyopathy	Aortic stenosis	Mitral incompetence
Valsalva	**Decreases:** • Venous return • Systemic vascular resistance • Cardiac output	**Increases:** Murmur	**Decreases:** Murmur	**Decreases:** Murmur
Squat and handgrip	**Increases:** • Venous return • Systemic vascular resistance • Cardiac output	**Decreases:** Murmur	**Increases:** Murmur	**Increases:** Murmur
Amyl nitrite	**Increases:** Venous return **Decreases:** • Systemic venous resistance • Left ventricular volume	**Increases:** Murmur	**Increases:** Murmur	**Decreases:** Murmur
Phenylephrine	**Increases:** • Systemic vascular resistance • Venous return	**Decreases:** Murmur	**Increases:** Murmur	**Increases:** Murmur
Extrasystole	**Decreases:** Left ventricular volume	**Increases:** Murmur	**Decreases:** Murmur	No change
Post-Valsalva release	**Increases:** Left ventricular volume	**Decreases:** Murmur	**Increases:** Murmur	No change

Management

Main goals of management are:

A. Treatment of symptoms of systolic and diastolic heart failure, arrhythmias, syncope or presyncope, and angina pain; following are the causes of above symptoms:

- **a.** Left ventricular outflow tract obstruction
- **b.** Diastolic dysfunction
- **c.** Ischemia
- **d.** Arrhythmias
- **e.** Mitral regurgitation

B. Prevention of sudden death

Medical therapy: It is based on the following:

- **a.** Drugs having negative chronotropic and ionotropic effects on heart leading to improvement in diastolic filling.
- **b.** Decrease in myocardial demand.

Drugs are the following:

A. Beta-blockers: These drugs will improve symptoms and exercise tolerance:

- **a.** Beta-blocker with additional alpha-blocking effects of drugs like carvedilol and labetalol should be avoided because of their vasodilatory properties.
- **b.** Mechanism of action:
  1. They inhibit sympathetic stimulation—negative ionotropic and chronotropic effects
  2. It will decrease the myocardial demand.
  3. It will augment diastolic filling of the ventricle.

B. Calcium-channel blocker: It is second line of agent.

Mechanism of actions:

- **a.** It reduces heart rate and blood pressure.
- **b.** It has negative chronotropic effect.
- **c.** It will improve rapid diastolic filling.

Beneficial effects are limited to verapamil and diltiazem—nondihydropyridine group. But nifedipine and amlodipine should be avoided because of their vasodilatory effects.

C. Disopyramide: It can be used as alternative to beta-blocker or CCB.

Mechanism of actions:

a. Strong negative ionotropic effect
b. It has ability to suppress the supraventricular and ventricular arrhythmias.

Potential disadvantages:

a. It has anticholinergic properties.
b. It will be accumulated in patients with hepatic and renal dysfunction.
c. It will augment conduction through the AV node during atrial fibrillation.
d. It has warning hemodynamic effects with time.

This drug should be given to those patients in whom surgical myectomy or alcohol-septal ablations are planned.

D. Angiotensin-converting enzyme inhibitor (ACEI) and angiotensin receptor blockers (ARBs) are avoided because of their potential vasodilatory effects.

E. Diuretics should be used with caution to reduce the circulatory overload in the setting of pulmonary edema as because overdiuresis may reduce the left ventricular volume and increase left ventricular outflow tract obstruction.

F. Digoxin should be avoided because it may worsen the left ventricular outflow tract obstruction.

Surgical Management

Indications

a. Symptomatic patients with symptomatic obstruction
b. Resting or latent pressure gradient of ≥50 mm Hg despite medical treatment
c. Younger patients with pressure gradient of ≥75 mm Hg and is of low surgical risk.

Procedures

A. Septal myectomy: It is the procedure of choice. It is effective in improving:

a. Left ventricular outflow gradient
b. Mitral regurgitation
c. Filling pressure

Following comitant surgeries are performed:

a. Papillary muscle attachment
b. Mitral valve regurgitation
c. Atrial fibrillation

B. Alcohol septal ablation: It is method of controlled infarction of septum and is of choice where septal myectomy cannot be done.

Result:

a. There is triphasic response:
   1. Immediate decrease in left ventricular outflow tract obstruction because of stunning
   2. Early reappearance
   3. Sustained fall by 3 months after the procedure is over because of remodeling of ventricular septum.

Risk of this procedure:

a. High-grade AV block requiring implantation of pace maker
b. Pericarditis
c. Coronary dissection
d. Large anterior wall myocardial infarction
e. Electrical instability of the scar

C. Dual chamber pacing: It should be done in those patients who are refractory medical symptoms and do not tolerate septal reduction therapy.

D. Special management: Atrial fibrillation:

a. It will worsen the heart failure.
b. It will increase the thromboembolic stroke.

In atrial fibrillation, there is acute hemodynamic decompensation along with pulmonary edema due to:

a. Loss of atrial systole
b. Decreased diastolic filling times

Therapeutic procedure:

a. All the patients having atrial fibrillation should be treated with anticoagulant.
b. Acute paroxysms of atrial fibrillation should be managed by prompt cardioversion.
c. Chronic atrial fibrillation—heart rate can be maintained by beta-blockers and CCBs.
d. Maze or radiofrequency ablation: It should be done who cannot maintain the heart rate with antiarrhythmic therapy. Otherwise, AV nodal ablation or dual chamber pacing should be done.

Q8. Refractory hypertension definition and its management.

DNBI/JUN2011 (10)

Causes of resistant hypertension.

MGR/OCT2011/MDII (7)

Resistant hypertension.

NTR UNIVERSITY OF HEALTH SC, VIJAYAWADA, ANDHRA, 2021 (10)

Resistant hypertension.

MAHARASHTRA UNI OF HEALTH SC, VIJAYAWADA, 2022 (10)

BHARATI VIDYAPEETH UNIVERSITY, WINTER 2017 (10)

BHARATI VIDYAPEETH UNIVERSITY, SUMMER 2018 (10)

RAJASTHAN UNIVERSITY, 2021 (08), 2019 (08)

Resistant hypertension: Diagnosis, mechanism, and updates in treatment.

BABA FARID UNI HEALTH SCIENCES, 2017 (10)

Work-up of a case of resistant hypertension.

BABA FARID UNI OF HEALTH SC, 2019 (10)

Approach to resistant hypertension.

SARDAR PATEL UNIVERSITY, 2019 (10)

RAJASTHAN UNIVERSITY, 2022 (25)

What do you understand by resistant hypertension? Discuss its management strategies.

AIIMS, BBS, 2023 (10)

How will you diagnose and manage resistant hypertension.

AIIMS (BHU), 2024 (10)

ANSWER

Definition of Resistant Hypertension

Hypertension can be defined as systolic blood pressure of >140 mm Hg and diastolic blood pressure of >90 mm Hg or those taking antihypertensive medications in patient above 18 years of age.

Resistant hypertension can be defined as blood pressure that will be above the 140/90 mm Hg in spite of use of three different classes antihypertensive medications at their best tolerated doses, one of which drugs must be diuretics.

Following are the characteristics of patients with resistant hypertension:

- **a.** Old age
- **b.** Black race
- **c.** Female sex
- **d.** Residents of Southeastern United States
- **e.** Excessive ingestion of salts: It produces resistant hypertension due to following factors:
  1. Direct increase in blood pressure
  2. Blunting the blood pressure lowering effects of antihypertensive drugs

  These effects are more pronounced in:
  1. African-American
  2. Elderly
  3. Patients with CKD
- **f.** Diabetes
- **g.** High blood pressure
- **h.** Obesity: It produces hypertension due to following factors:
  1. Impaired excretion of sodium
  2. Increased activity of sympathetic nervous system
  3. Increased activity of renin–angiotensin–aldosterone system
- **i.** Chronic kidney disease
- **j.** Left ventricular hypertrophy

Etiology

A. Genetic factors:

- **a.** Mutation of β and γ subunits of epithelial sodium channel may lead to Liddle's syndrome, a rare cause of monogenic hypertension.
- **b.** CYP3A5 enzyme is responsible for metabolism of cortisol and corticosterone. Mutation of the gene related to this enzyme is responsible for hypertension resistant to treatment.

B. Secondary causes of hypertension are the most common causes of resistant hypertension, these are the following:

- **a.** Common:
  1. Obstructive sleep apnea: Intermittent hypoxemia and/or resistance in the upper airway increases the sustained activity of sympathetic nervous system which in turn:
     - Increases cardiac output

- Increases peripheral resistance
- Increases fluid retention

It also increases reactive oxygen species along with decreased bioavailability of nitric oxide.

2. Primary aldosteronism
3. Renal parenchymal disease
4. Renal artery stenosis

b. Uncommon:

1. Cushing disease
2. Pheochromocytoma
3. Coarctation of aorta
4. Hyperthyroidism
5. Intracranial tumor

Confirm treatment resistance
Office blood pressure >140/90 or 130/80 mm Hg in patients with diabetes or chronic kidney disease
and
Patient prescribed 3 or more antihypertensive medications at optimal doses, including if possible a diuretic
or
Office blood pressure at goal but patient requiring 4 or more antihypertensive medications

↓

Exclude pseudoresistance
Is patient adherent with prescribed regimen? Obtain home, work, or ambulatory blood pressure readings to exclude white coat effect

↓

Identify and reverse contributing lifestyle factors
Obesity
Physical inactivity
Excessive alcohol ingestion
High salt, low fiber diet

↓

Discontinue or minimize interfering substances
Nonsteroidal anti-inflammatory agents
Sympathomimetics (diet pills, decongestants)
Stimulants
Oral contraceptives
Licorice
Ephedra

↓

Sereen for secondary causes of hypertension
Obstructive sleep apnea (snoring, witnessed apnea, excessive daytime sleepiness)
Primary aldosteronism (elevated aldosterone/renin ratio)
Chronic kidney disease (creatinine clearance <30 mL/min)
Renal artery stenosis (young female, known atherosclerotic disease, worsening renal function)
Pheochromocytoma (episodic hypertension, palpitations, diaphoresis, head ache)
Cushing's syndrome (moon facies, central obesity, abdominal striae, inter-scapular fat deposition)
Aortic coarctation (differential in brachial or femoral pulses, systolic bruit)

↓

Pharmacologic treatment
Maximize diuretic therapy, including possible addition of mineralocorticoid receptor antagonist
Combine agents with different mechanisms of action
Use of loop diuretics in patients with chronic kidney disease and/or patients receiving potent vasodilators (e.g., minoxidil)

↓

Refer to specialist
Refer to appropriate specialist for konwn or suspected secondary cause (s) of hypertension
Refer to hypertension specialist if blood pressure remains uncontrolled after 6 months of treatment

Treatment

A. Nonpharmacological treatment:

- **a.** Cessation of smoking
- **b.** Reduction of alcohol intake
- **c.** Restriction of dietary salt
- **d.** Increased physical activity
- **e.** Healthy dietary plan

B. Pharmacological treatment:

- **a.** ACEI under the age of 55 years and dehydropyridine CCB in case of older than 55 years. These drugs can be taken as combinations and thiazide as diuretic can be added as third drug.
- **b.** During choosing the combinations individual patient should be tailored and associated comorbidities should be considered.
- **c.** If the patient's presenting symptom is fluid overload, in that case diuretic should be added as first drug in place of CCB. Again, if patient complains of dry cough after initiation of ACEI then ARBs should replace ACEI.
- **d.** In case of resistant hypertension, chlorthalidone, a long-acting and most potent diuretic, should be given at a dose of 12.5 mg daily then in place of hydrochlorothiazide diuretics then it can be increased up to 50 mg daily.
- **e.** Indapamide, a potent thiazide-like diuretic, can be given in place of potent chlorthalidone as there is chance of renal impairment and hypokalemia. So, in elderly with renal impairment indapamide should be of choice at a dose of 1.5 mg controlled released tablet to be given in the morning.
- **f.** Blood pressure generally is low during night and nocturnal hypertension, i.e., nondipping hypertension is associated with cardiovascular disease and prognosis is poor. So, one hypertensive drug should be taken at night to prevent nocturnal hypertension and thus poor cardiovascular outcome.
- **g.** Spironolactone is considered as fourth anti-hypertensive drug to be added. It should be started at 25 mg/day and 2 weeks has to wait to get its full effect, then dose can be increased gradually over several months to 100 mg/day. In this high dose the adverse effects are gynecomastia, menstrual irregularities, tenderness in the breast, and sexual dysfunction.
- **h.** As alternative to spironolactone amiloride at a dose of 2.5–10 mg daily with proper and regular monitoring of potassium.
- **i.** ACEI and ARBs should not be given simultaneously. All the resistant patients under quadruple drugs should be re-evaluated to find secondary causes.
- **j.** Vasodilators like carvedilol or labetalol can be added as fifth drug as it will dilate vascular smooth muscles but these drugs are not cardioprotective. Carvedilol should be started as 12.5 mg daily for 2 days followed by weekly increasing 12.5 mg up to 50 mg/day. Labetalol can be started as 100 mg twice daily and should be increased up to 2.4 g daily, but it should not be increased >200 mg/day.
- **k.** Other drugs in line are alpha blockers like clonidine and methyldopa, vasodilator like hydralazine and minoxidil but these should be given as per expert's advice.

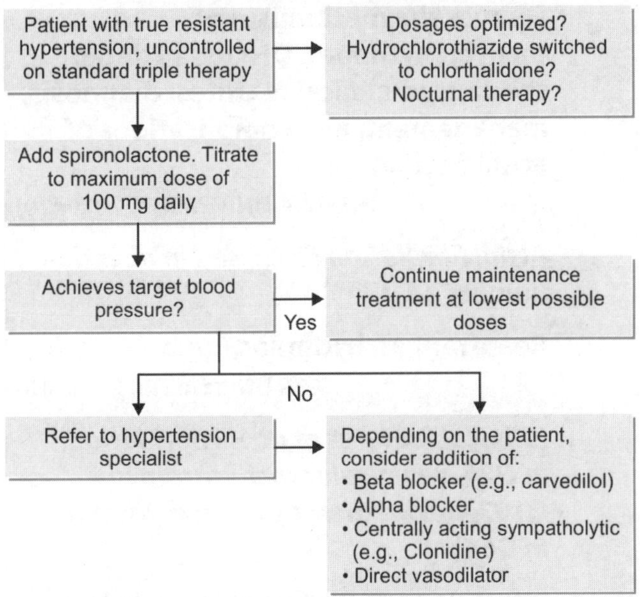

Q9. PSVT and its management.

DNBII/JUN2011 (10)

Discuss the pathophysiology of supraventricular tachycardia. Describe the management of PSVT.

DNBI/JUN2013 (10)

Reentrant arrhythmias

MGR/SEP2008/MDIV (6)

Mechanism and treatment of paroxysmal SVT. Management of infective endocarditis.

DNB, 2019, (3+2+5)

Pathogenesis of paroxysmal supraventricular tachycardia.

DNB, 2022 (5)

Etiology and clinical features of tachyarrhythmias. Device therapy for treatment of cardiac arrhythmias.

DNB, 2019 (5+5)

BHARATI VIDYAPEETH UNIVERSITY, WINTER 2017 (10)

AVNRT

BHARATI VIDYAPEETH UNIVERSITY, WINTER 2019 (10)

Discuss the mechanism of tachyarrhythmias. Discuss in detail the causes, clinical features, diagnosis, management, and complications of atrial fibrillation.

KERALA UNIVERSITY, 2019 (20)

Atrial fibrillation discussed in question number 14

Reentrant arrhythmias.

MGR UNIVERSITY, 2019 (10)

(Clinical features of atrial fibrillation in Q24, ventricular tachycardia in Q103, device therapy for arrhythmias in Q64)

Infective endocarditis answers in Q33.

Discuss tachycardia associated with accessary pathway.

NTR UNIVERSITY OF HEALTH SC, VIJAYAWADA, ANDHRA, 2022 (10)

Atrioventricular re-entry tachycardia.

GURU RAMDAS UNI HEALTH SC, AMRITSAR, 2022 (10)

Mechanism of cardiac arrhythmias.

AIIMS (DELHI), 2022, (10)

Discuss mechanism of tachyarrhythmias? Write down the treatment of AVNRT.

AIIMS, BBS, 2023 (10)

Treatment has been written in question number 13

Physiology of cardiac conduction system and its clinical significance in AV nodal re-entry mechanism.

AIIMS, BBS, 2022 (10)

Explain the ECG findings in WPW syndrome.

MGU, 2024 (5)

Cardiac conduction system has been described in question number 41.

Discuss genesis of supraventricular tachyarrhythmia. Write the management of PSVT.

WBUHS, 2024 (10)

ANSWER

Definition

Paroxysmal tachycardia can be defined as sudden onset of conduction and sudden termination of conduction requiring the atrial and/or AV node for its initiation and maintenance, consisting of narrow complex tachycardia except atrial fibrillation and multifocal atrial tachycardia.

Depending on the site of origin supraventricular tachyarrhythmias can be classified as following:

A. Atrial tachyarrhythmias:
- **a.** Sinus tachycardia
- **b.** Inappropriate sinus tachycardia
- **c.** Sinus nodal reentrant tachycardia
- **d.** Atrial tachycardia
- **e.** Multifocal atrial tachycardia
- **f.** Atrial flutter
- **g.** Atrial fibrillation

B. Atrioventricular arrhythmias:
- **a.** AV nodal reentrant tachycardia (AVNRT)
- **b.** AV reentrant tachycardia
- **c.** Junctional ectopic tachycardia
- **d.** Nonparoxysmal junction tachycardia

Mechanism of Paroxysmal Tachyarrhythmias

Abnormal Automaticity

Automaticity refers to ability of the cardiac tissue to generate activity spontaneously. It may be normal accelerated automaticity due to rapid firing rate of the pace maker, i.e., sinus node, AV node or Purkinje fibers due to ischemia, metabolic disturbance, exercise, etc. Examples are sinus tachycardia and junctional rhythm.

Abnormal automaticity refers to generation of automatic spontaneous pace maker activity in the setting of ischemia, metabolic disturbances, or pharmacologic interventions that control cardiac rhythm. Examples are accelerated idioventricular rhythm and multifocal atrial tachycardia.

Automatic Atrial Tachycardia

A. It will be generated from the ectopic focus in the crista terminalis present in the right atrium and in the left atrium around the base of the pulmonary vein occurring more in the younger patients.

B. It will not respond to vagal maneuver and is likely to be incessant and can be induced by treadmill test and isoproterenol administration.

Triggered Automaticity

It refers to the pace maker activity which is dependent on afterdepolarization of the prior impulse. Afterdepolarization is the membrane potential oscillation, if it will be the critical level of threshold for depolarization of the surrounding cardiac tissue, they will trigger action potential leading to precipitation of further afterdepolarization that perpetuating pace maker activity. Two types of afterdepolarization:

- **a.** Early afterdepolarization: It occurs in the plateau phase, i.e., phase 3 action potential prior to repolarization of the cardiac tissue, more evident at slow heart rate. Its examples are Long QT syndrome and Torsade de pointes (twisting of points). Its causes are:
  1. Class 1 antiarrhythmic drugs
  2. Class III antiarrhythmic activity
  3. Hypoxia
  4. Antibiotics like macrolides
  5. Psychotropic medications like haloperidol
  6. Nonsedative antihistaminic
- **b.** Delayed afterdepolarization: It refers to repolarization of the surrounding cardiac tissue in the phase 4 action potential and is demonstrated in conducting system of heart, myocardial cells, and valve tissues. It occurs in digitalis toxicity.

Triggered atrial tachycardia:

- **a.** It occurs in older individual and never incessant. Mechanism is due to delayed afterdepolarization due to sympathetic discharge or digitalis toxicity.

Re-entry Arrhythmia

It is the most common cause of arrhythmia. In order for re-entry to develop following three conditions must be met:

- **a.** Two functionally distinct conducting pathways must be met to form a single circuit.
- **b.** Unidirectional block in conduction in one of the pathways having longer refractory period due to difference of refractory period in the two pathways.
- **c.** Slow conduction of impulse along the unblocked pathway having shorter refractory period thus allowing the blocked pathway to regaining its excitability to sustain the arrhythmia.

This re-entry circuit occurs in:

- **a.** Sinoatrial node
- **b.** Atrium
- **c.** AV node
- **d.** By-pass tract in between the atrium and ventricle
- **e.** Ventricle

Multifocal Atrial Tachycardia

Here the mechanism is abnormal automaticity and abnormal triggered activity arising from different sites. Diagnostic criteria are:

- **a.** Atrial rate > 100 beats/min
- **b.** P waves having three or more different morphologies
- **c.** P-P, P-R, and R-R interval will vary.
- **d.** P waves are separated by isoelectric interval.

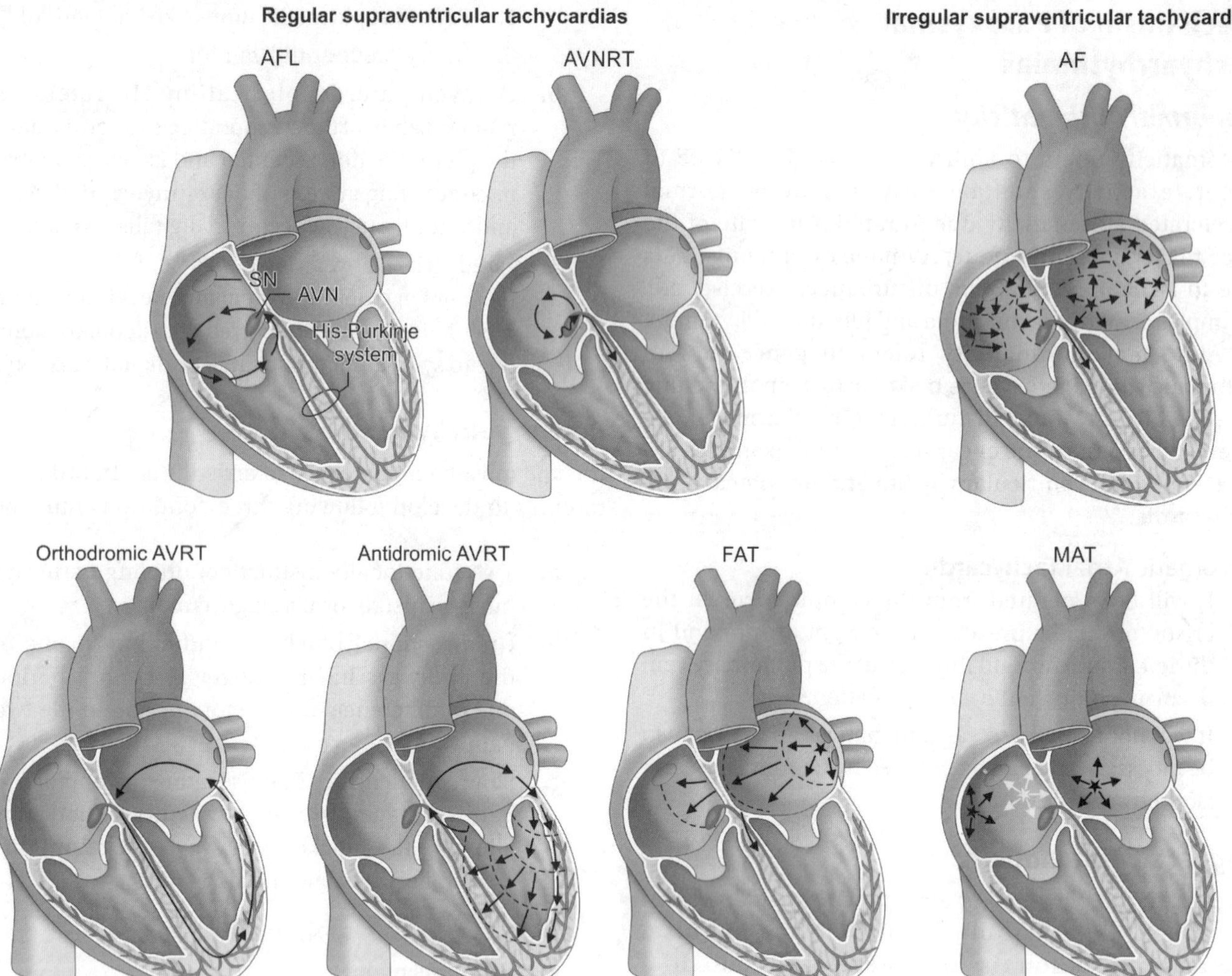

(AF: atrial fibrillation; AFL: atrial flutter; AVNRT: AV nodal reentrant tachycardia; AVRT: atrioventricular reentrant tachycardia; FAT: focal atrial tachycardia; MAT: multifocal atrial tachycardia)

Atrioventricular Nodal Re-entrant Tachycardia

It is characterized by narrow QRS complexes having ventricular rate of 150–250 beats/min.

Pathophysiology

Here, re-entrant circuit is composed of two separate pathways, fast and slow pathways in the atria including AV node. There are two types of AVNRT.

A. Typical AVNRT:

- **a.** Antegrade conduction through slow pathways to ventricles
- **b.** Retrograde conduction through fast pathway to the atria

Initiating event premature ventricular complex or premature atrial complex.

Premature atrial complex blocks the retrograde fast pathway but propagates along the antegrade pathway then back to retrograde fast pathway after it has repolarized.

Premature ventricular complex propagate passes through fast pathway retrogradely and returns to ventricle through the slow pathway.

B. Atypical AVNRT:

- **a.** Antegrade conduction through the fast pathway to the ventricles
- **b.** Retrograde conduction through the slow pathway to the atria

Here, the length of the cycle depends upon conduction velocity of the slow pathway, conduction through the fast path is very rapid. This type of tachycardia can be terminated by blocking the slow pathway. Sometimes,

AV dissociated can develop during this tachycardia when ventricle will not be involved in this circuit.

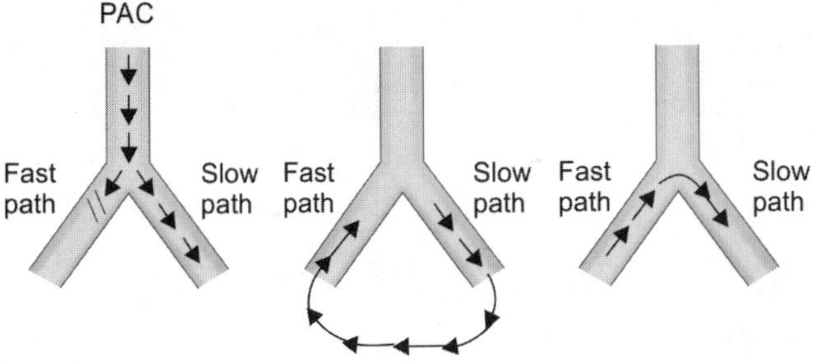

Clinical Features

A. Palpitations
B. Respiratory distress
C. Angina pain
D. Features of congestive heart failure
E. Rarely shock—which may be due to:
   a. Rapid ventricular rate
   b. Prolonged pause
   c. Bradycardia

Laboratory Features

A. P wave is hidden within or in the terminal portion of QRS complex—typical of AVNRT
B. In V1 it may be visible as small pseudo-R′ or in the inferior lead as negative deflection.
C. R-P segment is <100 ms.
D. Initiation and termination of AVNRT are abrupt.

Treatment

Treatment approach varies in different individuals, according to the characteristics of the patients and pattern of arrhythmias.

A. Medical therapy:
   a. Beta-blockers, CCBs, digoxin and adenosine—will block the antegrade slow pathway thus suppressing the AV nodal conduction.
   b. Class 1A and 1C antiarrhythmic drugs—slow the conduction in the retrograde pathway thus suppressing the AV nodal conduction.

   Drug of choice is adenosine for acute AVNRT termination, available in intravenous form with half-life is only 9 seconds. If adenosine is unsuccessful, beta-blocker or CCB is given. Digoxin is usually not given because of its limited usefulness.

   Recurrences may be prevented with any of the above drugs except adenosine.
B. Radiofrequency ablation can cure arrhythmias in majority of cases and thus eliminates the long-term suppressive therapy with medications.
C. Direct cardioversion should be done in unstable and symptomatic patients with low energy 10–50 J.

Atrioventricular Re-entrant Tachycardia

Pathophysiology

It relies on following paths:

A. Presence of accessory pathway as one portion of circuit
B. Presence of AV nodal path at other portion of circuit; atrium and ventricle are present on the same side of the accessory pathway.

Atrioventricular re-entrant tachycardia (AVRT) may be orthodromic or antidromic.

A. In case of orthodromic AVRT:
   a. AV node is used as antegrade limb.
   b. Accessory pathway as retrograde limb
   c. QRS complex is narrow.
B. In case of antidromic AVRT:
   a. Accessory pathway as antegrade limb
   b. AV node as retrograde limb
   c. QRS complex is wide.

Atrioventricular re-entrant tachycardia is mostly orthodromic type, here accessory pathway is concealed because of its retrograde conduction (ventricle to atrium) properties or it manifests as "delta" wave in ECG as in case of Wolff-Parkinson-White (WPW) syndrome.

In AVRT, unlike AVNRT, one ventricle must be involved hence bundle branch on the side of accessory pathway will prolong the atrial and ventricular conduction time.

Clinical Features

It is like that of AVNRT.

Laboratory Features

A. Because atrial and ventricular depolarization occurs in series rather than parallel, hence P wave is inscribed in ST segment or in T wave.
B. RP segment is >100 ms.
C. In orthodromic type—QRS is marrow whereas, in antidromic type QRS is wide.

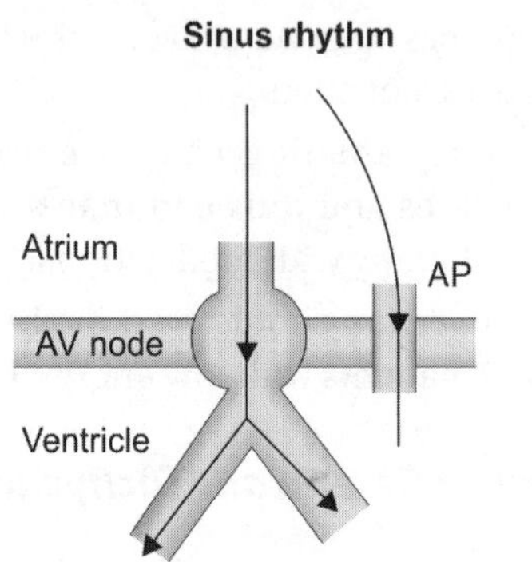

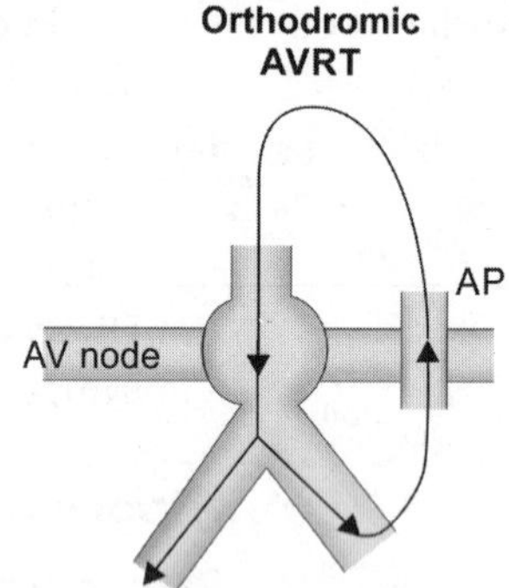

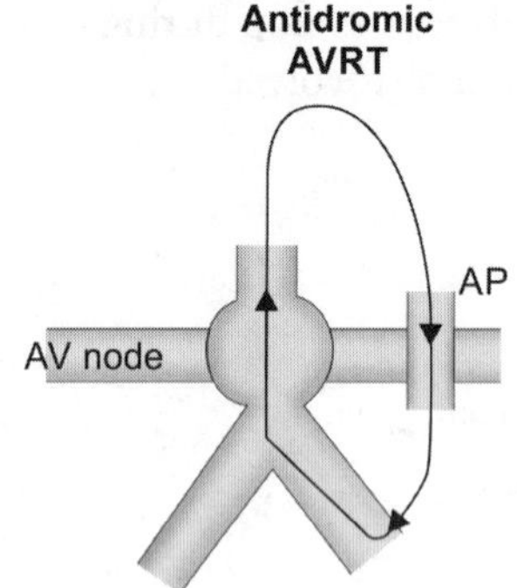

(AVRT: atrioventricular reentrant tachycardia)

Pre-excitation Syndrome

It refers to all the conditions where antegrade ventricular activation and retrograde atrial activation occur through wholly or partially through the anomalous pathway. Incidence is high in males with decreasing incidence with advancing age.

Pathophysiology

In this syndrome the accessory pathway runs between the atria and ventricles altering their conduction. The pathway may be congenital as there may be positive family history.

Wolff–Parkinson–White Syndrome

Here accessory pathway known as "Bundle of Kent" will permit atrial impulse to propagate to ventricles bypassing the normal pathways through the AV node. The impulse from the atria is conducted down the both accessory and AV nodal pathways to ventricle at near same time resulting pre-excitation of ventricle, which is really fusion beat having two components:

- **a.** A portion of ventricle activated via accessory pathway—give rise to "delta" wave
- **b.** Remainder portion of ventricle is activated through the normal activation pathway

If antegrade conduction occurs exclusively through accessory pathway, the resultant QRS complex will be wide. But this pathway has longer refractory period than AV node. The inciting event atrial premature complex is blocked in accessory pathway but propagates through the AV node to the ventricle as it has shorter refractory period, making normal width QRS complex. During this time accessory pathway will be recovered from its long refractory period, hence the impulse will be conducted retrogradely to atria. 5% patients have multiple accessory pathways.

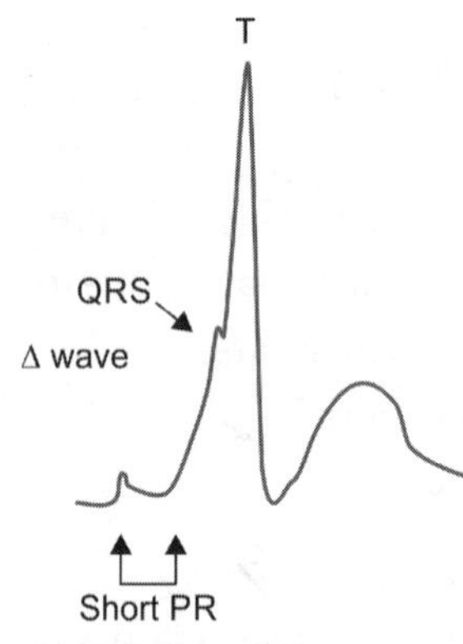

Mahaim Fiber Tachycardia

It is another form of reentrant tachycardia. There are two most common varieties:

A. Atriofascicular variety: Here the accessory pathway is located from right atrium to right bundle branch. As a result:

- **a.** Impulse will propagate antegradely via accessory pathways resulting left bundle branch block (LBBB) morphology along with left axis deviation.
- **b.** Impulse propagates through the AV nodal pathway retrogradely.

B. Fasciculoventricular variety: Here accessory pathway arises from His-Purkinje fibers to ventricle bypassing the distal conducting system. In this type there is no tachycardia; hence, therapy is not required.

Treatment

A. In case of paroxysmal supraventricular tachycardia (PSVT) with extreme hemodynamic instability or extreme symptomatic patients, stable patients are managed accordingly.

B. Normal QRS width: Both type, orthodromic and antidromic AV node dependent, are treated by:

- **a.** Vagal maneuvers
- **b.** AV nodal blocking drugs

c. Transvenous or transesophageal atrial pacemaker

d. Adenosine is effective in these AVRT but it may induce atrial fibrillation in 15% of patients.

e. In case of WPW syndrome having short refractory period of accessory pathway as it capable of rapid ventricular conduction—atrial fibrillation is a life-threatening complication; hence, it should be treated early.

C. Wide QRS width: In patients having accessory pathway usually present with wide QRS complex which results from any one of the following:

a. Antidromic AVRT

b. Orthodromic AVRT

c. Atrial arrhythmias like atrial fibrillation or atrial flutter where there is antidromic conduction occurring through antegrade pathway. Sometimes, it is not possible to diagnose the mechanism of wide QRS complex in the patients having accessory pathway, in that case drugs responsible for blocking the accessory pathway like procainamide should be given. Again in atrial arrhythmias if impulse propagates through accessory pathway antegradely, but not through AV nodal pathway, AV nodal blocking agents like beta-blocker, digoxin, and calcium blocking agents are avoided. If these drugs are given in wide complex atrial tachycardia, they will block AV nodal pathway and encourage the propagation of impulses through the accessory pathway leading to ventricular tachycardia and lastly ventricular fibrillation.

If tachycardia persists in spite of medical therapy, direct cardioversion with at least 200 Jules are required.

Long-term Management

A. Priority of therapy:

a. In asymptomatic patients with low risk of sudden death, no family history of sudden death, patient is not competitive athlete, or not at high occupation—usually no long-term therapy is required.

b. In symptomatic patient with history of atrial fibrillation, family history of sudden death, and have high risk occupation—long-term therapy is required.

B. Medical therapy: It is required in following conditions:

a. Patients with increased risk but no prior symptoms

b. In those patients whose accessory pathway is very close to normal conduction pathway that may precipitate AV block with radiofrequency ablation.

1. Single-drug therapy with amiodarone, flecainide, and sotalol as these drugs will slow the impulse conduction through the both pathways.

C. Combination therapy: Drugs acting AV node and the drugs blocking accessory pathway can be given in combination.

D. Percutaneous catheter ablation therapy: It is considered in following conditions:

a. Any patient with high risk

b. Patient having tachycardia refractory to medical therapy.

c. If patient is intolerant to medical therapy.

d. Patient is attached with high risk occupation like pilot.

Q10. Orthostatic hypotension, classification, and enumerate the various tests.

DNBIII/JUN2011 (10)

Pathophysiology and management of orthostatic hypotension.

DNB, 2022 (5)

RAJASTHAN UNIVERSITY, 2022 (11)

AIIMS (BBS), 2023 (10)

Define orthostatic hypotension. Enumerate the causes of neurogenic orthostatic hypotension. Describe the approach to the diagnosis and treatment of orthostatic hypotension.

DNB (OCT2024) (10)

Discuss the approach to a case of orthostatic hypotension.

WBUHS, 2025 (10)

ANSWER

Definition

Orthostatic hypertension can be defined as decrease in systolic blood pressure by 20 mm Hg decrease in diastolic blood pressure by 10 mm Hg within 3 minutes of standing as compared to blood pressure in sitting or supine position. It is present in 20% elderly patients.

Clinical Classification of Orthostatic Hypotension

A. Initial orthostatic hypotension: It can be defined as transient decrease in systolic blood pressure of >20 mm Hg and diastolic blood pressure of >20 mm Hg with symptom of cerebral hypoperfusion within 5–15 seconds after standing followed by resolution within 20 seconds.

B. Neurogenic orthostatic hypotension: It can be characterized as sustained decrease in systolic blood pressure by >20 mm Hg and diastolic blood pressure by >10 mm Hg with or without symptoms within 3 minutes of standing or head tilt. In this case sympathetic nervous system consistently fails to mediate reflex cardiovascular response to maintain normal blood pressure in response to orthostatic stress. This sympathetic noradrenergic failure occurs at sympathetic ganglia or postganglionic sympathetic neurons at vascular adrenergic receptors.

C. Delayed orthostatic hypotension: It can be characterized by hypotension fulfilling the criteria of neurogenic orthostatic hypotension but occurring after 3 minutes indicating milder form of adrenergic failure, causes are:

- **a.** Antihypertensive medications
- **b.** Venous pooling
- **c.** Transcapillary filtration of fluid
- **d.** Impairment of neurohumoral responses

D. Neurally mediated syncope or vasovagal syncope: It consists of complex phenomena which includes:

- **a.** Paroxysmal withdrawal of sympathetic vasomotor tone upon prolonged standing in a patients having otherwise normal functioning of autonomic nervous system.
- **b.** Following an interval of normal blood pressure in upright position
- **c.** Then decline in blood pressure within 1-3 minutes
- **d.** When the blood pressure decreases >50 mm Hg at cardiac level, patient becomes unconscious within 7 seconds.

E. Cardiovascular orthostatic hypotension: It will result from decrease in the circulatory blood volume leading to reflex tachycardia due to decreased cardiac output. The causes are:

- **a.** Dehydration
- **b.** Venous pooling:
  - **1.** Postprandial dilatation of splanchnic blood vessels
  - **2.** Sepsis
  - **3.** Prolonged recumbent or standing position
  - **4.** Vigorous exercises with dilatation of skeletal vessel bed
  - **5.** Alcohol
- **c.** Cardiac arrhythmias
- **d.** Cardiomyopathies
- **e.** Valvular cardiac diseases

F. Orthostatic pseudohypertension: It can be characterized by apparent orthostatic hypotension when baseline supine blood pressure will be elevated which may be due to:

- **a.** Concomitant recumbent hypertension
- **b.** Fluctuation of baseline blood pressure in patients having labile hypertension.

G. Metabolic orthostatic hypotension:

- **a.** Hypoaldosteronism
- **b.** Adrenocortical insufficiency
- **c.** Pheochromocytoma
- **d.** Severe potassium deficiency

H. Reduced intravascular volume:

- **a.** Burns
- **b.** Dehydration
- **c.** Emesis
- **d.** Diarrhea
- **e.** Hemorrhage
- **f.** Straining or heavy lifting

Different Tests to Diagnose Orthostatic Hypotension

A. Heart rate variation with deep breathing: It will test the parasympathetic component of cardiovascular reflexes through vagus nerve. Results are influenced by the following factors:

- **a.** Position of the patient—whether the patient is in standing, sitting, or in recumbent position.
- **b.** Rate and depth of the respiration—optimal measurement is 6 breaths per minute and FVC is >1.5 L.
- **c.** Medication
- **d.** Age
- **e.** Weight of the patient
- **f.** Degree of hypocapnia

Interpretation of the results is based on test data as compared to data of age-matched control in identical test conditions. For example:

1. Patient under 20 years of age, lower limit of normal heart rate variation is >15–20 beats/min
2. Patient >60 years of age, lower limit of normal heart rate variation is only 5–8 beats/min.

Interpretation: It will measure parasympathetic intactness. Muscarinic receptor antagonist like atropine will block variation of heart rate under deep breathing but sympathetic postganglionic blocker like propranolol has no affect.

B. Valsalva maneuver response:

a. Aim: It will assess the control between the parasympathetic tone in the form of heart rate and sympathetic adrenergic tone in the form of blood pressure, like:

1. Raised blood pressure will increase the vagal tone in the form of bradycardia through triggering of carotid bulb.
2. Decrease in blood pressure will decrease the vagal tone in the form of tachycardia.

b. In this method patient should be in supine position and asked to exhale fully against closed glottis or in a manometer which maintains 40 mm Hg expiratory pressure for 15 seconds during which time beat-to-beat blood pressure and change in heart rate are measured. There are four phases in Valsalva maneuver during which blood pressure and heart rate are measured. Following are the interpretation of results:

Phase	Maneuver	Blood pressure	Heart rates	Interpretations
I	Against partially closed glottis forced expiration	Raised due to aortic compression due to raised intrathoracic pressure	Decreased	Mechanical since it is related to intrathoracic and intra-abdominal pressure change
II early	Expiration should be continued	Decreased due to decreased venous return toward heart resulting reduced stroke volume	Reflex tachycardia	Vagal tone will be reduced
II late	Expiration should be continued	Raised toward or above baseline due to reflex increase in peripheral vascular resistance	Rate of increase will be slow	
III	Expiration end	Decreased due to increased capacitance of the pulmonary vascular bed	More increase in heart rate	Mechanical since it is related to intrathoracic and intra-abdominal pressure change
IV	Recovery	Raised temporarily above baseline due to: • Continued increase in pulmonary vascular resistance • Increased cardiac output	Compensatory bradycardia through the baroreceptor reflex	It requires intact sympathetic response

c. Interpretation:

1. During phase II recovery or phase IV if the blood pressure overshoots—it suggests dysfunction of sympathetic nervous system.
2. Parasympathetic function can be measured by heart rate changes during Valsalva maneuver. Valsalva ratio is defined as maximum tachycardia in phase II divided by maximum bradycardia in phase IV.

C. Sudomotor function:

a. Quantitative sudomotor axon reflex test: In normal subject sweating can be induced by release of acetylcholine from the sympathetic postganglionic fibers. This test can measure the regional acetylcholine-induced sweating as there is reduced or absent response which indicates postganglionic sudomotor axonic lesion. For example, in case of diabetic distal neuropathy there is decreased sweating in the feet.

b. Thermoregulatory sweat test: It will measure the global production of sweat in response to rise in body temperature and it can be demonstrated by placing the color change in indicator powder on the anterior surface of the body during raised temperature of the body. It will measure the intactness of both postganglionic and preganglionic sudomotor function.

Interpretation of the above two tests:

1. In case of postganglionic lesion—both the tests will show absent response.

2. In case preganglionic lesion—quantitative sudomotor axon reflex test will be normal but thermoregulatory sweat test demonstrates anhydrosis.

D. Orthostatic blood pressure recordings: In this test beat-to-beat recording of blood pressure is measured in supine, 70° tilt, and tilt-back position to determine the orthostatic failure of controlling blood pressure. The patient is asked to take rest in supine position for 20 minutes then beat to beat change in blood pressure and heart rate in different tilting position will be recorded for evaluation in a patient with unexplained syncope.

Tilt table is used in case of vasovagal syncope with specificity, sensitivity, and reproducibility. There is standard protocol for tilt apparatus, tilt-angle, and tilt-duration. Passive phase of 30–40 minutes with tilt-angle of 6–70° can detect reflex syncope, psychogenic syncope, or it may be nondiagnostic.

Treatment of Orthostatic Hypotension

Q11. Enumerate thrombolytic agents. Describe their indications, contraindications and complications in acute myocardial infarction.

DNBI/DEC2011 (10)

Newer thrombolytic agents in acute myocardial infarction.

BF/NOV2012/MDIV (10)

Discuss newer thrombolytic agents in acute myocardial infarction.

BF/NOV2013/MDIV (10)

Tenecteplase in acute myocardial infarction.

SNMC/MAY2013/MDIII (10)

ANSWER

Indication of Thrombolytic Agents

Acute myocardial infarction: In absence of any contraindication it has to be initiated within 30 minutes of presentation like door to needle time should be ≤30 minutes. These drugs promote conversion of plasminogen to plasmin which will lyse fibrin thrombi.

Angiographic flow pattern through the culprit coronary artery has been graded according to thrombolysis in myocardial infarction (TIMI) grading system:

a. Grade 0: Complete obstruction of the infarcted artery

b. Grade 1: There is some penetration of the contrast material beyond the point of obstruction.

c. Grade 2: There is evidence of perfusion of entire infarct vessel into the distal bed but the flow is delayed as compared to normal artery.

d. Grade 3: Evidence of full perfusion of the infarct vessel with normal flow. Later is the goal of reperfusion therapy, because full perfusion of the infarcted artery will provide better results to limit the size of infarct and reduce the short- and long-term mortality. Tissue plasminogen activator and other fibrin-specific plasminogen activators are more active than streptokinase in restoring full perfusion in the coronary circulation. Dose of tissue plasminogen activator is 15 mg bolus intravenously followed by 50 mg over 30 minutes followed by 35 mg over next 60 minutes.

Following thrombolytic agents used in case of myocardial infarction:

A. Fibrin-specific agents:

a. Reteplase—recombinant plasminogen activator: 10 unit + 10 units intravenous bolus at 30 minutes apart

b. Alteplase—tissue plasminogen activator: 15 mg intravenous bolus dose, followed by 0.75 mg/kg infusion over 30 minutes, then 0.5 mg/kg intravenous infusion over 60 minutes.

c. Tenecteplase—responsible for production of plasminogen conversion in absence of fibrin: It is given as single intravenous bolus dose according to the following criteria:

1. In case of <60 kg body weight—30 mg
2. If the body weight is <70 kg—35 mg
3. If the body weight is <90 kg—40 mg
4. If the body weight is >90 kg—50 mg

B. Nonfibrin-specific agents responsible catalyzing systemic fibrinolysis:

a. Urokinase

b. Streptokinase: 1.5 million units over 30–60 minutes

c. Urokinase

d. Prourokinase

e. Anisoylated purified streptokinase activator complex (anistrplase)

Short- and medium-term mortality to extent of ST segment resolution following thrombolytic therapy:

Categories of resolution	Resolution	30-day mortality	180-day mortality
Complete	≥70%	2.9%	4.8%
Partial	30–70%	5.8%	8.1%
None	≤30%	10.2%	11.1%

Contraindications of Thrombolytic Agents in STEMI

a. Absolute contraindications:
 1. Prior history of intracranial hemorrhage
 2. Known history of malignant intracranial neoplasm
 3. Known structural cerebral vascular lesion
 4. History of ischemic stroke in last 3 months
 5. History of bleeding diathesis with actively ongoing bleeding but excluding menstrual bleeding
 6. Suspected dissection of aortic aneurysm
 7. History of suspected closed head trauma or facial trauma within last 3 months
 8. History of intracranial or intraspinal surgery within last 2 months
 9. Severe uncontrolled hypertension not responding to emergency therapy
 10. In case of streptokinase history of prior treatment in last 6 months

b. Relative contraindications:
 1. History, chronic, severe, and poorly controlled hypertension
 2. Dementia
 3. Active diagnosed peptic ulcer
 4. Pregnancy or within 1 week of postpartum
 5. History of internal bleeding within last 2–4 weeks
 6. History of prior ischemic stroke in last 3 months
 7. Current use of anticoagulant increasing the INR >1.7 or prothrombin time more than 15 seconds.
 8. History of traumatic or >10 minutes cardiopulmonary resuscitation or major surgery within last 3 weeks
 9. At presentation significant systolic blood pressure of >180 mm Hg and diastolic blood pressure of >110 mm Hg
 10. Active cavitating pulmonary tuberculosis
 11. Infective endocarditis
 12. Puncture of noncompressible blood vessels in last 2 weeks

Potential Benefits of Late Perfusion

a. Scar formation will be improved and healing.
b. Infarct size will be reduced.
c. Expansion of infarct will be decreased.
d. Remodeling of noninfarct zone will be decreased.
e. Left ventricular volume will be decreased.
f. Incidence of arrhythmia will be decreased.
g. Mural thrombus formation will be reduced.
h. Provision of collateral flow to another infarct zone

Complications of Thrombolytic Therapy

a. Hemorrhage
b. Allergic reaction
c. Stroke
d. Embolism
e. Reperfusion arrhythmias

Following are the risk factors for above complications:

a. Increasing age >70 years
b. Low birth weight
c. Uncontrolled hypertension
d. Recent history of stroke or surgery
e. Presence of bleeding diathesis
f. Elevated pulse pressure
g. Severe congestive heart failure

Q12. Discuss causes, consequences of atherosclerosis and preventive strategies.

DNBIV/JUN2011 (10)

Discuss the risk factors of athero-sclerosis. Describe the management of hyperlipidemias.

DNBI/DEC2012 (10)

Describe the risk factors and preventive aspect of atherosclerosis.

ERA/MAY2011/MDII (10)

Enumerate the causes of secondary hyperlipidemias.

MGR/OCT2012/MDIV (7)

Anatomy and physiological changes in atheromatous plaques.

BABA FARID UNI OF HEALTH SC, 2019 (10)

ANSWER

Atherosclerosis

It is made up of patchy intimal plaque, atheroma, and most common sites being the large and medium sized arteries. The components of plaque are:

a. Cellular component—inflammatory cells and smooth muscle cells
b. Fibrous component—connective tissue
c. Fat component—lipid

Risk factors of atherosclerosis are:

a. Age
b. Family history
c. Male sex
d. Diabetes mellitus
e. Hypertension
f. Smoking
g. Hyperlipidemia
h. Alcohol intake
i. Hyperhomocysteinemia
j. Obesity
k. Sedentary lifestyle
l. Chlamydia infection

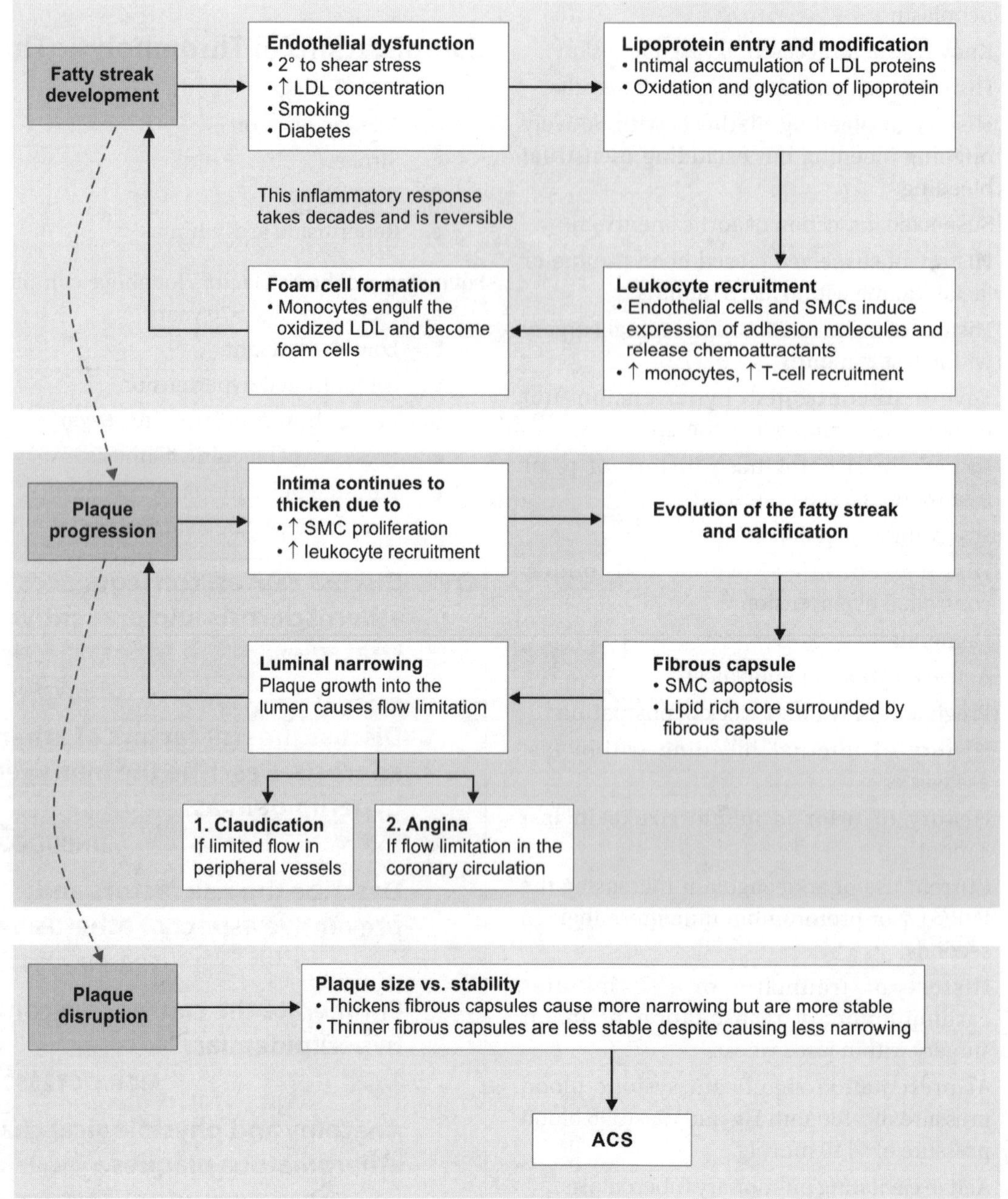

(ACS: acute coronary syndrome; LDL: low-density lipoprotein; SMCs: smooth muscle cells)

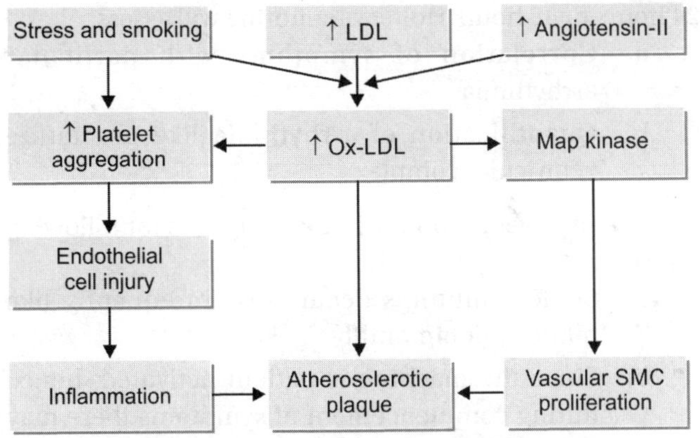

(LDL: low-density lipoprotein; SMCs: smooth muscle cells)

Causes of Secondary Hyperlipidemias

Pharmacological	• Corticoids • Alcohol • Oral contraceptives • Diuretics: β-blockers • Anabolic • Immunosuppressive drugs • Isotretinoin
Endocrine/ metabolic	• Obesity • Hypothyroidism • Hypopituitarism • Diabetes mellitus • Cushing syndrome • Idiopathic hypercalcemia • Pregnancy • Lipodystrophy • Acute intermittent porphyria
Liver diseases	• Hepatitis • Biliary atresia • Biliary cirrhosis • Alagille syndrome
Nephropathies	• Nephrotic syndrome • Hemolytic uremic syndrome • Chronic renal insufficiency
Infectious disease	• Acute viral/bacterial infection • HIV • Hepatitis • Pancreatitis
Inflammatory disease	• Systemic lupus erythematosus • Juvenile rheumatoid arthritis
Storage diseasea	• Glycogenosis • Sphingolipidoses • Gaucher disease • Cysteine storage disease • Juvenile Tay-Sachs disease
	• Niemann-Pick disease • Lipase acid deficiency
Others	• Kawasaki disease • Anorexia nervosa • Postsolid organ transplantation • Childhood cancer survivor • Progeria • Idiopathic hypercalcemia • Klinefelter syndrome • Werner syndrome

Q13. How do you approach a patient with cardiac arrhythmia? Classify antiarrhythmic drugs.

DNBIII/DEC2011 (10)

Antiarrhythmic drugs.

MGR/SEP2009/MDI (5) MGR/FEB2005/MDIII (5)

Diagnostic evaluation of tachyarrhythmias.

KUHS/MAY2013/MDII (10)

Treatment of tachyarrhythmias.

KUHS/MAY2013/MDIV (10)

Classify antiarrhythmic drugs. Etiology and management of atrial arrhythmias.

SAURASHTRA UNIVERSITY, 2022 (20)

Write about conduction system of heart. Write briefly about antiarrhythmic drugs

DR YSR UNI OF HEALTH SC, VIJAYAWADA, ANDHRA, 2022 (10)

Management of supraventricular tachycardia.

MGR UNIVERSITY, TAMIL NADU, 2021 (10)

Antiarrhythmic drugs.

MGR UNIVERSITY, TAMIL NADU, 2020 (10)

Etiopathogenesis of atherosclerosis. Mention early detection method for plaque and primary prevention.

SCBMCH, 2020 (20)

Classify anti-arrhythmic drugs. Describe their uses in different clinical scenario.

MANIPUR UNIVERSITY, 2019 (10)

ANSWER

Approach to arrhythmias is highly individualized, there are main two steps upon which the full diagnostic work-up and therapy are formed, and these are proper history and ECG. Arrhythmia can present with wide spectrum of presentation, it may be completely asymptomatic that can be diagnosed on routine ECG or the patient may undergo cardiac arrest. So, the more severe the clinical presentation the more aggressive is the evaluation followed by treatment.

Syncope may be due to cardiac origin, in that case extensive history should be taken regarding the family history of syncope or sudden death, past history of myocardial infarction or any other structural heart disease. Again family history of sudden death may influence the evaluation of heritable arrhythmias.

Palpitation in the absence of cardiopulmonary diseases may be of little clinical significance, but not always. Again, palpitation or syncope in presence of cardiac or pulmonary disease like atrial fibrillation or severe bradycardia has more ominous implications.

From the diagnosis point of view ECG is the only most important investigation that is required to diagnose arrhythmias provided it must be done at the time of presentation.

But another important investigation has to be done to confirm the specific diagnosis is electrophysiological study, by which following can be diagnosed:

- **a.** Delta wave in case of WPW syndrome
- **b.** Prolongation or shortening of QT interval
- **c.** Right precordial ST-segment abnormalities in case of Brugada syndrome
- **d.** Epsilon wave in case of arrhythmogenic right ventricular dysplasia.

Electrophysiological study is:

- **a.** Mostly interventional for diagnosis and therapy
- **b.** It can diagnose the mechanism of arrhythmia.
- **c.** It can deliver catheter-based ablative treatment.
- **d.** It can diagnose the etiology of symptoms like syncope, palpitation which occur due to arrhythmia.

The component of this study is baseline measurement during rest and understress or during maneuvers like pacing and pharmacotherapy.

Variants of body surface recordings like Holter monitoring with event recording, either continuous or intermittent body surface ECG recordings over long periods, may diagnose different cardiac arrhythmias during occurrence of symptoms.

24 hours or 48 hours Holter monitoring will assess:

- **a.** Correlation of symptoms with particular arrhythmia
- **b.** Quantification of arrhythmia like premature ventricular complex

Ambulatory event monitor is advantageous for following reasons:

- **a.** Some symptoms occur very infrequently like monthly or bimonthly.
- **b.** Since the machine is patient-activated, hence during commencement of symptoms there may be correlation with arrhythmias.

Implantable long-term monitor is of value in:

- **a.** Telemetric monitoring for diagnosis as well as efficacy of therapy
- **b.** Evaluating the infrequent but malignant symptoms which cannot be provoked at electrophysiological study.
- **c.** Assessing the presence of burden of atrial fibrillation (AF) in patients with stroke.

Exercise ECG is used in following circumstances:

- **a.** To determine the presence of myocardial ischemia.
- **b.** To analyze the morphology of QT interval during exercise as whether there is any chance of ventricular arrhythmias.
- **c.** To assess the appearance of symptom during activity.

Cardiac imaging can assess the any myocardial structural changes that may produce arrhythmia in future. For example:

- **a.** Ventricular arrhythmias usually occurs in following cases:
  1. Ventricular systolic dysfunction
  2. Dilatation of cardiac chambers
  3. Hypertrophic cardiomyopathy
  4. Infiltrative disease like sarcoidosis
- **b.** Supraventricular arrhythmias may occur in following conditions:
  1. Congenital conditions like AV reentry in Epstein anomaly

Echocardiography can diagnose:

- **a.** Structural abnormalities in the heart.
- **b.** Defect in the cardiac function.

MRI of heart can diagnose:

- **a.** Burden of scar in case of MI.
- **b.** Other structural abnormalities.

c. Arrhythmogenic right ventricular cardiomyopathy.

Head-up tilt test: It can evaluate a patient with history of syncope where there is suspicion of exaggerated vagal tone or vasodepression. Physiologically, during this test there is redistribution of blood volume along with increased ventricular contractility. But exaggerated activation of central reflex will lead to:

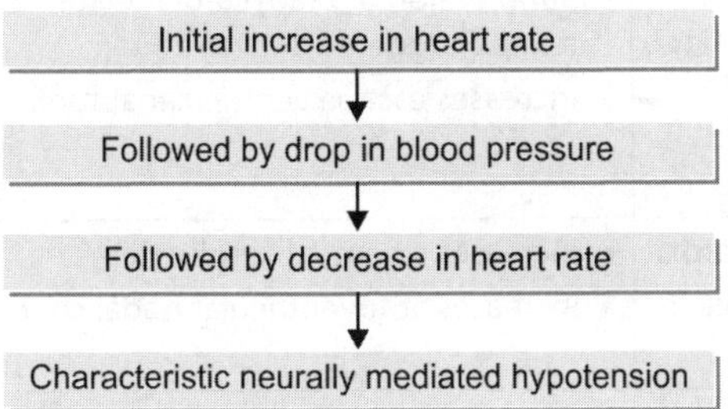

This test is useful for diagnosis of:

a. Orthostatic hypotension
b. Recurrent syncope or
c. Single episode of syncope with injury mainly in absence of structural heart disease
d. Syncope where other causes like ventricular arrhythmias has been excluded.

This test is contraindicated in following cases:

a. Severe coronary artery disease in presence of proximal coronary artery stenosis
b. In presence of severe mitral stenosis
c. In case of severe aortic stenosis producing obstruction to left ventricular outflow tract
d. Known case of severe cerebrovascular diseases.

Antiarrhythmic Drugs

Class	Subclass	Name of the drug	Clinical applications	Likely therapeutic mechanisms
Hyperpolarization-activated cyclic nucleotide-gated channel blocker				
0		Ivabradine	• Stable angina • CHF with heart rate ≥70 beats/min • Potential for new arrhythmias	Sinoatrial automaticity will be reduced
Voltage-gated sodium channel blockers				
1	1a	• Quinidine • Disopyramide • Ajmaline	• Supraventricular tachyarrhythmias • Recurrent AF • VT • VF • Brugada syndrome	• Reduction in ectopic atrial/ventricular automaticity • Accessory pathway conduction is reduced • Refractory period is increased • Reentrant tendency is reduced
	1b	• Lidocaine • Mexiletine	VT and VF mainly after MI	• Ectopic ventricular automaticity is reduced • Delayed afterdepolarization-induced triggered activity will be reduced • Reentrant tendency is reduced by converting unidirectional block to bidirectional block in ischemic partially depolarized myocardium
	1c	• Flecainide • Propafenone	• SVT, atrial flutter, AF and tachycardia involving accessory pathway • VT resistant to other treatment in absence of structural disease • Catecholaminergic polymorphic VT	• Ectopic ventricular automaticity is reduced • Delayed afterdepolarization-induced triggered activity will be reduced • Reentrant tendency is reduced by converting unidirectional block to bidirectional block • Reduction of excitability at rapid heart rate blocking reentrant pathways by depressing conduction
	1d	Ranolazine	• Stable angina • VT	• Decrease the action potential recovery time • Reduce early-after depolarization induced triggered activity

Continued

Continued

Class	Subclass	Name of the drug	Clinical applications	Likely therapeutic mechanisms
Autonomic inhibitors and activators				
II	IIa	Nonselective beta inhibitors like carvedilol, propranolol, nadolol	• Sinus tachycardia and other types of SVT • Rate control in AF and ventricular tachyarrhythmias	• Reduce sinoatrial and atrioventricular nodal automaticity • Reduce ectopic atrial/ventricular automaticity • Reduce DAD- and EAD-induced triggered activity
	IIb	Isoproterenol	• Increases the rate of ventricular escape rhythm in case of CHB prior to implantation of pacemaker • Drug-related bradycardia-dependent torsades de pointes	• Suppression of bradycardia-related EAD-related triggered activity • Increases escape ventricular automaticity
	IIc	• Atropine • Hyoscine • Scopolamine	• Mild-to-moderate sinus bradycardia • Super-HIS, AVN conduction block in inferior MI, vagal syncope	• Increases sinoatrial conduction • Increases atrioventricular nodal conduction
	IId	• Carbacol • Pilocarpine • Methacholine • Digoxin	SVT, sinus tachycardia	• Reduce sinoatrial automaticity • Reduce sinoatrial nodal entry • Reduce atrioventricular conduction
	IIe	• Adenosine • ATP	Acutely terminate AV nodal tachycardia and cAM-mediated triggered VT	• Reduce sinoatrial automaticity • Reduce sinoatrial nodal entry • Reduce atrioventricular conduction • Reduce of EAD- and DAD-induced triggered activity
Potassium channel blockers and openers				
III	IIIa	• Amiodarone • Ambasilide • Sotalol • Dofetilide • Ibutilide	• VT in case of structural heat disease or MI • WPW syndrome • AF with atrioventricular conduction through the accessory pathway • VF • Premature ventricular contraction • Tachyarrhythmias with AF or SVT	• Increases action potential recovery time • Increased refractory period with decreased reentry
		Vermakalant	Immediate conversion to AF	• Increases action potential recovery time • Increases refractory period with decreased reentry
	IIIb	• Nicorandil • Pinacidil	• Stable angina—Nicorandil • Pinacidil—in the treatment of hypertension	Decrease in action potential recovery time
	IIIc	Blockers under regulatory review in AF		Reduce sinoatrial automaticity
Calcium handling modulators				
IV	IVa	Bepridil	• Angina pectoris • SVT	• Reduce AV nodal conduction • Reduce reentry
		• Verapamil • Diltiazem	SVT and VT without structural heart disease	• Reduce AV nodal conduction • Reduce reentry • Reduce EAD- and DAD-induced triggered activity

Continued

Continued

Class	Subclass	Name of the drug	Clinical applications	Likely therapeutic mechanisms
	IVb	• Flecainide • Propafenone	Catecholaminergic polymorphic VT	Reduce EAD- and DAD-induced triggered activity
	IVc, IVd and IVe	No clinically approved drug		Reduce EAD- and DAD-induced triggered activity
Gap junction channel blockers				
V		Blocker under investigation		• Reduce ventriculoatrial conduction • Reduce accessory pathway conduction
Upstream target modulator				
VI		• ACEI • Captopril • Enalapril • Ramipril	• HTN • Symptomatic heart failure • Potential application in reducing arrhythmic substrate	Reduce structural and electrophysiological remodeling changes which compromise conduction of action potential
		• Losartan • Telmisartan • Olmesartan • Valsartan	• HTN • Symptomatic heart failure • Potential application in reducing arrhythmic substrate	Reduce structural and electrophysiological remodeling changes which compromise conduction of action potential
		• Omega-3 fatty acid • Eicosapentaenoic acid	• Post-MI reduction of risk factors of cardiac death. • MI • Stroke • Abnormal cardiac rhythms	Reduce structural and electrophysiological remodeling changes which compromise conduction of action potential
		Statins	• Post-MI reduction of risk factors of cardiac death • MI • Stroke • Abnormal cardiac rhythms	Reduce structural and electrophysiological remodeling changes which compromise conduction of action potential

(AF: atrial fibrillation; ACEI: angiotensin-converting enzyme inhibitor; ATP: adenosine triphosphate; AVN: atrioventricular node; CHB: complete heart block; CHF: congestive heart failure; DAD: delayed afterdepolarization; EAD: early afterdepolarization; HTN: hypertension; MI: myocardial infarction; VT: ventricular tachycardia; VF: ventricular fibrillation; SVT: supraventricular tachycardia; WPW: Wolff-Parkinson-White)

Classification of Atrial Arrhythmias

A. Sinus tachycardia
B. Atrial premature complexes
C. Atrial tachycardia
D. Atrial flutter
E. Atrial fibrillation
F. Atrioventricular reentrant tachycardia
G. Atrioventricular nodal reentrant tachycardia
H. Junctional ectopic tachycardia

Etiology of Atrial Arrhythmias

A. Structural heart disease:
- **a.** Coronary artery disease
- **b.** Valvular heart disease—stenosis or regurgitation
- **c.** Congenital heart disease
- **d.** Cardiomyopathies:
  - **1.** Dilated cardiomyopathy
  - **2.** Restricted cardiomyopathy
  - **3.** Hypertrophic cardiomyopathy

B. Hypertension leading to left atrial enlargement, cardiac remodeling resulting atrial fibrillation.

C. Pulmonary disease:
  a. Pulmonary embolism
  b. Pulmonary hypertension
  c. Chronic obstructive pulmonary disease

D. Infection and inflammation:
  a. Myocarditis
  b. Pericarditis

E. Electrolyte imbalance:
  a. Hyperkalemia
  b. Hypokalemia
  c. Hypomagnesemia

F. Thyroid diseases: Hyperthyroidism

G. Stimulants triggering arrhythmias:
  a. Alcohol
  b. Caffeine
  c. Nicotine
  d. Cocaine
  e. Amphetamine

H. Obstructive sleep apnea

I. Autonomic dysfunction:
  a. Increased vagal tone
  b. Sympathetic stimulation during stress and exertion

J. Genetic: Familial atrial fibrillation

K. Post-surgical:
  a. Cardiac surgery
  b. Coronary artery bypass graft
  c. Valve surgery
  d. Catheter ablation for treating other arrhythmias

L. Age-related degenerative changes in the electrical conduction system

Antiarrhythmic Drugs in Case of Atrial arrhythmias

A. Amiodarone:
  a. Orally 200–400 mg/day as leading dose followed by 600–800 mg daily for 1 to 2 weeks.
  b. Intravenously 150 mg over 10 minutes followed by 1 mg/min for 6 hours followed by 0.5 mg/min.
  c. Indications:
    1. Atrial flutter
    2. Atrial flutter
    3. Atrial tachycardia

B. Flecainide:
  a. Orally 50–200 mg twice daily.
  b. It is used in:
    1. Atrial fibrillation
    2. Atrial flutter

C. Propafenone:
  a. Orally 150–300 mg thrice daily.
  b. It is given in:
    1. Atrial flutter
    2. Atrial fibrillation

D. Sotalol:
  a. Orally 80–160 mg twice daily.
  b. It is indicated in:
    1. Atrial flutter
    2. Atrial fibrillation

E. Dofetilide:
  a. Orally it is given at a dose of 500 mg twice daily.
  b. It is indicated in atrial flutter and atrial fibrillation.

Beta-blockers: It is used to control rate in case of atrial arrhythmias.

A. Metoprolol:
  a. Orally 25–100 mg twice daily
  b. Intravenously 2.5–5 mg as bolus dose over 2 minutes followed by repetition every 5 minutes with total dose up to 15 mg.
  c. It is indicated in
    1. Atrial flutter
    2. Atrial fibrillation

B. Atenolol:
  a. Orally 25–100 mg once daily.
  b. It is given in atrial fibrillation to control rate.

C. Esmolol:
  a. It is given intravenously 500 mcg/kg as loading dose to be given over 1 minute followed by continuous infusion of 200 mcg/kg/min.
  b. It is given in critical care in atrial fibrillation to control rate.

Calcium channel blockers: It is used in atrial flutter and fibrillation to control rate.

A. Diltiazem:

a. Orally 120–360 mg daily.

b. Intravenously 0.25 mg/kg as bolus dose over a period of 2 minutes followed by 5–15 mg hourly as continuous infusion.

B. Verapamil:

a. Orally 120–360 mg daily as extended release tablet.

b. Intravenously 2.5–10 mg as bolus dose over 2 minutes and can be repeated after 15–30 minutes.

Digoxin: It is indicated to control the rate in case of heart failure, atrial flutter and atrial fibrillation.

a. Oral dose is 0.125–0.25 mg daily.

b. Intravenous dose is 0.25 mg bolus every 2 hourly up to total dose of 1.5 mg.

Anticoagulation: It is recommended in patient with atrial flutter or atrial fibrillation as there is risk of thrombo-embolism or stroke based on CHA_2DS_2-VASc score.

A. Warfarin:

a. Its dose is adjusted with PT or APTT and INR.

b. It is used as long term control.

B. Dabigatran:

a. Orally it is given as 150 mg twice daily and should be adjusted according to renal function.

b. It is indicated in non-valvular atrial fibrillation.

C. Rivaroxaban:

a. It is given as 20 mg once daily and in case renal impairment 15 mg daily.

b. It is indicated in non-valvular atrial fibrillation.

D. Apixaban:

a. It is given orally 5 mg twice daily and in renal impairment 2.5 mg twice daily.

b. It is given in non-valvular atrial fibrillation.

E. Edoxaban:

a. Orally 60 mg once daily, but in renal impairment dose should be half.

b. It is indicated for stroke prevention in non-valvular atrial fibrillation.

Catheter Ablation

In case drug refractory atrial arrhythmia radiofrequency catheter ablation should be done which involves heat applied destruction of small area of cardiac tissue leading to development of abnormal electrical signal with the aim to restoring of normal rhythm.

Electrical Cardioversion

In case of tachycardia resulting hemodynamic instability and refractory to medication direct cardioversion is given to restore the sinus rhythm.

Treatment of Underlying Cases

A. Hyperthyroidism
B. Hyperkalemia
C. Hypokalemia
D. Heart failure
E. Coronary artery disease

Treatment of Underlying Risk Related Factors

A. Alcohol
B. Caffeine
C. Cocaine
D. Hypertension
E. Obesity
F. Stress

Implantation of implantable cardioverter or pace maker.

Q14. Classify congenital cyanotic heart disease. Describe the clinical features and management of Fallot's tetralogy.

DNBIII/DEC2011 (10)

ANSWER

Classification of Congenital Heart Diseases

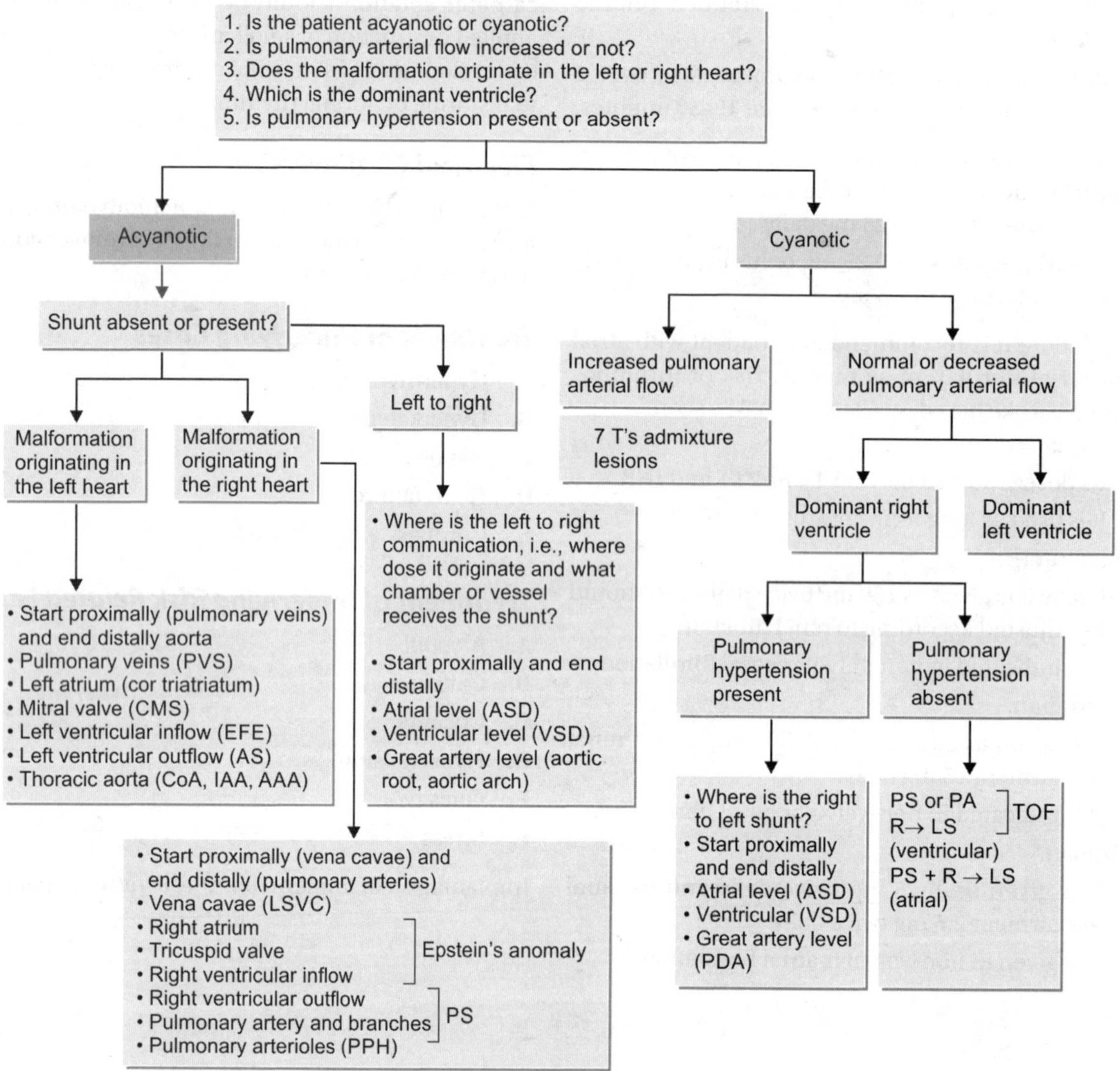

(AAA: abdominal aortic aneurysm; ASD: atrial septal defect; AS: aortic stenosis; CMS: congenital mitral stenosis; CoA: coarctation of the aorta; EFE: endocardial fibroelastosis; IAA: interrupted aortic arch; LS: left shunt; PA: pulmonary atresia; PDA: patent ductus arteriosus; PPH: primary pulmonary hypertension; PVS: pulmonary valvar stenosis; PS: pulmonary stenosis; TOF: tetralogy of Fallot; VSD: ventricular septal defect)

Fallot's Tetralogy

It is a common congenital heart disease, having 1 in 3,000 live births. Its pathology is composed of:

- **a.** Right ventricular outflow tract obstruction
- **b.** Nonrestrictive VSD
- **c.** Overriding of the aorta of ventricular septum involving >50% of right ventricle
- **d.** Right ventricular hypertrophy

All the above results from anterocephalad deviation of outlet septum.

Other associated lesions are the following:

a. Anomalous origin of the left anterior descending coronary artery from right coronary artery
b. Prominent conal branch from right coronary artery
c. Atrial septal defect of ostium secundum type
d. Presence of right aortic arch in 25% cases
e. Aortic insufficiency from long-term dilatation of aortic root
f. Other rare complications are:
    1. Pulmonary hypertension
    2. Supravalvular mitral stenosis
    3. Subaortic stenosis

Clinical Features

A. In case of patients who are not undergone surgical repair:
    a. Symptoms are:
        1. Central cyanosis
        2. Presence of "hypoxic spells" at 6 months of age characterized by:
            - Respiratory distress
            - Tachypnea
            - Cyanosis
            - Loss of consciousness
            - Death
        3. In case of mild obstruction shunt is left to right resulting "pink tet" along with minimal symptoms.
    b. On physical examination:
        1. Central cyanosis
        2. Clubbing
        3. Prominent right ventricular impulse due to equalization of right and left ventricular pressures
        4. Lift in right sternoclavicular junction in patients with right-sided aortic arch
        5. First heart sound is normal.
        6. Second heart sounds is single because pulmonary component is inaudible.
        7. Prominent systolic ejection murmur on left sternal border is associated with thrill due to infundibular stenosis—if the duration of murmur is short the severity will be increased.
        8. Early diastolic murmur along with aortic click due to dilated aortic root and overriding of aorta.
        9. Continuous murmur due to presence of aortopulmonary collateral vessels in the setting of pulmonary atresia.

B. In case of adult with undergone surgical repair with or without palliative repair: Last two shunt processes are abandoned now. Symptoms vary according to type of palliation:
    a. Brachial pulse on the anastomotic side is feeble or absent.
    b. There may be continuous murmur if pulse is present, it may also be due to aortopulmonary collaterals.
    c. Pulmonary artery stenosis prior to shunt insertion site may produce unilateral systolic or continuous murmur.
    d. Systolic ejection murmur—it will vary according to antegrade flow across the outflow tract.

C. In case of complete repair consisting of closure of VSD with patch along with variable degree of resection of right ventricular outflow tract.
    a. Symptoms:
        1. May be asymptomatic
        2. But they may present in late with:
            - Dyspnea
            - Exercise intolerance
            - Palpitations
            - Signs of right-sided heart failure
            - Syncope
        3. In absence of right ventricular dysfunction JVP is normal. But in presence of right ventricular dysfunction JVP will be increased with prominent "a" wave.
        4. Hyperdynamic pulse of aortic insufficiency
        5. Presence of lift at right sternoclavicular junction in case of right-sided aortic arch.
        6. Variable systolic ejection murmur with thrill at left sternal border with radiation to back and peripheral lung field.
        7. Presence of systolic murmur at lower left sternal border indicates presence of residual VSD.
        8. Continuous murmur due to presence of collaterals or prior shunt.

Treatment

A. If the patient has not undergone surgical repair or undergone palliative treatment, following problem may be expected:
   a. Chronic hypoxemia
   b. Pulmonary hypertension
   c. Erythrocytosis
   d. Long-term effect of right ventricular outflow tract obstruction
   e. Exposure of pulmonary circulation to systemic shunt flow
   f. Progressive infundibular pulmonary stenosis
   g. Paradoxical emboli
   h. Atrial arrhythmias
   i. Ventricular arrhythmias
   j. Endocarditis
   k. Increased risk of aortic insufficiency

B. Follow-up of the patients who already undergone surgical repair:
   a. They are increased risk of sudden death.
   b. Atrial and ventricular arrhythmias
   c. Pulmonary insufficiency—can be tolerated for many years, as a result of chronic right ventricular volume overload leads to right-sided heart failure. Hence is the most common indication of redo surgery after initial repair.
   d. Residual VSD
   e. Residual right ventricular outflow tract gradient
   f. Formation of right ventricular tract aneurysm at the site of repair by patch

C. Prophylaxis of infective endocarditis is required in patients with palliative treatment or who are unrepaired. Prophylaxis is recommended for only 6 months following prosthetic material or device placement or any residual defect. In case of pulmonary valve replacement with prosthetic material antibiotic prophylaxis is also required.

Surgical Intervention

It is either by repair or reintervention.

Goals of total repair are:
   a. Relieve the outflow tract obstruction
   b. Maintain the competency of preferably native pulmonary valve
   c. Closure of VSD

Processes of repair are the following:
   a. Classic Blalock–Taussig shunt: Anastomosis between native subclavian artery and right or left pulmonary artery
   b. Modified Blalock–Taussig shunt: Expanded polyfluoroethylene material shunt between innominate or subclavian artery and pulmonary artery
   c. Pott's shunt: Anastomosis between descending aorta and left pulmonary artery
   d. Waterston shunt: Anastomosis between ascending aorta and right pulmonary artery

Indications of reintervention are:
   a. Replacement of pulmonary valve in case of pulmonary valve insufficiency
   b. Replacement or revision of homograft in presence of residual symptoms of VSD.

Q15. Describe the principle and clinical uses of stress test. Differentiate between stress echocardiography and stress thallium.

DNBIII/DEC2010 (10)

Limitations of stress test.

BF/OCT2011/MDIV (10)

Stress echocardiography.

BF/OCT2011/MDIV (10)

ANSWER

Principle of Stress Test

A. Exercise stress testing: Standard stress testing has been replaced by nuclear imaging. In this method radioisotope has to be injected at the peak of exercise, the time is allowed for the circulation of this dye during exercise which is at least 1 minute before the termination of the exercise.

B. If the patient is not able to do exercise, in that case pharmacological intervention is followed by testing called pharmacologic stress testing—in this regard, following vasodilators are used:
   a. Adenosine: 140 μg/kg/min intravenous infusion over 6 minutes and radiotracer will be injected after 3 minutes of starting the infusion of adenosine.
   b. Dipyridamole: 0.142 mg/kg/min intravenous infusion over 4 minutes and maximum

vasodilatory effect is achieved after 4 minutes of complete transfusion and at that point radiotracer has to be injected. It will result slight increase in heart rate and decrease in blood pressure.

c. Regadenoson: It is selective A2A receptor agonist.
d. Dobutamine: It is β1 and β2 receptors agonist. It will increase the myocardial contractility and heart rate.

Interpretation of Test

A. Standard view of normal anatomy.
B. Review of sequence of image:
   a. Examination of unprocessed image to detect any artefact, extracardiac uptake, or evidence of increased uptake by lung.
   b. Rest image to be seen to detect extent and severity of defects.
   c. Stress image should be seen to detect the extent and severity of defect.
   d. Evaluation of polar map to compare with the pooled images which is derived from data base.
   e. Comparison between rest and stress images to detect any defect in the left ventricular cavity.
C. Characteristics of the defect:
   Here the defect is classified as:
   a. Fixed or nonreversible: Here decreased uptake of tracer is fixed and unchanged in both rest and during stress—it can be represented as scar.
   b. Reversible: Here the segment which is nonperfused during stress test will be normally perfused during rest—so it is ischemic myocardium but no scar.
   c. Partially reversible: Here the nonperfused area visible during stress test becomes partially resolved during rest—so it is an area of mixed ischemic and scarred myocardium.
   d. Reverse redistribution: Here the defect is absent in stress test but appears in rest image or appears larger in rest image as compared to stress image.

Indications of the Stress Test

A. Coronary artery disease:
   a. Detection of coronary artery disease
   b. Risk stratification
   c. Myocardial perfusion imaging
B. Assessment of ventricular function
C. Myocardial innervation imaging
D. Cardiac amyloidosis

Advantages of Stress Test

A. It can assess the ischemia, functional capacity, and prognosis.
B. Wide availability of equipment
C. It can be tested in different population accurately.

Disadvantages of Stress Test

A. Its sensitivity is lower as compared to stress imaging test.
B. It cannot localize the site and extent of myocardial ischemia which is immensely useful for revascularization.
C. Its specificity is poor with:
   a. Marked abnormalities in ST-T in the resting ECG
   b. Digitalis use
   c. LBBB or pace maker
   d. Female population

Stress Thallium Test

Here radiotracer is thallium-201 emitting gamma-ray and has half-life of 73 hours. It is actively transported into the cells by sodium-potassium adenosine triphosphatase (Na-K-ATPase) pump. Radionuclide is injected 1 minute before the peak exercise, sometimes it will be allowed for its redistribution. First image will be taken 5–10 minutes after injection and image for redistribution will be taken after 2.5–4 hours after first image.

a. Its initial uptake is related to regional blood flow. Myocardial extraction of thallium-201 is increased at low flow rate and decreased at high flow rate.
b. 85% of thallium is extracted by myocytes during first pass. Radiotracer distribution changes after administration and washout of thallium from myocytes—this process is called redistribution.
c. In case of ischemic myocardium uptake of thallium-201 is lower as compared to nonischemic segments, again, washout time is also slower than that from nonischemic segments.
d. This test is highly specific for scar at 2.5–4 hours after injection because this persistent defect sometimes may represent as viable myocardium. Hence, third image should be taken 18–24 hours after injection to see evidence of delayed imaging or late redistribution as uptake of radiotracer after revascularization.
e. Alternate approach is to inject thallium again to see the improved uptake due to neovascularization.

Advantages of This Test

- **a.** It is most available as well as most accurate test for diagnosis of coronary artery disease.
- **b.** It has high risk stratification capability, as abnormal perfusion scan is highly suggestive of coronary artery disease. It is very much sensitive to very small variation of blood flow.
- **c.** It is improved diagnostic accuracy as compared to stress echocardiography.

Stress Echocardiography

In this method echocardiography is done at resting condition and then immediately after exercise by treadmill walking or ride in a stationary bike till the achievement of target heart rate. During this point echocardiography will be done.

Causes of Incorrect Results in Stress Echocardiography

A. False positive results:
- **a.** Left bundle branch block prior to cardiac surgery
- **b.** Right ventricular pacing
- **c.** Nonischemic cardiomyopathy
- **d.** Overinterpretation
- **e.** Basal inferior or septal wall motion abnormality
- **f.** Poor image quality
- **g.** Hypertensive response to exercise, i.e., systolic blood pressure 220 mm Hg and diastolic blood pressure 110 mm Hg.

B. False negative results:
- **a.** Single vessel disease
- **b.** Inadequate level of stress
- **c.** Disease of left circumflex artery
- **d.** Poor image quality
- **e.** After maximum stress delay in capturing images

Advantages of Stress Echocardiography

A. Its sensitivity and specificity can be compared with the results of exercise nuclear imaging.

B. Results are immediately available.

C. It is portable.

D. It will provide information regarding presence and extent of the coronary artery disease.

E. Less time-consuming

F. Low cost as compared to exercise nuclear imaging

G. It can assess the following:
- **a.** Global wall motion
- **b.** Regional wall motion
- **c.** Wall thickness
- **d.** Size of the chamber
- **e.** Functions of the valves

H. It can diagnose new coronary artery disease in presence of baseline abnormalities.

Disadvantages of Stress Echocardiography

A. Interpretation is subject-orientated, not standardized.

B. In presence of resting wall motion abnormalities interpretation is difficult.

C. Images are nondiagnostic due to poor quality of images.

D. Prognostic potential is uncertain as there are very limited number of studies.

E. In patients with LBBB or paced ventricular rhythm there are very limited data, hence guidelines do not recommend this test.

Q16. Discuss the role of renin–angiotensin–aldosterone axis in the pathogenesis of essential hypertension. Discuss the direct renin inhibitors.

DNBIV/DEC2013 (10)

Describe pathophysiology in brief of primary hypertension. Discuss steps in evaluation of perioperative hypertension.

MGR/APR2012/MDII (7)

Discuss the role of renin–angiotensin–aldosterone system in blood pressure regulation. What are the pharmacological targets within this system for the treatment of hypertension?

AIIMS (BBS) 2024 (10)

Discuss about the renin–angiotensin–aldosterone system and the therapeutics of blocking the system at different levels. List the important side effects of each drug.

KERALA UNI, 2021 (20)

Discuss the regulation of blood pressure focusing on the role of renin–angiotensin–aldosterone system and baroceptor reflex.

WBUHS, 2025 (10)

ANSWER

Renin–angiotensin–aldosterone axis regulates blood pressure through two mechanisms:

- **a.** Vasoconstriction properties of angiotensin II
- **b.** Sodium-retaining properties of aldosterone

Renin is synthesized as enzymatically inactive precursor prorenin. Most of the renin is synthesized in the afferent arteriole in the kidney. Prorenin is directly secreted into the circulation or becomes activated in the secretary cells to renin and released into the circulation. There is no physiological activity of prorenin in the human being.

There are three stimuli responsible for renin secretion into circulation:

- **a.** Decreased transport of sodium chloride in the distal part of thick ascending limb of loop of Henle in the macula densa.
- **b.** Decreased pressure in the renal afferent arteriole through baroreceptor mechanism
- **c.** Stimulation of sympathetic nervous system of renin secreting cells via β1 adrenoceptors.
- **d.** Angiotensin II directly stimulates renin secretion through blockade of angiotensin-converting enzyme receptor and angiotensin type II receptors.

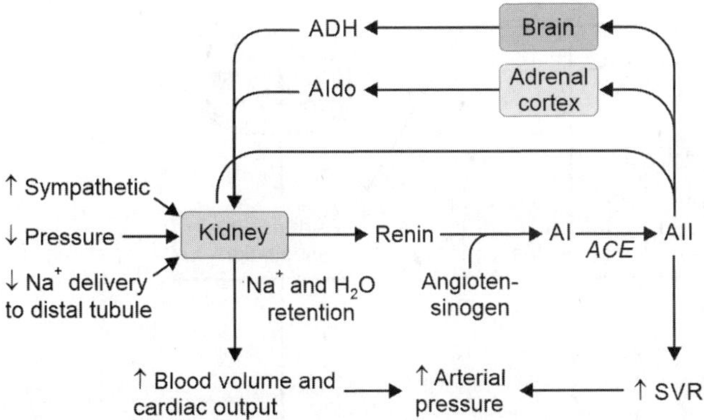

(ACE: angiotensin-converting enzyme; ADH: antidiuretic hormone; SVR: systemic vascular resistance)

Renin secretion is inhibited by following three factors:

- **a.** Increased transport of sodium chloride in the distal part of thick ascending limb of loop of Henle in the macula densa
- **b.** Increased pressure in the renal afferent arteriole through baroreceptor mechanism
- **c.** Inhibition of sympathetic nervous system of renin secreting cells via β1 adrenoceptors blockade
- **d.** Angiotensin II directly inhibits renin secretion through the stimulation of angiotensin II type 1 receptors.

After being released in to the circulation renin will cleave angiotensinogen to decapeptide angiotensin I which is again converted into octapeptide angiotensin II through the cleavage of C-terminal histidine-leucine dipeptide by the enzyme angiotensin-converting enzyme primarily but not exclusively located in the pulmonary circulation, at the same time this enzyme also inactivates vasodilator substance bradykinin to an inactive metabolite.

Angiotensin II acts through the angiotensin II type 1 receptors present on the cell membranes to release aldosterone from the zona glomerulosa of adrenal cortex. At the same time angiotensin II will stimulate type 1 receptor to secrete inositol 1,4,5-triphosphate (IP3) that stimulates vasoconstriction through release of intracellular calcium ion.

In addition angiotensin II directly acts on the cell of the vessel wall to play a role in the pathogenesis of atherosclerosis.

Angiotensin type 2 receptor is functionally opposite to that of type 1 receptor like, type 2 receptor stimulation leads to vasodilatation, increased excretion of sodium, and inhibition of cellular growth and formation of matrix through apoptosis of smooth muscle cells, and regulation of glomerular filtration rate (GFR).

Renin-secreting tumor in the kidney like benign hemangiopericytoma of juxtaglomerular apparatus, renal carcinoma, Wilm's tumor, and renin-producing tumor in lung, liver, colon, pancreas, and adrenal gland are responsible for hypertension.

In case of renal artery stenosis due to decreased perfusion pressure in the kidney stimulates secretion of renin.

Angiotensinogen, renin, and angiotensin II are present in the following tissues:

- **a.** Brain
- **b.** Aorta
- **c.** Arteries
- **d.** Heart
- **e.** Adrenal glands
- **f.** Kidneys
- **g.** Adipocytes
- **h.** Leukocytes
- **i.** Spleen
- **j.** Testes
- **k.** Ovaries
- **l.** Skin

Angiotensin II is formed in these tissues by the following proteases:

- **a.** Renin

b. Chymase
c. Tonin
d. Cathepsin

Tissue angiotensin II in excess is responsible for following:
a. Atherosclerosis
b. Cardiac hypertrophy
c. Renal failure

Aldosterone synthesis is stimulated by the following factors:
a. Angiotensin II
b. Potassium—aldosterone secretion will be decreased in potassium-depleted subject.
c. Adrenocorticotropic hormone (ACTH) level—but it is not the important tropic factor.

Functions of aldosterone in relation to cardiovascular system:
a. Aldosterone acts on amiloride-sensitive epithelial sodium channel present on the apical surface of principal cells of cortical collecting duct in kidney to increase the absorption of sodium in exchange of potassium and hydrogen ion leading to hypertension, hypokalemic metabolic alkalosis.
b. Aldosterone produces endothelial dysfunction, inflammation in the vascular wall, fibrosis, and oxidative stress leading to increased cardiovascular morbidity and mortality.

Cortisol has action on mineralocorticoid receptor, but cortisol will be converted into cortisone by 11-β-hydroxysteroid dehydrogenase type 2, and cortisone has no mineralocorticoid effect.

Primary hyperaldosteronism is mineralocorticoid-mediated hypertension; here aldosterone synthesis is independent of renin and angiotensin II.

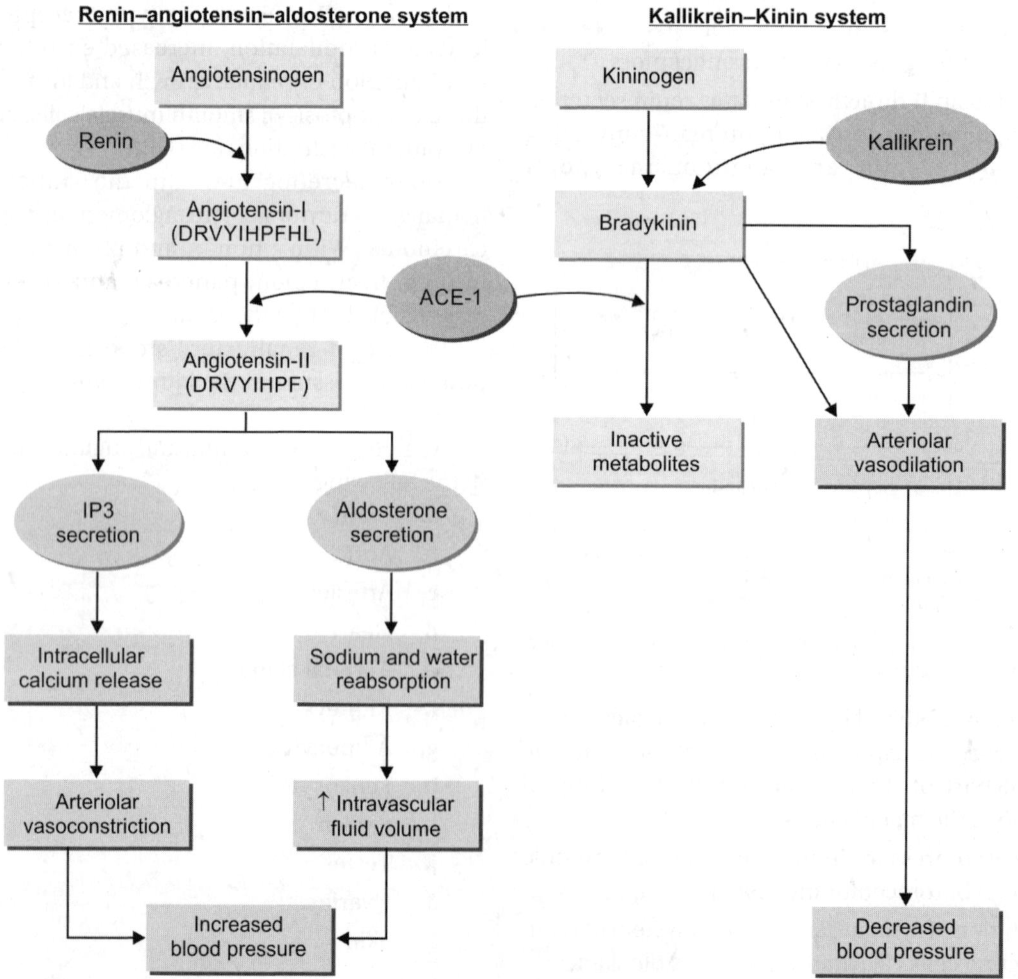

(ACEI: angiotensin-converting enzyme inhibitor; IP3: inositol 1,4,5–triphosphate)

Since mineralocorticoid receptors are present in different tissues, hence activation of these receptors is associated with structural and functional alteration of heart, kidney, and great vessels resulting myocardial fibrosis, vascular wall inflammation and remodeling, nephrocalcinosis leading to hypertension, and cardiovascular morbidity.

Intravascular Volume

Sodium is the main extracellular cation responsible for maintaining the extracellular fluid volume and it is excreted constantly to maintain sodium homeostasis. Now, if intake of sodium will exceed the capacity of the kidney to excrete it, then it will be retained in the blood increasing the blood volume and cardiac output. Many vascular beds have the capacity to autoregulate the blood flow. If the constant blood flow is to be maintained in the face of increased arterial pressure, resistance in those beds will be increased, since,

Blood flow = Pressure across the vascular bed/Vascular resistance

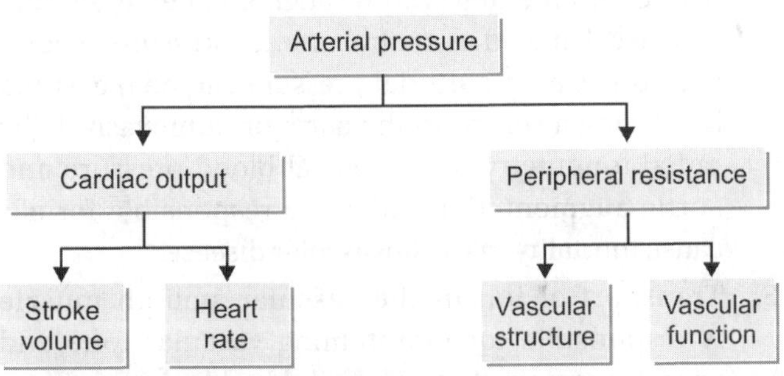

Initial increase in blood pressure is due to increased cardiac output. But later on, peripheral resistances will be increased and cardiac output returns to normal level.

Only chloride salt of sodium is responsible for increase in blood pressure, nonchloride salts have little effect. Sodium acts on neural, endocrine, and vascular system to increase the blood pressure. In case sodium intake-related hypertension "pressure-natriuresis" mechanism comes into play by which sodium will be excreted through kidney as a result of decreased absorption capacity of the renal tubules due to hormonal factor like atrial natriuretic factor but only subtle increase in GFR. So in case impaired capacity of the kidney to excrete sodium, arterial pressure has to be increased to get reasonable natriuresis.

Sodium-dependent hypertension may occur due to:

- **a.** Intrinsic renal disease
- **b.** Increased production of salt-retaining hormone like aldosterone
- **c.** Increased reabsorption of sodium by augmented neural activity to the kidney

In all the above conditions high blood pressure should be maintained to get sodium homeostasis.

Autonomic Nervous System

- **A.** Adrenergic reflexes responsible for short-term control of blood pressure
- **B.** Adrenergic system is responsible for long-term control of blood pressure in association with:
  - **a.** Volume-related factor
  - **b.** Hormonal factor—norepinephrine, dopamine, and epinephrine control tonic and phasic blood pressure

Adrenergic receptors' activities are mediated by:

- **a.** Guanosine nucleotide binding protein, i.e., G protein
- **b.** Intracellular concentration of second messenger

There are two main types of adrenergic receptors: α and β. Each receptor again is subdivided into two:

- **a.** α_1 and α_2
- **b.** β_1 and β_2

Other subtypes are also identified.

α receptor is activated by norepinephrine and β receptors are activated by epinephrine.

α_1 receptors are present on the postsynaptic cells on the smooth muscle and α_2 receptors are present on the presynaptic membrane of the postganglionic nerve endings synthesizing norepinephrine. During activation by catecholamine there is negative feedback from α_2 receptors thus inhibiting norepinephrine release. α_1 receptors increase reabsorption of sodium from the kidney. So, a class of antihypertensive drug will inhibit α_1 receptors and stimulates α_2 receptors, thus sympathetic outflow will be reduced.

β_1 receptors present in the myocardium are responsible for rate and strength of cardiac contraction.

β_1 receptors present in the kidney are responsible for renin release. One class of antihypertensive drug is responsible for inhibition of β_1 receptor.

Epinephrine stimulates β_2 receptors leading to relaxation of vascular smooth muscle resulting vasodilatation.

Again, high level of circulating catecholamine will downregulate the adrenergic receptors in various tissues that leads to decreased responsiveness to catecholamines—it is known as tachyphylaxis to catecholamine. As for example in case of pheochromocytoma results from downregulation of adrenergic receptors by orthostatic hypotension increased level of catecholamine.

On the other hand chronic low level of catecholamine there is upregulation of adrenergic receptors that leads to increased responsiveness to neurotransmitters.

Chronic administration of adrenergic receptor blocker will upregulate these receptors. So, abrupt withdrawal of this drug will lead to increased hypersensitivity of these receptors to sympathetic stimuli.

Several other reflexes can modulate the blood pressure. Stretch sensitive receptors are present in the carotid sinuses and aortic arch. As the arterial pressure increases these receptors will be stimulated, the net effects are:

a. Decreased sympathetic outflow
b. Decrease in blood pressure
c. Decreased heart rate

This reflex is responsible to control acute rise in blood pressure related to:

a. Postural changes
b. Physiological stress
c. Behavioral stress
d. Blood volume changes

But if the rise in blood pressure is sustained, baroreceptors are reset to higher pressure, so its activity will be declined. In case of autonomic neuropathy or impaired function of baroreceptors, patient may suffer from labile blood pressure along with blood pressure spike and tachycardia. Electrical stimulation of afferent nerve in the carotid sinus will lower the blood pressure in case of resistant hypertension.

Sympathetic outflow is increased in case obese individual and subject suffering from obstructive sleep apnea (OSA).

Vascular Mechanism

Main determinant of arterial pressure are:

a. Radius of the vessel
b. Compliance of the resistant vessel

A. Resistance to blood flow is inversely proportional to one-fourth of the radius of the vessel. So, small decrease in the radius of the vessel will give rise to significant increase in resistance to the blood flow. In case of hypertensive patient there are mechanical, structural, and functional changes in the vessels affecting arteries and arterioles.

B. There is also vascular remodeling—which is characterized by alteration of the vessel wall without any change in volume. But hypertrophic or eutropic remodeling lead to decrease in the size of the lumen and increase in the peripheral resistance. Again, low-grade inflammation, apoptosis, and lastly fibrosis—all of which affect the vascular remodeling.

C. Elasticity is another character of the vessel wall that will accommodate increased volume of blood with only little increase in blood pressure.

D. Arterial stiffness is another factor in hypertension. Slight rise in the blood flow cannot be buffered by the stiff artery. Due to this stiffness central blood pressure may not correspond to pressure in the brachial artery. During ejection of blood in the aorta a pressure is generated that will propagate at a given velocity; this wave will generate a reflected wave which travel back toward the aorta.

   Pulse pressure is related to:

   a. The functional properties of the large arteries
   b. Timing of incident waves
   c. Timing of the reflected wave

   So, pulse wave velocity of both incident and reflected waves will be increased in case of increased arterial stiffness. The result is augmentation of aortic systolic pressure and reduction in aortic diastolic pressure, i.e., increase in pulse pressure. The surrogate marker of arterial stiffening is aortic augmentation index that can be calculated as central arterial pressure to pulse pressure. Central arterial pressure can be measured by placing a sensor in the aorta or noninvasively by radial tonometry. Both central blood pressure and aortic augmentation index are responsible for all-cause mortality in cardiovascular disease.

E. Transport of ion in the vascular smooth muscle is responsible for maintaining vascular tone and vascular growth that are modulated by intracellular pH. There are three ion transport mechanisms for maintaining the intracellular pH:

   a. Na^+-H^- exchange: It is increased in hypertension due to increased vascular tone by two mechanisms:

      1. Activation of Na^+–Ca^{2+} exchange due to increased entry of sodium leads to increased intracellular calcium thereby increasing vascular tone.
      2. Increased pH will lead to increased sensitivity of the contractile apparatus to calcium causing increased contractility of the vascular smooth muscles.
      3. It increases sensitivity of smooth muscle cells to mitogen leading to growth of the cells.

   b. Na^+-dependent HCO_3–Cl^- exchange
   c. Cation-dependent HCO_3^- – Cl^- exchange

F. Several vasoactive substances are synthesized and released by vascular endothelium:

a. Nitric oxide: It is vasodilator substance; its action is impaired in hypertension.
b. Endothelin: It is potent vasoconstrictor; its action is amplified.

Immune Mechanism, Inflammation, and Oxidative Stress

A. In case of primary hypertension, there is increased level of circulating autoantibodies.
B. Aortic stiffness and hypertension are associated with activation of adaptive and innate immunity.
C. Generated reactive oxygen species by inflammation, angiotensin II, and vascular stretch:
   a. Stimulate and modify inflammatory response
   b. Attenuate the effect of endogenous vasodilator
   c. Control the pressure-natriuresis curve in the renal medulla

Gut Microbiota and Hypertension

Human gut contains nearly 300–500 species of microbes in the colon, these are mostly anaerobes. Composition of flora varies from individual to individual and it is affected by following factors:
   a. Genetic factors
   b. Vaginal or cesarean delivery
   c. Breastfeeding

Recently, it has been recognized that there is good correlation between the gut microbiota and hypertension, as correction of dysbiosis by probiotic can reduce hypertension.

Direct Inhibitors of Renin

A. Aliskiren:
   a. It will compete with angiotensinogen to get access to the active site of renin thereby reduces the serum concentration of angiotensin I and II and thus decreases the systolic and diastolic blood pressure.
   b. Dose is 150–300 mg/day
   c. Adverse effect: No obvious adverse effect, but in high dose it will produce diarrhea.
   d. Pharmacokinetics: Its bioavailability is poor, 90% of this drug is excreted unchanged in feces. ACEI, ARBs, and direct renin inhibitors cannot be used together.
   e. Contraindications:
      1. Renal artery stenosis
      2. Pregnancy
B. Enaikiren
C. Remikiren

These drugs are used in case of arterial hypertension. These will target the rate-limiting step in renin-angiotensin-aldosterone axis.

There will be hyperreninemia due to compensatory increased release of renin, but it is no clinically significant.

Target	Drug class	Name of the drug	Mechanism of actions
Renin	Direct renin inhibitors	Aliskiren	It prevents the conversion of angiotensin I to angiotensin II by inhibiting renin
Angiotensin-converting enzyme	Angiotensin-converting enzyme inhibitors	• Enalapril • Lisinopril • Ramipril	It prevents the conversion of angiotensin I to angiotensin II thereby reducing vasoconstrictor effect and secretion of aldosterone
Angiotensin receptor	Angiotensin receptor blockers	• Losartan • Valsartan • Telmisartan	It prevents the angiotensin II to attach with the receptor thereby reduces the vasoconstriction, sodium retention and effect of aldosterone
Aldosterone receptor	Mineralocorticoid receptor antagonists	• Spironolactone • Eplerenone	• It inhibits the activity of aldosterone • It will reduce sodium and water retention, but increases the serum potassium level
Angiotensinogen	It is under experimental stages	Not available in the market	It will target the protein precursor of the RAAS thereby reducing the overall activation of the system

Adverse effects of these above drugs:

Aliskiren	• Common side effects: Diarrhea, headache, hyperkalemia, hypotension, dizziness • Serious effects: Angioedema, severe hyperkalemia in case of diabetes, kidney disease, syncope
Angiotensin receptor blockers	• Common: Dizziness, hyperkalemia, hypotension, headache, back pain • Less common: Renal dysfunction, gastrointestinal symptoms like vomiting, diarrhea • Rare serious side effects: Severe hyperkalemia, hepatotoxicity
Mineralocorticoid receptor antagonists	• Common: Hyperkalemia, hypotension, nausea, vomiting diarrhea • Spironolactone specific side effects: Gynecomastia, menstrual disturbances, impotence, decreased libido • Eplerenone related side effects: Lower risk of gynecomastia

Q17. Discuss the vascular endothelial cell functions in health and diseases. Describe the clinical assessment of endothelial function.

DNBI/JUN2012 (10)

Endothelial cell dysfunction and atherogenesis.

PGI/NOV2012/MDI (10)

ANSWER

Endothelial cells act as a selectable permeable barrier to regulate the passage of molecules between blood and the tissue, following diseases intervene this barrier leading to "capillary leak":

- **a.** Atherosclerosis
- **b.** Hypertension
- **c.** Pulmonary edema
- **d.** Renal disease
- **e.** Sepsis

Following are the homeostatic properties of endothelium:

- **a.** Proper balance between vasoconstriction and vasodilatation: Following substances are responsible for vasodilatation:
  1. Prostacyclin
  2. Nitric oxide
  3. Hydrogen peroxide
  4. Endothelium-derived hyperpolarizing factor
- **b.** Anti-inflammatory properties
- **c.** Antithrombotic properties
- **d.** Profibrinolytic properties
- **e.** Antiproliferative properties
- **f.** Antioxidant properties
- **g.** Permselectivity

Following are the dysfunctional properties of endothelium:

- **a.** Impaired dilatation or vasoconstriction: It occurs due to:
  1. Excess catabolism or impaired production of nitric oxide
  2. Production of potent vasoconstrictor substances, i.e., endothelin
  3. Promotion of oxidative stress and inactivation of nitric oxide by endothelial cells and smooth muscle cells that produce reactive oxygen species and superoxide anion under pathologic conditions.
- **b.** Proinflammatory properties: Normally endothelial cells react little with circulating leukocytes. But during infection or injury released bacterial products like endotoxin and proinflammatory cytokines, activate endothelial cells to release a large number of adhesion molecules which bind to different classes of leukocytes.
  1. In case of acute bacterial infection adhesion molecules and chemokines will recruit granulocytes.
  2. In case of chronic infections like tuberculosis and atherosclerosis they will recruit monocytes.
- **c.** Prothrombotic properties
- **d.** Antifibrinolytic properties
- **e.** Proproliferative properties
- **f.** Pro-oxidant properties
- **g.** Impaired barrier function

Endothelial cells take part in different types of immune-mediated diseases. Examples are:

- **a.** Compliment-mediated lysis of endothelial cells
- **b.** In solid organ allograft endothelial cells present foreign histocompatibility complex antigen thereby promoting allograft arteriopathy.
- **c.** There is evidence of immune-mediated thrombotic thrombocytopenic purpura or hemolytic uremic syndrome.

Endothelium being activated by inflammatory cytokines, angiotensin II, and bacterial endotoxin produces:

a. Large quantities of major inhibitor of fibrinolysis
b. Large quantities of plasminogen activator inhibitor-1
c. Increased production of potent procoagulant factors

All the above factors will lead to local thrombus formation and disseminated intravascular coagulation.

Endothelial cells control the growth of adjacent smooth muscle cells.

A. Endothelial cells release heparan sulfate glycosaminoglycans that inhibits proliferation of smooth muscle
B. In case any injury or inflammation, endothelial cells produce growth factors and platelet-derived growth factor that promote migration as well as proliferation of vascular smooth muscle cells. Dysregulated production of these growth stimulatory molecules promotes accumulation of smooth muscle in atherosclerotic lesions.

Q18. Define sudden cardiac death. Describe initial evaluation and basic life support in such a situation.
DEC/JUN2012 (10)

Etiopathogenesis and prevention of sudden cardiac death.
PGI/APR2013/MDI (10)

Define sudden cardiac death.
DNB (DEC2018) (2)

Sudden cardiac death: Definition, risk factors, and secondary prevention.
DNB, 2024 OCT (5)

ANSWER

Definition

Sudden cardiac death (SCD) can be defined as death due to cardiac arrest in a patient with or without preexisting known heart disease and mode and time of death is unexpected, but if witnessed occurs within 1 hour of onset of symptoms. But if the patient can survive from circulatory arrest with return of spontaneous circulation with the help of cardiopulmonary resuscitation or defibrillation or spontaneously—this event is known as sudden circulatory arrest.

Etiology

Most common cause of SCD in nonischemic SCD is cardiomyopathy related to alcoholism, obesity, and fibrosis. According to age the common causes are:

A. From birth to 13 years—primarily form congenital cardiac abnormality.
B. From 14 to 25 years:
   a. HOCM
   b. Arrhythmogenic right ventricular cardiomyopathy
   c. Congenital coronary anomalies
   d. Genetic channelopathy
   e. Myocarditis
   f. WPW syndrome
   g. Marfan syndrome

Causes of Sudden Cardiac Death

A. Ischemic heart diseases (IHD):
   a. Myocardial infarction
   b. Coronary vasospasm
   c. Anomalous origin of the coronary artery
B. Inherited channelopathies:
   a. Short and long QT syndrome
   b. Early repolarization syndrome
   c. Brugada syndrome
   d. Catecholaminergic polymorphic ventricular tachycardia
C. Heart failure from nonpreserved ejection fraction systolic heart failure (ejection fraction < 35%)
D. Valvular disease—aortic stenosis
E. Congenital heart disease—tetralogy of Fallot
F. Cardiomyopathies:
   a. Alcoholic
   b. Obesity
   c. HOCM
   d. Myocarditis
   e. Fibrotic
   f. Arrhythmogenic right ventricular cardiomyopathy
D. Pulmonary causes:
   a. Massive pulmonary embolism
   b. Obstructive sleep apnea
   c. Bronchial asthma

E. Neurologic:
   a. Epilepsy
   b. Hereditary muscular dystrophy
   c. Friedreich ataxia

F. Situational: Intense exercise and athlete

Population-based Risk Factors

A. Black race
B. Male sex
C. Diabetes
D. Smoking
E. Hypertension
F. Changes in ECG: Prolongation of QT, QRS, early repolarization syndrome
G. Atrial fibrillation
H. Family history of SCD
I. Low magnesium level
J. Heavy alcohol intake
K. OSA
L. Diet low in PUVA

Triggering Factors

A. Heart failure
B. Electrolyte abnormality
C. Inflammation of myocardium
D. Vigorous exertion
E. Ischemia
F. Psychological stress

Evaluation of Patients of School or College Students and Athlete According to AHA Guidelines

Accordingly following two histories like family history and personal history and physical examination are very important.

A. Personal history:
   a. History of unexplained syncope or near syncope
   b. Chest pain or chest tightness or discomfort
   c. History of exertional dyspnea or unexplained dyspnea/fatigue or palpitation associated with exercise
   d. Elevated systolic blood pressure
   e. Prior recognition of heart murmur
   f. Prior restriction from participation in sports
   g. Prior testing of heart

B. From family history:
   a. Unexpected premature death before the age of 50 years having heart disease in more than 1 relative
   b. In close relative of <50 years history disability from the heart disease
   c. History of congenital cardiac diseases in the family:
      1. Brugada syndrome
      2. Long QT syndrome
      3. Short QT syndrome
      4. Hypertrophic cardiomyopathy
      5. Ion channelopathies

C. Physical examination:
   a. Evaluation of murmur in supine, standing, and with Valsalva maneuver
   b. Inequality of both radial and femoral pulses to detect coarctation of aorta
   c. Stigmata of Turner syndrome
   d. Blood pressure in both arms in supine and standing position
   e. Seizure activity

D. Investigations:
   a. Electrocardiography: IHD, MI, and inherited channelopathies
   b. Echography: Heart failure, cardiomyopathies, congenital heart disease, valvular heart and disease
   c. Exercise test for coronary artery disease, long QT syndrome, and catecholinergic ventricular tachycardia
   d. Coronary angiography: Coronary artery disease, congenital coronary artery abnormalities, and coronary spasm
   e. Electrophysiology in case of suspected arrhythmias
   f. Cardiac MRI can detect arrhythmogenic right ventricular cardiomyopathy
   g. Genetic testing in case Brugada syndrome, long QT syndrome
   h. Cardiac muscle biopsy

Basic Life Support in this Situation According to AHA Guidelines

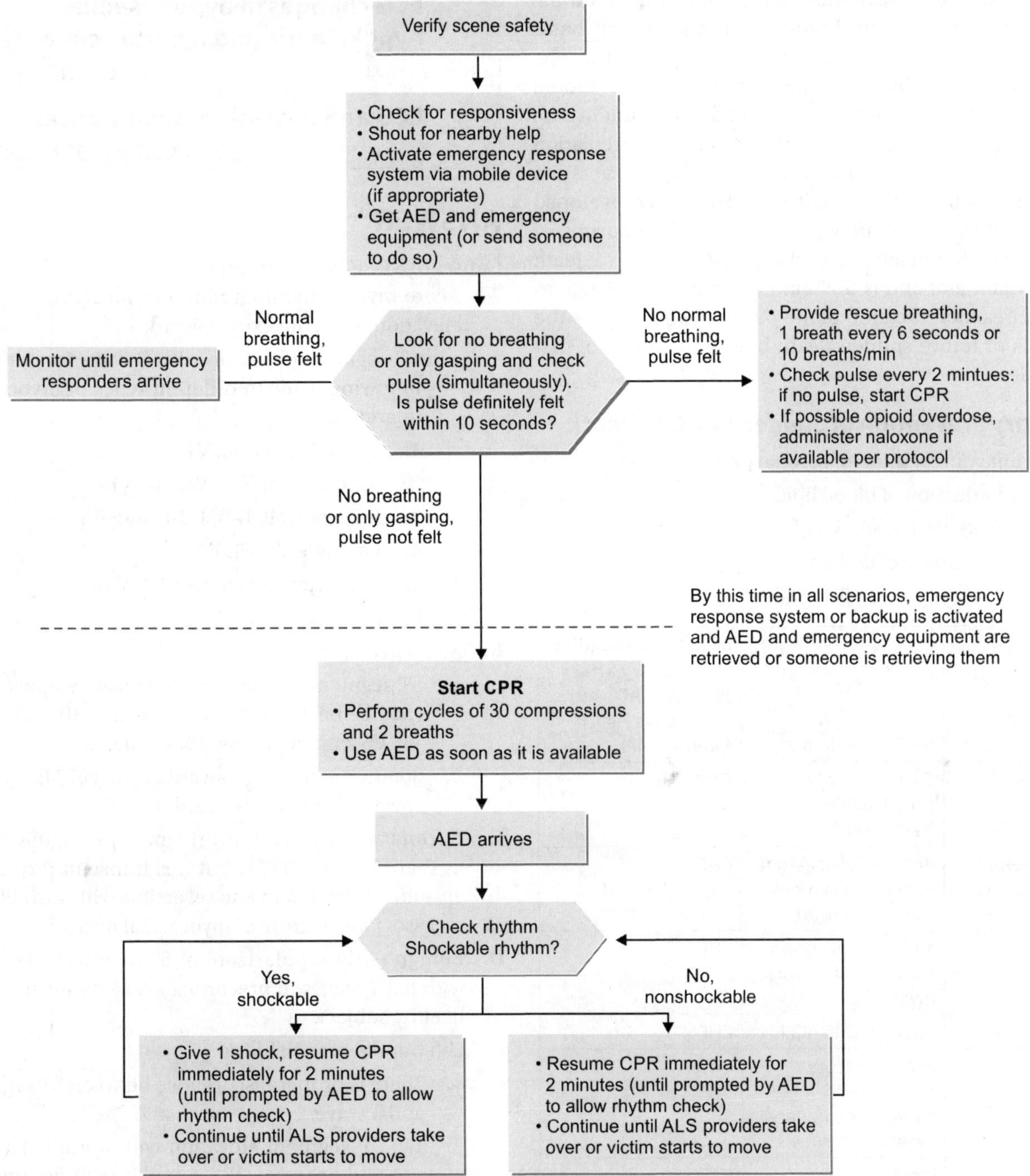

(AED: automated external defibrillator; ALS: advanced life support; CPR: cardiopulmonary resuscitation)

Prevention of Sudden Cardiac Death

Sudden cardiac death due to ventricular tachyarrhythmia requires primary prevention as it is mainly fatal; on the contrary, patients with bradyarrhythmias retain basal circulation, as for example, ventricular escape rhythm. So, in case of bradyarrhythmias, appropriate treatment should be given to prevent irreversible organ damage. But in case of ventricular fibrillation, there is rapid loss of circulation to the vital organs mainly brain resulting irreversible damage within few minutes. In spite of recently developed devices to treat these patients only a small proportion of patients go home alive. So, primary prevention of death is the main aim and is the main diagnostic challenge as it requires identification of the patients who may be the victims of future sudden death before the onset of first episode.

Primary Prevention of Sudden Cardiac Death

A. Primary prevention of coronary artery disease:

- **a.** Reduction of blood lipids
- **b.** Cessation of smoking
- **c.** Treatment of diabetes
- **d.** Treatment of hypertension

Drugs	Mode of action	Mortality reduction for coronary artery disease (CAD) and congestive heart failure (CHF)
Beta-blockers	Catecholinergic stimulation in the heart modifier	CAD/CHF
Aldosterone antagonists	Action of aldosterone is inhibited in the kidney and heart	CHF
ACEI	Inhibits angiotensin II to stimulate cardiac myocytes	CHF
ARBs	Alternative to ACEI	CHF
Angiotensin-receptor inhibitors	In case of acute coronary ischemia it prevents coronary events	CAD
HMG-CoA reductase inhibitor	It reduces LDL-C level with additional pleomorphic effect	CAD

(ACEI: angiotensin-converting enzyme inhibitor; ARBs: angiotensin receptor blockers; HMG-CoA: 3-hydroxy-3-methylglutaryl coenzyme A; LDL-C: low-density lipoprotein)

Q19. Discuss differential diagnosis of ST segment elevation. Describe ECG changes in hyperkalemia, hypokalemia and hypocalcemia.

DNBI/JUN2012 (10)

ECG and potassium significance.

MGR/OCT2012/MDIV (7)

ANSWER

Causes of ST-segment elevation:

A. Acute myocardial infarction producing ST segment elevation with convexity upward:

- **a.** ST-segment elevation with Q wave formation in following leads in different types of myocardial infarction:
  1. Septal infarction: V1–V2
  2. Anterior wall: V3–V4, LI, aVL
  3. Inferior wall: L-II, L-III, and aVF
  4. Lateral wall: V5–V6
  5. Right ventricular wall: V1, V4R
  6. Posterior wall: V7–V9

B. Acute pericarditis:

- **a.** ST segment elevation with concavity upwards or “Saddle back” involving L-I, L-II, L-III, aVF, AVL, V2–V6 with depressed PR segments.
- **b.** Spodick’s sign: Downward sloping of TP segment specific for acute pericarditis.

C. Coronary vasospasm in Prinzmetal’s angina: Same as that of acute STEMI but it is transient during the episode of chest pain and reversible with vasodilators no associated feature of myocardial necrosis.

D. Benign early repolarization: ST-segment elevation with tall T waves in precordial leads mainly in young healthy subject.

E. Left bundle branch block:

- **a.** There is proper discordance between ST segment and T wave:
  1. ST-segment elevation with upright T waves and negative QRS complex with dominant S wave—most prominent in V1–V3
  2. ST-segment depression with depressed T wave and positive QRS complex with dominant R wave—most prominent in L-I and aVL.

F. Left ventricular hypertrophy:
   a. ST segment elevation with deep S wave in V1–V3 and ST segment depression with tall R wave in L-I, aVL, and V5-V6
   b. Left axis deviation
G. Ventricular aneurysm:
   a. Elevation of ST segment with deep Q wave and inverted T waves in V1–V3
H. Brugada syndrome: Elevation of ST segment with partial right bundle branch block sign in V1–V3 with coved morphology
I. Ventricular paced rhythm: Similar features like that of LBBB but there is proper discordance with ST segment and T wave which is just opposite to that of QRS complex.
J. Raised intracranial pressure: Elevated ST segment like that of acute infarction or acute pericarditis with deep T wave inversion
K. Takotsubo cardiomyopathy: It is also called broken heart syndrome, it is associated with ST segment elevation or T wave inversion or moderate troponin rise.

ECG Features of Hypokalemia

A. Increased amplitude of P wave
B. PR interval will be prolonged
C. Widespread depression of ST segment and flattening or depression of T wave.
D. Prominent U wave in V2–V3
E. Apparently prolonged QT interval as a result of fusion of T with U waves (Long QU interval)

With worsening of hypokalemia:

F. Frequent supraventricular or ventricular ectopic
G. Atrial arrhythmia, atrial flutter, and atrial fibrillation
H. Ventricular tachycardia and ventricular fibrillation

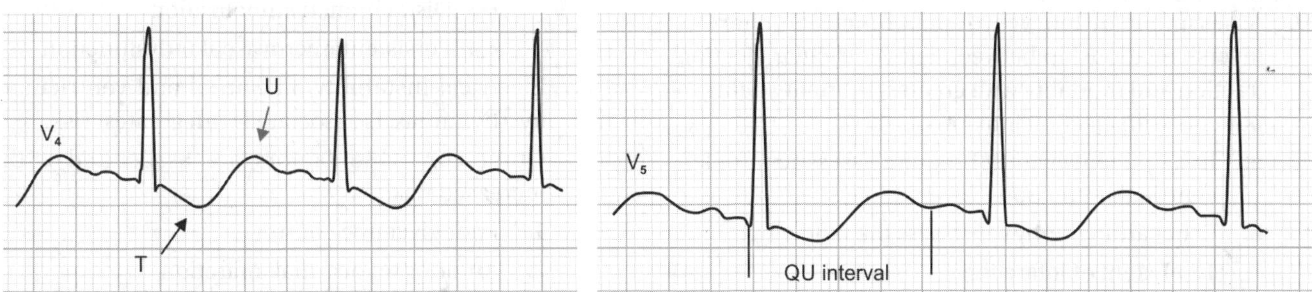

ECG Changes in Hyperkalemia

Potassium level (mmol/L)	Mechanism	ECG changes
5.5–6.5	Repolarization abnormalities	Peaked T waves
6.5–7.0	Progressive atrial paralysis	• P wave widening/ flattening • PR prolongation • P waves eventually disappear
7.0–9.0	Conduction abnormalities	Bradyarrhythmias: Sinus bradycardia; high-grade AV block with slow junctional and ventricular escape rhythms; slow AF Conduction blocks (bundle branch block, fascicular blocks) Prolonged QRS interval with bizarre QRS morphology
>9.0	All of above	• Development of sine wave appearance (preterminal rhythm) Asystole • Ventricular fibrillation • PEA with bizarre, wide complex rhythm

(PEA: pulseless electrical activity)

ECG Changes in Hypocalcemia

A. Prolongation of ST segment leading to QTc prolongation
B. Unchanged T wave
C. Arrhythmia is uncommon but there is report of atrial fibrillation
D. There may be torsades de pointes

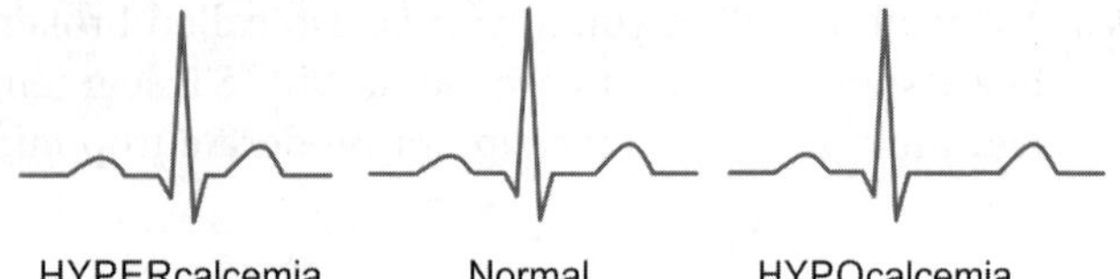

Q20. Discuss post myocardial infarction risk stratification, assessment, and secondary prevention.

DNBIII/JUN2012 (10)

ANSWER

Postmyocardial Infarction Risk Stratification

A. Age: Average age of the patient with myocardial infarction is 65 years but older patients may be at greatest risk

B. Assessment of left ventricular function: There is inverse relationship between left ventricular ejection fraction and mortality with greatest mortality being in patients with ejection fraction of <40%.

   a. In all patients with MI require assessment of left ventricular function.

   b. Echocardiography can assess the following:

      1. Extent of infarction
      2. Status of the remote myocardium
      3. Concomitant valvular function
      4. Mechanical complications of myocardial infarction like:
         - Ventricular septal rupture
         - Rupture of the ventricular free wall
         - Acute severe mitral regurgitation due to papillary muscle rupture
         - Ventricular pseudoaneurysm
         - Ventricular aneurysm
         - Dynamic left ventricular outflow tract obstruction
      5. Remodeling of the ventricle over time that may culminate in left ventricular dilatation.

   c. Left ventriculography: It is performed during diagnostic catheterization to estimate left ventricular function.

   d. Cardiac MRI: It is the gold standard for assessing the left ventricular function. With gadolinium contrast agent it can assess:

      1. Left ventricular ejection fraction
      2. Left ventricular volume
      3. Transmurality
      4. Extent of the scar
      5. Viability of the scar
      6. Integrity of the microvasculature.

C. Other indicators for prognostic information:

   a. Estimation of troponin levels

   b. C-reactive protein level

   c. B-type natriuretic peptide level

   d. ST segment elevation or depression indicates:

      1. High risk of death
      2. Heart failure
      3. Recurrent ischemia
      4. Severe coronary artery disease

      It is most important in case of persistent elevation of ST segment after neovascularization—it will indicate:

      - Distal branch embolization
      - Persistent microvascular dysfunction

   e. Electrical instability, like atrial and ventricular dysrhythmias, is associated with greatest risk.

   f. Other comorbid factors are associated with increased risk:

      1. Poor glycemic control
      2. Anterior myocardial infarction
      3. Renal insufficiency
      4. Anemia

D. Risk models: Following models are used which will utilize aforementioned risk factors to estimate and quantitate their future predictive score and subsequent risk cardiac events and mortality:

   a. TIMI score: It utilizes following criteria—

      1. Age ≥ 65 years
      2. Three or more risk factors for coronary artery disease: Hypertension, family history of coronary artery disease, tobacco use, diabetes mellitus, and hypercholesterolemia
      3. Known case of coronary artery disease with stenosis of ≥50%
      4. Use of aspirin in past 7 days
      5. Severe angina, i.e., ≥2 episodes in last 24 hours
      6. Elevation of ST segment of ≥0.5 mm
      7. Elevated cardiac marker level

      Risk of death by 14th day:

      - 0–1: 5%

- 2: 8%
- 3: 13%
- 4: 20%
- 5: 26%
- 6–7: 41%

b. Global Registry of Acute Coronary Events

E. Assessment of residual ischemia: Two most important predictors of mortality in patients those who had myocardial infarction:

a. Extent of coronary artery disease

b. Presence of residual ischemia:

1. In case of severe anatomical stenosis or in presence of perfusion ischemia in the noninfarct area either the patient should undergo additional revascularization or PCI of the noninfarct artery should be done in the same sitting.

2. Some patients should undergo stress test prior to discharge to see any need for additional neovascularization. In case of extensive anatomic disease the patient should undergo elective coronary artery bypass surgery during hospital stay or after discharge.

3. Majority of STEMI are treated with PCI or pharmacoinvasive therapy. But those who do not undergo PCI, they will undergo submaximal stress test within 2–3 days after onset of symptoms. Some of these patients not undergone angiography prior to discharge should undergo stress test. But in case of NSTEMI submaximal stress test is safe in those who have no sign of ischemia or heart failure.

4. Submaximal stress test provides following information:

- Prognostic information
- Assess the functional capacity
- Efficacy of medical therapy
- Guide to cardiac rehabilitation after discharge

The patients who are able to achieve the three metabolic equivalents of task are prognostically good. Those who cannot meet the task due to:

- Hypotension during exercise
- ST segment elevation or depression should undergo coronary angiography.

5. Where ECG cannot be interpretable, in that case stress echocardiography or radionuclide imaging should be recommended as these methods will increase the sensitivity and specificity of detecting coronary artery disease.

Secondary Prevention of Myocardial Infarction after Risk Assessment

A. Cessation of smoking as it will double the rate of reinfarction and death because:

a. It will produce coronary artery vasospasm.

b. It will reduce the effectiveness of beta-blocker therapy.

Smoking can be stopped by following methods:

a. Formal smoking cessation program

b. Hypnosis

c. Abstinence of smoking

d. Pharmacologic therapy:

1. Nicotine substitute can be given through the following vehicles:

- Transdermal patches
- Chewing gum
- Nasal spray
- Inhalers

But these nicotine substitutes should not be given in acute phases, it is safe in later phases.

Drugs are the following:

a. Bupropion: It is effective in cessation of smoking. Its dose is doubled in 3 days then it should be continued for 7–12 weeks, but patient should set a goal to stop smoking by 1–2 weeks.

b. Varenicline: It is partial agonist of nicotine receptors thus stimulates nicotine receptors but without any nicotine effect.

B. Management of lipid: All patients with myocardial infarction, 12 hours fasting lipid profile should be done and dietary and pharmacologic management should be given.

a. Diet: According to AHA guidelines diet should consist of:

1. <7% of total calorie will be saturated fat.

2. <200 mg—cholesterol

b. Therapy:

1. Drug of choice is statin in high dose.

2. If the patient is intolerant to statin therapy then proprotein convertase subtilisin/kexin type 9 (PCSK9) inhibitor or ezetimibe can be given.

According to recent data LDL level of <30 mg/dL is associated with no harm. If LDL level is <70 mg/dL with statin, then the second drug can be added.

3. Low level of high-density lipoprotein (HDL) is associated with increased risk for MI. Hence, its level should be increased by:
   - Aerobic exercise
   - Cholesteryl ester transfer protein inhibitors—evacetrapib or anacertrapib. These drugs will maintain sustained rise of HDL along with lowering of LDL.
4. Triglyceride level: High level is associated with increased risk of CAD. So, it should be lowered by:
   - Statin
   - Life style modification

C. Diabetic management: Blood sugar should be maintained to maintain the HbA1c at 7%.

D. Antiplatelet therapy:

a. Aspirin therapy:

1. Dose is 75–162 mg/day
2. Effects: It reduces:
   - The rate vascular mortality
   - Nonfatal stroke
   - Nonfatal myocardial infarction

b. Oral P2Y12 inhibitors therapy: These are platelet inhibitor via adenosine diphosphate (ADP) antagonism.

- Drugs are: Clopidogrel—75 mg/day
- Prasugrel—10 mg/day. It is absolutely contraindicated in case of prior stroke. It is relatively contraindicated in the patient of >75 years of age and weight of <60 kg.
- Ticagrelor—90 mg twice daily. It should be used with aspirin with low dose.

E. Warfarin sodium: In case large myocardial infarction with left ventricular thrombus patient is at risk of embolic stroke and it should be treated with 6 weeks warfarin therapy as it will help in stabilization and endothelialization of thrombus. But now warfarin is recommended only in following conditions:

a. Deep venous thrombosis

b. Atrial fibrillation

c. Prosthetic heart valves

d. Left ventricular thrombus

F. Newer oral anticoagulants like rivaroxaban can be given.

G. Beta-blockers: These drugs are:

a. Antihypertensive

b. Anti-ischemic

c. Antiarrhythmic

d. Reduce the left ventricular wall stretch

Effects:

a. Decreases the risk of sudden death

b. Decreases the risk of nonsudden cardiac death

c. Nonfatal infarction

These drugs are effective in:

a. Patient is at high risk

b. Patient with anterior infarction

c. Complex ventricular ectopy

d. Advanced age of the patient

e. Left ventricular dysfunction

These drugs should be started as soon as the patient will be stable.

Drugs having intrinsic sympathomimetic activity are:

a. Metoprolol

b. Propranolol

c. Carvedilol

d. Atenolol

e. Timolol

Contraindications:

a. Relative contraindications:

1. Second or third degree heart block
2. Severe asthma
3. Severe chronic obstructive pulmonary disease (COPD)
4. Severe decompensated congestive cardiac heart failure
5. Heart rate of <60 beats/min
6. Hypotension with systolic blood pressure <120 mm Hg
7. Other signs of low output state
8. In case of frequent episodes of hypoglycemia in diabetic patient it should not be given though diabetes mellitus is itself is not a contraindication.

b. Absolute contraindication:

1. Heart rate >100 beats/min
2. Cardiogenic shock

H. ACEI and ARBs:

a. Indications: These drugs reduce the congestive cardiac failure and ventricular dilatation leading to ventricular remodeling.

b. According to AHA class I recommendation patients with left ventricular ejection fraction of <40% with diabetes, CKD, and hypertension and according to class II recommendation all patients with cardiovascular disease should be treated with these drugs.

c. Adverse effects are:

1. In case of ACEI: Cough, rash, and disturbance in taste, hypotension

2. In case of ARBs: In case of CKD, it is contraindicated.

I. Aldosterone antagonists:

a. There will be risk of death in patients with low ejection fraction and congestive cardiac failure.

b. It is contraindicated in hyperkalemia and chronic renal failure with creatinine level of >2.5 mg/dL.

J. Calcium channel blocker:

a. Indications:

1. Refractory angina

2. Rapid atrial arrhythmia

3. In patients having clear contraindication against the use of beta-blockers

b. Contraindications:

1. In case of nifedipine:

- Increased risk of sudden death or reinfarction after myocardial infarction
- Hypotension
- Tachycardia
- Induction of coronary steal syndrome increasing myocardial oxygen demand

2. In case of verapamil and diltiazem:

- Left ventricular dysfunction
- Congestive cardiac failure

These drugs are useful in patients having no sign of congestive cardiac failure (CCF) or left ventricular dysfunction but contraindication to beta-blocker.

Q21. Describe the clinical features, diagnosis, differential diagnosis and treatment of angina pectoris.

DNBIII/JUN2012 (10)

Describe the pathophysiology, diagnosis and management of chronic stable angina.

DNBIII/DEC2012 (10)

Describe a typical attack of angina pectoris. Mention all possible clinical findings during the attack and briefly the causative mechanism. What is angina equivalent?

DNBII/APR2016 (10)

Describe blood supply to the heart. Discuss non-invasive myocardial testing in patient with coronary artery disease.

SCBMCH, 2018 (15)

Blood supply to the heart described in question number 39.

ANSWER

Pathophysiology

Under normal condition at a given level of oxygen myocardium controls the blood flow to supply adequate amount of oxygen to prevent myocardial ischemia. Three major determinants of myocardial oxygen demand:

A. Heart rate

B. Myocardial oxygen tension

C. Myocardial contractility

Adequate supply of oxygen to the myocardium requires:

A. Satisfactory level of oxygen carrying capacity of the blood—it can be determined by:

a. Inspired level of oxygen

b. Pulmonary function

c. Concentration and functional level of hemoglobin

B. Adequate level of coronary blood flow, majority of blood flow occurs through diastole. 75% of coronary vascular resistance occurs in three sets of arteries:

a. Large epicardial coronary arteries (R1)

b. Prearteriolar vessels (R2)

c. Arteriolar and intramyocardial capillary vessels (R3)

Amongst above sets of vessels major determinant of flow-limiting coronary atherosclerotic obstruction in main coronary vascular resistance is found in R2 and R3. Normal coronary vessels will control the supply of oxygen to the myocardium by varying their resistance and thereby flow and myocardium is able to extract the oxygen according to its need. Intramyocardial vessels normally have a capacity to dilate in response to exercise or emotional stress to supply oxygen and other substrates regularly—it is known as metabolic regulation. On the other hand coronary vessels have their capacity to alter their resistance to maintain coronary flow—it is autoregulation.

In case of atherosclerosis coronary arterial lumen will be reduced to limit the myocardial perfusion in response to myocardial demand in case of exercise or emotional stress. In case of severe lumen obstruction myocardial oxygen supply in basal state will be reduced.

This blood supply is also reduced in following cases like:

- **a.** Severe coronary vasospasm
- **b.** Coronary artery emboli
- **c.** Arterial thrombi
- **d.** Ostial narrowing in case of aortitis
- **e.** Congenital abnormality like left anterior descending coronary artery from pulmonary artery rarely produces myocardial ischemia or infarction.
- **f.** In case of aortic stenosis
- **g.** In left ventricular hypertrophy with limited coronary arterial flow.

Reduction in the oxygen carrying capacity of blood can occur in:

- **a.** Anemia
- **b.** Presence of carboxyhemoglobin

So, myocardial ischemia can occur due to presence of two or more causes, like:

- **a.** Increased myocardial demand in case of left ventricular hypertrophy due to hypertension
- **b.** Reduced supply of oxygen due to anemia
- **c.** Coronary arterial narrowing in case of atherosclerosis
- **d.** Failure of normal dilatation of coronary resistance vessels

Coronary Atherosclerosis

Major site of atherosclerosis is epicardial coronary arteries. Following are the risk factors:

- **a.** Low level of HDL
- **b.** High level of LDL
- **c.** Cigarette smoking
- **d.** Hypertension
- **e.** Diabetes mellitus

The functions that will be disturbed by the above factors are:

- **a.** Local control of tone of the vessels
- **b.** Maintenance of antithrombotic surface thereby controlling the adhesion of inflammatory surface as well as diapedesis.

When the above factors will be disturbed this will lead to:

- **a.** Inappropriate constriction of the vessels
- **b.** Formation of thrombus in the lumen
- **c.** Abnormal interactions between the monocytes and platelets and activated vascular endothelium

Above actions in the vascular milieu leads to subintimal collection of:

- **a.** Smooth muscle cells
- **b.** Fibroblasts
- **c.** Intercellular matrix defining atherosclerotic plaque

So, when the vessels are vulnerable, flowing blood is also vulnerable in the following form:

- **a.** Hyperglycemia
- **b.** Increased level of LDL cholesterol
- **c.** Tissue factor fibrinogen
- **d.** von Willebrand factor
- **e.** Coagulation factor VII
- **f.** Platelet microparticles

Vulnerable vessels and vulnerable blood ultimately lead to hyperfibrinogenemia and hyperfibrinolysis.

Atherosclerotic plaques are developed in the following areas of the epicardial coronary arteries:

- **a.** Different segment of the artery
- **b.** At the sites of increased turbulence in the coronary flow like branch point of the epicardial arteries

When the luminal diameter will be reduced to 50% there will be reduction of blood flow to limit the supply of oxygen to myocardium. If reduction of luminal diameter is reduced to 80%, coronary flow will be further reduced to ischemia at rest or at minimal activity.

Plaque is subject to rupture or erosion at the site of cap, as a result plaque is exposed to two interrelated factors:

- **a.** Platelet being activated will aggregate.
- **b.** Activation of coagulation cascade that will lead to deposition of fibrin strands. Ultimately thrombus will be formed by aggregated platelets, fibrin strand, and red blood cells—it will compromise the vessel lumen leading to reduction of blood

flow and thus myocardial ischemia. Myocardial ischemia depends upon the following:

1. Quantity of myocardium involved
2. Severity of obstruction
3. Whether the obstruction is acute or chronic:
    - In case of acute obstruction of left main coronary artery or proximal left anterior descending artery will be hazardous.
    - In case of chronic obstruction or gradual narrowing of the vessels large amount of collateral vessels are developed which will provide sufficient blood flow to sustain the viability of the myocardium.
    - In case of progressive worsening of the stenosis of the proximal part of the coronary vessel, vessel distal to the lesion will dilate to reduce the vascular resistance to maintain coronary blood flow. There is also pressure gradient across the stenosis in the vessel leading to fall in poststenotic vessel. With the maximum dilatation of resistance vessels, myocardial blood flow will be completely dependent upon the coronary artery pressure distal to obstruction.

As a result, myocardial ischemia will be developed due to following:

a. Increased myocardial oxygen demand:
    1. Increased physical activity
    2. Excessive emotional stress
    3. Tachycardia

Clinical Features

Constellation of symptoms in >50 years in male and >60 years in female includes four following features:

A. Location: In the retrosternal area radiating to shoulder, ulnar surface of both arms, forearms, and hand. It can also radiate to back, interscapular region, jaw, teeth, root of the neck, epigastrium but rarely above the neck and below the epigastrium. But it will never transmit to trapezius muscles—it is typical of acute pericarditis.

B. Radiation to trigger:
    a. It is triggered by:
        1. Exertion:
            - Exercise
            - Sexual activity
        2. Emotions:
            - Fright
            - Frustration
            - Stress
            - Anger
        3. Exposure to cold
        4. Consumption of heavy meal
    b. Angina may resolute in spite of continued exertion—"Walk through phenomenon".
    c. Initial exertion produces angina pain but second similar exertion will not produce angina—"Warm-up phenomenon"—this may be due to recruitment of collateral blood vessels during first episode.
    d. Angina may be developed with the change of position due to shift in blood volume—"Decubitus angina".
    e. Angina frequently occurs at night triggered by tachyarrhythmias or nightmares—"Nocturnal angina". It may be due to:
        1. Respiratory pattern changes during sleep leading to diminished oxygenation of blood
        2. Expansion of intrathoracic volume in recumbency increasing end-diastolic volume and increasing myocardial demand thereby left ventricular failure.

C. Character:
    a. Pain may be described as squeezing, tight chocking, and smothering, choking and rarely frank pain.
    b. Some patients experience profound fatigue, dyspnea, lightheadedness, diaphoresis, nausea, altered mental status, and syncope in absence of chest discomfort—it is "angina equivalent".
    c. Fixed threshold angina: It occurs at certain level of activity. Here, there is fixed coronary stenosis and fixed myocardial demand for oxygen, so ischemia will develop when oxygen requirement increases—this is stable exertional angina.
    d. In some patients angina pain varies throughout the day or day to day—it may be due to varying changes in the vasomotor tone. These patients experience angina pain with minor effort in the morning but in the evening may not experience same angina pain with heavy exertion.

D. Duration:
    a. Chest pain usually lasts for 3–5 minutes by slowing or cessation of activities, rest, and by sublingual

nitroglycerin; its diagnosis should be suspected when the pain is not relieved by above measures.

b. Women may present these features in different location or quality as compared to men or may present with angina equivalent.

As coronary atherosclerosis is associated with involvement of other arteries, patient should be asked about the following organs:

a. Intermittent claudication—peripheral arterial disease
b. Transient unconsciousness—transient ischemic attack (TIA)

Family history of premature IHD:

a. <55 years in first degree male relatives, <65 years in female relative
b. Hyperlipidemia
c. Diabetes mellitus
d. Cigarette smoking

Physical Findings

A. Signs associated with high risk of coronary artery disease:
   a. Increased blood pressure
   b. Features of anemia
   c. Features of thyroid disease
   d. Nicotine stain in the fingers—smoking
   e. Features of hypertensive vascular disease like retinal arteriopathy
   f. Features of hyperlipidemia like corneal arcus xanthelasma
   g. Evidence of carotid and peripheral vascular disease
   h. Blood pressure between the arms and between arms and legs (ankle-brachial index)
   i. Fundoscopy reveals:
      1. Increased light reflex
      2. Arteriovenous nicking
B. Physical examination during the episode of chest pain:
   a. Tachycardia
   b. Hypertension
   c. Palpation reveals:
      1. Abnormal contraction of cardiac impulse—left ventricular dyskinesia
   d. Auscultation reveals:
      1. Systolic murmur
      2. S3 and S4 gallop
      3. Ischemic mitral regurgitation
      4. Pulmonary edema

Diagnosis

A. Baseline ECG:
   a. Baseline ECG monitoring for initial screening:
      1. Majority of patients demonstrate normal ECG.
      2. Presence of pathological Q has, along with persistent ST segment depression, unfavorable outcome.
      3. Other abnormalities are LVH, bundle branch block, and pre-excitation syndrome.
   b. It is useful to assess the chest pain and stratify the risk.
   c. At the time of chest pain it can identify the cause of chest pain, like:
      1. Changes of T wave
      2. Changes in ST segment
      3. Change in conduction pattern
B. Diagnostic testing:
   a. Stress testing with ECG: In this test ischemia is provoked by graded exercise test or pharmacologic testing followed by functional assessment by echocardiography or radionuclide imaging to detect ischemia in myocardium.
      1. Methods to induce ischemia: Graded exercise should be done at age-predicted maximum heart rate (220-age). It provides objective assessment of functional capacity and also prognostic information. Exercise duration is symptoms-limited:
         - Evidence of chest discomfort
         - Severe shortness of breath
         - Dizziness
         - Severe fatigue
         - ST segment depression of >2 mm
         - Fall in systolic blood pressure >10 mm Hg
         - Development of ventricular arrhythmias

         This test is used to:
         - Discover any limitation in exercise performance
         - Detect ECG changes of myocardial ischemia
         - Detect its relationship with chest discomfort

It is also important to measure the following during stress test:

- Total duration of exercise
- Time to onset of ischemic ST segment change and chest discomfort
- External work performed
- Internal cardiac work performed, i.e., heart rate-blood pressure product
- Depth of ST segment depression and time needed for recovery

2. Methods to assess ischemia: Ischemic ECG changes response can be defined as:
   - Flat or downsloping depression of ST segment of >0.1 mV below baseline (PR segment)
   - Lasting for 0.08 second
   - Any evidence of conduction disturbances, ventricular arrhythmia developed during exercise

   There may be false positive or false negative results in one-third of cases.

   False positive results occur in following conditions:
   - Asymptomatic men of <40 years of age
   - Premenopausal women with no risk factor for premature atherosclerosis
   - Patients taking digitalis or other antiarrhythmic drugs
   - Patients with intraventricular conduction disturbances
   - Resting ST and T abnormalities
   - Ventricular hypertrophy
   - Abnormal serum potassium levels

   False negative test:
   - Obstruction in the left circumflex artery, because lateral portion of the heart supplied by this vessel is not presented in ECG.

   Normal response to graded exercise:
   - Progressive increase in blood pressure and heart rate—if there is failure of increase in blood pressure or actual decrease along with sign of ischemia in this test—it is adverse prognostic sign.
   - Development of angina
   - With or without severe >0.2 mV depression of ST segment before stage II completion of Bruce protocol
   - With or without depression of ST segment persisting for >5 minutes after exercise termination

b. Stress echocardiography: It can identify extent and location of regional motion abnormalities by assessing:

1. Regional or global wall motion abnormalities
2. Dilatation of left ventricle with stress

If the patient is unable to perform exercise test, then dobutamine stress test should be performed. Here, there is biphasic response with dopamine:

1. Contractility initially increases with low dose
2. Contractility decreases with higher dose of dopamine
3. Augmentation of contractility of hypokinetic segment of myocardium—suggests presence of hibernating myocardium in the distribution of the specific coronary artery.

Results of echo are difficult to interpret because of:

1. Hypertensive response to exercise
2. Presence of severe mitral regurgitation
3. Preexisting abnormalities of wall motion

Radionuclide imaging: It is done by positron-emission computed tomography with thallium-201 or technetium-99m-lebeled radiotracer.

Positron emission tomography is performed with rubidium 82 or 13N ammonia. It can perform:

1. Greater spatial resolution and diagnostic accuracy
2. Quantify coronary blood flow
3. Assess the coronary blood flow

c. Resting echocardiography: It will provide useful information:

1. Regional wall motion abnormalities of left ventricle
2. Impairment of left ventricle
3. Left ventricular hypertrophy
4. Presence of substantial mitral regurgitation
5. Quantification of aortic stenosis
6. Presence of hypertrophic cardiomyopathy

d. MRI: Using gadolinium contrast it evaluates following abnormalities:

1. Regional wall motion abnormalities
2. Ejection fraction
3. Myocardial perfusion

4. Direct visualization of coronary arteries
5. Delayed gadolinium phase will demonstrate:
   - Location of scar in the myocardium
   - Transmurality of scar

e. Electron beam computed tomography: It can demonstrate calcification of coronary artery. It will provide "calcium score." Increased calcium score is with increased risk of cardiovascular events.

f. Multidetector computed tomography: It evaluates epicardial coronary artery; it assesses coronary artery stenosis with 97% specificity.

g. Coronary angiography:

Indications:

1. In patient with chronic stable angina but severely symptomatic in spite of medical therapy who are being considered for PCI or CABG.
2. In patents with troublesome symptoms and diagnostic difficulties there is need to rule out or confirm the diagnosis.
3. In patients with known possible angina and survived cardiac arrest
4. In patients with angina with evidence of ischemia on noninvasive testing along with clinical and laboratory evidence of ventricular arrhythmia.
5. High-risk patients of sustaining coronary events which is based on signs of severe ischemia on noninvasive testing regardless of severity of symptoms.

h. Intravascular ultrasound: It will help in the following assessments:

1. Quantitate plaque area
2. Artery size
3. Luminal stenosis
4. Assess hazy areas in coronary angiogram
5. Questionable areas and extent of stenosis
6. Calcium content of plaque

i. Optical coherence tomography: It provides better resolution better than intravascular ultrasound. It can visualize:

1. Thrombus
2. Thin cap atheroma
3. Better characteristic of stent and arteriolar remodeling

By this method following three important physiological indices are identified:

1. Diastolic to systolic average peak coronary blood flow velocity ratio of <1.8 distal to obstruction.
2. Diastolic to systolic average peak coronary blood flow velocity ratio of >1.7 proximal to obstruction.
3. Coronary flow reserve, i.e., increase in coronary arterial blood flow with adenosine.

Direct measurement of pressure gradient:

1. Ratio of mean pressure distal and proximal to lesion after maximal vasodilatation of <0.75–0.8—hemodynamically significant lesion.

Treatment

A. Treatment of risk factors:

a. Hypertension

b. Diabetes mellitus

c. Cigarette smoking

d. Obesity: Low saturated fat diet, trans-unsaturated fatty acid diet, and low calorie intake

e. Hyperlipidemia: Aim is:

1. Long-term relief from angina
2. Reduced need for vascularization
3. Reduced need for vascularization

Method:

1. Low-fat diet
2. Weight loss
3. Exercise

Drugs:

1. Statin reduces LDL-C by 25–50%, increases HDL by 5–9%, and decreases triglyceride (TG) by 5–30%.
2. Ezetimibe reduces LDL level.
3. PCSK9 dramatically reduces LDL level in statin-intolerant patient.
4. Fibric acid and qmega-3 fatty acids may lower residual hypertriglyceridemia.

Guidelines:

1. In case of established CAD in the age of >75 years and under 75 years with moderate and high-intensity statin with a goal of ≥50% lowering of LDL, but recent evidence suggests LDL should be <70 mg/dL.

Following patients should be taken care of in following high risk of developing clinical events:

1. Older subject of >65 years
2. Smoker
3. Symptomatic peripheral arterial disease with prior stroke or MI
4. History of non-MI-related coronary revascularization
5. Presence of residual CAD with >40% residual stenosis in two major epicardial vessels
6. HDL level < 40 mg/dL in men and <50 mg/dL in female
7. High sensitivity CRP > 2 mg/L
8. Presence of metabolic syndrome

B. Pharmacologic therapy:

a. Nitrates:

Mechanism of actions:

1. After being metabolized it will release nitric oxide that binds with guanylyl cyclase present in the smooth muscle cells to produce increased amount of cyclic guanosine monophosphate that will be responsible for relaxation of smooth muscles.
2. Nitric oxide activates platelet guanylyl cyclase leading to impairment of flux of calcium and activates platelet.

Actions:

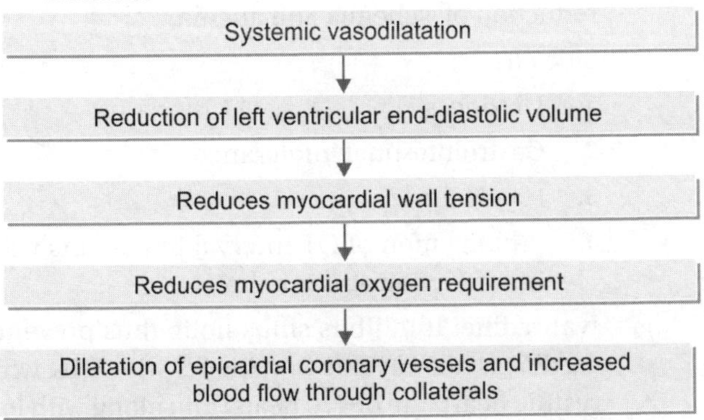

It will improve exercise tolerance in patients with chronic angina.

It will relieve ischemia in patients with Prinzmetal's angina and unstable angina.

Side effects:

1. Oral drug has to be taken with meals to prevent heart burn.
2. Headache—but its severity can be reduced with its continued use.
3. Transient episodes of flushing, dizziness, and postural hypotension.

Drugs are:

Drug		Dose	Schedule
Nitroglycerin	Ointment	0.5–2 inch	2–3 times daily
	Transdermal patch	0.2–0.8 mg/h	Daily, remove at bed time
	Sublingual tablet	0.3–0.6 mg	• Up to three doses • 5 minutes apart
Isosorbide dinitrate	Oral	10–40 mg	2–3 times daily
	Oral sustained release	80–120 mg	Once-twice daily
Isosorbide mononitrate	Oral	20 mg	2 times daily
	Oral sustained release	30–240 mg	Once daily

b. Beta adrenergic blocker:

Action:

1. It decreases the rate-pressure product.
2. Decreases myocardial oxygen demand.
3. Decreases left ventricular wall tension helping redistribution of blood flow from epicardium to endocardium.

Relative contraindications:

1. Asthma and reversible airway obstruction in patients with COPD
2. Atrioventricular conduction disturbances
3. Severe bradycardia
4. Raynaud's phenomenon
5. History of mental depression

Side effects:

1. Reduced exercise tolerance
2. Reduced exercise tolerance
3. Nightmares
4. Fatigue
5. Cold extremities
6. Left ventricular failure
7. Bronchial asthma
8. Worsening of claudication
9. Intensification of hypoglycemia in patient taking oral hypoglycemic drugs and insulin

Drugs	Selectivity	Doses in angina
Acebutalol	B1	200–600 mg twice daily
Atenolol	B1	50–200 mg/day
Bisoprolol	B1	10 mg/day

Continued

Continued

Drugs	Selectivity	Doses in angina
Esmolol	B1	50–300 μg/kg/min
Labetalol	None	200–600 mg twice daily
Metoprolol	B1	50–200 mg twice daily
Nebivolol	B1	5–40 mg/day
Propranolol	None	80–120 mg twice daily
Timolol	None	10 mg twice daily

c. Calcium channel blockers:

There are four types of calcium channels:

1. L: This channel enhances the calcium entry into the cell during phase III action potential.
2. T: This channel is located in the atria and SA node and affects the phase I depolarization.
3. N and P channels: These are present in nervous system.

Three types of CCBs:

1. Dihydropyridines—Nifedipine: It binds to extracellular portion of L channels at specific site but does not bind to T channel.
2. Benzothiazepines—diltiazem
3. Phenylalkylamines—verapamil: It binds to intracellular part of L channel and inhibits T channel.

Drug	Dose	Duration of action	Side effect
Amlodipine	5–10 mg four times daily	Long acting	Headache, edema
Felodipine	5–10 mg four times daily	Long acting	Headache, edema
Nifedipine	30–90 mg	Short acting	Hypotension, dizziness, flushing, nausea, constipation
Nicardipine	20–40 mg thrice daily	Short acting	Hypotension, dizziness, flushing, nausea, constipation
Diltiazem	30–80 mg four times daily	Short acting	Hypotension, flushing, bradycardia, edema
Verapamil	80–160 mg	Short acting	Hypotension, heart failure, edema, bradycardia

d. Antiplatelet drugs:

1. Aspirin: It inhibits irreversibly platelet cyclo-oxygenase and inhibits activation of platelet. Dose is 75–325 mg orally daily. It is used in stable angina, unstable angina, and myocardial infarction. It can reduce the cardiac events in adult men over 50 years of age.
2. Clopidogrel: It will block P2Y12 ADP receptor-mediated aggregation of platelet. Dose is 300–600 mg as loading dose followed by 75 mg daily. It is used in chronic stable angina. It combines with aspirin to reduce the death from coronary ischemic events. It also reduces formation of thrombus.

e. ACE inhibitors: It decreases the preload and afterload to some extent; it decreases the myocardial oxygen demand.

It is used in stable angina, myocardial infarction, and diabetes mellitus.

f. Ranolazine:

Mechanism of action:

It reduces late sodium entry into the myocytes thus reducing sodium-dependent calcium entry into the cytosol. As a result there is downstream reduction of intracellular calcium levels which leads to reduction of diastolic stiffness and improvement of diastolic blood flow resulting in reduction of ischemia and angina.

Side effects:

1. Dizziness
2. Gastrointestinal intolerance
3. Headache
4. Prolongation of QT interval in patients with liver function abnormality.

g. Ivabradine: It inhibits sinus node thus prevents cardiovascular events in patients with IHD with resting heart rate of ≥70 beats/min along with left ventricular dysfunction.

Q22. Describe the basic mechanisms of systolic dysfunction, diastolic dysfunction, and ventricular remodeling.

DNBI/JUN2012 (10)

Define heart failure. Describe its pathophysiology, diagnosis, and treatment.

DNBIIIA/DEC2013 (10)

Etiologies of chronic heart failure. Pathogenesis of heart failure with depressed ejection fraction. Drugs treatment of chronic heart failure.
DNBIIIA/JUN2015 (10)

Enumerate factors that can decompensate chronic heart failure. Cardiac biomarkers for diagnosing chronic heart failure. Explain how ACEI improve the quality of life of patients with chronic heart failure.
DNBIIIA/DEC2015 (10)

Ventricular remodeling.
MGR/APR2014/MDI (5)

Describe etiology, clinical features, diagnosis and management of primary diastolic dysfunction of the heart.
MGR/SEP2009/MDIII (20)

Recent advances in the management of heart failure.
MGR/APR2015/MDIV (7)

Neurohumoral activation and compensatory mechanisms in heart failure.
MGR/MAR2006/MDI (6)

Etiopathogenesis, clinical features and recent trends in the management of chronic heart failure.
MGR/SEP2006/MDIV (20)

Define cardiac failure. Describe the management of cardiac failure.
RGUHS/APR2003/MDII (20)

Destination therapy in heart failure.
MUHS/NOV2013/MDIV (10)

Principles of management of chronic heart failure.
PGI/APR2013/MDII (10)

Describe heart failure with normal ejection fraction.
BF/MAY2013/MDIV (10)

What are the modalities of non-pharmacological treatment of congestive cardiac failure?
BF/OCT2011/MDIII (20)

Discuss the current concepts in the management of heart failure.
BF/OCT2010/MDIV (20)

Discuss the advances in the diagnosis and management of early heart failure.
BF/MAY2010/MDIII (25)

Diastolic dysfunction.
BF/MAY2009/MDIV (10)

Markers in heart failure.
BF/JUN2016/MDII (10)

Describe the pathophysiology, diagnosis and management of diastolic heart failure.
GMC/2016/MDI (25)

New concepts in cardiac failure.
MGR/APR2016/MDIV (7)

How will you approach a case of heart failure? What are the types and recent trends in the management of heart failure?
MLB/MAY2009/MDII (20)

Recent advances in the management of heart failure.
KERALA UNIVERSITY, 2022, (10)

Define diastolic dysfunction. What is the difference between diastolic dysfunction and diastolic heart failure? What are the strategies and how would you manage diastolic dysfunction?
WEST BENGAL HEALTH UNI, 2022 (10)

Briefly outline the neurohumoral activation in heart failure. What are the novel heart failure markers? Write the role of SGLT-2 inhibitors in the management of heart failure.
WEST BENGAL HEALTH UNI, 2022 (10)

Discuss recent advances in the management of cardiac failure

VEER NARMAD SOUTH GUJARAT UNIVERSITY, 2022 (25)

Define, classify, and describe etiology, pathophysiology of heart failure. How would you manage the case of chronic heart failure?

MAHARASHTRA UNIVERSITY OF HEALTH SC, VIJAYAWADA, 2021 (10)

Biomarkers in heart failure

MAHARASHTRA UNIVERSITY OF HEALTH SC, VIJAYAWADA, 2021 (5)

TEERTHANKER MAHAVEER UNI, 2017 (10), MGR UNI, TAMIL NADU, 2018 (10)

BHARATI VIDYAPEETH DEEMED UNI, JHELUM, 2019 (10)

AIIMS, 2023 (10)

Describe pulsus alternans. Clinical features and management of left ventricular failure.

DNB, 2019 (2+4+4)

Etiology and pathogenesis of heart failure. Treatment of heart failure with reduced ejection fraction.

DNB, 2019 (2+3+5)

Management of heart failure.

BHARATI VIDYAPEETH UNIVERSITY, SUMMER 2016 (10)

Discuss types and common causes of heart failure. How can heart failure be diagnosed and managed effectively?

BHARATI VIDYAPEETH UNIVERSITY, WINTER 2016 (10)

Recent advances in the management of heart failure

BHARATI VIDYAPEETH UNIVERSITY, SUMMER 2017 (10)

Management of heart failure.

BABA FARID UNI OF HEALTH SC, 2017 (10)

Resistant heart failure and its management.

BABA FARID UNI OF HEALTH SC, 2017 (10)

Brain natriuretic peptides.

MGR UNI, TAMIL NADU, 2018 (10)

Classify heart failure. Discuss investigations, and management of heart failure.

BHARATI VIDYAPEETH UNIVERSITY, SUMMER 2017 (15)

Describe in detail the risk factors, pathophysiology, stages, evaluation and management of heart failure.

TEERTHANKER MAHAVEER UNI, JUNE, 2018 (10)

Pharmacologic and invasive cardiac care support in acute heart failure.

TEERTHANKER MAHAVEER UNI, 2018 JUNE (20)

Classify heart failure. Describe its pathophysiology. Write briefly on evidence based updates in the management of heart failure with reduced ejection fraction.

BHARATI VIDYAPEETH UNIVERSITY, WINTER 2019 (15)

Add answers from question 95

Diagnosis and management of heart failure with decreased ejection fraction.

BABA FARID UNI OF HEALTH SC, 2018 (10)

Recent advances in the management of heart failure.

KERALA UNIVERSITY, 2019 (10)

Discuss etiology, pathophysiology, diagnosis and evidence based advances in management in heart failure with preserved ejection fraction.

SARDAR PATEL UNIVERSITY, 2019 (25)

Describe and classify cardiomyopathies. Discuss the various drugs used in the treatment of chronic congestive heart failure.

NTR UNIVERSITY OF HEALTH SC, VIJAYAWADA, ANDHRA, 2020 (10)

Classifications of cardiomyopathies described in question number 60.

RAAS in the cardiovascular system.

SAURASHTRA UNIVERSITY, 2020 (20)

Preserved ejection fraction heart failure.

AIIMS (NEW DELHI), 2022 (10)

Discuss Frank–Starlings law and its clinical significance. Describe mechanisms of various types of heart failure. Write a note on mechanisms of action of different drugs used in management of heart failure.

AIIMS, 2023 (20)

HFpEF.

SCBMCH, 2022 (10)

HFpEF definition, pathophysiology, clinical features laboratory diagnosis and management.

SCBMCH, 2018 (10)

Clinical features and laboratory diagnosis of chronic heart failure.

SCBMCH, 2019 (10)

Etiopathogenesis and management of heart failure.

SCBMCH, 2021 (10)

Discuss the pathophysiology of heart failure. What are the distinctive phenotypes of acute decompensated heart failure, their presentations, and management principles?

DNB (JUN2022) (10)

Define asymptomatic left ventricular dysfunction and its pathogenesis. Outline the protocol for its screening. Discuss the role of SGLT-2 inhibitors and devices therapy in ASLVD.

DNB (OCT2024) (10)

Describe the classification of heart failure. Discuss the management of heart failure with preserved ejection fraction.

AIIMS, BBS, 2023 (10)

Define heart failure. Enumerate the stages of heart failure. How will you diagnose and manage "heart failure with reduced ejection fraction".

MGU, 2024 (20)

Preload and afterload heart failure.

MANIPUR UNIVERSITY, 2018 (10)

Describe recent advances in the management of heart failure with reduced ejection fraction.

MANIPUR UNIVERSITY, 2019 (10)

Heart failure with reduced ejection fraction.

MAHATMA UNIVERSITY, 2018 (10)

What is diastolic dysfunction? How do you manage a patient with diastolic dysfunction?

WBUHS, 2023 (10)

Discuss the ventricular abnormalities in heart failure. How do you investigate and treat a case HFpEF.

WBUHS, 2024 (10)

ANSWER

Definition

Heart failure can be defined as a progressive disease of heart muscles which are progressively damaged by index event leading to loss of myocytes or prevent the myocardium to generate the force to contract normally. Inciting event may be acute as in case of myocardial infarction or it may be chronic as in case of volume overloading or hereditary cardiomyopathies.

Definition of asymptomatic left ventricular dysfunction: It can be defined as presence of left ventricular systolic and diastolic dysfunction in absence of any clinical symptom but detected by echocardiography or cardiac MRI or nuclear imaging.

Cardiac dysfunction can be divided into two types:

A. Systolic dysfunction:

- **a.** It is characterized by reduced with enlarged left ventricular chamber.
- **b.** It is clinically associated with left ventricular failure with cardiomegaly.
- **c.** It is also called as heart failure with reduced ejection fraction.

B. Diastolic dysfunction:

   a. It is characterized by increased resistance to filling and increased filling pressure.

   b. It is associated with pulmonary congestion with normal or slightly associated ventricle. It is also known as heart failure with preserved ejection fraction.

Causes of Chronic Heart Failure

A. Ischemic cardiomyopathy

B. Dilated cardiomyopathy:

   a. Subclinical viral myocarditis

   b. Familial dilated cardiomyopathy

   c. Hypertensive cardiomyopathy

   d. Diabetic cardiomyopathy

   e. Cardiotoxic agents:

      1. Anthracycline

      2. Alcohol

      3. Stimulant drugs

      4. Toxin exposure

   f. Inflammatory cardiomyopathy

   g. Tachyarrhythmia-induced cardiomyopathy

   h. Peripartum cardiomyopathy

   i. Valvular disorders

   j. Hypothyroidism

   k. Thiamine and other nutritional deficiency

   l. Anemia

   m. Inherited myopathy

   n. Chagas disease

   o. Sarcoidosis

Systolic Dysfunction with Reduced Ejection Function

The patient is asymptomatic or minimally symptomatic in spite of initial decline in cardiac pumping capacity. It is due to several compensatory mechanisms that will be acted upon to modulate the left ventricular function for several months or years. These include:

   a. Renin–angiotensin–aldosterone system (RAAS) and adrenergic system which through increased salt and water retention maintains the cardiac output.

   b. Increased contractility of myocardium

   c. Factors of setting the peripheral resistance:

      1. Brain natriuretic peptides—ANP and BNP

      2. Bradykinin

      3. Prostaglandins—PGE2 and PGI2

      4. Nitric oxide

      Bradykinin and natriuretic peptides are degraded by neprilysin, a membrane bound peptidase.

As a result of above compensatory mechanisms the function of left ventricle will be within the physiologic range and the patients remains minimally asymptomatic for months or years. But at some point of time the patients become progressively increasing symptomatic with increased morbidity and mortality, this transition from asymptomatic to symptomatic condition is accompanied by adrenergic, neurohumoral, and cytokine systems that lead to several adaptive changes in the myocardium known as left ventricular remodeling.

As a result of following complex events occurring from cellular and molecular level left ventricular remodeling develops:

   a. Alteration of contractile properties of cardiac myocyte.

   b. Progressive loss of myocyte as a result of cellular necrosis, apoptosis, and autophagic cell death.

   c. Hypertrophy of myocyte

   d. Desensitization of beta-adrenergic receptors

   e. Myocardial metabolism becomes abnormal

   f. Recognition and dissolution of organized structured collagen of extracellular matrix surrounding the myocytes which will be replaced by interstitial collagen matrix having no capability of giving support to myocytes. Stimuli for these changes are:

      1. Mechanical stretch of myocytes

      2. Circulating neurohormones:

         - Angiotensin II
         - Norepinephrine

      3. Inflammatory cytokines:

         - Tumor necrosis factor
         - Other peptides
         - Growth factor like endothelin
         - Reactive oxygen species like superoxide.

Progressive overexpression of these biological molecules exerts their deleterious effect to depress the cardiac function. By the following process the cardiac myocyte can alter the biological activity to depress the cardiac function.

Neurohumoral activation is responsible for following transcriptional and posttranscriptional changes regulating excitation-contraction coupling and cross-bridge interactions:

Decreased function of sarcoplasmic reticulum calcium adenosine triphosphatase leading to:

   a. Decreased uptake calcium into sarcoplasmic reticulum.

b. Leakage of calcium from sarcoplasmic reticulum due to hyperphosphorylation of ryanodine receptor.

As a result following changes occur in the cross-bridges:

a. Decreased expression of alpha-myosin heavy chain
b. Increased expression of beta-myosin heavy chain
c. Myocytolysis
d. Cytoskeleton link between sarcomeres and extracellular matrix.

All the above changes will lead to impairment of the ability of the monocytes to contract which in turn leads to depressed left ventricular systolic function with reduced ejection fraction.

Neurohumoral activation also leads to cardiac systolic dysfunction in following mechanisms:

A. Activation of sympathetic nervous system:

Chronic activation of sympathetic nervous system results:

a. Decreased responsiveness of beta-adrenergic receptors
b. Decreased store of norepinephrine
c. Sympathetic innervation of the myocardium

As a result of the above changes lead to hypertrophy, necrosis followed by fibrosis of the cardiac myocytes.

Extracardiac effects of the above mechanisms include:

a. Increased tubular reabsorption of sodium
b. Activation of RAAS
c. Neurogenic and systemic vasoconstriction
d. Vascular hypertrophy

B. Activation of RAAS:

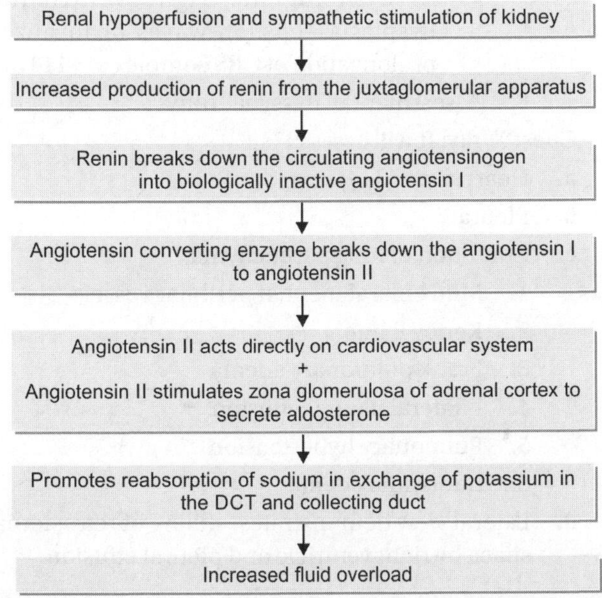

Other effects of aldosterone: It promotes:

a. Vascular hypertrophy
b. Myocardial hypertrophy followed by fibrosis
c. Endothelial dysfunction
d. Inhibition of uptake of norepinephrine

Diastolic Dysfunction with Preserved Ejection Fraction

Relaxation of myocardial muscle cells is ATP-dependent process that is regulated by following mechanisms:

a. Uptake of calcium by sarcomere by SARC2A
b. Extrusion of calcium by sarcolemmal pump.

In case of myocardial ischemia decreased concentration of ATP leads to slowing to myocardial contraction.

Again, in case of myocardial stiffness secondary to ventricular hypertrophy or fibrosis left ventricular pressure will be elevated at end-diastole.

In case of noncompliant ventricle, if tachycardia occurs, there is disproportionate shortening in time of ventricular filling leading to increased left ventricular filling pressure—that in turn increases pulmonary capillary pressure resulting dyspnea.

All the causes culminate lead to diastolic dysfunction with preserved ejection fraction.

But both systolic and diastolic dysfunction may be present in patients with heart failure.

Left Ventricular Remodeling

Ventricular remodeling refers to following changes in the left ventricle after cardiac injury:

a. Shape
b. Size
c. Mass
d. Volume
e. Composition of heart

All the above changes will lead to abnormal hemodynamic and mechanical burden which lead to remodeling of the ventricles leading to progression of heart failure. Along with increase in the left ventricular end-diastolic volume there is progressive thinning of left ventricular wall leading to dilatation of left ventricle—it has following effects:

A. There is increase in the afterload leading to functional afterload mismatch, which in turn further decreases the stroke volume. Increased stress of left ventricular end-diastolic wall may lead to:

a. Worsening of left ventricular function due to hypoperfusion of subendocardium.

  b. Activation of family of genes that are sensitive to free radicals generated such as TNF, interleukin 1β.
  c. Sustained expression of stretch activation of pathways of hypertrophic signaling.

B. There is increased tethering of the papillary muscles leading to incompetence of mitral valve apparatus resulting functional mitral regurgitation. As a result hemodynamic load will be increased thus further worsening of heart failure.

According to recent studies reversal of left ventricular remodeling by medical and device therapy can lead to improve in clinical outcome in patients with systolic dysfunction with reduced ejection fraction, so main aim in heart failure is left ventricular remodeling reversion or prevention.

Genetic and Epigenetic Factors

Genetic predisposition to cardiomyopathy like familial cardiomyopathy and epigenetic factors like DNA methylation, modification of histones, etc., may lead to asymptomatic left ventricular dysfunction.

Dysfunction at the Microvascular Level

Coronary endothelial dysfunction leads to coronary microvascular dysfunction results decreased perfusion of the myocardium. This results in subclinical myocardial ischemia leading to myocardial fibrosis and left ventricular dysfunction.

Diagnosis

A. Comprehensive metabolic panel:
  a. Hyponatremia: It portends worse prognosis
  b. Hypokalemia: It occurs in patients under diuretic therapy
  c. Hyperkalemia—It occurs in:
    1. Overaggressive potassium repletion
    2. Treatment with RAAS
    3. Use of potassium sparing diuretics
    4. Diabetic patients with type IV renal tubular acidosis (RTA)
  d. Anemia: It may be due to iron deficiency or chronic renal disease.
  e. Liver function test
  f. Lipid profile
  g. Blood urea nitrogen, creatinine
  h. Fasting blood glucose and postprandial blood glucose
  i. Thyroid function test
  j. Serum B-natriuretic peptide or N-terminal pro-B natriuretic peptide:
    1. It can differentiate cardiac from non-cardiac cause of dyspnea.
    2. It is an independent predictor of elevated left ventricular end diastolic pressure.
    3. It will assess the mortality risk in patient with heart failure.
    4. It correlates with NYHA classification
    5. It will assess the efficacy of treatment.

    These may be elevated in renal dysfunction, atrial fibrillation and in elderly.

    It will be falsely negative in:
    1. Hypothyroidism
    2. Advanced heart failure due to myocardial fibrosis.
    3. Obesity
  k. Troponin T and I: Its persistent elevation indicates adverse outcome and increased mortality.

B. ECG:
  a. It can provide cause and treatment of heart failure (HF).
  b. It can evaluate the patients with HF.
  c. It is essential to look for the evidence of:
    1. Myocardial infarction (MI)
    2. Hypertrophy of heart chambers
    3. Conduction disease
    4. Different types of arrhythmias
    5. Specific diagnosis in case of amyloidosis:
      - Low voltage complexes with pseudo-infarction pattern in anterior leads.
      - Arrhythmogenic right ventricular dysplasia—epsilon waves or localized prolongation of QRS complex of >110 ms.
    6. Assessment of dyssynchrony

C. Chest X-ray: It will assess:
  a. Heart size
  b. Pleura
  c. Condition of lung parenchyma:
    1. Mild enlargement of perihilar vessels
    2. Kerley B line
    3. Frank pulmonary edema
    4. Bilateral pleural effusion
    5. Pulmonary hypertension
    6. Interstitial edema
  d. Lateral view demonstrates—filling of retrosternal space by right ventricle and pleural effusion.

D. Assessment of left ventricular function:

a. Two-dimensional (2D) and Doppler echocardiography: It can evaluate the following:

1. Etiology of heart failure:

- Regional wall motion abnormalities—ischemic and nonischemic cardiomyopathies
- Presence and severity of valvular dysfunction like stenosis or regurgitation.

2. Prognosis of HF: Following parameters are very useful to assess the mortality and morbidity:

- Ejection fraction (EF) and left ventricular dimension: EF ≥ 50%—suggests adequate systolic function whereas EF of <30–40%—suggests depression of cardiac contractility.
- Left ventricular mass: Eccentric hypertrophy leading to cardiac remodeling increases left ventricular mass. Eccentric hypertrophy means >95 g/m^2 in women and >115 g/m^2 with regional motion thickness of ≤0.42.

3. Myocardial performance index (Tei index): Tei index of >0.77 in patients with DCM is highly predictive of increased morbidity and mortality.

4. Measures of diastolic dysfunction

b. Magnetic resonance imaging (MRI): It will provides following information:

1. Cardiac anatomy and functions for assessing left ventricular mass and volumes.

2. It can diagnose specific cardiomyopathies.

3. Late gadolinium hyperenhancement demonstrating scar: It will discriminate between the ischemic and nonischemic causes of fibrosis.

c. Nuclear imaging: Single-photon emission computed tomography and positron emission tomography (PET) imaging can rule out myocardial ischemia, viability, and metabolic activity. Viability can be assessed critically in patients with coronary artery disease (CAD) and potential for recovery in case of revascularization by radiotracers such as 18F fluorodeoxyglucose and thallium 201.

E. Right ventricular catheterization: It combined with exercise testing or addition of vasodilator agents can evaluate impact of hemodynamics. Indications of catheterization are following:

a. Short-term management of cardiogenic shock.

b. Evaluation of patients for cardiac transplantation.

c. Clarification of hemodynamics in the context-specific comorbidities, i.e., right ventricular infarction.

d. Clarification or optimization of medical therapy in case of refractory symptoms.

F. Exercise testing:

a. It is done for assessing the need for cardiac transplantation in case of advanced HF.

b. Peak oxygen uptake of <14 mL/kg/min: It is associated with poor prognosis.

G. Biomarkers:

Both BNP and N-terminal pro-BNP released from failing heart–sensitive markers for HF with depressed ejection fraction, but may be increased in case of preserved ejection fraction but to a lesser extent. It is also useful to establish the diagnosis, prognosis, and severity of chronic HF, and optimal dose of medical therapy. It can also be elevated in following cases:

a. Age of the patients

b. Renal impairment

c. Sex: It is more elevated in women

d. In right HF from any cause

e. Patients taking angiotensin receptor-neprilysin inhibitor (ARNI) therapy

It can also falsely be elevated in obesity.

Other biomarkers such as ST-2 and galectin-3: These can determine the prognosis.

H. Genetic testing: It should be done in different causes of cardiomyopathies like

a. Titin

b. Laminin A and C

c. Myosin heavy chain

d. Cardiac troponin T mutation

Diagnostic Criteria for Heart Failure with Preserved Ejection Fraction

A. Presence of symptoms and signs typical of heart failure:

a. Note that the signs are not always evident in patients with HF with preserved ejection fraction, as filling pressure may only increase with exercise and the jugular venous pressure may not be elevated at rest.

b. Typical signs and symptoms included are:

1. Breathlessness,

2. Reduced exercise tolerance

3. Fatigue

4. Swelling in the ankle

5. Displaced apex beat

6. Absent third heart sound

B. A preserved ejection fraction of ≥50%:

a. Previous studies have included patients with left ventricular ejection fraction of ≥40%.

b. According to new guidelines a gray zone between left ventricular ejection fractions 40% and 50%.

C. Elevated levels of natriuretic peptide:

a. Brain natriuretic peptide level of ≥35 pg/mL.

b. Amino terminal pro-BNP level of ≥125 pg/mL.

D. Objective evidence of other cardiac structural or functional alteration:

a. Either left ventricular hypertrophy (increased left ventricular mass index) or left atrial enlargement.

b. Diastolic dysfunction on echocardiography (increased E/e′ or decreased e′) or cardiac catheterization (increased left ventricular end-diastolic pressure or pulmonary capillary wedge pressure, particularly with exercise).

According to commonly used Framingham Diagnostic criteria following 2 major or 1 major and 2 minor criteria can make the diagnosis of heart failure:

Major criteria:

A. Acute pulmonary edema

B. Cardiomegaly

C. Distension of neck vein

D. Hepatojugular reflux

E. Paroxysmal nocturnal dyspnea or orthopnea

F. Pulmonary crepitations

G. Third heart sound

Minor criteria:

A. Ankle edema

B. Dyspnea on exertion

C. Nocturnal cough

D. Hepatomegaly

E. Pleural effusion

F. Heart rate more than 120 beats/min.

Treatment

A. Acute decompensated typical heart failure:

a. High-risk features are:

1. Renal insufficiency

2. Biomarker of injury

3. Acute coronary syndrome

4. Arrhythmia

5. Hypoxia

6. Pulmonary embolism

7. Infection

b. In normotensive patients: Diuretics

c. In case of hypertensive patients: Vasodilators

B. Acute decompensated "pulmonary edema":

a. Risk factors are:

1. New-onset arrhythmias

2. Valvular heart disease

3. Inflammatory heart disease

4. Myocardial ischemia

5. Drug toxicity

6. Central nervous system (CNS) injury

b. Opiates and vasodilators

c. Administration of oxygen through noninvasive ventilation.

C. Acute decompensated "low output" failure:

a. Features are:

1. Hypoperfusion

2. Dysfunction of end-organ

b. Risk-factors:

1. Low pulse pressure

2. Extremities cool

3. Cardiorenal syndrome

4. Hepatic congestion

c. Treatment:

1. Vasodilators

2. Inotropic therapy in case of low blood pressure or refractory to diuretic therapy.

3. Hemodynamic monitoring

D. Acute decompensation "cardiogenic shock":

a. Features are:

1. Hypotension

2. Low-cardiac output

3. End-organ failure

b. Risk-factors:

1. Extreme distress

2. Pulmonary congestion

3. Renal failure

c. Therapy:

1. Ionotropic therapy with catecholamines

2. Mechanical ventilatory support
3. Intra-aortic balloon pump
4. Percutaneous ventricular assist device
5. Ultrafiltration

E. **Treatment of acute decompensated heart failure:**

Drug	Dose	Caution	Comments
Ionotropic drug			
Use: Hypotension, end-organ hypoperfusion or shock			
Dobutamine	2–20 μg/kg/min	Increased demand of myocardium for oxygen	Adverse effects: Hypersensitivity carditis, clinical tolerance to prolonged infusion
Milrinone	0.375–0.75 μg/kg/min	• Hypotension • Arrhythmia	Caution: • Decrease dose in renal insufficiency • Effective in presence of beta-blocker
Levosimendan	0.1 μg/kg/min	Hypotension, arrhythmia	Caution: Should not be used in case of blood pressure
Vasodilators			
Indications: Pulmonary congestion to get rapid relief from dyspnea in presence of preserved blood pressure			
Nitroglycerin	10–20 μg/min increased up to 200 μg/min	• Headache • Flushing • Tolerance	It is effective in high dose
Nesiritide	Bolus 2 μg/kg followed by 0.01 μg/kg/min infusion	Hypotension	• There may be decrease in perfusion pressure in kidney • Bolus may increase hypotension
Nitroprusside	0.3 μg/kg/min to be titrated to 5 μg/kg/min	In case of renal insufficiency chance of thiocyanate toxicity	Placement of arterial line for titration to maintain normal blood pressure
Serelaxin	• Not available • Tested at 30 μg/kg/day	Baseline blood pressure be >125 mm Hg	It is ineffective in confirmatory trials
Ularitide	15 ng/kg/min for 48 hours	Baseline blood pressure >116 mm Hg	Aggravation of hypotension
Diuretics			
In case of volume overload with pulmonary congestion first-line therapy can be used as bolus or continuous infusion Initial low dose is 1 × home dose Or, high dose–2.5 × high dose Are equally effective, high risk of renal worsening in case of high dose			
Furosemide	20–240 mg daily	Electrolyte monitoring	In case of severe infusion, continuous infusion is required
Torsemide	10–100 mg daily	Continuous electrolyte monitoring	It is given orally, it is more effective in advanced heart failure
Bumetanide	0.5–5 mg daily	Electrolyte monitoring	Orally used, immediate bioavailability

Treatment of Cardiorenal Syndrome

It is most dreaded complication of acute decompensated heart failure. It is the complex interplay between heart and renal abnormalities resulting from deterioration of one organ while proper therapies are administered to preserve the function of the other organ. Nearly 30% of patients with acute decompensated heart failure suffer from abnormal renal function. But different studies fail to demonstrate the correlation between:

a. Deterioration of renal function
b. Cardiac output
c. Left-sided filling pressure
d. Reduced renal perfusion

So, in patients with acute decompensated heart failure this syndrome may result from complex interplay of neurohumoral factors that will be exacerbated by "backward failure" resulting from:

a. Increased intraabdominal pressure

b. Impaired return of renal venous blood flow

So, in the face of elevated right-sided filling pressure, continuous diuretic therapy may be responsible for reduction of glomerular filtration rate (GFR) and worsening of cardiorenal syndrome.

In the later stage of heart failure, ionotropic therapy or mechanical support of circulation may improve the renal function.

Ultrafiltration

Ultrafiltration may supplement the need for diuretic therapy. Following are the proposed benefits of ultrafiltration:

a. Controlled rate of fluid removal

b. No effect on serum electrolytes

c. Decreased neurohumoral activity

But different studies failed to demonstrate the advantages of ultrafiltration over conventional diuretic therapy as ultrafiltration may decrease the weight but there is worsening of serum creatinine.

F. Treatment of chronic heart failure with reduced ejection fraction:

Drug	Initiation	Target dose
ACEI		
Lisinopril	2.5–5 mg four times daily	20–35 mg four times daily
Enalapril	2.5 mg twice daily	10–20 mg twice daily
Captopril	6.25 mg thrice daily	50 mg twice daily
Trandolapril	0.5–1 mg four times daily	4 mg four times daily
ARBs		
Losartan	50 mg four times daily	150 mg four times daily
Valsartan	40 mg twice daily	160 mg twice daily
Candesartan	4–8 mg four times daily	32 mg four times daily
Aldosterone antagonists		
Eplerenone	25 mg four times daily	50 mg four times daily
Spironolactone	12.5–25 mg four times daily	25–50 mg four times daily
Beta-blockers		
Metoprolol	12.5–25 mg four times daily	200 mg four times daily
Carvedilol	3.125 mg twice daily	25–50 mg twice daily
Bisoprolol	1.25 mg four times daily	10 mg four times daily
Arteriovenous vasodilators		
Hydralazine/ Isosorbide dinitrate	37.5/20 mg thrice daily	75/40 mg thrice daily
Fixed-dose hydralazine/ Isosorbide dinitrate	37.5/20 mg thrice daily	75/40 mg four times daily
Angiotensin receptor-neprilysin inhibitor		
Sacubitril; l-valsartan	100 mg twice daily	200 mg twice daily

(ACEI: angiotensin-converting-enzyme inhibitor; ARBs: angiotensin receptor blockers)

Other drugs used are the following:

a. Heart rate modification:

Ivabradine, inhibitor of I_f current in SA node inhibitor will slow the heart rate without any negative chronotropic effect. It should be considered in:

1. Symptomatic patients with heart rate of 70 beats/min after guideline-based beta-blockers, ACEI, and mineralocorticoid receptor antagonists.
2. Patients who are intolerant to beta-blocker.

b. Digoxin:

Action:

1. Mild inotropic effect
2. Attenuate carotid sinus baroreceptor activity
3. It is sympathoinhibitory

As a result it will decrease:

1. Plasma renin level
2. Plasma norepinephrine level
3. Serum aldosterone level

It should be started with low dose because at high dose therapeutic safety is very low.

c. Oral diuretics:

Loop diuretics are used for its increased potency, frequent adjustment of dose due to its variable oral absorption, and fluctuating kidney function.

d. Calcium channel blocker:

1. First-generation drugs such as diltiazem and verapamil are not used as because these drugs may destabilize the patients who are asymptomatic.
2. Second-generation drugs such as amlodipine and felodipine can safely reduce the blood pressure with reduced ejection fraction, but without affecting morbidity and mortality.

e. Inflammation:

1. Anticytokine agents such as infliximab and etanercept are unsuccessful rather they will worsen the heart failure.
2. Intravenous immunoglobulin therapy has no beneficial outcome.
3. Nonspecific immunomodulation—where blood sample from HF patient is exposed to controlled oxidative stress followed by intramuscular injection of the treated sample to the same patient to initiate apoptosis of leukocytes. Result of physiologic response of the apoptotic cells is reduction of production of inflammatory cytokines with increasing production of anti-inflammatory cytokines.

f. Statin should be used to reduce the major cardiovascular events along with improved survival of nonheart failure patients.

g. Anticoagulation and antiplatelet therapy:

Heart failure with reduced ejection fraction is associated with hypercoagulable state leading to thromboembolic phenomena such as stroke, peripheral arterial disease, and pulmonary embolism. According to recent guideline aspirin can be used in patient with ischemic cardiomyopathy.

h. Fish oil: Long-chain omega-3 polyunsaturated fatty acid enrich the circulating eicosapentaenoic acid, and as the later one has inverse relationship with mortality in these HF patients, this oil obviously help these patients.

i. Micronutrients: There is strong association of HF with reduced ejection fraction with thiamine and selenium. Thiamine deficiency occurs in malnutrition and diuretic therapy. So thiamine supplementation may improve the HF.

j. Enhanced external counterpulsation: In CAD patients graded external pneumatic compression at high pressure each for 1 hour session for 35 sessions in 7 weeks will reduce the angina pain and also extend the time of exercise-induced ischemia of the limb.

k. Exercise: It can be recommended in patients with HF but after improvement of cardiac condition.

Triggering Factors for Decompensation in Heart Failure

a. Excessive salt and water intake
b. Excessive physical exertion
c. Nonadherence to treatment
d. Different types of arrhythmias
e. Pulmonary thromboembolism
f. Systemic hypertension
g. Myocardial ischemia/MI
h. Fever/infection
i. Elevated room temperature
j. Anemia
k. Nutritional deficiencies
l. Excessive consumption of alcohol
m. Depression
n. Pregnancy
o. Renal failure
p. Use of illicit drugs like cocaine
q. Inappropriate prescription/inappropriate dose
r. Factors related to physician:

1. Intravenous fluid overload
2. Undetected volume overload
3. Failure to provide adequate advice to the patient regarding diet and physical activity.
4. Lack of training in the management of patients with HF.

s. Factors related to medication:

1. Digitalis intoxication
2. Water-retaining or prostaglandin inhibiting drugs
3. Negative ionotropic drugs

Mechanism of Action of ACEI

A. Activation of RAAS:

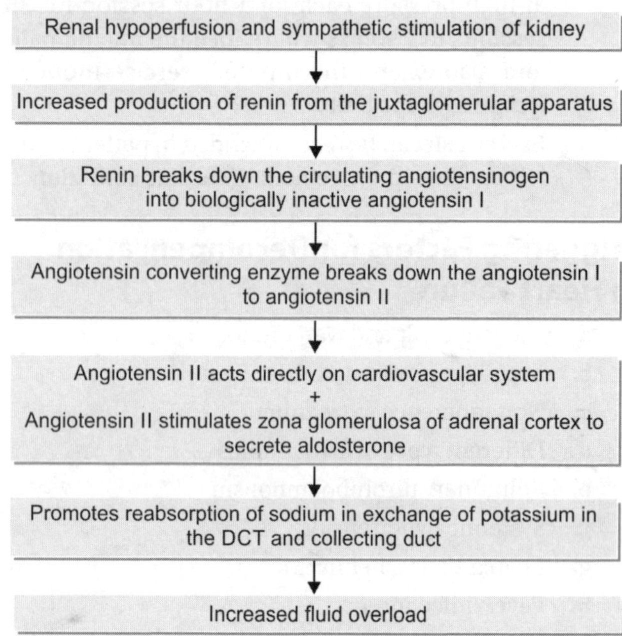

Other effects of aldosterone: It promotes:

- **a.** Vascular hypertrophy
- **b.** Myocardial hypertrophy followed by fibrosis
- **c.** Endothelial dysfunction
- **d.** Inhibition of uptake of norepinephrine

Angiotensin-converting-enzyme will be blocked by ACEI leading to reduced formation of angiotensin-II thus aldosterone secretion from the adrenal gland will be reduced. So fluid retention will be decreased.

Emerging Treatment of Heart Failure

A. Empagliflozin:

It is sodium-glucose cotransporter-2 inhibitor. It has following positive effects:

- **a.** On markers of arterial stiffness
- **b.** Vascular resistance
- **c.** Visceral adiposity
- **d.** Albuminuria
- **e.** Plasma urate

  As per European Society of Cardiology (ESC) 2016, metformin is the drug of choice in HF and when associated with empagliflozin it will reduce hospitalization for HF.

B. Iron therapy:

According to ESC 2016 guideline it is class IIB recommendation. Intravenous iron is useful in HF patients with reduced ejection fraction along with iron deficiency with serum ferritin of <100 μg/L or in between 100 and 299 μg/L and saturation of transferrin of <20% to:

- **a.** Improve the HF symptoms
- **b.** Improve the exercise capacity
- **c.** Improve the quality of life

C. Omecamtiv mecarbil:

It is cardiac-specific myosin activator. It will increase the rate of binding of actin with myosin leading to increase in stroke volume without the increase in oxygen consumption or increasing the intracellular calcium.

D. Ularitide (Urodilatin):

It is secreted by distal tubular cells in the kidney, binds to natriuretic peptide receptor-A (NPR-A) in the inner medullary collecting duct, then via cyclic GMP inhibits reabsorption of sodium. It has also vasodilatory, neurohumoral effects.

E. Influenza vaccination:

Patients with chronic HF are at high risk of complication due to influenza virus. Influenza vaccine trial demonstrated that this vaccine will provide benefit in HF.

F. Serelaxin:

Relaxin is a polypeptide, released from the female endometrium. Serelaxin is a recombinant human relaxin 2, in pregnancy it:

- **a.** Increases the cardiac output
- **b.** Increases arterial compliance
- **c.** Increases renal blood flow

G. Rivaroxaban:

It is well-known anticoagulant that reduces morbidity and mortality in HF in chronic heart disease.

H. Vericiguat:

It is soluble guanylate cyclase stimulator molecule on natriuretic peptide in patients whose HF is gradually worsening.

I. Patiromer calcium and sodium zirconium cyclosilicate:

Hyperkalemia is one and very important risk factor in HF with reduced ejection fraction patients. These two novel drugs will increase the loss of potassium through gastrointestinal tract thereby reducing the side effects of hyperkalemia produced by many antihypertensive drugs. Patiromer suspension helps in exchange of potassium at the expense of calcium and other drug sodium zirconium traps potassium in the small bowel in crystalline lattice.

J. Istaroxime: It inhibits the action of Na/K ATPase and reverses the Na/Ca exchanger thereby increases the calcium entry leading to contraction of cardiac muscle cells. It may be the rising star in the new modalities of management of HF.

Invasive cardiac care support in acute heart failure:

A. Intra-aortic balloon counter pulsation:

a. Indications:
1. Post myocardial infarction cardiogenic shock
2. Acute mitral regurgitation
3. Severe failure with reduced cardiac output
4. Post infarction VSD
5. As a bridge to more definitive treatment.

b. Advantages:
1. It improves coronary perfusion by increasing the left ventricular diastolic pressure
2. It will reduce the cardiac afterload leading to increase in the cardiac output.
3. It will provide short term hemodynamic support in critical situation.

c. Contraindications:
1. Aortic dissection
2. Aortic regurgitation
3. Severe peripheral disease
4. Uncontrolled bleeding
5. Coagulopathy

d. Complications:
1. Aortic dissection or aortic rupture
2. Ischemia of the involved limb
3. Thrombosis
4. Infection
5. Embolization.

B. Veno-arterial extracorporeal membrane oxygenation:

a. Indications:
1. Severe cardiogenic shock
2. Acute heart failure unresponsive to pharmacologic therapy
3. As a bridge to cardiac transplantation
4. Cardiac arrest
5. Acute decompensated heart failure
6. As a bridge to ventricular assisted device.

b. Advantages:
1. It will provide fulltime cardiopulmonary support
2. As a bridge to transplant or recovery.
3. It will improve the oxygen delivery to increase tissue perfusion.

c. Contraindications:
1. Severe neurological injury
2. Irreversible multiorgan failure
3. Advanced age
4. Poor prognosis
5. End stage heart failure without transplant.

d. Complications:
1. Vascular complications
2. Bleeding at the cannulation site
3. Infection
4. Hemolysis
5. Thrombosis
6. Liver dysfunction
7. Renal failure

C. Left ventricular assisted device:

a. Indications:
1. Acute heart failure
2. As a bridge to transplant
3. Cardiogenic shock unresponsive to therapy
4. Refractory heart failure
5. End stage heart failure no a candidate for cardiac transplant

b. Advantages:
1. It will provide long term circulatory support
2. It will improve the left ventricular after-load
3. It will improve the cardiac output and tissue perfusion
4. It acts as a bridge to cardiac transplant

c. Contraindications:
1. Irreversible neurological injury
2. Multiorgan failure
3. Severe peripheral arterial disease
4. Infection
5. Coagulopathy
6. Poor candidacy for cardiac transplant

d. Complications:
1. Infection
2. Thrombosis leading to stroke
3. Failure of the device
4. Right ventricular failure

5. Bleeding as a result of administration of anticoagulant

D. Percutaneous coronary intervention:

a. Indications:

1. Acute coronary syndrome
2. Coronary artery occlusion leading to cardiogenic shock

b. Advantages:

1. It will improve the myocardial function by restoring the coronary perfusion
2. It will reduce the size of the infarct by increasing the coronary artery perfusion
3. It can be performed quickly in any lab.

c. Contraindications:

1. Severe coagulopathy
2. Diffuse coronary artery disease
3. Recent stroke
4. Recent major surgery

d. Complications:

1. Hematoma at the insertion site
2. Infection
3. Dissection of the coronary artery
4. Stent thrombosis
5. Contrast induced nephropathy
6. Restenosis
7. Procedural arrhythmia

E. Ultrafiltration:

a. Indications:

1. Diuretic resistant acute fluid overload leading to acute heart failure
2. Severe pulmonary congestion leading to pulmonary edema
3. Significant renal impairment leading decreased responsive to diuretics.

b. Advantages:

1. Removes the fluid leading to decreased fluid overload and decreased pulmonary congestion.
2. It can be useful in case of renal dysfunction

c. Contraindications:

1. Hypotension
2. Severe electrolytic imbalances
3. Where cardiac condition is unstable

d. Complications:

1. Infection
2. Electrolyte imbalance
3. Hypotension leading to worsening of renal function
4. Hemorrhage at the insertion site

Management of Selected Comorbidity

A. Sleep disordered breathing: Frequent period of hypoxic episode with evidence of micro- or macroarousal will trigger adrenergic surge that leads to impaired both systolic and diastolic function and worsening of hypertension. So, in patients with difficulty to treat hypertension or worsening of function of right heart in presence of improved left ventricular function will trigger for search of sleep disordered breathing. This feature can be treated by positive airway pressure which can improve:

a. Oxygenation
b. Left ventricular ejection fraction
c. 6-minute walk test

B. Anemia: It is common and is associated with increased proclivity for admission in hospital or increased mortality. It is more common in following cases:

a. Renal insufficiency
b. Women
c. African-Americans
d. Advanced stage of HF
e. Gastrointestinal bleeding
f. Iron deficiency
g. Dysregulated metabolism of iron

Treatment by intravenous iron in the form of iron-sucrose or carboxymaltose can improve anemia.

C. Depression: It is very common in HF with reduced ejection fraction. It is associated with:

a. Poor quality of life (QOL).
b. Limited functional reserve.
c. Increased risk of mortality and morbidity.

It can be treated by sertraline but cannot provide greater reduction of depression and cannot improve cardiovascular status.

D. Atrial arrhythmias: Atrial fibrillation is common and carries worse prognosis. Rhythm control can be achieved by:

a. Pharmacotherapy with amiodarone and dofetilide—these both are safe and effective but cannot alter the natural history of the disease.
b. Catheter-induced ablation and pulmonary vein isolation are also safe and effective.

E. Diabetes mellitus: Empagliflozin can decrease the cardiovascular mortality and hospitalization in HF.

According to American Heart Association the treatment of Heart Failure

Stage A or at risk of heart failure:

A. Its case hypertensive patient guideline directed medical therapy should be administered.

B. In case of type II diabetes mellitus SGLT-2 inhibitor should be given to reduce hospitalization.

C. Life style modification should be recommended.

D. Optimum management of cardiovascular disease in case of coronary heart disease.

E. Screening of heart failure by natriuretic peptide evaluation should be recommended.

Stage B or pre-heart failure:

A. In case of left ventricular ejection fraction ≤ 40% ACEI should be administered to prevent clinical heart failure or reduction of mortality.

B. In case of left ventricular ejection fraction ≤ 40% with evidence of acute coronary syndrome and myocardial infarction statin and beta blocker should be given to reduce mortality, heart failure and adverse cardiovascular events.

C. In case of left ventricular ejection fraction ≤ 30% receiving medical therapy and NYHA class I, primary prevention intracoronary device is recommended.

D. In case of left ventricular ejection fraction ≤ 40% beta blocker is recommended irrespective of etiology to prevent symptomatic heart failure.

E. In case of left ventricular ejection fraction ≤ 50% thiazolidinedione and non-dihydropyridine calcium channel blockers increase the risk of hospitalization for heart failure should be avoided.

F. Repair of valve repair, replacement or intervention should be done according to recommended guidelines.

Stage C or heart failure:

A. Vaccination should be administered for respiratory illness to reduce mortality.

B. Multidisciplinary management should be done for improving self-care and reducing the mortality.

C. Low sodium diet is recommended.

D. Psychiatric evaluation should be done

E. Exercise training is recommended to improve the functional class

F. In case of congestion thiazide diuretics should be given to improve symptoms.

G. In case of heart failure with reduced ejection fraction, ARNi is recommended if the patient is intolerant to ACEI and ARB should be given. ARNi should not be administered within 36 hours of last dose of ACEI. ARNi should not be given to a patient with history of angioedema.

H. In heart failure with reduced EF beta blocker carvedilol, bisoprolol or sustained release metoprolol should be given to reduce mortality.

I. In case of heart failure with reduced ejection fraction, NYHA class III or IV, eGFR of more than 30 mL/min/m^2 and serum potassium less than 5 meq/L, MRA is recommended. If serum potassium more than 5 meq/L, MRA will be harmful.

J. In case of heart failure with reduced ejection fraction SGLT-2 inhibitor should be administered to reduce mortality irrespective of the diabetic status of the patient.

K. In case of heart failure with reduced ejection fraction, NYHA class III to IV and patient is receiving optimum medical therapy, hydralazine and nitrate should be recommended.

L. All the medications should be titrated to achieve the proper outcome.

M. Ivabradine should be given in patient already receiving optimum medical therapy and heart rate 70 beats/min to improve mortality benefits.

N. Device therapy:

- **a.** Implantable cardioverter defibrillator is indicated as primary prevention of sudden cardiac death in patient with heart failure with reduced ejection fraction of ≤ 35% and NYHA class II or III and on goal directed medical therapy.
- **b.** Cardiac resynchronization therapy is recommended in patient with biventricular pacing with heart failure with reduced ejection fraction of ≤ 35% and NYHA class II or III, QRS duration ≥ 150 milliseconds, sinus rhythm with LBBB.

O. Revascularization therapy is indicated in patient with CAD and with heart failure with reduced ejection fraction and on goal directed medical therapy.

Stage D or advanced heart failure:

A. The patient should be referred to heart failure specialist.

B. Ionotropic support and device therapy.

C. Mechanical cardiac support like durable left ventricle assist device or ECMO as it makes a bridge to cardiac transplantation.

D. Cardiac transplantation.

Novel Biomarkers of Heart Failure

A. Suppression of tumorigenicity 2 (ST2): It is a member of interleukin 1 receptor family existing in both soluble and transmembrane forms. Its high level is associated with:

a. Myocardial stress and fibrosis.

b. Adverse outcome in patient with heart failure

c. Prognostic information independent of natriuretic peptides.

B. Galectin-3: It is beta-galactoside binding lectin secreted by macrophages and is involved in myocardial inflammation and fibrosis. Its high level is associated with:

a. Worst outcome in heart failure.

b. Progression of heart failure with and increased mortality.

C. Growth differentiation factor 15: It is member of transforming growth factor beta superfamily and is associated with increased oxidative stress as well as inflammation. Its level is increased in:

a. Severity of heart failure

b. Adverse clinical outcome

D. Soluble urokinase plasminogen activator receptor: It will reflect immune activation and inflammation. Its level is increased in:

a. Worst outcome in case of heart failure

b. Poor prognostic information that complements natriuretic peptides.

E. Midregional pro-adrenomedullin: It is stable fragment of adrenomedullin, it is involved in maintaining the vascular integrity and vasodilatation. Its high level is associated with:

a. Severity of heart failure

b. Prognosis in heart failure

c. Prediction of short term and long term outcome in heart failure

d. Assessing the risk of hospitalization and mortality.

F. MicroRNAs: These are small non-coding RNA regulating post-transcriptional gene expression. These are associated with:

a. Progression of myocardial injury in heart failure

b. Myocardial remodeling and apoptosis.

SGLT-2 Inhibitor in Heart Failure

A. The drugs are:

a. Empagliflozin

b. Dapagliflozin

c. Canagliflozin

B. Mechanism of action:

a. Diuresis and natriuresis: These drugs produce osmotic diuresis and natriuresis leading to decreased plasma volume and preload.

b. Reduction of interstitial fluid: These drugs will reduce the interstitial fluid and intravascular volume leading to reduction of vascular congestion without the activation of neurohumoral activation.

c. Modulation of cardiac metabolism: These drugs will shift the utilization of myocardial substrate from glucose to ketone bodies thereby improving the myocardial energetics and function.

d. Reduction of oxidative stress and inflammation: It will reduce the oxidative stress and inflammation thereby protect the heart.

e. These drugs reduce the afterload through reduction of systemic vascular resistance.

Role of SGLT-2 Inhibitors in case of Asymptomatic Left Ventricular Failure

A. In case of heart failure with reduced ejection fraction, clinical trial demonstrated that there is reduced risk of hospitalization and reduced risk of cardiovascular death through the following mechanisms:

a. Natriuresis

b. Reduction of pre and afterloads

c. Improved metabolism of the myocardium

B. In case of heart failure with preserved ejection fraction, by the improvement of diastolic function, and reduction of left ventricular mass the cardiovascular death rate will be reduced.

Frank–Starling Law

Frank–Starling law can be defined as relation between the filling of the ventricle during diastole, i.e., ventricular end diastolic volume and force of subsequent ventricular contraction. So if the end diastolic ventricular volume is high the subsequent ventricular contraction will be forceful leading to increased stroke volume.

The background of the phenomenon is stretching of the cardiac muscle fibers during filling of the ventricle which aligns the actin and the myosin filaments to an optimum position to form cross-bridge thereby enhances the contraction of the ventricles.

Frank–Starling Relationship

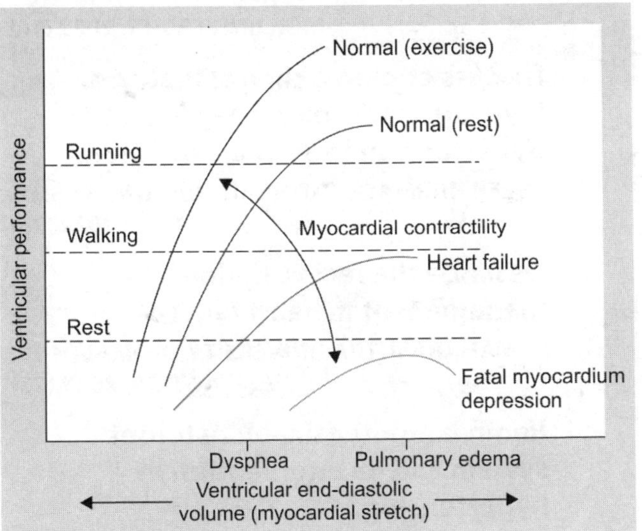

Clinical Significance of this Law

a. Normal physiology:

1. Maintenance of the cardiac output according to the body's physiological demand, i.e., during exercise due to increased metabolic demand the venous return will be increased and the cardiac output will be increased.
2. It will balance between the left and right ventricular output and thereby reduces the pulling of blood in the pulmonary vascular bed.

b. Heart failure:

1. Decompensated heart failure where the ventricle will operate on the flattened part of the curve, so, in spite of increased preload the stroke volume will not be increased, as a result of increased preload there is pulmonary vascular congestion in case of left ventricular failure and peripheral edema in case of right ventricular failure. So diuretics should be administered to reduce the vascular congestion.

c. Stage of shock:

1. In case of hypovolemic shock, there is decreased preload leading to reduced contraction of the ventricles and it will reach in the lower portion of the curve. This can be replenished by administration of the fluid that can increase the preload and heart muscle contraction will reach a favorable point of the curve. But in case of cardiogenic shock curve will be flattened due to cardiac muscle dysfunction, in spite of administration of intravenous fluid there will be limited benefit.

d. In case of pulmonary hypertension, contraction ability of the right ventricle is determined by the Frank–Starling curve. As a result of chronically increased pressure right ventricle will fail.

e. Effect of the left ventricular compliance: As a result of left ventricular hypertrophy there will be reduced compliance of left ventricular cavity leading to decreased stroke volume.

f. In case of trained athlete increased venous return to the heart along with the ventricular dilatation both the stroke volume and cardiac output will be increased.

Frank–Starling's Mechanism

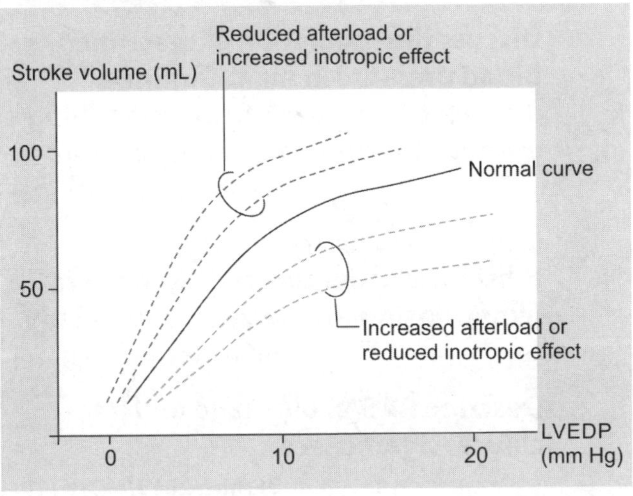

Clinical Monitoring of the Frank–Starling Curve

a. Pressure-volume loops is used to visualize the combined relation between preload, afterload and stroke volume and cardiac output.

b. Echocardiographic monitoring of the ventricular end diastolic volume and stroke volume which can assess the position of the heart on the Frank–Starling curve.

c. Pulmonary capillary wedge pressure can be monitored to measure the left ventricular preload.

Q23. Define hypertension. Classify and enumerate the causes of secondary hypertension. Describe hypertensive emergencies and their management.

DNBI/DEC2012 (10)

Classify the antihypertensive drugs. Add a note on latest one antihypertensive drug.

MGR/SEP2007/MDI (5)

Newer guidelines on hypertension.

MJPRU/2014/MDIV (10) MJPRU/2015/MDIV (10)

Discuss the classification, etiology, clinical features, diagnosis, investigation, and management of hypertension in adult.

MGR/MAR2006/MDI (15)

Discuss the regulation of systemic blood pressure in man. Outline a diagnostic approach to an underlying etiology in secondary hypertension.

BF/OCT2011/MDI (23)

Define and classify systemic hypertension. Discuss clinical approach to hypertension in a 20 years young lady.

BF/MAY2013/MDIII (10)

Describe RASAS blockage and its clinical significance.

BF/MAY2013/MDIV (10)

Discuss the causes of secondary hypertension. What are hypertensive emergencies and discuss the drugs used in the treatment of a case of hypertensive emergency.

BF/OCT2011/MDII (30)

Discuss various homeostatic mechanisms of blood pressure control. Enumerate the causes of secondary hypertension.

BF/OCT2010/MDI (25)

Classify antihypertensive drugs.

MGR UNIVERSITY, TAMIL NADU, 2022 (5)

ARNI.

MGR UNIVERSITY, 2022 (10)

Discuss etiology, clinical features, investigation, and management of hypertension in 30 years old man.

VEER NARMAD SOUTH GUJARAT UNIVERSITY, 2022 (25)

Describe the recent updates in management in heart failure

MAHARASHTRA UNIVERSITY OF HEALTH SC, VIJAYAWADA, 2021 (25)

Renin–angiotensin–aldosterone system and its intervention in hypertension.

KERALA UNIVERSITY, 2017 (10)

Hypertensive emergencies.

NTR UNIVERSITY OF HEALTH SC, VIJAYAWADA, ANDHRA, 2022 (10)

Secondary hypertension.

BABA FARID UNI OF HEALTH SC, 2017 (10)

Approach to a patient with hypertension.

BABA FARID UNI OF HEALTH SC, 2018 (10)

Vascular remodeling in hypertension.

BABA FARID UNI OF HEALTH SC, 2018 (10)

Enumerate secondary hypertension. Describe clinical features and management of secondary hypertension.

VEER NARMAD SOUTH GUJARAT UNIVERSITY, 2019 (25)

Management of hypertensive emergencies.

NTR UNIVERSITY OF HEALTH SC, VIJAYAWADA, ANDHRA, 2020 (10)

Secondary hypertension.

RAJASTHAN UNIVERSITY, 2021 (8)

Classify anti-hypertensive drugs. Outline the management of hypertension in pregnancy.

SAMS (ODISHA), 2023 (10)

Hypertension in pregnancy described in question number 106.

Recent guidelines of hypertension.

SCBMCH 2023 (5)

Enumerate the causes of secondary hypertension. Outline the approach to a patient with resistant hypertension.

DNB (OCT2024) (10)

Resistant hypertension described in question number 8.

Etiology of hypertension in young was described in question number 79.

What is nocturnal hypertension? Discuss the management of hypertensive emergencies.

DNB, 2024 MAY (10)

Masked hypertension.

MAHATMA UNIVERSITY, 2019 (10)

ANSWER

According to JNC-8 Guideline Definition of Hypertension

Classification of blood pressure in adults (age ≥18 years)			
Classification	**Systolic blood pressure (mm Hg)**		**Diastolic blood pressure (mm Hg)**
Normal	<120	and	<80
Prehypertension	120–139	or	80–89
Stage 1 HTN	140–159	or	90–99
Stage 2 HTN	≥160	or	≥100

(HTN: hypertension)

Etiology of Hypertension

A. Primary hypertension:

a. Genetic causes: 20–60% hypertension is inherited as familial. Large number of genes are responsible for hypertension, but single gene-related hypertension is less common.

b. Different intermediate phenotypes are responsible. These are:

1. Familial dyslipidemia
2. Metabolic syndrome
3. Insulin resistance
4. Abnormal distribution of fat
5. Sodium hypersensitivity
6. Modulation of aldosterone and renal blood flow
7. Abnormal ion transport system

B. Causes of secondary hypertension:

Age groups	Percentage of patients who have hypertension with an underlying cause	Most common etiologies
Children (birth to 11 years)	70–85	• Renal parenchymal disease • Coarctation of the aorta
Adolescents (12–18 years)	10–15	• Renal parenchymal disease • Coarctation of the aorta
Young adults (19–39 years)	5	• Thyroid dysfunction • Fibromuscular dysplasia • Renal parenchymal disease
Middle-aged adults (40–64 years)	8–12	• Hyperaldosteronism • Thyroid dysfunction • Obstructive sleep apnea • Cushing syndrome • Pheochromocytoma
Older adults (65 years and older)	17	• Atherosclerotic renal artery stenosis • Renal failure • Hypothyroidism

Causes of Secondary Hypertension with Special Features

Possible secondary hypertension cause	Suggestive features
	Vascular causes
Renal artery stenosis	• Renal bruit • Increase in creatinine level after starting ACE inhibitor or ARB

Continued

Continued

Possible secondary hypertension cause	Suggestive features
Coarctation of aorta	Differential blood pressure >20 mm Hg between arm and leg Delayed or absent femoral pulse
Endocrine causes	
Thyrotoxicosis	• Heat intolerance • Menstrual disturbance • Tachycardia and tremor
Hyperaldosteronism	Hypokalemia
Pheochromocytoma	• Episodic sweating and pallor • Palpitations • Blood pressure elevation in paroxysms
Cushing's syndrome	• Central obesity • Abdominal striae, width >1 cm and violaceous (reddish-purple) Facial plethora, round facial appearance • Easy bruising
Other causes	
Obstructive sleep apnea	• Snoring • Daytime somnolence
Drug-induced	Potential offending medication

(ACE: angiotensin converting enzyme; ARB: angiotensin II receptor blockers)

Hypertension Criteria

Criterion	Systolic blood pressure	Diastolic blood pressure
Office blood pressure	≥140 mm Hg	≥90 mm Hg
Ambulatory blood pressure (daytime)	≥130 mm Hg	≥80 mm Hg
Ambulatory blood pressure (night time)	≥120 mm Hg	≥70 mm Hg
Home blood pressure	≥135 mm Hg	≥85 mm Hg

Hypertension Emergencies

Definition

It is characterized by spectrum of clinical presentation due to abrupt rise in blood pressure above 180 mm Hg systolic blood pressure and 120 mm Hg diastolic blood pressure with evidence of acute target organ damage in an otherwise stable patient without any evidence of acute target organ damage.

Hypertensive urgency: It can be defined as severe hypertension but without damage of any organ.

Following are the precipitating factors of hypertensive emergencies:

- **a.** Essential hypertension from poorly controlled hypertension.
- **b.** Renovascular disease
- **c.** Nonadherence to antihypertensive medication
- **d.** Preeclampsia
- **e.** Pheochromocytoma
- **f.** Acute and chronic renal parenchymal disease
- **g.** Ischemic stroke
- **h.** Intracranial hemorrhage
- **i.** Drug induced:
  1. Drug interaction
  2. Idiosyncratic reaction
  3. Sudden withdrawal
  4. Collagen vascular disease
  5. OSA

Organ Involved with Clinical Presentation

A. Nervous system:
- **a.** Hypertensive encephalopathy
- **b.** Cerebral infarction
- **c.** Cerebral hemorrhage
- **d.** Subarachnoid hemorrhage

B. Cardiovascular system:
- **a.** Myocardial ischemia
- **b.** Unstable angina pectoris
- **c.** Myocardial infarction
- **d.** Acute left ventricular dysfunction
- **e.** Acute pulmonary edema
- **f.** Aortic dissection

C. Kidney:
- **a.** Acute renal failure

D. Eye:
- **a.** Arteriolar spasm
- **b.** Hemorrhage
- **c.** Exudates
- **d.** Papilledema

E. *Hematology*: Microangiopathic hemolytic anemia

F. *Pregnancy*: Eclampsia and preeclampsia. It may lead to:
- **a.** Maternal stroke
- **b.** Cardiopulmonary decompensation to pulmonary edema
- **c.** Fetal decompensation
- **d.** Abruption placenta
- **e.** Stillbirth

G. Others:

a. Perioperative hypertension

b. Pheochromocytoma crisis

c. Sympathomimetic hypertensive crisis following cocaine, amphetamine or abrupt cessation of clonidine.

Pathology

a. Diffuse necrotizing vasculitis

b. Thrombi in the arteriole

c. Deposition of the fibrin in the arteriolar walls in the kidney, brain, retina, uterus, and other organs.

Treatment According to Organ Involved

Name of the disease	Drugs used
Hypertensive encephalopathy	Nitroprusside, labetalol, and nicardipine
Stroke	Nicardipine, nitroprusside, and labetalol
Malignant hypertension	Nitroprusside, labetalol, and enalaprilat
Myocardial infarction, unstable angina	Labetalol, nitroprusside, esmolol, and nicardipine
Acute left ventricular failure	Loop diuretic, nitroprusside, and enalaprilat
Aortic dissection	Labetalol, esmolol, and nitroprusside
Postoperative hypertension	Nitroprusside, nitroglycerin, labetalol, and nicardipine
Adrenergic crisis	Nitroprusside and phentolamine
Preeclampsia, eclampsia	• Labetalol, hydralazine, and nicardipine • ACEI and ARBs should be avoided due to possible fetal/placental toxicity • Magnesium sulfate should be given to decrease convulsion

(ACEI: angiotensin-converting-enzyme inhibitors; ARB: angiotensin II receptor blockers)

Drugs with Dose of the Drugs

Name of the drug	Doses of the drugs intravenous use	Toxicity
Nitroprusside	Initially 0.3 µg/kg/min intravenously, that can be increased every 5 minutes until desired level of blood pressure	• Cyanide toxicity. Prophylactic transfusion of vitamin B12 to decrease the concentration of cyanide, tissue hypoxia • Hypotension, nausea, vomiting, and twitching
Labetalol (alpha- and beta-adrenergic blocking agents)	2 mg/min up to 300 mg, Or, 20 mg over 2 minutes followed by 40–80 mg at 10 minutes interval up to total 300 mg	It should not be used in case of heart failure, atrioventricular block, COPD, and bronchial asthma
Hydralazine—direct relaxation vascular smooth muscle cells along with reflex increase in stroke volume and heart rate	Initially 10–20 mg at 30 minutes interval. Hypotensive effect starts within 10–30 minutes	Hirsutism, reflex tachycardia, headache, nausea, vomiting, and aggravation of angina
Nitroglycerin—it is arterial and vasodilator with more effect on large arteries	Initially 5 µg/min followed by 5 µg/min at 3–5 minutes intervals In case of nonresponse, it should be increased to 20 µg/min with incremental increases of 10–20 µg/min may be used	Headache, flushing at high dose, and tolerance after prolonged use
Nicardipine	Initially 5 mg/hour it should be titrated by 2.5 mg/h at 5–15 minutes interval, maximum up to 15 mg/h	
Enalaprilat	0.625–1.25 mg over 5 minutes 6–8 hourly, maximum up to 5 mg/dose	Renal failure and hypotension
Esmolol	Initially 80–500 µg/kg over 1 minute followed by 50–300 µg/kg/min	Hypotension, asthma, and heart block
Phentolamine	5–15 mg bolus	

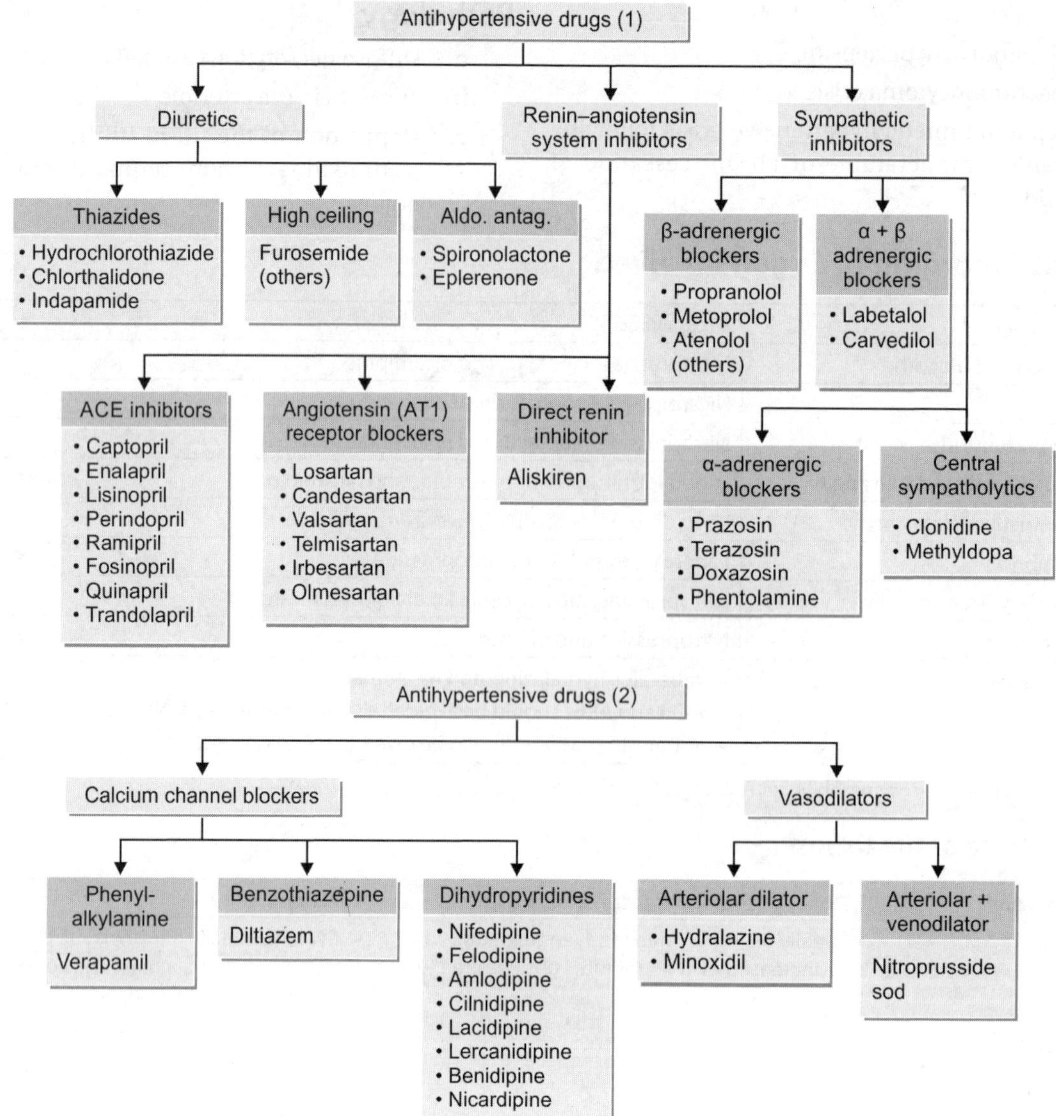

(ACE: angiotensin-converting-enzyme)

Direct Inhibitors of Renin

A. Aliskiren:

a. It will compete with angiotensinogen to get access to the active site of renin thereby reduces the serum concentration of angiotensin I and II and thus decrease the systolic and diastolic blood pressure.

b. As monotherapy it is as effective as ACEI or ARBs.

c. It is also effective with amlodipine and hydrochlorothiazide.

d. Dose is 150–300 mg/day

e. Adverse effect: No obvious adverse effect, but in high dose it will produce diarrhea.

f. Pharmacokinetics: Its bioavailability is poor, 90% of this drug is excreted unchanged in feces. ACEI, ARBs, and direct renin inhibitors cannot be used together.

g. Contraindications:

1. Renal artery stenosis
2. Pregnancy

B. Enalkiren

C. Remikiren

These drugs are used in case of arterial hypertension. They will target the rate-limiting step in renin–angiotensin–aldosterone axis.

There will be hyperreninemia due to compensatory increased release of renin, but it is not clinically significant.

Clinical Features

Hypertension can be documented when there is evidence of increased blood pressure at least three occasions which is based on average of two pressure readings taken in each of more than equal totwo follow-up visits after initial screening. Following related history to be taken:

A. Extent of the damage of end-organs such as heart, brain, and kidney.

B. History relating to the cardiovascular status of the patients.

C. Exclusion of the secondary causes of hypertension.

In case of undiagnosed hypertension, patients may present with the following features of end-organ damage:

D. History regarding the risk factors:
- **a.** Obesity: Body mass index (BMI) ≥ 30 kg/m^2
- **b.** Smoking or chewing of tobacco
- **c.** Diabetes
- **d.** Hyperlipidemia: Elevated low-density lipoprotein-cholesterol (LDL-C)
- **e.** Age > 55 years for men and > 65 years for women.
- **f.** Chronic kidney disease with GFR of <60 mL/minute
- **g.** Lack of exercise
- **h.** Family history of premature cardiovascular disease.

E. History-related to organ involvement:
- **a.** Evidence of myocardial infarction like severe chest pain
- **b.** History-related to angina like central chest pain
- **c.** History-related to HF such as exertional dyspnea, cough, and hemoptysis
- **d.** History-related to cerebral stroke such as headache, vomiting, and altered consciousness
- **e.** History of chronic renal disease

F. History-related to secondary hypertension:
- **a.** History of known renal disease, anemia, and urochrome presentation
- **b.** History suggestive of pheochromocytoma such as labile hypertension, sweating, and palpitation
- **c.** History of hyperthyroidism such as heat intolerance, sweating, and tachycardia
- **d.** History of obstructive sleep apnea
- **e.** Weakness, fatigability suggestive of hyperaldosteronism
- **f.** Presence of renal stones of hyperparathyroidism

Physical Examinations

A. Nervous system:
- **a.** Hypertensive encephalopathy
- **b.** Cerebral infarction
- **c.** Cerebral hemorrhage
- **d.** Subarachnoid hemorrhage

B. Cardiovascular system:
- **a.** Myocardial ischemia
- **b.** Unstable angina pectoris
- **c.** Myocardial infarction
- **d.** Acute left ventricular dysfunction
- **e.** Acute pulmonary edema
- **f.** Aortic dissection

C. Kidney:
- **a.** Acute renal failure

D. Eye:
- **a.** Arteriolar spasm
- **b.** Hemorrhage
- **c.** Exudates
- **d.** Papilledema
- **e.** Hematology: Microangiopathic hemolytic anemia

E. *Pregnancy*: Eclampsia and preeclampsia. It may lead to:
- **a.** Maternal stroke
- **b.** Cardiopulmonary decompensation to pulmonary edema
- **c.** Fetal decompensation
- **d.** Abruption placenta
- **e.** Stillbirth

F. Evidences of peripheral arterial disease

Laboratory Evaluation

A. Initial work:
- **a.** Fasting blood sugar
- **b.** Glycosylated hemoglobin
- **c.** *Serum electrolytes*: Sodium, potassium, and calcium
- **d.** Serum creatinine and urea
- **e.** Estimated GFR
- **f.** Uric acid
- **g.** Urine analysis, microalbumin

B. Investigations-related to secondary hypertension:
- **a.** Chronic kidney disease (CKD):
  1. Estimated GFR,

2. Cystatin C,
3. *Serology*: Antinuclear antibody (ANA), antidouble stranded DNA (anti-DS-DNA), and C3 and C4.
4. Ultrasonography of kidney:
   - *In CKD*: Small scarred kidney
   - *In case of diabetes*: Enlarged kidney
   - Renal biopsy

b. *Coarctation of aorta*: Aortography, computed tomography (CT) angiography

c. *Drug-induced hypertension*: Drug screening

d. *Cushing syndrome*: Dexamethasone suppression test, 24 hours urinary cortisol, and late-night salivary cortisol

e. *Pheochromocytoma*: 24-hour urinary metanephrines, normetanephrine estimation, and plasma free metanephrines

f. Primary aldosteronism:
   Plasma aldosterone-to-renin activity ratio,
   1. Ours urinary aldosterone level,
   2. Saline infusion to determine low serum aldosterone level whether it is suppressed or not.

g. Renovascular hypertension:
   1. Doppler flow ultrasonography
   2. MR angiography
   3. CT angiography

h. *Sleep apnea*: Sleep study with oxygenation, polysomnography, and night time pulse oximetry

i. Thyroid or parathyroid disease: Thyroid-stimulating hormone (TSH) level and serum parathyroid level

C. Investigations to rule out emergencies:

a. Complete blood count along with peripheral blood smear: Microangiopathic hemolytic anemia

b. Dipstick urine analysis, red blood cell cast, and microscopic hematuria: Chronic renal impairment

c. Other tests as above

D. Imaging studies:

a. In case of suspected renal artery stenosis:
   1. CT angiography
   2. *MR angiography*: But if the estimated GFR is <30 mL/min, then gadolinium should not be used as it may further damage the kidney by producing fibrosis.
   3. Invasive renal arteriography

b. *Digital subtraction angiography*: In case of renal or pulmonary causes of hypertension it can evaluate the disease, but there is risk of dye-induced nephrotoxicity or atheroemboli in case of chronic renal disease and diabetes mellitus.

c. *Echocardiography*: It can detect the following features:
   1. Left ventricular hypertrophy
   2. Left atrial dilatation
   3. Diastolic left ventricular dysfunction
   4. Systolic left ventricular dysfunction

d. Stress echocardiography can detect the prognosis in patients with systemic hypertension.

E. Holter monitoring

F. Cerebral evaluation:

a. Fundus examination:
   1. Hypertensive retinopathy
   2. Diabetic retinopathy

b. Residue of cerebrovascular accident by CT and MRI

c. CT and MRI

d. Assessment of peripheral arterial disease:
   1. *Ankle-brachial index*: It can be measured by lower extremity systolic pressure/upper extremity systolic pressure
   2. *Duplex Doppler studies*: It can detect anatomic site of stenosis. It should be routinely after femoral-tibial-pedal bypass and femoral-popliteal bypass with venous conduit.
   3. CT or MR angiography
   4. Arteriography

Nonpharmacological Therapy

A. *Reduction of sodium intake*: Recommended dose is 100 mEq/L/day in all patients with hypertension or prehypertension. In case of white, black, and Asian subjects it will improve the vascular compliance, but in black pulse wave velocity will be reduced.

B. *Exercise*: It will increase the blood flow that will increase the shearing stress on the endothelium leading to release of vasodilator, nitric oxide. Even after brisk walking blood pressure fall of nearly 22 mm Hg. This exercise-induced improvement is more in case of hypertensive patients as compared to normotensive patients. It is enhanced in young athlete but in case of elderly with systolic hypertension such improvement in vascular compliance is not seen.

C. Dietary factors:

a. Dietary approaches to stop hypertension (DASH) diet which is enriched with vegetables and fruits and low in saturated fat and total fat as this diet will reduce the blood pressure by 12/6 mm Hg. This reduction in blood pressure is due to its natriuretic effect. Its high content of potassium and ascorbic acid will lower the blood pressure.

b. Lowering the sugar content in the diet will lower the blood pressure.

c. Dark brown chocolate will release nitric oxide thus improving the endothelial function leading to lowering of blood pressure.

d. Nuts reduces the peripheral resistance that will lead to lowering of blood pressure.

e. Coffee:

1. In case of habitual drinker, it will increase the sympathetic nerve activity but no change in blood pressure.

2. In case of nonhabitual drinker, due to its active ingredients, it will increase sympathetic nerve activity as well as blood pressure.

D. *Alcohol*: Moderate white as well as red wine will reduce the blood pressure. Within few hours of alcohol intake there is reduction of blood pressure peripherally and centrally. But in case of heavy drinker, there is increase in arterial stiffness.

E. *Stress relief method*: Yoga, meditation as well as music

a. Will decrease sympathetic activity

b. Will reduce the variability in blood pressure

Pharmacologic therapy in hypertension:

Drug	Initial dose	Dose range	Adverse effects
Renin inhibitors			
Aliskiren	150 mg once daily	150–300 mg once daily	• Angioedema • Hypotension • Hyperkalemia • Contraindication: Pregnancy
Aliskiren + hydrochlorothiazide	150/12.5 mg once daily	150/12.5–300/25 mg once daily	
ACE inhibitors			
Benazepril	10 mg once daily	5–40 mg once or twice daily	• Hypotension • Dry cough • Dizziness • Hyperkalemia • Kidney dysfunction • Angioedema • Alteration in taste • Rash • Rarely blood dyscrasia • Contraindication: Pregnancy
Benazepril + hydrochlorothiazide	5/6.25 mg once daily	5/6.25–20/25 mg once daily	
Benazepril + amlodipine	10/2.5 mg once daily	10/2.5–40/10 mg once daily	
Captopril	25 mg twice daily	50–450 mg in 2–3 doses	
Captopril + hydrochlorothiazide	25/15 twice daily	25/15–50/25 mg twice daily	
Enalapril	5 mg once daily	5–40 mg 1–2 doses	
Enalapril + hydrochlorothiazide	5/12.5 mg once daily	5/12.5–10/25 mg	
Fosinopril	10 mg once daily	10–80 mg once or twice daily	
Fosinopril + hydrochlorothiazide	10/12.5 mg once daily	10/12.5–20/12.5 mg once daily	
Lisinopril	5–10 mg once daily	5–40 mg once daily	
Lisinopril + hydrochlorothiazide	10/12.5 mg once daily	10/12.5–20/12.5 mg once daily	
Perindopril	4 mg once daily	4–16 mg in 1–2 doses	
Perindopril + amlodipine	3.5/2.5 mg once daily	14/10 mg once daily	
Ramipril	2.5 mg once daily	2.5–20 mg in 1–2 doses	
Trandolapril	1 mg once daily	1–8 mg once daily	

Continued

Continued

Drug	Initial dose	Dose range	Adverse effects
Angiotensin II receptor blocker			
Azilsartan	40 mg once daily	40–80 mg once daily	• Hypokalemia • Renal dysfunction • Angioedema • Contraindication: Pregnancy
Azilsartan + chlorthalidone	40/12.5 mg once daily	40/12.5–40/25 mg once daily	
Candesartan	16 mg once daily	8–32 mg once daily	
Candesartan + hydrochlorothiazide	16/12.5 mg once daily	32/12.5 mg once daily	
Eprosartan	600 mg once daily	400–800 mg 1–2 doses	
Irbesartan	150 mg once daily	150–300 mg once daily	
Irbesartan + hydrochlorothiazide	150/12.5 mg once daily	150/12.5–300/50 mg once daily	
Losartan + hydrochlorothiazide	50/12.5 mg once daily	50/12.5–100/25 mg once daily	
Olmesartan	20 mg once daily	20-40 mg once daily	
Olmesartan + hydrochlorothiazide	20/12.5 mg once daily	20/12.5–40/25 mg once daily	
Olmesartan + amlodipine	20/5 mg once daily	20/5–40/10 mg once daily	
Telmisartan	40 mg once daily	20–80 mg once daily	
Telmisartan + hydrochlorothiazide	40/5 mg once daily	40/5–80/10 mg once daily	
Valsartan	80 mg once daily	80–320 mg once daily	
Valsartan + hydrochlorothiazide	80/12.5 mg once daily	80–320 mg once daily	
Nondihydropyridine agents			
Diltiazem	90 mg once daily	180–360 mg in two doses	• Edema • Headache • Bradycardia • GI disturbance • AV block • Heart failure • Urinary frequency
Verapamil	80 mg thrice daily	80–480 mg in three divided doses	
Amlodipine	2.5 mg once daily	2.5–10 mg once daily	• Edema • Palpitation • Headache • Hypotension • Tachycardia • GI disturbance
Felodipine	5 mg extended release once daily	5–10 mg once daily	• Myopathy • Hepatotoxicity • Edema
Isradipine	2.5 mg twice daily	2.5–5 mg twice daily	
Nicardipine	20 mg thrice daily	20–40 mg thrice daily	
Nifedipine	30 mg extended release once daily	30–90 mg extended release once daily	
Nisoldipine	17 mg once daily	17–34 mg once daily	

Continued

Continued

Drug	Initial dose	Dose range	Adverse effects
Thiazide and related diuretics			
Hydrochlorothiazide	12.5–25 mg once daily	12.5–50 mg once daily	• Hyponatremia • Hypokalemia • Hypocalcemia • Hypomagnesemia • Hyperuricemia • Hyperglycemia • Hyperlipidemia • Erectile dysfunction
Chlorthalidone	12.5–25 mg once daily	12.5–50 mg once daily	
Metolazone	1.25–2.5 mg once daily	1.25–2.5 mg once daily	
Indapamide	2.5 mg once daily	2.5–5 mg once daily	
Bendroflumethiazide	2.5 mg once daily		
Loop diuretics			
Furosemide	20 mg twice daily	40–320 mg in 2–3 doses	• Hyponatremia • Hypokalemia • Hypocalcemia • Hypomagnesemia • Hyperuricemia • Hyperglycemia • Hyperlipidemia • Erectile dysfunction
Ethacrynic acid	50 mg once daily	50–100 mg once or twice daily	
Bumetanide	0.25 mg twice daily	0.5–10 mg in 2–3 doses	
Torsemide	5 mg once daily	5–10 mg once daily	
Aldosterone receptor antagonists			
Spironolactone	12.5–25 mg once daily	12.5–100 mg once daily	• Hyperkalemia • Metabolic acidosis • Gynecomastia
Amiloride	5 mg once daily	5–10 mg once daily	
Eplerenone	25 mg once daily	25–100 mg once daily	
Beta-adrenergic blocking agents			
Acebutolol	400 mg once daily	200–1200 mg in 1–2 doses	
Atenolol	25 mg once daily	25–100 mg once daily	
Betaxolol	10 mg once daily	10–40 mg once daily	
Bisoprolol	5 mg once daily	5–20 mg once daily	
Carvedilol	6.25 mg twice daily 20 mg extended release once daily	12.5–50 mg in two doses 20–80 mg extended release once daily	
Labetalol	100 mg twice daily	200–2,400 mg in two doses	
Metoprolol	50 mg twice daily 25 mg slow release once daily	50–200 mg twice daily 25–400 mg slow release once daily	
Nadolol	20 mg once daily	20–320 mg once daily	
Nebivolol	5 mg once daily	40 mg once daily	
Pindolol	5 mg twice daily	10–60 mg in two doses	
Propranolol	20 mg twice daily 80 mg extended release once daily	40–600 mg in two doses 120–640 mg extended release once daily	
Timolol	5 mg twice daily	10–60 mg in two doses	
Alpha-adrenergic blocking agents			
Doxazosin	1 mg at bed time	1–16 mg once daily	• Postural hypotension • Dizziness • Headache

Continued

Continued

Drug	Initial dose	Dose range	Adverse effects
Prazosin	1 mg at bed time	2–20 mg in 2–3 doses	• Sexual dysfunction • Drowsiness • Urinary incontinence • Syncope with first dose
Terazosin	1 mg at bed time	1–20 mg in 1–2 doses	
Central sympatholytics			
Clonidine	0.1 mg twice daily	0.2–0.6 mg in two doses	• Dry mouth • Sexual dysfunction • Bradyarrhythmias • Contact dermatitis with clonidine patch • Methyldopa: o Hepatitis o Hemolytic anemia
Guanfacine	1 mg once daily	1–3 mg once daily	
Methyldopa	250 mg twice daily	500–2,000 mg in two doses	
Direct vasodilator			
Hydralazine	25 mg twice daily	50–300 mg in 2–4 doses	• GI disturbances • Headache • Nasal congestion • LE like syndrome • Tachycardia
Minoxidil	5 mg once daily	10–40 mg once daily	• Tachycardia • Fluid retention • Hirsutism • Pericardial effusion • Thrombocytopenia

(ACE: angiotensin-converting-enzyme; GI: gastrointestinal)

Vascular Remodeling in Hypertension

Vascular remodeling in the large and medium sized arteries in case of hypertension occurs due to complex interplay between molecular and cellular mechanisms.

A. Structural changes in the blood vessels:

- **a.** Wall of the blood vessels will be thick, less elastic leading to decrease in the overall diameter of the vessels in response to increased pressure.
- **b.** Big vessel like aorta will become stiff, less compliant leading to increase in the systolic blood pressure.
- **c.** In the small arteriole there:
  - **1.** Hypertrophy of the wall due to thickening of the vessel wall
  - **2,** Hyperplasia of the vascular smooth muscles
  - **3.** Inward remodeling leading to decrease in the internal diameter of the vessels.

B. Dysfunction of the vascular endothelium:

- **a.** Damage of the endothelial layer due to hypertension
- **b.** Decreased production of the nitric oxide, a potent vasodilator and increased production of potent vasoconstrictor endothelin-1 leading to worsening of the vascular tone.
- **c.** It will promote further oxidative stress and inflammation leading to further remodeling of the blood vessels.

C. Changes in the smooth muscle cells:

- **a.** Vascular smooth muscle cells proliferate, migrate leading to transition of contractile phenotype to synthetic one.
- **b.** Increased production of collagen, elastin and their accumulation in the vessel wall leading to thickening of the vessel wall and decreased elasticity.
- **c.** Dysregulated production of matrix metallo-proteinase, leading to decreased breakdown of the extracellular matrix protein resulting incre-ased accumulation of these protein contributing to increased thickness of the vascular wall.

D. Inflammatory cytokines and oxidative stress:

a. There is chronic low grade inflammation leading to release of inflammatory cytokines and increased accumulation of macrophages and T cells in the vessel wall.

b. The inflammatory cells also release proinflammatory cytokines and reactive oxygen species leading to endothelial dysfunction as well as proliferation of the smooth muscle cells contributing accelerated remodeling of the vascular wall.

E. Genetic modifications:

a. Certain genetic expression alters proliferation of smooth muscle cells and promotes endothelial dysfunction.

b. DNA methylation, modification of histones lead to genetic changes which alter vascular tone and remodeling.

Nocturnal Hypertension

It can be defined as excessive rise in the blood pressure in the nighttime. Normally, blood pressure can be decreased by 20% or more in the nighttime as compared to day-time blood pressure. So, the criteria are:

A. Failure to dip the blood pressure at night, i.e., dip in the blood pressure to less than 10%.

B. Presence of excessive rise in the blood pressure during sleep.

C. At night, systolic blood pressure is ≥ 120 mm Hg and diastolic blood pressure ≥ 70 mm Hg.

Diagnosis of nocturnal hypertension:

A. Ambulatory blood pressure monitoring—it is the gold standard. It will monitor blood pressure every 15–30 minutes and can identify the dip at night. In this procedure following types of dipping pattern can be observed:

a. Normal blood pressure drop by 10–20%.

b. Non dipper, i.e., less than 10% drop in the blood pressure.

c. Reverse dipper, i.e., nighttime blood pressure is more than day time blood pressure.

d. Extreme dipper, i.e., drop in nighttime blood pressure more than 20%

B. If the ambulatory blood pressure monitoring, home blood pressure monitoring procedure is required.

Treatment of Nocturnal Hypertension

Pharmacological therapies—should be admitted at night.

A. ACE inhibitors and ARBS—these will inhibit nocturnal blood pressure.

B. CCB: It will be effective in case of non-dippers

C. Beta blockers—these drugs will blunt the activity of beta receptors at night.

Other types of therapies are described already in this question.

Masked Hypertension

Definition: It can be defined as elevation of systolic blood pressure in office 120–129 mm Hg and diastolic blood pressure by less than 80 mm Hg but raised blood pressure on ambulatory or home measurement (130/80 mm Hg).

White coat hypertension can be defined as office blood pressure of 130/80 mm Hg or more but less than 160/100 mm Hg that comes down to 130/80 mm Hg or less at least 3 months after the antihypertensive therapy. Here ambulatory blood pressure monitoring can clinch the diagnosis in this case.

Q24. Discuss the electrophysiology, etiology, and management of atrial fibrillation.

DNBI/DEC2012 (10)

Electrophysiology of atrial fibrillation and its medical and surgical management.

DNBIIIA/DEC2014 (10)

Discuss the mechanism of tachyarrhythmias. Discuss in detail the causes, classification, clinical features, diagnosis, management, and complications of atrial fibrillation.

MGR/APR2015/MDII (15)

Enumerate the causes of atrial fibrillation with a note on paroxysmal atrial fibrillation.

MGR/APR2012/MDIV (7)

Management of paroxysmal atrial fibrillation.

GMC/2015/MDIV (10)

Treatment of atrial fibrillation.

MJPRU/2015(S)/MDIII (10)

Principles of management of atrial fibrillation.

PGI/NOV2012/MDII (10)

Define cardiac arrhythmia. Enumerate supraventricular tachyarrhythmias and describe their clinical presentation. How will you manage a case of permanent atrial fibrillation in patients with mitral valve disease?

BF/MAY2012/MDII (30)

Recent trends in treatment of atrial fibrillation.

BF/MAY2011/MDIV (10)

Describe the important arrhythmias and their treatment.

BF/JUN2016/MDI (10)

Discuss lone atrial fibrillation.

BF/JUN2016/MDI (10)

Discuss newer anticoagulants in nonrheumatic atrial fibrillation management.

ERA/MAY2012/MDIII (15)

Clinical approach to atrial fibrillation and treatment modalities.

NTR UNIVERSITY OF HEALTH SC, VIJAYAWADA, ANDHRA, 2022 (10)

Newer anticoagulants.

NTR UNIVERSITY OF HEALTH SC, VIJAYAWADA, ANDHRA, 2022 (10)

GURU GOBIND SINGH (PGIMER), NEW DELHI, 2019 (10)

Atrial fibrillation in normal heart.

NTR UNIVERSITY OF HEALTH SC, VIJAYAWADA, ANDHRA, 2022 (10)

Discuss newer oral anticoagulants in atrial fibrillation.

TEERTHANKER MAHAVEER UNI, 2020 (20)

Atrial fibrillation.

NTR UNIVERSITY OF HEALTH SC, VIJAYAWADA, ANDHRA, 2022 (10)

BHARATI VIDYAPEETH UNIVERSITY, SUMMER 2017 (10)

Treatment of atrial fibrillation.

BHARATI VIDYAPEETH UNIVERSITY, SUMMER 2016 (10)

Describe pathogenesis of atrial fibrillation and outline of treatment.

RAJIV GANDHI UNIVERSITY OF HEALTH SC, KARNATAKA, 2017 (10)

Dabigatran.

BHARATI VIDYAPEETH UNIVERSITY, SUMMER 2018 (10)

Antiplatelet agents.

NTR UNIVERSITY OF HEALTH SC, VIJAYAWADA, ANDHRA, 2022 (10)

BABA FARID UNIVERSITY OF HEALTH SCIENCES, 2018 (10)

Management of a case of atrial fibrillation.

BABA FARID UNIVERSITY OF HEALTH SCIENCES, 2018 (10)

Target specific oral anticoagulants.

BHARATI VIDYAPEETH UNIVERSITY, SUMMER 2019 (10)

Management of atrial fibrillation.

AIIMS, 2023 (10), AIIMS, 2020 (10)

Describe atrial fibrillation etiology and management in elderly.

AIIMS, 2020 (8)

Management of atrial fibrillation.

SCBMCH, 2021 (10)

Describe conducting system of the heart with diagram. Describe mechanism of arrhythmia and pharmacological and nonpharmacological management of arrhythmia.

SCBMCH, 2010 (20)

Anticoagulant to prevent stroke in patient with atrial fibrillation.

DELHI UNI, 2024 (10)

Etiology and management of atrial fibrillation.

ODISHA UNI, 2022 (10)

Describe the causes of atrial fibrillation. Discuss the strategies of management of AF. Outline the recent advances on pulsed field ablation system.

DNB, OCT 2024 (10)

Discuss the recent management of atrial fibrillation.

MANIPUR UNIVERSITY, 2021 (10)

Explain the management of atrial fibrillation, including anticoagulation strategies and rate versus rhythm control.

WBUHS, 2025 (10)

ANSWER

Definition

It can be defined as totally disorganized rapid, irregular activation of atria leading to loss of atrial contraction with rapid ventricular rate of 120–200 beats per minutes in absence of AV nodal conduction defect and slower ventricular rate in presence of increased vagal tone or AV conduction disease.

Classification According to Patterns

A. *New-onset atrial fibrillation (AF)*: It is the first presentation. Irrespective of duration.

B. Paroxysmal AF: These episodes are self-limiting within 48 hours usually may be up to 7 days. It may be initiated by:

- **a.** Small rapidly firing wavelets in atrial muscle around the pulmonary veins which can be abolished by catheter ablation.
- **b.** Triggering points from nonpulmonary vein area occurring in older patients and in patients with underlying severe cardiac disease.

C. *Persistent AF*: These episodes will persist for >7 days and requires termination by direct current or pharmacological cardioversion and it will be followed by prolonged cardiac sinus rhythm. Here, the rapidly firing foci originate from within pulmonary vein or other nonpulmonary vein sites such as myocardial sleeves, superior venacava or coronary sinus. Persistence of AF is facilitated by structural abnormalities like fibrosis which uncouples atrial fibers leading to automaticity and reentry of electrical signal.

D. *Long-standing persistent AF*: These last for ≥12 months when adaptation of strategy of rhythm control is decided. It is due to extensive fibrosis due to aging and atrial hypertrophy secondary to hypertension and other structural cardiac disease leading to remodeling of electrophysiology affecting conduction as well as refractoriness.

E. *Permanent AF*: These arrhythmias are accepted by physician.

F. *Lone AF*: It is characterized by presence of AF in patients of younger than 60 years of age having no structural heart disease as demonstrated in ECG.

Classification According to Types

A. *AF secondary to structural heart disease*: It occurs in patients with—

- **a.** Long-standing hypertension along with left ventricular hypertrophy
- **b.** Left ventricular systolic dysfunction
- **c.** Left ventricular diastolic dysfunction
- **d.** Other structural heart disease

B. *Focal AF*: In patients with repetitive atrial runs frequent short episodes of paroxysmal AF.

C. *Monogenic AF*: It occurs in patients with cardiomyopathies or channelopathies.

D. *Polygenic AF*: Common genetic variants carry AF.

E. *Postoperative AF*: It occurs after cardiac surgery who showed sinus rhythm prior surgery.

F. AF in patients with prosthetic valves and mitral stenosis.

Causes

- **a.** Advanced age
- **b.** Male sex are more vulnerable than female sex.
- **c.** Valvular heart disease
- **d.** Hypertension
- **e.** CAD
- **f.** CHF
- **g.** Physiological stress
- **h.** Hyperthyroidism
- **i.** Pulmonary embolism
- **j.** Chronic lung disease
- **k.** Infectious disease
- **l.** Caffeine
- **m.** Various metabolic disturbances
- **n.** OSA
- **o.** Preexcitation syndrome

- **p.** Cardiomyopathies
- **q.** Pericarditis
- **r.** Postcardiac surgery

Pathophysiology

Mechanism of AF is the complex interaction between the triggering factor and the substrate. Triggering factor is action potential that induces after-depolarization but strong enough to overcome the recovering depolarization. This after-depolarization is discharged with high frequency and starts as extrasystole but is not persistent. As this impulse of extrasystole encounters myocardium with variable refractoriness and excitability it gives rise to electrical block. As a result, reentry circuit will arise giving rise to new impulse waves will again produces new reentry circuit—so multiple reentry circuits are produced to maintain persistence of arrhythmias.

Most common site of origin of trigger is muscular sleeves in the left atrium extending to pulmonary vein as refractory period in this region is very short as compared to surrounding myocardium in absence of AF.

Triggering areas are:

- **a.** Catheter ablation isolating the pulmonary vein from surrounding myocardium for AF may further induces AF. Other triggering factors are atrial premature complexes, atrial flutter, and AVNRT.
- **b.** Atrial myocardial remodeling due to electrical, autonomic, and structural changes.

All triggering factors are responsible for:

- **a.** Altering sympathomimetic activity
- **b.** Shortening the refractory period
- **c.** Increases propensity to propagate AF.
- **d.** Oxidative and inflammatory changes at molecular level.

Clinical Features

A. Clinical consequences depend upon:

- **a.** Rapid ventricular rate
- **b.** Loss of atrial contribution
- **c.** Predisposition to thrombus formation
- **d.** Potential embolization

B. Clinical presentation varies according to:

- **a.** Ventricular rate
- **b.** Underlying heart disease
- **c.** Associated comorbidities

C. Rapid ventricular rate predisposes to:

- **a.** Hemodynamic collapse
- **b.** Exacerbation of HF in patients with impaired cardiac function, HOCM, and systolic function compromised HF.
- **c.** Patient may present with:
  - **1.** Easy fatigability
  - **2.** Exercise intolerance
  - **3.** Syncope
  - **4.** Dizziness
- **d.** Depressed ventricular function with cardiomyopathy in response to chronic tachycardia may not present with palpitations so do not require medical consultation.

Electrophysiology

A. P wave is absent and it will be replaced by fibrillary waves.

B. Ventricular response is irregularly irregular.

C. Atrial rate is 400–700/minute

D. Ventricular rate is 120–180/minute in absence of drug therapy.

E. Following features should be identified to give special attention:

- **a.** Left ventricular hypertrophy
- **b.** Ventricular preexcitation
- **c.** Ischemic heart disease

F. Measurement of PR, QRS, and QT interval prior to treatment with antiarrhythmic agents.

G. *Ashman phenomenon*: In AF usually morphology of QRS complexes is normal, but in case of LBBB, aberrant ventricular conduction, QRS morphology will change due to abrupt changes in cardiac cycle. The QRS morphology looks like right bundle branch morphology.

Treatment

Treatment of AF depends upon:

- **a.** Symptoms of the patients
- **b.** Hemodynamic effect of AF
- **c.** Risk of stroke
- **d.** Underlying heart disease

A. In case of new-onset AF which can produce pulmonary edema, angina, and severe hypertension:

- **a.** QRS synchronized cardioversion with 200 Jules under sedation or anesthesia.

- **b.** If the shock fails, greater shock energy with different electrode is required.
- **c.** Intravenous ibutilide may be given prior to cardioversion because it will lower the energy requirement. It is used in case of reinitiation of AF. But it should not be used in case of prolonged QT interval because chance of torsades de pointes.

B. If the patient is stable:

- **a.** Rate control to give relief from the symptoms
- **b.** Administration of anticoagulation to reduce the risk of stroke
- **c.** Now decision should be taken whether:
  1. Therapy is required to restore sinus rhythm
  2. AF is allowed to be continued only with rate control measurement.

C. *Anticoagulant strategies in AF*: There is increased risk of thromboembolism in case of electrical, pharmacologic or spontaneous cardioversion within 10 days following restoration to sinus rhythm. Hence following factors should be considered:

- **a.** Duration of AF:
  1. If AF is >48 hours of duration:
     - Transthoracic echocardiography should be done to exclude left atrial thrombus.
     - Or, 3 weeks therapeutic anticoagulation prior to cardioversion regardless of CHA_2DS_2-VAC score.
  2. *If AF is <48 hours duration*: Since there is high risk of thromboembolism—anticoagulation is recommended immediately before and after cardioversion.
  3. *Duration of anticoagulation*: Therapy should be continued for 4 weeks after cardioversion, but long-term anticoagulation is individualized according to risk and benefit of therapy.
  4. Patients with AF are prone to develop different types of ischemic stroke. In these patients recommendation of anticoagulant depends upon the following scores, i.e., CHA_2DS_2VaSc:
     - Congestive HF with ejection fraction of <40%
     - Hypertension
     - Age > 65 years
     - Diabetes mellitus
     - History of stroke or TIA
     - Vascular disease (peripheral vascular disease)
     - Age > 75 years
     - Female sex

     If score is <0: No aspirin or anticoagulant based on individual assessment.

     If score is 1: Anticoagulant or aspirin based on individual assessment.

     If score is 2 or more: Anticoagulation is recommended if the patient is not at high risk of bleeding.
  5. Choice of anticoagulant:
     - *In case of nonvalvular AF*: Intravenous heparin, LMWH, warfarin, and new oral anticoagulants.
     - *In case of mitral stenosis*: Warfarin
     - *In case other valvular heart disease*: Noncoumadin anticoagulant
  6. In following cases long-term anticoagulation is required:
     - *Thromboembolic risk*: According to current guideline CHA_2DS_2-VAC score is recommended to assess the risk. But pattern of AF is not considered.
     - *Bleeding risk*: Most commonly used score (HAS-BLED) is taken to assess the bleeding risk.
       - Hypertension
       - Renal and liver function
       - Stroke
       - Bleeding tendency
       - Labile international normalized ratio
       - Elderly
       - Drugs/alcohol
     - *Choice of oral anticoagulant*: In case of severe kidney disease most new oral anticoagulants should be avoided. In case of patients with AF antithrombotic drugs can be started considering following factors:
       - Drug interactions
       - Cost
       - Tolerability
       - Preference of the patients
       - Dose frequency
       - Clinical characteristics
       - Comorbidities

- *Nonpharmacologic prevention of stroke*: In case of unacceptable risk of bleeding after anticoagulation device like "WATCHMAN" is most commonly used to occlude left atrial appendage followed by 6 weeks oral anticoagulation and aspirin treatment followed by aspirin and clopidogrel.

D. Rate control:

Here it is most important to recognize the sins of preexcitation of ventricle in patients with AF because AV nodal blocking agents will enhance the conduction through the accessory pathway leading to 1: 1 AV conduction. Ideal ventricular rate should be set to 100/minutes, but <110/minute can be accepted in absence of symptoms. Drugs used are:

a. *Beta-blocker*: Oral and intravenous form can be used.

b. Nondihydropyridine CCB such as verapamil and diltiazem. But these drugs should not be used in case of decompensated HF or cardiac amyloidosis.

c. *Digitalis*: In patients having contraindication to beta-blocker or CCB and left ventricular systolic dysfunction digitalis should be used or it can be used as adjunct to beta-blocker. It can reduce the resting heart rate but cannot reduce the heart rate in case of increased sympathetic tone. There are chances of digitalis toxicity like all the arrhythmias except rapidly conducted atrial tachyarrhythmias. Digitalis toxicity can be treated by digoxin-specific antibody.

d. In case of chronic rate control beta-blockers, CCB, and digoxin are used in combination, but dose should be adjusted according the activity, goal being <80/minute or <110/minute without symptoms. Periodic function of ventricular function should monitored periodically.

e. If all the drugs fail to control and to restore the sinus rhythm, then catheter ablation at AV junction to create heat block and followed by permanent pacemaker for life-long pacing should be of choice.

f. Right ventricular apical pacing can depress the right ventricular function by inducing dyssynchronous ventricular activation.

g. Biventricular pacing will minimize the degree of ventricular dyssynchrony by directly pacing the bundle of His.

E. Rhythm control:

a. Risk factors associated with AF such as obesity, alcoholism, hypertension, and sleep apnea should be treated first as it may reduce the episodes of AF.

b. Dugs such as beta-blockers, CCB or digoxin or catheter-induced AV node ablation can control rhythm also. It is usually indicated in case of stable patients with AF.

c. But in case of unstable patients with AF producing great hemodynamic instability direct current cardioversion is required.

1. Electrical cardioversion by direct current cardioversion
2. Pharmacologic cardioversion by flecainide, propafenone, dofetilide, amiodarone, and intravenous ibutilide.
    - Class-I sodium channel blocking agents such as flecainide, propafenone, and disopyramide can be given in patients without significant structural heart disease.
    - Class-II agents such as sotalol and dofetilide can be given in patients with CAD and structural heart disease, but there is 3% chance of getting QT prolongation and torsades de pointes. Hence these drugs should be started in hospital setting with continuous monitoring.
    - Amiodarone can be administered in patients with HF and CAD.

Complications of Atrial Fibrillation

A. Thromboembolism including stroke

B. Acute myocardial infarction

C. New-onset HF

D. Worsening of HF

E. Hemodynamic instability resulting cardiogenic shock

F. Tachycardia-induced cardiomyopathy

G. Sudden death from Wolff-Parkinson-White (WPW) syndrome

Classification of Arrhythmias

A. *Tachyarrhythmias*:

a. *Supraventricular arrhythmia*: Here arrhythmias originate from above the AV node.

1. Atrial tachycardia

2. Atrial premature complexes
3. Atrioventricular nodal reentrant tachycardia
4. Atrioventricular reentrant tachycardia
5. AV junctional extrasystoles
6. Atrial flutter
7. Atrial fibrillation

b. *Ventricular tachyarrhythmias*: Here the arrhythmia originates from below the AV node.
1. Ventricular premature beats
2. Atrial flutter
3. Atrial fibrillation

B. Bradyarrhythmias:
a. Sinus bradycardia
b. First-degree AV block
c. Second-degree AV block
d. Third-degree AV block or complete AV block

Tachyarrhythmias can also be classified according to the duration of QRS complexes:

A. Narrow QRS complex tachycardia where duration of QRS complex is <120 milliseconds.
a. Sinus tachycardia
b. Atrial flutter
c. Atrial tachycardia
d. Atrioventricular nodal reentrant tachycardia
e. Atrioventricular reentrant tachycardia
f. Junctional ectopic tachycardia
g. Sinoatrial nodal reentrant tachycardia

B. *Wide QRS complex tachycardia*: Here duration of QRS complex is ≥120 milliseconds
a. Monomorphic or polymorphic ventricular tachycardia
b. Ventricular premature complexes
c. Ventricular fibrillation

Clinical Presentation and Management of Supraventricular Tachyarrhythmia

A. Atrioventricular reciprocal tachycardia like WPW syndrome:
a. Palpitation
b. Shortness of breath
c. Syncope
d. ECG findings:
1. Slurred upstroke of QRS complex
2. Delta wave
e. Management:
1. Amiodarone or procainamide
2. If fails synchronized cardioversion
3. Definite therapy is ablation of accessory pathways.

B. Atrioventricular nodal reentrant tachycardia:
a. Sudden tachycardia
b. Chest tightness
c. Palpitation
d. Shortness of breath
e. Syncope
f. ECG findings:
1. Narrow complex tachycardia along with P waves hidden in the T waves.
2. Heart rate 150–160 beats/min
g. Treatment:
1. Carotid sinus pressure
2. Adenosine
3. Cardioversion
4. Ablation or chronic suppressive treatment with beta-blockers or diltiazem and verapamil.

C. Atrial flutter:
a. Usually asymptomatic
b. Hypotension
c. Palpitation
d. Dyspnea
e. ECG findings:
1. Regular tachycardia
2. Sawtooth appearance of P wave
3. Variable degree of heart block
f. Treatment:
1. Control of ventricular rate with beta-blockers and CCBs
2. Reversion to sinus rhythm by ablation or cardioversion.

D. Multifocal atrial tachycardia:
a. Usually asymptomatic
b. Features of underlying disease
c. Dyspnea
d. ECG findings:
1. Different morphologies of P waves
2. Varying PR interval
e. Treatment:
1. Oxygen therapy

2. Treatment of underlying causes
3. In refractory cases:
   - Rate control with CCBs in case of COPD
   - Later on beta-blockers

Newer Anticoagulants

These are orally active anticoagulants actively used in case of atrial fibrillation, pulmonary embolism and deep vein thrombosis. The drugs are:

Direct thrombin inhibitors:

a. Dabigatran: It inhibits factor IIa (thrombin) which converts fibrinogen to fibrin.

Factor Xa inhibitors: Factor Xa helps in generation of thrombin. The drugs are

a. Rivaroxaban
b. Apixaban
c. Edoxaban

Advantages of Newer Anticoagulants

A. These drugs do not require regular monitoring of INR.
B. Dose will be fixed.
C. Faster onset of action.
D. Fewer dietary restrictions
E. Low risk of intracranial hemorrhage as compared to warfarin
F. Drug interactions and food interactions are few.
G. Now a days antidotes to the oral anticoagulants are available like:
   a. Idarucizumab for dabigatran
   b. Andexanet alfa for factor Xa inhibitors.

Disadvantages

A. These drugs are costly as compared to warfarin.
B. Their use in certain types of patients like renal impairment, mechanical heart valves or pregnancy are limited.

Contraindications

A. Active bleeding
B. Coagulopathy
C. Major trauma
D. Recent major surgeries
E. Acute intracranial hemorrhage

Antiplatelet Agent

These drugs inhibit platelet activation or platelet aggregation. These drugs can be classified according to their mechanism of actions:

A. *Cyclooxygenase inhibitors*: These drugs inhibit the cyclooxygenase enzyme leading to reduced synthesis of thromboxane A2 which promotes platelet aggregation. The drug is aspirin which inhibits COX1 irreversibly leading to long lasting inhibition of platelet aggregation.
B. *P2Y12 receptor inhibitors*: This group of drugs inhibit P2Y12 receptor present on the platelet leading inhibition of platelet aggregation.
   a. Clopidogrel: It is thienopyridine group of drug that inhibits this receptor irreversibly.
   b. Prasugrel: It is thienopyridine group of drug which inhibits this receptor irreversibly. It is more potent as compared to Clopidogrel.
   c. Ticagrelor: It is non-thienopyridine that inhibits this enzyme reversibly. It has rapid onset of action.
   d. Cangrelor: It inhibits this enzyme reversibly. This drug is given intravenously. Due to its short half-life it is used during percutaneous coronary intervention.
C. Glycoprotein IIb/IIIa inbihibtor

Pulse Field Ablation System

Definition

It a technology used to treat atrial fibrillation where short high voltage electrical impulses is passed to the cardiac tissue to damage their cell membranes thereby damage of the tissues through the conversion of the electrical energy to thermal energy.

Required Components

A. Pulse field ablation catheter containing electrodes that will be introduced through the femoral vein into the heart.
B. Pulse generator: It will send high voltage electrical current in pulses, each pulse persisting for few microseconds to milliseconds to damage and disrupt the cell membrane.
C. Target areas in the heart to prevent damage of the surrounding tissues.

Mechanism of Action

Here the electrical impulses propagate to the cell membranes in the heart to create a hole in the cell membrane in the targeted tissue thereby damaging the cells to prevent damage of the surrounding tissues—this method is known as electroporation.

Indications:

A. Persistent and paroxysmal atrial fibrillation to damage the abnormal electrical pathways. As the most common site of origin of abnormal pathways is pulmonary vein, hence isolation of the pulmonary vein is most essential in this regard.

B. Ventricular tachycardia

C. Atrial flutter

Benefits of this Method

A. As this procedure is target oriented, fewer complication of this procedure may occur from this procedure.

B. Patient will recover from this procedure very early.

C. This method is targeted and very precise, hence negligible tissue damage can occur from this procedure.

D. In this procedure there is no need of cooling.

> **Q25. Enumerate and classify beta-blockers. Discuss the indications of beta-blockers in medicine.**
>
> **DNBIII/DEC2013 (10)**
>
> **BHARATI VIDYAPEETH UNIVERSITY, SUMMER 2018 (10)**
>
> **Newer beta blockers in hypertension.**
>
> **BABA FARID UNIVERSITY OF HEALTH SC, 2018 (10)**

ANSWER

Classification of Beta-blockers

A. Selective beta-blockers:
- **a.** With intrinsic sympathomimetic activity:
  1. Acebutolol
  2. Celiprolol
- **b.** Without sympathomimetic activity:
  1. Atenolol
  2. Esmolol
  3. Metoprolol
  4. Bisoprolol
  5. Betaxolol
  6. Bevantolol

B. Nonselective beta-blockers:
- **a.** With intrinsic sympathomimetic activity:
  1. Pindolol
  2. Carteolol
  3. Penbutolol
  4. Alprenolol
  5. Oxprenolol
- **b.** Without intrinsic sympathomimetic activity:
  1. Propranolol
  2. Nadolol
  3. Sotalol
  4. Timolol
  5. Tertalolol

C. With alpha-blocking activity:
- **a.** Labetalol
- **b.** Carvedilol
- **c.** Bucindolol

Actions of beta-blockers:

A. *Beta-1 receptors*: It is primarily present in the heart responsible for cardiac activity like reduction of:
- **a.** Heart rate
- **b.** Blood pressure
- **c.** Myocardial contractility
- **d.** Myocardial oxygen consumption

B. *Beta-2 receptor blocker*: It will inhibit relaxation of smooth muscles of:
- **a.** Bronchus
- **b.** Vessels
- **c.** Gastrointestinal tract
- **d.** Genitourinary tract

C. Other functions of beta-blockers are antagonism of:
- **a.** Glycogenolysis
- **b.** Gluconeogenesis

All the above will lead to hypoglycemia.

Uses of Beta-blockers

Cardiac	Noncardiac
• Hypertension • Angina pectoris • Myocardial infarction • Cardiac arrhythmias • CCF • Hypertrophic obstructive cardiomyopathy • Dissecting aortic aneurysm	• Pheochromocytoma • Thyrotoxicosis • Migraine prophylaxis • Anxiety • Essential tremors • Glaucoma • Portal hypertension

(CCF: congestive cardiac failure)

Organ system/ tissue	Side effects
Cardiovascular	• Bradycardia • Heart failure • Decreased atrioventricular conduction

Continued

Continued

Organ system/ tissue	Side effects
	• Intensification of existing atrioventricular block • Postural hypotension • Cold hands and feet • Worsening of peripheral vascular disease
Pulmonary	Worsening of chronic obstructive bronchopulmonary disease asthma may be precipitated
Neurologic	• Fatigue • Sleep disturbances (insomnia, nightmares) • Depression • Hypotonia
Gastrointestinal	• Nausea, vomiting, diarrhea, and constipation • Stomach cramps
Ocular	• Rare: Dry eves, visual disturbances
Hematologic	• Rare: Thrombocytopenia
Metabolic	• Very rare: hypoglycemia in at-risk patients • Reduced high-density lipoprotein (HDL) cholesterol and increased triglycerides level

Newer Beta Blockers

A. Nebivolol:
- **a.** Mechanism of actions:
  - **1.** It is selective beta-1 blockers.
  - **2.** It has vasodilatory properties as it will release nitric oxide
- **b.** Its functions:
  - **1.** It will lower the blood pressure
  - **2.** It will improve the endothelial function.
- **c.** Dosage: Starting dose is 5 mg once daily orally and it can be increased up to 40 mg daily based on the response of the patient.

B. Carvedilol:
- **a.** Mechanism of actions:
  - **1.** It is selective beta-1 blocker
  - **2.** It is alfa-1 blocking drug
- **b.** Function:
  - **1.** Hypertension associated with heart failure
  - **2.** Hypertension associated with left ventricular dysfunction
- **c.** Dosage: Starting dose is 6.25 mg once daily orally and can be increased up to 25 mg daily.

C. Bisoprolol:
- **a.** Mechanism of action: It is highly selective beta blocker.
- **b.** Function: It will control hypertension.
- **c.** Dosage: Starting dose is 5 mg daily orally and it can be increased up to 20 mg once daily.

Q26. Discuss the etiology, diagnosis, and management of peripheral arterial disease.

DNBIII/JUN2013 (10) DNBIIIA/JUN2016 (10)

What is intermittent claudication? What are the clinical types of claudication seen in the lower limbs? Brief outline the management strategies.

WBUHS, 2023 (10)

ANSWER

Definition

It can be defined as a clinical disorder characterized by stenosis, occlusion of the aorta or the arteries of limbs leading to features of ischemia of the affected limb or limbs.

Causes of Peripheral Arterial Disease

A. Thrombosis
B. Vasculitis
C. Embolism
D. Fibromuscular dysplasia
E. Entrapment
F. Cystic adventitial disease
G. Trauma

Risk Factors

A. *Age*: It occurs at any age but risk is higher with advancing age.
B. *Sex*: Both sex are equally affected. But in case of PAD men are more symptomatic as comparted to women.
C. *Race*: African-American are more affected than other ethnicities.
D. Coronary artery disease or stroke
E. Hypertension
F. Hyperlipidemia
G. *Use of tobacco*: It will damage the blood vessels and unhealthy cholesterol level.

H. Diabetes mellitus
I. Advanced chronic kidney disease
J. Tobacco use
K. In 20–40% families genetic predisposition.
L. Stress
M. Obesity
N. Metabolic syndrome

Pathology

Segmental stenosis or occlusion involves following arteries:

a. Abdominal aorta and iliac arteries in 30% of arteries—these are the primary sites.
b. Femoral and popliteal arteries—80% of patients.
c. More distal vessels—tibial and peroneal arteries.

Atherosclerotic lesions involve in the arterial branching points due to following:

a. These are sites of increased turbulence
b. Altered shear stress
c. Intimal injury

Pathology of the lesion includes:

a. Presence of atherosclerotic plaques with deposition of calcium
b. Thinning of media
c. Patchy destruction of muscles and elastic fibers
d. Fragmentation of internal elastic lamina
e. Thrombi composed of fibrin and platelets

Clinical Evaluation

A. Symptoms:
   a. Fewer than 50% are asymptomatic except slow or impaired gait
   b. Intermittent claudication—most common symptom. It is described as cramp, pain, ache or sense of fatigue in the muscles mainly occurs during exercise and relieved by rest.
   c. Site of claudication depends upon the location of arterial obstruction:
      1. In case of aortoiliac obstruction—buttock, hip, thigh, and calf pain occurs.
      2. In case of femoral-popliteal artery involvement—calf muscles are involved.
   d. Lower limb is involved more than the upper extremity muscles due to higher incidence of obstruction mainly in lower limb.
   e. In case of inability of the flow of blood to meet the metabolic demand of the muscles in resting position due to critical vascular obstruction—it will lead to critical limb ischemia in that case patients complain of rest pain at night as the limb is in horizontal position but relieve when the limb is in dependent position. But in severe cases rest pain will persist.

B. Physical examination:
   a. Distal to obstruction:
      1. In case of partial obstruction—bruit will be present.
      2. In case of complete obstruction—absent pulse.
   b. Muscle atrophy.
   c. In more severe cases:
      1. Loss of hair
      2. Pallor or cyanosis
      3. Reduced temperature of the skin
      4. Thickened nails
      5. Smooth and shiny skin
   d. In critical ischemia—ulcer or gangrene.
   e. Elevation of limb and repeated flexing of calf muscles—pallor of the foot and soles. But in the dependent position of the limb there is rubor secondary to reactive hyperemia, but it depends upon:
      1. Severity of obstruction
      2. Presence of collateral vessels.
   f. In case of severe ischemia—edema develops because these patients try to keep their limb at dependent position to alleviate pain.

Noninvasive Testing

Normally classical history and classical physical findings can establish the diagnosis but presence and severity of the vascular disease can be recorded by following noninvasive tests:

A. Sphygmomanometric calf is placed at the ankle and Doppler device is used to record the flow of blood or auscultate from the arteria dorsalis pedis and posterior tibial arteries.
   a. Normally, systolic blood pressure in arms and legs is similar.
   b. Due to amplification of pulse-wave ankle pressure is slightly higher than pressure in the arm.

c. In presence of hemodynamically significant stenosis in the leg systolic blood pressure will be increased.

d. Ankle to brachial index, i.e., ratio of ankle to brachial artery pressure:

1. *In normal subject*: 1.00–1.40
2. *In case of borderline obstruction*: 0.91–0.99
3. *In case of peripheral arterial disease*: <0.90
4. >1.40-noncompressable disease.

B. Pulse volume recordings:

It refers to graphical representation of volume change in the pulse in extremities during each cardiac cycle. It can be obtained by placing the blood pressure calf and measuring the pressure at high thigh, lower thigh, calf, ankle, mid foot, and toe, and it should be used in conjunction with measurement of segmental blood pressure. It is used to:

a. Localize the disease
b. Follow-up postrevascularization
c. Noncompressable vessels

C. *Exercise testing*: In this test in case of suspected PAD:

Patient is asked to go for fixed treadmill settings of 2 mile/h at 2% grade for 5 minutes. Pre-exercise and postexercise blood pressure are measured—abnormal result is defined as decrease of >20% in postexercise blood pressure.

D. *Duplex ultrasound*: It combines B-mode imaging and Doppler flow velocity waveform analysis. It can detect the stenotic lesion of native arteries and also bypass graft.

E. Transcutaneous oximetry

Treatment

Aim of giving therapies:

a. To reduce the risk of cardiovascular events such as myocardial infarction and death.
b. To improve limb symptoms
c. To prevent progression of the disease to critical ischemia
d. To preserve the viability of limb.
e. To initiate antiplatelet therapy to improve cardiovascular symptoms

Lifestyle modifications:

A. Smoking:

a. Counseling
b. *Drug therapy*: Nicotine patch, bupropion, and varenicline—these will increase the cessation of smoking and reduce recidivism.

B. Control of blood pressure by:

a. ACEI and ARBs
b. In patients with coexistent CAD beta-adrenergic blocker as it may not worsen the claudication.

C. In case of hypercholesterolemia—statin to reduce the risk of stroke, myocardial infarction, and death.

D. In patients with atherosclerosis to reduce the cardiovascular events platelet inhibitor including aspirin, ADP antagonist, and clopidogrel as it will also improve intermittent claudication, critical limb ischemia prior to revascularization.

E. If along with aspirin other antiplatelet drug such as protease-activated receptor-1 antagonist, vorapaxar to inhibit thrombin-mediated activation of platelets,

a. It will decrease the cardiovascular events in atherosclerotic heart disease.
b. It reduces ischemia and peripheral revascularization.

F. Since warfarin is associated with increased risk of bleeding, hence it is not used in case of chronic PAD. Combination of low dose oral factor Xa inhibitor, rivaroxaban along with aspirin though improves PAD, CAD in case of atherosclerosis, but there is risk of bleeding.

G. Therapy of intermittent claudication and critical limb ischemia:

a. Supportive medications:

1. Care of feet:
   - Feet should be kept clean.
   - Avoidance of excessive drying by moistening cream.
   - Well-fitted protective shoes to protect the feet from trauma.
   - Avoidance of elastic support hose to prevent reduction of blood flow.
   - In case of critical ischemia in the limb shocks blocks under the head of the bed along with canopy over the feet to improve perfusion pressure.
   - In patients with claudication, supervised exercise training program of 30–45 minutes sessions to be done 3–5 times per weeks for at least 12 weeks—it will increase the threshold level for ischemia. During exercise vasodilators should not be used as it will dilate vessels distal to the obstruction leading decrease in perfusion pressure.

b. *Cilostazol*: It is phosphodiesterase inhibitor with vasodilator along with antiplatelet properties improves claudication by 40–60%.
c. Pentoxifylline increases the blood flow through microcirculation to improve tissue oxygenation.
d. *Statin*: It is effective in intermittent claudication.
e. No growth factor can show improvement in critical limb ischemia.
f. *Revascularization*: In disabling, progressively severe symptoms catheter-based or surgical intervention should be done to improve:
   1. Walking distance and functional capacity.
   2. Ischemia to relieve pain and to prevent loss of limb.

   Conventional angiography, MRI or CTA should be done to assess the vascular anatomy to know whether the patient is a perfect candidate for revascularization surgery. Endovascularization should include:
   1. Percutaneous transluminal balloon angioplasty including drug-coated balloon
   2. Placement of stent including drug-eluting stent
   3. Stent graft
   4. Atherotomy

   Percutaneous transluminal angioplasty (PTA) and stenting of iliac artery are associated with higher success rate as compared to stenting in femoral and popliteal arteries because patency rate is higher in proximal case.

   Prognosis depends upon the length of the lesion and severity of lesion. Prognosis is worse in case of occlusive lesion as compared to nonocclusive lesion.

   Stenting of distal arteries along with proximal artery can be done to prevent loss of limb.
g. Operative procedures of femoral-popliteal and aortoiliac artery depend upon:
   1. Location of the lesion
   2. Size of the lesion
   3. Associated general conditions of the patient.

   In case of aortoiliac artery disease the procedures are the following:
   1. *Aortobifemoral bypass*: It is most common bypass using Dacron graft, immediate patency approaches 99%.
   2. Axillofemoral bypass
   3. Aortoiliac endarterectomy

   Operative complications:
   1. Myocardial infarction
   2. Stroke
   3. Infection of the graft
   4. Peripheral embolization
   5. Sexual dysfunction from interruption of the autonomic nerves in the pelvis

   Operative mortality is 1–3%.

   Operative therapy for femoral-popliteal artery disease includes:
   1. In situ and reverse autogenous saphenous vein bypass graft
   2. Placement of polytetrafluoroethylene or other synthetic graft.

   Long-term patency depends upon:
   1. Type of the graft used
   2. Location of distal anastomosis
   3. Patency of the run-off vessels. Beyond the anastomosis.

Q27. Describe significance of serum cardiac biomarkers in STEMI. What is the strategy of prehospital management of STEMI?

DNBIIB/DEC2013 (10)

Cardiac biomarkers.

NTR UNIVERSITY OF HEALTH SC, VIJAYAWADA, ANDHRA, 2022 (10)

ANSWER

Cardiac Biomarkers

Serum biomarkers after being released into interstitium from the cardiac infarct zone after ST-elevation myocardial infarction (STEMI) are cleared by cardiac lymphatics. Rate of liberation of cardiac biomarkers depends upon:

a. Intracellular location of markers
b. Their molecular weight
c. Local blood flow
d. Rate of lymphatic flow

When liberation of markers exceeds the clearing capability of the cardiac lymphatics then it will enter the venous circulation. Criteria of acute myocardial infarction is rise or fall of values of cardiac biomarkers with at least one value above 99th percentile of upper reference limit in case of normal individual.

A. *Cardiac-specific troponin T and cardiac-specific troponin I*: Its amino acid sequence is different from those present in the skeletal muscle. These proteins are quantitatively estimated with highly specific monoclonal antibodies. In case of STEMI these will be elevated many times upper limit of normal and it has definite diagnostic value. With highly sensitive assay technique cardiac-specific troponin value of <1 ng/L in nonischemic heart disease (IHD) patients can be measured. Other than acute myocardial infarction it is positive in following cases:

a. Non-STEMI

b. Congestive cardiac failure

c. Aortic dissection

d. Hypertrophic cardiomyopathy

e. Pulmonary embolism

f. Cardiac contusion

g. Acute neurologic disease

h. Drug toxicity

In case of very small STEMI where creatine phosphokinase-myocardial band (CPK-MB) value is normal, cardiac-troponin is of diagnostic value.

B. *High-sensitivity cardiac troponin*: It is recently approved by the United States of America (USA) as an early and accurate detector of myocardial injury. According to definition, it must be able to detect the concentration below 99th percentile above the lower limit of detection of assay in >50% of healthy population and at this 99th percentile it should have coefficient of variance of <10%. In patients with chest pain this assay is utilized rapidly and reliably to detect myocardial ischemia. If the first value is negative, second estimation should be done after 1–3 hours without compromising sensitivity of negative predictive value.

C. *Creatine kinase and creatine kinase-myocardial band (CK and CK-MB)*: CK will rise within 4–8 hours and will return to normal by 48–72 hours. But it is not specific for cardiac injury because it is also elevated in:

a. Disease of skeletal muscles

b. Trauma in the skeletal muscles

c. Intramuscular injection

Creatine kinase-myocardial band is released from the cardiac muscles but not in extracardiac tissue. A ration of CK-MB mass to CK activity of ≥2.5 is diagnostic of myocardial infarction. But initial normal values cannot exclude recent complete occlusion.

D. *Copeptin*: It is C-terminal of vasopressin prohormone—it can quantify the endogenous cardiac stress in myocardial infarction in addition to cardiac-specific troponin. According to ESC 2015, where high-sensitivity cardiac troponin estimation is not available, in that case it can rule out MI very early as compared to hs-cTn.

E. *Myoglobin*: It is released from necrotic myocardium more rapidly than serum glutamic oxaloacetic transaminase (SGOT), lactate dehydrogenase (LDH) or CK. But it is less specific making it inferior to hs-cTn. It is elevated within 2 to 3 hours of myocardial injury. But it is less specific as its level will be increased in case of any muscle injury.

F. C-reactive protein: It is an inflammation marker. It is not specific as it will rise in any type of cardiac inflammation. High sensitivity CRP can assess the risk of future cardiovascular events.

G. Lactate dehydrogenase: It is secreted from red blood cells including cardiac tissue. Hence its level is elevated in any type of tissue injury including heart, hence it is not specific for cardiac injury.

H. Add novel biomarkers in heart failure from question number.

Strategies of Prehospital Management of STEMI

Prognosis of STEMI is related to following two complications:

a. Electrical complication—arrhythmias

b. Mechanical complications—pump failure

Most common cause of death in STEMI is ventricular fibrillation that occurs within 24 hours, it is more serious when occurs in first hour. Hence major elements of prehospital care in STEMI include:

A. Prompt symptoms recognition and prompt seeking of medical attention by the patients—this is the area where there is possible greatest delay—this can be reduced by educating the patients regarding the importance of chest discomfort by health personnel.

B. Emergency medical team should be deployed very rapidly that can perform urgent resuscitation and defibrillation if required.

C. Expeditious transportation of the patients from the home to hospital having best possible care to be given by physicians and nurses in the form of advanced cardiac life support (ACLS) and management of arrhythmias.

D. Rapid implementation of reperfusion therapy.

Regular office visit in case patients with history of chest discomfort or those are at risk of IHD.

In the ambulance patients should be monitored and treated if required by trained personnel in the ambulance thus shortening the time interval between onset of symptoms and initiation of treatment. In the prehospital treatment general guidelines in initiation of fibrinolysis are the following:

- **a.** 12-lead ECG monitoring to confirm the diagnosis
- **b.** Presence of paramedics in the ambulance
- **c.** Paramedical should be trained to interpret ECG
- **d.** Management of STEMI
- **e.** Online medical command and control which can authorize the initiation of treatment.

Q28. Physiology of circulation in the third trimester of pregnancy.

DNBIB/JUN2015 (10)

ANSWER

A. Maternal hemodynamic changes:

Systemic vasodilatation occurs in first trimester which again decreases to normal in the middle of second trimester then gradually increases in the third trimester, ultimately systemic vascular resistance increases to prepregnancy level near term and 2 weeks after delivery maternal hemodynamics will come to normal to prepregnant level.

B. Cardiac output:

Cardiac output will remain increased throughout the pregnancy and it can be assessed by echocardiography in maternal left lateral position

C. Blood pressure:

During pregnancy there is decrease in systolic, diastolic blood pressure, mean arterial pressure, and central systolic blood pressure, but diastolic blood pressure and mean arterial pressure will decrease more. Arterial pressure gradually increases in third trimester and returns to preconception level in postpartum.

D. Heart rate:

Heart rate is progressively increased throughout the pregnancy as 10–20 beats/min to reach maximum at third trimester. So overall increase is 20–30% over the baseline.

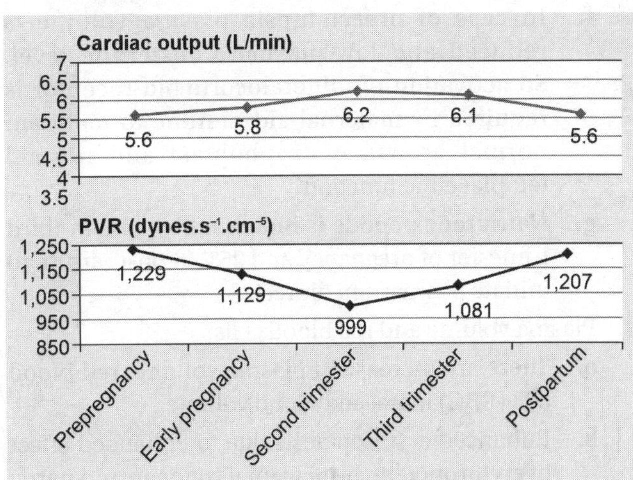

Serial blood pressures before, during, and after pregnancy

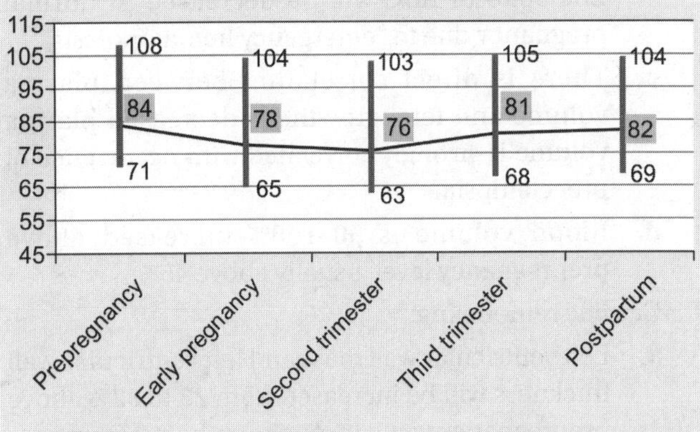

E. Myocardial contractility:

Myocardial contractility, left and right ventricular ejection fractions will not change throughout the pregnancy.

F. Renin–angiotensin–aldosterone system:

- **a.** In pregnancy substantial activation of RAAS lead to increase in plasma volume starting from 6–8 weeks to maximal at 30th week.
- **b.** There is also salt and water retention in the body due to stimulation of this axis to maintain blood pressure normal.
- **c.** In the third trimester there is increase in exchangeable sodium of 500 meq with net gain of 1,000 meq.
- **d.** Relaxin stimulates vasopressin and drinking leading to increased water retention in the body and decrease in plasma osmolarity and hypervolemic hyponatremia of pregnancy ensues.
- **e.** Progesterone on the other hand acts on mineralocorticoid receptor to prevent sodium retention and to protect against hypokalemia.

f. In case of preeclampsia plasma volume is reduced and low plasma aldosterone level. So activation of mineralocorticoid receptor is required by maternal aldosterone to maintain normal growth of trophoblast and normal fetoplacental function.

g. Natriuretic peptide is increased by 40% in third trimester of pregnancy and 25% at postpartum to initiate postpartum diuresis.

G. Plasma volume and red blood cells:

a. There are increase in plasma volume, red blood cell (RBC) mass, and blood volume.

b. Enhanced erythropoiesis due to enhanced effect of erythropoietin by placental lactogen and partly by iron deficiency that occurs in pregnancy. Life span of RBC will be decreased in normal pregnancy due to "emergency hematopoiesis".

c. There is direct correlation between plasma volume and fetal growth, as decreased plasma volume is strongly correlated with occurrence of preeclampsia.

d. Blood volume is 50–100% increased above prepregnancy level, usually above 45%.

H. Cardiac remodeling:

a. Left ventricular wall mass and left ventricular wall thickness will be increased from 28 to 52% above prepregnancy value throughout the pregnancy.

b. Aortic augmentation index, a marker of aortic stiffness that decreases during first trimester but gradually increases in the third trimester.

Q29. Role of fibrin-specific thrombolytic therapy in ST-elevated acute myocardial infarction. Contraindication for thrombolysis. Complications of thrombolytic therapy.

DNBIIIA/DEC2015 (10)

Fibrinolytic system.

MGR/OCT2013/MDI (5)

ANSWER

Role of Fibrinolytic Therapy in ST-segment Elevated Acute Myocardial Infarction

In absence of any contraindication, fibrinolytic therapy should be started within 30 minutes of presentation of symptom with the aim of making full restoration of coronary artery patency. Fibrinolytic drugs convert plasminogen to plasmin which in turn lyses fibrin meshes to dissolve the clot. ECG justifying fibrinolytic therapy:

a. New ST segment elevation at J point greater than 0.1 mV in two adjacent leads other than V2–V3, where the following cut points apply.

b. ≥0.2 mV in men of >40 years and ≥0.25 mV in men of <40 years or ≥0.15 mV in women.

c. New or presumably new LBBB.

d. 12 lead ECG consistent with true posterior myocardial infarction.

Thrombolysis in myocardial infarction grading system:

A. *Grade 0*: Complete occlusion of coronary artery.

B. *Grade 1*: Some penetration of contrast material beyond the point of obstruction but without any perfusion of distal coronary bed, but flow is delayed as compared to normal artery.

C. *Grade 2*: Perfusion of entire intact vessel into the distal bed but flow is delayed as compared to the normal artery.

D. *Grade 3*: Full perfusion of the intact vessels but with normal flow.

Full perfusion of the infarct-related coronary artery with fibrinolytic agents is the goal because it:

a. Limits infarct size

b. Maintain normal left ventricular function

c. Reduce short and long term mortality rate.

Absolute Contraindications

A. History of cerebrovascular hemorrhage at any time

B. Nonhemorrhagic stroke or other cerebrovascular events within the past year

C. Marked hypertension having systolic pressure of >180 mm Hg and diastolic pressure of >110 mm Hg at any time during the acute presentation.

D. Suspicion of aortic dissection

E. Significant closed-head or facial trauma within 3 months

F. Active internal bleeding including menses

Relative Contraindications

A. It requires assessment of risk benefit ratio, including current use of anticoagulants (INR of ≥2)

B. Any invasive or surgical procedure within 2 weeks

C. Cardiopulmonary resuscitation time is >10 minutes.

D. Known bleeding diathesis

E. Pregnancy

F. Hemorrhagic ophthalmic condition like hemorrhagic diabetic retinopathy
G. Active peptic ulcer disease
H. History of severe hypertension that has been adequately controlled now.
I. Recent internal bleeding within 2–4 weeks.
J. Dementia

Complications

A. Allergic reaction to streptokinase
B. Hypotension in 4–10% of patients
C. Hemorrhage is the most serious complication. So unnecessary venous and arterial procedures should be avoided in these patients. Most serious complication is hemorrhagic stroke. It will be increased if the age of the person is >70 years.

Q30. Peripartum cardiomyopathy.

DNBI/APR2016 (10)

Peripartum cardiomyopathy.

DNB, 2022 (5)

RAJIV GANDHI UNIVERSITY OF HEALTH SC, KARNATAKA 2016 (10)

TEERTHANKER MAHAVEER UNI, 2017 (10)

MGR UNI, TAMIL NADU, 2018 (10)

ANSWER

Definition

It occurs during the last trimester or within first 6 months of postpartum.

Criteria of Peripartum Cardiomyopathy

1. Development of heart failure in last month of pregnancy or 5 months postpartum
2. Absence of preexisting heart disease
3. Indeterminant cause
4. Echocardiographic findings (a, together with b or c; or all of these)
   a. Left ventricular end-diastolic dimension >2.7 cm/m^2
   b. M-mode fractional shortening <30%
   c. Left ventricular ejection fraction <0.45

Pathophysiology

There are 11 hypothesis as a causal factors responsible for cardiomyopathy:

A. Viral myocarditis during peripartum period due to coxsackievirus, echovirus, parvovirus B19, Epstein-Barr virus, human cytomegalovirus, and herpes virus 6.
B. Autoimmune myocarditis as a result of cross-reaction of cardiac muscle antigen with antiuterine antibodies.
C. Aggressive apoptosis of cardiac cells.
D. Inadequate response to hemodynamic stress.
E. Selenium deficiency in case of malnutrition
F. Inflammatory response to cytokines
G. *Increased prolactin effect on the heart*: Abnormal 16 kDa prolactin fragment induced by oxidative stress affects angiogenesis.
H. *Genetic mode of transmission in case of familial predisposition*: Truncating mutation in TTN is present in 15% of PPCM.
I. Effect of estrogen and progesterone
J. Myocardial stunning due to adrenergic surge
K. Ischemia of myocardium

Risk Factors

A. Increased maternal age
B. Increased parity
C. Twin pregnancy
D. Malnutrition
E. Use of tocolytic therapy for premature labor
F. Preeclampsia
G. Cocaine abuse
H. Poverty
I. African descent

Several of the above risk factors are responsible for antiandrogenic signaling through secreted vascular endothelial growth factor like soluble FLT1. Hence decreased angiogenic reserve may be a pathogenic factor in postpartum cardiomyopathy.

New mothers who ingested salts while reclining on a warm bed along with impaired mobilization of excess circulating volume after delivery may predispose to PPCM.

Clinical Manifestations

Most of the patients present with symptoms just after delivery or in the first week of postpartum. Symptoms are:

a. Dyspnea
b. Orthopnea
c. Paroxysmal nocturnal dyspnea

On physical examination reveals:

a. Tachycardia

b. Elevated pulsatile jugular vein
c. Third heart sound
d. Displaced apical impulse
e. Basal crackles reflecting pulmonary edema
f. In severe cases evidence of cardiogenic shock or acute respiratory failure.

Evaluation

A. *Cardiac biomarkers*: B-type natriuretic peptide and N-terminal natriuretic peptide are raised.
B. *ECG demonstrated*: Sinus tachycardia, interventricular conduction delay or sometimes LBBB pattern.
C. Echocardiography demonstrates:
  a. Variable degree of left ventricular dilatation
  b. Left ventricular systolic dysfunction
  c. Right ventricular or biventricular enlargement
  d. Mitral regurgitation
  e. Tricuspid regurgitation
  f. Pulmonary hypertension
  g. Intracardiac thrombus
  h. Echocardiographic criteria as described above.
D. Cardiac MRI can estimate ejection fraction accurately.
E. Cardiac biopsy to diagnose giant cell myocarditis or cardiac sarcoidosis.

Complications

A. Progression to severe HF
B. Arrhythmia
C. Cardiogenic shock
D. Thromboembolic events such as stroke, TIA
E. Death

Treatment

A. Optimization of patient's volume status.
B. Drugs used are:
  a. Beta-1 blockers
  b. ACEI—but it is contraindicated in pregnant patients.
  c. Diuretics are used to control symptoms related to HF.
  d. Sacubitril/valsartan can improve HF in case of pregnancy-induced cardiomyopathies.
  e. Bromocriptine being a dopaminergic agonist having prolactin blocking properties will decrease the effect of 16-kDa prolactin present on the cardiac myocyte.
C. Cardiac resynchronization therapy improve ejection fraction and outcomes when medical therapy is ineffective.

Q31. What is effective circulatory volume? Enumerate conditions with increased and decreased effective circulatory volume states and basic management strategies for each.

DNBII/APR2016 (10)

ANSWER

Effective circulating volume is a part of extracellular fluid remain in the arterial system that is normally 700 mL in 70 kg subject and is responsible for proper tissue perfusion to maintain adequate cellular metabolism through provision of nutrients and removal of waste products. But the better physiologic definition is the pressure perfusing the baroreceptors in the carotid sinus as well as glomerular afferent arteriole because it is the change in pressure rather than volume.

Effective circulatory volume varies with the extracellular fluid volume and these are proportional to total body sodium stores as it holds water in the extracellular spaces. Sodium loading leads to volume expansion, on the other hands, sodium loss leads to volume depletion.

Clinical conditions	Effective volume	Extracellular volume	Plasma volume	Cardiac output
Volume depletion	Low	Low	Low	Low
Heart failure	Low	Increased	Increased	Low
Arteriovenous fistula	No change	High	High	High
Advanced cirrhosis	Decreased	High	High	Normal or high

In case of congestive cardiac failure due to low cardiac output effective circulatory volume will be low thus lowering the pressure on the baroreceptors which in turn induces compensatory retention of fluid by kidney leading to expansion of extracellular fluid, the result is low effective circulating volume along with increased extracellular and plasma volume.

Control of effective circulating volume by renal excretion:

Kidney is the primary regulator of body sodium and volume balance. Through the urinary sodium excretion in an appropriate manner. When there is increased in volume after sodium overload or after closure of arteriovenous fistula, excretion of sodium will be raised through the kidney to lower the volume toward normal. On the other hand in case of volume depletion kidney will retain sodium. So volume regulation should be efficient because small changes in sodium intake are associated with parallel changes in sodium excretion.

In patients with low sodium diet, intake of sodium is suddenly increased, half of the excess intake is excreted in urine, but remaining sodium will increase the body sodium store thus elevating plasma osmolality and stimulates thirst center increasing water intake and stimulates the secretion of ADH which stimulates reabsorption of water from distal renal tubule and collecting duct to reabsorb sodium. As a result there is fluid retention, effective circulating volume, body weight, and plasma osmolality will return to normal. So on subsequent 3–4 days only small fraction of orally taken sodium will be retained. At the end of 3–4 days, a steady state will be reached when there is mildly increased fluid retention due to retention of both sodium and water in first 4 days. There is correlation between total amount of retained sodium and increment in sodium intake above the baseline.

Clinical implications:

There is implication of steady state in pathogenesis and treatment of disease state.

As for example in patient with volume overload, to decrease the extracellular fluid volume diuretics are given that inhibit reabsorption of sodium from different parts of nephron to lower the ECF volume. The initial loss of volume activates renin-angiotensin system to limit the fluid losses. These counter-regulatory processes are so efficient that if the dose of the diuretic is constant, all fluid and electrolyte will be within first 7–14 days of therapy but maximum natriuretic effect occurs with the first dose.

Same occurs in case of potassium also. With the increased intake of potassium, body potassium store will be elevated but with little rise in serum potassium. This will also mediate through increased excretion of aldosterone to excrete the potassium in increased quantity. Again excess water suppresses the antidiuretic hormone leading to excretion of dilute urine. Hence, in normal subject excess sodium, excess fluid, potassium or bicarbonate will not persist in presence of normal renal function.

Treatment:

Treatment of HF is the same with impaired systolic function with reduced ejection function.

Treatment of volume depletion is fluid administration.

In case of advanced cirrhosis dose of the diuretics should be reduced.

Q32. A 20 years old male has a blood pressure of 180/110 mm Hg.

Enumerate the possible causes of hypertension in this patient. Outline the diagnosis and treatment of renal artery stenosis.

DNBIIIA/JUN2016 (10)

ANSWER

Definition

It is a major cause of renovascular hypertension.

Most common cause of renal artery stenosis is atherosclerosis in older individual. In younger than 50 years woman the cause is fibromuscular dysplasia. As the lumen of the renal artery decreases blood flow to kidney also decreases with decrease perfusion of kidney structure and function.

Diagnosis

A. Laboratory studies:

- **a.** Serum creatinine—assess the renal function
- **b.** 24 hours collection of urine or protein-creatinine ratio on randomly collected urine can also assess the renal function and also assess the degree of proteinuria. In case of vascular disease there is minimal to moderate degree of proteinuria.
- **c.** Urine analysis should be done to detect RBC or cast
- **d.** Serological test for vasculitis such as ANA, C3, C4, and ANCA.
- **e.** Peripheral renin activity is increased in case of renal vascular disease.

B. *Ultrasonography*: It can suggest the asymmetry of kidney size.

C. *Duplex ultrasonography*: It shows renal arteries and assess the flow velocity to assess the severity of the stenosis. It is inexpensive and widely available. Velocities in renal artery of >200 cm/sec will predict the lesion as hemodynamically important, i.e., lumen is 60% occluded. But if the velocity is >300 cm/sec can be taken to avoid false positivity.

D. *Radionuclear scanning by captopril renography with technetium-99mTc mertiatide*: Captopril-mediated fall in filtration pressure will amplify the differences in renal perfusion.

E. *Spiral CT scan and MRI*: Both will demonstrates renal arteries and perirenal aorta. It provides excellent images. Only gadolinium toxicity will occur if the GFR is <30 mL/min/1.73 m^2. MRI will demonstrates the following also:

a. Absolute blood flow rate
b. Glomerular filtration rate
c. Renal perfusion rate
d. Provide accurate renal size serially with volume measurement.

F. *Blood oxygen-dependent MRI*: It can give functional assessment by evaluating kidney tissue perfusion in patient with atherosclerotic renal artery stenosis.

G. *Arteriography*: Following are the different types of arteriography:

a. *Conventional aortography*: It requires arterial puncture and there is risk of arterial emboli. It can also produce contrast-induced tubular necrosis.
b. Intravenous subtraction angiography:
   1. It can demonstrate stenosis in the main renal artery but it cannot show accessory renal artery.
   2. It will avoid the use of high volume of contrast material into the artery.
c. *Intra-arterial digital subtraction angiography*: It will locate theseverity of the vascular lesion. It is associated with fewer complications. It is considered as a gold standard for the diagnosis of large vessel disease.
d. *Carbon-dioxide angiography*: It is alternative contrast agent used combining digital subtraction angiography to avoid contrast-induced nephropathy.

Treatment

A. In case of normal or near normal renal function revascularization of the kidney is recommended to preserve normal renal function:

a. Degree of stenosis is >80–85%.
b. Stenosis is 50–80% and captopril-enhanced arteriography demonstrates activation of intrarenal renal artery stenosis.

B. Observation instead of revascularization with serial duplex scanning every 6 months with accurate correction of dyslipidemia along with the use of drugs that prevent platelet aggregation is recommended in case of following criteria:

a. Degree of stenosis is <50%.
b. Stenosis is 50–80%, scintigraphy is negative.

C. In case of renal impairment when the objective is recovery of kidney function along with prevention of further kidney function impairment, following are the prerequisites for revascularization:

a. Serum creatinine is <4 mg/dL.
b. Serum creatinine is >4 mg/dL but with possible renal artery thrombosis.

If the either of the above two conditions is satisfied in that case revascularization can be done in following cases:

a. Stenosis is >80%.
b. Rise in serum creatinine level after administration of ACEI.
c. Stenosis is 50–80% and scintigraphy is positive.

In case of atherosclerotic renal artery stenosis if the blood pressure and kidney function are controlled by medical therapy, then it should be continued.

Medical therapy should include:

a. Blockade of renin–angiotensin system
b. Attainment of goal of blood pressure
c. Cessation of smoking,
d. Administration of statins
e. Administration of aspirin

Surgery:

A. Younger female patients with fibromuscular dysplasia with otherwise normal vessels can be treated by percutaneous renal artery angioplasty.

B. Surgical revascularization will improve the renal function in patients with ischemic nephropathy.

Following are the operative bypass procedures with saphenous veins, autologous arteries or prosthetic material:

a. Aortorenal
b. Hepatorenal
c. Lienorenal
d. Ileorenal
e. In case of atherosclerotic arterial disease atherotomy is done to improve the blood flow.
f. In case of nonatheromatous renal artery disease reconstruction renal arteries.

C. In case of revascularization of the totally occluded renal artery following features can predict whether it will salvage the kidney function:

a. Length of the kidney is >9 cm.
b. Localization of renin secretion
c. Collateral circulation and nephrogram on angiographic studies
d. Split function study results to demonstrate different concentration of urine.

e. Viable renal tissue in biopsy examination

f. After arteriotomy during surgery, there is spontaneous back-bleeding.

Complications of surgery:

A. Renal artery dissection

B. Capsular perforation

C. Hemorrhage

D. *Atheroembolic disease*: It may be catastrophic producing

According to recent guidelines following clinical factors determining the role of revascularization in addition to medical therapy:

A. During the treatment of systemic hypertension progressive decline in GFR.

B. In spite of adequate medical therapy blood pressure is difficult to control.

C. Recurrent or rapid decline in GFR associated with systemic blood pressure reduction.

D. During the therapy with ACEI or ARBs there is decline in GFR.

E. Recurrent congestive cardiac failure cause cannot be explained by left ventricular function.

According to recent guidelines favoring medical therapy and surveillance of renal artery stenosis:

A. Very advanced age and/or limited life expectancy

B. Controlled blood pressure with stable renal function

C. Stable renal artery stenosis without progression on surveillance studies

D. Extensive comorbidity that make revascularization too risky.

E. High risk for or previous experience with atheroembolic disease.

F. Other concomitant renal parenchymal diseases that leads to progressive renal dysfunction.

Q33. Etiology of infective endocarditis. Outline the diagnosis (clinical and laboratory) of infective endocarditis.

DNBIIIA/JUN2016 (10)

Discuss etiopathogenesis, clinical manifestations, diagnosis, and management of infective endocarditis.

MGR/AUG2004/MDIII (15.
MGR/MAR2002/MDIII (25)

Bacterial endocarditis.

GMC/2015/MDIII (10)

Diagnosis and complications of infective endocarditis.

PGI/APR2013/MDII (10)

Discuss the etiopathogenesis, clinical manifestations, diagnosis, and management of a case of acute infective endocarditis.

BF/MAY2011/MDII (30)

Recent advances in laboratory diagnosis in infective endocarditis.

BF/MAY2009/MDIII (10)

Management of infective endocarditis.

MLB/MAY2013/MDII (20)

Mechanism and management of paroxysmal SVT. Management of infective endocarditis.

DNB, 2019 (5+5)

Diagnosis and management of infective endocarditis.

MAHARASHTRA UNIVERSITY OF HEALTH SC, VIJAYAWADA, 2021 (10)

Etiology and clinical features of infective endocarditis. Treatment of subacute bacterial endocarditis.

DNB, 2019 (2+3+5)

Etiology, clinical manifestations, diagnosis, and management of infective endocarditis.

DNB, 2018 (10)

PSVT management answers in Question number 9.

Blood culture in infective endocarditis.

MGR UNIVERSITY, 2017 (5)

Describe the etiology, clinical features and management of infective endocarditis.

NTR UNIVERSITY OF HEALTH SC, VIJAYAWADA, ANDHRA, 2020 (10)

Diagnosis and management of infective endocarditis.

WEST BENGAL UNIVERSITY OF HEALTH SCIENCE, 2020 (10)

Prosthetic valve endocarditis.
KERALA UNIVERSITY, 2020 (10)

Differences between native valve and prosthetic valve endocarditis.
AIIMS (DELHI) 2022 (10)

How can you diagnose and treat a case of infective endocarditis.
SCBMCH, 2019 (10)

Describe the criteria for diagnosis of infective endocarditis. Discuss in brief the etiology, complications, and management of right sided infective endocarditis.
DNB (OCT2024) (10)

Clinical features, management of infective endocarditis.
ODISHA UNI, 2022 (10)

Cardiac surgical treatment in patients with endocarditis—indications, timing, antibiotic therapy after cardiac surgery for endocarditis.
ODISHA UNI, 2022 (10)

Discuss the pathophysiology, clinical features and diagnostic approach to infective endocarditis. Outline the principles of management.
WBUHS, 2024 (10)

Write the diagnosis and management of infective endocarditis.
MANIPUR UNIVERSITY, 2019 (10)

Enumerate the organisms causing major clinical forms of endocarditis mentioning specifically in injection drug users. Describe the clinical manifestations and approach of management.
WBUHS, 2024 (10)

Discuss the pathophysiology, clinical features and diagnostic approach to infective endocarditis. Outline the principles of management.
WBUHS, 2024 (10)

ANSWER

70–75% of infective endocarditis has associates preexisting cardiac abnormalities, mitral valve regurgitation or prolapse being the leading conditions.

A. In case of native valve endocarditis:

- **a.** *S. aureus*:
  - **1.** In case of catheter-induced bacteremia.
  - **2.** In case of intravenous drug users with opioid. Valves most commonly affected are tricuspid valve in 70% cases followed by mitral valve then aortic valve.
- **b.** Coagulase-negative staphylococci
- **c.** Enterococci in patients with genitourinary and obstetric procedure, in these patients may not have underlying heart disease.
- **d.** *Streptococcus pneumoniae*—these patients may present as "Osler triad" that also includes pneumococcal pneumoniae, meningitis.
- **e.** *Streptococcus* viridans,
- **f.** HACEK organisms—it includes *Haemophilus* species, *Aggregatibacter* species, *Cardiobacterium hominis*, *Eikenella corrodens*, and *Kingella kingae*.
- **g.** *S. bovis* originating from gastrointestinal tract—it is associated with colonic polyp and colonic tumors.
- **h.** Other members of Enterobacteriaceae such as *Salmonella*, *Klebsiella*, *Enterobacter*, *Escherichia coli*, proteus, *Serratia*, *Citrobacter*, *Shigella* and *Yersinia*.
- **i.** *Staphylococcus lugdunensis*—it is rare cause of endocarditis.

B. Prosthetic valve endocarditis:

- **a.** There is greatest risk of infection in first 2 months of implantation of mechanical and bioprosthetic valves—it is called early prosthetic valve endocarditis due to nosocomial and intraoperative contamination of coagulase-negative staphylococci.
- **b.** If it occurs after 2 months of surgery—it is known as late prosthetic valve endocarditis. The organisms involved are:
  - **1.** *S. aureus*
  - **2.** Coagulase-negative *Staphylococcus*
  - **3.** Facultative gram-negative bacilli
  - **4.** Diphtheroids
  - **5.** Fungi

  Portal of entry is similar to that of native valve endocarditis.

C. *Pacemaker and defibrillator endocarditis*: It involves devices or endothelium at the point of contact with device.

   a. One-third of cases within 3 months of device implantation—it occurs due to direct intraoperative microbial seeding.

   b. One-third of cases within 4–12 months of implantation

   c. One-third of cases after 1 year of implantation.

   d. *The organisms are*: *S. aureus*, coagulase-negative staphylococci, and methicillin-resistant *S. aureus* (MRSA).

   e. In case of late infection there is thinning of overlying tissue followed by erosion of the device, ultimately infection involves electrodes and endocardium.

D. Other causes of endocarditis are:

   a. *Pseudomonas aeruginosa*

   b. *Candida albicans*

   c. *Bacillus*

   d. *Lactobacillus*

   e. *Corynebacterium*

E. 5–15% cases of infective endocarditis are culture negative due to prior exposure of antibiotics. Remainder of cases are due to fastidious organisms:

   a. *Granulicatella*

   b. *Abiotrophia*

   c. *C. burnetii* has a predilection for prosthetic valves.

   d. *Bartonella* species—in Europe.

   e. HACEK

   f. *Corynebacterium* species—involves intracardiac devices.

   g. *Propionibacterium acne*—involves intracardiac devices

Clinical Picture

A. *Acute infective endocarditis*: Patients become toxic, progresses to valvular destruction and metastatic infection within several days to weeks. It usually involves normal valves or it may be absent.

B. *Subacute infective endocarditis*: Patients become mild to moderately toxic within several weeks to months, metastatic infection is rare.

C. Rate of progression depends upon:

   a. Age of the patients

   b. Underlying health of the patients

   c. Nature and extent of the underlying valvular disease.

D. Hallmark of infective endocarditis are fever and appearance of new murmur. Fever may be absent in following cases:

   a. Elderly patients

   b. Uremic patient

   c. Immunosuppressed

   Murmur may be absent in following cases:

   a. Right-sided endocarditis

   b. Mural involvement

   c. Involvement of intracardiac devices

E. Features of congestive cardiac failure as a consequences of dysfunction of valve or intracardiac fistulae. It will progress more aggressively in case of aortic valve as compared to mitral valve.

F. If infection spreads to adjacent annulus or myocardial infarction, it may lead to perivalvular abscesses and intracardiac fistulae with appearance of new murmur.

G. Spreading of infection from abscesses in the aortic valve annulus to upper ventricular septum leading to interruption of conduction system producing varying degrees of heart block.

H. Mitral perivalvular abscesses—rare cause of conduction abnormalities

I. Features of myocardial infarction from emboli in the coronary artery in 2% patients.

J. Other nonspecific symptoms are—weight loss, fatigue, malaise, chills and night sweat, and bodyache.

Noncardiac manifestations:

A. Peripheral features due to embolic phenomenon:

   a. Janeway lesion—erythematous, macular, and nontender lesions on the fingers, soles, and palm.

   b. Clubbing

   c. Osler nodes—painful tender erythematous nodules present on the pads of the fingers or toes.

   d. Roth's spot—retinal hemorrhage

   e. Splinter hemorrhage—subungual dark linear streaks

   f. Petechial lesion

B. Hematogenous spread of focal infection into the following organisms:

   a. Skin

   b. Spleen

   c. Kidney

   d. Skeletal system

   e. Meninges

C. Arterial emboli originate from endocarditis caused by:

a. *S. aureus*

b. Mobile vegetation of >10 mm in diameter

c. Infections involving anterior leaflet of mitral valve

D. Arterial emboli produce following features:

a. Ischemia to spleen, bowel, and extremities

b. Central nervous system:

1. Stroke

2. Seizures

3. Encephalopathy

4. Aseptic meningitis

5. Purulent meningitis

6. Intracranial hemorrhage

7. Hemorrhagic infarction

8. *Mycotic aneurysms*: It is characterized focal dilated arteries at the points weakened by lodgment of septic emboli in the vasorum.

9. Microabscesses in case of staphylococcal endocarditis.

c. Immune complex deposition on the glomerular basement membrane leading to hypocomplementemic glomerulonephritis and renal infarction.

d. Embolic infarction in kidney leads to flank pain and hematuria.

Investigations

A. Blood culture:

a. In case of native valve, prosthetic valve endocarditis, and cardiovascular implantable electronic device endocarditis and if the patients not received antibiotics during past 2 weeks, three groups of bottle culture sets that should be separated by at least 2 hours and should be taken from different sites over 24 hours.

If culture is negative, then two additional culture set should be taken:

1. In case of hemodynamically stable patients with suspected endocarditis and patient already received antibiotics within last 2 weeks, empirical antibiotics should not be administered. This delay helps to take additional blood to be taken for culture.

2. In case of hemodynamically unstable patients or patients requiring urgent surgery, empirical antibiotics can be administered after taking three sets of blood for culture.

B. Nonblood culture test:

a. Serological tests for following organisms which are very difficult to recover from blood culture:

1. *Brucella*

2. *Bartonella*

3. *Legionella*

4. *Chlamydia psittaci*

5. *C. burnetii*

b. From vegetations which can be obtained during surgery or embolectomy

c. Microscopic examination with special stains

d. Polymerase chain reaction:

1. Recovery of microbial DNA—identify bacteria.

2. DNA encoding ribosomal subunit 16S or 28S—identify fungi.

C. Cardiac imaging:

a. Echocardiography:

1. Confirms vegetables

2. Detects intracardiac complications

3. Assesses the cardiac functions

b. Transthoracic echocardiography:

1. It is safe and noninvasive.

2. It can detect vegetations in >95% patients with definite endocarditis.

3. It cannot evaluate prosthetic valves and cannot detect intracardiac complications.

4. It cannot detect vegetations of <2 mm in size.

5. In case of suspected endocarditis negative study cannot exclude the diagnosis rather it should be repeated after 7–10 days.

6. It is optional method of diagnosis in following cases:

- Prosthetic valve endocarditis
- Intracardiac devices
- Myocardial abscess
- Valve perforations
- Intracardiac fistula

c. Three-dimensional transesophageal echocardiography (TEE) will enhance the findings of standard TEE.

d. 18-fluorodeoxyglucose PET or CT can evaluate and identify:

1. Perivalvular infection

2. Perigraft infection

3. Prosthesis-aorta graft infection

e. In case of nosocomial staphylococcal bacteremia there is increased risk of endocarditis if any of the following is present, hence these patients should be investigated by TEE:
   1. Positive for blood culture for 2–4 days.
   2. Patient depends on dialysis
   3. Infection in the spine
   4. Nonvertebral osteomyelitis
   5. Abnormalities in endocarditis-predisposing valves.

D. Other studies:
   a. Complete blood count
   b. Renal function tests
   c. Liver function tests
   d. Chest X-ray
   e. Electrocardiography
   f. *CRP*: Increased
   g. Rheumatoid factor

Treatment

Organisms	Drugs and dosage
Penicillin susceptible streptococci	• Penicillin G 2–3 MU intravenously 4 hourly for 4 weeks • Ceftriaxone 2 g intravenously as single dose for 4 weeks • Vancomycin 15 mg/kg intravenously 12 hourly for 4 weeks • Penicillin G 2–3 MU intravenously 4 hourly **or** • Ceftriaxone 2 g intravenously four times daily for 2 weeks **Plus** • Gentamicin 3 mg/kg four times daily intravenously as a single dose or 8 hourly in divided doses
Relatively penicillin-resistant streptococci, *Streptococcus gallolyticus*	• Penicillin G 4 MU 4 hourly or ceftriaxone 2 g intravenously 6 hourly for 4 weeks **Plus** • Gentamicin 3 mg/kg 6 hourly intravenously or intramuscularly as a single dose or 8 hourly in equally divided doses for 2 weeks • Vancomycin 15 mg/kg intravenously 12 hourly for 4 weeks
Moderately penicillin-resistant streptococci, *Granulicatella, Abiotrophia*, or *Gemella*	• Penicillin G 4–5 MU 4 hourly or ceftriaxone 2 g intravenously 6 hourly for 6 weeks Plus • Gentamicin 3 mg/kg 6 hourly intravenously or intramuscularly as a single dose or 8 hourly in equally divided doses for 6 weeks • Vancomycin 15 mg/kg intravenously 12 hourly for 4 weeks
Enterococci	• Penicillin G 4–5 MU intravenously 6 hourly **Plus** • Gentamicin 1 mg/kg intravenously 8 hourly • For 4–6 weeks both
	• Ampicillin 2 g intravenously 4 hourly **Plus** • Gentamicin 1 g/kg intravenously 8 hourly • Both for 4–6 weeks
	• Vancomycin 15 mg/kg intravenously 12 hourly **Plus** • Gentamicin 1 g/kg intravenously 8 hourly • For 6 weeks both
	• Ampicillin 2 g intravenously 4 hourly **Plus** • Ceftriaxone 2 g intravenously 12 hourly • Both for 6 weeks

Continued

Continued

Organisms	Drugs and dosage
	Staphylococci
Methicillin-sensitive *Staphylococcus aureus* infecting native valves	• Nafcillin, oxacillin or flucloxacillin 2 g intravenously 4 hourly for 4–6 weeks • Cefazolin 2 g intravenously 8 hourly for 4–6 weeks • Vancomycin 15 mg/kg intravenously 12 hourly for 4–6 weeks
Methicillin-resistant *S. aureus* infecting native valves	15 mg/kg vancomycin intravenously 8–12 hourly for 4–6 weeks
Methicillin-sensitive *S. aureus* infecting prosthetic valves	• Nafcillin, oxacillin or flucloxacillin 2 g intravenously 4 hourly for 6–8 weeks **Plus** • Gentamicin 1 mg/kg intravenously or intramuscularly 8 hourly for 2 weeks **Plus** • Rifampin 300 mg orally 8 hourly for 6–8 weeks
Methicillin-resistant *S. aureus* infecting prosthetic valves	• Vancomycin 15 mg/kg intravenously 12 hourly for 6–8 weeks **Plus** • Gentamicin 1 mg/kg intravenously or intramuscularly 8 hourly for 2 weeks **Plus** • Rifampin 300 mg orally 8 hourly for 6–8 weeks
HACEK organisms	• Ceftriaxone 2 g daily intravenously as a single dose for 4 weeks • Ampicillin/sulbactam 3 g intravenously 6 hourly for 4 weeks
Coxiella burnetii	• Doxycycline 100 mg orally 12 hourly **Plus** • 200 mg hydroxychloroquine orally 8 hourly • Both for: • In case of native valve 18 months • In case of prosthetic valves 24 months
Bartonella species	• Doxycycline 100 mg 12 hourly for 6 weeks **Plus** • Gentamicin 1 mg/kg intravenously 8 hourly for 2 weeks

Diagnosis: Follow the modified Duke criteria (for more details see Question number 6).

Difference between Native Valve and Prosthetic Valve Endocarditis

Criteria	Native valves	Prosthetic valves
Site of involvement	Natural valves of the heart are affected	Both mechanical and bioprosthetic valves are affected
Incidence	Incidence is high as compared to prosthetic valve	Incidence is low as compared to native valves
Mortality and morbidity	Less risk of mortality and morbidity	High risk of mortality and morbidity
Onset of the disease	It is acute or may be subacute	• In early case: Within 60 days of valve implantation • In late case it occurs after 60 days of implantation
Causative organisms	• *Streptococcus viridans*—most common • *Staphylococcus aureus*—in acute cases • *Enterococcus* • HACEK organisms	In early case: • Coagulase negative staphylococci • *Staphylococcus aureus* • Gram negative bacilli and fungi In late case: • Similar to native valve involvement • *Streptococcus viridans* • *Staphylococcus aureus* • HACEK organisms

Continued

Continued

Criteria	Native valves	Prosthetic valves
Pathogenesis	• Bacteremia from • Urinary tract infection • Dental procedure • Gastrointestinal infections	In early case: • Either intraoperative or perioperative procedures. In late case: • Hematogenous seeding • Preceding bacteremia
Risk factors	• Congenital cardiac defect • Rheumatic valvular diseases • Intravenous drug users • Poor dental hygiene	• Recent valve replacement • Immunosuppression • Prolonged stay in the hospital • Invasive procedures
Clinical features	• Fever, malaise, fatigue • Worsening of the existing murmur • Different embolic events • Presence of immune phenomena like Roth spot, Osler nodes, janeway lesion	• The presentation is similar to native valve endocarditis but it is more severe • Para-valvular leak • In case of late infective endocarditis • Signs of chronic infections • Embolic phenomenon
Diagnosis	• Blood culture is positive in more than 90% of cases • In echocardiography there is presence of vegetation or abscesses	• Blood culture to detect the pathogens • Echocardiography may demonstrate the vegetation, para-valvular leak
Complications	• Heart failure • Embolic phenomena like stroke and pulmonary embolism. • Septicemia	• Same as that of native endocarditis but it is severe. • Para-valvular abscesses • Para-valvular leak • Prosthetic valve dehiscence • Intra-cardiac fistula • Systemic embolism
Treatment	• Based on antibacterial sensitivity administration of the antibiotics • Indications of surgery: ○ Heart failure ○ Large vegetation ○ Uncontrolled infection ○ Recurrent infection	• Duration of administration of the antibiotic is high • Surgery in case of dysfunction of the prosthetic valves
Prognosis	In case of early diagnosis and treatment with antibiotics according the sensitivity, prognosis is good	Due to prosthetic valve involvement the prognosis is worse
Mortality	15–20%	20–40%

Right Sided Endocarditis Involves Most Commonly Tricuspid Valves, Less Commonly Pulmonary Valves

Risk factors are the following:

A. Intravenous drug user

B. Intravenous catheters like central venous catheter, hemodialysis catheter, catheter required for parenteral nutrition

C. Congenital endocarditis

D. Cardiac devices like cardioverter defibrillators.

E. Prosthetic tricuspid valve

F. Immunosuppressive therapy

Causative organisms responsible are:

A. *Staphylococcus aureus*—most common

B. In case of catheter induced infection, coagulase negative streptococci

C. *Enterococcus* species

D. *Streptococcus viridans*

E. *Streptococcus pneumoniae*

F. Gram negative bacilli:
   a. *Pseudomonas aeruginosa*
   b. *Serratia*
   c. *Klebsiella*

G. Fungi—*Candida*

Clinical features:

A. General features:
   a. Fever
   b. Malaise
   c. Anorexia
   d. Weight loss
   e. Night sweat

B. Cardiac symptoms:
   a. New onset of right sided murmur or sudden change in the character of the murmur during inspiration.
   b. Features of right sided heart congestive hepatomegaly and peripheral edema failure like enlarged pulsatile neck vein.
   c. Pulmonary features from septic right sided emboli leading to development of pulmonary infarction or pulmonary embolism.
   d. Dermatological manifestation are same as described above.

Complications:

A. Tricuspid regurgitation leading to right sided heart failure

B. Septic pulmonary embolism or infarction

C. Pulmonary infarction

D. Metastatic infarction like mycotic aneurysm, abscess in the spleen

Diagnosis: Same as above already described.

Treatment as already described above in this question.

Indications of surgery in case of infective endocarditis are the following:

A. Heart failure due to
   a. Aortic regurgitation leading to decompensated heart failure
   b. Prosthetic valve dysfunction

B. Uncontrolled infection due to:
   a. Abscess formation
   b. Pseudoaneurysm
   c. Development of fistula in the heart
   d. In case of recurrent embolization, vegetation of more than 100 mm in size.
   e. Infection with multidrug resistant organisms
   f. Sepsis refractory to antibiotic treatment

C. Prevention of recurrent embolization as in case of large vegetation of more than 10 mm in size.

D. Prosthetic valve endocarditis if:
   a. If it will develop within 2 months of surgery
   b. Paravalvular abscess
   c. Valve dehiscence

Timing of surgery:

A. Surgery within 24 hours of disease:
   a. Acute severe aortic regurgitation leading to cardiogenic shock.
   b. Hemodynamic instability due to large destructive lesions
   c. Severely resistant infection or fungal infection

B. Surgery within few days in following conditions:
   a. Large vegetation of more than 10 mm in diameter
   b. Recurrent vegetation
   c. Valvular dysfunction leading to heart failure
   d. Paravalvular abscess
   e. Valve dehiscence

C. Elective surgery after 1 to 2 weeks of antibiotic treatment:
   a. Persistent vegetations
   b. Residual valvular dysfunction after endocarditis

Antibiotic treatment after surgery:

A. Duration of therapy:
   a. In case of native valve endocarditis: 4 to 6 weeks of intravenous antibiotics
   b. In case of prosthetic valve endocarditis: ≥ 6 weeks

B. Empiric antibiotic treatment prior to result of blood culture:
   a. In case of native valve: Vancomycin + Ceftriaxone + Gentamicin
   b. In case of prosthetic valve: Vancomycin + Rifampicin + Gentamicin

C. Based on the blood culture results definite therapy:
   a. *Staphylococcus aureus*: Oxacillin/nafcillin + in case of prosthetic valve rifampin
   b. Methicillin resistant *Staphylococcus aureus*: Vancomycin + Rifampicin + Gentamicin
   c. *Streptococcus viridans*: Penicillin G ± Gentamicin
   d. *Enterococcus*: ceftriaxone + Gentamicin or ampicillin
   e. Fungal endocarditis: Amphotericin B + vlave surgery

Q34. Classify dyslipidemias and describe various management strategies.

DNBIV/DEC2011 (10)

ANSWER

Classification of Dyslipidemia

Classification	Diseases	Genetic defect	Lipid abnormalities	Clinical features
Type 1 Chylomicronemia	Deficiency of lipoprotein lipase	Autosomal recessive	Triglyceride > 1,000 mg/dL to >10,000 mg/dL	• Pancreatitis • Eruptive xanthoma
	Apo CII deficiency	Autosomal recessive	Partial genetic defect Triglyceride > 500 mg/dL	
Type IIa (Increased LDL cholesterol level and/or particles	Polygenic hypercholesterolemia	Multiple genetic defect	LDL-C level > 130 mg/dL	Increased risk of atherosclerotic coronary vascular disease
	Heterogenic hypercholesterolemia	Dysfunction or absence of LDL receptor Autosomal dominant	LDL-C level > 190 mg/dL	• Increased risk of atherosclerotic coronary vascular disease • Tendon xanthoma
	Homogenic hypercholesterolemia		LDL-C level > 350 mg/dL	• Increased risk of atherosclerotic coronary vascular disease • Tendon xanthoma
Type IIb Increased LDL, VLDL-C, and triglyceride level and/or particle	Familial combined hyperlipidemia	Multiple genetic defect of various apolipoprotein and/or lipoprotein genes	LDL-C level > 160 mg/dL Triglyceride level > 300 mg/dL	Increased risk of atherosclerotic coronary vascular disease
Type III Increased triglyceride level, IDL-C level, and/or particles	Familial dysbetalipoproteinemia	Defect in ApoE gene Autosomal recessive	LDL-C level > 220 mg/dL Triglyceride level: > 300 mg/dL	• Increased risk of atherosclerotic coronary vascular disease • Palmar xanthoma • Skin creases become orange-colored • Tuberoeruptive xanthoma in knee and elbows
Type IV Increased triglyceride/VLDL-C levels	Familial hypertriglyceridemia	Unknown genetic defect Autosomal dominant	TG level > 150 mg/dL	Increased risk of atherosclerotic coronary vascular disease
Type V Increased triglyceride level, increased chylomicron, and VLDL-C level	Hyperprebetalipoproteinemia	Unknown genetic defect	Triglyceride level > 500 mg/dL LDL-C level > 130 mg/dL	• Increased risk of atherosclerotic coronary vascular disease • Pancreatitis • Eruptive xanthoma

(LDL: low-density lipoprotein; VLDL: very low-density lipoproteins)

Treatment of Hyperlipidemia

Primary target is LDL-C Secondary target is raised HDL-C	
LDL-C: High risk patients: <100 mg/dL Very high risk patients: <70 mg/dL Moderately high risk patients: <130 mg/dL Low risk patients: <160 mg/dL	High risk patients: • Life style modification plus LDL-C lowering drugs Very high risk patients: • If baseline level is ≥100 mg/dL—lipid-lowering drugs. Combination of drugs may be used • If the baseline level is <100 mg/dL, LDL lowering drug should be started as per clinical judgment Moderately high risk patients: • If LDL level is ≥160 mg/dL—life style modification plus LDL-C lowering agents • If LDL level is ≥130 mg/dL—life style therapy plus lipid-lowering therapy • If LDL level is between 100 and 129—then life style therapy plus lipid-lowering therapy depending upon the risk of the patients In case of low risk patients: • If LDL level is ≥190 mg/dL—life style therapies plus LDL-C lowering agents • If LDL level is 160–189 mg/dL—only life style modification, LDL-lowering therapy will be optional • Statin should be prescribed in all patients with diabetic age of 40–79 years and LDL level of 60–189 mg/dL • For diabetes with atherosclerotic cardiovascular disease—**atorvastatin** 40–80 mg/day and **rozuvastatin** 20–40 mg daily • Statin will lower the LDL level by 6% • Side effects are myopathy and hepatotoxicity • **Cholesterol absorption inhibitor ezetimibe** can be used as second-line of drug, and lower LDL by 15–20% • **Proprotein convertase subtilisin/kexin type 9** inhibitors can lower LDL by 45–60%, but it is needed in metabolic syndrome. But in case of familial hypercholesterolemia if LDL cannot be decreased by statin and ezetimibe, then PCSK 9 can be given • **Bile acid binding resin cholestyramine, colestipol, and colesevelam** are more effective but they will increase the triglyceride level, hence it should be given with caution in case of metabolic syndrome with fasting triglyceride level >300 mg/dL • Side effects are gastrointestinal symptoms • Nicotinic acid can be used as lipid lowering agent • Fibrates are used to lower LDL level
Triglyceridemia	
Reduction of triglyceride level to <150 mg/dL	• If triglyceride level is >500 mg/dL, it must be treated to prevent serious hypertriglyceridemia and acute pancreatitis. But, it should be treated even when level is >200 mg/dL to prevent cardiovascular disease • **Fibrate like gemfibrozil or fenofibrate** is the drug of choice to reduce the fasting triglyceride level by 30–50%, LDL level by 10–15%, and increases the HDL level by 15–20%. Concomitant administration of the drugs that use 3A4 cytochrome for their metabolism should not be given with fibrate as the fibrate may precipitate myopathy in this case • Intermittent high-dose of statins reduce triglyceride level • **Nicotinic acid** reduces fasting triglyceride level by nearly 35%, VLDL particle with secondary LDL reduction, and increases in HDL, but the effect is less pronounced than fibrate. But in case of metabolic syndrome with diabetes mellitus nicotinic acid can increase the fasting blood glucose level • **Omega-3 fatty acid preparations such as eicosapentaenoic acid ± docosahexaenoic acid** at a dose of 1.5–4.5 g/day will lower the fasting triglyceride level by 25–40%. There is no drug interaction but the side effects are eructation with fishy taste

Continued

Continued

HDL cholesterol	
Rising the HDL level	• Statins, fibrates, and bile acid binding resins have modest effect • Omega-3 fatty acid has no effect • Nicotinic acid has only the capability of rising the HDL cholesterol

(HDL: high-density lipoprotein; LDL: low-density lipoprotein; VLDL: very low-density lipoproteins)

Indications of High-intensity and Moderate-intensity Statins According to 2018 AHA Specific Guidelines

Treatment recommendation	Indications
High-intensity statin Or, Moderate-intensity statins if age is >75 years	Presence of clinical atherosclerotic coronary vascular disease
High-intensity statin	Primary elevation of LDL-C is ≥190 mg/dL
Moderate-intensity statin Or, High-intensity statin if 10 years cardiovascular risk ≥7.5% or other risk-enhancing criteria	• Age: 40–75 years • Presence of diabetes • LDL ≥ 70 mg/dL
Treat with moderate-to-high-intensity statin	• Age: 40–75 years • No clinical atherosclerotic cardiovascular disease or diabetes • LDL-C: 70–189 mg/dL • Estimated 10 years cardiovascular disease risk ≥7.5% or coronary artery calcium > 0 and >75th percentile

(LDL-C: Low-density lipoprotein cholesterol)

Q35. Restrictive cardiomyopathy.

MGR/APR2014/MDI (5)

BABA FARID UNI OF HEALTH SC, 2017 (10)

ANSWER

Definition

Restrictive cardiomyopathy is characterized by abnormal diastolic function leading to impaired diastolic filling but with mildly decreased ejection fraction as well as contractility.

Causes of Restrictive Cardiomyopathy

A. Amyloidosis:
- **a.** Primary—light chain amyloid
- **b.** Familial—abnormal transthyretin
- **c.** Senile—normal transthyretin

B. Storage diseases:
- **a.** Hemochromatosis—iron
- **b.** Inherited metabolic disorders
  - **1.** Fabry's disease
  - **2.** Glycogen storage disease type II and III

C. Fibrotic:
- **a.** Radiation
- **b.** Scleroderma

D. Endomyocardial:
- **a.** Carcinoid syndrome
- **b.** Radiation
- **c.** *Drugs*: Serotonin, ergotamine

E. Overlapping with other cardiomyopathies:
- **a.** Early stage DCM
- **b.** Partial recovery from DCM

Clinical Features

A. Subtle exercise intolerance: It may be the first symptom.

B. Features of right-sided symptoms:
- **a.** Abdominal discomfort
- **b.** Edema
- **c.** Ascites

C. Other symptoms related to amyloidosis are:
- **a.** Syncope
- **b.** Stroke
- **c.** Peripheral neuropathy
- **d.** Angina

D. Clinical findings:
- **a.** Jugular venous pressure demonstrates rapid Y decent

b. Presence of inspiratory increase in jugular venous pressure: Kussmaul's sign.
c. Pulse usually in sinus rhythm but may atrial fibrillation.
d. Cardiac impulse is less displaced like DCM and less dynamic than hypertrophic obstructive cardiomyopathy (HOCM).
e. In case of sinus rhythm fourth heart sound is more common.
f. Other features related to etiologies like:
   1. Thickened tongue
   2. Periorbital purpura
   3. Hepatomegaly

Diagnosis

A. ECG:
   a. Conduction disturbance
   b. Low-voltage complexes
B. Echocardiography:
   a. Thickened left ventricle with left ventricular hypertrophy
   b. Bright myocardium
   c. Rapid early diastolic filling as evidenced by mitral inflow in Doppler study.
   d. Biatrial enlargement
   e. Characteristic longitudinal strain suggestive of amyloidosis
   f. Normal left ventricular size with reduced ejection fraction
   g. Thickening of atrial septum
C. Technetium pyrophosphate imaging demonstrates amyloid deposition in the myocardium. It is the modality of choice of diagnosing transthyretin amyloidosis.
D. Cardiac MRI demonstrates:
   a. Distinctive pattern of diffuse hyperenhancement of gadolinium—suggests amyloidosis.
   b. Late gadolinium enhancement suggests extensive cardiac involvement.
E. Demonstration of tissue infiltration in the tissue biopsy by special stain demonstrates amyloid.
F. Genetic testing: *TTR* gene sequencing in case of suspected TTR mutant patients.

Treatment

A. In case of transthyretin amyloidosis—tafamidis can act by following mechanisms:
   a. It improves survival
   b. It reduces hospitalization
   c. It improves quality of life
B. In light-chain amyloidosis: Alkylator-based chemotherapy or melphalan in high dose which is followed by autologous stem cell transplantation.
C. In case of immunoglobulin light chain amyloidosis: Standard or high dose chemotherapy along with stem cell transplantation.
D. In acute case:
   a. In case of right-sided HF loop diuretics, thiazides, and aldosterone antagonists are useful but in high dose it may worsen the renal function.
   b. Digoxin should not be used because of chance of arrhythmias.
   c. Beta-blockers:
      1. Reduce the heart rate
      2. Improve diastolic filling by increasing the diastolic time.
   d. Verapamil works by:
      1. Improving myocardial relaxation
      2. Increasing diastolic filling time
   e. ACEI can be given in case of adequate blood pressure by improving the diastolic filling time.
   f. Corticosteroid can improve the conduction abnormalities in sarcoidosis.
E. In case of primary cardiac amyloidosis cardiac transplantation.

Q36. Drug therapy in resistant hypertension.

MGR/APR2014/MDI (5)

ANSWER

Following issues associated with resistance to treatment	Considerations in treatment
Edema resolution, edema control	Thiazide to chlorthalidone to Loop diuretics

Continued

Continued

Following issues associated with resistance to treatment	Considerations in treatment
Inadequate control of heart rate	Beta-blocker, alpha and beta-blocker, verapamil, and diltiazem
Aldosterone normal to high normal, renin is low	Mineralocorticoid
Renin and aldosterone levels are low	Night shift work should be avoided Low salt diet Amiloride
Medication can be splitted to control effectively	BP pattern should be evaluated according to home and ambulatory blood pressure monitoring
Questionable medicine adherence	Indirect or direct method should be initiated to detect nonadherence, if it is found then it should be discussed with the patient's party
Pattern of blood pressure response to medications outside clinician visit	Meal effect on blood pressure should be identified Duration of medication defect
Sleep disordered breathing Presence of significant anxiety that is associated with highly variable hypertension	Nondrug strategies should be initiated that should be separated from hypertensive education

Management of Resistant Hypertension

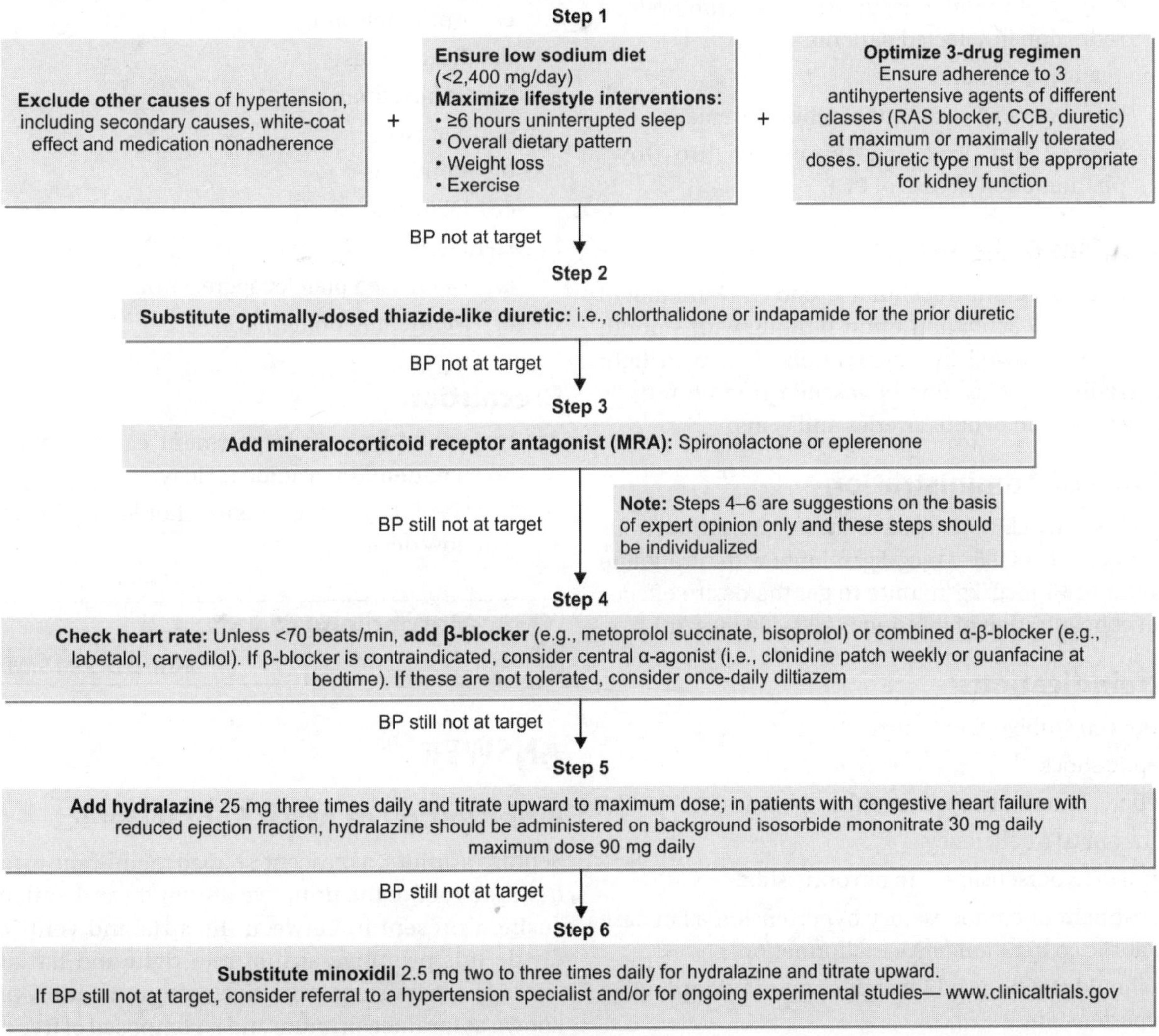

Step 1

Exclude other causes of hypertension, including secondary causes, white-coat effect and medication nonadherence

+

Ensure low sodium diet (<2,400 mg/day)
Maximize lifestyle interventions:
- ≥6 hours uninterrupted sleep
- Overall dietary pattern
- Weight loss
- Exercise

+

Optimize 3-drug regimen
Ensure adherence to 3 antihypertensive agents of different classes (RAS blocker, CCB, diuretic) at maximum or maximally tolerated doses. Diuretic type must be appropriate for kidney function

BP not at target

Step 2

Substitute optimally-dosed thiazide-like diuretic: i.e., chlorthalidone or indapamide for the prior diuretic

BP not at target

Step 3

Add mineralocorticoid receptor antagonist (MRA): Spironolactone or eplerenone

BP still not at target

Note: Steps 4–6 are suggestions on the basis of expert opinion only and these steps should be individualized

Step 4

Check heart rate: Unless <70 beats/min, **add β-blocker** (e.g., metoprolol succinate, bisoprolol) or combined α-β-blocker (e.g., labetalol, carvedilol). If β-blocker is contraindicated, consider central α-agonist (i.e., clonidine patch weekly or guanfacine at bedtime). If these are not tolerated, consider once-daily diltiazem

BP still not at target

Step 5

Add hydralazine 25 mg three times daily and titrate upward to maximum dose; in patients with congestive heart failure with reduced ejection fraction, hydralazine should be administered on background isosorbide mononitrate 30 mg daily maximum dose 90 mg daily

BP still not at target

Step 6

Substitute minoxidil 2.5 mg two to three times daily for hydralazine and titrate upward.
If BP still not at target, consider referral to a hypertension specialist and/or for ongoing experimental studies— www.clinicaltrials.gov

(BP: blood pressure; CCB: calcium channel blocker; RAS: renin–angiotensin system)

Q37. Sodium nitroprusside.
MGR/OCT2013/MDI (5)

ANSWER

Indications

A. Food and Drug Administration (FDA) approved indication of nitroprusside:
  a. Acute hypertensive crises
  b. Acute decompensated HF
  c. Induction of perioperative hypertension

B. Other uses of nitroprusside:
  a. Hypertension in case of acute ischemic stroke
  b. In case of acute mitral regurgitation afterload reduction
  c. In cardiogenic shock with raised systemic vascular resistance to increase cardia output.
  d. In case of valvular aortic stenosis acute preload reduction in selected patients.

C. Emergency treatment:
  a. Symptomatic treatment of schizophrenia.
  b. Prevention and treatment of "no-flow" phenomenon in case of PCI.

Mechanism of Actions

Nitric oxide triggers intracellular cyclic GMP-mediated protein kinase G activation upon binding with smooth muscle cells followed by inactivation of myosin light chains leading to relaxation of vascular smooth muscle resulting dilatation of both arteries and veins.

Methods of Administration

It should be mixed in 5% dextrose water for intravenous infusion at a rate of 0.5–4 mcg/kg/minute with titration to maximum of 10 mcg/kg/minute to get the desire effects. Typical concentration of infusion is 200–400 mcg/mL.

Contraindications

A. Tobacco amblyopia
B. Septic shock
C. Leber's hereditary optic atrophy
D. Vitamin B12 deficiency
E. Known hypersensitivity to nitroprusside
F. Treatment of compensatory hypertension as in case of aortic coarctation or AV malformation.
G. It should not be used for induction of perioperative hypertension.

Adverse Effects

A. Cardiovascular effects:
  a. Bradycardia
  b. Tachycardia
  c. Flushing
  d. Palpitation
  e. Substernal chest pain
  f. Shortness of breath

B. Endocrine:
  a. Hypothyroidism

C. Dermatologic:
  a. Skin rash
  b. Diaphoresis
  c. Erythematous streaking

D. Central nervous system:
  a. Headache
  b. Dizziness
  c. Apprehension
  d. Restlessness

E. Gastrointestinal:
  a. Nausea
  b. Vomiting
  c. Diarrhea

F. Hematologic:
  a. Decreased platelet aggregation
  b. Methemoglobinemia

Precaution

A. In case of hepatic impairment caution should be taken to monitor cyanide toxicity.
B. In case of renal impairment it should be administered with low dose.

Q38. Morphology of ASD.
MGR/OCT2013/MDI (5)

ANSWER

Embryology of Atrial Septal Defect

Septum primum, a crescent-shaped membrane extending from the roof of the primitive atrium toward endocardial cushion present in between the atria and ventricles to divide this primitive atrium into right and left atrium. There is a persistent primitive communication present known as foramen primum and is composed of free edge of septum primum and endocardial cushion. Before closure of this foramen there develop multiple fenestrations in the septum primum that coalesce to form septum secundum. When septum primum fuses with endocardial cushion, ostium secundum will maintain the right to left atrial flow which is important for fetal circulation. Failure of fusion this septum primum with the endocardial cushion—it is known as ostium primum.

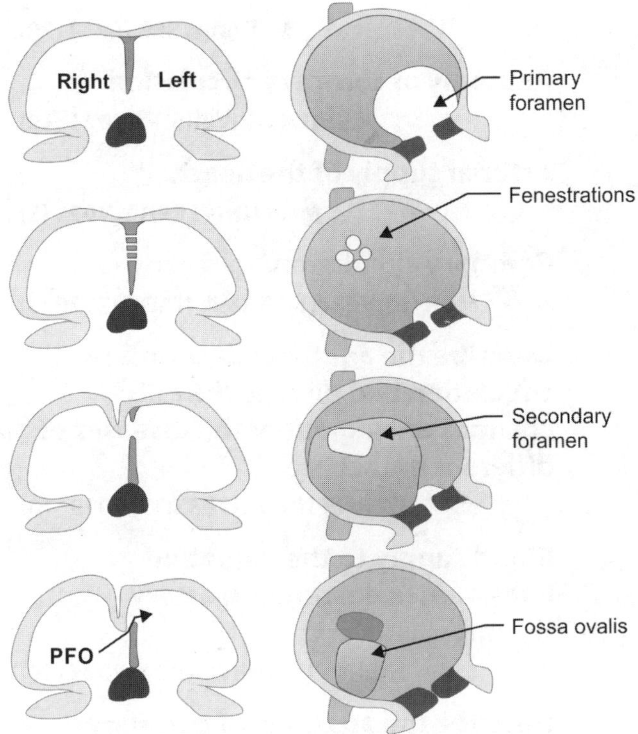

(PFO: patent foramen ovale)

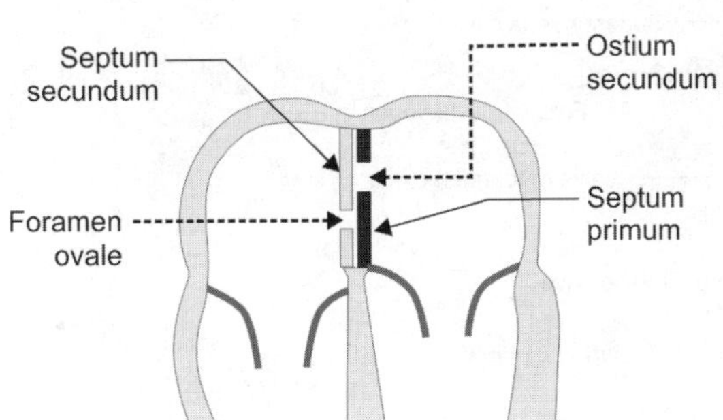

When second septum known as septum secundum is formed to the right of the septum and again grows toward the endocardial cushion thereby closing the ostium secundum. Failure of closure of ostium secundum is known as foramen secundum atrial septal defect (ASD).

There are three types of atrial septal defect:

A. Ostium secundum type ASD: It is 70–75% of ASD. It is located in the mid-portion of atrial septum within the fossa ovalis. It is twice more common in females. Isolated ostium secundum ASD may be associated with:
   - **a.** Mitral valve prolapse
   - **b.** Other congenital heart disease
   - **c.** Mitral stenosis—known as Lutembacher syndrome

B. Ostium primum defect: It is present in 15–20% of ASD. It is a part of spectrum of AV defect. It is present in the inferoanterior portion of atrial septum, it is associated with:
   - **a.** A cleft in the anterior leaflet of mitral valve leading to mitral regurgitation.
   - **b.** In the complete form there is large VSD or common aortic valve.

C. Sinoseptal defect or sinus venosus defect: It is 5–10% of ASD. In this lesion the defect is either junction between right superior vena cava—atria and right upper pulmonary veins, so here there is no direct communication between right and left atria. This defect occurs at the orifice of superior vena cava at right atrial junction.

D. Coronary sinus defect: It is characterized by an opening between coronary sinus and left atrium.

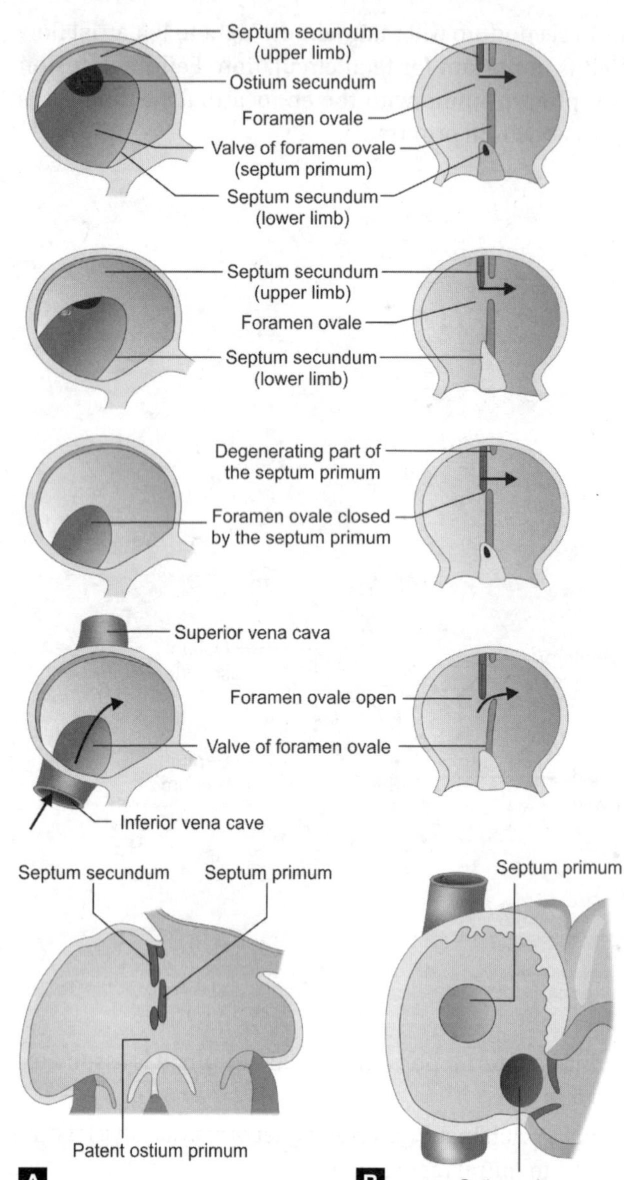

Q39. Coronary arteries and its branches—clinical importance.

MGR/APR2013/MDI (5)

Coronary circulation.

MGR2010/MDI (5)

Blood supply to the heart.

MGR/OCT2013/MDI (5)

Describe the course, relation, and branches of coronary arteries.

MGR/MAR2007/MDI (5)

Describe coronary circulation. Which artery is affected in different walls of myocardial infarction? How would you suspect the artery involved by seeing EKG?

MLB/MAY2009/MDI (20)

Anatomy of coronary circulation.

KERALA UNIVERSITY, 2021 (10)

Arterial supply of the heart.

MGR UNIVERSITY, 2021 (5)

Coronary circulation.

MGR UNIVERSITY, TAMIL NADU, 2020 (5)

Describe the anatomy of coronary circulation and discuss the ECG changes arising out of the diseases of different branches.

MANIPUR UNIVERSITY, 2019 (10)

Blood supply to the heart and left anterior descending artery thrombosis.

MANIPUR UNIVERSITY, 2024 (10)

Describe the anatomy of coronary arteries and discuss the significance of their anatomical variations.

WBUHS, 2025 (10)

ANSWER

Coronary arteries arise from coronary sinuses of valsalva just next to origin of aorta.

A. Right coronary artery originates from anterior aortic sinus and supplies:
- **a.** Right atrium
- **b.** Right ventricle
- **c.** Sinoatrial node
- **d.** Atrioventricular node
- **e.** Selected portion of left ventricle

B. Left coronary artery just after originating from left posterior aortic sinus divides into:
- **a.** Left circumflex artery
- **b.** Left anterior descending artery

This artery supplies left atrium and left ventricle.

There is extensive overlaps between these two arteries due to presence of extensive collaterals.

Coronary arteries are divided into two types:

a. Epicardial vessels: These are superficial, larger, and act as conductors of blood flow.

b. Intramuscular vessels: These vessels are smaller run through the myocardium, their different branches are of high resistance but fine-tuned and then control the blood flow into myocardium and endocardium.

Arterioles from coronary arteries branch into numerous capillaries lying adjacent to cardiac myocytes. High cardiac myocytes to capillary ratio associated with short diffusion distance are responsible for adequate supply of oxygen delivery to these myocytes and removal of metabolic products from these cells.

Now capillary will flow the blood into the venules which joins to form cardiac veins which ultimately drain into coronary sinus present in the posterior side of the heart, from the coronary sinus blood lastly drains into right atrium. Following table indicates the wall of the heart supplied by different coronary arteries:

Cardiac anatomical regions	Coronary arteries supplied
Inferior wall	Right coronary artery
• Anterior wall of the left ventricle • Anterior 2/3rd of the interventricular septum • Apex of the heart	Left anterior descending artery
Anteroapical wall	Left anterior descending artery distal part
Lateral wall of the left ventricle In some case posterior wall	Left circumflex artery
• Right ventricle • Inferior wall of the left ventricle • Sinoatrial node • Atrioventricular node	Right coronary artery
Posterior wall of the left ventricle	Posterior descending artery

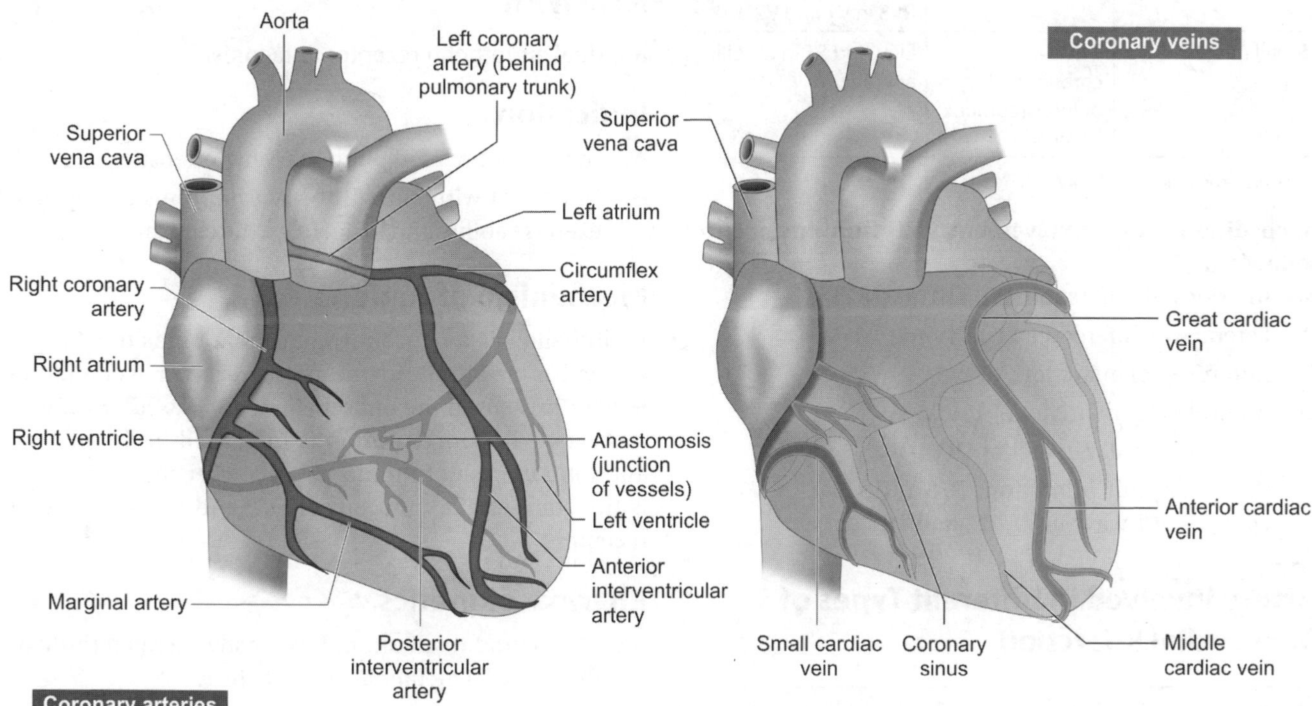

Variation in the Coronary Arteries

A. Origin of branches:

a. Conus branch sometimes may arise from right aortic sinus directly which is known as third coronary artery or preinfundibular artery

b. Sometimes sinuatrial nodal artery may arise from right coronary artery, left circumflex artery or coronary sinus.

c. Atrioventricular nodal artery supplying the atrioventricular node usually arises from right coronary artery, but it may also arise from left circumflex artery.

Arterial Involvement According to EKG Findings

Category	Site of occlusion	ECG features
Proximal left anterior descending artery	Proximal to first left perforator	Elevated ST in V1–V6, aVL, fascicular or bundle branch block
Mid left anterior descending artery	Proximal to large diagonal but distal to first septal perforator	Elevated ST in V1–V6, aVL
Distal left anterior descending artery	Distal to large diagonal or diagonal itself only	Elevated ST in V1–V6 Or, L1, aVL, and V5–V6
Moderate to large inferior, posterior, and lateral, right ventricular infarction	Proximal right coronary artery or left circumflex artery	Elevated ST in LII, LIII, aVF, And, any of the following three: V1, V3R, V4R V5, V6, R>S in V1 and V2
Small inferior	Distal right coronary artery or left circumflex branch	Elevated ST in LII, LIII, and aVF

(ECG: electrocardiogram)

According to wall involvement EKG findings are the following:

A. Inferior wall infarction: LII, LIII, and aVF
B. Lateral wall infarction: LI, aVL, and V4–V6
C Anteroseptal infarction: V1–V3
D. Anterolateral infarction: V1–V6.
E. Right ventricular infarction: RV4–RV5
F. Posterior wall infarction: R/S ratio > 1 in V1–V2, changes of T wave in V1, V8, and V9

Artery Involved in Different Types of Myocardial Infarction

Leads with ST segment elevation	Myocardium affected	Affected coronary artery
V1–V2	Anterior	Proximal LAD
V3–V4	Septal	LAD
V5–V6	Apical, lateral	Distal LAD, left circumflex or right coronary artery
LI, Avl	Anterior, anterolateral	Left circumflex artery
LII, LIII, and Avf	Inferior	• 90% by right coronary artery • 10% by left circumflex artery
V7, V8, and V9 (Reciprocal ST segment elevation in V1–V3)	Posterolateral	• Right coronary artery • Left circumflex artery

(LAD: left anterior descending)

Q40. Discuss Bosentan.

MGR/APR2013/MDI (5)

ANSWER

It is dual endothelin receptor antagonist.

Indications

A. In the treatment of pulmonary hypertension.
B. In patient with class III or IV symptoms to improve exercise ability and to decrease the clinical worsening.

Mechanism of Actions

Endothelin—is a neurohormones that binds to ET_A and ET_B with more affinity for the former receptor as compared to later present in the endothelium and vascular smooth muscles. ET_A concentration is increased in the plasma and lung in case of pulmonary hypertension. Bosentan is the competitive inhibitor of ET_A and ET_B endothelin receptors.

Pharmacokinetics

It is 98% bound to albumin. It is mostly excreted through bile following its metabolism in the liver.

Adverse Effect

A. Dizziness
B. Joint pain
C. Respiratory tract infection
D. Headache
E. Hypotension
F. Syncope
G. Flushing

Uses:

A. In case of <40 kg of body weight—62.5 kg 12 hourly.

B. In case of >40 kg of body weight—62.5 mg twice daily for 4 weeks followed by 125 mg 12 hourly.

Dose modification:

A. In case of liver impairment its use should be restricted. If AST/ALT level is more than three times upper limit of normal this drug should be stopped.

Q41. Conducting system of the heart.

MGR/OCT2012/MDI (5)

MGR/SEP2010/MDI (5)

Conductive system of the heart and ECG.

MGR/SEP2009/MDI (5)

Describe conduction system of the heart and add a note on pacemaker potential.

KERALA UNIVERSITY, 2018 (10)

Pacemaker potential in question number 111

Conduction system of the heart and electrocardiogram.

NTR UNIVERSITY OF HEALTH SC, VIJAYAWADA, ANDHRA, 2022 (10)

Anatomy of the conduction system of the heart.

BABA FARID UNI OF HEALTH SC, 2018 (10)

Conduction system of the heart.

MGR UNIVERSITY, TAMIL NADU, 2019 (5)

NTR UNIVERSITY OF HEALTH SC, VIJAYAWADA, ANDHRA, SEPTEMBER, 2020 (10)

NTR UNIVERSITY OF HEALTH SC, VIJAYAWADA, ANDHRA, NOVEMBER, 2020 (10)

Describe the conduction system of the heart. Write in brief on the management of bradyarrhythmias.

MANIPAL UNIVERSITY, 2021 (10)

Bradyarrhythmias have been describe in question number 141, 136.

ANSWER

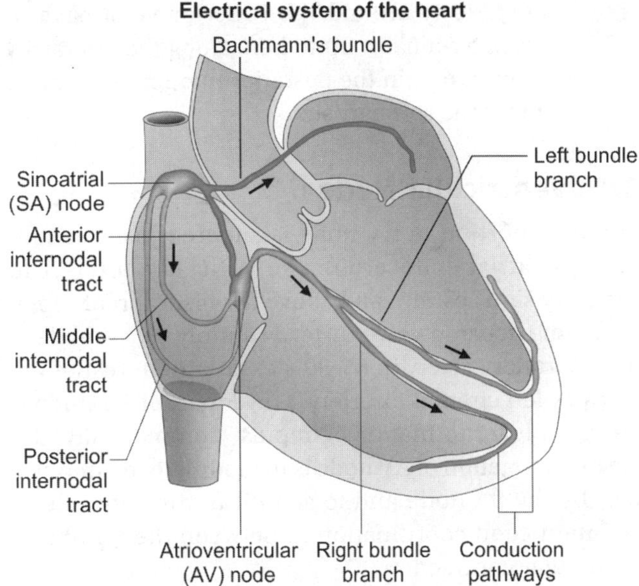

Sinoatrial Node

It is spindle-shaped fibrous structure having 10–20 mm long and 2–3 mm wide situated < 1 mm from epicardial surface at the junction of anteromedial aspect of superior vena cava and right atrium laterally in the right atrial sulcus. It is deeply innervated by postganglionic cholinergic and adrenergic nerves releasing neurotransmitters that stimulates muscarinic and beta-1 and beta-2 adrenergic receptors, respectively.

Arterial supply to SA node is right coronary artery in 55% of cases and 45% of case by left circumflex artery.

Intra-atrial and Intermodal Pathways

There are three intra-atrial pathways:

a. Anterior intermodal pathway: It originates from anterior margin of SA node then curving anteriorly around the superior vena cava to enter anterior interatrial band known as Bachmann bundle. This bundle will carry the impulse from right atrium to left atrium.

b. Middle intermodal pathway: It originates from superior and posterior margins of the sinus node, runs posterior the superior vena cava to crest of interatrial septum and from there it will descend along the septum to join superior margin of AV node.

c. Posterior intermodal pathway: It originates from posterior margin of the SA node then runs posteriorly around the superior vena cava to crista terminalis, from there along the interatrial septum to join the posterior margin of AV node above the coronary sinus.

Atrioventricular Node

Compact portion of AV node is situated just beneath the right atrial endocardium superficially anterior to coronary sinus ostium and above the insertion of septal leaflet of tricuspid valve. Arterial supply to AV node is right coronary artery in 85–90% cases and in rest of the cases by left circumflex artery. Lower part of AV node is responsible for formation of impulse automatically. But the main function of AV node is to modulate the impulse sent by the SA node and to send it to the ventricle to maintain good coordination in between the atrial and ventricular contraction.

Bundle of His

It originates from distal part of compact AV node progress distally perforating central fibrous body then runs through the annulus fibrosus and penetrates membranous septum as nonbranching portion. Penetrating portion of AV bundle is enclosed by central fibrous body and membranous septum and it will send extension to central fibrous body. Proximal part of penetrating portion of AV bundle is heterogenous like that of compact AV node and distal penetrating portion is similar to that proximal bundle branches. Upper muscular interventricular septum is supplied by anterior and posterior descending coronary artery making the conduction system to more impervious to ischemia at this site.

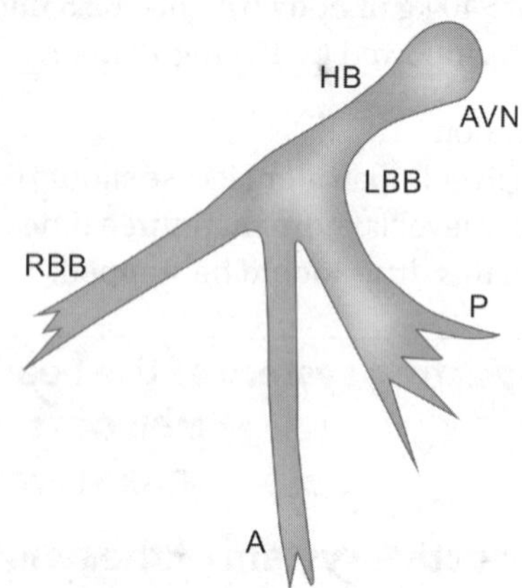

(AVN: atrioventricular node; HB: his bundle; LBB: left bundle branch; RBB: right bundle branch)

Bundle Branches

It originates from superior margin of muscular part of interventricular septum just below the membranous part of septum. Cells of left bundle branch extends downward as a continuous sheet beneath the noncoronary aortic cusp. But right bundle branch extends as unbranched sheet intramyocardially along the right side of interventricular septum to the base of anterior papillary muscles and apex of the right ventricle.

Terminal Purkinje Fibers

These fibers connect terminal bundle branches and form extensive interweaving networks on the endocardial surface of both the ventricles that transmit impulses simultaneously into both the ventricular myocardium. These ventricles are less concentrated at the base of the ventricles.

Conducting System and ECG

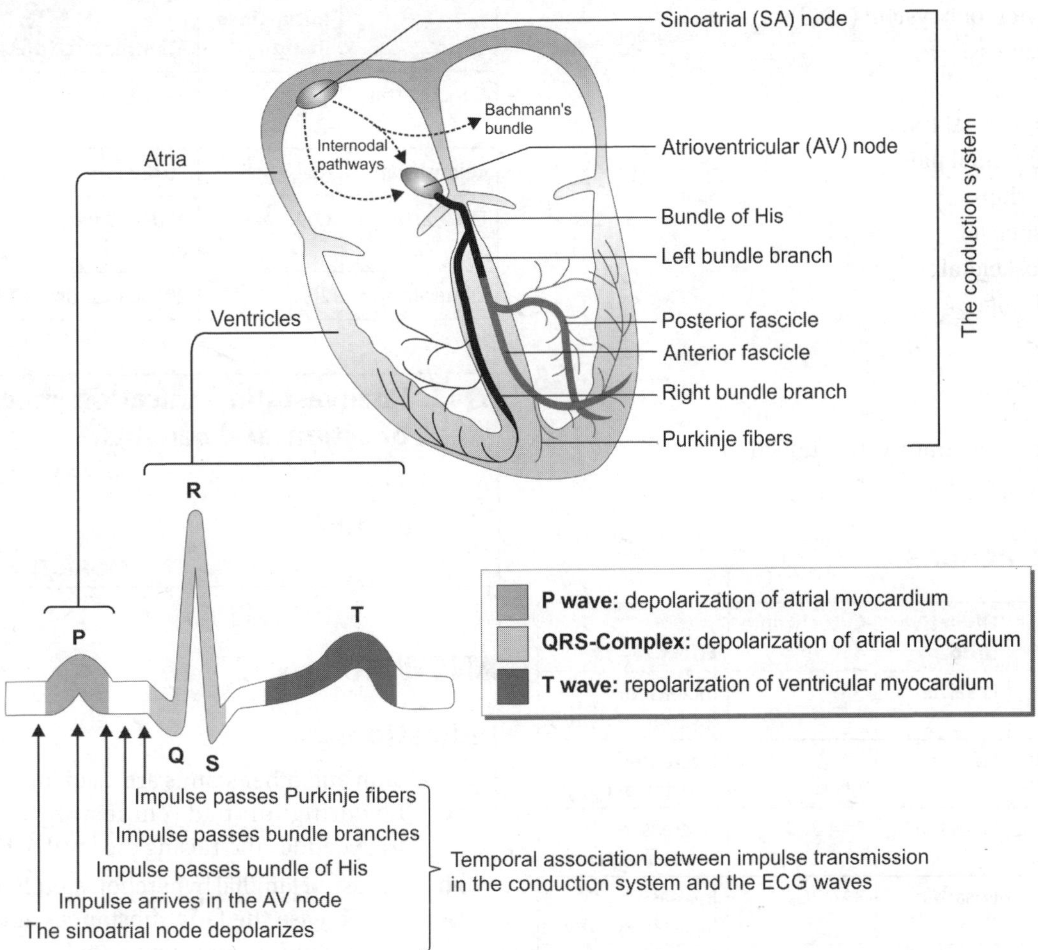

(ECG: electrocardiogram)

Pacemaker structures	Intrinsic frequency
Sinoatrial node	70 beats/min
Atrial myocardium	60 beats/min
Atrioventricular node	40 beats/min
Bundle of His	20–40 beats/min
Purkinje fibers	20–40 beats/min

Q42. ARB: Clinical use.

MGR/OCT2012 (5)

ANSWER

These are new classes of antihypertensive agents.

Mechanism of Actions

It selectively inhibit angiotensin II by competitive inhibition of angiotensin II receptors. Angiotensin II receptor blockers (ARB) displaces angiotensin II from angiotensin I receptors thereby inhibiting:

- **a.** Angiotensin II-mediated vasoconstriction
- **b.** Aldosterone release
- **c.** Release of catecholamine
- **d.** Release of arginine vasopressin
- **e.** Water intake

All the above factors contribute to lowering of blood pressure.

Pharmacokinetics

Losartan's metabolite EXP-3174 is 10–20 times more potent as compared to losartan and is responsible for its long duration of action. Olmesartan and candesartan are the prodrug, their active metabolites are produced during absorption from the gastrointestinal tract. Once olmesartan is converted into its active metabolite it will never be metabolized further.

Adverse Effects

A. Central nervous system (CNS):
- **a.** Dizziness
- **b.** Fatigue

B. Gastrointestinal tract:
- **a.** Abdominal pain
- **b.** Diarrhea
- **c.** Dyspepsia

C. Musculoskeletal:
- **a.** Arthralgia
- **b.** Pain

D. Pulmonary:
- **a.** Cough
- **b.** Upper respiratory tract infection
- **c.** Viral infection

Drug Interactions

Precipitant drug	Objective drug	Cytochrome 450	Effect
Cimetidine	Losartan		Increased losartan activity
Indomethacin	Losartan		Decreased losartan activity
Rifampin	Losartan	3A4 2C9	Decreased losartan activity
Fluconazole	Losartan	3A4 2C9	Increased losartan activity
Phenobarbital	Losartan		Decreased losartan activity
Digoxin	Telmisartan		Increased activity of digoxin

Drugs with Doses

Drug	Initial dose in mg	Maintenance dose in mg
Losartan	50	25–100 twice daily
Valsartan	80	80–320 four times daily
Irbesartan	150	150–300 four times daily
Candesartan	16	8–32 twice daily or four times daily
Telmisartan	40	20–80 four times daily
Eprosartan	600	400–800 twice or four times daily
Olmesartan	20	20–40 four times daily

Q43. Rozuvastatin: indication, mechanism of action, and benefits.

MGR/OCT2012/MDI (5)

Statins.

MGR/SEP2010/MDI (5)

ANSWER

Indications

Rozuvastatin and other statins are used for:

- **a.** Lowering of bad cholesterol, LDL-C and triglyceride, and raising the level of HDL.
- **b.** In case of familial hypercholesterolemia it is given to decrease the fatty substances and cholesterol in the children and young adult.

Mechanism of Actions

Statin is HMG-CoA reductase inhibitor. Hence it inhibits the rate limiting enzyme in cholesterol synthesis. Cholesterol is synthesized in the liver, so this drug will reduce the cholesterol synthesis thereby increasing the LDL receptor in the liver that leads to reduction of LDL level in the circulation. There is also decrease in triglyceride level and increase in HDL level. Statin has been divided into high intensity and moderate intensity statins. Rozuvastatin is under high-intensity group thereby indicated as follows.

Statin Treatment in Hyperlipidemia

Primary target is LDL-C Secondary target is raised HDL-C	
LDL-C: High risk patients: <100 mg/dL Very high risk patients: <70 mg/dL Moderately high risk patients: <130 mg/dL Low risk patients: <160 mg/dL	High risk patients: • Lifestyle modification plus LDL-C lowering drugs *Very high risk patients:* • If baseline level is ≥100 mg/dL—lipid-lowering drugs. Combination of drugs may be used • If the baseline level is <100 mg/dL, LDL lowering drug should be started as per clinical judgment • Moderately high risk patients: • If LDL level is ≥160 mg/dL—lifestyle modification plus LDL-C lowering agents • If LDL level is ≥130 mg/dL—lifestyle therapy plus lipid-lowering therapy • If LDL level is between 100 and 129—then lifestyle therapy plus lipid-lowering therapy depending upon the risk of the patients • In case of low risk patients: • If LDL level is ≥190 mg/dL—lifestyle therapies plus LDL-C lowering agents • If LDL level is 160–189 mg/dL–only lifestyle modification, LDL-lowering therapy will be optional • Statin should be prescribed in all patients with diabetic age of 40–79 years and LDL level of 60–189 mg/dL • For diabetes with atherosclerotic cardiovascular disease—**atorvastatin** 40–80 mg/day and **rozuvastatin** 20–40 mg daily • Statin will lower the LDL level by 6% • Side effects are myopathy and hepatotoxicity • **Cholesterol absorption inhibitor ezetimibe** can be used as second-line of drug, and lower LDL by 15–20% • **Proprotein convertase subtilisin/kexin type 9** inhibitors can lower LDL by 45–60%, but it is needed in metabolic syndrome. But in case of familial hypercholesterolemia if LDL cannot be decreased by statin and ezetimibe, then PCSK 9 can be given • **Bile acid binding resin cholestyramine, colestipol, and colesevelam** are more effective but they will increase the triglyceride level, hence it should be given with caution in case of metabolic syndrome with fasting triglyceride level > 300 mg/dL • Side effects are gastrointestinal symptoms • Nicotinic acid can be used as lipid-lowering agent • Fibrates are used to lower LDL level
Triglyceridemia	
Reduction of triglyceride level to <150 mg/dL	• If triglyceride level is >500 mg/dL, it must be treated to prevent serious hypertriglyceridemia and acute pancreatitis. But it should be treated even when level is >200 mg/dL to prevent cardiovascular disease • **Fibrate such as gemfibrozil or fenofibrate** is the drug of choice to reduce the fasting triglyceride level by 30–50%, LDL level by 10–15%, and increases the HDL level by 15–20%. Concomitant administration of the drugs that use 3A4 cytochrome for their metabolism should not be given with fibrate as the fibrate may precipitate myopathy in this case • Intermittent high dose of statins reduce triglyceride level • **Nicotinic acid** reduces fasting triglyceride level by nearly 35%, VLDL particle with secondary LDL reduction, and increases in HDL, but the effect is less pronounced than fibrate. But in case of metabolic syndrome with diabetes mellitus nicotinic acid can increase the fasting blood glucose level • **Omega-3 fatty acid preparations such as eicosapentaenoic acid ± docosahexaenoic acid** at a dose of 1.5–4.5 g/day will lower the fasting triglyceride level by 25–40%. There is no drug interaction but the side effects are eructation with fishy taste
HDL cholesterol	
Rising the HDL level	• Statins, fibrates, and bile acid binding resins have modest effect • Omega-3 fatty acid has no effect • Nicotinic acid has only the capability of rising the HDL cholesterol

(HDL: high-density lipoprotein; LDL: low-density lipoprotein; VLDL: very low-density lipoproteins)

Treatment recommendation	Indications
High-intensity statin Or, Moderate-intensity statins if age is >75 years	Presence of clinical atherosclerotic coronary vascular disease
High-intensity statin	Primary elevation of LDL-C is ≥190 mg/dL
Moderate-intensity statin Or, High-intensity statin if 10 years cardiovascular risk ≥7.5% or other risk-enhancing criteria	• Age: 40–75 years • Presence of diabetes • LDL ≥ 70 mg/dL
Treat with moderate-to-high-intensity statin	• Age: 40–75 years • No clinical atherosclerotic cardiovascular disease or diabetes • LDL-C: 70–189 mg/dL • Estimated 10 years cardiovascular disease risk ≥7.5% or coronary artery calcium > 0 and > 75th percentile

Q44. Left ventricle.

MGR/APR2012/MDI (5)

ANSWER

Left ventricle is situated posterior to the right ventricle. Its inlet portion is incorporated by mitral valves and its outlet portion leads to aortic valve area which is bounded anterosuperiorly by interventricular septum and posteroinferiorly by aortic leaflet of mitral valve. Left ventricle forms the sternocostal, left, and diaphragmatic cardiac surfaces via its obtuse margin. Its territories are designated by anterior and inferior interventricular grooves indicating the lines of attachment of ventricular septum. Different parts of left ventricle:

A. Apex: It is the conical part of left ventricle present in the left fifth intercostal space near the midclavicular line having direction anteroinferior to the left.

B. Base: It is extended from the papillary muscle to the plane of AV groove being separated superiorly by AV groove from left atrium, posteriorly by coronary sinus.

C. Free wall: It is area of ventricular wall which is not contact with interventricular septum and apex.

D. Myoarchitecture: Muscles of left ventricle starts from AV junction and continues up to ventriculoarterial junction. At the obtuse margin wall is three times thicker, i.e., 12–15 mm than right ventricle excluding contribution of trabeculae, at the apex muscle is 1–2 mm thick.

E. Internal features:

a. Inlet portion: Left ventricle is described as tripartite of inlet portion, outlet portion, and apical trabeculae. Inlet portion is limited my mitral valve and tension apparatus extending from bicuspid annulus to the papillary muscles that anchor tendinous cord and leaflets to the ventricular wall.

b. Mitral valve annulus: It is smaller than tricuspid annulus. All the valve annulus are connected by central fibrous body.

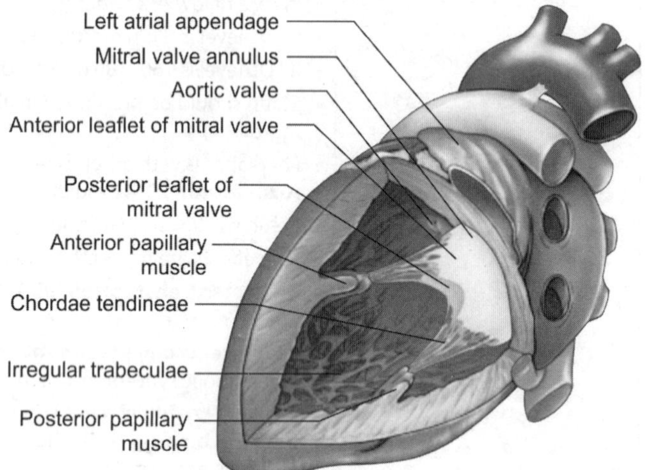

c. Mitral valve: It is composed of annulus, leaflets, and chordae tendinae. Mitral valve leaflet is composed of anterior and posterior leaflets which are linked together by inferoseptal and superolateral commissures. Leaflets can be divided into scallops separated by indentations or slits formed by free edges of leaflets supported by chordae tendinae. Posterior leaflet has three scallops but anterior leaflet has no scallop. Anterior leaflet also known as anteromedial leaflet is located posterior to aortic root. It has thick rough zones due to attachment of chordae tendinae attached on the ventricular surface. Posterior leaflet positioned posteroinferiorly has three zones such as rough, clear, and basal zones according to the attachment of chordae tendinae.

d. Papillary muscles: The muscle that arising from sternocostal mural myocardium is known as anterolateral papillary muscle and that arising from diaphragmatic surface is posteromedial papillary muscle.

e. Mitral chordae tendinae: These arise from papillary muscle tips to mitral valve leaflets.

F. Outlet portion: It is the aortic vestibule leading to aortic valve that has bordered by anterosuperiorly by muscular part of ventricular septum and posteroinferiorly by aortic leaflet of mitral valve.

a. Aortic root: It refers to the location of aortic valve in between left ventricular outflow tract and ascending portion of aorta. It is composed of sinuses of valsalva, annulus, interleaflet trigones, aortic valve leaflets, commissures, and sinotubular junction.

b. Aortic valve annulus is a semilunar crown like structure providing structural support to the aortic valve.

c. Aortic sinus of valsalva: It is present just above the aortic leaflets, from here aortic roots bulge outward. Two of the three sinuses known as right and left facing sinuses giving rise to left and right coronary arteries. Third one is named as nonfacing aortic sinus.

d. Coronary and nonadjacent leaflets: Aortic valve is composed of three semilunar leaflets: Based on link between the leaflets and sinuses to the origin of the coronary artery:

1. Right coronary leaflet
2. Left coronary leaflet
3. Noncoronary leaflet

Between the leaflets commissures are evenly spaced around the valve with an angle toward apex of the annulus. They are made of collagen fibers.

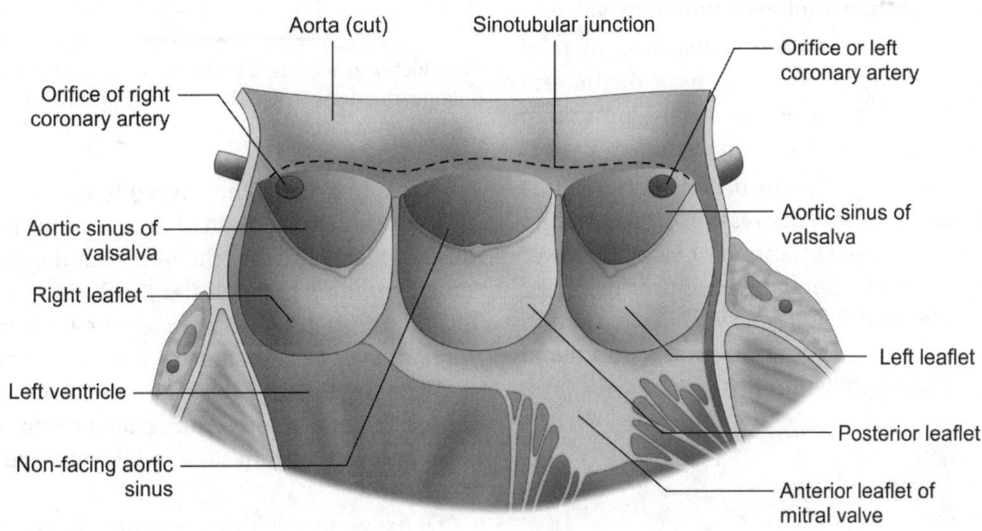

Function of Left Ventricle

Left ventricle pumps out the blood to throughout the body to maintain oxygenation and it depends upon the cardiac output and it is influenced by preload, afterload, and left ventricular contractility. Cardiac output is defined as amount of blood ejected out of the heart at a given heart rate.

Cardiac output = stroke volume × heart rate
Stroke volume = End-diastolic volume – End-systolic volume

Left ventricular ejection fraction can be defined as amount of blood ejected out of the heart during systolic phase relative to the volume in the left ventricle at the end of diastolic phase.

Left ventricular ejection fraction = Systolic volume/End-diastolic volume

Q45. Right atrium.

MGR/MAY2011/MDI (5)

ANSWER

It is the first chamber of the heart where the deoxygenated blood enters into the heart from systemic circulation through superior and inferior vena cava. Deoxygenated blood also come through the coronary sinus carrying the venous blood from coronary arteries, there are also venae cordis minimae, i.e., tiny cardiac veins that open directly into right atrium. Right atrium is composed of two pouches:

a. Right atrial main cavity
b. Small chamber projecting toward left just like ear—this is called auricle.
c. There is a shallow groove known as sulcus terminalis present on the outside at the junction between right atrium and right ventricle—this will form a ridge in the inner portion known as crista terminalis separating main part of right atrium posteriorly from sinus venosus from anterior part that is derived from primitive atrium. Its anterior part is marked by bundle of muscle fibers known as musculi pectinati.
d. Coronary sinus opens into the right atrium in between the inferior vena cava and AV valve guarded by nonfunctioning rudimentary valve.
e. In the right atrium there is features of fetal development in the form of fossa ovalis and annulus ovalis present on the atrial septum that separates right atrium from left atrium.
f. Fossa ovalis, the remnant of foramen ovale is represented as shallow depression, upper margin of this fossa is formed by annulus ovalis and lower margin represents persistent septum primum. Annulus is formed from the lower edge of septum secundum. During right atrial contraction blood is pumped into right ventricle.

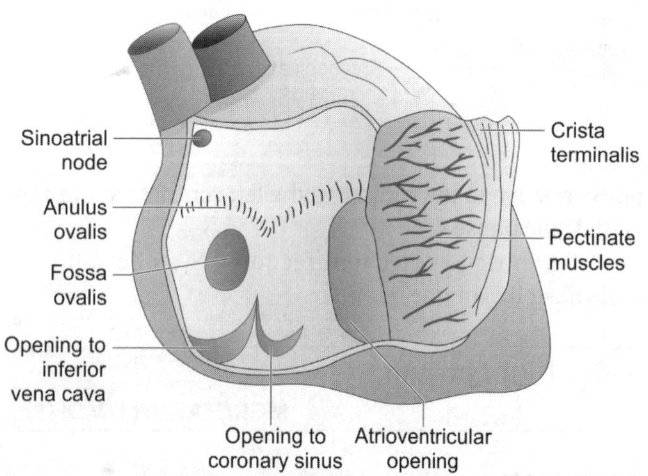

Q46. Fetal circulation.
MGR/OCT2011/MDI (5) MGR/SEP2007/MDI (5)

ANSWER

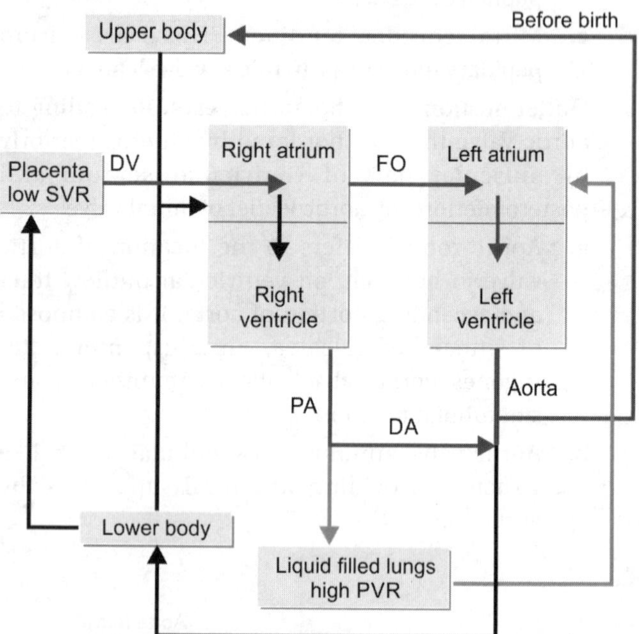

(DA: ductus arteriosus; DV: ductus venosus; FO: foramen ovale; PA: pulmonary artery; PVR: pulmonary vascular resistance; SVR: systemic vascular resistance)

Placenta accepts the oxygen free blood from the fetus through the two umbilical arteries that passes through the umbilical cord. On the other hand oxygen rich blood returns to fetus through the third vessel umbilical vein. This oxygen rich blood entering the fetus passes through the fetal liver to right side of the heart. This oxygen rich blood passes through the one of the two extraconnections between right and left atrium called patent foramen ovale toward the left atrium then to left ventricle and lastly out of the aorta.

Deoxygenated blood coming from the fetal body also enters the right atrium where it is mixed with highly oxygenated blood and enter the left ventricle that chamber sends the blood into the lungs. Most of the blood leaves the right ventricle bypass the lungs through the second of the two extraconnections which is known as ductus arteriosus. This ductus arteriosus sends the oxygen-poor blood to the lower half of the fetal body. This oxygen-poor blood leaves the fetus through the umbilical arteries and will back to placenta to pick up oxygen.

Patent foramen ovale and ductus arteriosus both are the normal findings in the fetus as these pathways in the fetal circulation make fetus possible to survive in pregnancy in spite of complex heart problems, but that will be closed just after birth in case of normal fetal heart.

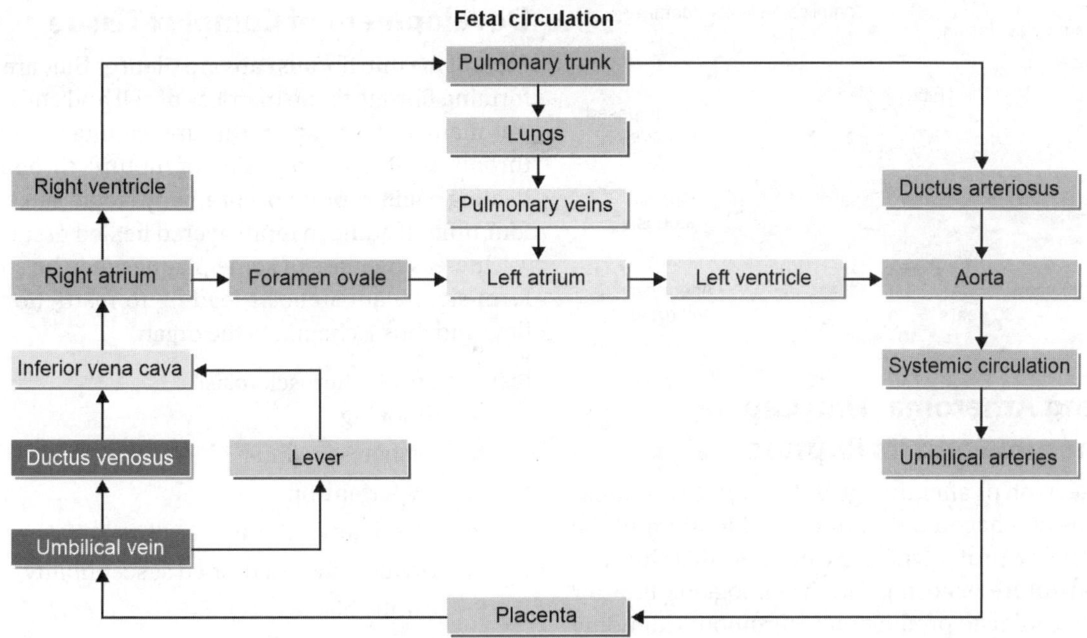

Scheme of fetal circulation

Q47. Atherosclerotic plaque.

MGR/APR2012/MDI (5)

Discuss the pathogenesis of atherosclerosis. How would you manage a case of dyslipidemia to prevent coronary artery disease?

MUHS/MAY2010/MDII (25)

Describe the pathogenesis of atherosclerosis.

MJPRU/2015/MDI (10)

ANSWER

Atheromatous plaques are mainly in the branching points of the arteries and also in the inner curvature where laminar flow will be disturbed or insufficient to support quiescent state of endothelium. As a result endothelium will be activated leading to increased permeability allowing extracellular matrix proteins causing diffuse thickening of intima along with ApoB lipoprotein retention. There is recruitment of monocytes originating from spleen and bone marrow which is governed by up-regulation of molecules of endothelial cells arresting them at the luminal surface.

At the beginning of the inflammation endothelial cells secrete adhesion molecules and smooth muscle cells secretes chemokines and chemoattractant both of which draw monocytes, lymphocytes, mast cells, and neutrophils into the arterial wall along with secretion of proteoglycans, collagen, and elastic fibers into the extracellular matrix by smooth muscle cells. Upon entry in the arterial wall monocytes will be transformed into macrophages which again transformed into foam cell after taking lipid as multiple small inclusions—degree of the accumulation of lipid is critical for early diagnosis of atherosclerosis. This changes can be reversed. Atherosclerosis will start when lipid accumulation appears as:

- **a.** Confluent extracellular lipid pool
- **b.** Extracellular lipid cores
- **c.** Decreased cellularity

Atherosclerosis is a chronic inflammatory disease beginning with accumulation of fat in the macrophages or lipid laden foam cells in the intimal wall known as fatty streak. This is followed by evidence of chronic inflammation at the susceptible sites that progresses to fibroatheroma. Both fatty streaks and fibroatheroma are formed and evolved in the same sites. There is increased accumulation of macrophage foam cells along with other inflammatory cells along with binding of extracellular proteoglycans with lipid in increasing capacity. Some factors provoke death of the macrophages and smooth muscle cells perpetuating further inflammation. Increased extracellular lipid along with further cellular necrosis lead to distortion and disruption of normal intimal architecture. This lipid laden necrotic core will be dominated in the central part of intima. Fibrous tissue will be added as fibrous cap at the top of lipid laden necrotic core just beneath the endothelium. This will start at the age of 15 years and persist throughout the life.

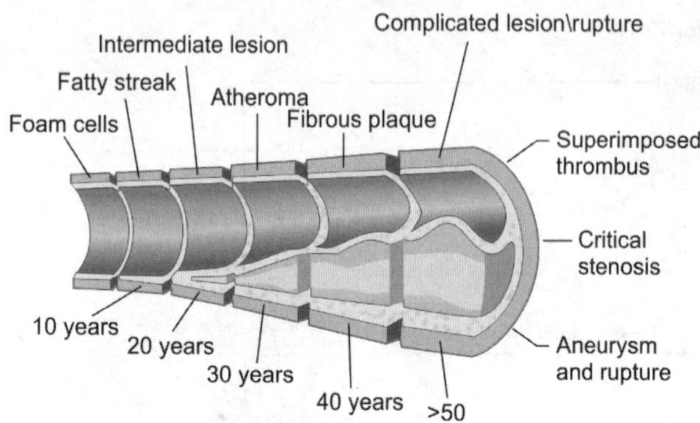

Advancing Atheroma: Thin Cap Fibroatheroma and its Rupture

This stage seen on or after the age of 55 years. In few areas thick fibrous cap become thin due to dissolution of the fibrous tissue by proteolytic enzymes and this thin cap is liable to rupture exposing the thrombogenic interior arterial wall leading to production of thrombus extending into arterial lumen. This type of plaque is known as vulnerable plaque because of there is risk of rupture leading to thrombosis which is started at in 55–65 years of age, the year of chances of myocardial infarction or stroke. Thin cap atheroma and ruptured plaques involve epicardial portion of coronary arteries mainly involving proximal portion of major coronary arteries.

There are two types of plaques:

- **a.** Stable plaque: Stable plaques regress or static or grows slowly.
- **b.** Unstable plaques: It is complicated by erosion, fissure, rupture, and lead to stenosis, thrombosis or infarction.

Now plaque also advances and distorts adjacent media and adventitia. With further growth of plaque local segment of the arterial wall will grow in caliber along with compensatory threatened reduction of caliber of the lumen. This compensation will be stopped when 40% of the lumen will be occupied and remodeling starts. Any further plaque enlargement will block the lumen which is hemodynamically significant. New fragile vasa vasorum will invade the distorted intima from the media, they may leak due to loss of pericytes supports and fragility of the endothelium leading to hemorrhage in the arterial wall which will perpetuates inflammation and fibrous tissue.

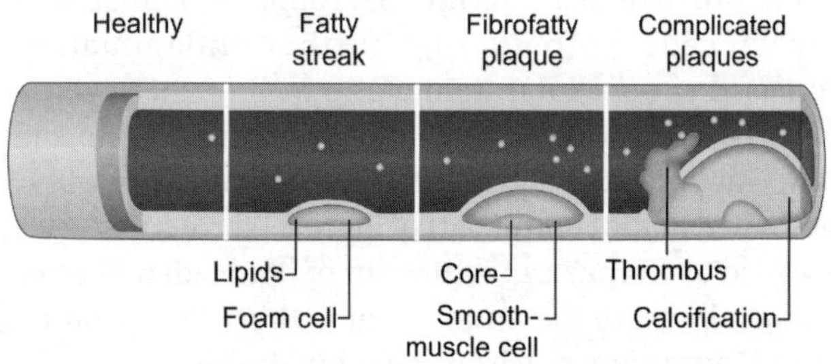

Development of Complex Tissue

Most of the thin fibrous caps are silent as they are healed by forming fibrous tissue matrices of cell and collagen fibers, but many of them again rupture leading to formation of thrombus. So cyclic occasion of rupture, thrombosis, and healing again rupture occur in any single site as many as four times leading to multilayered healed tissue.

Increasing mass of some plaques may be sufficient to form significant stenosis leading to restriction of blood flow and thus ischemia to the organ.

Risk factors of atherosclerosis:

- **a.** Smoking
- **b.** Diabetes mellitus
- **c.** Hypertension
- **d.** Blood flow pattern
- **e.** Genetically determined susceptibility
- **f.** Family history
- **g.** Age
- **h.** Male sex
- **i.** Hyperhomocysteinemia
- **j.** Alcohol ingestion
- **k.** Obesity
- **l.** Chlamydia infection
- **m.** Sedentary lifestyle

Stages of Atherosclerosis

Lipid modification

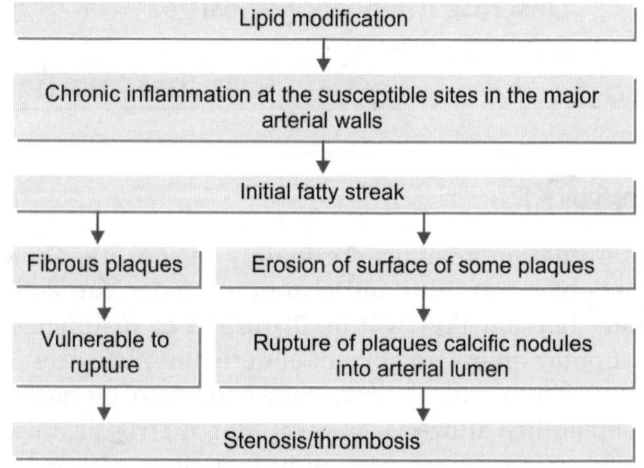

Management of hyperlipidemia (please see answer in question number 34).

Q48. Side effects of beta-blockers.

MGR/SEP2010/MDI (5)

ANSWER

Side Effects of Beta-blockers

A. Cardiovascular effects:
- **a.** Bradycardia
- **b.** AV block
- **c.** Raynaud's phenomenon
- **d.** Severe decompensated cardiac failure

B. Pulmonary effect:
- **a.** Bronchial asthma
- **b.** Bhronchospastic chronic obstructive pulmonary disease

C. Drug interactions:
- **a.** Decreased absorption of cholestyramine, colestipol, and aluminum salts
- **b.** Decreased plasma concentration of alcohol, phenytoin, and phenobarbital,
- **c.** Increased bioavailability of hydralazine, cimetidine
- **d.** Depress sinus node function by diltiazem, verapamil

D. Others:
- **a.** Fatigue
- **b.** Headache
- **c.** Sleep disturbances
- **d.** Depression
- **e.** Insomnia

Q49. Pericarditis.

MGR/SEP2009/MDI (5)

Discuss etiology, clinical features, and management of pericarditis.

MUHS/MAY2012/MDII (25)

ECG changes in acute pericarditis.

DNB, 2020 (5)

Discuss the etiology, clinical features, and diagnosis of acute pericarditis.

SAMS (ODISHA), 2023 (10)

ANSWER

Inflammation of pericardium is known as acute pericarditis. It mostly affects males between 16 and 65 years of age.

Etiology of Acute Pericarditis

A. Infection:
- **a.** Viral:
  1. Echovirus
  2. Coxsackie virus
- **b.** Bacterial infections following pneumonia:
  1. *Staphylococcus*
  2. *Streptococcus*
  3. Tubercular
- **c.** Fungal infection:
  1. Histoplasma
  2. *Aspergillus*
  3. *Candida*
  4. Blastomycosis

B. Noninfectious:
- **a.** Idiopathic
- **b.** Postmyocardial infarction
- **c.** Dressler syndrome
- **d.** Postcardiotomy syndrome
- **e.** Uremic
- **f.** Neoplastic
- **g.** Autoimmune cause
- **h.** Inflammatory
- **i.** Drugs:
  1. Hydralazine
  2. Procainamide
  3. Doxorubicin
  4. Phenytoin
  5. Penicillin

Clinical Features

A. Chest pain: It usually occurs at rest, sudden in onset, retrosternal, continuous, sharp or stabbing in character, it varies with respiration and posture, radiating to trapezius relieved by sitting up and leaning forward.

B. On examination: Pericardial rub—there is scratchy high pitch sound described like "creaking of new leather" best heard on lower left sternal border or sometimes anywhere in the chest, intensified during respiration, while patient in leaning forward, it may be fleeting recurring after few hours. Commonly rub is biphasic having atrial and ventricular systolic components.

C. ECG changes: There are four stages of ECG changes:
- **a.** Stage 1: Diffuse-ST segment elevation with concavity upward with upright T and depression

of PR segment seen in all the leads except V_1 and aVR. But in some cases PR segment elevation and ST segment depression in aVR.

b. Stage 2: Resolution of PR and ST segments along with flattening of T wave.
c. Stage 3: It is characterized by inversion of T wave.
d. Stage 4: Upright T wave follows after several days to weeks.

If pericarditis remains after 4–6 weeks.

Diagnosis

A. Tests for suspected myocardial disease: Following should be recommended:
   a. Routine blood tests:
      1. Total leukocyte count
      2. Liver function test
   b. ECG
   c. Chest X-ray: Enlarge water-bottle configuration in case of large pericardial effusion.
   d. Transthoracic echocardiogram: Within a day of symptomatic presentation:
      1. In 40% cases effusion
      2. Cardiac tamponade/constrictive histology
      3. Increased pericardial brightness
      4. Wall motion abnormality
   e. Inflammatory markers:
      1. ESR
      2. CRP
      3. Ultrasensitive CRP
   f. To detect underlying etiology:
      1. Culture
      2. Tuberculin test
      3. Viral serology
      4. Fungal tests
      5. Thyroid function test
      6. Immunology panel
      7. Cardiac biomarkers
      8. Cytology
B. Echocardiography: It is considered in the following cases: It will demonstrate:
   a. May be normal
   b. Pericardial effusion with or without pericardial tamponade
   c. Increased pericardial brightness
   d. In 5% cases of myopericarditis wall motion abnormalities
C. Cardiac computerized tomography: It will demonstrate:
   a. Noncalcified thickened pericardium with effusion
   b. Sign of inflammation: Irregular pericardium
   c. Iodine contrast enhancement in favor of inflammation
D. Cardiac MRI: It is considered in following situations:
   a. Atypical presentation
   b. Failure of medical therapy
   c. Equivocal echocardiogram along with poor prognostic features.
   d. Concern for chronic pericarditis

   It will demonstrate:
   a. Noncalcified thickened pericardium with effusion
   b. Exudative signal is present with high T1W signal intensity
   c. Increased T2 short-tau inversion recovery time suggestive of pericardial edema.
   d. Increased late gadolinium enhancement suggests organization of pericarditis.

Medical Therapy

A. First-line of therapy is nonsteroidal anti-inflammatory drugs (NSAIDs). Choice of aspirin/NSAIDs depends upon:
   a. Tolerance of the patients
   b. Side effects
   c. Comorbidities of the patients
   d. Physician expertise
B. Colchicine: Dose of the colchicine is 0.5 mg twice daily for 3 months if the weight of the patient is >70 kg and 0.5 mg daily if the weight of the patient is <70 kg.
C. Steroids if used in the first episode it will increase the recurrence by four fold. Hence it is not recommended as first-line of treatment. It can be considered with colchicine at a dose of 0.2–0.5 mg/kg for 1 month.

Complications

A. Recurrent pericarditis: It can be defined as episode of pericarditis after a period of symptom free interval of 4–6 weeks which is 15–30% after first episode.
B. Pericarditis with myocardial involvement, i.e., myopericarditis: It can be defined as pericardial involvement secondary to myocardial involvement.

Q50. Rheumatic fever.

MGR/MAR2009/MDI (5)

Describe the epidemiology, pathogenesis, diagnosis, and treatment of rheumatic fever.

MGR/MAR2010/MDII (20)

Describe pathogenesis of rheumatic fever.

MJPRU/2015(S)/MDI (10)

Revised Duckett-Jones criteria for acute rheumatic fever. Infections in post-splenectomy patients.

DNB, 2020 (5+5)

Acute rheumatic fever.

KERALA UNIVERSITY, 2018 (10)

RAJASTHAN UNIVERSITY, 2021 (25)

Diagnostic criteria of acute rheumatic fever.

BHARATI VIDYAPEETH UNIVERSITY, SUMMER 2019 (10)

Discuss rheumatic fever. How can you diagnose rheumatic fever?

SCBMCH, 2014 (15)

Describe the clinical features and preventive aspects of rheumatic fever.

MANIPUR UNIVERSITY, 2019 (10)

Discuss management of rheumatic fever.

MAHATMA UNIVERSITY, 2022 (10)

ANSWER

Introduction

It is a poststreptococcal infection autoimmune disorder occurring under 40 years of age.

Epidemiology

Incidence of rheumatic fever vary in different countries worldwide. In developing countries incidence is 200/100,000 population whereas, in United States it is <1/100,000 population.

It is more common in populations between the ages of 5 and 18 years susceptible to streptococcal pharyngitis. It affects both sexes equally, but Sydenham chorea is common in female after the age of puberty.

Etiopathogenesis

There is strong evidence of association of group A *Streptococcus* (GAS) and occurrence of acute and recurrent attack of rheumatic fever. It is due to hyperimmune response to GAS and its level strongly correlates with severity of manifestation of rheumatic fever. It will start approximately 3 weeks following upper respiratory infection but it is rare before the age of 5 years when the immune system is immature. This immune response is due to molecular mimicry between the streptococcal cellular antigen and human connective tissue protein.

a. Most important antigens present in the external layer of the bacterial cell wall are M, T, and R proteins.
b. M-protein has following actions:
   1. Type specific immunity
   2. Powerful antiphagocytic action: It is known as marker of streptococcal rheumatogenic potential.

Patients suffering from acute rheumatic fever possess high level of antibodies against M protein of GAS but not those serotypes which are associated with impetigo and pyoderma as these serotypes are associated with glomerulonephritis.

3% of untreated patients with streptococcal pharyngitis are associated with acute rheumatic fever. But 50% patients with acute rheumatic fever develops recurrence.

There is familial and genetic predisposition of rheumatic fever as evidenced by the following:

a. Monoclonal antibody to B-cell alloantigen (D8/17) is detected in rheumatic fever patients but it is present in <14% of general population only.
b. Patients with HLA-D 1, 2, 3, and 4 are associated with rheumatic fever.

Diagnosis

GAS infection	Major Jones criteria		Minor Jones criteria	
Culture	**Low risk**	**High risk**	**Low risk**	**High risk**
ASO titer	Carditis (clinical or subclinical)	Carditis (clinical or subclinical)	Polyarthralgia	Monoarthralgia
Anti-DNAase B	Polyarthritis only	Monoarthritis or polyarthritis or polyarthralgia	Fever ≥ 38.5°C	Fever ≥ 38.5°C
Other	Chorea	Chorea	ESR ≥ 60 mm/first hour and/or CRP ≥ 3.0 mg/dL	ESR ≥ 30 mm/first hour and/or CRP ≥ 3.0 mg/dL
Antistreptococcal antibodies	Erythema nodosum	Erythema nodosum	Prolonged PR interval	Prolonged PR interval
Streptococcal antigens	Subcutaneous nodules	Subcutaneous nodule		

A. Carditis:

a. It ranges from asymptomatic to severe congestive HF to death. The typical manifestations are:

1. Tachycardia
2. Arrhythmia
3. Murmur
4. Pericardial rub
5. Cardiomegaly
6. Heart failure in there is associated myocarditis.

b. Most characteristic of component endocarditis involving mitral and aortic valves:

1. Hallmark is mitral regurgitation
2. Aortic regurgitation if present, it is always associated with mitral regurgitation.
3. According to rule of thumb MI occurs under the age of 30 years, MS in 3rd decade, and mixed valvular disease thereafter.
4. In case of subclinical carditis valvular thickening in echocardiography is present in absence of any murmur.
5. In case of acute mitral regurgitation apical systolic murmur is associated with mid-diastolic Carey-Coombs murmur due to rheumatic valvulitis.

c. Pericarditis may present with chest pain, friction rubs, and distant heart sound.

B. Arthritis:

Asymmetrical painful, migratory, and transient arthritis involving large joints such as knee, ankle, elbow, and shoulders present commonly in elderly and improved with salicylates within 48 hours. But monoarthritis or oligoarticular arthritis, involvement of first metatarsophalangeal joints, enthesopathy and cervical spine involvement may occur.

C. Sydenham chorea:

It is an extrapyramidal disorder characterized by quasipurposive involuntary movement involving face and limbs, hypotonic muscles, and initial liability.

a. It is late manifestation appearing 3 months after upper respiratory tract infection. It runs benign course and resolves within 2–3 months.

b. Initial manifestations are difficulty in walking, talking, and writing.

D. Subcutaneous nodules:

It is characterized by 0.5–2 cm, firm, and painless, freely movable isolated or clustered nodules present on the extensor surface of wrists, knee and elbow, over the bony prominences, dorsum of the foot, tendons, occipital regions, and cervical processes.

E. Erythema marginatum:

It is characterized by evanescent erythematous non-pruritic macular rash of varying sizes having pale center disappearing within few days.

Laboratory Investigations

A. Regarding GAS infection:

a. Culture of throat—negative report is sufficient to stop the treatment in case of low suspicion of rheumatic fever.

b. Elevated or greater than twofold rising titer of ASO titers as compared to convalescent titer.

c. Previous GAS infection probability can be increased by measuring antibodies to antideoxyribonuclease B.

B. Biopsies:

a. Aschoff nodules: In the proliferative stage it is a granulomatous inflammation present in the interventricular septum, left atrial appendages, and left ventricle pathognomonic of rheumatic carditis.

b. Histologic findings in case of endocarditis are:

1. Cellular infiltration
2. Hyaline degeneration of the affected valve leading to formation verrucae at the edge that will prevent co-optation of valvular leaflets.
3. Endomyocardial biopsy: It is not indicated in acute rheumatic fever but is helpful in case of chronic inactive rheumatic carditis.

C. Other laboratory studies:

a. Hematological:

1. Hypochromic or normochromic anemia
2. Leukocytosis
3. Thrombocytosis
4. High ESR

b. Biochemical:

1. Raised CRP

c. Radiography:

1. Cardiac size
2. Increased pulmonary vasculature
3. Pulmonary edema

d. ECG:

1. Prolonged PR interval
2. Increased rate

e. Echocardiography

Treatment

A. Patients with carditis should get secondary prophylaxis for at least 10 years after the first attack or till 25 years of age.

B. Congestive cardiac failure should be treated accordingly.

C. For inflammatory manifestations:

a. Aspirin: 80–100 mg/kg/day 4 hourly in case of children and 4–8 g/day every 4–6 hours in adults.

b. If the patient can produce Reye's syndrome after taking aspirin, in those cases NSAIDs like naproxen 10–20 mg/kg/day should be given daily every 12 hours with maximum dose of 1,250 mg for adult.

c. In case of intolerance to aspirin, 1–2 mg/kg/day corticosteroid can be given. In case of severe carditis steroid has some role. Duration of anti-inflammatory therapy should be continued till the normalization of clinical and laboratory findings of disease activity.

Prevention of Rheumatic Fever

Primary prevention	Dosage	Route	Duration
Benzathine penicillin	• 600,000 U ≤ 27 kg • 1.2 million U ≥ 27 kg	IM	Once
Penicillin V	500 mg (two to three times/day)	Oral	10 days
Penicillin allergic patients			
Erythromycin ethyl succinate	40 mg/kg/day–two to three times/day	Orally	10 days
Erythromycin estolate	20–40 mg/kg/day two to four times/day	Orally	10 days
Secondary prevention			
Benzathine penicillin	1.2 million U	IM	3–4 weeks
Or Penicillin V	250 mg	Orally	Twice daily
Penicillin allergic patients			
Erythromycin	250 mg	Orally	Twice daily

Duration of Therapy for Secondary Prevention

State of the disease	Duration of therapy
RF + Carditis + Residual valvular defect	• At least 10 years after first episode and at least 25 years of age • In case of more severe valvular heart disease lifelong prophylaxis
RF + Carditis in absence of any valvular disease	10 years after first episode or 25 years of age whichever is long duration
RF without carditis	5 years after first episode or 18 years of age
RF after valve surgery	Lifelong

Infections in post-splenectomy patients.

Q51. Pericardium.

MAR/SEP2008/MDI (5)

ANSWER

Definition

Pericardium is a fibrous sac enclosing the heart and great vessels keeping in a stable location in the mediastinum separating from the lungs and other mediastinal structures allowing the heart and the great vessels to move as per requirement.

Pericardium consists of two layers:

A. Fibrous pericardium: It is conical in shape with its apex fused with the great vessels at the base of the heart and broader base fused with the central fibrous area of the diaphragm. Sternopericardial ligament attaches anterior aspect of the pericardium to the sternum.

B. Serous pericardium lines the inner surface of fibrous pericardium as parietal layer and is reflected around the root of the great vessels to cover the outer surface of the heart as visceral layer. In between the visceral and parietal layer of pericardium there is small amount of fluid known as pericardial fluid. A small part of visceral layer that covers the visceral surface but not the great vessels is known as epicardium.

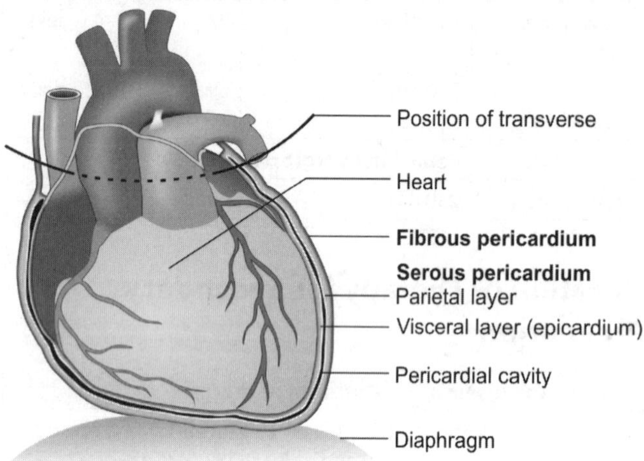

Serous pericardium forms two sinuses while it reflecting of various cardiac structures: Transverse sinus and oblique sinus. Actions of pericardial sac:

- **a.** It limits its motion.
- **b.** It will promote lubricating surface for the heart to beat inside.
- **c.** It will prevent excessive dilatation of the heart.
- **d.** It can limit overfilling of the heart.
- **e.** It will influence the pressure-volume relationship of cardiac chamber by giving limited space for the heart as a whole.

Q52. Constrictive pericarditis.

MGR/APR2015/MDII (7)

Discuss, pathophysiology, clinical features, diagnosis, and management of constrictive pericarditis.

MGR/SEP2010/MDIV (20)

Discuss the etiology, clinical features, diagnosis, and management of constrictive pericarditis.

MGR/MAR2008/MDIII (20)

Constrictive pericarditis.

KERALA UNIVERSITY, 2021 (10)

NTR UNIVERSITY OF HEALTH SC, VIJAYAWADA, ANDHRA, 2022 (10)

Explain the waves in JVP in chronic pericarditis.

MGU, 2024 (5)

ANSWER

Definition

It can be defined as noncompliant pericardium as a result of consequence of inflammation, fibrosis, and calcification encasing the heart in rigid cavity leading to HF with diastolic ventricular filling.

Classification

A. Transient constrictive pericarditis: It follows following events:

- **a.** Episodes of acute pericarditis with effusion.
- **b.** Pericarditis
- **c.** Pericardiotomy
- **d.** Chemotherapy

It is called transient because inflammation can be resolved by itself by anti-inflammatory drugs within 3–6 months.

B. Effusive-constrictive pericarditis: It occurs in patients with pericardial tamponade in whom in spite of pericardiocentesis intrapericardial pressures remain elevated with predominant involvement of visceral pericardium which is also known as constrictive epicarditis.

C. Chronic constrictive pericarditis: It occurs if constriction persists after 3–6 months.

Pathophysiology

A. Nondistensible pericardium limits the cardiac filling to fixed volume.

- **a.** In case of early diastole ventricle will expand normally and fills rapidly secondary to increased systemic and pulmonary pressures.
- **b.** But diastolic filling comes to abrupt halt when both the ventricles will reach the extremes of confines of rigid pericardium. So most of the

ventricular filling in the second phase of diastole, i.e., early filling.

c. Very little contribution from the third phase or diastasis or fourth phase or atrial systole.

So hallmark of constrictive pericarditis is equalization of end-diastolic pressure in all four cardiac chambers.

B. Transmission of intrathoracic pressures to the cardiac chambers is prevented by stiff pericardium throughout the respiratory cycle—it is called intrathoracic-intracardiac pressure dissociation. As a result there is significant respirophasic variation of ventricular preload which is associated with enhanced ventricular interdependence.

C. During respiration due to increased intrathoracic pressure right heart preload and velocity of blood inflow through the tricuspid valve are increased, on the other hand there is decrease in left atrial preload and inflow velocity through the mitral valve as a consequence of transmission of full negative intrathoracic pressure to pulmonary vein but with little or no transmission to left-sided chambers. Net result of respiration is right-sided chambers loaded with blood and partially empty left-sided chambers within stiff pericardium along with leftward shifting of interventricular septum.

D. During expiration there is positive intrathoracic pressure that reduce right-sided preload and inflow through the tricuspid valve. But pressure on the pulmonary vein will be increased leading to increased left-sided filling and increased blood flow through the mitral valve. So, net result is full left-sided chambers and emptier right-sided chambers within stiff pericardium lead to shifting of ventricular septum toward right and reversal of late diastolic flow in the hepatic veins.

E. Myocardial systolic function and myocardial relaxation are usually spared. But due to teethering myocardium to pericardium myocardial function is compromised.

Clinical Presentation

A. Early symptoms: It is insidious, symptoms are nonspecific consisting of fatigue, malaise, and decreased exercise tolerance.

B. Patients may present with right-sided HF such as nonpulsatile engorged neck vein, enlarged and tender liver and ascites and Kussmaul's sign, i.e., lack of inspiratory fall venous distension.

C. Distant heart sound due to decreased transmission through the thickened pericardium.

D. Soft first heart sound because of closing of mitral as well as tricuspid valve by the end of diastole.

E. Pericardial knock in early diastole due to abrupt cessation of diastolic filling when rigid pericardium impedes the ventricular filling.

F. Vesicular breath sound is decreased at bases due to pleural effusion.

G. Key features in JVP are:

a. Prominent deep and rapid Y decent due to rapid emptying of the right atrium into the right ventricle in early systole but the rapid filling of the right atrium is halted by the constricted pericardium.

b. Prominent X decent which occurs due to downward displacement of the atrioventricular valves into the right ventricle during ventricular systole.

c. In case of normal sinus rhythm a wave may be visible and in case of reduced right ventricular compliance, "a" wave may be accentuated.

d. Combination of prominent "X" and "y" decent leads to "M" or "W" shaped contour of the venous wave.

Diagnosis

A. Routine work-up in case of suspected constrictive pericarditis:

a. Total white blood cell count

b. Liver function test

c. Echocardiogram: Transthoracic echocardiography is the first-line imaging. Following are the characteristics of echocardiographic findings:

1. Pericardial thickening as indicated by parallel motion of visceral and parietal pericardium.
2. Flattening of left ventricular posterior wall endocardium.
3. Oscillatory diastolic beat-to-beat ventricular septal movement: Septal bounce shudder.
4. Septal wall motion variation with respiration.
5. Plethora of inferior vena cava
6. Increased respirophasic variation of AV inflow.
7. Inspiratory reduction of >25% in velocities of peak mitral E-wave velocities.
8. Respiratory variation in flow through pulmonary veins during diastole.
9. Reversal of expiratory hepatic diastolic flow, and during diastole hepatic diastolic reversal-to-forward flow velocity ratio of >20%.

10. Annulus paradoxus or inverse relationship of E/e′.
11. Annulus reversus or reverse relationship between lateral and medial mitral annuli.
12. Key echocardiographic criteria for chronic constrictive pericarditis are:
    - Abnormal septal wall motion

      Plus
    - Elevated e′ velocity of medial mitral annulus of >8 cm/sec

      And/or
    - Hepatic vein expiration flow ratio of >0.79

      Plus
    - Increased respirophasic variation in AV inflow.

      Plus
    - Plethora of inferior vena cava.

d. Doppler echocardiography can exclude restrictive cardiomyopathy.

e. ECG

f. Cardiac MRI: It will demonstrate:
1. Abnormal septal wall motion
2. Septal bounce
3. Respirophasic variation in septal excursion.
4. It can assess the pericardial thickening—>4 mm thickening is supportive of diagnosis.
5. It can quantify systolic function of left and right ventricle.

g. Inflammatory marker: ESR, CRP, and hsCRP.

h. Chest X-ray: It will demonstrate:
1. Pericardial calcification best seen in right ventricle and AV groove in left lateral position.
2. Pleural effusion

i. Cardiac catheterization: It will differentiate restrictive cardiomyopathy from pericardial effusion.
1. Right atrial pressure waveform demonstrates:
    - Prominent "a" wave due to contraction of atria against elevated pressure in the ventricle.
    - Exaggerated "x" descent
    - Sharp "y" descent
2. Ventricular pressure waveform: It will demonstrate:
    - Square-root sign, i.e., dip-and-plateau wave—initial downward wave is due to drop in ventricular pressure during isovolumic relaxation period which is followed by early diastolic filling as indicated by upward deflection.
    - Equalization of elevated left and right ventricular end-diastolic pressure within 5 mm Hg.
    - Right ventricular systolic pressure of <55 mm Hg which is contradictory to right ventricular systolic pressure of >55 mm Hg.

Medical Therapy

The treatment of constrictive pericarditis is pericardiectomy, but in some cases medical therapy is appropriate.

A. In case of constrictive pericarditis with evidence of inflammation should be treated by anti-inflammatory drugs for 3–6 months like colchicine, in some refractory cases steroids followed by pericardiotomy.

B. In case of effusive-constrictive pericarditis pericardiocentesis along with trial of medical treatment followed by pericardiectomy.

C. In case of patients with New York Heart Association (NYHA) class I symptoms they should be treated by diuretics plus low-sodium diet, in some cases pericardiectomy.

D. In case of severe morbidity they should be treated with medical therapy because of high postoperative mortality.

E. In more than 90% of patients pericardiectomy is responsible for symptomatic improvement. But, there is postoperative mortality is 6–12%.

Q53. Pacemakers in AV conduction diseases.

MGR/OCT2013/MDII (7)

Describe the guidelines for various pacemaker implantations in acquired AV block.

MGR/APR2012/MDII (7)

Pacemaker therapy in cardiac practice.

MUHS/MAY2010/MDII (10)

ANSWER

Guideline for Various Pacemakers in Case of Acquired AV Block

A. Class I recommendation:

- **a.** Third degree or high grade AV block at any anatomic level associated with:
  1. Symptomatic bradycardia
  2. Essential drug therapy that produce symptomatic bradycardia
  3. Periods of asystole > 3 seconds or any escape rate < 40 beats/min while awake or an escape rhythm originating below AV node.
  4. Postoperative AV block not expected to resolve.
  5. Catheter ablation of AV junction
  6. Neuromuscular diseases such as myotonic dystrophy, Kearns–Sayre syndrome, Erb dystrophy, and peroneal muscular atrophy regardless of the presence of symptoms.
- **b.** Second degree AV block with symptomatic bradycardia.
- **c.** Type II second degree AV block with a wide QRS complex with or without symptoms.
- **d.** Exercise-induced second or third degree AV block in absence of ischemia.
- **e.** Atrial fibrillation with bradycardia and pauses > 5 seconds.

B. Class IIa:

- **a.** Asymptomatic third degree AV block regardless of level.
- **b.** Asymptomatic type II second degree AV block with a narrow QRS complex.
- **c.** Asymptomatic type II second degree AV block with block within or below the His at electrophysiological study.
- **d.** First or second degree AV block with symptoms similar to pacemaker syndrome.

C. Class IIb:

- **a.** AV block in the setting of drug use/toxicity, when the block is expected to recur even with drug discontinuation.
- **b.** Neuromuscular diseases such as myotonic dystrophy, Kearns–Sayre syndrome, Erb dystrophy and peroneal muscular atrophy with any degree of AV block regardless of the presence of symptoms.

D. Class III:

- **a.** Asymptomatic first degree AV block
- **b.** Asymptomatic type I second degree AV block at the AV node level.
- **c.** AV block that is expected to resolve or is unlikely to recur (Lyme disease, drug toxicity).

Q54. Indications and principles of cardiac revascularization therapy.

MGR/OCT2012/MDII (7)

Coronary revascularization.

NTR UNIVERSITY OF HEALTH SC, VIJAYAWADA, ANDHRA, 2022 (10)

Iatrogenic injuries during percutaneous coronary intervention. Proprotein convertase subtilisin/kexin type 9 (PCSK9) inhibitors.

DNB, 2024, OCT (10)

Indications of cardiac catheterization and angiography.

MANIPUR UNIVERSITY, 2018 (10)

ANSWER

Indications of Coronary Revascularization (Percutaneous Coronary Intervention)

A. In case of patients in whom there is objective evidence of substantial ischemia of myocardium or symptoms related to ischemia and angiographic of obstructive coronary artery disease.

B. In case of ST-segment elevated myocardial infarction within 3 hours of symptoms onset. But, in patients presenting within 3–12 hours of symptom onset of coronary vascularization or superior in terms of therapy.

C. Unstable angina and non-ST segment myocardial infarction are subject to future morbidity and mortality, hence early cardiac catheterization followed by revascularization is essential.

D. A large proportion of cases of stable angina.

E. Symptoms-limiting angina pectoris despite optimum medical therapy and it is accompanied by evidence of ischemia on stress test.

Contraindications of Revascularization

A. Absolute contraindication: Only one is significant in active bleeding.

B. Relative contraindication:

- **a.** Bleeding diathesis
- **b.** Unstable or high-risk coronary artery anatomy
- **c.** Recurrent in-stent restenosis
- **d.** Short-life expectancy because of different comorbid conditions.

Clinical Predictors of Adverse Outcome

A. Older age
B. Acute myocardial infarction
C. Cardiogenic shock
D. Unstable angina
E. Congestive HF
F. Multivessel coronary artery disease
G. Left ventricular function
H. Diabetes mellitus
I. Peripheral vascular disease
J. Renal impairment
K. Small body size

Angiographic Predictor of Adverse Outcome

A. Presence of thrombus
B. Bypass graft
C. Lesion of >20 mm in length
D. Extremely angulated lesion of >90°
E. Excessive tortuosity of proximal segment
F. Total occlusion of >3 months old and/or bridging collaterals
G. Unprotected left main trunk
H. Inability to protect major side branches
I. Degenerated vein grafts with friable lesions

Success

A. Angiographic success can be defined as presence of a residual stenosis < 50% with percutaneous transluminal coronary angioplasty or <20% with stenting along with TIMI 3 flow has been achieved in 96–99% of patients.

B. Procedural success is just angiographic success in absence of major-in-hospital complications.

C. Clinical success can be defined as procedural success along with relief from clinical features of myocardial ischemia.

Complications

A. Abrupt closure is most common and major adverse cardiac event and it occurs within 6 hours of coronary intervention. Most common causes of abrupt closure is suboptimal stent expansion or dissection which is followed by vasospasm, thrombus formation, and occlusion of side branch. Risk factors are:

- **a.** Acute myocardial infarction
- **b.** Poor coronary flow postintervention
- **c.** Complex lesion morphology

B. Atheroembolism: It occurs in all types of interventions, but mostly occurs in case of:

- **a.** Degenerated vein graft
- **b.** Patients presenting with acute coronary syndrome
- **c.** Directional rotational atherectomy

Iatrogenic Complications during Percutaneous Coronary Intervention

A. Complications in the coronary artery:

- **a.** Dissection due to injury by the guidewire, catheter and balloon leading to tear in the intimal layer of the artery and formation of a false lumen.
- **b.** There may be perforation in the coronary artery during rapid intervention by the inflated balloon or stent requiring urgent surgery.
- **c.** The ischemia may be persistent ischemia as a result of interrupted microcirculation be the embolism or spasm.
- **d.** There may be chance of restenosis due to less expansion of the stent or wrong position or inadequate antiplatelet therapy.

B. Vascular complications:

- **a.** Hematoma at the site of arterial puncture mainly in the femoral artery.
- **b.** Pseudoaneurysm in case of inadequate sealing of the puncture site in the artery.
- **c.** In case of puncture in the high femoral artery there may be chance of retroperitoneal hemorrhage leading to hypovolemic shock.
- **d.** Radial artery may be occluded in case of transradial artery puncture due to presence of collateral circulation.
- **d.** Excessive manipulation of the catheter leads to tear in the aortic wall intima leading to aortic dissection.

C. Cardiac complications:

a. Inflation of the balloon in the left anterior descending artery leading to papillary muscle dysfunction resulting mitral regurgitation.

b. There may be retrograde coronary total occlusion leading to injury in the coronary sinus.

D. Systemic complications:

a. In patients with high serum creatinine or suffering from chronic kidney disease leading to contrast induced nephropathy if the dose of dye will be high.

b. Due to improper flushing of the catheter air embolism can occur.

PCSK9 inhibitors has been written in general chapter question number 169.

Q55. Clinical manifestations and management of cardiac tamponade.

MGR/APR2012/MDII (7)

Cardiac tamponade.

KERALA UNIVERSITY, 2022, (10)
VEER NARMAD SOUTH GUJARAT UNIVERSITY, 2021 (20)
BHARATI VIDYAPEETH UNIVERSITY, 2017, WINTER (10)
BHARATI VIDYAPEETH UNIVERSITY, SUMMER 2016 (10)
BHARATI VIDYAPEETH UNIVERSITY, SUMMER 2016 (10)
SARDAR PATEL UNIVERSITY, 2019 APRIL (5)
SAMS (ODISHA) 2021 (10)

ANSWER

Introduction

It is a severe condition characterized by impaired ventricular filling due to increase in intrapericardial pressure as a result of accumulation of blood, pus, and fluid or gas as evidenced by spectrum of presentation from compensated to decompensated pericardial tamponade leading to cardiogenic shock. Features of cardiac tamponade are determined by interplay between the following:

a. Stiffness of pericardium due to:

1. Infiltration

2. Fibrosis

3. Calcification

b. Size of effusion

c. Rate of accumulation of pericardial fluid

Pathophysiology

A. Pericardium is gradually stretched due to fluid accumulation, ultimately it will reach a limit beyond which little increased accumulation of pericardial fluid is associated with large increase in pericardial pressure.

B. As a result there is equalization of intracardiac diastolic pressure within the distended pericardium—this will lead to absolute decrease in:

a. Intracardiac volumes

b. Ventricular diastolic filling

c. Stroke volume

C. Initially cardiac output will be maintained by increased adrenergic tone leading to resting tachycardia along with peripheral vasoconstriction.

D. There is competition for maintaining fixed right and left ventricular volumes.

a. During inspiration due to increased negative intrathoracic pressure there is increased right ventricular venous return with concomitant reduction of the left ventricular filling due to decreased pulmonary vein to left ventricular pressure gradient leading to decreased inflow velocity of blood through the mitral valve and delayed opening of mitral valve. Due to decreased velocity of blood flow through the mitral valve the interventricular septum will be deviated into left ventricular cavity leading to further reduction of left ventricular stroke volume causing further lowering of systolic blood pressure which is known as pulsus paradoxus. Just the opposite changes occur during expiration.

b. Finally all the above compensatory mechanism fails leading to decrease in cardiac output with cardiogenic shock.

Clinical Features

Features are due to decreased cardiac output. These are the following:

a. Restlessness

b. Agitation

c. Syncope or near-syncope

d. Drowsiness

e. Decreased urine output

f. Respiratory distress

g. Chest discomfort
h. Weakness
i. Anorexia
j. Weight loss

On physical examination reveals Beck triad—which is characterized by the following:

a. Jugular venous distension
b. Hypotension
c. Distant heart sound

Other features are also found:

a. Compensatory tachycardia
b. Tachypnea
c. Elevated central venous pressure with prominent "x" descent and absent "y" wave.
d. Diminished heart sound or distant heart sound due to large amount of pericardial effusion.
e. Pulsus paradoxus, i.e., inspiratory drop in systolic blood pressure of >10 mm Hg.

Investigations

A. Transthoracic and Doppler echocardiography will demonstrate:
   a. Presence of pericardial effusion
   b. Right atrial diastolic collapse mainly in late diastole continuing into ventricular systole.
      Duration of diastolic collapse directly correlates with severity of cardiac tamponade.
   c. Right ventricular early diastolic collapse—mostly found in anterior right ventricular free wall and infundibulum when the patient is in supine position.
   d. Left atrial diastolic collapse—though rare but more specific sign of cardiac tamponade.
   e. Abnormal increase in right ventricular dimension during inspiration.
   f. Exaggerated respiratory variation in case of atrioventricular inflow.
   g. Tricuspid E-wave velocity during expiration will decrease to >60%.
   h. Plethora of inferior vena cava
   i. Expiratory blunting or reversal of diastolic flow through hepatic veins.
B. Transthoracic echocardiography will detect pericardial hematoma.
C. Cardiac MRI and CT scan will be reserved for subacute complex cases such as:
   a. Equivocal postsurgical case
   b. Regional tamponade
   c. Loculated pericardial effusion
D. Right heart catheterization: It can confirm:
   a. Cardiac tamponade
   b. Quantification of hemodynamic comprise
   c. Assess conditions after pericardiocentesis
   d. Equalization of average diastolic pressure in all the chambers. Which will be raised between 10 and 30 mm Hg.

Treatment

A. Drainage of pericardial fluid is very important to give urgent relief to the patients. Timing and method of drainage depends upon:
   a. Etiology of effusion
   b. Patient's level of acuity
   c. Availability of trained physician

   Different methods of pericardiocentesis are:
   a. Pericardiocentesis under echocardiographic or fluoroscopic guidance
   b. Surgical drainage: It is preferred in case of:
      1. Recurrence
      2. Purulent effusion
      3. Loculated effusion
      4. Urgent bleeding into the pericardium
   c. In case of loculated pericardial effusion drainage through the pericardial window.
   d. Other medical support are:
      1. Inotropic support if the patients are hypotensive.
      2. Avoidance of vasodilators and diuretics.

Q56. Pharmacology of levosimendan and its usefulness in heart failure.
MGR/APR2012/MDII (7)

ANSWER

This drug, ionodilator given intravenously for acute decompensated HF has following pharmacological effects:

A. Cardiac contractility is increased which is mediated by calcium sensitization of troponin C.
B. Opening of potassium channels present on the sarcolemma of vascular smooth muscle cells.
C. Opening of potassium channels present in the mitochondria of cardiomyocytes.

It is given as a short-term treatment in case of acute decompensated HF that cannot be controlled by conventional therapy or inotropic therapy. It has also some positive effects in following conditions:

a. Right ventricular failure: It acts through following mechanisms:
   1. It reduces right ventricular afterloads
   2. It improves right ventricular contractility
   3. It improves diastolic function of right ventricle
b. Cardiogenic shock
c. Takotsubo cardiomyopathy
d. Other conditions requiring inotropic therapy

Therapeutic Effects

A. Hemodynamics:
   a. It will produce dose-dependent increase in:
      1. Stroke volume
      2. Cardiac output
      3. Heart rate
   b. It will decrease in:
      1. Pulmonary capillary wedge pressure
      2. Peripheral vascular resistance
      3. Mean right atrial pressure

   These features are obtained at the end of 5 minutes of bolus infusion and will be maintained for 7–9 days after stopping the infusion of this drug due to presence of active metabolite OR-1896 in the blood.
B. It should be used with caution in case of low baseline elevated blood pressure. It will improve dyspnea. It will decrease rapidly sustained decrease in natriuretic peptides.
C. Renal function: In case of decompensated HF there is deterioration of renal function leading to adverse outcome. Estimated GFR will be increased. But severe renal failure is a contraindication for this drugs.
D. This drug has positive effects on liver, splanchnic, and diaphragmatic function.

Clinical Effects of this Drugs

Hemodynamic and neurohumoral effects	Clinical effects
Severely decreased pulmonary capillary wedge pressure	Heart failure symptoms are relieved
Highly increased cardiac output and cardiac index	Also, other beta-blockers maintain the effects
Increased stroke volume	Its active metabolite maintains the sustained effects
Highly decreased systemic vascular resistance	Tolerance will not be developed
Highly decreased pulmonary vascular resistance	Myocardial oxygen consumption is not increased
Severely decreased natriuretic peptide levels	Anti-ischemic effect
	Diastolic dysfunction is not impaired

Dose in Case of Acute Decompensated Heart Failure

A. To maintain systemic blood pressure of >100 mm Hg and if immediate effect is needed 6–12 μg/kg to be given intravenously over 10 minutes as a loading dose.
B. Maintenance dose is 0.05–0.2 μg/kg/min, but varies from individual to individual.
C. Duration of infusion is up to 24 hours.
D. Before and during the treatment hypovolemia should be avoided.
E. One should also avoid hypokalemia.

Q57. Refractory heart failure.

MGR/MAY2011/MDII (7)

MGR UNIVERSITY, 2019 (10)

Resistant heart failure.

MUHS/NOV2013/MDII (10)

Management of refractory heart failure.

MUHS/NOV2010/MDIV (10)

Classification of heart failure and treatment of refractory heart failure.

DR YSR UNI OF HEALTH SC, VIJAYAWADA, 2022 (10)

Management of refractory heart failure.

NTR UNIVERSITY OF HEALTH SC, VIJAYAWADA, ANDHRA, 2022 (10)

KERALA UNIVERSITY, 2017 (10)

Classification of heart failure in Q22

Management of intractable heart failure.

SCBMCH, 2019 (10)

Discuss refractory heart failure.

SCBMCH, 2020 (10)

Discuss the management of refractory heart failure.

MANIPUR UNIVERSITY, 2021 (10)

ANSWER

Definition

It can be defined as persistence of symptoms limiting daily life, i.e., NYHA functional class III and IV in spite of previous treatment with the drugs, i.e., ACE inhibitors, angiotensin II receptor antagonists, digoxin, beta-blockers, and diuretics. These patients have advanced structural heart disease as well as severe features of heart disease and these candidates are in absence of any contraindications for different specialized interventions such as vascular remodeling, implantation of intracardiac devices or intravenous administration of inotropic drugs.

Following are the Factors for Causing Cardiac Decompensations

- **a.** Anemia
- **b.** Infections: Common viral infections
- **c.** Pulmonary embolism
- **d.** Thyroid dysfunction
- **e.** Excessive alcohol consumption
- **f.** Atrial fibrillation with rapid ventricular rate
- **g.** Obesity
- **h.** Presence of underlying heart disease
- **i.** Nonischemic-dilated cardiomyopathy

Pathophysiology Along with Clinical Features

Symptoms of refractory HF are due to following mechanisms:

- **a.** Congestion in the lung due to left atrial pressure—it produces:
  1. Exertional dyspnea,
  2. Orthopnea,
  3. Cough with decubitus
  4. Dyspnea at rest
- **b.** Low cardiac output.
- **c.** Systemic congestion due to right atrial filling pressure. It produces:
  1. Ascites
  2. Edema
  3. Easy satiety
  4. Anorexia
  5. Undernutrition discomfort when the patient tries to stoop forward or backward.

Other nonspecific features:

- **a.** Asthenia
- **b.** Lack of energy
- **c.** Depression
- **d.** Easy fatigue

Due to low cerebral perfusion:

- **a.** Changes in the nocturnal sleep patterns
- **b.** Difficulties in concentration
- **c.** Drowsiness

Hemodynamic profile of these patients are subdivided into four categories depending upon systemic or pulmonary congestion and low cardiac output. Following clinical assessments have prognostic value as these will guide the treatment, these are:

- **a.** Normal venous pressure
- **b.** Systolic blood pressure of >80 mm Hg
- **c.** Stable renal function
- **d.** Capacity to walk on leveled surface without fatigue

Following table demonstrates assessment of hemodynamic profile in refractory HF:

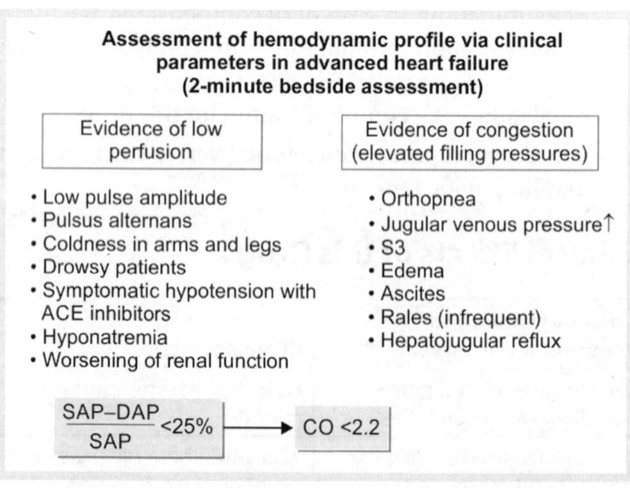

There are four types of hemodynamic profiles:

Hemodynamic profile in advanced heart failure

Low perfusion at rest? / Congestion at rest?	No	Yes
No	Warm and dry (A)	Warm and wet (B)
Yes	Cold and dry (L)	Cold and wet (C)

A. Profile A: Here there is no evidence of elevated filling pressure or low cardiac output. Here the treatment aims:

a. Maintenance of adequate filling pressure.

b. Prevention of disease progression.

B. Profile B: Here the patients present with congestion without low cardiac output. They should be treated with:

a. Diuretics as out-patient basis or decompensation are of recent onset.

b. If the patients will not respond, intravenous diuretics or potent oral diuretic like metolazone, but these drugs require close monitoring of serum potassium level.

c. Nesiritide, a recombinant form of endogenous type B natriuretic peptide is used in case of decompensated HF to improve symptoms of congestion by:

1. Binding with the receptors present in the vessels in the kidney, brain, and adrenal glands and thus reversing the resistance to endogenous peptide.
2. Vasodilatation
3. Increasing natriuresis
4. Activation of renin–aldosterone–adrenal axis.

d. Antidiuretic hormone arginine-vasopressin (AVP): It is powerful vasoconstrictor and modulator of transportation of free water through the kidney. There are two types of AVP receptors:

1. V_{1A} receptors: It is responsible for vasoconstriction and mitogenesis of the vascular smooth muscles.
2. V_2 receptors: It reduces the free water excretion and modify the reabsorption of urea and sodium through the kidney. Tolvaptan, V_2 receptor antagonist increases free water clearance and thus reduces congestion.

e. Inotropic drugs are not required in these type of patients. But, if they are already on beta-blocker,

C. Profile C: These patients are both having congestion along with low cardiac output. So, here is aimed at to improve congestion and at the same time to improve perfusion. So treatment should be the following:

a. Patients should be treated with inotropic agents to improve the cardiac output then this patient should be dried with diuretics.

b. Nesiritide should be given in these patients.

c. Levosimendan has been recently used through the following mechanisms:

1. Cardiac contractility is increased which is mediated by calcium sensitization of troponin C.
2. Opening of potassium channels present on the sarcolemma of vascular smooth muscle cells.
3. Opening of potassium channels present in the mitochondria of cardiomyocytes.

d. If hypotension impedes withdrawal of inotropic drugs, ACE inhibitors has to be stopped. Intravenous infusion of inotropic drugs will provide hemodynamics stable. If the patient suffers from chronic decompensated HF with worsening of renal function and elevated urea and creatinine levels in spite of high dose of diuretic therapy, then this inotropic agents are also useful. It may act as "bridging therapy" in these patients who are awaiting for cardiac transplantation or for recovering from severe infections.

D. Profile L: These patients have low output and absence from congestion due to absence of elevated left ventricular filling pressure. So treatment should be following:

a. In patients with low filling pressure volume therapy should be started or vasodilator therapy should be reduced or stopped.

b. In absence of these two conditions treatment should not be difficult. Inotropic drug should not be given. Beta-blockers can be given to reduce the heart rate.

Terminal Heart Failure

It can be defined as an incurable disease due to refractory to conventional as well as recent advancing treatment for HF or no curative treatment at all and threatens the patient's life in <6 months, can produce serious symptoms affecting the functional capacity and mental status of the patients. Following prognostic factors that helps to predict the survival time of the decompensated HF patients are:

A. Clinical:
   a. Ischemic heart disease
   b. Sustained arterial hypotension
   c. NYHA class III and IV
   d. Absence of triggering factors recognizable for treatment
   e. Presence of other concomitant diseases
B. Hemodynamic:
   a. Left ventricular ejection fraction of <20%
   b. Arterial hypotension
   c. Diminished cardiac output
   d. Sinus tachycardia
   e. Renal failure
C. Biochemical:
   a. Hyponatremia
   b. High level of natriuretic peptide
   c. Norepinephrine
D. Electrophysiological:
   a. Presence of potentially serious arrhythmias

Treatment of Terminal Heart Failure

A. 3–5 mg morphine subcutaneously 4 hourly or orally 10–20 mg immediate release morphine should be started 4 hourly followed by gradual increase of the dose to get desired response.
B. Intravenous diazepam should be started at a dose of 5–10 mg 12 hourly, it will reduce anxiety-associated dyspnea as it will perpetuate dyspnea.
C. Oxygen therapy to reduce dyspnea as its effect is psychological.
D. Cardiac transplantation. Indications according to AHA 2001 are the following:
   a. Absolute contraindications:
      1. Hemodynamic involvement due to heart failure:
         - Refractory cardiogenic shock
         - Documented dependency on intravenous inotropic
         - Drugs to maintain adequate perfusion
      2. Peak VO_2 < 10 mL/kg/min after reaching anaerobic metabolism.
      3. Severe symptoms of ischemia that consistently limit normal activity and are not suitable for surgery, coronary revascularization, or PTCA.
      4. Recurrent ventricular arrhythmias that are refractory to all therapeutic modalities.
   b. Relative contraindications:
      1. Peak VO_2 11–14 mL/kg/min or 55% of expected with significant impairment of daily activity.
      2. Unstable and recurrent ischemia that are not suitable for other interventions.
      3. Recurrent instability of fluid balance/renal function not due to poor compliance of the patient with medical therapy
   c. Insufficient indications:
      1. Reduced ejection fraction of left ventricle
      2. History of symptoms of functional class III NHYA class IV HF.
      3. Peak VO_2 15 mL/kg/min or 55% overpredicted without other indications.

Q58. Hypotension.

MGR/SEP2009/MDII (6)

ANSWER

Causes

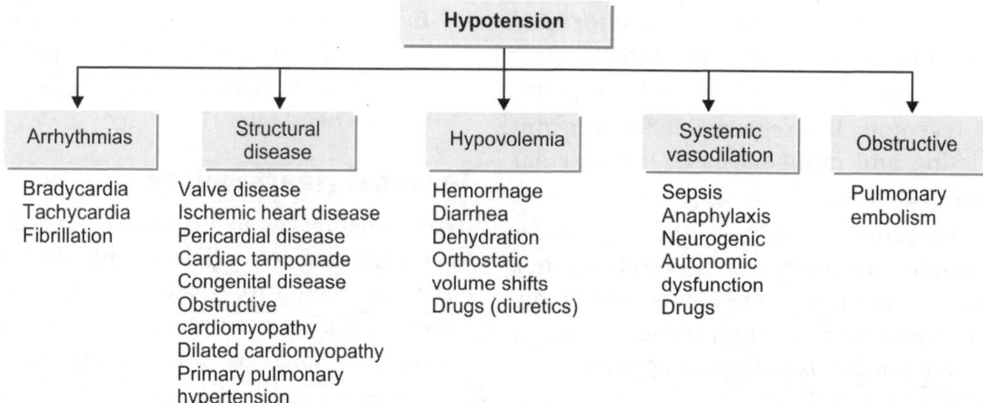

Medications that are Responsible for Low Blood Pressure

a. Diuretics: Furosemide and hydrochlorothiazide
b. Alpha-blockers: Prazosin
c. Beta-blockers: Atenolol and propranolol
d. Drugs in Parkinson's disease: Pramipexole, other drugs containing levodopa
e. Antidepressant: Tricyclic antidepressant, imipramine, and doxepin
f. Drugs for erectile dysfunction: Sildenafil and tadalafil

Types of Low Blood Pressure

a. Orthostatic hypotension: Orthostatic hypertension can be defined as decrease in systolic blood pressure by 20 mm Hg decrease in diastolic blood pressure by 10 mm Hg within 3 minutes of standing as compared to blood pressure in sitting or supine position. It is present in 20% elderly patients.
b. Postprandial hypotension: It is characterized by drop of blood pressure occurred 2–3 hours after eating mostly affecting adult. Blood will flow toward gastrointestinal tract after eating leading to increase in heart rate and constriction of the blood vessels with the aim to stabilize the blood pressure, hence these subjects feel dizziness. It mostly occur in hypertensive patients or patients with Parkinson's disease. It can be corrected by:
    1. Low carbohydrate meals
    2. Drinking more and more water
    3. Avoidance of alcohol
c. Neurally-mediated hypotension: It is characterized by lowering of blood pressure after standing for a long periods affecting mostly adults and children.
d. Low blood pressure due to nervous system damage known as multiple system atrophy with orthostatic hypertension or Shy-Drager syndrome: It occurs due to damage of autonomic nervous system controlling involuntary function such as blood pressure, digestion, and heart rate.

Risk Factors

A. Age: >65 years of age
B. Patients on medication
C. Certain diseases

Clinical Features

a. Faintness
b. Dizziness
c. Lightheadedness
d. Nausea
e. Depression
f. Cold and calmy skin
g. Blurring of vision
h. Loss of consciousness

Diagnosis

A. Laboratory studies:
    a. Fasting blood sugar
    b. Low hemoglobin
B. Electrocardiogram
C. Test for orthostatic hypotension
D. Echocardiogram

Treatment

A. Use of more salts: Excessive use of sodium can rise the blood pressure or can lead to HF.
B. Drinking more and more water: Fluid intake should be increased to prevent dehydration and also hypotension.
C. Compression stockings: Elastic stocking should be used to get relief of pain, swelling of varicose vein, and prevent the accumulation of blood into the legs. Some patients wear abdominal binders.
D. Medications should be taken to increase blood pressure.
E. Treatment of orthostatic hypotension: **To be seen in question number 6**

Q59. Mitral valve prolapse.

MGR/MAR2009/MDII (6)

Mitral valve prolapse.

MAHARASHTRA UNIVERSITY OF HEALTH SCIENCE, 2020 (10)

Importance of DICK in cardiac auscultation and clinical features of MVP.

NTR UNIVERSITY OF HEALTH SC, VIJAYAWADA, ANDHRA, 2022 (10)

ANSWER

Definition

Mitral valve prolapse is characterized by protruding of mitral leaflets > 2 mm beyond the annulus encroaching the left atrium during systole having coaptation points of leaflets lying superior to the annular plane. It is equally prevalent in both sexes.

Etiopathogenesis

There are two types of prolapse:

A. Primary prolapse: It is associated with:
   a. Marfan syndrome
   b. Osteogenesis imperfecta
   c. Ehlers–Danlos syndrome
   d. Loeys–Dietz syndrome
   e. Thoracic skeletal abnormalities:
      1. High-arched palate
      2. Pectus excavatum
      3. Straight back
      4. Scoliosis
   f. Other associated features are:
      1. Bruisability
      2. Meniscal tears
      3. Dislocation of joints
      4. Inguinal hernias
   g. Autosomal dominant mode of inheritance with variable penetrance. There are three loci on chromosomes 11, 13, and 16.
   h. There is myxomatous degeneration of mitral valve leaflets. There is reduced production of type III collagen which can be shown in electron microscopy as fragmented collagen fibrils.

B. Secondary mitral valve prolapse (MVP): Here there is disproportion between size of left ventricular cavity and mitral leaflet, as a result mechanical forces will lead to prolapse of leaflets. It occurs in younger women. It is associated with the following diseases:
   a. ASD
   b. Hyperthyroidism
   c. Emphysema
   d. HOCM

Clinical Features

A. Symptoms:
   a. More common in women of 15–30 years of age, but may occur in older of >50 years of age.
   b. No symptom, these patients can be diagnosed by routine examination or echocardiography.
   c. Chest pain, panic attacks, and instability of autonomic nervous system.
   d. Atrial or ventricular arrhythmias
   e. Transient ischemic attack or stroke

B. Physical findings:
   a. Typical finding is mid-systolic click with late systolic blowing murmur. Systolic click occurs at least 0.14 seconds after first heart sound.
   b. But the dynamic changes like decrease in the size of left ventricle such as decreased venous return, decreased systemic volume, and increased contractility leads to occurrence of earlier click with increased duration of murmur in following cases:
      1. Valsalva maneuver
      2. Standing
      3. Amyl nitrate inhalation
      4. Dehydration
   c. Increase in size of the left ventricle such as increased venous return, increased systemic flow, and decreased contractility leads to occurrence of late systolic click with decreased duration of murmur in following cases:
      1. Squatting
      2. Infusion of phenylephrine
   d. MVP varies in clinical expression. In some cases there is only systolic click and murmur due to mild prolapse of posterior leaflets. In severe cases severe murmur due to rupture of chordae tendineae with flail leaflet.

Investigations

A. ECG: It will demonstrate:
   a. Biphasic or inverted T waves in lead II, III, and aVF.
   b. Ventricular premature beats.

B. Transthoracic echocardiography demonstrates:
   a. Abnormal position and prolapse of mitral valve leaflets.
   b. Systolic displacement of the mitral leaflet bell by at least 2 mm into the left atrium superior to the plane of mitral valve annulus.
   c. One or both leaflets are involved.

C. Color Doppler study measures the color flow and continuous wave can assess the severity. In many cases prolapse is eccentric, in that case assessment of effective regurgitant orifice area and volume is very difficult.

D. Transesophageal echocardiography can assess more accurate anatomic information.

E. Three dimensional echocardiography or cardiac magnetic resonance provides accurate information regarding left ventricular dimension.

Treatment

A. Antibiotic prophylaxis is given in case of infective endocarditis.

B. Beta-blockers can relieve chest pain and it will control palpitation.

C. According to CHA_2DS_2-VASc score stroke can be prevented in case of atrial fibrillation and bleeding risk can be assessed.

D. Indications of surgery:
- **a.** Symptomatic severe MR
- **b.** Signs of established or progressive systolic dysfunction of left ventricle.
- **c.** Pulmonary hypertension
- **d.** Recent onset of atrial fibrillation.

E. Type of surgery:
- **a.** Repair of mitral valve: Transcatheter edge-to-edge repair of the anterior and posterior leaflets in case of symptomatic patients.
- **b.** Mitral valve replacement of flail leaflet or MVP

F. Technical success depends upon:
- **a.** Anatomical defect
- **b.** Skill as well as experience of the surgeon.

G. Reported hospital mortality rate is 2%.

Importance of DICK in Cardiac Auscultation

DICK is a special diastolic sound heard in diastolic phase of the cardiac cycle. It is heard in the following conditions:

A. Mitral stenosis: Opening snap indicating the opening of the mitral valve leaflets during diastole and the leaflets are pliable.

B. Tricuspid stenosis: Opening snap indicating the opening of the tricuspid valve leaflets during diastole and the leaflets are pliable.

C. Constrictive pericarditis: Early pericardial knock in early diastole indicating constrictive pericarditis due to abrupt cessation of ventricular filling as a result of rigid pericardium.

Q60. Discuss in detail the etiopathogenesis of dilated cardiomyopathy, its clinical features, diagnosis, and management.

MGR/APR2015/MDIII (15)

MGR/APR2013/MDIII (15)

Etiopathogenesis of dilated cardiomyopathy. Clinical approach to peripartum cardiomyopathy. Clinical approach to peripartum cardiomyopathy.

NTR UNIVERSITY OF HEALTH SC, VIJAYAWADA, ANDHRA, 2022 (10)

Classify cardiomyopathy. Discuss pathophysiology, clinical features, lab diagnosis, and management of dilated cardiomyopathy.

MGR UNIVERSITY, TAMIL NADU, 2019 (15)

Dilated cardiomyopathy—etiology, clinical features, and management.

MGR UNIVERSITY, TAMIL NADU, 2020 (10)

Discuss briefly cardiomyopathies.

SAMS (ODISHA), 2021 (10)

Question number 07, 60, 125, 106

ANSWER

Definition

It can be defined as enlargement as well as dilatation of the both ventricles due to heart muscle disease leading to impaired contractility as evidenced by reduced ejection fraction, i.e., <40% seen by echocardiography.

Etiological Classification

A. Primary or idiopathic dilated cardiomyopathy:
- **a.** Familial or genetic predisposition due to mutation of following genes:
  1. Desmin (cytoskeletal)
  2. Lamin C (nuclear membrane)
  3. Myosin (contractile protein)

B. Secondary dilated cardiomyopathy:
- **a.** Infectious myocarditis:
  1. Viral
     - Adenovirus

- Rabies
- Echovirus
- Hepatitis
- Yellow fever
- Influenza virus A and B
- Coxsackie virus

2. Chagas disease
3. Lyme disease
4. Whipple's disease

b. Ischemic disease due to coronary artery disease
c. Hypertension
d. Metabolic and endocrine related:
   1. Hyperthyroidism
   2. Hypothyroidism
   3. Acromegaly
   4. Hypoparathyroidism
   5. Hyperparathyroidism
   6. Diabetes mellitus
   7. Electrolyte imbalance—potassium, phosphate, and magnesium
e. Nutritional deficiency:
   1. Thiamine deficiency
   2. Protein deficiency
   3. Starvation
f. Toxins:
   1. Medicine-induced (anthracycline), vascular endothelial growth factor.
   2. Poisons
   3. Anesthetic drugs
   4. Heavy metals
g. Alcohol abuse
h. HIV
i. Peripartum cardiomyopathy
j. Connective tissue diseases:
   1. Rheumatoid arthritis
   2. Scleroderma
   3. Systemic lupus erythematosus (SLE)
k. Infiltrative disease:
   1. Hemochromatosis
   2. Amyloidosis
l. Stressed cardiomyopathy (Takotsubo cardiomyopathy)
m. Broken heart syndrome
n. Physical agents:
   1. Extremes of temperature
   2. Electric shock
   3. Ionizing radiation
o. Immunologic:
   1. Postvaccination
   2. Transplant rejection
   3. Serum sickness

Pathophysiology

It is characterized by enlargement of left ventricular cavity along with enlargement of the cavity size but with little or no hypertrophy which can be estimated by decreased ratio of left ventricular mass to size of the cavity. It is associated with both left ventricular systolic and diastolic dysfunction but primary abnormality being systolic dysfunction due to abnormal left ventricular remodeling which ultimately leads to increased end-diastolic and end-systolic volumes.

Enlargement of the other chambers is mainly secondary to enlargement of left ventricular cavity. Progressive ventricular dilatation will lead mitral and tricuspid regurgitation that will lead to further decrease in cardiac output and increase in end-systolic volume and increases the myocardial wall stress.

In early phase systolic dysfunction is compensated by increasing the stroke volume and heart rate along with increase in peripheral vascular resistance, all of which are responsible for maintaining the blood pressure within normal limit.

In case of systolic decompensation entire pressure-volume loop will be shifted to right side along with increase in end-diastolic pressure and end-diastolic volume.

Coronary arterial flow will also be decreased by:

a. Hypotension
b. Elevated wall stress
c. Decreasing the perfusion gradient

According to Frank-Starling law when myocardial force at end-diastole is compared with end-systole, there will be increase in muscle length, as result greater amount of force is required. So overstretching of the myocardial unit will lead to failure of that unit.

Compensatory mechanisms will be blunted and additionally these will lead to further myocardial injury as well as myocardial dysfunction through eccentric or concentric remodeling.

Neurohumoral Activation

Low cardiac output will lead to decreased organ perfusion resulting:

a. Activation of adrenergic nervous system: It will increase the circulating level of dopamine, norepinephrine. It will increase the sympathetic tone and decrease the parasympathetic tone, all of which will lead to increased cardiac output through the beta-adrenergic receptors and peripheral vascular tone through alpha-adrenergic receptors. Long time exposure to these catecholamine will ultimately lead to down-regulation of the receptors present in the myocardium resulting blunting of all the responses. Stimulation of alpha-adrenergic receptors increases the myocardial workload by increasing the peripheral vascular resistance.

b. Activation of renin–angiotensin–aldosterone system: In this system increased level of angiotensin II will perform following functions:
   1. Increased secretion of catecholamine leads to increased systemic vascular resistance.
   2. Increases the secretion of aldosterone leading to retention of sodium and water.
   3. It will aggravate myocardial fibrosis.

c. Release of vasopressin: It will be released from hypothalamus and controlled by hyponatremia through osmotic stimuli and hypotension and diuresis through nonosmotic stimuli. It will perform following functions:
   1. It will aggravate peripheral vascular resistance.
   2. It will reduce free water clearance through kidney.

d. Secretion of neuropeptides: There are three natriuretic peptides:
   1. Atrial natriuretic peptide: It will be released from atria due to stretching of atrial muscles. Its effects are the following:
      - Vasodilatation
      - Attenuation of cell growth
      - Inhibition of aldosterone
      - Diuresis
   2. Brain natriuretic peptide: It is secreted from ventricles as a result of volume and pressure overload, mainly in chronic HF. Its effects are:
      - Vasodilatation
      - Natriuresis
   3. C-type natriuretic peptide

Body's compensatory mechanisms ultimately will be overwhelmed leading to further decompensation of myocardial function.

Circulating cytokine function acting as a factor of injury to myocardium:

a. Tissue necrosis factor-alpha is responsible for dysfunction of left ventricle, it may be due to apoptosis myocardial muscle cells or by direct depression of myocardial function.
b. Interleukin-1b will depress the myocardial function.
c. Interleukin-2R is increased in case of congestive cardiac failure activated by T-lymphocytes.
d. Interleukin-6 stimulates hepatic production of CRP, a marker of inflammation. IL-6 will correlate with hemodynamic function that occurred as a result of left ventricular dysfunction.

Clinical Features

A. History:
   a. Following symptoms are indicator of severity of the disease:
      1. Dyspnea on exertion
      2. Orthopnea
      3. Paroxysmal nocturnal dyspnea
      4. Increasing weight gain
      5. Increasing weight
      6. Fatigue
   b. Medical history related to this disease:
      1. Angina
      2. Anemia
      3. Hypertension
      4. Breast cancer
      5. Coronary artery disease
      6. Prior history of myocardial injury
      7. Addition of new medication or noncompliant to old medications
      8. Social history relating to alcohol and smoking
      9. Family history of sudden cardiac death or cardiomyopathy.

B. Physical signs:
   a. Vital signs:
      1. Tachycardia
      2. Tachypnea
      3. Hypertension
   b. Other findings related to this disease:
      1. Engorged pulsatile jugular vein
      2. Signs of hypoxia:
         - Cyanosis
         - Clubbing
      3. Pedal edema
      4. Crepitation at the bases of lungs
      5. Tender and enlarged liver

c. Following findings in the neck are important in regard to the decompensation:
   1. Jugular venous distension
   2. A wave
   3. Large CV wave indicating the presence of tricuspid regurgitation.
   4. Presence of hepatojugular reflex.

d. Examination of heart:
   1. Shifting of apical impulse
   2. Right ventricular heave
   3. There may be paradoxical splitting of second heart sound with loud P2
   4. S3 or S4 may be noted—these are low frequency sound best heard with the bell.
   5. Gallop may be heard in case of cardiac decompensation.

Investigations

Following are the work-up of dilated cardiomyopathy:

A. Complete blood count: Documentation of anemia

B. Comprehensive metabolic panel: To detect:
   a. Hyponatremia
   b. Raised creatinine from parent disease or secondary to drug like ACE inhibitors.
   c. Contraction alkalosis secondary to diuretic therapy.
   d. Hypomagnesemia because it may produce refractory hypokalemia which can be corrected by administration of magnesium.

C. Liver function test: It will be done to detect:
   a. Alcoholic liver disease
   b. Hemochromatosis
   c. Hepatic congestion—nutmeg liver

D. Thyroid function test

E. Cardiac biomarkers: Serum markers of myocardial necrosis such as troponin, creatine kinase, and creatine kinase-B are elevated in myocarditis.

F. Iron studies

G. B-type natriuretic peptide: It is helpful to monitor the presence as well as overload of fluid. Its serial level can monitor the treatment.

H. Chest radiography:
   a. Enlargement of heart and increased cardiothoracic ratio.
   b. Pulmonary vascular congestion along with interstitial edema suggests acute decompensated HF.
   c. Concave hilar shadow with prominent vasculature in upper lung field.
   d. Right-sided or bilateral pleural effusion.
   e. Presence of abnormal calcification in valve or in pericardium.

I. Echocardiography:
   a. Pulmonary embolism can be differentiated from the pulmonary hypertension by presence of right ventricular enlargement.
   b. M-mode study measures:
      1. Left ventricular end-diastolic dimension of >65 mm.
      2. Hypertrophy can be measured left ventricular mass index >115 g/m^2 in men and >95 g/m^2 in women.
   c. Doppler study can measure:
      1. The flow velocity through the mitral and tricuspid valves.
      2. Evaluating left ventricular filling to pulmonary venous flow by assessing E to A ratio: This provides the information on left ventricular diastolic function and pressure in the left atrium.
      3. Tissue Doppler interrogation: It will measure velocity of a portion of ventricular wall mainly the left ventricular basilar annular area.
      4. Segmental wall motion abnormalities suggests ischemic etiology.

J. Cardiac MRI with gadolinium contrast can evaluate extent of mid-wall fibrosis as it may correlate with the risk of arrhythmias and failure to get improved following treatment. In future it will be used for risk stratification in patients with dilated cardiomyopathy.

K. CT scan:
   a. It can assess the biventricular volume and ejection fraction.
   b. To assess the ischemic cardiomyopathy Agatston coronary calcium score of 0–100% specificity to exclude coronary artery disease.
   c. CT angiography can detect:
      1. Infiltrative disease as evidenced by heterogenous attenuation of myocardium.
      2. Location of HOCM
      3. Right ventricular arrhythmogenic dysplasia
      4. Left ventricular decompensation
      5. Congenital malformation

L. Electrocardiography:
  - **a.** Atrial fibrillation
  - **b.** Left ventricular hypertrophy
  - **c.** Premature ventricular complexes
  - **d.** Left bundle branch block
  - **e.** Varying degrees of AV block

M. Cardiac catheterization: It can demonstrate the following:
  - **a.** Central venous pressure
  - **b.** Pulmonary artery wedge pressure
  - **c.** Right ventricular end-diastolic pressure
  - **d.** Pulmonary vascular resistance
  - **e.** Mixed venous saturation
  - **f.** Adequacy of cardiac output

N. Toxicology screening for screening of drugs, poison, metals, cocaine, and methamphetamine

O. Endomyocardial biopsy: Class II indications are:
  - **a.** Rapidly deteriorating cardiac function of recent onset.
  - **b.** Patients on chemotherapy with doxorubicin.
  - **c.** Possibility of cardiac involvement in patients with systemic diseases such as sarcoidosis, hemochromatosis, amyloidosis, and endomyocardial fibroelastosis.

Staging: It is based on the NYHA system:

A. Stage A (high risk of developing HF): Hypertension, diabetes mellitus, coronary artery disease, and family history of cardiomyopathy

B. Stage B (asymptomatic HF): Previous history of myocardial infarction, asymptomatic valvular disease, and left ventricular systolic dysfunction

C. Stage C (symptomatic left ventricular failure): Structural heart disease, fatigue, dyspnea, and reduced exercise tolerance

D. Stage D (refractory end-stage HF): In spite of maximal treatment marked symptoms at rest, recurrent hospitalization

Treatment

According to 2016 AHA following are the update of HF therapies:

A. ACE inhibitors

B. ARBs

C. Beta-blockers

D. Aldosterone antagonists

E. Cardiac glycosides

F. Diuretics

G. Nitrates

H. Vasodilators

I. Sacubitril-valsartan combination should be used in case of HF with reduced ejection fraction of <40% and NYHA class ≥ II to reduce mortality, reduce period of hospitalization as compared to enalapril treatment.

J. Ivabradine

K. Human B-type natriuretic peptide: It is produced through the recombinant DNA technology with same amino acid sequence as that of human BNP. It will effectively correct the hemodynamic derangement in decompensated HF through its vasodilating and diuretic effect.

L. Inotropic agents: Phosphodiesterase inhibitor milrinone is reserved for following patients:
  - **a.** During acute decompensation of HF hemodynamic directed treatment
  - **b.** Those who are refractory to medical therapy
  - **c.** Palliation of end-stage HF
  - **d.** Act as bridging to transplantation of heart

M. Anticoagulants: It is used in patients with:
  - **a.** Atrial fibrillation,
  - **b.** Mural thrombus
  - **c.** Artificial valves

N. Left ventricular-assisted device: It is used in case of advanced HF as a bridge to transplantation. It is also approved as a permanent implantation.

O. Cardiac resynchronization therapy (biventricular pacing): Here pulse generator is placed under the skin with leads positioned in the right atrium, right ventricle, and through coronary sinus to pace left ventricle. This therapy also has defibrillating capabilities.

Current indications of class-I resynchronization therapy are:
  - **a.** NYHA class I symptoms of longer than 40 days following myocardial infarction, left ventricular ejection fraction of ≤30%, sinus rhythm, and LBBB with duration of QRS complex ≥ 150 ms.
  - **b.** NYHA class II or greater on guideline-directed medical therapy with persisting symptoms of longer than 40 days after myocardial infarction, left ventricular ejection fraction of ≤35%, sinus rhythm, and LBBB with QRS duration of ≥150 ms.

P. Automatic implantable cardioverter-defibrillators: It has a potential to detect and correct ventricular tachycardia/ventricular fibrillation. Programmable therapies are:

a. Antitachycardia pacing for ventricular tachycardia
b. Defibrillatory shock

Indications of ICD: According to AHA/ACC 2013 guidelines:

a. Class IA: Primary prevention of sudden death in patients with HF with reduced ejection fraction 40 days after myocardial infarction having left ventricular ejection fraction of ≤35% or NYHA class II and III symptomatic patients on guideline-directed medical therapy and expected to live >1 year.
b. Class IB: Primary prevention of sudden death in patients with HF with reduced ejection fraction 40 days after myocardial infarction having left ventricular ejection fraction of ≤30% with NYHA class I symptoms receiving goal-directed medical therapy and expected to live >1 year.

Q. Ventricular restoration surgery

R. Transplantation of heart:

a. Absolute indications are:
   1. Refractory cardiogenic shock.
   2. Patient is dependent on inotropic infusion for organ perfusion.
   3. Severe ischemia not responding to any intervention.
   4. Peak oxygen consumption of <1 mL/kg/min with achievement of anaerobic threshold.
   5. Symptomatic ventricular arrhythmias which is refractory to therapy.
b. Relative contraindications:
   1. Peak oxygen consumption of 11–14 mL/kg/min along with major limitation in the daily activity.
   2. Recurrent unstable chronic HF neither due to noncompliance nor suboptimal medical therapy.

S. Gene therapies:

a. This therapy is under investigation. Recombinant adeno-associated viral gene therapy along with transfer of phospholamban has been successfully prevented left ventricular systolic and diastolic dysfunction.
b. Vascular endothelial growth factor has beneficial effect on ischemic cardiomyopathies, improving angina, and reducing revascularization.

T. Myoblast transplantation: It involves injection of skeletal myoblast as autograft into the myocardial scar. It is under trial.

U. Stem cell transplantation: Autologous stem cell when injected intracardially or intravenously in patients with congestive cardiac failure it demonstrated to prevent the abnormal cardiac remodeling.

V. CardioMEMS: It is wireless pulmonary artery pressure monitoring system that will guide management as well as reduction of hospital stay. According to ESC 2016 guidelines, it should be done in class IIB recommendations in patients with HF to reduce the risk of recurrence.

Drug	Initiation	Target dose
ACE inhibitors		
Lisinopril	2.5–5 mg four times daily	20–35 mg four times daily
Enalapril	2.5 mg twice daily	10–20 mg twice daily
Captopril	6.25 mg thrice daily	50 mg twice daily
Trandolapril	0.5–1 mg four times daily	4 mg four times daily
ARBs		
Losartan	50 mg four times daily	150 mg four times daily
Valsartan	40 mg twice daily	160 mg twice daily
Candesartan	4–8 mg four times daily	32 mg four times daily
Aldosterone antagonists		
Eplerenone	25 mg four times daily	50 mg four times daily
Spironolactone	12.5–25 mg four times daily	25–50 mg four times daily
Beta-blockers		
Metoprolol	12.5–25 mg four times daily	200 mg four times daily
Carvedilol	3.125 mg twice daily	25–50 mg twice daily
Bisoprolol	1.25 mg four times daily	10 mg four times daily
Arteriovenous vasodilators		
Hydralazine/ Isosorbide dinitrate	37.5/20 mg thrice daily	75/40 mg thrice daily

Continued

Continued

Drug	Initiation	Target dose
Fixed-dose hydralazine/ Isosorbide dinitrate	37.5/20 mg thrice daily	75/40 mg four times daily
Angiotensin receptor-neprilysin inhibitor		
Sacubitril–valsartan	100 mg twice daily	200 mg twice daily

Peripartum cardiomyopathy: Answers to be taken from question 30.

Q61. Pleiotropic effects of statins and the latest controversies associated with its use.

MGR/MGR/APR2015/MDIV (7)

Statins.

MUHS/MAY2013/MDIV (10)

ANSWER

Introduction

There is clear association between atherosclerosis and elevation of plasma cholesterol. Cholesterol is the prime component of cell wall, steroid hormones, and bile acids. Rate-limiting enzyme hydroxymethylglutaryl CoA reductase catalyzing the conversion of HMG-CoA to mevalonic acid which is inhibited by statins.

A. **Effects of statins and isoprenylated proteins**:

By inhibiting L-mevalonic acid synthesis it will decrease the synthesis of intermediates of biosynthetic pathway of cholesterol which is helpful in post-translational modification of different proteins such as heme-a, heterotrimeric G-protein, nuclear lamins, and GTP-binding proteins.

B. **Statin and endothelial function**:

Vascular endothelium is responsible for contractile function as well as cellular composition of the vascular wall. Hypercholesterolemia produces endothelial dysfunction, the earliest manifestation of atherosclerosis leading to impaired synthesis, release, and activity of nitric oxide. As nitric oxide is responsible for vascular relaxation, inhibits aggregation of platelets, vascular smooth muscle proliferation as well as interaction between leukocyte-endothelial, so absence of bioavailability of nitric oxide leads to vasoconstriction and hypertension. Statin improves the endothelial function by:

a. Lowering the serum cholesterol level
b. It decreases angiotensin II-induced production of free radicle in the vascular smooth muscle cells by downregulating AT II receptors expression and Rac-1-mediated NADH activity.
c. Increases the endothelial nitric oxide production by increasing the nitric oxide synthetase activity via posttranslational activation of phosphatidylinositol 3-kinase pathway.
d. Increases the expression of tissue plasminogen activator.
e. Inhibits the potent vasoconstrictor endothelin-1 expression.
f. Caveolin, it binds to endothelial nitric oxide synthetase to downregulate the enzyme. Statin inhibits caveolin.
g. It inhibits the production of reactive oxygen species like superoxide thereby enhancing the endothelium-dependent relaxation of smooth muscle cells.

C. **Statin and progenitor cells**:

a. It increases angiogenesis through proliferation, migration, and survival of circulating endothelial progenitor cells.

D. **Statin and proliferation of smooth muscle cells**:

a. Smooth muscle cells proliferation plays a central role in any vascular lesions, such as postangioplasty restenosis, transplant atherosclerosis. Statin inhibits isoprenoid synthesis decreases platelet-derived growth factor-induced hyperphosphorylation and cyclin-dependent kinase activities.
b. Statin arrests cell cycle at G1/S phase transition thereby inhibiting vascular smooth muscle cells proliferation.

E. **Statin and function of platelets**:

At the site of rupture of plaque there is formation of platelet-associated thrombus which is accompanied by hypercholesterolemia is responsible for acute coronary syndrome—it is due to increased cholesterol/ phospholipid ratio in the platelet. Other mechanisms of ACS are increased biosynthesis of thromboxane A2 level, increased density of α_2 receptor, and cytosolic calcium in the platelet. Statin effects are:

a. Increased endothelial nitric oxide synthesis inhibits platelet aggregation.
b. There is downregulation of platelet reactivity markers. Reduction of production of thromboxane A_2.

c. It reduces content of the cholesterol in the platelet.

F. **Platelet and plaques**:

Atherosclerotic lesion in the blood vessels is formed centrally by highly thrombogenic material surrounded by fibrous cap separating it from blood stream. Plaque rupture occurs as a result of fissuring, erosion, and ulceration of the fibrous cap which leads to thrombosis eventually. Collagen being the main component of the fibrous cap is responsible for tensile strength of the fibrous cap. Activated macrophages secretes proteolytic enzyme metalloproteinase weakens the fibrous cap at its shoulder region at the sites of its joining with the arterial wall leading to plaque instability, rupture followed by thrombosis. Statin stabilizes the plaques and reduces the incidence of acute coronary syndrome by:

a. Reducing the size of the plaques
b. Altering the physicochemical properties of the lipid core
c. Inhibiting the expression of matrix metalloproteinase and tissue factors by both cholesterol-independent and cholesterol-dependent pathways.

G. **Statin and vascular inflammation**:

Cytokines secreted by macrophages, T-lymphocytes will modify the functions of endothelial cells, proliferation of smooth muscle cells, cellular degradation, and thrombosis. In the early stage monocytes adhere to endothelium and penetrate into subendothelial cells.

a. Statin reduces the number of inflammatory cells by inhibition of adhesion molecules like intracellular adhesion molecule-1 that is responsible for recruitment of inflammatory cells.
b. Statin decreases the expression of P-selectin and leukocyte adhesion by increased production of nitric oxide.
c. Major histocompatibility complex class II (MHC-II) and CD40/CD40L activates T-lymphocytes thereby controlling immune response, important regulator in this pathway being transactivator CIITA. Statin inhibits the promotors IV of transactivator CIITA leading to inhibition of MHC-II expression present on the endothelial cells and monocytes and macrophages.
d. In case of low-grade inflammation cytokines like interleukin-6 produced in the liver produces high sensitivity-CRP, acute phase reactant, and predictive of acute coronary artery disease. Statin will lower this hs-CRP

All the above effects will lead to decreased evidence of stroke, acute coronary artery diseases, and dementia.

Q62. Drug-eluting stents.

MGR/MAR2010/MDIV (6)
MGR/MAR2006/MDI (5)
MUHS/MAY2011/MDIV (10)

Discuss bare-metal stents versus drug-eluting stent, advantages and disadvantages.

BF/NOV2013/MDIV (10)

Drug eluting stents.

MGR UNIVERSITY, TAMIL NADU, 2020 (10)

ANSWER

Bare-metal Stent

This stent is flexible, polished, laser-cut, balloon-mounted, and expandable tube which is composed of stainless steel or metal like chromium-cobalt.

Advantages being:

a. Very effective in treatment of dissection
b. Reduces the incidence of sudden closure
c. Reduces restenosis
d. Can be used during CABG.

Disadvantages are:

a. High incidences of subacute closure in spite of intensive anticoagulation regimen.
b. There is increased incidence of bleeding complications requiring hospitalization.

These have been minimized by:

a. Improvement in periprocedural antithrombotic regimen
b. Use of high pressure implantation of stents
c. Evolution of stent design
d. Easy delivery of the stent

Restenosis rate is increased with this stent because of the following reasons:

a. Small reference vessel size
b. Small postprocedural luminal diameter
c. Long lesion length
d. Diabetes
e. Lesions located in the left anterior descending artery
f. Presence of untreated edge dissection during the procedure

Drug-eluting Stent

These are the vascular prostheses used to reopen and maintain the atherosclerotic coronary arteries. There are three characteristics of drug-eluting stent (DES), these are:

A. Scaffold
B. Drug-delivery mechanism, i.e., polymer
C. Therapeutic agents used

There are several generations of DES:

A. First-generation of DES: Here the scaffold is stainless steel coated with sirolimus and paclitaxel.

B. Second-generation of DES: Here the scaffold is cobalt-chromium made with different polymer coating that allows:
  - **a.** Decreased strut thickness
  - **b.** Improved flexibility
  - **c.** Deliverability
  - **d.** Enhanced bioavailability
  - **e.** Better eluting profile
  - **f.** Superior neo-endothelialization

C. Third-generation DES: Here scaffold is entirely bioabsorbable coated with biodegradable polymer: This is under clinical testing. In this bioabsorbable polymer DES everolimus is allowed to be eluted from platinum-chromium polymer which is absorbed overtime.

First bioabsorbable polymer DES is synergy stent—here it elutes everolimus from the platinum-chromium platform, later on the polymer will also be absorbed overtime, then only the effect of bare-metal stent will remain.

But in case of DES, polymer will be on the stent surface after drug elution.

Scaffoldings

Stents can be classified according to metallic basis and design. Different metallic compounds are further characterized by their unique physical properties like:

- **a.** Radial strength: It measures the resistance to external compression.
- **b.** Ferromagnecity
- **c.** Material fatigue
- **d.** Radiolucency: It means visibility of the stent during angiography.

Stainless steel has good radiolucency and lack of ferromagnetism.

Therapeutic Agents

Antiproliferative agents prevent proliferation of vascular smooth muscle cells and neointimal hyperplasia.

Paclitaxel inhibits microtubules thus inhibits cell cycle leading to its arrest in G0–G1 and G–M phase.

Sirolimus binds to FKBP12 thus inhibiting mTOR and P13 pathway leading to cell cycle arrest in G1 phase.

Zotarolimus and everolimus will arrest cell division during mitotic division in the growth phase.

Other therapeutic agents under investigation are:

- **a.** Dual DES carrying two therapeutic agents: Antiproliferative and antithrombotic agents.
- **b.** Phytocide has antiproliferative and anti-inflammatory effects.
- **c.** Glucocorticoid has anti-inflammatory effect which leads to prevention of restenosis.
- **d.** Gene-eluting stents delivering plasmid DNA that appreciated proteins inside the cells. Example is vascular endothelial growth factor helps proper and healthy endothelialization in the luminal surface of the stent.
- **e.** Tacrolimus
- **f.** Galangin
- **g.** Probucol
- **h.** Radioactive stent

Coating

It serves following for different purposes:

- **a.** It facilitates adhesion of stent.
- **b.** It helps in release of drugs.
- **c.** It increases bioavailability.
- **d.** It modulates thrombogenicity.

Polymers help in drug delivery in following methods:

- **a.** Diffusion
- **b.** Dissolution
- **c.** Ion exchange

Most important complication is stent thrombosis: It is defined as:

- **a.** Early, i.e., within 30 days
- **b.** Late, i.e., 30 days to 1 year
- **c.** Very late, i.e., >1 year

It may be related to the following factors:

A. Stent-related factors: Following implantation of DES re-endothelialization takes several weeks due to antiproliferative effects of the polymer. Incidence of stent thrombosis is 0.5–1% per year.

B. Procedure-related factors:

a. Incomplete apposition of stent to plaque or vessel wall

b. Inadequate expansion of stent

c. Dissection of stent edge

Risk factors are:

a. Intravascular ultrasound imaging to optimize the stent length

b. Long length of the lesion

c. Diameter of small artery

d. Complex lesion morphology

C. Patient-related factors:

a. Diabetes

b. Renal disease

c. Impaired left ventricular function

d. Premature cessation of dual antiplatelet therapy due to:

1. Nonadherence
2. Need for surgery
3. Bleeding complication
4. Financial consideration

D. Duration of antiplatelet therapy: In case of patients with acute coronary syndrome 12 months dual antiplatelet therapy is recommended to reduce major adverse cardiac events. In case of DES early cessation of dual antiplatelet therapy will lead to significant number of stent thrombosis.

Q63. Ebstein's anomaly.
MGR/SEP2008/MDIII (6)

ANSWER

Anatomic Abnormality

In this anomaly anterior leaflet can be redundant or fenestrated or sail like or it may be adherent to underlying myocardium along with apical displacement of the septal and posterior leaflets along with failure of reabsorption of the valve tissue. As a result there is distortion and displacement of tricuspid valve leaflets, the result is artialization of right ventricle. Associated congenital, structural, or conduction abnormalities.

Hemodynamic Consequences

a. Tricuspid regurgitation due to leaflet abnormalities and its severity depends upon extent of displacement—it may be minimum to severe displacement.

b. Atrialized right ventricle will contract and relaxe with right ventricle, but during discordant contraction of right ventricle it will lead to stagnation of blood in the right atrium.

c. During right ventricular contraction blood will be regurgitated into right atrium and accentuates regurgitation.

Etiology

A. It is congenital disease of uncertain origin.

B. But following maternal environmental factors can influence the etiology:

a. Benzodiazepine use

b. Exposure to varnishing substances

c. History of previous fetal loss

d. Ingestion of lithium in first trimester of pregnancy

Epidemiology

It is more common in child of white females. It may present in the following stages:

A. Fetal life: It can be accidentally diagnosed by echocardiography.

B. Neonatal life and in infancy: Patients present with cyanosis and HF: It is typically present in infancy but it will improve with increased resistance in pulmonary vasculature.

C. Adult life: In this age patients present with fatigue, cyanosis, dyspnea evidence of tricuspid regurgitation, and/or right-sided HF.

Clinical Features

A. Related to anatomic abnormalities of this diseases:

a. Cyanosis

b. Fatigue and dyspnea

c. Symptoms-related to right-sided HF

d. Palpitations

e. Sudden cardiac death

B. Other less common presenting features are:

a. Bacterial endocarditis

b. Brain abscess as a result of right to left heart shunt

c. Paradoxical embolism such as stroke, TIA

Physical Findings

a. Cyanosis

b. Clubbing

c. Asymmetry of the precordium

d. Jugular venous pulse

e. Arterial pulses: Normal, but may be diminished in late course.

f. Heart sound:

1. Wide split first heart sound: Loud tricuspid component and soft mitral component.
2. Presence of prolonged PR interval
3. Normal second heart sound, occasionally wide split and delayed pulmonary component due to RBBB
4. Third and fourth heart sounds are commonly present.

Laboratory Testing

A. ECG:

a. Normal sinus rhythm

b. Arrhythmias:

1. Intermittent and paroxysmal supraventricular tachycardia
2. Atrial flutter
3. Atrial fibrillation
4. Ventricular tachycardia

c. Abnormal P-wave indicating right atrial enlargement.

d. Prolonged PR interval

e. RBBB

f. Low voltage QRS complexes

B. Chest X-ray:

a. Normal features

b. Cardiomegaly

c. Large right atrium

d. Small aortic root and main pulmonary artery shadow

e. Decreased pulmonary vasculature

C. Echocardiography:

a. M-mode echocardiography:

1. Paradoxical septal wall motion
2. Dilated right ventricle
3. Delayed closure of tricuspid valve which is >65 msec than mitral valve closure

b. Two dimensional (2D) echocardiography:

1. Eccentric coaptation of leaflet.
2. Dilated right atrium.
3. Dilated right ventricle with its decreased contractile performance.
4. Abnormal morphology and septal attachment of anterior and septal tricuspid leaflets.

c. Doppler studies:

1. Varying degrees of tricuspid regurgitation.
2. Associated shunts have to be excluded.

D. MRI

Management

A. Pharmacotherapy:

a. Diuretic therapy like furosemide

b. Administration of cardiac glycosides like digoxin

c. ACE inhibitors like enalapril

B. Surgical therapy:

a. Correction of tricuspid valve abnormalities and right ventricular abnormalities.

b. Any associated cardiac abnormalities should be corrected.

c. Palliative procedures to be done in the early days of life that act as bridging procedure to definite surgical procedure to be done in adult life.

d. Cardiac transplantation.

Prognosis

A. Male sex

B. Presentation in early age

C. Cardiothoracic ration of >0.65 in chest radiograph

D. Ratio of distance between AV ring and distal attachment of septal leaflet to septal; leaflet length is >0.45

E. Increasing ration of right atrium and atrialized right ventricle to functional right ventricle is:

a. Grade 1: <0.5

b. Grade 4: >1.5

F. NHYA class: It is linked with mortality rate.

Q64. Enumerate the therapeutic procedure of recurrent arrhythmia. Add a note on catheter ablation.

MGR/OCT2012/MDIV (7)

Device therapy in cardiac arrhythmias.

DNB, 2019 (5)

ANSWER

Following are the procedures for recurrent arrhythmia:

A. Invasive therapies:

a. Electrical cardioversion: It is performed in a patient after administration of short-acting anesthesia. The electrical impulse is delivered through the chest wall to synchronize the heart and thus normal rhythm to restart.

b. Catheter ablation

c. Pulmonary vein isolation: In case of persistent or paroxysmal atrial fibrillation the aim to isolate the foci around the pulmonary vein in the form of ring or scar by ablation.

B. Different devices:

a. Permanent pacemaker

b. Implantable cardioverter-defibrillator: It can prevent ventricular tachycardia or ventricular fibrillation by constant monitoring of cardiac rhythm. There are three ways by which it can restore normal rhythm:

1. Antitachycardia pacing: In case of very fast rhythm it will deliver energy to the cardiac muscles to beat the heart in normal rhythm again.
2. Cardioversion/Defibrillation: When heart beats very fast and in very irregular way then it will deliver a shock to the cardiac muscles to restore the cardiac muscles again.
3. Antibradycardia pacing: It acts as back-up pacing to prevent too slow heart rate.

c. Biventricular pacemakers and defibrillators, i.e., cardiac resynchronization therapy.

Catheter Ablation

In this method radiofrequency energy is delivered through the catheter to destroy a small area of connective tissue in order to restore normal sinus rhythm.

Indications of Ablation

A. Typical right atrial flutter

B. Atrioventricular nodal reentrant tachycardia

C. Atrioventricular reentrant tachycardia

D. Atrial tachycardia

E. Paroxysmal atrial fibrillation in structurally normal heart.

F. Ventricular tachycardia in structurally normal heart.

Contraindications and Precautions

A. Patient should be hemodynamically stable.

B. Decompensated HF should be converted into compensated HF.

C. Active managed infection

D. Ongoing bleeding should be managed.

E. Respiratory difficulty, airway problem, and difficulty in lying in flat positions should be addressed because this procedure take several hours to perform.

F. Consultation and preanesthetic consent is required from the anesthetics because it should be performed under general anesthesia.

Vascular Access

A. Right atrial and ventricular ablation through the femoral venous access.

B. Left atrial ablation through femoral venous access then through transseptal puncture from right to left atrium.

C. Left ventricle ablation through femoral venous or femoral arterial access.

Anticoagulation

A. In patients having arrhythmias on oral anticoagulation, no interruption of anticoagulation is required.

B. In case of catheters requiring ablation in left atrium and left ventricle should require heparin infusion after the vascular access being established with a goal of activated clotting time of 300–450 seconds.

C. In case arterial access INR should be 1.5–2.0.

Different Methods Used in Ablation

A. Radiofrequency ablations: Here the energy is delivered to raise the temperature to over 50°C to produce irreversible tissue injury. Amount of energy delivered depends upon degree of tissue resistance.

B. Irrigated-tip catheters are done for atrial fibrillation and scar-mediated ventricular tachycardia as it requires larger area of ablation and also requires longer time to ablate.

C. Contact force catheter: It is force-sensing catheter having a sensor at the tip to provide feedback regarding the direction as well as force of the catheter tip.

D. Phased-array catheter: It has a goal of delivering two pattern of ablation such as circular and linear in more efficient manner.

E. Cryoablation:

a. In this method, cryorefrigerant is used to the targeted tissue to reduce the temperature to –40°C both in extracellular and intracellular compartments to produce mechanical destruction.

b. Cryoballoon catheter: It is done to isolate pulmonary vein by positioning the catheter with balloon-tipped containing cryorefrigerant within the ostium of pulmonary vein.

Postprocedural Complications

A. Major complications:

- **a.** Overall mortality rate is 3–6%.
- **b.** Vascular access:
  1. Hematoma
  2. Retroperineal bleeding
  3. Pseudoaneurysm
  4. AV fistula
- **c.** Cardiac perforation
- **d.** Cardiac tamponade
- **e.** Thromboembolism
- **f.** Death
- **g.** Others:
  1. Atrial-esophageal fistula
  2. Injury to conduction system
  3. Genitourinary system
  4. Pulmonary edema
- **h.** Complications unique to ablation of ventricular tachycardia:
  1. Coronary artery injury
  2. Hemodynamic instability
- **i.** Epicardial ablation produces:
  1. Pericardial bleeding
  2. Coronary artery injury
  3. Phrenic nerve injury

B. Management of anticoagulation:

Appropriate management before, during, and after the ablations will lead to very low rates of thromboembolic events.

- **a.** Oral anticoagulants should be started for a period of 3–4 weeks prior to ablation procedure.
- **b.** During the procedure therapeutic oral anticoagulation should be continued with little interruption to maintain the INR within typical therapeutic window. Oral dabigatran and apixaban should be hold on the morning on the day of procedure and should be started immediately after the procedure.
- **c.** During the procedure in case of ablation of left atrium and left ventricle intravenous infusion of heparin bolus should be started through the vascular access and continued to maintain ACT of 350–400 seconds.

Q65. Discuss pathophysiology, etiology, clinical features, diagnosis, and management of aortic stenosis.

MGR/SEP2010/MDIV (20)

MGR/MAR2008/MDIV (20)

Aortic stenosis.

RGUHS/MAR2008/MDII (20)

ANSWER

Aortic stenosis is obstruction of blood flow across the aortic valve.

Etiologies

A. If age is <70 years:

- **a.** Bicuspid aortic valve—50%
- **b.** Degenerative disease—18%
- **c.** Postinflammatory
- **d.** Hypoplastic
- **e.** Unicommissural
- **f.** Indeterminate cause

B. If age is >70 years:

- **a.** Degenerative disease—50%
- **b.** Bicuspid aortic valve—27%
- **c.** Postinflammatory
- **d.** Hypoplastic

Pathophysiology

In aortic stenosis, there is resistance to blood flow through the ostium leading to increased pressure gradient between the left ventricle and aorta, gradual increase left ventricular systolic pressure. To normalize the left ventricular wall stress as a compensatory mechanism there is parallel increased replication of sarcomeres leading to concentric hypertrophy of left ventricle, so at this stage:

A. Chamber will not be dilated

B. Preserved ventricular function

C. Diastolic compliance is reduced leading to increase in left ventricular end-diastolic pressure.

With the increase in left ventricular end-diastolic pressure there is increase in pulmonary capillary pressure and decrease in cardiac output due to diastolic dysfunction along with decreased cardiac contractility leading eventually to HF.

Patients with aortic stenosis will maintain normal cardiac output for many years with preserved left ventricular function but during exercise fails to maintain required cardiac output leading arise of exercise-induced symptoms.

Diastolic dysfunction occurs due to impaired left ventricular relaxation with/or without decreased left ventricular compliance as a consequence of:

A. Increased afterload

B. Hypertrophy of left ventricle

C. Myocardial ischemia

Following relief of valvular obstruction, left ventricular hypertrophy may regress but the amount of regression depends upon the amount of fibrosis.

In severe aortic stenosis diastolic filling of left ventricle is maintained by left atrial contraction. So if atrial fibrillation develops, cardiac output cannot be maintained leading to HF.

There is increase in oxygen requirement in the subendocardial region due to:

A. Increased left ventricular muscle mass.

B. Increased left ventricular systolic pressure.

C. Prolonged systolic ejection phase.

In this condition coronary blood flow will be maintained when corrected for left ventricular muscle mass, but there is reduced coronary flow reserve.

In case of elevated left ventricular end-diastolic pressure myocardial perfusion will be decreased leading to subendocardial ischemia as a consequence of:

A. Decline in the capillary density in the myocardium.

B. Decreased diastolic transmyocardial pressure gradient.

Angina occurs due to increased oxygen requirement occurs as a consequence of the following:

A. Hypertrophy of the myocardium.

B. Diminished delivery of oxygen due to diminished coronary flow reserve.

C. Decreased diastolic perfusion pressure.

D. Relative subendocardial myocardial ischemia.

Presentations

A. Patient is asymptomatic for 10–20 years, during this time left ventricular outflow tract obstruction and left ventricular systolic pressure gradually rise.

B. Exertional dyspnea secondary to abnormal left ventricular diastolic dysfunction.

C. Chest pain precipitated by exertion and relieved by rest.

D. Lightheadedness.

E. Easy fatigability.

F. Features of HF due to left ventricular systolic dysfunction due to mismatched afterload, subendocardial myocardial ischemia, and diastolic dysfunction from left ventricular hypertrophy:

- **a.** Paroxysmal nocturnal dyspnea
- **b.** Dyspnea on exertion
- **c.** Orthopnea
- **d.** Shortness of breath

G. Syncope during exertion results from decreased arterial pressure as a consequence of systemic vasodilatation in the face of fixed cardiac output.

H. Syncope at rest due to:

- **a.** Ventricular tachycardia
- **b.** Atrioventricular block
- **c.** Atrial fibrillation
- **d.** Abnormal vasodepressor reflexes secondary to increased left ventricular intracavitary pressure.

I. Syncope may be associated with convulsions.

J. Gastrointestinal bleeding from angiodysplasia (Heyde syndrome).

K. Features of infective endocarditis more in younger women having milder valvular deformity.

L. Increased incidence of aortic root dilatation and aortic dissection in case of bicuspid aortic valve.

M. Features due to emboli of calcium in various organ such as kidney, heart, and brain in case of calcific aortic stenosis.

Physical Examination

A. Pulsus tardus—delayed and plateau peak having decreased amplitude with gradual downslope.

B. There may be coexistence of systolic blood pressure but level >200 mm Hg will never occur.

C. Pulsus alternans due to left ventricular systolic dysfunction

D. Raised jugular venous pressure with prominent "a" wave due to hypertrophy of interventricular septum reducing right ventricular compliance.

E. Heaving apical impulse, if there is hyperdynamic impulse, there may be associated aortic regurgitation.

F. Heart sound:

- **a.** First heart sound is normal.
- **b.** Aortic component of second heart sound is soft or absent due to:
  1. Calcified aortic valve
  2. Immobile aortic valve

3. Prolonged ejection systolic murmur obscuring the aortic component of second heart sound.

c. Paradoxical splitting of second heart sound due to late closure of aortic valve

d. Pulmonary component may be loud due to presence of pulmonary hypertension.

G. Ejection click: It is common in children 40–60 msec after onset of first heart sound due to congenital aortic stenosis along with pliable aortic valve leaflet, but it is rare in adult due to calcific aortic stenosis with calcified valve. It is best heard in the lower left sternal border and may be transmitted toward apex making confusion with split of first heart sound.

H. S4 may be heard due to forceful atrial contraction into hypertrophied ventricle. Its presence in young adult signifies severe aortic stenosis.

I. Murmur: Crescendo-decrescendo harsh low-pitched systolic murmur beginning shortly after first heart sound, gradually increasing the intensity followed by decrease to end just prior to second heart sound, best heard in the right second intercostal space at sternal border radiating to both or single carotid arteries. In case of elderly, the murmur is more prominent at the apex due to radiation of high-frequency component of the murmur—this is Gallavardin phenomenon. This makes confusion with mitral regurgitation murmur. But, there is accentuation of murmur of aortic stenosis following long R-R interval which will distinguish it from mitral regurgitant murmur as later will not change.

Severity of murmur is best correlated with duration and timing of peak of the murmur rather than intensity of murmur, increase in duration, and late systolic peak is associated with severe aortic stenosis.

Murmur intensity is reduced with Valsalva maneuver, whereas murmur intensity of HOCM will be reduced by Valsalva maneuver. Murmur of aortic stenosis is augmented by squatting.

Murmur of aortic stenosis will be muffled or inaudible in following conditions:

a. Left ventricular failure

b. Decreased cardiac output

c. Atrial fibrillation

J. Presence of high-pitched blowing murmur in diastole—suggestive of aortic regurgitation.

K. Sometimes features of right ventricular failure characterized by raised jugular venous pressure, tender hepatomegaly, and pedal edema due to bulging of interventricular septum into right ventricle impeding the right ventricular filling.

Investigations

A. Echocardiography: Following are the three echocardiographic findings found in aortic stenosis:

a. Decrease in maximal separation of aortic cusp of <8 mm in adult with no motion of the cusp.

b. Presence of an echo-dense aortic valve with no motion of the cusp

c. Presence of otherwise unexplained left ventricular hypertrophy

Criteria for determining the severity of aortic stenosis:

Severity	Transvalvular pressure gradient	Aortic valvular area in cm^2
Mild	<25	>1.5
Moderate	25–40	1–1.5
Severe	>40	<1
Critical	>80	<0.5

Color Doppler echocardiography can accurately diagnose bicuspid aortic valve in patients with severe symptomatic aortic stenosis. Major limitation is underestimation of the gradient if the beam of the sound is not parallel to the velocity of aortic jet.

Overestimation of severity of aortic stenosis by Doppler ultrasound in case of the following:

a. Severe anemia—hemoglobin of 8 g/dL

b. Small aortic root

B. Cardiac catheterization: It can measure the left ventricular end-diastolic volume and systolic volume by calculation of ejection fraction as it can quantitate the status of pump function of left ventricle. But in presence of severe aortic stenosis, ejection fraction may underestimate the performance of left ventricle.

C. Coronary angiography: It should exclude coronary artery disease in all the patients over 35 years of age prior to consideration for surgery. It should also be performed in all the patients under 35 years of age if they have the following:

a. Left ventricular dysfunction

b. Symptoms suggestive of coronary artery disease

c. Two or more coronary risk factors for coronary artery disease excluding sex.

D. Radionuclide ventriculography: It can evaluate the myocardial perfusion—

a. During rest

b. During exercise
c. During exertion

E. Exercise stress testing: It should be contraindicated in case of severe aortic stenosis but may be indicated in asymptomatic severe aortic stenosis.

Provocative stress testing by infusion of dobutamine can be done to assess the severity in case where the severity is uncertain due to small stroke volume and small mean aortic valve gradient because it will increase the stroke volume and heart rate.

a. In case of low pressure gradient with severe aortic stenosis aortic valve area does not change but mean pressure gradient will be increased significantly.
b. In patient of low cardiac output as a result of concomitant myocardial infarction but not due to aortic stenosis, small increase in aortic valve area, and aortic valve gradient.

F. Cardiac MRI: It can assess the aortic valve area.

G. Chest X-ray: In anteroposterior view—

a. Normal cardiac size
b. Rounding of left border and the apex
c. Posterior dilatation of ascending aorta
d. Left atrium is slightly enhanced.
e. Pulmonary venous hypertension

In lateral view:

a. Presence of calcification

In severe cases:

a. Left atrial enlargement
b. Enlargement of pulmonary artery
c. Enlargement of right atrium
d. Calcification of aortic valve
e. Presence of pulmonary congestion

H. Electrocardiography:

a. T-wave inversion with ST-segment depression with predominantly positive QRS complexes.
b. More than 0.3 mV depression of ST segment indicates left ventricular strain is suggestive of severe left ventricular hypertrophy.
c. Predominantly negative "p" wave in V1 indicates left atrial enlargement.
d. Normally, there is sinus rhythm but there may be atrial fibrillation in case of associated mitral valve disease and hyperthyroidism. There may be AV block due to extension of calcification of conduction system.

I. B-natriuretic peptide: It gives prognostic information in asymptomatic patients with severe aortic stenosis. It will also provide prognostic information on the outcome in postoperative patients.

Treatment

A. Medical treatment:

In patients with uncontrolled heart failure:

a. Oxygen support
b. Cardiac monitoring
c. Oximetry monitoring
d. Intravenous access
e. Loop diuretics
f. Nitrates
g. Morphine
h. Vasodilator therapy is contraindicated as it lowers the systemic vascular resistance in the face of fixed cardiac output leading to syncope. But in patients of severe heart failure with left ventricular dysfunction and severe aortic stenosis can be benefited from administration of nitroprusside with concomitant pulmonary artery catheter monitoring.
i. Treatment of hyperlipidemia as it will retard the progression of aortic stenosis.
j. Invasive or noninvasive ventilatory support

In patients with angina:

a. Administration of nitrate
b. Oxygen
c. Morphine
d. Nitroglycerine-induced syncope
In case of atrial fibrillation sinus rhythm should be restored.

B. Surgical therapy:

a. **Percutaneous balloon valvoplasty should be done in:**
1. Critically ill patients who are not the candidate of valve replacement
2. As a bridge to replacement of aortic valve

Valvoplasty is considered in severe heart failure or patients with cardiogenic shock:

1. Patients who refuse surgery
2. Pregnant patients with critical aortic stenosis
3. Comorbid patients having very low life expectancy
4. Patients with heart failure but requiring

Mortality in children and adolescent is 1% and it may be an alternative to surgical valvotomy.

Restenosis is common in:

1. Unicuspid aortic valve
2. Severely dysplastic valve

b. **Total aortic valve replacement**:

In case of associated coronary artery disease both valve replacement along with coronary artery bypass graft should be done simultaneously. Successful replacement will improve the patient hemodynamically.

Choice of valve replacement can be guided by the following:

1. Longevity of the patient
2. Ability of the patients to tolerate anticoagulation

Risk in patient with normal left ventricular function and no comorbidity is <5%. Following are the risk factors:

1. High NYHA class
2. Older age
3. Associated with aortic regurgitation
4. Preoperative left ventricular dysfunction

Overall 5-year mortality in adult patients after valve replacement is 80–94%. Following are the risk factors for late death:

1. Left ventricular systolic dysfunction
2. High perioperative NYHA class
3. Atrial fibrillation
4. Concomitant aortic regurgitation
5. Preoperative ventricular arrhythmias
6. Coronary artery disease with previous history of myocardial infarction

Two types of aortic valve replacement:

a. Transcatheter aortic valve replacement:

Indications:

1. Symptomatic severe aortic stenosis with prohibitive risk of surgical aortic valve replacement
2. Severely symptomatic aortic stenosis with high-grade surgical risk
3. Severely symptomatic aortic stenosis with intermediate surgical risk

Types of valve:

1. Edwards Sapien valve: This is a self-expandable bovine pericardial valve.
2. Medtronic valve: This is porcine pericardial valve.
3. Boston scientific: It is controlled mechanical expanding bovine pericardial valve.
4. St Jude valve: It is a self-expanding bovine pericardial valve.

Indications of surgical aortic valve replacement:

1. Symptomatic patients with severe aortic stenosis
2. Asymptomatic patients with severe aortic stenosis and left ventricular ejection fraction of <50%
3. Severe aortic stenosis having heart surgery for another indication

Bioprostheses: These include porcine heterografts and pericardial prosthesis of bovine origin.

Q66. Systolic murmurs.

MJPRU2015(S)/MDI (10)

ANSWER

Systolic murmur has been classified in detail below.

Classification

It can be classified according to time of onset and termination:

A. Early systolic murmur: This high-pitched decrescendo murmur starts with first heart sound and it will confine to early systole by ending prior to mid systole. These are regurgitant murmurs that occur due to retrograde flow of blood from high pressure to low pressure chamber.

Causes are:

a. Acute severe mitral regurgitation: In this case regurgitation of flow occurs into normal size but limited distensible left atrium, as a result pressure gradient between left ventricle and left atrium will be abolished. This murmur will radiate to axilla increased during expiration.

1. Spontaneous rupture of chordae tendinae
2. Subacute bacterial endocarditis (SBE) of the mitral valve
3. Rupture of papillary muscles secondary to AMI
4. Disruption of mitral apparatus

b. Acute tricuspid regurgitation: Murmur is soft, medium-pitched best heard at the lower left border of sternum, aggravated during inspiration. It is associated with right ventricular S4 and tall "v" wave in jugular venous pulse. Causes are:

1. Infective endocarditis
2. Right ventricular infarction
3. Carcinoid tumor
4. Carcinoid syndrome

c. Small VSD: This murmur is high-pitched ejection murmur, the size of the murmur gradually decreases as the ventricular septum thickens and ultimately will be sealed off.

B. Mid systolic murmur: This murmur is:

a. High- to medium-pitched.

b. Crescendo–decrescendo in configuration, i.e., diamond-shaped.

c. Occurs after first sound and ends before second heart sound.

Causes are:

a. Acquired aortic stenosis:

1. It is high-pitched, harsh in quality, heard in the right second intercostal space and occasionally at the apex, and radiating along carotid.
2. According to its severity its peak occurs early or late and short or long duration respectively.
3. Intensity is increased during expiration.
4. In case of associated aortic regurgitation, its intensity will be increased.
5. In case of associated systemic hypertension, coarctation of aorta intensity of the murmur will be decreased due to rapid obliteration of the gradient.
6. In case of aortic sclerosis due to fibrocalcific changes in the aortic valve, there are two distinct mid-systolic murmurs due to "Gallavardin dissociation" are heard:
   - Noisy medium-pitched murmur heard at right base due to high velocity jet at the aortic root
   - High-frequency musical murmur heard at the apex due to high frequency vibration of the aortic cap.

b. Congenital valvular aortic stenosis:

1. It is best heard at right second intercostal space.
2. Associated systolic ejection sound is present suggestive of bicuspid aortic stenosis.
3. S2 is single.
4. S4 in presence of AR

c. Hypertrophic obstructive cardiomyopathy:

1. Murmur is best heard at the apex or lower left sternal edge.
2. It is associated with pulsus bisferiens along with double or triple apical impulse.
3. A2 is of normal intensity.

d. Pulmonary stenosis: It may be valvular, subvalvular, or supravalvular.

1. This murmur is heard at left second intercostal space, aggravated during inspiration, radiated to left side of the neck or may be localized.
2. It is accentuated during inspiration.
3. It begins with pulmonary ejection sound.
4. According to its severity, its peak occurs early or late and short or long duration respectively.
5. It is associated with prominent "a" wave in jugular venous pulse.

In case of supravalvular stenosis:

1. Murmur is best heard at the apex.
2. It is shorter in duration and increased in intensity with severity of obstruction and it is accompanied by ejection sound due to dilatation of aorta.
3. P2 may be absent.

In case of supravalvular aortic stenosis:

1. Murmur is less harsh with variable intensity, high-pitched.
2. It is best heard in upper left sternal border at upper left sternal border and infraclavicular region.

e. Functional mid-systolic murmur:

1. Idiopathic dilatation of pulmonary artery
2. Dilatation of aortic root dilatation
3. Due to increased flow into the aorta:
   - Pregnancy
   - Anemia
   - Thyrotoxicosis
   - Exercise
   - Fever
   - Peripheral AV fistula
4. Due to increased flow into the pulmonary artery. Causes are:
   - Atrial septal defect
   - Ventricular septal defect
   - Straight-back syndrome

f. Innocent mid-systolic murmur: It occurs due to increased flow normal left ventricular outflow tract.
   1. Still's murmur—occurs in young children, but disappears in puberty.
   2. It is related to small diameter of ascending aorta.
   3. Character is "croaking" or "buzzing" in quality.
   4. It is best heard along the third and fourth left sternal border.

g. Innocent mid-systolic murmur: It occurs due to increased flow normal left ventricular outflow tract.
   1. It occurs in children, adolescent as well as in adults.
   2. Murmur is of blowing in quality with low-medium frequency.
   3. It is best heard in the pulmonary area with radiation along the border of left sternum.

C. Holosystolic murmur:
   a. Chronic mitral regurgitation:
      1. It is blowing type best heard at the apex radiating to left axilla, angle of left scapula.
      2. Occasionally, it will radiate to vertebral column from cervical spine to lumbar spine in case regurgitation within left atrium posterolaterally due to involvement of anterior cusp.
      3. In case of posterior cusp involvement, murmur may be heard in the left sternal border, and radiates into neck if the direction of jet is forward against interatrial septum.
   b. Tricuspid regurgitation:
      1. It is blowing in character, and best heard in the lower left sternal edge.
      2. It is usually secondary to pulmonary stenosis or pulmonary hypertension.
      3. Its intensity is increased during inspiration—Carvallo's sign, but it is absent in case of associated organic TR.
   c. Restrictive VSD:
      1. It occurs when there is systemic vascular resistance and that exceeds right ventricular systolic pressure and there is associated pulmonary vascular resistance from the onset of systole to end of systole.
      2. Its intensity is ≥4/6 grade in intensity.
      3. It is best heard in the third to fifth intercostal space on the left border of sternum.
      4. Valsalva maneuver and inhalation of amyl nitrate will decrease the intensity of murmur.

Q67. Ventricular assist device.

MGR/SEP2008/MDIV (6)

ANSWER

Main aim of ventricular device is to unload the failing heart that helps to maintain the circulation of blood to vital organs in the body.

Types of Devices

There are three generations of devices according to principle of operation:

A. First generation device—it is pulsatile positive displacement pumps requiring.
   a. Extensive surgical dissection
   b. Large diameter lead
   c. Audible pump

   The name of the instruments:
   a. Heartmate 1
   b. Thoratec PVAD
   c. Novacor

B. Second generation devices—these are axial flow pump devices, used increasingly nowadays. These are smaller devices consisting of continuous-flow rotary pump having only rotor, only moving part.

C. Third generation devices: These magnetic devices tested for clinical use.

Indications for Use

A. It acts as bridging to transplant.
B. It acts as bridging to recovery from refractory heart failure.
C. It acts as lifetime of destination therapy.
D. It acts as bridge to candidacy.

Following parameters are to be checked for the purpose of risk stratification:

A. Critical cardiogenic shock in case of crash and burn
B. Progressive decline in spite of inotropes
C. Patient is stable but inotrope dependent.
D. Patients have resting symptoms or on oral therapy at home.
E. Patient has exercise intolerance.

F. Patient has limited exertion capacity.

G. Patient suffering from NYHA class III

Complications of Ventricular Assisted Devices

A. Increased risk of bleeding in the form of hematemesis or melena or epistaxis. Contributory factors are:
  - **a.** Anticoagulation
  - **b.** Antiplatelet therapies
  - **c.** Nonpulsatile blood flow that leads to malformation of blood vessels in the gut
  - **d.** Pump-related changes in the clotting factors

B. Right heart failure characterized by engorged neck vein, enlarged tender liver, and pedal edema. Inadequate filling of the device and reduced cardiac output will lead to poor appetite and fatigue organ dysfunction. These patients can be treated by diuretics and intravenous fluid.

C. Stroke: It occurs due to—
  - **a.** Blood clots leaving the pump
  - **b.** High blood pressure
  - **c.** Bleeding into the brain
  - **d.** Those who have past history of previous stroke

D. Infection: It usually occurs in first few weeks or months after implant. Common bacteria is *S. aureus* which gains entry through the exit site. Bacteria from genitourinary tract or gastrointestinal tract secondarily infect the devices. Patients with immunosuppression and diabetes mellitus are at increased risk.

E. Device failure:

The full team of performing successful implantation of devices and follow-up:

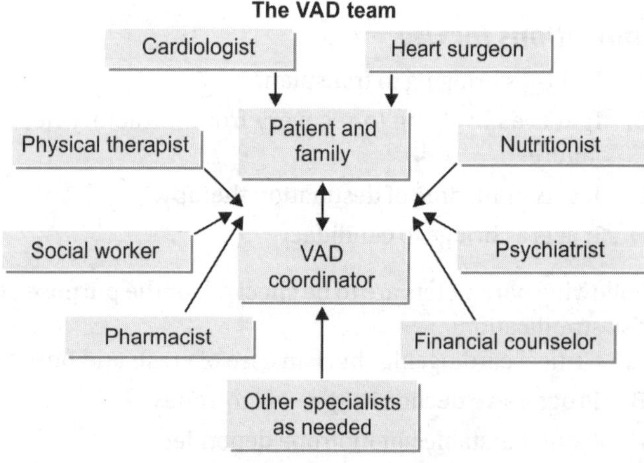

(VAD: ventricular assist device)

Q68. Swan–Ganz catheter.
MGR/SEP2008/MDIV (6)

ANSWER

Introduction

In this procedure, catheter is inserted through the central vein such as femoral, jugular, and antecubital or brachial vein into the right side of the heart and proceed toward the pulmonary artery. It can assess:
  - **a.** Right-sided cardiac chamber filling pressure
  - **b.** Estimation of cardiac output
  - **c.** Evaluation of intracardiac shunt
  - **d.** Valvular studies
  - **e.** Vascular resistance

Anatomy and Physiology

Catheter is to be inserted through the central vein then through the superior or inferior vena cava to reach to right atrium. Now from the right atrium through the tricuspid valve into right ventricle, from there the catheter is allowed to pass through the right ventricular outflow tract into the pulmonary artery. Tip will be laid into the pulmonary artery where catheter balloon can be inflated or deflated to measure the pulmonary artery pressure. Balloon will be inflated to measure the pulmonary capillary wedge pressure that can indirectly assess the left-sided filling pressure.

Indications for Catheterization

A. Pulmonary hypertension can be evaluated or can be assessed.

B. In severe shock, volume status can be assessed.

C. In case of septic or cardiogenic shock, these can be differentiated by measuring the mixed venous oxygen saturation.

D. Cardiac tamponade and constrictive pericarditis can be evaluated.

E. In case of any planning of surgical repair right-sided valvular disease, cardiac shunts and congenital heart disease can be assessed.

Contraindications in Case of Right Heart Catheterization

A. Lack of consent

B. Presence of right-sided ventricular assisted devices

C. Presence of infection at the site of insertion

Complications

A. Infections at the site of catheter insertion

B. Pneumothorax or hemithorax

C. Entrapment of air from infusion pump leading to air embolism

D. Cardiac wall perforation or rupture of the valve

E. Atrial or ventricular arrhythmias due to irritation of the wall of the heart by catheter

F. Misplacement of catheter due to long looping of the catheter in the right atrial chamber

G. During inflation of the balloon of the catheter, there is chance of vessel rupture.

H. There is a chance of pulmonary infarction if the balloon is kept in inflated position for long time or it can migrate into the distal branches.

I. Thromboembolism secondary to infection or inflammation of the catheter

Clinical Significance

A. It can determine the causes of shock such as cardiogenic, septic, or distributive shock.

B. It can determine the causes of pulmonary hypertension for proper treatment after the classification of this pulmonary hypertension.

C. It can detect the intracardiac pressure and valvular abnormalities.

D. It can determine the intracardiac shunts as well as hemodynamic status prior to procedure.

E. It is the procedure of diagnosis and management of different conditions in spite of its underuse of this procedure.

F. It can estimate the pulmonary capillary wedge pressure which can indirectly provide the estimation of left-sided filling pressure.

Q69. Acute coronary syndrome in first 2–4 hours.

GMC/2015/MDIII (10)

Interventional management of coronary artery disease.

MGR/SEP2010/MDIV (6)

MGR/MAR2008/MDIV (6)

Discuss the recent advances in acute coronary syndrome.

MGR/MAR2007/MDIV (20)

What are the indications of percutaneous coronary interventions? Discuss the advantages and disadvantages of bare and drug eluting stents.

MJPRU/2016/MDIV (20)

Primary percutaneous coronary intervention versus fibrinolysis in acute ST-elevated myocardial infarction.

PGI/APR2014/MDIII (10)

Discuss etiopathogenesis, diagnosis, and management of acute coronary syndrome.

SNMC/MAY2008/MDIII (20)

Acute coronary syndrome.

BF/MAY2009/MDIII (15)

Revascularization in acute arterial ischemia.

BF/JUN2016/MDIV (10)

A 60 years old man presented with severe retrosternal pain and diaphoresis for 1 hour and ECG revealed marked ST segment elevation in the anterior chest leads. Discuss the laboratory diagnosis, management and acute complications during first 24 hours.

MJPRU/2015(S)/MDII (20)

Enumerate the risk factors of ischemic heart disease. Clinical features and management of acute coronary syndrome.

DNB, 2018 (2+4+4)

Pathophysiology of acute coronary syndrome.

KERALA UNIVERSITY, 2017 (10)

A 65 years old man is brought to the casualty with acute onset of chest pain. If the clinical features point to acute myocardial infarction, how will you manage the patient?

KERALA UNIVERSITY, 2020 (20)

Write on etiopathogenesis, diagnosis, and clinical management of acute coronary syndrome. Write briefly on acute complications of acute myocardial infarction.

RAJASTHAN UNIVERSITY, 2021 (50)

Acute coronary syndrome in young.

SCBMCH, 2020 (10)

Acute complication of acute myocardial infarction answer in question number 155.

Discuss etiopathogenesis, clinical features laboratory findings and management of acute myocardial infarction.

SCBMCH, 2012 (20)

Discuss the management of acute myocardial infarction under the heads—prehospital, in-hospital, and post-hospital.

DNB, 2024 MAY (10)

Management of STEMI.

MANIPAL UNIVERSITY, 2018 (10)

Discuss the role of percutaneous coronary intervention in the management of myocardial infarction.

MANIPUR UNIVERSITY, 2019 (10)

Discuss the role of percutaneous coronary intervention in the management of acute coronary syndrome.

MANIPUR UNIVERSITY, 2021 (10)

ANSWER

Just after getting the patients with acute myocardial infarction with suspected STEMI the goal of treatment includes:

- **a.** Control of cardiac discomfort
- **b.** Rapid identification of patients who is the proper candidate of reperfusion therapy.
- **c.** Triage of patients who are at low-risk in the proper location in the hospital.
- **d.** Inappropriate discharge of the patients with STEMI from the hospital.

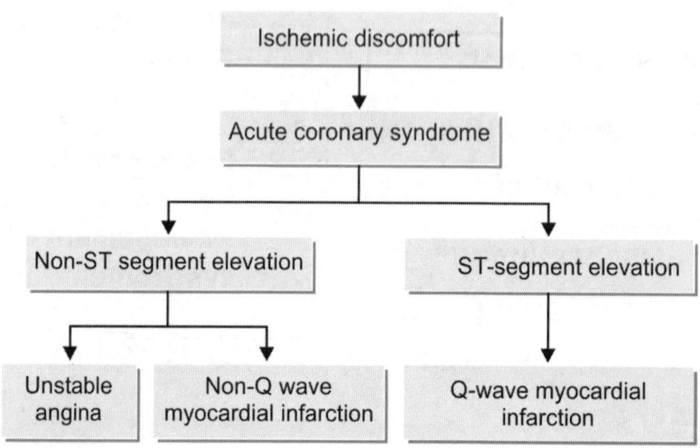

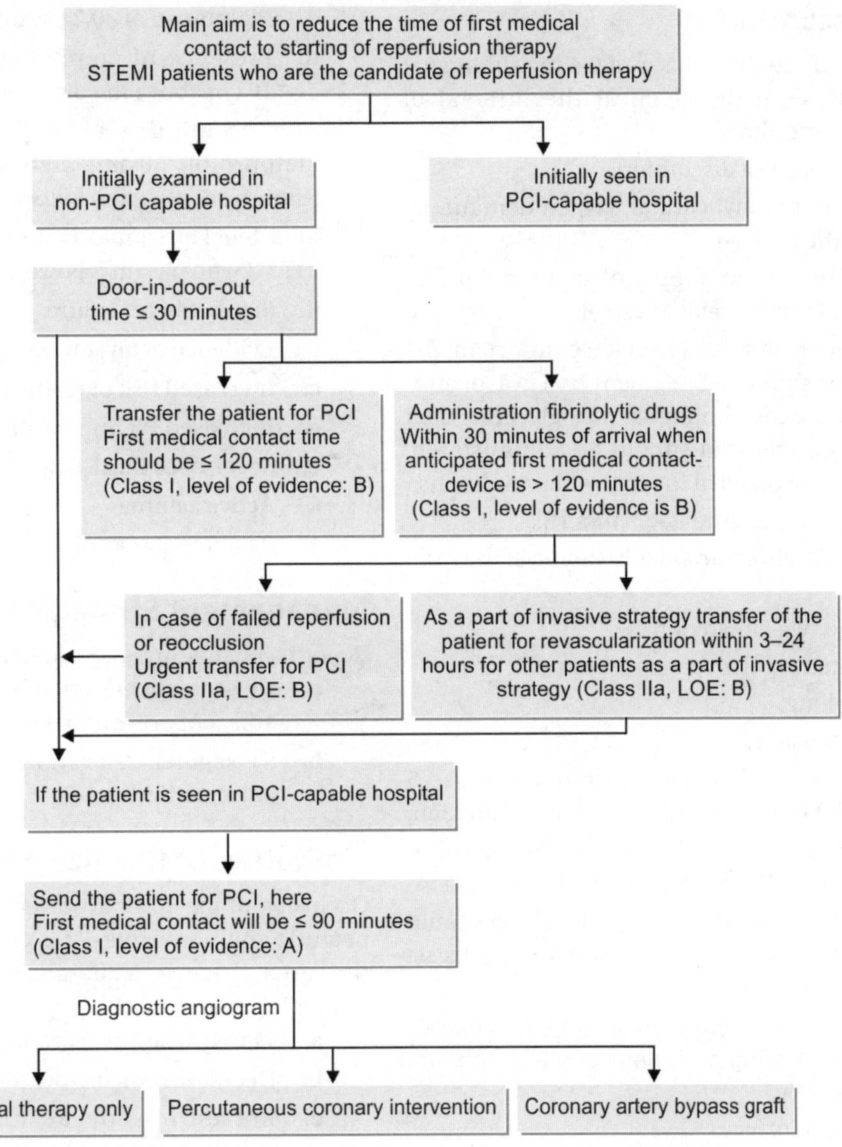

(LOE: level of evidence; PCI: percutaneous coronary intervention; STEMI: ST-elevation myocardial infarction)

Management in the Emergency Department

A. Aspirin 325 mg chewable tablet to be given so that it after absorption through buccal mucosa inhibits cyclooxygenase in platelets to inhibit level of thromboxane A_2. It is then continued at 75–162 mg daily.

B. If the oxygen saturation is within normal limit, then oxygen administration will provide limited benefit. But if the oxygen saturation is low, the oxygen has to be administered at a rate of 2–4 L/min for 6–12 hours after infarction, then it should be continued if saturation level is <90%.

C. Intravenous access should be maintained through the slow transfusion of normal saline or 5% of dextrose solution.

D. Continuous ECG monitoring to see any evidence of new arrhythmias as well as deviation of ST segment.

E. At every 1.5 hours vital signs should be monitored till the patient is stable then at every 4 hours, if required.

F. Until the patient is stable, oral feed should be given in the form of water. Then, diet containing sodium 2 g, <200 mg/day cholesterol, and <7% total calorie low-saturated fat should be given.

G. Complete bed rest in acute case

Control of Discomfort

A. Nitroglycerin: Up to three doses of 0.4 mg sublingual nitroglycerin has to be given at the interval of 5 minutes with the aim of:

a. Reduction of chest discomfort

b. Decrease in the myocardial oxygen demand by reducing the preload

c. Increase in oxygen supply of myocardium by dilatation of infarct related vessels

B. If there is recurrence of chest discomfort in the form of further shift of ST segment or T wave, after favorable response to sublingual nitroglycerin, then intravenous nitroglycerin should be administered. But, it should be avoided in the following conditions:

a. Systolic blood pressure is <90 mm Hg.

b. Evidence of right ventricular ischemia in the form of:

1. Inferior wall infarction
2. Elevated jugular venous pressure
3. Clear lung
4. Hypotension

c. Patients who are taking phosphodiesterase-5 inhibitor for the treatment of erectile dysfunction.

d. Idiosyncratic reaction like severe hypotension which can be relieved by intravenous atropine.

C. Morphine: Small dose like 2–4 mg morphine should be administered intravenously to provide analgesic effect in STEMI. Effects are—

a. Systemic arteriolar and venous sympathetic vasoconstriction leading to venous pooling. This can be corrected by:

1. Elevation of legs
2. Intravenous administration of fluid

b. Diaphoresis and nausea which will be corrected by itself and replaced by sense of well-being.

c. Bradycardia mainly in case of inferior wall myocardial infarction through its vagotonic effect. This can be recovered by administration of intravenous 0.5 mg atropine.

D. Beta-blockers: It will—

a. Reduce the pain by reducing the diminishing the myocardial oxygen demand.

b. Reduce the risk of reinfarction.

c. Reduce the risk of ventricular fibrillation.

Drug is intravenous metoprolol 5 mg at every 2–5 minutes for total three doses provided:

a. Heart rate is >60 beats/min.

b. Systolic pressure of >100 mm Hg

c. PR interval of <0.24 seconds

d. Presence of crepitation which is not present 10 cm above the diaphragm

After 15 minutes of the last intravenous dose of metoprolol, 50 mg metoprolol should be given 6 hourly for 48 hours followed by 100 mg 12 hourly.

Beta-blocker should be initiated within 24 hours of STEMI who has no following contraindications:

a. Signs of heart failure

b. Evidence of low output

c. Increased risk of cardiogenic shock

d. Increased PR interval of >0.24 hours

e. Second- or third-degree heart block

f. Active asthma

g. Reactive airway disease

Management Strategies

Reperfusion therapy is considered in following conditions:

a. ST-segment elevation of at least 2 mm in the two adjacent precordial leads

b. ST-segment elevation of at least 1 mm in two adjacent limb leads

Limitation of the Size of the Infarct

Occlusion of the coronary artery makes the myocardium necrotic and nonviable—it is central zone. Surrounding this area there is ischemic myocardium, known as ischemic penumbra which can be corrected by:

a. Timely restoring coronary perfusion

b. Decreasing the myocardial oxygen demand

c. Prevention of accumulation of noxious metabolites

d. Blunting the effect of inflammatory mediators induced reperfusion-perfusion injury

Nearly one-third patients with STEMI within 24 hours develop spontaneous reperfusion of the infarcted artery and these patients demonstrate improved healing of the infarcted tissue.

Reperfusion can be done through the following two methods:

a. Fibrinolysis—pharmacotherapy

b. Percutaneous coronary intervention

Restoration of epicardial infarcted artery along with improved perfusion of the downstream zone of myocardium will ultimately limit the size of the infarct. Now ischemic myocardium can be protected by maintaining the optimum balance between the myocardial oxygen demand and supply through:

a. Control of pain
b. Treatment of congestive cardiac failure
c. Decreasing the hypertension
d. Minimizing the arrhythmia

Corticosteroid and NSAIDs should be avoided in STEMI because of the following reasons:

a. Healing of the myocardium will be hampered leading to increased scar size.
b. Increased incidence of myocardial rupture
c. Increased resistance to coronary blood flow leading to decreased flow to myocardium

Following are the recommendations of reperfusion therapy according to the ESC 2017 guideline:

Criteria	Class
Reperfusion therapy is indicated in patients with ischemic symptoms of ≥12 hours duration and persistent elevation of ST segment	IA
Primary PCI strategy is recommended over fibrinolysis within indicated timeframes	IA
If timely primary PCI cannot be performed after the diagnosis of STEMI, fibrinolytic therapy is recommended within 12 hours of onset of symptoms in patients having no contraindication	IA
In patients with time from the onset of symptom of >12 hours, a primary PCI is indicted in presence of ongoing symptoms suggestive of ischemia, hemodynamic instability, or life-threatening arrhythmias	IC
A routine primary PCI strategy should be considered in patients presenting 12–48 hours after onset of symptoms	IIAB
In asymptomatic patients, routine PCI of an occluded infarct-related artery > 48 hours after the onset of STEMI is not indicated	IIIA

(PCI: percutaneous coronary intervention; STEMI: ST-elevation myocardial infarction)

Fibrinolytic therapy: Follow the answers in question number 29.

Percutaneous Coronary Intervention

Rescue Percutaneous Coronary Intervention

It is characterized by emergency PCI in patients in whom reperfusion has been failed with fibrinolytic therapy. Success rate of rescue PCI in case of moderate to large infarction can be determined in terms of left ventricular function. More than 30% patients receiving fibrinolytic therapy demonstrate TIMI 0–1 at 90 minutes and it is associated with long-term survival. But, if the reperfusion is not evident 90 minutes even after fibrinolytic therapy especially in case of large myocardial infarction, in that case emergency angiography followed by mechanical reperfusion should be done.

As guidelines of the AHA/ACC 2004, indications of PCI are the following:

A. Class I indication for rescue PCI:
   a. Cardiogenic shock in patients of <75 years of age but are unsuitable for revascularization [Level of evidence (LOE): B]
   b. Severe congestive heart failure and/or pulmonary edema (Killip Class III) (LOE: B)
   c. Hemodynamically compromised ventricular arrhythmias (LOE: C)
B. Class IIa indications for rescue PCI:
   a. Cardiogenic shock in patients of >75 years of age.
   b. Patients with failed perfusion and a moderate or large myocardium at risk (anterior)
   c. Patients with hemodynamic or electrical instability or persistent ischemic symptoms

Clinical Indicators of Reperfusion

Resolution of chest pain is not the accurate indicator of reperfusion, because pain may be blunted by:

a. Narcotic analgesia by morphine
b. Partial denervation in case of severe MI

So, it can be measured by:

a. Serial changes in ECG is more reliable indicator
b. Accelerated idioventricular rhythm is fairly specific indicator of reperfusion. But, other supraventricular or ventricular arrhythmias may be seen in patients with nonperfused infarct related artery.

So, successful reperfusion is indicated by following combinations:

a. Resolution of chest pain
b. More than 70% resolution of ST-segment elevation as it suggests effective perfusion at tissue level
c. Run of accelerated idioventricular rhythm

Benefit of Rescue Revascularization

Patients with failed reperfusion by thrombolytic therapy can be benefited from rescue angioplasty with or without PCI as it will reduce 50% of death, heart failure, reinfarction, or stroke.

Facilitated Percutaneous Coronary Intervention

It is characterized by immediate pharmacologic therapy followed by prompt mechanical perfusion of the infarcted related artery. Pharmacotherapy includes:

- **a.** Full dose lytic therapy, or
- **b.** Half-dose lytic therapy and half-dose GPIIB/IIIA inhibitor, or
- **c.** GP IIB/IIIA only

Addition of Anti-platelet Drugs with Reperfusion Therapy

A. Aspirin:

- **a.** Primary PCI: Loading dose is 150–300 mg orally followed by 75–100 mg daily indefinitely.
- **b.** With fibrinolytic therapy: To start with 150–500 mg orally followed by 75–100 mg as maintenance dose.
- **c.** In case of CKD, no dose adjustment is required.

B. Clopidogrel:

- **a.** Primary PCI: Loading dose is 600 mg orally followed by 75 mg daily as maintenance dose.
- **b.** With fibrinolytic therapy:
  - **1.** If age is <75 years, then 300 mg loading dose orally followed by 75 mg as maintenance dose for 1 year.
  - **2.** If age is >75 years, loading dose is not given, but maintenance dose is 75 mg orally daily for 14 days (class IA) or up to 1 year in absence of bleeding [interstitial cystitis (IC)].
  - **3.** If PCI is performed in ≤24 hours after fibrinolytic therapy, 300 mg clopidogrel orally should be given before or during PCI.
  - **4.** If PCI is performed in >24 hours after fibrinolysis, 600 mg clopidogrel orally should be given before or during PCI.
- **c.** In CKD, no dose adjustment is required.

C. Prasugrel:

- **a.** Primary PCI: 60 mg loading dose orally should be given followed by 10 mg as maintenance dose for up to 1 year.
- **b.** If the age of the patient is >75 years, this drug is not recommended. If deemed necessary, 5 mg dose should be given. Loading dose is not required.
- **c.** In case of PCI performed >24 hours after fibrinolytic therapy, 60 mg prasugrel should be given at the time of PCI.

D. Ticagrelor:

- **a.** Primary PCI (class B): Loading dose is orally 180 mg followed by 90 mg twice daily for 1 year.

E. GP IIB/IIIA inhibitors:

- **a.** It should be given for bailout therapy in case of angiographic evidence of:
  - **1.** Massive thrombus
  - **2.** Slow or no flow through the coronary artery
  - **3.** Thrombotic complications (IIa recommendation)
- **b.** Routine use of this drug along with unfractionated heparin as an adjunct to primary PCI in patient in absence of any contraindication (class IIb recommendation)
- **c.** Upstream use of this drug can be considered in high-risk patients who are being transferred for primary PCI.

Risk Factors of Ischemic Heart Disease

A. Non-modifiable risk factors:

- **a.** Age: Incidences are increased above 35 years of age in both male and female.
- **b.** Sex: Males are more vulnerable as compared to females.
- **c.** Ethnicity: Black, Hispanics, Southeast Asian people are at increased risk of developing coronary artery disease.
- **d.** Family history: Patient with family history of cardiac disease in less than 50 years of age are at increased risk as compared to patient without family history of CAD.

B. Modifiable risk factors:

- **a.** Hypertension: It develops CAD through both mechanical and oxidative stress on the arterial wall.
- **b.** Hyperlipidemia: Hypercholesterolemia, low HDL and hypertriglyceridemia
- **c.** Diabetes mellitus: Heart disease is more common in diabetic male as compared to female.
- **d.** Obesity: It is an independent risk factor, but increases the risk when it is associated with hypertension, diabetes mellitus or hyperlipidemia.
- **e.** Smoking
- **f.** Poor diet:
  - **1.** Trans fat
  - **2.** Saturated fat

  All the above factors produce endothelial dysfunction, insulin resistance, and inflammation.
- **g.** Sedentary life style

C. Following diseases may be responsible for ischemic heart disease:

- **a.** Chronic kidney disease through the inflammatory mediators, oxidative stress, decreased production of nitric oxide.
- **b.** Nonalcoholic fatty liver disease
- **c.** Systemic lupus erythematosus through the pro-inflammatory effect on coronary circulation.
- **d.** Rheumatoid arthritis through its pro-inflammatory effect.
- **e.** Inflammatory bowel disease as its chronic inflammatory effect.
- **f.** Thyroid disease through its dyslipidemia, atherosclerosis, cardiac function, vascular compliance and arrhythmias
- **g.** Increased level of testosterone
- **h.** Vitamin D deficiency

Clinical features are written in question number 76.

Acute complications of acute myocardial infarction written in question number 155.

Q70. Measurement of cardiac output.

MGR/MAR2008/MDI (4)

ANSWER

Following are the measurement methods of cardiac output:

A. Fick principle:

a. Direct Fick method:

1. Principle: Total uptake of oxygen by the body is equal to product of difference between the arterial venous oxygen content and cardiac output, i.e.:

   Cardiac output X $(C_a - C_v) = VO_2$
2. Advantage:
   - It is accurate.
   - It is the gold-standard method.
   - Necessary invasive device is available in the intensive care unit.
3. Disadvantages:
   - It requires stability of cardiac output for several minutes.
   - It is highly invasive requiring pulmonary arterial catheter and arterial line.
   - It also requires cumbersome VO_2 measuring machine.

b. Indirect Fick method:

1. Principle: It measures the cardiac output by Fick equation, but it requires substitution of the estimated values for some measured variables. Here, the equation is:

   Cardiac output = Dose of the indicator/Area under the concentration-time curve, which can be simplified by Stewart–Hamilton equation.

   V = m/ct,

   where,

   V = Cardiac output

   C = Concentration

   M = Dose of the indicator

   T = Time
2. Advantages:
   - Access to mixed venous blood and arterial blood are not essential.
   - Numerous options of indicator like saline at cold or at room temperature, dye, and lithium
   - It is less invasive as compared to direct method.
   - It can correlate with gold-standard measurements of cardiac output.
3. Disadvantages:
   - This method is highly technique dependent.
   - It is rendered inaccurate by valvular disease and intracardiac shunts.
   - Its accuracy is reduced by estimated coefficients in the equation.

B. Left ventricular Doppler measurement of the cardiac output:

a. Principle: Here, cardiac output can be measured by measuring the cross-sectional area of the left ventricular outflow tract and integrating the area under the velocity/time curve that can be measured from the aorta by Doppler study.

b. Advantages:

1. It is easily available.
2. It is noninvasive.
3. In case of experienced hand it is accurate.

c. Disadvantages:

1. It is limited by availability of ultrasound window.
2. Its accuracy depends upon the beam angle.
3. It is poorly reproducible.

C. Indicator dilution technique

D. Arterial pulse contour analysis:

  a. Principle: Here, stroke volume can be measured from the area present under the flow/time curve that is derived from arterial pressure waveform with the use of calibration factor.

  b. Advantages:

    1. It is less invasive and it does not require mixed venous blood—only arterial and central venous catheter is required.

    2. It is convenient.

    3. Analysis of pulse contour is automated and continuous.

  c. Disadvantages:

    1. It depends upon good arterial waveform

    2. It is confused by atrial fibrillation and intra-aortic balloon counterpulsation.

    3. Calibration factors should be measured.

E. Bioimpedance

F. Flow measuring rotameter

G. Electromagnetic flow probe

H. Transthoracic impedance

I. Magnetic susceptibility plethysmography

Q71. Nonbacterial thrombotic endocarditis.
MGR/SEP2007/MDI (5)

ANSWER

Definition

It is characterized by appearance of vegetations on the cardiac valves consisting of aggregates of platelets and fibrin but devoid of bacteria or any inflammation.

Pathogenesis

There is evidence of endothelial damage followed by exposure of the subendothelial tissue to circulating platelets. Whole pathogenesis has been divided into following factors that initiate nonbacterial thrombotic endocarditis (NBTE) followed by complete formation of verrucae:

A. Immune complexes: In Libman-Sacks endocarditis platelet-fibrin rich thrombi will be formed on the rough ventricular surface of the mitral valve—this is typically warty, sessile, and wart-like, size is pin-head to 3–4 mm.

B. Hypoxia: It activates tissue-factor leading to hypercoagulable state that ultimately produces NBTE.

C. Hypercoagulability: Following are the clotting factor abnormalities—

  a. Hyperfibrinogenemia

  b. Hypofibrinogenemia

  c. Thrombocytopenia

  d. Decreased concentration of factors V, VII, XIII, decreased anti-thrombin III

D. Carcinomatosis

Clinical Features

A. Diseases that is known to be associated with murmur, like malignancy, disseminated, SLE, features of antiphospholipid syndrome

B. Presence of heart murmur or appearance of new murmur or change of pre-existing murmur

C. Evidence of multiple systemic emboli—recurrent emboli is a hallmark of NBTE. Systemic embolization occurs in kidney, spleen, and mesenteric bed.

Diagnosis

A. Comprehensive hematological studies:

  a. Complete blood count

B. Coagulation studies:

  a. Activated partial thromboplastin time

  b. Prothrombin time

  c. Thrombin time

  d. Fibrinogen level

  e. D-Dimer

C. Multiple blood cultures should be taken to exclude infective endocarditis.

D. Immunological assay for anti-phospholipid syndrome

E. Echocardiography: There is evidence of small <1 cm in diameter with broad base and irregular in shape.

F. Cardiac MRI: It will demonstrate stroke pattern of multiple small, medium, or large disseminated lesions.

Management

A. Treatment of the etiology

B. In case of advanced noncurable cancer, surgery neither improves the final outcome nor prevents recurrent embolization.

C. In case of curable cancer, coagulability should be corrected followed by consideration of surgery as per priority. In absence of any contraindication anticoagulation with heparin should be considered.
D. In case of acute congested heart failure due to dysfunction of the valve or history of recurrent thromboembolism in spite of continuous anticoagulation, surgery should be of choice in absence of severe comorbid conditions.

Q72. Prevention of infective endocarditis.
MGR/SEP2007/MDI (5)

Indications for infective endocarditis prophylaxis and the drugs used.
DR YSR UNI OF HEALTH SC, VIJAYAWADA, ANDHRA, 2022 (10)

Infective endocarditis prophylaxis guidelines.
DNB, 2022 (3)

ANSWER

Prophylaxis is required for the following heart diseases:
A. Prosthetic heart valves
B. Congenital heart disease
C. Past history of infective endocarditis
D. Congenital heart disease that has not been repaired including palliative shunts or conduits
E. Presence of residual defect at or adjacent to the site of repair in case of repaired congenital heart disease
F. During first 6 months after the repair of congenital heart disease with prosthetic material or device
G. Cardiac valvulopathy in case of recipients of cardiac transplantation

In the following procedures antibiotic prophylaxis are required:
A. Oropharyngeal procedure
B. Dental procedure involving manipulation of gingival tissue, perforation of oral mucosa or periapical region of the teeth.
C. Tonsillectomy and/or adenoidectomy
D. Respiratory procedures
E. Miscellaneous
F. Invasive procedures involving incision
G. Procedures on infected skin or musculoskeletal system

Prophylactic regimen are the following:

Clinical circumstances	Antibiotics	Doses
Standard prophylaxis	Amoxicillin	2 g orally prior to procedure
If the patient cannot take orally	Ampicillin Or Ceftriaxone	2 g intravenously within 30 minutes before the procedure Or 1 g intravenously or intramuscularly within 30 minutes before the procedure
In case of allergy to penicillin	Clindamycin Or Cephalexin Or Azithromycin or clarithromycin	600 mg orally 1 hour before the procedure Or 2 g orally 1 hour before the procedure Or 500 mg orally 1 hour prior to procedure

Pneumococcal vaccine is recommended in all patients with prosthetic valves.

Q73. Pulsus paradoxus.
MLB/MAT2009/MDII (20)

Describe pulsus paradoxus using labeled diagram. Discuss the clinical examination findings and list the conditions causing it.
DNB, 2020 (4+3+3)

ANSWER

Definition

It can be defined as an exaggerated decrease in the arterial pulse amplitude during quiet respiration as a result of exaggerated normal inspiratory decline of systolic pressure of >10 mm Hg leading to 7% inspiratory decline of left ventricular stroke volume.

It is apparent paradox because there is disappearance of pulse during inspiration in spite of presence of heart beat.

If the decline in the systolic blood pressure of >20 mm Hg, it can be detected in the radial artery or brachial artery during palpation.

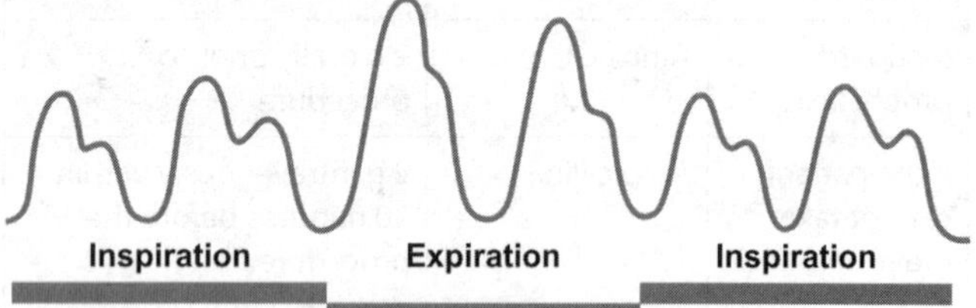

Causes of Pulsus Paradoxus

A. Physiological:
   a. Pregnancy
   b. Extreme obesity
   c. Student's paradox in case voluntary exaggerated inspiration
B. Cardiovascular causes:
   a. Pericardial tamponade
   b. Effusive-constrictive pericarditis
   c. Massive pulmonary embolism
   d. Restrictive cardiomyopathy
   e. Severe hypovolemic shock
C. Pulmonary cause:
   a. Chronic obstructive pulmonary disease

Mechanism of Pulsus Paradoxus

In normal condition, the inspiratory fall in the intrapericardial pressure (IPP) is: 3–6 mm Hg causing increase in the transmural pressure as well as venous return but only with slight change in the size of right and left ventricles.

In pulsus paradoxus, exaggerated decline in intrapericardial pressure as well as right atrial pressure leads to increase in right ventricular transmural diastolic pressure (distending pressure) thereby augmenting venous returns toward heart. As a result:

a. There is an increase in dimension of right ventricle that shifts the interventricular septum toward left ventricle leading to decrease in both dimension and compliance of left ventricle hence impeding left ventricular filling, cardiac output, and arterial pressure.
b. Increase in intrapericardial pressure decreases the left ventricular transmural pressure which further declines in left atrial and left ventricular filling leading to decrease in left ventricular output and thus decreases the systolic arterial pressure.

Following are the additional factors for pulsus paradoxus:

a. During inspiration there is pooling of blood in the pulmonary bed including pulmonary veins and capillaries produces further decline in left atrial and ventricular filling thus decreasing left ventricular output.

In case of chronic obstructive pulmonary disease as a result of decrease in lung compliance, there is magnification of inspiratory decease in left ventricular volume, and during expiration there is excessive rise in systolic pressure above normal.

Causes and Types of Pulsus Paradoxus

A. Total pulsus paradoxus: Here, there is complete disappearance of pulse during inspiration that occurs in case of very severe cardiac tamponade and cardiac tamponade associated with severe hypovolemia.
B. Reverse pulsus paradoxus: It is characterized by inspiratory increase and expiratory decrease in systolic arterial pressure. It is found in the following conditions:
   a. Positive pressure breathing with artificial ventilator: Here, intrathoracic pressure will be increased during inspiration and decreased during expiration, i.e., it is reversal of normal phenomena.
   b. Isorhythmic AV dissociation: During inspiration, atrial activity increases stroke volume and decreases during expiration.

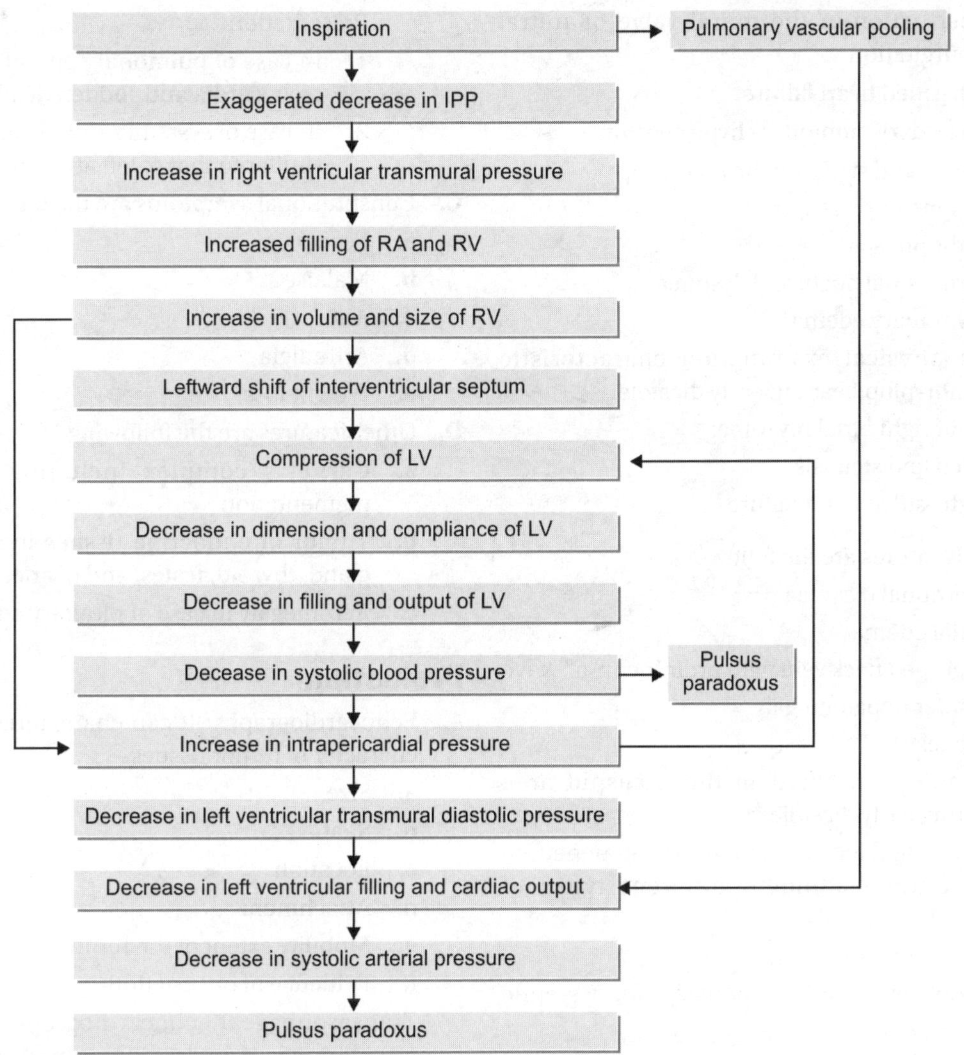

Q74. Atrial myxoma.

MGR/FEB2005/MDI (5)

ANSWER

Introduction

It is the most common primary cardiac tumor, >75% of myxoma originates from the left atrium at:

- **a.** Fossa ovalis border of the interatrial septum
- **b.** Mitral annulus

20% originates from right atrium and 5% from both atria and ventricle.

Etiology

Myxoma cells originate from multipotent mesenchymal cells that can differentiate into neural and endothelial cells. 10% of myxoma patients are autosomal dominant known as Carney's complex and rest 90% are sporadic in origin.

Pathophysiology

This tumor is pedunculated, soft, having friable or smooth or villous surface.

Smooth surfaced tumor is responsible for obstructive features where friable and villous surface are associated with embolic phenomenon.

This tumor produces following factors:

- **A.** Vascular endothelial growth factor is responsible for angiogenesis.
- **B.** Cytokines and growth factors are responsible for constitutional symptoms.

Clinical Features

- **A.** Obstructive features:
  - **a.** In case of left atrial myxoma produces:

1. Obstruction in the mitral valve or mitral regurgitation
2. Left-sided heart failure
3. Secondary pulmonary hypertension

Symptoms and signs are the following:

1. Dyspnea
2. Orthopnea
3. Paroxysmal nocturnal dyspnea
4. Pulmonary edema
5. On physical examination characteristic tumor-plop heard in early diastole.

b. In case of right atrial myxoma:

1. Tricuspid stenosis
2. Right-sided heart failure

Clinical features are the following:

1. Exertional dyspnea
2. Pedal edema
3. Engorged neck vein with prominent "a" wave
4. Tender hepatomegaly
5. Ascites
6. Tumor-plop heard in the tricuspid area during early diastole

c. Both right- and left-sided myxoma can penetrate myocardium leading to different types of arrhythmias.

B. Thromboembolic symptoms:

a. Left atrial myxoma is responsible for systemic embolization in:

1. Central nervous system
2. Kidney
3. Spleen
4. Adrenal gland
5. Abdominal aorta
6. Iliac arteries
7. Femoropopliteal arteries

Different features are:

1. Transient ischemic attack
2. Hemiplegia
3. Loss of vision
4. Chest pain
5. Dyspnea

b. Right atrial myxoma produces:

1. Pulmonary embolization
2. Systemic embolization in case of atrial septal defect or patent foramen ovale

Presentation:

1. In case of pulmonary embolization hypoxia, tachycardia and sudden death
2. In case of systemic embolization features are similar to that of left atrial myxoma.

C. Constitutional symptoms are the following:

a. Fever
b. Malaise
c. Anorexia
d. Arthralgia
e. Weight loss

D. Other features are the following:

a. Carney's complex including unusual skin pigmentation
b. Tumor of endocrine tissues including adrenal gland, thyroid, testes, and ovaries
c. Acromegaly in case of pituitary adenoma

Evaluation

A. Echocardiography: It can characterize the following character of tumor tissues—

a. Size
b. Shape
c. Location
d. Attachment
e. Mobility extent of the tumor
f. Evidence of obstruction

Transesophageal echocardiography is better than transthoracic echocardiography in delineating the tumor.

B. Cardiac MRI: It can delineate the anatomy and microenvironment of the tumor.

C. PET-scan: It can also characterize the tumor.

D. Coronary angiography: It can assess the blood supply of the tumor as this investigation has to be done prior to resection of the tumor.

Treatment

Prompt surgical resection of the tumor is the treatment of choice followed by repair of the defect by pericardial patch and the tumor should be sent for biopsy.

Q75. Describe the clinical picture, diagnosis and management of dissection of aorta.

MGR/FEB2005/MDIII (5)

Classification and management of aortic dissection.

DNB, 2022 (5)

ANSWER

Introduction

As a result of tear in the wall of the intima there is separation of intima from media resulting dissection of the aorta. It can progress in antegrade direction and less commonly in retrograde direction producing a false lumen in the wall of the aorta.

Atypical variants are intramural hematoma, aortic ulcer due to pathologic weakening of the wall of the aorta due to medial necrosis, inflammation or atherosclerosis.

Risk factors are:

- **a.** Hyperlipidemia
- **b.** Smoking
- **c.** Cocaine use
- **d.** Coarctation of aorta
- **e.** Bicuspid aortic valve

Etiologies

A. Genetic syndrome associated are:

- **a.** Marfan syndrome
- **b.** Loeys-Dietz syndrome: Autosomal dominant, triad features are—
  - **1.** Arterial tortuosity along with aneurysm
  - **2.** Hypertelorism
  - **3.** Bifid uvula
- **c.** Ehlers-Danlos syndrome type IV (vascular form)
- **d.** Familial thoracic aortic aneurysm and dissection syndrome

B. Hereditary conditions and congenital anomalies

C. Vasculitides are associated with inflammation of large vessels such as giant cell arteritis, syphilis, Takayasu's arteritis and Behçet's disease, and aortitis.

D. Association with 3rd trimester of pregnancy and during early postpartum in women of <40 years of age.

E. Direct trauma to chest produces aortic transection and hematoma.

Classification

A. According to involvement of anatomic site:

- **a.** Stanford classification:
  - **1.** Type A: Any dissection involving ascending aorta
  - **2.** Type B: Any dissection not involving ascending aorta
- **b.** DeBakey classification:
  - **1.** Type I: Entry point is in the ascending aorta, extends into aortic arch, and often beyond.
  - **2.** Type II: Confines entirely to the ascending aorta.
  - **3.** Type III: Entry in the descending aorta (distal to left subclavian artery) extending distally (usually) or proximally (rarely).

B. According to severity:

- **a.** Acute (<2 weeks from onset)
- **b.** Chronic (>2 weeks from onset)

Clinical Features

A. Symptoms:

- **a.** In case of proximal dissection: Chest pain, tearing, stabbing, ripping in character, radiating to interscapular region, back, and abdomen.
- **b.** In case of descending aorta dissection: Pain occurs in back, chest, and abdomen.

  It is less common in elderly.

B. Physical findings:

- **a.** Murmur of severe of aortic insufficiency—it is associated with aortic dissection, and may lead to acute heart failure.
- **b.** Hypotension and shock—it is associated with cardiac tamponade.
- **c.** Syncope
- **d.** Myocardial infarction—it occurs due to retrograde extension of dissection into the coronary artery ostium.
- **e.** Cerebrovascular accident—it occurs due to extension to cephalad carotid arteries.
- **f.** Paraplegia—due to extension into intercostal and spinal arteries
- **g.** Pulse deficit and acute ischemia of the limb—due to dissection of arterial supply in the limbs
- **h.** Cardiac arrest

Evaluation

The aims are:

A. Defining the extension of dissection

B. Clinical management:

- **a.** Site of intimal tear
- **b.** Ascending versus descending aortic involvement
- **c.** Presence or absence of aortic regurgitation

d. Presence or absence of pericardial effusion and/or cardiac tamponade
e. Involvement of coronary artery
f. Involvement of visceral arterial supply

Investigations

A. Electrocardiography: It is done to exclude ACS.
B. Chest X-ray can detect the dissection, but negative chest X-ray cannot exclude the dissection, hence further imaging is required.
C. CT scan: It can detect aortic dissection with 100% sensitivity and specificity.
D. MRI: It should be done with gadolinium contrast and black blood imaging technique for evaluation of anatomy and morphology of the aorta. Advantages are the following:
   a. It can identify anatomic variants.
   b. It can assess the branch arterial involvement.
   c. It will provide information about aortic valve involvement.
   d. It can assess the left ventricular systolic function.
E. Transthoracic echocardiography: It can evaluate proximal aorta with high sensitivity and specificity. It is limited by obesity, emphysema, mechanical ventilation that can be overcome by esophageal approach.
F. Invasive aortography: It will give following information—
   a. Location of dissection
   b. Visualization of false lumen and intimal flap
   c. Involvement of branch vessels
   d. Communication between true and false lumen
   e. It can visualize penetrating aortic ulcer—it is characterized by protrusion of endovascular contrast into atherosclerotic plaque.

Therapy

Following are the indications of aortic dissection:

Medical therapy	Surgical therapy	Endovascular therapy
Uncomplicated type B dissection	Acute type A dissection	Type B dissection associated with malperfusion syndrome
Stable aortic arch only dissection	Alternative to endovascular therapy in case of complicated type B dissection	Complicated type B dissection in thoracic artery dissection including which is characterized by: • Propagation • Compromise of major branches of aorta • Impending rupture • Continued pain
Stable chronic type B dissection	Dysfunction of end organ	Alternative to medical treatment in case of uncomplicated type B dissection
	Aortic valve insufficiency with Marfan syndrome with retrograde extension toward ascending aorta	Fenestration of the intimal flap along with stenting of narrowed vessel branch in order to increase the flow through these vessels

Medical Therapy

Patient should be admitted in intensive therapy unit for hemodynamic monitoring. In absence of hypotension, treatment should be given to:

a. Reduce cardiac contractility
b. reduce systemic arterial pressure
c. reduce the shear stress.

In case of acute dissection:

Drugs	Loading dose	Maintenance dose
	First-line agent	
Propranolol	1 mg intravenously for 3–5 minutes	2–6 mg intravenously 4–6 hourly
Labetalol	10 mg intravenously over 2 minutes, followed by 20–80 mg over 10–15 minutes	2 mg/min as intravenous infusion which can be titrated to 5–20 mg/min
Esmolol	500 μg/kg intravenously as bolus dose	50–200 μg/kg/min continuous intravenous infusion
Metoprolol	5 mg intravenously over 5 minutes	5–10 mg intravenously 4–6 hourly
	Second line of drugs	
Enalaprilat	0.625 mg intravenously	0.625 mg intravenously 4–6 hourly
Verapamil	0.075 = 0.1 mg/kg—2.25–5 mg/kg intravenously over 2 minutes	5–15 mg/h intravenous infusion

Continued

Continued

Drugs	Loading dose	Maintenance dose
Diltiazem	0.25 mg/kg intravenously over 2 minutes, there is no effect, 0.35 mg/kg after 15 minutes	5 mg/h

The aim is to maintain the heart rate at 60 beats/min.

To maintain systolic blood pressure ≤ 120 mm Hg level, sodium nitroprusside. But, intravenous vasodilator is contraindicated as it may propagate dissection by increasing the hydraulic shear.

Surgical Therapy

It is the preferred treatment in acute aortic dissection of ascending aorta and in case of intramural hematoma.

Procedure includes:

- **a.** Intimal flap excision
- **b.** Obliteration of false lumen
- **c.** Placement of interposition graft
- **d.** Aortic valve replacement in case of involvement of aortic valve

Postoperative mortality is 15–25%. Major causes of postoperative mortality are:

Postoperative complications

- **A.** Respiratory failure
- **B.** Stroke
- **C.** Bleeding requiring reoperation
- **D.** Heart failure
- **E.** Infections
- **F.** Myocardial infarction
- **G.** Ventricular arrhythmias
- **H.** Acute postoperative renal failure
- **I.** Mesenteric ischemia
- **J.** Paraplegia

Hybrid procedure involving both surgery and endovascular repair is required if the dissection involves both aortic arch and descending thoracic aorta.

Q76. Outline the management of strategy for patients with unstable angina and non-ST segment elevation myocardial infarction (NSTEMI). Add a note on the pathophysiology of cardiogenic shock.

MGR/OCT2003/MDIII (15)

MGR/SEP2007/MDIV (20)

Discuss the advances in the management of unstable angina and non-ST segment elevation myocardial infarction.

BF/OCT2010/MDIII (25)

Evaluation of cardiac pain in its initial stages.

ERA/MAY2011/MDII (10)

Discuss the management of unstable angina.

ERA/MAY2012/MDIII (15)

Management of unstable angina.

KERALA UNIVERSITY, 2017 (10)

Management of non-ST elevated acute coronary syndrome.

BABA FARID UNI OF HEALTH SC, 2018 (10)

RAJIV GANDHI UNI OF HEALTH SC, 2018 (10)

Risk stratification in non-ST elevation acute coronary syndrome.

BABA FARID UNI OF HEALTH SC, 2019 (10)

ANSWER

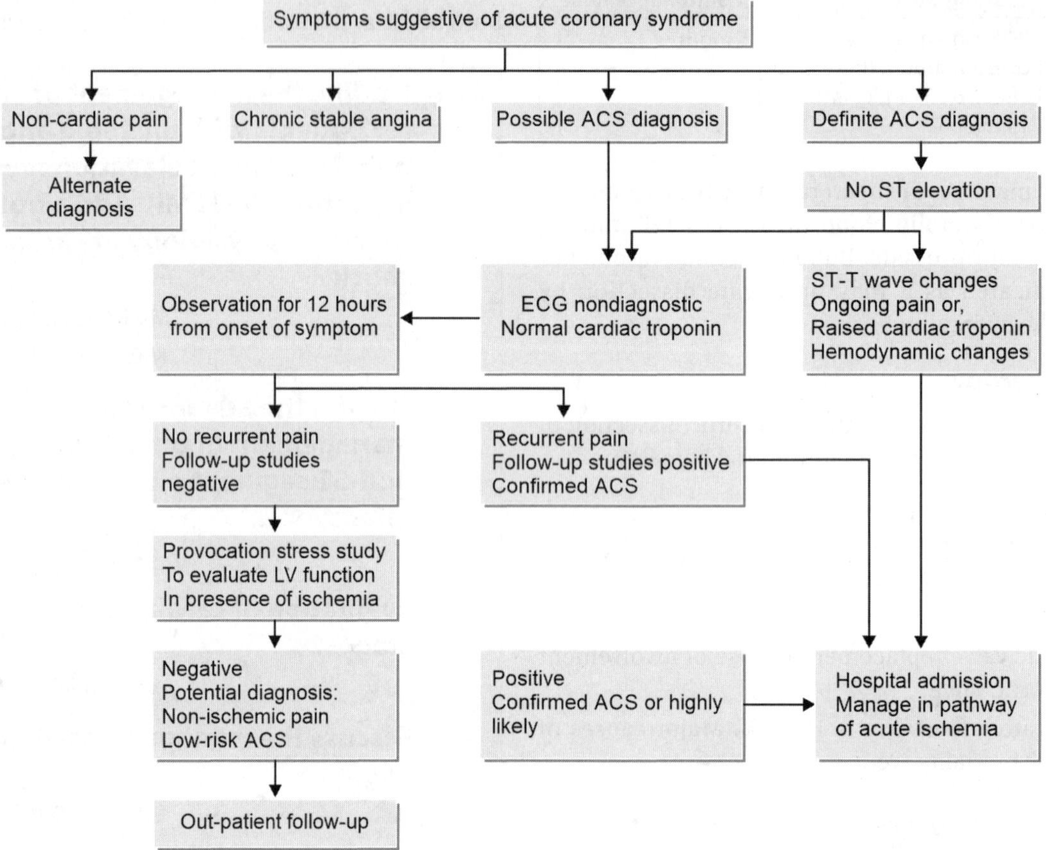

(ACS: acute coronary syndrome)

A. From history and physical examination:

a. Severe chest pain has any one of the three characteristic features:

1. Occurs at rest or with minimal exertion and lasting for >10 minutes.
2. Relatively recent onset or within prior 2 weeks

   Along with or without

3. Crescendo pattern of pain, i.e., pain is more severe, prolonged, or frequent as compared to previous episodes.

Diagnosis of non-STEMI can be established if the patient has any of the three features along with absence of ST segment elevation in ECG plus the evidence of myocardial necrosis ion the form of elevated biomarkers in the blood.

Chest pain is located in the substernal region radiating to left shoulder, left arm with or without radiation superiorly to jaw and neck.

b. There may be angina equivalent like:

1. Dyspnea
2. Epigastric discomfort
3. Nausea
4. Weakness

It is more common in:

1. Elderly
2. Women
3. Diabetes mellitus

Physical findings are unremarkable, but in case of large areas of ischemia following may be present:

a. Pale
b. Cool skin
c. Sinus tachycardia
d. Third heart sound
e. Fourth heart sound
f. Basal crepitation
g. Hypotension occasionally

B. Electrocardiogram:

It should be done within 10 minutes of the first contact. It may be normal, in that case it should be done within 15–30 minutes in case of persistent symptoms. In some cases V_7–V_9 and V_3R and V_4R lead should be taken to rule out the involvement of left circumflex artery as well as right ventricular myocardial infarction. It will demonstrate:

a. Evidence of new ST-segment depression which may be transient or persists for several days following the event.
b. T wave changes—though it is more common but less specific unless it is:
   1. Newly developed
   2. Inversion of ≥3 mV

C. Cardiac biomarkers:

a. Cardiac troponin: According to AHA 2015 guideline, dynamic elevation of cardiac troponin above the 99th percentile of the healthy individual is the diagnostic of myocardial infarction. It will be elevated within 1 hour of onset of the event and persistently elevated for 7–14 days. These assays when compared with standard troponin assays it has following advantages:
   1. 20% increase relatively in type 1 MI and twofold increase in case of type 2 MI.
   2. It will reduce the troponin blind interval for AMI.
   3. It has a higher negative predictive value for MI.

Following are the causes of cardiac troponin in absence of IHD:

Cardiac causes	Noncardiac causes
Congestive cardiac failure	Pulmonary embolism
Tachyarrhythmias	Renal failure
Aortic dissection	• Trauma • Electric shock • Burns
Coronary spasm	Hyper- or hypothyroidism
Cardiac procedures	Sepsis
Infiltrative diseases	Shock
Hypertensive emergencies	Stroke
Myocarditis/Pericarditis	Rhabdomyolysis
Structural disease like aortic stenosis	Toxicity

b. Creatine kinase—myocardial band: It will be elevated within 4–8 hours and peak for 18–24 hours. Hence, it is 50% less sensitive, serial testing can increase its sensitivity and specificity. False positive results are found in following cases:
   1. Renal failure
   2. Peripartum period
   3. Skeletal muscle injury
   4. Postsurgery
c. Copeptin: It is C-terminal part of vasopressin, and it has a promising role in the diagnosis of MI when it is used in association with cardiac troponin. So according to ESC 2015, when high sensitive cardiac troponin assay is not available it can be recommended.
d. Myoglobin: It is leaked from the damaged myocardium more rapidly as compared to AST, creatine kinase and LDH, hence it will be raised very early and highly sensitive.
e. C-reactive protein: It will be elevated as general marker of inflammatory process.

D. Coronary computed tomography:

In equivocal cases it should be done to improve the accuracy as well as speed of evaluation with the following goals:

a. To exclude or recognize the myocardial infarction by using cardiac troponin
b. To detect ischemia at rest by serial ECG.
c. To detect significant coronary obstruction at rest or evidence of myocardial ischemia by stress testing.

Risk Stratification

This can be done by following scoring:

A. TIMI risk scoring tool: It is composed of seven risk indicators that is rated during presentation, it can predict mortality for both 30 days and 1 year.

History	Presentation
Age ≥65 years	• Recent severe angina • Evidence of at least two episodes over last 24 hours
≥3 coronary artery disease risk factors	Elevated cardiac biomarkers
Known case of coronary artery disease	Deviation of ST segments ≥ 0.5 mm
ASA for 7 days	

a. TIMI score: 0–2—Low risk
b. TIMI score: 3–4 points—intermediate risk
c. TIMI score: 5–7 points—High risk

Additional risk factors are:

a. Diabetes mellitus
b. Left ventricular dysfunction
c. Renal dysfunction
d. Elevated level B-type natriuretic peptide

B. GRACE score:

Medical history		Findings at initial hospital presentation		Findings during hospitalization	
Age in years	**Points**	**Resting heart rate in beats/ minute**	**Points**	**Initial serum creatinine in mg/dL**	**Points**
≤29	0	<49.9	0	0–0.39	1
30–39	0	50–69.9	3	0.4–0.79	3
40–49	18	70–89.9	9	0.8–1.19	5
50–59	36	90–109.9	11	1.2–1.59	7
60–69	55	110–149.9	23	1.6–1.99	9
70–79	73	150–199.9	35	2–3.99	15
80–89	91	>200	43	>4	20
≥90	100	**Systolic blood pressure in mm Hg**		**Elevated cardiac enzymes**	15
History of CCF	24	<79.9	24		
History of MI	12	80–99.9	22		
		100–119.9	18		
		120–139.9	14		
		140–159.9	10		
		160–199.9	4		
		>200	0		
		ST segment depression	11	**No. in-hospital percutaneous intervention**	14

Continued

Continued

Total risk score = sum of points

GRACE risk score	In-hospital risk stratification	GRACE risk score	Post-discharge 6 months stratification
<108	Low	<108	Low
109–140	Intermediate	89–118	Intermediate
>104	High	>118	High

Medical Management

Patient should be admitted in ICU with continuous monitoring of pulse, respiratory rate, temperature, and blood pressure and moist oxygen should be administered.

Anti-ischemic Treatment

Drugs	Indications	Dosage	Contraindications/Adverse effects
Nitrates	ACS patients with chest discomfort	To start with 0.3–0.6 mg sublingually or buccal spray if symptoms persists In case of persistence of symptoms in spite of giving three doses at 5 minutes apart, nitroglycerin should be given intravenously at a rate of 5–10 µg/min, followed by gradual increase by 10 µg/min at every 3–5 minutes until: • Relief of symptoms • Fall of systolic blood pressure to <90 mm Hg • Dose will reach 200 µg/min	• Hypotension • Severe aortic stenosis • Right ventricular infarction • Patient receiving phosphodiesterase type 5 inhibitor such as sildenafil, vardenafil, and tadalafil
Beta-blockers	ACS patients	Intravenous beta-blockers: • Metoprolol 5 mg every 5 minutes • Esmolol 50–300 mg/kg/min • Atenolol 5 mg intravenously with monitoring blood pressure, heart rate, crepitation on auscultation	• Acute or severe heart failure • Low cardiac output • Systolic pressure < 90 mm Hg • Contraindication to therapy to beta-blocker like active broncho-spasm, high-degree AV block

Continued

Continued

Drugs	Indications	Dosage	Contraindications/Adverse effects
		Oral beta-blocker: • Metoprolol: 50–200 mg twice daily • Propranolol: 80–320 mg for 2–4 doses • Atenolol: 25–100 mg once daily • Bisoprolol: 5–20 mg daily • Target heart rate: 50–60 beats/min	• Shock • Heart rate of <50 beats/min
Calcium-channel blocker	• Patients with ACS not relieved by or intolerant to nitrates, beta-blockers • Variant angina	Verapamil or diltiazem is used	• Pulmonary edema • Left ventricular dysfunction
Morphine sulfate	• Symptoms not relieved by three serial sublingual nitroglycerin tablet • Recurrence of ischemic symptoms	2–5 mg intravenously and it can be repeated every 5–30 minutes as required to get relief	• Respiratory depression • Hypotension • Obtundation • Confusion

(ACS: acute coronary syndrome)

Antiplatelet Drugs

Drug	Mechanism of action	Doses	Adverse effects/ Contraindications
Aspirin	It irreversibly inhibits thromboxane A2 production by cyclo-oxygenase enzyme	Initial dose is 325 mg nonenteric tablet, it is followed by 75–100 mg nonenteric tablet	Risk of bleeding if the dose is exceed 200 mg. Contraindications are: • Allergy to aspirin • Active bleeding • Platelet disorder
Clopidogrel	It is prodrug, it is converted into active metabolite R130964 by cytochrome P and irreversibly blocks plate-P2Y12 receptor	Loading dose is 300–600 mg, it is followed by 75 mg/day. If it is given with aspirin as dual anti-platelet therapy, there is 20% reduction of cardiovascular death, myocardial infarction and stroke as compared to aspirin	Bleeding
Prasugrel	• Thienopyridine, it has action more rapid onset of action and inhibits platelet as compared to clopidogrel • It should be given as pre-PCI	Loading dose is 60 mg orally followed by 10 mg/day	Contraindicated in prior history of stroke, TIA, or high risk of bleeding
Ticagrelor	It is reversible platelet P2Y inhibitor	Loading dose is 180 mg followed by 90 mg twice daily	Transient development of dyspnea, but not exacerbation of CHF or COPD
Cangrelor	• It is P2Y inhibitor, acts as an adjunct to PCI to reduce the risk of periprocedural cases of stable angina, non-STEMI, and STEMI • It reduces the risk of stent thrombosis	30 µg/kg intravenous dose followed by immediate infusion of 4 µg/kg/min	
Abciximab	It is a Fab fragment of chimeric-human-murine monoclonal antibody c7E3	0.25 µg/kg as bolus dose followed by infusion of 0.125 µg/kg/min (maximum up to 10 µg/min) for 12–24 hours	

Continued

Continued

Drug	Mechanism of action	Doses	Adverse effects/ Contraindications
Eptifibatide	It is derived from structure of barbourin, platelet GPIIb/IIIa inhibitor received from venom of southern pygmy rattlesnake	180 µg/kg bolus dose, it is followed by 10 minutes later by next 2nd bolus of 180 µg/kg along with 2 µg/kg/min for 72–96 hours following 1st dose	
Tirofiban	It is tyrosine derivative, nonpeptide inhibitor of platelet GP IIb/IIIa receptor		

(CHF: congestive heart failure; COPD: chronic obstructive pulmonary disease; GP: glycoprotein; PCI: percutaneous coronary intervention; STEMI: ST-segment elevation of myocardial infarction; TIA: transient ischemic attack)

Anticoagulants

Drugs	Doses	Contraindications/Adverse effects
Unfractionated heparin	• Bolus dose is 70–100 U/kg (maximum 5,000 U), it is followed by 12–15 U/kg/h infusion (maximum 1,000 U/h) • It should be titrated to activated clotting time 250–300 seconds	• Duration is 48–72 hours, but weaning is required so that rebound thrombin generation can be minimized • Heparin-induced thrombocytopenia occurs in 5% of patients due to formation of antibodies against complex heparin as well as platelet factor 4 resulting DIC. It can be treated by stopping heparin • Lepirudin: intravenous bolus 0.4 mg/kg followed by 0.15 mg/kg/h continuous infusion
Enoxaparin	• 1 mg/kg subcutaneously 12 hourly • 1st dose is preceded by 30 mg intravenous bolus • Renal adjustment to 1 mg/kg once daily in case of creatinine clearance/min	In case of renal insufficiency severe obesity, its level should be monitored
Fondaparinux, inhibitor of factor Xa activity	2.5 mg subcutaneously four times daily	Low risk of major bleeding
Bivalirudin, direct thrombin inhibitor	Initial intravenous bolus dose of 0.75 mg/kg followed by infusion of 1.75 mg/kg/h	Low risk of major bleeding

(DIC: disseminated intravascular coagulation)

Additional drugs are:

A. HMG-CoA Inhibitor—statin 80 mg/day prior to PCI will reduce periprocedural MI and ACS recurrences. If the patient will not demonstrate adequate response to statin, 10 mg ezetimibe should be given to further reduce the LDL-C level.

B. Angiotensin-converting enzyme inhibitor

C. Angiotensin receptor blockers

Q77. Angiotensin receptor blockers.

MGR/OCT2003/MDIII (5)

ANSWER

Mechanism of Actions

Renin–angiotensin system is implicated in the pathogenesis of:

a. Essential hypertension

b. Reno-vascular hypertension

c. Congestive cardiac failure

d. Renal diseases associated with albuminuria

Selective inhibition of angiotensin II by competitive inhibition of angiotensin receptors by displacing the angiotensin II from angiotensin I receptor that leads to reduction of blood pressure through:

a. Antagonizing the angiotensin-I induced vasoconstriction
b. Inhibition of aldosterone release
c. Inhibition of catecholamine release
d. Inhibition of arginine vasopressin release
e. Decreasing water intake
f. Increased renal loss of water

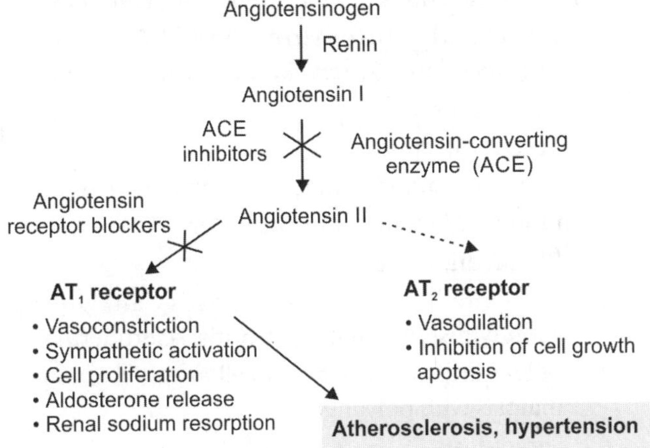

Name of the drugs are:

a. Losartan
b. Telmisartan
c. Valsartan
d. Olmesartan
e. Irbesartan
f. Candesartan
g. Eprosartan

Candesartan and olmesartan are pro-drugs, only become metabolically active during the absorption through the gastrointestinal tract.

Adverse Effect

A. Upper respiratory tract infection
B. Headache
C. Occasional dizziness
D. Inability to sleep
E. Dyspnea
F. Heart burn
G. Nasal congestion
H. Back pain
I. Fatigue
J. Diarrhea
K. Angioedema
L. Renal failure
M. Rarely hyperkalemia

Therapeutic Effects

A. Hypertension
B. Prevention of stroke
C. Diabetic nephropathy
D. Myocardial infarction
E. Migrainous headache

Contraindications

A. Bilateral renal artery stenosis
B. Drugs causing hyperkalemia
C. Woman not practicing contraception
D. Angioedema to ACE inhibitors

Uses

Active ingredient	Daily maintenance dosage (min–max)	Indications approved by FDA
Losartan	25–100 mg in 1 or 2 doses	• Hypertension • Left ventricular hypertrophy • Diabetic nephropathy
Irbesartan	150–300 mg in 1 dose	• Hypertension • Nephropathy in type 2 diabetes mellitus patients
Candesartan	8–32 mg in 1 dose	• Hypertension • Heart failure
Eprosartan	400–800 mg in 1 or 2 doses	Hypertension
Olmesartan	20–40 mg in 1 dose	• Hypertension • Pediatric hypertension
Telmisartan	40–80 mg in 1 dose	• Hypertension • Cardiovascular risk in diabetic patients
Valsartan	80–320 mg in 1 dose	• Hypertension • Heart failure • Postmyocardial infarction

(FDA: Food and Drug Administration)

Q78. Discuss the etiology, pathophysiology, clinical features, complications and management of pericardial effusion.
MGR/MAR2008/MDIV (20)

Define and describe causes of pericardial effusion. Clinical features and echocardiographic diagnosis of cardiac tamponade.

DNB 2018 (2+3+3+2)

A 35 years old male patient has suddenly developed chest pain on the left side followed by worsening of breathlessness. On examination he has hypotension and pulsus paradoxus.

What is the most likely diagnosis?

How will you confirm the diagnosis?

What intervention is required to save his life?

(Answer in Q55)

GURU RAMDAS UNI OF HEALTH SC, 2022 (10)

ANSWER

Definition

Accumulation of >50 mL of fluid in the pericardial cavity is called pericardial effusion.

It can be classified according to the following:

A. Onset:
- **a.** Acute: Less than 3 months
- **b.** Chronic: More than 3 months

B. Size:
- **a.** Mild pericardial effusion—50–100 mL, echo-free space is <10 mm.
- **b.** Moderate pericardial effusion—100–500 mL, echo-free space is 10–20 mm.
- **c.** Large pericardial effusion—More than 500 mL, echo-free space is >20 mm.

C. Localization of accumulation:
- **a.** Circumferential
- **b.** Loculated

D. Composition of the pericardial fluid:
- **a.** Transudate
- **b.** Exudate
- **c.** Hemopericardium
- **d.** Pyopericardium

E. Hemodynamic impact:
- **a.** None
- **b.** Effusive-constrictive
- **c.** Tamponade

Causes of Pericardial Effusion

A. Idiopathic

B. Infections:
- **a.** Viral infections—echo-virus, adenovirus, mump virus, infectious mononucleosis, and influenza
- **b.** Bacterial infection—*Staphylococcus, Streptococcus, Hemophilus influenza, Salmonella*
- **c.** Tuberculosis
- **d.** Fungal infection
- **e.** Other infections—amebiasis, *Echinococcus*

C. Immunologic/inflammatory disorders:
- **a.** Rheumatic fever
- **b.** Systemic lupus erythematosus, ankylosing spondylitis, rheumatoid arthritis, scleroderma
- **c.** Polyarteritis nodosa, giant cell arteritis, granulomatosis with polyangitis
- **d.** Sarcoidosis
- **e.** Inflammatory bowel disease, Whipple disease
- **f.** Behçet's syndrome, Reiter syndrome

D. Acute myocardial infarction
- **a.** Delayed postmyocardial—pericardial injury syndrome
- **b.** Postmyocardial infarction syndrome

E. Trauma

F. Metabolic:
- **a.** Myxedema
- **b.** Uremia
- **c.** Hypoalbuminemia

G. Neoplastic:
- **a.** Primary:
  1. Teratoma
  2. Fibroma
  3. Sarcoma
  4. Angioma
- **b.** Secondary:
  1. Breast carcinoma
  2. Bronchogenic carcinoma
  3. Leukemia
  4. Melanoma
  5. Lymphoma

H. Drugs:
- **a.** Hydralazine
- **b.** Minoxidil
- **c.** Warfarin
- **d.** Phenytoin
- **e.** Methysergide
- **f.** Procainamide

Clinical Presentations

Spectrum of clinical presentation is from asymptomatic presentation to cardiac tamponade. Clinical presentation depends upon:
- **a.** Etiology of pericardial effusion
- **b.** Volume of effusion
- **c.** Rate of accumulation:
  - **1.** Rapid accumulation will lead to early symptom like tamponade.
  - **2.** Slow accumulation may develop symptoms only after accumulation of large amount of pericardial fluid.

Following are the symptoms:
- **a.** Chest discomfort
- **b.** Chest fullness
- **c.** Progressive dyspnea
- **d.** Orthopnea
- **e.** Nausea/Vomiting
- **f.** Different types of compressive symptoms:
  - **1.** Compression on esophagus leads to dysphagia.
  - **2.** Compression on recurrent laryngeal nerve leads to hoarseness of voice.
  - **3.** Compression on phrenic nerve leading to hiccups
- **g.** Physical examination reveals:
  - **1.** Muffled heart sound in case of large pericardial effusion
  - **2.** Ewart's sign:
    - Dullness on percussion
    - Bronchial breath sound
    - Egophony below the angle of left scapula
  - **3.** Sinus tachycardia along with low blood pressure—are ominous sign of pericardial tamponade. In case of cardiac tamponade:
    - Pulsus paradoxus of >10 mm Hg
    - Beck triad—Muffled heart sound, jugular venous distention, and hypotension.

Management

Following are the high-risk features:
- **a.** Signs of tamponade:
  - **1.** Tachycardia
  - **2.** Tachypnea
  - **3.** Hypotension
- **b.** Large effusion
- **c.** Chronic effusion
- **d.** Suspicion for neoplastic process or bacterial process

Following are the work-up for suspected pericardial effusion:
- **a.** Routine work-up for pericardial disease
- **b.** Echocardiogram
- **c.** Exclusion of the chronic diseases:
  - **1.** Hypothyroidism
  - **2.** Chronic kidney disease
  - **3.** Cancer screening

Indications of imaging: Following are the echo-findings in case pleural effusion—
- **a.** There is evidence of persistent intrapericrdial echo-free space throughout the cardiac cycle, but presence of echo-free space only during the systolic phase is suggestive of normal amount of pericardial fluid—it is trivial effusion.
- **b.** Small amount of pericardial fluid of <10 mL present posteriorly distal to AV ring.
- **c.** Moderate effusion means echo-free space: 10–20 mm surrounding the heart.
- **d.** Large effusion having echo-free space of >20 mm—it is circumferential with greater anterolateral expansion.
- **e.** Loculated pericardial effusion—presence of echo-densities, stranding or presence of adhesions—suggests exudate over transudate.
- **f.** There is presence of echo-free space between descending aorta and heart as evidenced by 2D echocardiography in parasternal view—suggestive of left pleural effusion.
- **g.** Anterior effusion can be differentiated from anterior epicardial fat which is based on:
  - **1.** High echo-densities
  - **2.** Synchronous with the heart

CT and MRI can be considered in case of suspicious cases like:
- **a.** Pericardial masses

b. Pericardial thickening
c. Complex effusion

CT scan characterizes the effusion based on CT attenuation:

a. <10 HU—indicates simple transudate
b. 20–60 HU—indicates:
    1. Purulent effusion
    2. Malignant effusion
    3. Myxedematous effusion
c. 60–80 HU—
    1. Hemopericardium
    2. Chylopericardium

Features of pericardial thickening on CT scan are:

a. Similar attenuation to effusion
b. High-attenuation nodularities
c. Lack of movement with change of position
d. Enhancement of pericardium with contrast

Medical Therapy

A. Treatment of the etiologies
B. Following are the recommendation of pericardiocentesis:
    a. Large chronic effusion
    b. Presence of significant symptoms
    c. Suspicion of etiology—whether it is bacterial or neoplastic.
    d. Presence of features of tamponade
C. Slow drainage at a rate of 30 mL/day decreases the risk of reaccumulation.
D. Pericardiotomy is needed in the following cases:
    a. Effusion with recalcitrant symptoms
    b. Effusion is loculated.
    c. Need for biopsy

Prognosis

A. Small pericardial effusion is associated with worse prognosis adjusted for age and sex and underlying condition.
B. Moderate and large pericardial effusion are associated with worse prognosis as these are caused by neoplastic process and bacterial infection.
C. Following are the echocardiographic follow-up in case of pericardial effusion:
    a. In case of small asymptomatic effusion—no follow-up is usually required.
    b. Follow-up is required every 6 months in case of moderate pericardial effusion.
    c. Follow-up is required every 3–6 months in case of large pericardial effusion.

Q79. Causes of hypertension in young.

MGR/MAR2007/MDIV (5)

A 20 years old male presented with BP of 170/110. He has breathlessness and severe headache. Answer the following:

What are the causes of hypertension in young age group? How will you investigate in this patient? Outline the pharmacological management of this case?

KERALA UNIVERSITY, 2017 (20)

Define hypertension. Discuss the approach of management in a newly diagnosed young hypertensive patient.

RAJIV GANDHI UNIVERSITY OF HEALTH SC, KARNATAKA, 2017 (10)

ANSWER

Hypertension in young can be defined as hypertension diagnosed in patients younger than 40 years of age. These patients tend to have other medical problems, such as diabetes mellitus, dyslipidemia, obesity, etc.

Category	Systolic pressure in mm Hg	Diastolic pressure in mm Hg
Optimal	<120	<80
Normal	<130	<85
High normal	130–139	85–89
	Hypertension	
Stage 1	140–159	90–99
Stage 2	160–179	100–109
Stage 3	≥180	≥110

Prior to diagnose the patients as young hypertensive, accurate measurement of blood pressure should be done. He should be asked regarding diet and intake of medicines.

Following medicines are responsible for young hypertension:

Drugs	Examples
Estrogen	Oral contraceptives
Herbal	Ephedra, ginseng
NSAIDs	Ibuprofen, COX-2 inhibitor, naproxen
Psychiatric medications	Clozapine, lithium, TCA, carbamazepine, and buspirone
Sympathomimetic	Decongestant and diet pills
Illicit medicines	Cocaine and amphetamine

(COX-2: cyclooxygenase 2; NSAIDs: nonsteroidal anti-inflammatory drugs; TCA: tricyclic antidepressant)

Causes of secondary hypertension in young:

Diseases	History	Clinical features
Primary aldosteronism	Excessive urination, muscle spasm, weakness, and headache	Blood pressure not controlled
Pheochromocytoma	Palpitations, headache, diaphoresis, skin sensations, and weight loss	Fluctuating blood pressure, orthostatic hypotension
Cushing syndrome	Weight gain, insomnia, weakness, depression, easy bruising, and arthralgia	Thinning of skin, proximal myopathy, reddish-purple striae, Cushingoid appearance
Acromegaly	Visual disturbance, increasing size of ring and/or shoe	Frontal bossing, macroglossia, hyperpigmentation, enlarged hand and feet, and prognathism
Hyperthyroidism	Hyperactivity, weight loss, irritability, palpitation, diarrhea, and oligomenorrhea	Warm and moist skin, tremors, tachycardia, different eye signs, and goiters
Hypothyroidism	Tiredness, cold intolerance, weight gain, hoarseness of voice, poor appetite, and constipation	Dry coarse skin, edema, diffuse alopecia, goiter, delayed relaxation of tendon reflexes, myxedematous facies, and puffiness of hand
Hyperparathyroidism	Kidney stones, polyuria, depression, joint/bone pain, epigastric pain	Depression and muscle weakness
Renal parenchymal disease	Low urine output, dizziness, weakness, and facial/lower limb swelling	Edema, anemia, and facial edema
Renal artery stenosis	Uncontrollable blood pressure, sudden deterioration of renal function	Renal bruit
Polycystic kidney disease	Flank pain, hematuria, recurrent urinary tract infection	Kidneys are palpable and ballotable
Coarctation of aorta	Chest pain, hypertension	• Presence of systolic murmur at left infraclavicular area • Difference in blood pressure between arms and legs is 20 mm Hg
OSA	Daytime somnolence	Morbid obesity

(OSA: obstructive sleep apnea)

Algorithm for Management of Hypertension in Young Adults

I. Introduction

A. Purpose

B. Definition of 'young' (e.g., < 40 or < 50 years)

II. Confirmation of Hypertension

1. Office BP measurement technique
2. Repeat measurements on ≥ 2 visits
3. Use out-of-office BP (home, ABPM) to confirm

III. Risk Assessment and Evaluation

1. Cardiovascular risk factors (lipids, diabetes, smoking, family history)
2. Target organ damage assessment
3. Screen for secondary hypertension causes

IV. Lifestyle (Nonpharmacologic) Therapy—For All

1. Dietary changes (DASH, low salt, potassium)
2. Weight loss/BMI optimization
3. Physical exercise

4. Alcohol restriction, smoking cessation
5. Stress, sleep hygiene

V. Treatment Decision Based on BP Category

A. High-normal/Borderline: Lifestyle changes and follow-up in 3–6 months.

B. Stage 1 hypertension:
   - Low risk: Lifestyle + Observe
   - Moderate/High risk or TOD: Start drug therapy + Lifestyle

C. Stage 2 hypertension: Initiate combination therapy (2 drugs) + Lifestyle

VI. Pharmacologic Therapy

Preferred drug classes: ACE inhibitors (ACEi), angiotensin receptor blockers (ARB), calcium channel blockers (CCB), thiazide/thiazide-like diuretics. Beta-blockers for specific indications.

Common antihypertensives with dosage and duration

Drug class and example	Typical dosage range	Duration/Notes
ACE inhibitor—Enalapril	5–20 mg/day (once or divided bid)	Long-term; monitor renal function, potassium
ARB—Losartan	25–100 mg/day (once or divided bid)	Long-term; useful in ACEi intolerance
CCB—Amlodipine	5–10 mg once daily	Long-term; monitor for edema, headache
Thiazide diuretic—Hydrochlorothiazide	12.5–25 mg once daily	Best in morning; monitor electrolytes
Thiazide-like—Chlorthalidone	12.5–25 mg once daily	Preferred for longer duration of action
Beta-blocker—Metoprolol	25–100 mg bid	Indicated in IHD, arrhythmias; not first-line in young without comorbidity

VII. Follow-up and Titration

Monitor BP every 4–8 weeks initially. If not controlled, escalate drugs. Assess adherence, lifestyle, secondary causes. Once stable, follow-up every 3–6 months.

VIII. Resistant Hypertension and Referral

If BP uncontrolled on ≥ 3 drugs (including diuretic), re-evaluate for secondary causes, refer to specialist, and consider advanced therapies (e.g., renal denervation).

IX. Flowchart (Simplified Diagram)

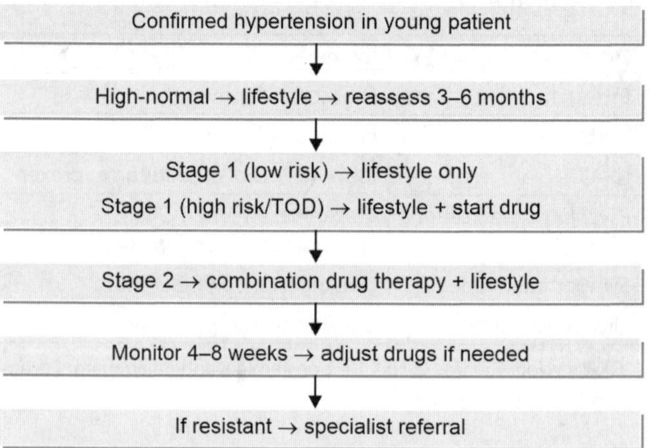

Algorithm for Management of Hypertensive Emergencies in Young Adults

I. Introduction

Hypertensive emergency is defined as severely elevated blood pressure (usually >180/120 mm Hg) with evidence of acute target organ damage (brain, heart, kidneys, aorta, eyes). It requires immediate reduction of blood pressure with intravenous agents under monitored settings.

II. Initial Assessment

1. Confirm severe BP elevation with proper technique.
2. Assess symptoms and signs of target organ damage: neurological deficits, chest pain, dyspnea, oliguria, retinal changes.
3. Obtain baseline investigations: ECG, troponin, renal function, urinalysis, fundoscopy, chest X-ray, CT/MRI brain if indicated.
4. Admit to ICU/monitored setting.

III. Treatment Goals

- Reduce mean arterial pressure (MAP) by no more than 25% within the first hour.
- Then, if stable, reduce to 160/100–110 mm Hg over the next 2–6 hours.
- Gradual normalization over 24–48 hours, unless specific conditions (aortic dissection, eclampsia, etc.) require faster reduction.

IV. Intravenous Antihypertensive Drugs (Commonly Used in Emergencies)

Drug	Typical dose and administration	Notes/Duration
Nicardipine	Start 5 mg/h IV infusion, titrate by 2.5 mg/h every 5–15 min, max 15 mg/h	Onset 5–15 min; duration 30–60 min; preferred in neurologic emergencies
Clevidipine	1–2 mg/h IV infusion, double every 90 sec until goal, then titrate; max 32 mg/h	Ultra-short acting; rapid titration possible
Labetalol	IV bolus 20 mg over 2 min, then 40–80 mg every 10 min (max 300 mg); or infusion 1–2 mg/min	Onset 2–5 min; duration 2–6 h; avoid in asthma/heart failure
Esmolol	IV bolus 500 mcg/kg over 1 min, then infusion 50–100 mcg/kg/min (max 300 mcg/kg/min)	Ultra-short acting β1-blocker; duration 10–20 min; useful in aortic dissection
Nitroglycerin	Start 5 mcg/min IV infusion, increase by 5 mcg/min every 5–10 min to 20–200 mcg/min	Onset 2–5 min; duration 5–10 min; useful in ACS, pulmonary edema
Sodium Nitroprusside	Start 0.3–0.5 mcg/kg/min IV, titrate up to 10 mcg/kg/min	Immediate onset; duration 1–2 min; risk of cyanide toxicity—short-term use only
Hydralazine	IV bolus 10–20 mg every 4–6 h	Onset 10–20 min; duration 3–8 h; often used in pregnancy-related emergencies
Fenoldopam	Start 0.1 mcg/kg/min IV infusion, titrate by 0.05–0.1 mcg/kg/min every 15 min (max 1.6 mcg/kg/min)	Dopamine-1 agonist; improves renal perfusion; duration 30–60 min

V. Special Considerations in Young Adults

1. Higher prevalence of secondary hypertension (renal, endocrine, coarctation of aorta).
2. Careful evaluation of etiology after stabilization.
3. Consider pregnancy-related emergencies in young women (preeclampsia/eclampsia).

VI. Follow-up after Stabilization

- Transition to oral antihypertensives once stable (within 24–48 h).
- Tailor regimen according to underlying cause and comorbidities.
- Outpatient follow-up within 1–2 weeks after discharge, then every 1–3 months until stable.
- Investigate and treat secondary causes if suspected.
- Long-term lifestyle modification and adherence monitoring are essential.

VII. Simplified Algorithm Flow (Text Representation)

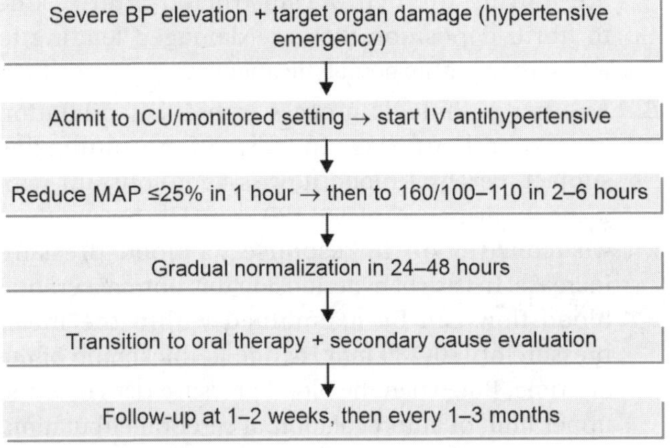

Q80. Pathogenesis of malignant hypertension.

MGR/MAR2008/MDIV (6)

ANSWER

Definition

This is hypertensive emergency that leads to target organ damage including central nervous system, kidney, and cardiovascular system. Accelerated hypertension is defined as sudden increase in blood pressure over the baseline associated with damage of target organs. Hypertensive urgency can be defined as systolic blood pressure of >220 mm Hg and diastolic blood pressure of >120 mm Hg but without any target organ damage.

Causes:

A. Essential hypertension

B. Any form of secondary hypertension

C. Complication of pregnancy like pre-eclampsia, eclampsia

D. Cocaine

E. Monoamine-oxidase inhibitors

F. Oral contraceptives

G. Withdrawal of β-blockers, alcohol and α-stimulant
H. Renal artery stenosis
I. Pheochromocytoma
J. Coarctation of aorta
K. Hyperaldosteronism

Etiopathogenesis

A. Main vascular lesion is fibrinoid necrosis of arterioles and small arteries. While red blood cells are flowing through the obstructed arteries due to fibrin deposition they are damaged leading to microangiopathic hemolytic anemia.
B. Another pathologic process in brain is dilatation of cerebral arteries. In case of normotensive subject, cerebral blood flow is kept constant with a mean pressure of 60–120 mm Hg by cerebral vasoconstriction in response to blood pressure increase. In case of hypertension this normal cerebral blood flow can be maintained within the mean pressure of 110–180 mm Hg due to thickening of the arteriole. But, when the blood pressure rises over the upper limit of autoregulation of cerebral circulation, cerebral blood vessels will dilate leading to cerebral hyperperfusion and cerebral edema producing hypertensive encephalopathy.
C. The characteristic finding in malignant hypertension is albuminuric retinitis that differs from atherosclerotic retinitis by the presence of neuroretinal edema due to increased intracranial pressure as a consequence increased diastolic pressure.
D. In kidney, there is acute tubular necrosis that leads to rapid deterioration of renal function and eventually death.

   All the above eye, renal changes are seen in essential hypertension, acute and chronic nephritis, polycystic kidney disease, pyelonephritis, Cushing syndrome, and toxemia in pregnancy will lead to malignant hypertension.
E. Measures taken for the blood pressure reduction can reverse the malignant phase to benign phase.

Q81. Heart transplantation.
MJPRU/2015/MDI (10)

Heart lung transplant.
MGR/APR2016/MDIV (7)

ANSWER

Following are the candidates of cardiac transplantation:

A. Accepted criteria: Heart failure survival score: High risk—
   a. Peak oxygen consumption < 14 mL/kg/min (<12, if the patient is on β-blocker)
   b. Predicted peal oxygen consumption < 50%.
   c. New York Heart Association Class III/IV heart failure refractory to maximum medical treatment
   d. Severely limiting ischemia not amenable to maximal interventional or surgical treatment
   e. Recurrent symptomatic ventricular arrhythmias refractory to medical, ICD, and surgical treatment.
B. Probable criteria: Heart failure survival score—medium risk:
   a. Peak oxygen consumption < 14 mL/kg/min and severe functional limitation
   b. Instability of the status of the fluid in the body and renal function despite good compliance, daily weight, salt and fluid restriction, and flexible diuretics
   c. Recurrent unstable ischemia not amenable to revascularization procedure
C. Inadequate criteria: Heart failure survival score—low risk:
   a. Peak oxygen consumption 15–18 mL/kg/min without other indication
   b. Left ventricular ejection fraction of <20% only
   c. History of NYHA of class III/IV only
   d. History of ventricular arrhythmia only

Contraindications to Cardiac Transplantation

A. History of pulmonary infarction within last 6–8 weeks
B. Active or recently diagnosed malignancy
C. Significant chronic renal impairment with persistent serum creatinine of >2.5 mg/dL or creatinine clearance < 25 mL/min.
D. Significant chronic hepatic impairment with persistent serum bilirubin level of >2.5 mg/dL or serum AST/ALT is more than two times normal.
E. History of systemic amyloidosis
F. Presence of significant lung disease
G. Presence of significant coagulopathies

H. Recent history of peptic ulcer disease
I. History of major chronic disabling disease
J. Excessive obesity with body mass index of >30%
K. History of carotid or peripheral vascular disease
L. Brittle diabetes
M. Diabetes mellitus with end-organ damage
N. Age: >65 years
O. Psychosocial causes:
   a. Active mental illness
   b. Psychosocial imbalances refractory to medical intervention
   c. Evidences of tobacco, alcohol abuse within last 6 months refractory to medical intervention

Following pretransplantation investigations should be done:

A. Laboratory evaluation:
   a. Complete blood count including total WBC, platelet count
   b. Serum biochemistry including liver function test, urea, creatinine, serum electrolytes, lipid profile, thyroid function test, uric acid, prothrombin time, activated partial thromboplastin time, and iron profile.
   c. Blood grouping and cross matching
   d. Serology including IgM and IgG antibodies against hepatitis B and C, cytomegalovirus, herpes-zoster, toxoplasmosis, HIV and as when required.
   e. Prostate specific antigen in male of >50 years
   f. Pap smear and mammogram in female of >40 years of age
   g. Screening against panel of donor antigen (panel reactive antibodies) and HLA phenotype
   h. 24 hours urine for creatinine clearance and total protein
   i. Urine culture for bacteria, fungus if indicated.
B. Cardiac evaluation:
   a. ECG
   b. Echocardiography
   c. 24 hours Holter monitoring
   d. If indicated Thallium scan
   e. Exercise stress test with measurement of oxygen uptake
   f. Right and left heart catheterization study
   g. In case of suspicion of heart failure myocardial biopsy in selected cases.
C. Renal study: Intravenous pyelogram if indicated.
D. Vascular study:
   a. Study of peripheral vascular system
   b. Transcranial Doppler study
   c. If the age is >55 years, carotid Doppler study
E. Pulmonary evaluation:
   a. Chest X-ray
   b. Pulmonary function test
   c. In case of age of >55 years, chest computerized tomogram for thoracic aorta
F. Gastrointestinal study:
   a. If age is >55 years, abdominal ultrasound
   b. If indicated upper gastrointestinal series
   c. If required barium enema
   d. If indicated liver biopsy
G. Bone: Bone densitometry
H. Neurologic screening
I. Psychiatric screening
J. Complete dental evaluation
K. Cardiothoracic evaluation

Allocation of donor heart depends upon:

A. Urgency of the clinical situation: If the patient is on mechanical support devices or under constant daily hemodynamic evaluation and under intravenous inotropic support should be given prior importance, whereas ambulatory patients living in their home has lower urgency status.
B. Time spent on the waiting list
C. Total distance from the recipient center: Total transit time from donor center to recipient center should be limited to 4 hours.

Donor-recipient Matching

A. In case of sensitized individual having circulating antibodies should have virtual or prospective cross match
B. Donor-recipient size match
C. Age of the donor should be restricted to 55 years.
D. Presence or absence of coronary artery disease, left ventricular hypertrophy in case of donor
E. Excessive leak of injury markers like troponin for donor
F. Poor cardiac contractile performance in donor heart

Classic heart can be derived from a patient with brain death, but now-a-days heart from a patient with circulatory death is evaluated increasingly for cardiac reanimation by variety of techniques such as ex-vivo reanimation followed by transplantation.

Contraindication in Case of Donor

A. Age is >55–60 years
B. Diffuse coronary artery disease
C. Evidences of myocardial infarction
D. Evidence of other heart disease
E. Refractory ventricular arrhythmias
F. Malignancy of any organ except central nervous system
G. Generalized infection refractory to treatment

Surgery for Cardiac Transplantation

Most common operation is "bi-caval orthotopic cardiac transplant" as it mimics normal anatomy—in this method:

A. Superior vena cava, inferior vena cava, aorta and pulmonary great vessels of both donor and recipient are connected.
B. Roof of the left atrium with draining pulmonary veins of the recipient is retained which will be connected with the donor left atrium—as this technique will maintain the function of right atrium of the donor—it governs the early postoperative right heart output thus preventing atrial arrhythmias.
C. Recipient is now left with surgical denervation, so the transplanted heart is not under sympathetic and parasympathetic control. So in early postoperative phase, high dose of catecholamine is required for maintaining adequate functioning of transplanted heart.
D. Bradycardia of the allograft cannot be treated with atropine as the heart is already denervated; hence, here the drug of choice is isoproterenol.
E. As the transplanted heart will adapt to the circulation of the host, it starts normal functioning at rest and later on with physical activity.

Following immunosuppressive drugs are used in case of cardiac transplantation:

Class of drugs	Generic drug	Cellular target	Side effects
Calcineurin inhibitors	Cyclosporine	Binds to cyclophilin and inhibits calcineurin	Hypertension, dyslipidemia, DM, and alopecia
	Tacrolimus	Binds to immunophilin and inhibits calcineurin	
ATG	Rabbit ATG	Deplete T cells in blood and peripheral lymphoid tissues	Cytokine release syndrome, thrombocytopenia, and leukopenia, serum sickness
	Horse ATG		
IL-2 receptor antagonists	Basiliximab	It will inhibit CD-25 present on the IL-2 receptor	Increased risk of infection
Anti-metabolites	Azathioprine	Its active metabolite 6-mercaptopurine is cell cycle inhibitor	• Pancreatitis • Bone marrow suppression • Hepatitis
	Mycophenolate mofetil	It will inhibit T and B cell proliferation	• Gastrointestinal toxicity • Leukopenia
Proliferation-signal inhibitors	Sirolimus	It will inhibit mechanistic target of rapamycin	• Nonspecific pneumonia • Pericardial effusion
	Everolimus	It inhibits mTORC1	• Hyper-lipidemia

(ATG: antithymocyte globulin; DM: diabetes mellitus; IL-2: interleukin 2; mTORC1: mammalian target of rapamycin complex 1)

Heart–Lung Transplantation

It is characterized by simultaneous replacement of heart and lung in patients suffering from end-stage cardiac and pulmonary diseases.

Causes of cardiopulmonary diseases requiring heart–lung transplantation:

A. Irreparable congenital heart diseases leading to pulmonary hypertension (Eisenmenger syndrome)
B. Primary pulmonary hypertension with irreversible right-sided heart failure
C. Sarcoidosis of heart and lung
D. In cystic fibrosis and irreversible bronchiectasis, both lungs should be transplanted along with heart if the function of the heart is also compromised.

Contraindications of Heart–Lung Transplantation

A. Relative contraindication is age: It should be not >60 years.
B. HIV positivity

Preclinical Evaluation

A. History and physical evaluation:
   a. History of cardiopulmonary diseases
   b. Exposure to infectious diseases
   c. Exposure to environment
   d. Family history
   e. Genetic history
   f. Substance-abuse history
B. On physical examination:
   a. Gastrointestinal bleeding
   b. Vascular insufficiency
   c. Occult carcinoma
C. Laboratory examinations:
   a. Serology
   b. Tests foe Epstein–Barr virus, cytomegalovirus, herpes-simplex virus
   c. History of immunization against hepatitis, rubella
   d. Serologic testing for fungus and tuberculin skin tests in attention to exposure to environment as this can indicate past exposure.
   e. In male patients with PSA positivity, appropriate work-up is required prior to transplantation.
   f. In case of PAP stain positive patients, proper evaluation and therapy are required prior to transplantation.
   g. Results of the following tests have to be in the normal ranges, otherwise therapy should be required prior to transplantation:
      1. Complete blood count
      2. Platelet count
      3. Prothrombin time
      4. Activated partial thromboplastin time
      5. Following biochemistry profile:
         - Liver function test
         - Lipid profile
         - Pulmonary function test
      6. Urine analysis
   h. Following should be used to determine the immunogenic stability of that patients for transplantation and donor matching:
      1. Blood grouping and screening
      2. Panel antibody typing
      3. Tissue typing
C. Imaging studies:
   a. CT scan of thorax to determine the size of the thorax for the donor and the diseases that prohibit transplantation.
   b. Echocardiography as well as dynamic MRI should be done to estimate the right ventricular ejection fraction. Ejection fraction of >30% indicates recovery of heart function if lung will be transplanted.
   c. In females, bilateral mammogram should be done to exclude any abnormality.
   d. PA view and lateral view of chest should be done to detect the size of the chest and to assess the suitability of the donor.
D. Evaluation of function of heart and lung:
   a. Diffusion capacity of the lung for carbondioxide
   b. Maximum venous oxygen consumption

   If FEV_1 is >1 L and maximum venous oxygen consumption is >15 mL/dL/min, patient can be treated conservatively other than transplantation.

   c. Pulmonary vascular resistance: If it is >4 Woods units—it indicates that patients can be corrected from cardiac transplantation only.

Post-transplantation Follow-up

A. Endomyocardial biopsy to be done at weekly interval for 2–4 weeks for assessing the rejection of the heart.
B. To evaluate the signs of rejection or infection of lung, chest X-ray, and spirogram should be performed. Bronchoalveolar lavage and transbronchial biopsy should be performed to streamline the diagnosis.
C. Depending upon the condition of the patients, timing of long-term follow-up should be fixed. Following investigation is required in case of outpatient visit:
   a. Serum electrolytes, sugar, liver function test, lipid profile, and the serum level of immunosuppressant drugs
   b. Pulse oximetry
   c. Spirometry
   d. Cardiac evaluation in the form of echocardiography to assess the cardiac function

Donor Selection

A. Donor should be a subject who developed brain death after catastrophic accident.
B. If the patients are under mechanical ventilation, lung becomes susceptible to infection, fat embolism,

neurogenic pulmonary edema, and atelectasis. These types of lungs having underlying pulmonary diseases are not considered for transplantation. Lung tissue should be viable for 4–6 hours; hence, it has to be transplanted within these hours.

C. Current donor criteria are the following:
   - **a.** Age < 50 years
   - **b.** Chest X-ray demonstrates clear lung fields
   - **c.** Low peak-inflation pressure
   - **d.** Arterial oxygen saturation of >100 mm Hg on 40% inspired oxygen and >300 mm Hg on 100% inspired oxygen.
   - **e.** On bronchoscopy, there is no evidence of tracheobronchial infection.

D. After fulfilling the above criteria, donor should be matched against recipients based on ABO compatibility and size of the organs.

E. Measurement of chest should be done by following methods:
   - **a.** Chest circumference
   - **b.** Chest wall dimension on chest X-ray
   - **c.** Height-and-weight estimated lung volumes

Ideally to prevent postoperative atelectasis donor heart-lung should be slightly smaller than those of the recipients. During storage and transportation, care has to be taken to occlude trachea.

Technique

In Case of Donor

By median sternotomy, heart and lungs are mobilized with minimal handling, heart should be flushed with cold cardioplegic solution and lung by cold modified Colin solution after infusion of prostaglandin through the pulmonary artery. Then both the organs should be removed en bloc and will be placed in a cold electrolyte solution for transit for destination.

In Case of Recipient

Operation should be done by cardiopulmonary bypass, heart and lung are removed, phrenic nerve should be preserved, and bronchial artery should be addressed to postoperative bleeding complications.

Now, donor heart and lung are inserted, anastomosis of trachea has to be done first followed by anastomosis of right atrium and it is followed by aortic anastomosis. It should be checked that trachea of the donor has to be short due to its limited vascularity in this area.

Following transplantation of diabetes mellitus, hypertension of the recipient should be taken care of.

Complications

A. Rejection of transplantation: The treatment is methylprednisolone 500–1,000 mg/day for 3–5 days, monoclonal antibody, or polyclonal antibody.

B. Implantation response: This is transient but reversible deterioration of compliance, pulmonary vascular resistance, and gas exchange starts occurring just after transplantation and continues for 1 week. Treatment is:
   - **a.** Preservation technique
   - **b.** Judicious postoperative diuresis

C. Infection: Early mobilization and aggressive pulmonary therapy of the recipient will reduce this pulmonary complication. Tracheal fluid should be cultured for pathogens, proper history of the exposure of the patients, and by bronchoalveolar lavage.

D. Allograft vascular disease and bronchiolitis obliterans: These are the main causes of late graft rejection and death.
   - **a.** In the coronary arteries, there is concentric myointimal hyperplasia.
   - **b.** In the bronchiole of the lungs, there are squamous metaplasia and fibrous replacement.

Immunosuppressants

A. Cyclosporine: It will suppress both humoral immunity and to greater extent cell-mediated immunity like delayed hypersensitivity response, allergic encephalitis, and allograft rejection.

B. Prednisolone decreases inflammation by:
   - **a.** Reversing the increased capillary permeability
   - **b.** Suppressing the activity of polymorphonuclear leukocytes

C. Methylprednisolone: It decreases inflammation by—
   - **a.** Reversing the increased capillary permeability
   - **b.** Suppressing the activity of polymorphonuclear leukocytes

D. Tacrolimus: This calcineurin inhibitor is two to three times more potent than cyclosporine.

E. Mycophenolate mofetil:

a. It inhibits inosine monophosphate dehydrogenase and reduces synthesis of purine by lymphocytes that inhibits its proliferation.

b. It will inhibit antibody production.

F. Azathioprine:

a. It antagonizes purine metabolism.

b. It inhibits synthesis of DNA, RNA, and protein.

c. It decreases proliferation of immune cells resulting lowering of autoimmune activity.

Q82. Atrial septal defect in adult.

MGM/MAR2006/MDIV (5)

Describe the etiology, classification and complications and consequences of congenital heart disease. Mention clinical features, diagnosis and management of patients with atrial septal defect.

MGR/SEP2006/MDIV (20)

Enumerate the common congenital heart diseases. Discuss atrial septal defect.

SAMS (ODISHA), 2023 (10)

ANSWER

Classification of Congenital Heart Diseases

A. Acyanotic heart disease:

a. Left to right shunt:

1. Atrial septal defect
2. Ventricular septal defect
3. Atrioventricular septal defect
4. Endocardial cushion defect
5. Persistent ductus arteriosus

b. Obstructive lesion:

1. Pulmonary stenosis
2. Aortic stenosis
3. Coarctation of aorta

c. Cyanotic heart disease:

1. Tetralogy of Fallot
2. Transposition of great arteries
3. Tricuspid atresia
4. Truncus arteriosus
5. Total anomalous pulmonary venous drainage

Etiology

Etiology of congenital heart disease is unknown.

Most of the cases are multifactorial because the combined genetic predisposing factors and environmental factors may be responsible for this.

Critical congenital heart disease is usually sporadic and isolated, sometimes these diseases are associated with genetic syndrome.

10–15% of congenital heart diseases are related to chromosomal abnormalities, most of them are aneuploidies like trisomy-21, trisomy-13, and Turner syndrome.

Potential environmental factors are:

a. Diabetes mellitus

b. Mental exposure to toxin or drugs

c. Viral infection during pregnancy

d. Phenylketonuria

Cardiac Complications of Congenital Heart Diseases

A. Heart failure

B. Growth failure

C. Pneumonia

D. Recurrent respiratory tract infection

E. Cerebral abscess

F. Paradoxical embolism

Noncardiac Complications in case of Congenital Heart Disease

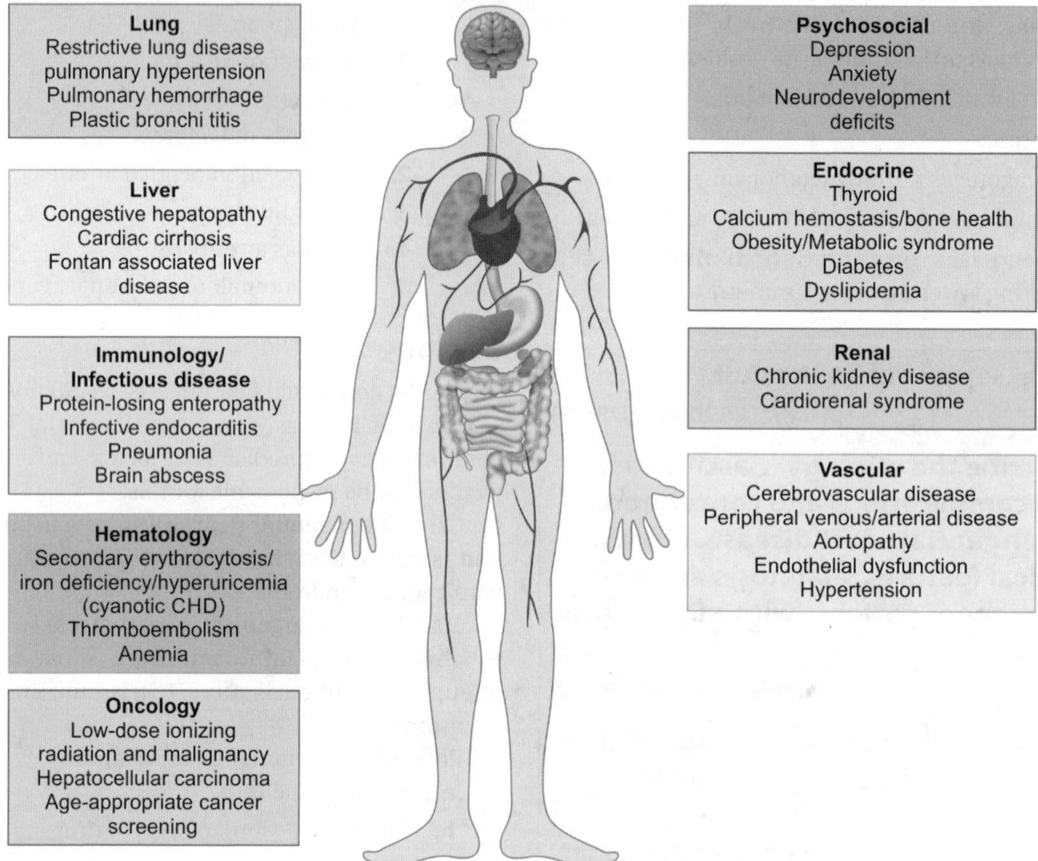

Clinical Features of Atrial Septal Defect

Most of the patients are undetected over decades due to lack of symptoms other than fatigability, recurrent respiratory tract infections, or exertional respiratory distress.

If it is undetected in childhood, symptoms can develop over decades as a result of changing compliance with age, atrial arrhythmias, pulmonary hypertension and sometimes mitral valve disease in case of ostium primum defect.

In case of older patients, clinical deterioration occurs due to following mechanisms:

A. Decrease in left ventricular compliance will enhance left-to-right shunt.

B. Different types of supraventricular arrhythmias like atrial fibrillation, atrial flutter, and paroxysmal atrial tachycardia are increased in frequency after 4th decade and may produce right ventricular failure.

C. Mild-to-moderate pulmonary hypertension in presence of large left-to-right shunt leads to volume and pressure overload of right ventricle.

So, presenting symptoms are:

a. Dyspnea
b. Easy fatigability
c. Palpitation
d. Syncope
e. Stroke
f. Heart failure
g. Sustained atrial arrhythmias

Physical Examinations

A. Left parasternal heaves due to hyperdynamic right ventricle due to increased diastolic filling and large stroke volume

B. Palpable pulsation of pulmonary artery

C. Ejection click due to dilated pulmonary artery

D. Splitting of first heart sound with increased intensity of tricuspid component due to:
  a. Forceful right ventricular contraction
  b. Delayed closure of tricuspid leaflets

E. Wide and fixed split of second heart sound due to delayed closure of the pulmonary valve.

F. In case of ASD with moderate left-to-right shunt results increased right ventricular stroke volume across the pulmonary valve produces crescendo-decrescendo murmur which can be heard left two intercostal space on the left sternal border.

G. There may be mid-diastolic rumbling murmur at the lower left sternal border due to increased flow of blood across the tricuspid outflow tract.

H. In case of ostium primum defect with cleft in the mitral valve leaflet, there may be systolic regurgitant murmur which can be heard at the apex.

I. If the patient develops pulmonary hypertension along with right ventricular hypertrophy:

- **a.** Absence of pulmonary ejection murmur
- **b.** Absence of tricuspid flow murmur
- **c.** Presence of right ventricular S4

J. In case of reversal of shunt, there is clubbing and cyanosis.

Diagnosis

A. Laboratory studies:

- **a.** Complete blood count
- **b.** Type and screen
- **c.** Metabolic profile
- **d.** Coagulation studies—PT and APTT

B. Chest X-ray:

- **a.** Cardiomegaly due to dilatation of right atrium and right ventricle
- **b.** Prominent pulmonary artery
- **c.** Pulmonary vascular markings are enhanced.
- **d.** In case of sinus venosus defect, proximal dilatation of superior vena cava

C. Transthoracic echocardiography: It can visualize the atrial septal defect along with evaluation of right atrium, right ventricle, pulmonary arteries, and other abnormalities.

D. Doppler echocardiography demonstrates biphasic pattern in systole and diastole with small right to left heart shunt in the beginning stage of systole.

E. Continuous wave Doppler echocardiography can estimate right ventricular systolic pressure in presence of tricuspid regurgitant jet.

F. Contrast echocardiography can detect right to left heart shunt by demonstrating microcavitation bubbles in the left atrium and left ventricles.

G. Cardiac MRI can demonstrate size and position of ASD in more specific manner.

H. Electrocardiography:

- **a.** In ostium secundum defect:
  1. Normal sinus rhythm
  2. Right axis deviation
  3. rSR′ pattern in V_1
- **b.** In ostium primum defect:
  1. Left axis deviation
  2. rSR′ pattern in V_1
- **c.** In sinus venosus defect:
  1. Left axis deviation
  2. Negative P wave deflection
- **d.** In case of associated pulmonary hypertension:
  1. rSR′ pattern in V_1
  2. Tall monophasic R wave with deep inverted T wave

I. Cardiac catheterization:

- **a.** Measurement of serial oxygen can estimate magnitude of the shunt.
- **b.** In case young right heart pressure may be normal in spite of large shunt.
- **c.** If there is high oxygen saturation in the superior vena cava or catheter directly enters into pulmonary vein from right atrium, the defect is sinus venosus defect.

Treatment

Surgery is the treatment of choice.

Decision of Surgery

A. Clinical and echocardiographic information regarding size and location of defect

B. Hemodynamic impact of the left to right heart shunt

C. Presence and degree of pulmonary hypertension

Elective closure of the defect is required in presence of right ventricular loads and clinically significant shunt.

In childhood spontaneous closure of the ostium secundum may occur but in adult spontaneous closure is unlikely hence proper monitoring is required.

Contraindication for intervention is required in following conditions:

- **a.** Diagnosis during pregnancy
- **b.** Presence of severe pulmonary hypertension
- **c.** Small size of the defect and shunt
- **d.** Severe left to right ventricular dysfunction

Mortality in case repair of ostium secundum defect is 1–3%. Since there is chance of paradoxical embolization even in case of small shunt continuous evaluation is required. Long-term prevention of death and complications can be avoided by doing operations before 25 years of age and when the pressure in the pulmonary artery is <40 mm Hg.

There are no significant differences between transcatheter and surgical closure of defect in terms of:

- **a.** Survival
- **b.** Functional capacity
- **c.** Atrial arrhythmias
- **d.** Embolic neurological events

Risk factors for unsuccessful transcatheter septal defect closure are:

- **a.** Smaller retroaortic and inferior rims
- **b.** Morphological atrial septal variations
- **c.** Malattached septum primum

Following are associated with transcatheter occlusion of devices:

- **a.** Device embolization and malpositioning
- **b.** Postimplantation arrhythmias
- **c.** Formation of thrombus
- **d.** Cardiac perforation
- **e.** Device erosion
- **f.** Increased level of cardiac troponin I
- **g.** Residual shunt
- **h.** Pericardial effusion
- **i.** Transient ischemic attack
- **j.** Sudden death

Q83. Atherosclerosis: etiopathogenesis, primary and secondary prevention.

MGR/SEP2008/MDII (20)

ANSWER

Risk factors for atherosclerosis are:

A. Conventional factors:

- **a.** Cigarette smoking
- **b.** Hypertension
- **c.** Dyslipidemia
  - **1.** High LDL < 40 mg/dL
  - **2.** Low HDL
  - **3.** High triglyceride
- **d.** Diabetes mellitus
- **e.** Chronic kidney disease stage 3/4
- **f.** Obesity
- **g.** Physical inactivity
- **h.** Family history of chronic kidney disease
- **i.** Evidence of calcification in coronary artery in men ≥45 years and women ≥55 years of age

B. Nonconventional factors:

- **a.** Homocysteine
- **b.** Polycystic ovarian disease
- **c.** Inflammation
- **d.** Lipoprotein A
- **e.** Psychological stress:
  - **1.** Depression
  - **2.** Anger
  - **3.** Hostility
  - **4.** Distress

Category	Risk factors or 10 years risk of atherosclerotic cardiovascular diseases	Target of LDL
Extreme risk	Progressive atherosclerotic cardiovascular diseases in spite of LDL < 70 mg/dL	<55 mg/dL
	Established clinical atherosclerotic cardiovascular diseases in patients with DM, CKD ¾ or heterogenous familial hypercholesterolemia	
	History of premature atherosclerotic cardiovascular diseases (<55 years for male and <65 years for female)	
Very high risk	Established or recent hospitalization for ACS, coronary, carotid or peripheral vascular disease, 10 years' risk is >20%	<70 mg/dL
	DM or CKD stage ¾ or more risk factor(s)	
	Heterogenous familial hypercholesterolemia	
High risk	≥2 risk factors and 10 years' risk is 10–20%	<100 mg/dL
	DM and CKD stage ¾	
Moderate risk	≤2 risk factors and 10 years' risk is <10%	<100 mg/dL
Low risk	No risk factor	<130 mg/dL

Note: Subtract 1 risk factor if HDL is >60 mg/dL.

Primary Prevention

Primary prevention:

A. Reduces the risk of myocardial infarction as well as heart failure.

B. Decreases the need for coronary revascularization procedure.

C. Extends and improves the quality of life.

Primary prevention starts with:

A. Smoking: Goal is complete cessation of smoking and not exposure to environmental tobacco smoke. Following are the 5 "A":

- **a.** Patient is asked about the status of tobacco use at every visit.
- **b.** Every patient is advised to quit tobacco who uses tobacco.
- **c.** Willingness to quit tobacco is assessed in every patient.
- **d.** Each patient is assisted for counseling and developing plan how to quit.
- **e.** Follow-up is arranged referral to special programs or pharmacotherapy like replacement of nicotine and bupropion.

B. Diet: DASH diet is advised. It is high in vegetables, fruits, whole grains, poultry, fish, low fat or fat-free dairy product, beans, nuts, and nontropical vegetable oils, rich in calcium, potassium, magnesium, protein and fibers, low sweets, and sugar-sweetened beverages. Total daily target is 2,000 calorie. This diet reduces:

- **a.** Blood pressure can be reduced by 5–6/3 mm Hg in case of adult with blood pressure 120–159/80–95 mm Hg for both male and female, white and black, older and adult, and hypertensive and nonhypertensive subjects.
- **b.** LDL-C by 11 mg/dL and increases HDL by 4 mg/dL. But no effect on triglyceride in case of adult having total cholesterol < 260 mg/dL and LDL-C < 160 mg/dL.

C. Alcohol intake of 5–25 g/day will reduce the cardiovascular incidence and all-cause mortality.

D. Physical activity: According to Physical activity Advisory Committee of US department—

- **a.** Regular physical activity reduces the excessive weight gain and helps the subject to maintain within healthy range.
- **b.** In case of pregnancy, it will reduce:
  1. Excessive weight gain in pregnancy
  2. Risk of developing gestational diabetes
  3. Postpartum depression
- **c.** Regular physical activity:
  1. Improves cognitive function.
  2. Reduces the risk of dementia.
  3. Reduces fall and fall-related injuries.
  4. Reduces cancer of the breast, esophagus, colon, bladder, lung, kidney, and endometrium.
  5. Retards the osteoarthritis progression.
  6. Retards the progression of hypertension and diabetes mellitus.
- **d.** In case of adult:
  1. 150–300 minutes of moderate intensity aerobic activity per week
  2. 75–150 minutes of vigorous intensity aerobic physical activity per week
  3. Equivalent aerobic moderate and vigorous intensity physical activity per week
- **e.** Older adult will do:
  1. Aerobic activity
  2. Balance training
  3. Muscle strengthening activity
- **f.** Pregnant woman can do 150 minutes moderate intensity physical activity per week.
- **g.** Adult disable person can perform both aerobic and muscle strengthening activity.

Following general principles should be considered during recommendation of increasing activity:

- **a.** Increased physical activity will start with walking.
- **b.** Complete exercise program consists of:
  1. Stretching
  2. Aerobic exercise
  3. Resistance training
- **c.** More frequent exercise will provide more benefit.
- **d.** Excellent benefit can be obtained from 40 minutes of daily exercise.
- **e.** More strenuous exercise like jogging will provide more benefit.

E. Weight management:

According to 2019 AHA guideline, following recommendation regarding weight loss has to be followed:

- **a.** Over-weight or obese adults maintain weight loss with the help of counseling as well as lifestyle modification including calorie restriction.
- **b.** In case of type 2 diabetes mellitus through the dietary plan with 150 minutes of moderate intensity aerobic exercise per week or 75 minutes of vigorous intensity exercise per week can:
  1. Improve glycemic control
  2. Achieve the ideal weight
  3. Improve other risk factors

Secondary Prevention

A. In 75 years or below, patients with clinical atherosclerotic cardiovascular disease should be started with statin therapy.

B. If the patient is intolerant to statin but can get benefit from it, moderate intensity statin therapy should be started.

C. Blood pressure control: Goal of blood pressure is 140/90 mm Hg or in case of diabetes mellitus or chronic kidney disease 130/80 mm Hg.

For all patients:

a. Lifestyle modification
b. Daily physical activity
c. Sodium restriction
d. Alcohol moderation
e. Increased fresh fruits consumption
f. Low-fat dairy products

If the blood pressure is more than the above range, then

a. Angiotensin-converting enzyme inhibitors
b. Angiotensin II receptor blockers
c. Beta-blockers

D. Management of lipid:

a. Dietary therapy:
   1. Saturated fat: <7% of total calories
   2. Trans-fatty acids: <7% of total calories
   3. Cholesterol: <200 mg/dL

b. Add:
   1. Plant sterol 2 g/day
   2. Viscous fiber > 10 g/day

c. Daily physical activity

d. Increase consumption of omega-3 fatty acids like fish in capsule form—1 g/day to reduce the risk.

e. Treatment of high triglyceride level

f. In case of hospitalized patients prior to discharge following medications should be recommended:
   1. LDL-C should be <100 mg/dL, but <70 mg/dL is reasonable.
   2. If baseline LDL level is 100 mg/dL, lipid lowering drug should be started.
   3. If the patient is on treatment and LDL-C level is 100 mg/day, intensification of the therapy should be done.
   4. If LDL-C is 100 mg/dL, LDL-C level should be lowered to 70 mg/dL reasonably.
   5. If triglyceride level is 200–4,990 mg/dL, and non-HDL-C level is <130 mg/dL, more and more reduction of non-HDL-C to 100 mg/dL is reasonable.

Following are the options for lowering non-HDL-C level:

1. More intensification of LDL-C lowering therapy
2. Niacin (after LDL-C lowering therapy)
3. Fibrate (after LDL-C lowering therapy)

If triglyceride level is >500 mg/dL:

1. Fibrate or niacin should be administered to prevent acute pancreatitis before starting LDL-C lowering therapy.
2. Patients with hypertriglyceridemia should not take alcohol.
3. If triglyceride level is >200 mg/dL, then bile-acid sequestrating resin should not be prescribed.

E. Management of diabetes—the goal is to maintain HbA1c at 7%. It can be done by:

a. Lifestyle modification
b. Pharmacotherapy
c. Vigorous modification of other risk factors such as blood pressure control and cholesterol treatment
d. Coordinate diabetic care along with patient's primary care

F. Antiplatelet agents and anticoagulants:

a. According to AHA guidelines, aspirin at a dose of 75–150 mg/day should be started and continued indefinitely unless it is contraindicated. In case of CABG, 100–325 mg aspirin should be started within 6 hours of operation to reduce the incidence of saphenous vein closure followed by more the 162 mg of aspirin and it should be continued for up to 1 year.

b. Clopidogrel 75 mg/day should be started with aspirin in case of ACS or PCI with stent placement and should be continued for 1 year.

c. In case of PCI with stent placement, high dose of aspirin for 1 month for metal stent, 3 months for sirolimus-eluting stent, and 6 months for paclitaxel-eluting stent followed by 75–150 mg aspirin should be continued indefinitely.

d. International normalized ratio should be maintained to 2–3 for paroxysmal AF or flutter and in postmyocardial infarction patients.

G. Renin, angiotensin, and aldosterone system blockers:

a. In absence of any contraindication, ACE inhibitors should be continued indefinitely in case of patients with left ventricular ejection fraction of ≤40% in patients with hypertension, diabetes, and chronic kidney disease.

b. Angiotensin-converting enzyme inhibitor is considered in case of low-risk patient with normal left ventricular ejection fraction where cardiovascular risk factors are well-controlled.

c. Angiotensin II receptor blockers are used where ACE inhibitors are intolerant and in patients with heart failure.

H. Beta-blockers should be started in patients who had myocardial infarction, acute coronary syndrome, and left ventricular dysfunction unless contraindicated.

I. Patients with cardiovascular disease should receive influenza vaccine every year.

Q84. Acute aortic regurgitation.

RGUHS/APR2001/MDII (10)

Aortic regurgitation.

RAJIV GANDHI UNIVERSITY OF HEALTH SC, 2019 (10)

ANSWER

Definition

Aortic regurgitation can be defined as diastolic flow of blood from the aorta to left ventricle due to incompetence of aortic valve leaflet or annulus of the aorta.

Causes of Acute Aortic Regurgitation

A. Abnormalities of leaflet:
  a. Acute infective endocarditis
  b. Traumatic rupture of the valve
  c. Postaortic balloon valvoplasty
  d. Acute prosthetic valve dysfunction
  e. Perivalvular leak
  f. Dehiscence of prosthetic valve

B. Aortic root and ascending root abnormalities:
  a. Acute aortic root dissection
  b. Traumatic injury to aortic root

Causes of Chronic Aortic Valvular Insufficiency

A. Rheumatic heart disease—most common cause
B. Infective endocarditis
C. Myxomatous degeneration of the aortic valve
D. Bicuspid aortic valve
E. Age related dilatation of the aorta
F. Ectasia of aortic annulus
G. Aortic dissection
H. Dilatation of aortic root secondary to syphilis

Pathophysiology

Acute Aortic Regurgitation

In acute aortic regurgitation left ventricle has not sufficient time to increase adapt the increased left ventricular volume, left ventricle fails to produce adequate stroke volume, as a result cardiac output falls acutely leading to development of hypotension and cardiogenic shock.

Acute increase in left ventricular diastolic pressure causes mitral valve to preclose in early diastole, as a result pulmonary vasculature will be protected from left ventricular elevated diastolic pressure at early phase.

But, further decompensation of left ventricle will lead to diastolic mitral regurgitation, as a result diastolic pressure will be transmitted into pulmonary vascular bed leading to development of pulmonary edema.

In case of hypotension, there is compensatory tachycardia which shortens the diastolic filling period when mitral valve opens.

Chronic Aortic Regurgitation

During aortic regurgitation, blood will flow into the left ventricle during diastole due to eccentric hypertrophy of cardiomyocytes. As left ventricle dilates, large amount of blood will be accumulated in the ventricle-blood from left atrium and regurgitated blood from aorta. But as the left ventricular end diastolic volume and pressure will be increased to such extent that the sarcomere will be stretched maximally. So, left ventricular remodeling and compensatory mechanism fail leading to decline in the initially compensated left ventricular stroke volume.

Clinical Features

Physical findings:

A. Hypotension
B. Tachycardia
C. Pallor
D. Cyanosis
E. Diaphoresis
F. Cool extremities
G. Pulmonary congestion
H. Altered mental status
I. Peripheral examination:
  a. Pulse pressure is normally slightly widened.
  b. In case of suspicion of aortic dissection, blood pressure differences should be measured.

J. Heart size is normal.

K. Apex beat will not be shifted laterally.

L. Heart sounds:
   a. Mitral component of first heart sound is soft due to early closure of mitral leaflet.
   b. Third heart sound can be heard in case of cardiac decompensation.

M. Murmur:
   a. Early diastolic murmur of acute aortic regurgitation is shorter and low in intensity.
   b. In case of acute severe case, murmur may not be audible in case of equilibrium of both left ventricular and aortic pressure.
   c. There may be systolic murmur in the aortic area due to increased blood flow across the aortic valve.
   d. If mid-diastolic murmur is heard—it is short, known as Austin-Flint murmur.

In Chronic Aortic Regurgitation

A. Wide pulse pressure

B. Laterally and inferiorly displaced apical impulse

C. Blowing type decrescendo diastolic murmur in the neoaortic area, i.e., 3rd and 4th intercostal spaces just lateral to left sternal border

D. Muffled S2

E. Presence of Austin flint murmur in the apical area

F. In case of early heart failure presence of S3.

Peripheral signs of aortic regurgitation:

A. Quincke sign: Repeated alternating blanching and blushing of the nail fold capillaries.

B. Water-hammer pulse: Bounding pulse of the radial arteries

C. Pulsus bisferiens or double peak pulse

D. Corrigan sign: Bounding pulse in the carotid arteries demonstrating sudden expansion followed by sudden collapse.

E. De Musset sign: Nodding of the head with each heartbeat.

F. Müller sign: Systolic pulsation in the uvula

G. Traube sign: Presence of pistol shot sound heard during pressing the femoral artery by the diaphragm of the stethoscope.

H. Duroziez's sign: Appearance of a diastolic murmur heard when pressure is applied distal to stethoscope and systolic murmur when the pressure is applied proximally.

I. Hill's sign: Presence of high systolic pressure in the lower limb is more than 20 mm of Hg as compared to upper limb.

J. Becker's sign: During funduscopic examination, presence of retinal pulsation.

K. Mayne's sign: When the arm is raised the diastolic blood pressure will be decreased by more than 15 mm Hg.

L. Landolfi's sign: Presence of rhythmic constriction and dilatation of the pupil with each heartbeat.

Laboratory Investigation

A. Electrocardiography: Only nonspecific ST-T changes are seen.

B. Chest X-ray:
   a. Dimension of left atrium and left ventricle is normal.
   b. In case aortic dissection widened mediastinum
   c. Widened cardiac silhouette due to pericardial effusion
   d. There may be pulmonary congestion.

C. Echocardiography:
   a. Evaluation of aortic root
   b. Assessment of overall size of left ventricle and its function
   c. Doppler echocardiography can also assess the severity of the AR.
   d. M-mode echocardiography can demonstrate premature closure of mitral valve.
   e. M-mode also detects evidence of regurgitant jet striking the mitral valve leaflet.

Based on 2017 American society of Echocardiography aortic insufficiency classified into following types:

A. Type 1 aortic insufficiency: Normal function of aortic valve leaflet but there is dilatation of aortic root or perforation of valve cusp.
   a. Type 1a: Sinotubular junction and the ascending aorta is enlarged.
   b. Type 1b: Sinus of Valsalva and sinotubular junction are dilated.
   c. Type 1c: Aortic annulus is dilated.
   d. Type 1d: Perforation of aortic cusp is present.

B. Type 2 aortic insufficiency: Aortic cusp prolapse due to excessive tissue in the leaflet or disruption of commissure.

C. Type 3 aortic insufficiency: Restriction of the motion of the aortic leaflets due to various processes.

Chronic aortic regurgitation can be classified into four stages:

A. Stage A: Patient is at risk of aortic insufficiency

B. Stage B: Patient with progressive mild to moderate aortic insufficiency

C. Stage C: Patient with asymptomatic severe aortic insufficiency:

 a. Stage C1: Patient with left ventricular ejection fraction of more than 50%, mild to moderate left ventricular dilatation and end-systolic dimension less than 50 mm.

 b. Stage C2: Left ventricular ejection fraction less than 50%, severe left ventricular dilatation, end-systolic dimension more than 50 mm or indexed left ventricular end-systolic dimension more than 25 mm/m^2.

D. Stage D: Severely symptomatic patient with severe aortic regurgitation.

Treatment

A. Medical therapy:

 a. In patients presenting with cardiogenic shock—intravenous vasodilators are given to:

  1. Reduce the afterload of the ventricle.

  2. Lower left ventricular end-diastolic pressure.

  3. Augment the forward cardiac output.

 b. In severe cases: Temporary transvenous atrial/ventricular pacing with or without intravenous inotropic drugs to provide temporary hemodynamic support.

 c. Beta-blockers are used with caution in case of associated aortic dissection. It will reduce dP/dt reflecting transmission of force from left ventricular ejection to arterial wall. Though it is helpful in case of aortic dissection, but this drug will slow the heart rate that leads to increase the length of the diastole, as a result there is exacerbation of aortic regurgitation leading to cardiovascular collapse.

 d. In case of associated with endocarditis, antibiotic should be given after getting the proper culture/sensitivity report.

 e. Patients those are being triaged for surgery can be treated with rapid pacing with the aim to reduce the duration of diastole if intravenous vasodilators fail to produce tachycardia.

B. Surgical therapy:

 a. Treatment of the etiology such as aortic dissection, acute severe aortic regurgitation is always surgical emergency.

In case of chronic aortic regurgitation:

A. Medical therapy depends upon the stage of aortic regurgitation.

 a. For stage B and C aortic regurgitation: Angiotensin-converting enzyme inhibitors, dihydropyridine calcium channel blockers, angiotensin receptor blockers—class I recommendation.

 b. For stage C2 and D aortic regurgitation with symptoms of left ventricular dysfunction and in whom surgery cannot be done due to presence of co-morbidities—angiotensin-converting enzyme inhibitors, dihydropyridine calcium channel blockers, angiotensin receptor blockers, beta-blockers—class II recommendation

Indications of Aortic Valve Replacement

A. In symptomatic patient—severe symptoms like dyspnea, angina pain or heart failure.

B. In asymptomatic patient:

 a. Severe aortic regurgitation with ejection fraction of less than 50%.

 b. Severe aortic regurgitation with end-systolic dimension more than 50 mm or indexed to body surface area 25 mm/m^2

 c. Severe aortic regurgitation with end-diastolic dimension less than 65 mm

 d. On serial imaging progressive left ventricular dilatation

C. Acute severe aortic regurgitation: In case of acute aortic regurgitation with hemodynamic instability from trauma, infective endocarditis

D. Concomitant cardiac surgery: If the patient is undergoing surgery for coronary artery bypass or operation for aortic aneurysm.

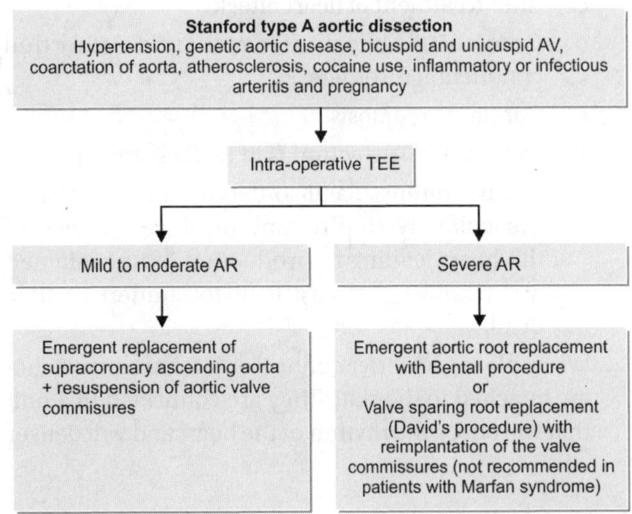

(AR: aortic regurgitation; AV: aortic valve; TEE: transesophageal echocardiography)

Q85. Defibrillators.

MGR/SEP2008/MDII (6)

ANSWER

Defibrillators are the machines which can restore the normal beat by sending the electrical impulses or shock to the heart. It can correct different types of arrhythmias or prevent sudden cardiac death due to sudden stoppage of the heart.

There are different types of defibrillators:

A. Automated external defibrillator: It is of light-weight and portable battery-operated that will check the rhythm of the heart and send electrical impulses to restore normal rhythm. Electrodes also will send the information to the computer to analyze the rhythm whether electrical shock is needed or not; if yes, send the shock impulse. It is required in following cases:
   - **a.** In patients with sudden unexpected stoppage of the heart.
   - **b.** It can be used in adult and children of at least 1 year of age.
   - **c.** It can be used during the time of cardiopulmonary resuscitation as there is chance of cardiac arrest.

B. Implantable cardioverter defibrillator (ICD): It is placed surgically in the chest or abdomen for checking arrhythmias. If arrhythmia is detected it will automatically send low energy electrical impulses to slow down or speed up the abnormal heart rate to restore the blood flow to different organs. It can be used in the following circumstances:
   - **a.** It can correct dangerous arrhythmias.
   - **b.** It can keep an irregular heartbeat to trigger sudden cardiac arrest.
   - **c.** After treatment of heart attack
   - **d.** Congenital heart diseases and inherited conduction disorders
   - **e.** Cardiac sarcoidosis
   - **f.** Detection of arrhythmias in ECG or stress test
   - **g.** Few neuromuscular disorders such as progressive muscular dystrophy may produce damage of the heart leading to production of unexplained arrhythmias that can lead to sudden cardiac death.

C. Wearable cardioverter defibrillator: It has sensors that are attached to the skin. They are connected to a unit that will check the rhythm of the heart and will deliver the shock as per requirement. It can deliver both high and low energy shock. Sensors detect arrhythmias and make the clinician alert. In case of nonresponse, device will automatically send impulses to correct the rhythm. This can be used in the following circumstances where there is risk of arrhythmias for a short time:
   - **a.** If the patient is recovering from heart attack.
   - **b.** If the patient is waiting for cardiac transplant.
   - **c.** If the patient is suffering from severing infection in case of severe sepsis.
   - **d.** If you are removing ICD or waiting for implantation of ICD.

Expectation from electrical shock:

A. Light shock: It is unnoticed, not at all painful, one cannot feel it or feel it as sudden fluttering of chest.

B. High-energy shock: It will last for fraction of second but it is strong and painful like someone thumping or kicking the chest.

C. Unnecessary shock: Just after surgery during adjustment device may deliver unnecessary shock. Again, in case of exercise induced tachycardia device may trigger unnecessary shock. If the patient forgets to take the medicine, he will feel phantom shock even in absence of undetectable arrhythmias by the device.

Contraindications of cardioversion:

A. Known atrial thrombus and no emergency

B. Sinus rhythm or sinus tachycardia

C. Tachycardia along with increased automaticity
   - **a.** Junctional tachycardia
   - **b.** Multifocal atrial tachycardia

D. Toxicity of digitalis

E. Severe electrolyte disturbances

F. If the patient cannot be sedated satisfactorily.

Q86. Intra-aortic balloon counterpulsation.

MGR/SEP2008/MDII (20)

ANSWER

Its main functions are as follows:

A. In case of cardiogenic shock to provide hemodynamic support.

B. In patients with severe coronary artery disease to provide relief from medically refractory ischemia.

It should be given for a short period as there is risk of complication after its prolonged use.

Indications for Intra-aortic Balloon Counterpulsation

A. Acute myocardial infarction with cardiogenic shock. But, AHA/ACC recently downgraded the recommendation Ib (i.e., should be used) to IIa (i.e., can be used).

B. Refractory angina or myocardial ischemia awaiting revascularization:

- **a.** In patients with severe unrevascularized severe coronary artery disease suffering from symptoms of ischemia and hemodynamic instability which is refractory to medical therapy can be benefited from IABP counterpulsation.
- **b.** Class I recommendation in case of STEMI and class IIa recommendation of NSETMI or unstable angina who are suffering from severe ischemic symptoms in spite of intensive medical therapy and class IIb recommendation for pulmonary edema for IABP counterpulsation placement.

C. High-risk PCI: Those patients with high risk of complications during PCI including—

- **a.** Unprotected left main coronary artery disease
- **b.** Left ventricular dysfunction with ejection fraction of ≤30%
- **c.** Severe multivessel coronary artery disease
- **d.** Target vessel supplying >40% of the territory of myocardium
- **e.** Active congestive heart failure

D. Mechanical complications of acute myocardial infarction: Two important complications of acute myocardial infarction are acute mitral regurgitation and VSD—these may produce rapid hemodynamic deterioration leading to cardiogenic shock. IABP acts as an adjunct to medical afterload reduction in case of STEMI in ACC/AHA class I recommendation.

E. Refractory ventricular arrhythmias: Incessant VT—

- **a.** Compromises filling of left ventricle.
- **b.** Reduces stroke volume.
- **c.** Causes cerebral ischemia.

IABP placement will improve hemodynamics, controlled refractory ventricular arrhythmias, and lessen ischemia.

F. End-stage cardiomyopathy/bridging to heart transplantation: IABP placement will improve cardiac hemodynamics, improves cardiac output and lowers the filling pressures in patients with ischemic and dilated cardiomyopathy, and also acts as bridging to cardiac transplantation.

Disadvantages for prolonged use of IABP are infection and prolonged bed rest. But now-a-days IABP is infrequently used for prolonged mechanical support because ICD with inotropic therapy is used for those patients awaiting for transplantation.

G. Decompensated severe aortic valvular stenosis or severe mitral regurgitation: IABP can improve stroke volume along with reduction of transvalvular pressure gradient prior to aortic valve replacement. IABP also acts as bridge to specific surgical treatment in case of acute MI complicated by mitral regurgitation.

H. Low cardiac output after cardiopulmonary bypass: In case of severe left ventricular dysfunction or in case of prolonged runs on cardiopulmonary bypass due to stunning of the myocardium from prolonged cardioplegic arrest IABP support will improve hemodynamics and thus it facilitates weaning from bypass.

I. Support during noncardiac surgery: Patients with coronary artery disease. Recent myocardial infarction or severe left ventricular dysfunction may develop complications during noncardiac surgery. These patients may be helped from IABP as it will maintain the hemodynamics throughout the surgical procedure.

Contraindications

A. Type A and B aortic dissection

B. Abdominal or thoracic aneurysms as these will precipitate acute aortic dissection, atheroemboli dislodgment or rupture of aorta.

C. Severe peripheral vascular disease:

- **a.** It is caused by vascular insufficiency in the accessed limb due to large size of the balloon sheath and catheter. So this process is contraindicated in case of iliofemoral diseases.
- **b.** Balloon catheter and sheath can compromise peripheral perfusion leading to limb ischemia and threatened visibility of the limb.

D. Descending aortic and peripheral vascular graft are relative contraindications and permission from vascular surgeon is required prior to insertion in these patients.

E. Coagulopathy or contraindication to heparin: Heparin-induced thrombocytopenia can be anticoagulated by direct thrombin inhibitors like bivalirudin.

F. Moderate-to-severe aortic insufficiency: IABP usually inflates during diastole and deflates during systole. In case of aortic insufficiency inflation during diastole it will worsen the aortic insufficiency when the blood will be displaced into the proximal aorta. Severe insufficiency is a contraindication.

Hemodynamics of Balloon Pump Function

A. Decrease in the afterload: At the beginning of the systole IABP will deflate to produce following actions:

a. It will reduce the afterload.
b. It will reduce the end-diastolic pressure.
c. It will improve the stroke volume.
d. It will improve the ejection fraction of left ventricle.
e. It will increase the cardiac output by 20%.
f. It will decrease the mean pulmonary capillary wedge pressure by 20%.
g. It will reduce the hemodynamic stress of the left ventricular wall.

B. Augmentation of coronary perfusion: Just prior to dicrotic notch IABP will inflate leading to—

a. Displacement of blood to proximal aorta
b. Augmentation of aortic diastolic pressure
c. Increase in the coronary perfusion pressure. It is more dramatic in presence of systemic hypotension.
d. Increase in peak coronary flow velocity

Following cannot be improved:

a. No improvement in coronary flow through the narrowed coronary artery unless prior angioplasty is done.
b. Collateral flow cannot be increased.

So, in case of coronary artery disease IABP will relieve ischemia by decreasing the stress of left ventricular wall and decreasing the myocardial oxygen demand. By reducing afterload.

Timing of Balloon Pump

Ideal balloon pump deflates just prior to dicrotic notch on the downslope of systolic pressure waveform and it deflates before the onset of next systolic pressure waveform—it should be adjusted manually.

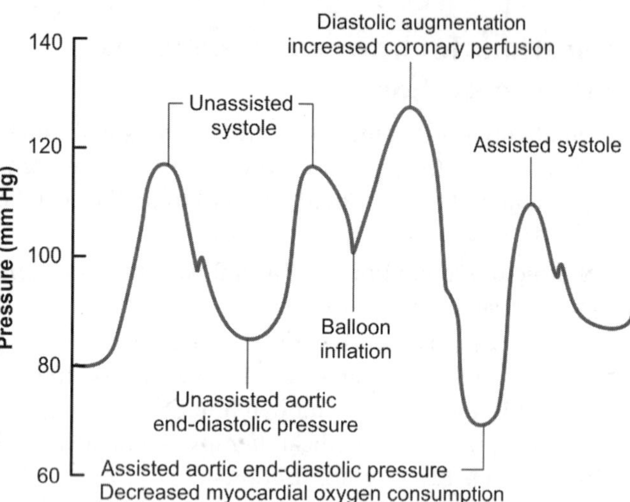

A. Early inflation: It can be defined as IABP inflation before the closure of AV valve (dicrotic notch). There may be premature closure of AV valve in following cases:

a. Increased afterload
b. Stress of the left ventricular free wall
c. Myocardial oxygen demand
d. Decrease in stroke volume

It can be corrected by delay in the inflation until AV valve will be closed.

B. Late inflation: It can be defined as IABP inflation after AV valve closure. It will decrease coronary perfusion as well as diminished augmentation of diastolic pressure.

It can be corrected by adjustment of inflation just prior to dicrotic notch.

C. Early deflation: It can be defined as IABP deflation prior to isovolumic left ventricular contraction. As a result:

a. There is suboptimal diastolic augmentation
b. Suboptimal augmentation of coronary perfusion
c. Suboptimal reduction of afterload

Result is increase in myocardial oxygen demand.

It can be corrected by adjustment of deflation before the onset of systole.

D. Late deflation: It can be defined as IABP deflation after the onset of systole. As a result there is:

a. Impaired emptying of left ventricle
b. Increased preload and afterload

c. Increased consumption of myocardial oxygen
d. Reduction of stroke volume

It can be corrected by making the deflation before the onset of systole.

Complications

A. Vascular complications:
   a. Limb ischemia
   b. Hematoma around the access site
   c. Bleeding form the access site
B. Ischemia
C. Bleeding
D. Pseudoaneurysm
E. Infection:
   a. Access site infection
   b. Catheter infection
   c. Bacteremia
F. Balloon rupture
G. Balloon entrapment
H. Red blood cell and platelet destruction
I. Rare complications due to plaque embolization in renal, mesenteric, and spinal arteries:
   a. Acute renal failure
   b. Mesenteric ischemia
   c. Paraplegia

Q87. Describe structure and function of normal mitral valve. Describe the etiology, clinical features, diagnosis and management of mitral incompetence.

RGUHS/NOV2001/MDII (25)

Mitral valve apparatus.

NTR UNIVERSITY OF HEALTH SC, VIJAYAWADA, ANDHRA, 2021 (10)

ANSWER

Mitral valve connects left atrium with left ventricle.

Gross anatomy: Mitral apparatus is composed of—

A. Left atrial wall: It extends over the proximal portion of posterior leaflet. Hence, in case of left atrial enlargement there will be mitral regurgitation due to involvement of posterior leaflet.
B. Mitral valve annulus: It is a fibrous ring but no continuous around the orifice, hence it is "D"-shaped. It connects with the leaflets. The straight border of the annulus presents posterior to the aortic valve. It will contract to reduce the surface of the area of the valve in the phase of systole so that complete closure of mitral valve is ensured. Dilatation of this annulus will lead to mitral regurgitation.
C. Mitral valve leaflet: These are attached around the circumference of the mitral orifice. There free edges have multiple indentations, among these anteromedial and posterolateral commissures will divide the leaflets into anterior and posterior cusps. These commissures can be identified by the attachment of chordae tendinae with leaflets.
   a. Anterior leaflet: It is located posterior to aortic root and anchored to the aortic root. It is large and semilunar having free edge that may or may not have indentations. It is also known as anteromedial leaflet. There are two zones namely rough and clear zones separated by prominent ridge on its atrial surface which is the line of closure of leaflets.
   b. Posterior or posterolateral leaflet having wide attachment as compared to anterior leaflet. It is located posterior to two commissural areas. It has been divided into three scallops by two indentations, middle scallop being larger of them. Rough zone of this leaflet is distal ridge of the line of leaflet closure. Clear zone of this leaflet has no attachment of chordae tendinae. Basal zone is present in-between the clear zone and annulus, here chordae are attached.
D. Chordae tendinae: These are fibrous ring that that either originates from apical areas of papillary muscles and/or from ventricular wall and ultimately are attached with the valve leaflets or muscles. These are of two types:
   a. False chordae
   b. True chordae
E. Papillary muscles: These arise from the middle-third and the apex of the ventricular wall, anteromedial papillary muscle is larger than the posterolateral papillary muscles. Anteromedial and posterolateral papillary muscles are supplied by left anterior descending or circumflex artery and right coronary artery respectively. Rupture of this muscle leads to mitral regurgitation and fusion of these muscles leads to mitral stenosis.

F. Left ventricular wall

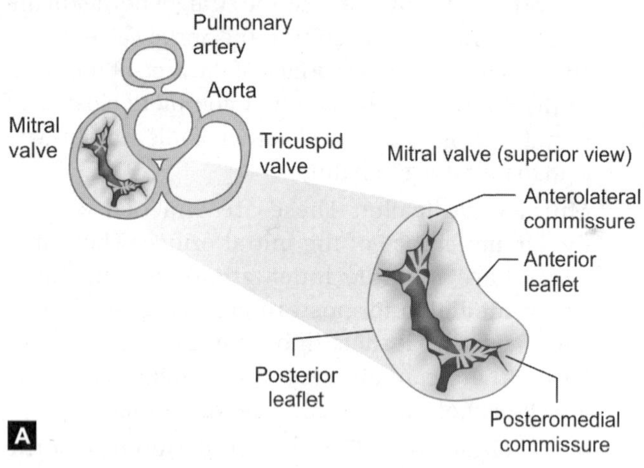

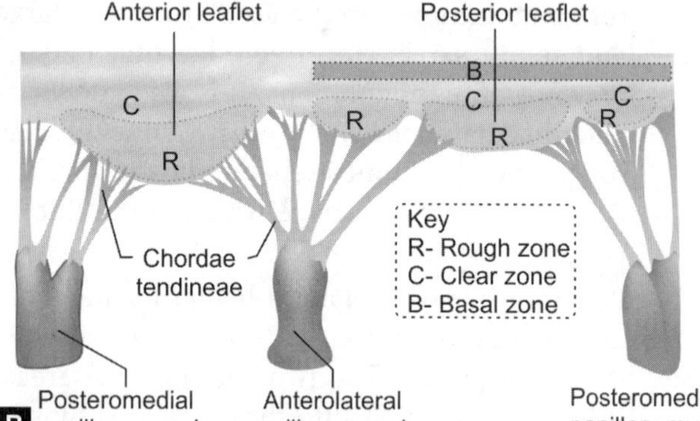

Superior view of mitral valve and and surrounding structures

Functions of the Mitral Valve

Normally during diastole of ventricle mitral valve opens thus allowing the oxygenated blood to flow from the high pressure area left atrium to decompressed left ventricle and pressure in the left ventricle will gradually rise. When the left ventricle contracts, pressure in the cavity will rise more than that of left atrium leading to closure of mitral valve and prevents leaking of blood into left atrium, as a result all the blood will enter into the aorta.

Etiologies of Mitral Regurgitation

A. Abnormalities of leaflets:
- **a.** Myxomatous degeneration
- **b.** Rheumatic disease leading to scarring and contraction of leaflets
- **c.** Cleft in the leaflets
- **d.** Double orifice mitral valve
- **e.** Endocarditis leading to perforation of leaflets and retraction in the healing phase

B. Mitral annular abnormalities:
- **a.** Dilatation of annulus due to left ventricular dilatation, DCM, IHD
- **b.** With surface dilatation, loss of adequate coaptation of leaflets
- **c.** Mitral annular calcification due to:
  1. Degenerative disorders in elderly
  2. Hypertension
  3. Diabetes
  4. Dystrophic calcification in CKD
  5. Marfan syndrome

C. Abnormalities in chordae:
- **a.** Ruptured chordae due to myxomatous degeneration producing flail leaflet
- **b.** Rheumatic heart disease due to fibrosis of chordae and calcification

D. Abnormalities in papillary muscles:
- **a.** Rupture in myocardial infarction
- **b.** Dysfunction due to ischemia
- **c.** Infiltrative disease: Amyloidosis and sarcoidosis
- **d.** Parachute mitral valve

Clinical Features

A. Symptoms:
- **a.** In case of acute severe mitral incompetence:
  1. Dyspnea
  2. Orthopnea
  3. Features of cardiogenic shock
- **b.** In case of chronic mild-to-moderate MR patient may be asymptomatic as here left ventricular overload will be well-tolerated.
- **c.** In case chronic severe MR patients may present with fatigue, exertional dyspnea, and orthopnea.
- **d.** In case of right-sided heart failure due to pulmonary hypertension in case of long-standing MR: pedal edema, ascites, and tender right upper abdomen.

B. Physical findings:
- **a.** Carotid upstroke is sharp but of low volume due to low cardiac output.
- **b.** Pedal edema in case of right-sided heart failure
- **c.** In case of acute MR, arterial pressure is reduced
- **d.** In late phase, neck vein is pulsatile and engorged due to right ventricular failure secondary to pulmonary hypertension.

e. In the apical area:
   1. Apex beat: It is hyperdynamic, sometimes it may be displaced laterally due to left ventricular dilatation.
   2. Systolic thrill
   3. Palpable rapid filling wave (S3)

f. In the parasternal area, late systolic thrust may be felt due to systolic expansion of left atrium, sometimes it may be difficult to differentiate it from right ventricular heave due to right ventricular hypertrophy.

g. In the pulmonary area palpable P2 due to pulmonary hypertension

h. Tender hepatomegaly

i. Ascites

C. On auscultation:

a. In the mitral area:
   1. First heart sound is soft or absent or buried under the murmur.
   2. Low-pitched S3 heard 0.12–0.17 seconds after closure of aortic second sound—it is due to sudden tensing of papillary muscles, chordae, and valvular leaflet.
   3. Holosystolic blowing murmur of grade III/IV intensity is heard at the apex with diaphragm of stethoscope radiating to axilla best heard during expiration.
   4. In case of acute severe MR, the murmur is decrescendo and ceases in the mid-to-late systolic phase.
   5. If chorda tendinae is ruptured or posterior leaflet involvement with prolapse murmur is eccentric and anteriorly thus striking left atrium adjacent to root of the aorta, so the systolic murmur will be radiated to the base of the heart confusing with the murmur of aortic stenosis. In case of ruptured chordae, the quality of murmur has "seagull" or cooing quality. In case flail leaflet murmur is musical in quality.
   6. Murmur of MI is intensified by isometric handgrip but will be reduced during straining phase of Valsalva maneuver.

Investigations

A. Electrocardiography:

a. Features of left or biventricular enlargement

b. Feature of left atrial enlargement, but there may be feature of right atrial enlargement.

c. In case of chronic MI, features of atrial fibrillation

B. Chest X-ray:

a. In case of chronic MI, left atrium and left ventricle are enlarged.

b. In late phase, left atrium is massively enlarged forming the right border of the heart.

c. Feature of left ventricular failure like pulmonary congestion, Kerley B line, and interstitial edema.

d. Calcification of mitral valve leaflet. Or annulus—best seen in left lateral view of chest.

e. In case of acute MR asymmetric pulmonary edema due to occurrence of regurgitant jet into the orifice of upper lobe pulmonary vein.

C. Echocardiogram:

a. Transthoracic echocardiography assesses:
   1. Mechanism of MR
   2. Hemodynamic severity
   3. Function of left ventricle from:
      - Left ventricular end-systolic volume
      - Left ventricular end-diastolic volume
      - Ejection fraction
   4. Structure and function of leaflets
   5. Integrity of chordae
   6. Size of left atrium and left ventricle
   7. Global left ventricular systolic function

b. Doppler echocardiography can demonstrate:
   1. Width and area of color flow mitral regurgitant jet within the left atrium
   2. Pulmonary venous flow contour
   3. Duration as well as intensity of continuous wave Doppler signal
   4. Early peak mitral flow velocity
   5. Quantitative measurement of regurgitant volume
   6. Effective regurgitant orifice area
   7. Velocity of tricuspid regurgitant velocity—it can estimate pulmonary artery pressure.

c. Exercise testing with transthoracic echocardiography assesses:
   1. Exercise capacity
   2. Dynamic changes in the severity of MR
   3. Systolic pressure in the pulmonary artery
   4. Functions of both ventricles

Treatment

A. Medical treatment: It depends upon the cause of MR.

- **a.** In chronic MR with atrial fibrillation anticoagulation with warfarin or oral apixaban or rivaroxaban
- **b.** If associated with rheumatic mitral stenosis, oral anticoagulant should not be used, here cardioversion should be considered in case of chronicity of atrial fibrillation, size of left atrium.
- **c.** In case of DCM or ischemic cardiomyopathy treatment of heart failure like:
  1. Diuretics
  2. Beta-blockers
  3. Angiotensin-converting enzyme inhibitor
  4. Digitalis
  5. Cardiac synchronization therapy
- **d.** In case of prior history of infective endocarditis, antibiotic prophylaxis should be used as preventive therapy.
- **e.** Isometric form of exercise should be avoided in patient with severe MR having sinus rhythm, normal left ventricular size, and systolic function.
- **f.** In case of severe acute regurgitation due to postmyocardial infarction papillary muscle rupture, prior to preparation of surgery, diuretics, intravenous vasodilators, and mechanical support are considered.

B. Surgical therapy: In case of slowly progressive MR, there should be balance between the nature of the disease and postoperative complications. Risk is lower in case of valve repair as compared to valve replacement. Repair consists of:

- **a.** Valve reconstruction by different valvoplasty technique
- **b.** Insertion of annuloplasty ring

Valve repair:

- **a.** Prevents complications of mechanical valve replacement like hemorrhage and thromboembolism and failure of bioprosthesis requiring repeat valve replacement in case of bioprosthesis.
- **b.** Preserves papillary muscle integrity and subvalvular apparatus
- **c.** Preserves chordae tendinae
- **d.** Maintains left ventricular function

Surgery should be recommended in asymptomatic patients with:

- **a.** Left ventricular dysfunction characterized by:
  1. Ejection fraction of <60%
  2. Left ventricular end-systolic dimension of >40 mm
- **b.** Recent onset atrial fibrillation of <3 months
- **c.** Pulmonary hypertension as defined by pulmonary artery pressure of ≥50 mm Hg. At rest and ≥60 mm Hg with exercise.
- **d.** Progressive decrease in ejection fraction or increase in end-systolic dysfunction that is evident on serial imaging.

In case of myxomatous degeneration of mitral valve with normal left ventricular function and absence of coronary artery disease can be treated surgically by:

- **a.** Chordal transfer
- **b.** Creation of neochords
- **c.** Resection of limited leaflet
- **d.** Insertion of annuloplasty band

In case of associated atrial fibrillation following treatments are considered:

- **a.** Biatrial maze surgery
- **b.** Radiofrequency isolation of pulmonary veins

In case of ischemic MR, coronary revascularization should also be considered. Current method includes annuloplasty repair with undersized rigid ring.

In case of ischemic MR with significant left ventricular systolic dysfunction having ejection fraction of <30%, risk of surgical repair is very high, reduced left ventricular performance, and reduced long-term survival.

Q88. Paradoxical stroke.

MGR/SEP2008/MDII (6)

ANSWER

Introduction

It is an uncommon cause of arterial occlusion when a thrombus will cross the intracardiac defect to enter into the systemic circulation and the patient will present with symptoms relating to the affected organ.

Etiology

A. Patent foramen ovale: Here, the shunt occurs between the septum primum and septum secundum. Valsalva maneuver such as coughing, sneezing, and squatting will increase the right atrial pressure increasing the chance of transfer of potential thrombi into systemic circulation.

B. Atrial septal defect: Normally, there is no chance of paradoxical embolism because left atrial pressure is more than the right atrial pressure resulting left to right heart shunt, but as the right atrial pressure increases with ages resulting from secondary pulmonary hypertension, there will be reversal of shunt leading to chance of paradoxical embolism.

C. Ventricular septal defect: Normally, there is no chance of paradoxical embolism because left ventricular pressure is more than the right ventricular pressure resulting left to right heart shunt, but as the right ventricular pressure resulting from secondary pulmonary hypertension increases with ages, there will be reversal of shunt leading to chance of paradoxical embolism.

D. Pulmonary arterio-venous malformation: Here, there is pathological connection between pulmonary artery and pulmonary veins returning to left atrium resulting permanent right to left atrial shunt.

Pathophysiology

Important risk factor is deep venous thrombosis as the thrombus will be dislodged from the deep vein, enters into right atrium and/or ventricle from there it will enter into left atrium and/or ventricle or through the pulmonary arterio-venous malformation, and lastly in systemic circulation to produce paradoxical embolism.

History

A. History of coughing or straining

B. History of diabetes mellitus, deep vein thrombosis, cardiovascular diseases, atrial fibrillation, hypercholesterolemia, and syncope or hypertension

C. History related to migraine as 50% patients of intracardiac shunt may present with migraine.

D. History of congenital heart disease, patent foramen ovale, atrial septal defect, and VSD

E. Social history—tobacco use

F. Family history

Physical Signs

A. Signs of congenital heart defect like:

- **a.** Digital clubbing
- **b.** Right ventricular hypertrophy
- **c.** Wide fixed splitting

B. Neurological evaluation:

- **a.** Speech abnormality
- **b.** Visual abnormality
- **c.** Unilateral weakness
- **d.** Difficulty in swallowing
- **e.** Seizures

C. Peripheral pulses evaluation to detect the ischemia of peripheral limb

Evaluation

A. Electrocardiography to evaluate atrial fibrillation or other arrhythmias

B. Transthoracic echocardiography with color Doppler studies can evaluate:

- **a.** Intracardiac shunt
- **b.** Cardiac myxoma
- **c.** Formation of thrombus

C. Transcranial Doppler sonography: It can evaluate—

- **a.** Any shunt
- **b.** Pulmonary arteriovenous malformation
- **c.** Microemboli in the intracranial artery

D. Ear oximetry: It can detect intracardiac shunt. When Valsalva maneuver will produce transient right to left heart shunt resulting transient decrease in arterial oxygen saturation that can be detected by this method.

E. Coagulation studies for measurement of protein C and protein S level

F. D-Dimer level if there is suspicion of pulmonary embolism.

G. Ultrasound to evaluate deep venous thrombosis

H. CT angiography of the chest to evaluate in case of suspected pulmonary embolism

I. Arterial blood gas measurement: It can determine oxygenation and ventilation status.

J. Noncontrast MRI can detect intracranial hemorrhage.

K. CT angiogram can evaluate embolization in the extremities, kidney.

Treatment

A. Elimination of the pathways of embolization through the percutaneous or surgical approach to occlude intracardiac shunt and pulmonary arteriovenous malformation

B. Medical management to control recurrent venous thrombosis including antithrombotic therapy, like clopidogrel, aspirin, as monotherapy or combination

C. Combination of above

Initial treatment should be anticoagulation. Then if there is any intracardiac communication, it should be closed percutaneously or by open surgery.

Q89. Cardiac cycle.

RGUHS/MDI (10)

Describe cardiac cycle.

NTR UNIVERSITY OF HEALTH SC, VIJAYAWADA, ANDHRA, 2022 (10)

Cardiac cycle.

NTR UNIVERSITY OF HEALTH SC, VIJAYAWADA, ANDHRA, 2022 (10)

DNB, 2019 (3)

KERALA UNIVERSITY, 2018 (10)

Discuss the physiological basis of the cardiac cycle. Explain in brief the changes in the cardiac cycle and cardiac output during submaximal and maximal exercises.

DNB (OCT2024) (10)

ANSWER

Cardiac cycle is the series of pressure changes taking place within the heart that lead to movement of pressure changes through the different chambers of the heart.

Function

Regarding the events in the cardiac cycle, the sequences should be compartmentalized. Contraction of both atria occurs prior to contraction of the both ventricles. Cardiac cycle has been divided into two phases:

a. Diastole represents ventricular filling. It begins with closure of aortic and pulmonary valves and ends with closure of mitral and tricuspid valves. It is comprised of ventricular relaxation and ventricular filling. It represents the return of blood in the preparation of next ventricular contraction.
b. Systole represents ventricular contraction or ejection. Systole begins with closure of the mitral and tricuspid valves and ends with closure of aortic and pulmonary valves. It comprises ventricular contraction with increase in the pressure in the ventricles.

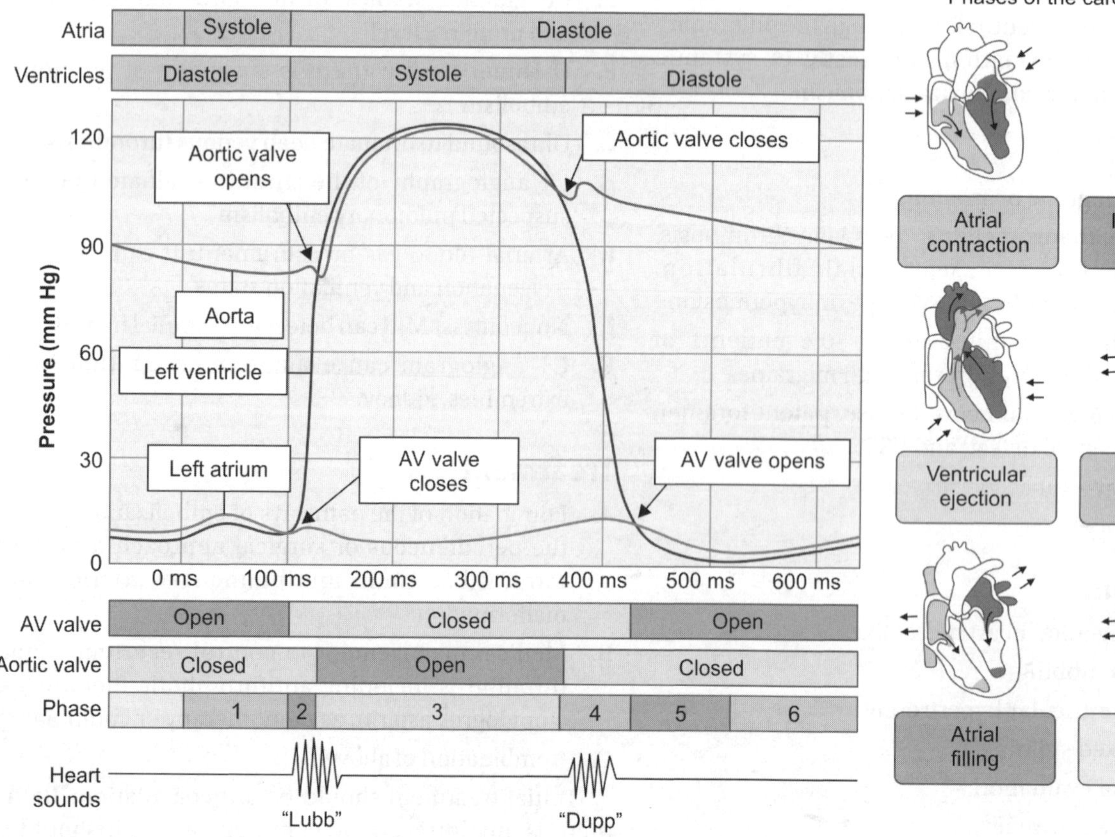

(AV: atrioventricular)

Hemodynamic Mechanism

A. Ventricular function has been subdivided into four phases:

a. Isovolumic relaxation: It is the period of relaxation of ventricles when aortic and pulmonary valves are closed and mitral and pulmonary valves are yet to be opened. This period creates very pressure within the ventricle creating a gradient which helps to open the mitral valve leaflets.

b. Ventricular filling: This is the period when mitral and tricuspid valves open and large amount of blood from right and left atria force into the right and left ventricles respectively according to the pressure gradient.

c. Isovolumic contraction: As both the ventricles fill and transition to contracting, as a result ventricular pressure exceeds that of the systemic and pulmonary vessels. As a result mitral and tricuspid valves begin to close—it is the beginning of the systole and makes the first heart sound which can be denoted as S1. This is the period between the closing of the mitral and tricuspid valves and prior to the opening of the aortic and pulmonary valves. In the last phase of isovolumic contraction, i.e., in last 0.1 second atria forcefully contract to push last amount of blood into the ventricles—this phase is known as protodiastole.

d. Rapid ventricular ejection phase: This is the phase when pressure in both the ventricles exceeds the intra-aortic and intrapulmonary artery pressure, both aortic and pulmonary valves open with ejection of blood into the aortal and pulmonary artery from the ventricles. A healthy ventricle will eject 60% of its volume, pressure within the ventricles gradually decreases as compared to the aorta and pulmonary arteries leading to closure of these valves that coincide with second heart sound (denoted by S2).

Total cardiac cycle is 0.8 seconds—Total timing of ventricular diastole is 0.5 seconds and total timing of ventricular diastole is 0.3 seconds. Among the total time of ventricular diastole 0.1 second is atrial systole.

Maximum and minimum pressures in different heart chambers:

A. Left ventricle: 120/15 mm Hg
B. Right ventricle: 25/5 mm Hg
C. Right atrium: 4–5 mm Hg
D. Left atrium: 25/10 mm Hg
E. Pulmonary artery: 25/10 mm Hg
F. Aorta: 120/80 mm Hg

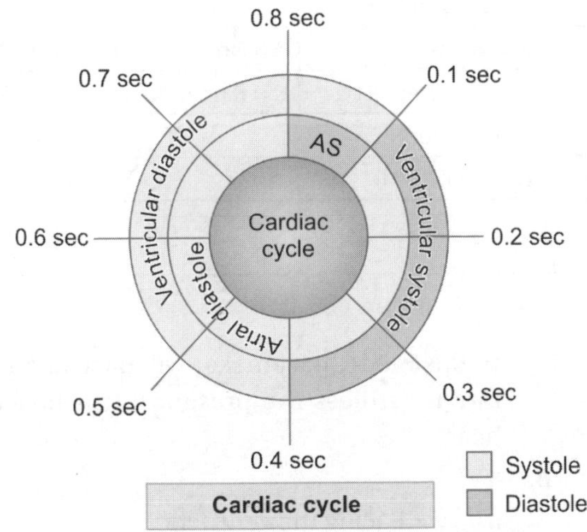

Cardiac cycle

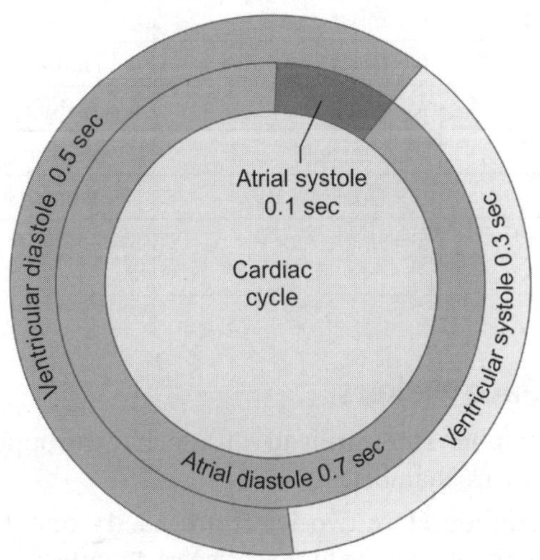

Changes in the cardiac cycle and cardiac output during submaximal exercise:

Parameter	Effect of submaximal exercise
Stroke volume	Increases
End-diastolic volume	Increases as a result of increased venous return
End systolic volume	Increased contractility leading to decreased end-systolic volume
Ejection fraction	Increased
Duration of diastolic period	Decreased
Stroke volume	Increased
Cardiac output	Increased

Changes in the cardiac cycle and cardiac output during maximal exercise:

Parameter	Effect of maximal exercise
Heart rate	200–220 beats/min
Cardiac output	6–8 times of normal rate. In trained athlete 35–40 L/min
Stroke volume	Increased up to 100–200 mL/beat
End-diastolic volume	Increased due to increased venous return
End-systolic volume	Decreased as a result of increased contractility
Ejection fraction	Increased from 60 to 85%
Duration of diastole	Decreased due to increased heart rate
Duration of systole	It is relatively preserved
Preload	Increased due to the following causes: • Increased venous return • Increased sympathetic activity • Increased muscle pump
Systemic vascular resistance	Decreased due to vasodilatation of the muscles
Contractility of the myocardium	Increased due to sympathetic over-activity

Q90. Indications and types of pace makers.

RGUHS/MDII (10)

ANSWER

Indications are described in question number 53.

Types of Pace Makers

North American Society of pacing and electrophysiology published a code "pacemaker code" in 1983 and it has been revised in 2002. Five position codes are accepted for pacemaker therapy:

A. First position—chamber paced

B. Second position—chamber sensed

C. Third position—Device response to sensed events labeled as I, T, D.

D. Programmability and rate modulation

E. Multisite pacing:

Position	I	II	III	IV	V
Category	Chamber paced	Chambers sensed	Response to sensing	Programmability	Multisite pacing
Letters	0 = None	0 = None	0 = None	0 = None	0 = None
	A = Atrium	A = Atrium	T = Triggered	R = Rate modulation	A = Atrium
	V = Ventricle	V = Ventricle	I = Inhibited		V = Ventricle
	D = Dual (A + V)	D = Dual (A + V)	D = Dual (T + I)		D = Dual (A + V)
Manufacturers' designation	S = Single A or V	S = Single A or V			

Types of Pace Makers

A. Single chamber: Here one lead will attach to the upper or lower heart chamber.

B. Dual chamber: Here two leads are used—one for upper chamber and one for lower heart chamber.

C. Biventricular pacemaker

Single Chamber Mode

A. VOO:

- **a.** V = Pacing the ventricle
- **b.** O = sensing is off.
- **c.** O = Response to sensing is off.

In this mode, pacemaker will pace at a programmed rate regardless the present intrinsic activity of the heart.

B. VVI:

- **a.** V = Pacing the ventricle
- **b.** V = Sensing the ventricle
- **c.** I = Inhibit

In this mode, pacemaker senses the electrical activity and holds the pacing as when required.

C. AOO:

- **a.** A = Atrial pacing
- **b.** O = Sensing is off.
- **c.** O = Response to sensing is off.

In this mode, pacemaker will pace at a programmed rate regardless the present intrinsic activity of the heart.

D. AAI:

a. A = Atrial pacing

b. A = Atrial sensing

c. I = Inhibit

In this mode, the pacemaker can adapt intrinsic atrial rate and is able to pace whenever required and able to inhibit when required.

Dual-chamber Pacemaker

A. DDD:

a. D = Pacing both atria and ventricles

b. D = Sensing both atria and ventricles

c. D = Inhibits or triggers

B. VDD:

a. V = Pacing the ventricle

b. D = Sensing both atria and ventricles

c. D = Inhibit or trigger

Nontracking Mode

A. DDI:

a. D = Pacing both atria and ventricles

b. D = Sensing both atria and ventricles

c. I = Inhibit

B. DOO:

a. D = Pacing both atria and ventricles

b. O = Sensing is off.

c. O = Inhibit

Q91. Describe pathophysiology of deep vein thrombosis. Describe its clinical features, investigations, and measures to prevent pulmonary thromboembolism from the same.

MUHS/MAY2010/MDII (25)

Deep vein thrombosis.

SNMC/MAY2013/MDI (15)

ANSWER

Pathophysiology of Deep Vein Thrombosis

Virchow's triad consists of:

a. Venous stasis

b. Endothelial injury

c. Hypercoagulable state

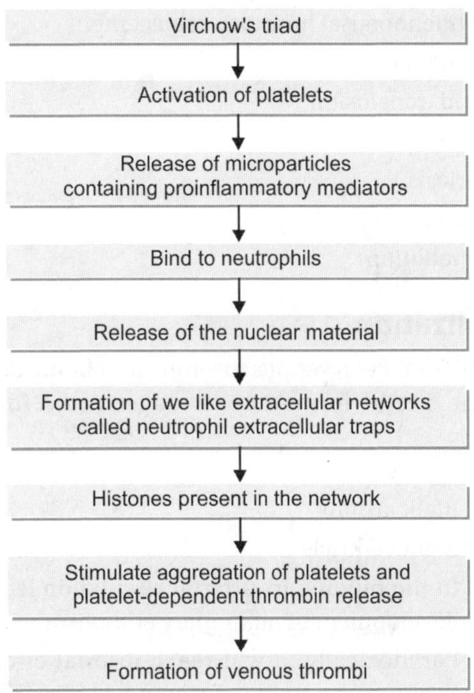

Thrombi will be upregulated in:

a. Environment of stasis

b. Low oxygen tension

c. Upregulation of proinflammatory genes

Prothrombotic State

Antithrombin, protein C, and protein S are naturally occurring circulating coagulation inhibitor. Deficiency of these factors is associated with prothrombotic state.

Two most common autosomal dominant mutations are:

A. Factor V Leiden produces resistance to endogenous anticoagulant and activated protein C.

B. Mutation of prothrombin gene leads to increased concentration of plasma prothrombin.

As a result, prothrombotic state will be produced.

Antiphospholipid syndrome is the acquired cause of thrombophilia.

Following are the associated risk factors:

A. Cancer

B. Obesity

C. Smoker

D. Systemic arterial hypertension

E. Chronic obstructive pulmonary disease

F. Long air travel

G. Chronic kidney disease

H. Surgery

I. Estrogen-containing contraceptives

J. Postmenopausal hormone replacement

K. Pregnancy

L. Blood transfusion

M. Inflammatory bowel disease

N. Psoriasis

O. Trauma

P. Air pollution

Embolization

Thrombi from deep venous thrombi after being detached from the site of formation to lodge in the following vessels:

- **a.** Vena cava
- **b.** Right atrium
- **c.** Right ventricle
- **d.** In the pulmonary arterial circulation leading to development of pulmonary embolism.
- **e.** Paradoxically, it will reach arterial circulation through the patent foramen ovale and atrial septal or VSD.

In some patients with pulmonary embolism, there may be no feature of thrombosis as total clot has already been dislodged.

Physiology

Most common abnormalities in gas exchange include:

A. Arterial hypoxemia

B. Increased alveolar-arterial oxygen difference

Above two factors are responsible for:

- **a.** Inadequate transfer of oxygen into the lungs
- **b.** Increase in anatomical dead space due to absence of contact of breathed oxygen with exchange unit of the lung
- **c.** Increase in physiological dead space because ventilation of the gas exchange unit will exceed the pulmonary venous flow through the pulmonary capillaries.

C. Increased pulmonary vascular resistance:

- **a.** Obstruction to the vessels
- **b.** Serotonin secreted by platelets

Vasoactive mediators are responsible for ventilation-perfusion mismatching in the areas remote from embolus.

D. Impaired gas exchange resulting increased anatomical dead space due to the following:

- **a.** Obstruction to the vessels
- **b.** Alveolar hypoventilation resulting from hypoxemia relative to perfusion in nonobstructed lung.
- **c.** Right to left heart shunting
- **d.** Due to loss of gas exchange surface, there is impairment of transfer of carbon monoxide.

E. Alveolar hyperventilation due to stimulation of irritant receptors

F. Constriction of the airways distal to bronchi resulting increased airway resistance

G. Pulmonary compliance will be decreased due to:

- **a.** Edema of the lung
- **b.** Hemorrhage in the lung
- **c.** Loss of surfactant

Pulmonary Hypertension, Right and Left Ventricular Dysfunction and Right Ventricular Microinfarction

- Pulmonary arterial resistance rises from obstruction in the pulmonary artery and neurohumoral mediators leading to development of pulmonary arterial hypertension.

  As a result, there is a rise in right ventricular wall tension leading to right ventricular dilatation which ultimately produces right ventricular dysfunction.
- Due to stretching of right ventricular wall there is release of biomarkers like BNP.
- Due to increased wall tension of right ventricle interventricular septum bulges into left ventricle and thus compresses this cavity leading to decreased distensibility and thus impaired filling of left ventricle resulting left ventricular dysfunction.
- Increased tension of the right ventricular wall compresses the right coronary artery resulting right ventricular ischemia and microinfarction along with release of cardiac biomarkers like troponin.
- Left ventricular underfilling results low cardiac output that leads to systemic hypotension, if untreated culminates circulatory collapse and death.

Classification of Deep Venous Thrombosis

A. Lower extremity DVT: It is 10 times more common than other DVT. It will start in the calf vein then extends proximally to popliteal vein, then to femoral and ileac vein.

B. Upper extremity DVT: It occurs due to the following—

- **a.** Placement of pace makers

b. Internal cardiac defibrillators
c. Indwelling central venous catheter

It is aggravated by:
a. Increasing the diameter of the catheter
b. Increasing the number of the lumen

C. Superficial venous thrombosis: It will present with erythematous tender palpable cord. There is a chance of extension of thrombosis into the deep veins.

Clinical Evaluation

Most common symptom is cramp or "Charley horse" in the calf muscles and it will increase over several days. Wells Point Score criteria can help in clinical diagnosis of DVT.

Clinical variables	DVT score
Active cancer	1
Paralysis, paresis or recent cast	1
Bedridden for >3 days, major surgery for <12 weeks	1
Tenderness along the distribution of deep veins	1
Entire leg swelling	1
Unilateral calf swelling	1
Pitting edema	1
Collateral superficial nonvaricose vein	1
Alternative diagnosis at least as likely as DVT	−2

a. Low likelihood of DVT: Score is 0 or less.
b. Moderate likelihood of DVT: Score is 1–2.
c. High likelihood of DVT: Score is ≥3.

Diagnosis

A. Blood test:
a. Quantitative D-dimer assay in plasma by ELISA: It will be raised due to breakdown of fibrin by plasmin. It is >80% sensitive in DVT that also includes isolated DVT in the calf but >95% for pulmonary embolism. Normal value can rule out the DVT. This level is also increased in following conditions:
1. Sepsis
2. Pneumonia
3. Myocardial infarction
4. Cancer
5. Postoperative state
6. Second or third trimester of pregnancy

Hence, it is rarely of highly valuable in hospitalized patients.

b. Cardiac biomarkers are elevated in right ventricular microinfarction. The biomarkers are:
1. Troponin
2. Plasma heart-type fatty acid binding protein
3. B-type natriuretic peptide
4. N-terminal pro-brain natriuretic peptide

B. Electrocardiogram:
a. Sinus tachycardia
b. S1Q3T3 pattern—this is specific for right ventricular strain.

C. Noninvasive imaging modalities:
a. Venous ultrasonography:
1. Noncompressibility of the involved vein due to passive distention by thrombus
2. Direct visualization of low echogenic homogenous material
3. Absence of collateral channels

b. Doppler ultrasonography:
1. Absence of augmentation of Doppler flow pattern on manual compression
2. Loss of respiratory variation due to obstruction by DVT

c. MR venography: It can visualize the thrombus by gadolinium contrast.
d. Contrast plethysmography: It is a principal diagnostic test in case of suspected DVT.

Treatment

A. Primary therapy: In case of extensive iliofemoral, femoral, and upper extremity DVT low dose catheter directed thrombolysis should be the treatment of choice.

B. Secondary prevention:
a. Administration of low-dose anticoagulant
b. Placement of inferior venacaval filter "Angel filter" at bedside under ultrasonographic visualization of the internal jugular or femoral vein
c. In case of lower limb acute DVT, below knee gradual compressive stockings with pressure of 30–40 mm Hg for lessening the discomfort and due to its gradual loss of elasticity it should be replaced by every 3 months.

Q92. Baroreceptor activation therapy in hypertension.

AMU/2011/MDI (10)

ANSWER

Hypertension is a major contributory factor for morbidity and mortality as it is poorly controlled despite lifestyle modification therapy and pharmacological measures by three drugs. According to ESC resistant hypertension can be defined as office blood pressure of >140/90 mm Hg in spite of administration of three antihypertensive drugs, which is ≥130/80 mm Hg with ≥3 antihypertensive drugs and <130/80 mm Hg with ≥4 drugs according to AHA. Hypertension is associated with clinical or subclinical cardiovascular disease.

Baroreceptor activation therapy pathway:

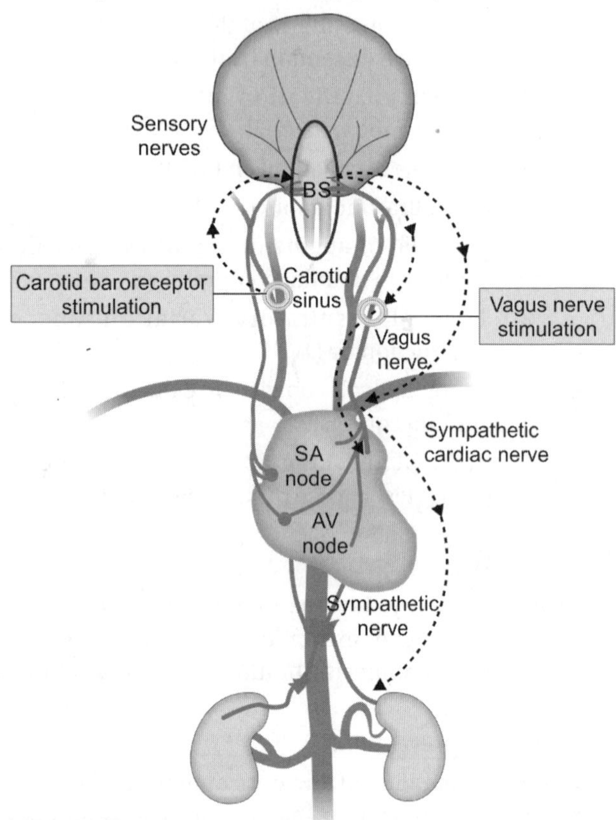

(AV: atrioventricular; BS: baroreceptor stimulation; SA: sinoatrial)

Role of Sympathetic Nervous System in Hypertension

Pathogenesis of essential hypertension is multifactorial. In case of resistant hypertension sympathetic nervous system is overactive thereby exerts its direct effect on the:

- **a.** Heart and its vasculature
- **b.** Renin–angiotensin–aldosterone system
- **c.** Glomerular filtration rate
- **d.** Renal tubular sodium reabsorption

So, impairment of baroceptors acts as a crucial role due to its reduced ability to control sympathetic nervous system. Imbalance of autonomic nervous system may lead to impaired left ventricular function thereby precipitating heart failure. Compensatory mechanisms will lead to excessive activity of sympathetic nervous system that may lead to:

- **a.** Adverse cardiac remodeling
- **b.** Increased heart rate
- **c.** Salt and water retention

Concept of Baroreflex Activation Therapy

Carotid baroreflex activation therapy consists of:

- **a.** Lead placed adjacent to carotid sinus
- **b.** Implantable pulse generator
- **c.** External programming system

As a result of arterial distention by increased blood flow and pressure carotid sinus is stimulated, then baroreceptors are stimulated, from there reflex arc passes through the afferent fibers to brainstem resulting reduced sympathetic discharge and increased parasympathetic discharge leading to:

- **a.** Reduction of systolic and diastolic blood pressure
- **b.** Improvement in cardiac structure
- **c.** Improvement of cardiac structural tissue
- **d.** Inhibition of renin-angiotensin-aldosterone system
- **e.** Decreased renal sodium reabsorption

Now second generation minimally invasive device Barostim Neo^{TM} system also reduces blood pressure. Its efficacy in case of resistant hypertension has been demonstrated in many trials, but due to its high risk bias and small sample size it has not become well-popularized.

Complications

- **a.** Pocket hematoma
- **b.** Pneumothorax
- **c.** Pain chest

Q93. Immunomodulation therapy in heart failure.

AMU/2011/MDI (10)

Pharmacologic and invasive cardiac care support in acute heart failure.

TEERTHANKER MAHAVEER UNI, 2018 JUNE (20)

ANSWER

Following are the comorbidities associated with heart failure with preserved ejection fraction:

A. Hypertension: It is the most common comorbidity and angiotensin is responsible for hypertension induced inflammation that leads to subsequent damage of vascular wall and myocardium.

B. Type 2 diabetes mellitus: It increases the mortality and morbidity by following mechanisms—

- **a.** Insulin resistance leads to:
  1. Increased free fatty acid metabolism
  2. Reduced uptake of glucose by myocardium

  This will lead to production of increased amount of toxic intermediates and reactive oxygen species. As a result proinflammatory cytokines are secreted by epicardium and myocardium and attract macrophages leading to impairment of myocardial and vascular function.
- **b.** Hyperglycemia increases retention of sodium.
- **c.** There is increased neurohumoral activation.

C. Obesity and lipid metabolism: Weight loss will lead to—

- **a.** Improved exercise capacity
- **b.** Reduction of hs-CRP

Statin prescribed in hyperlipidemia produces following actions:

- **a.** Antioxidant function
- **b.** Improved endothelial function
- **c.** Anti-inflammatory properties
- **d.** Immunomodulatory property leading to reduced expression of MHCII
- **e.** Reduces T-cell response

Immunomodulation on Heart Failure with Reduced Ejection Fraction

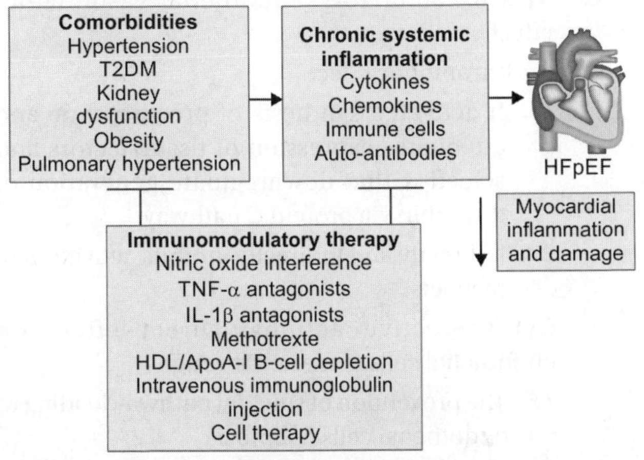

Nitric Oxide Signaling

Nitric oxide is produced by cardiac microvascular endothelial cells

↓

Results activation of soluble guanylate cyclase in the vascular smooth muscle cells and cardiac myocytes

↓

Production of cyclic guanosine monophosphate

↓

It regulates protein kinase G

In case of heart failure with preserved ejection fraction protein kinase G activity is defective leading to hypertrophy of cardiac myocytes which in turn produces left ventricular diastolic dysfunction.

Phosphodiesterase inhibitor: It activates protein kinase G resulting decreased myocardial stiffness and left ventricular ejection time.

Nitrate and nitrite: These increase the bioavailability of nitric oxide that contributes vascular integrity.

Soluble guanylate cyclase stimulator: It has anti-inflammatory, anti-fibrotic, and anti-proliferative effects.

Tumor Necrosis Factor-alpha antagonists

Tumor necrosis factor-alpha, IL-6, and IL-1 lead to cardiac remodeling through alterations in extracellular matrix, left ventricular dysfunction, cardiomyopathy, and pulmonary edema.

Pentoxyphylline: It will improve the left ventricular ejection fraction and reduce TNF-alpha production and Fas/Apo-1 in heart failure with preserved ejection fraction.

Aldosterone antagonists for TNF receptor and chimeric antibodies: Etanercept improves left ventricular function, and increases 6-minute walk test.

Interleukin-1β Antagonist

It is produced by inflammatory cells and it is a product of cytoplasmic innate immune complexes namely inflammasomes.

Decreased uric acid production: It will activate NLRP3 inflammasome leading to triggering IL-1β mediated inflammation. Oxypurinol inhibits xanthine oxidase and thus improves left ventricular function.

Methotrexate

It will improve the left ventricular function in patients with high inflammatory risk profile.

High-density Lipoprotein and Apolipoprotein A-1

Heterogenicity of HDL particle is due to difference in content in lipid and apolipoprotein. Earlier studies demonstrated that larger particle of HDL is more protective. Cholesterol ester transfer protein inhibitors and niacin will increase HDL-C level substantially without significant reduction of cardiovascular risk. Different studies demonstrated that in spite of very high HDL-C level, very high HDL-C particles were associated with high risk of cardiovascular diseases. On the other hand, high level of ApoA-I is associated with lower risk of cardiovascular disease.

More dense HDL particles are more functional as these particles promote efflux of cholesterol from lipid laden-macrophages more effectively, other functions are:

- **a.** Anti-inflammatory activity
- **b.** Anti-infective
- **c.** Cytoprotective
- **d.** Antioxidative
- **e.** Anti-thrombotic

B-cell Depletion

B-cell response is tightly regulated by immune system of the body. In heart failure with preserved ejection fraction, systemic inflammation along with exposed cardiac proteins as a result of damaged cardiomyocytes breaks immune tolerance leading to activation of autoreactive B and T cells. Monoclonal antibody rituximab by depleting B cells leads to improvement in heart failure.

Intravenous Immunoglobulin Injection

Main feature of B cells is the production of immunoglobulin targeting against myocardial proteins. As a result cardiac protein will combine with antibodies which lead to lysis of cardiomyocytes and it is associated with end-stage heart failure. Intravenous injection of immunoglobulin will clear these antibodies leading to improvement of left ventricular ejection fraction in chronic heart failure.

Cell Therapy

Stem cells like cardiac progenitor cells and mesenchymal cells produce cardiac myocytes that lead to improvement of cardiac functions in spite of poor cardiac engraftment. It is due to immunosuppressive properties of these cells.

Q94. HDL-C functionality and cardiovascular risk.

AMU/2011/MDI (10)

ANSWER

Introduction

Cardiovascular disease is the leading cause of death in the world and there is clear inverse relationship between blood level of HDL-C and atherosclerotic cardiovascular disease even in presence of LDL-C level below 70 mg/dL. It has been shown that for each 1 mg/dL decrease of HDL-C level is associated with 2% and 3% reduced risk of atherosclerotic cardiovascular disease in men and women, respectively.

High-density lipoprotein-C apolipoprotein consists of two ApoA-I and ApoA-II that are required for HDL-C synthesis. ApoA-I is synthesized in the liver and intestine and responsible for 70% HDL protein and present in almost all HDL-C particle whereas, ApoA-II is synthesized by the liver only and responsible for 20% of HDL protein and present in about two-thirds of HDL-C particle. According to mass spectrometry studies HDL-C protein carries multiplicity of proteins which involved in following actions:

- **a.** It affects metabolism of lipids.
- **b.** It regulates complement.
- **c.** It regulates acute phase response.
- **d.** It regulates proteinase inhibition.

Lipidomic approaches identified nearly 200 species molecular lipid in normolipidemic HDL including phospholipids, steroids, sphingolipid, monoacylglycerides, diacylglycerides, triglycerides, cholesterol esters, and free-fatty acids.

High-density lipoprotein-C has following beneficiary functions leading to provision of protection against cardiovascular diseases:

- **a.** High-density lipoprotein-C removes cholesterol from the peripheral vessel wall back to liver—called reverse cholesterol transport.
- **b.** Antioxidative effect
- **c.** Anti-inflammatory endothelial-vasodilatory effect
- **d.** Antithrombotic effect:
  1. It activated synthesis of prostacycline and attenuates expression of tissue factors and selectins that downregulate generation of thrombin via protein C pathway.
  2. It directly and indirectly inhibits activation of platelets.
- **e.** Cytoprotective actions: Direct effect on endothelial cells is exerted through—
  1. The prevention of suicidal pathway leading to endothelial cells apoptosis

2. Decrease the protease activity cysteine protease-32

f. It protects LDL from oxidative damage in the intima induced-free radicals along with consequent inhibition of generation of proinflammatory lipid peroxides and short chain oxidized phospholipids.

g. It will decrease the recruitment of monocytes in the arterial wall by inhibiting adhesion molecular expression in the endothelial cells.

h. It upregulates the expression of endothelial nitric oxide synthetase and maintains lipid environment in the caveolae containing the presence of nitric oxide synthetase and nitric oxide both of which will lead to increased production of nitric oxide, antiprotective signaling molecule.

i. It also stimulates the production of nitric oxide as a result of activation of kinase cascade by high-affinity HDL receptor and class B type I scavenger receptor.

In case of genetic Milano mutation of ApoA-I substitution of arginine to cysteine at position of 173 leads to formation of homodimers and heterodimers with ApoA-II, as a result very low HDL-C and hypertriglyceridemia without any evidence of premature coronary atherosclerosis. Weekly infusion of recombinant ApoA-I Milano will significantly regress the coronary atherosclerosis in acute coronary syndrome and this proves functionality of HDL which plays an important role in reduction of premature atherosclerosis as compared to HDL-C.

High-density Lipoprotein Particle Substitution and HDL Functionality

Heterogenicity of HDL particle is due to difference in content in lipid and apolipoprotein. Earlier studies demonstrated that larger particle of HDL is more protective. Cholesterol ester transfer protein inhibitors and niacin will increase HDL-C level substantially without significant reduction of cardiovascular risk. Different studies demonstrated that in spite of very high HDL-C level, very high HDL-C particles were associated with high risk of cardiovascular diseases. On the other hand, high level of ApoA-I is associated with lower risk of cardiovascular disease.

More dense HDL particles are more functional as these particles promote efflux of cholesterol from lipid laden-macrophages more effectively, other functions are:

a. Anti-inflammatory activity
b. Anti-infective
c. Cytoprotective
d. Anti-oxidative
e. Anti-thrombotic

Factors Affecting the HDL-C Functionality

A. Proteins of HDL are the following proteins other than ApoA-I and ApoA-II:

a. ApoC-I
b. ApoC-II
c. ApoC-III
d. ApoE
e. ApoJ
f. ApoL
g. Lecithin-cholesterol acyl transferase
h. Serum paroxonase-1
i. Platelet activating factor acetyl hydrolase

Oxidative environment of acute phase response in case of myocardial infection, systemic inflammation, chronic inflammation, surgery can convert HDL particle from anti-inflammatory to proinflammatory and proatherogenic particle by binding with amyloid A and ceruloplasmin and thus limit the ability to promote reverse cholesterol transport and prevents modification of LDL.

Apo-A-1 containing 2-OH-Trp-72 accounts for 20% Apo-A-1 in atherosclerotic arteries.

B. In case of type 2 diabetes mellitus glycation impairs the function of HDL and may lead to accelerated atherosclerosis.

C. In case of metabolic syndrome small dense HDL particles becomes dysfunctional having impaired antioxidative property.

D. Carbamylation of HDL leads to formation of foam cells in the atherosclerotic lesion.

E. Myeloperoxidase-mediated HDL oxidation makes it dysfunctional in regard to reverse cholesterol transfer, anti-inflammatory, and antioxidative properties.

F. Ethnicity:

a. Black South African women are more protective from cardiovascular disease as compared to men due to their improved HDL antioxidant functionality as compared to white women in spite of the greater prevalence of obesity in women than white women.

G. Obesity impairs HDL-C structure and functionality which can be improved after bariatric surgery.

H. Dietary factors:
   - **a.** Saturated fat consumption will impair anti-inflammatory and arterial endothelial function.
   - **b.** Polyunsaturated fat consumption improves anti-inflammatory activity of HDL.

High-density Lipoprotein Cholesterol Efflux Capacity

Cholesterol efflux from lipid laden macrophages occurs via following receptors:
   - **a.** ABCA1
   - **b.** ABCG1
   - **c.** Scavenger receptor SR-B1

It is a very important marker of protection from atherogenicity and it is an excellent surrogate for functionality of HDL. Cholesterol efflux capacity from lipid laden macrophages present in the arterial wall has inverse relationship with carotid intima-medial wall thickness and angiographic coronary artery disease independent of level of HDL-C.

Cholesterol efflux capacity is impaired in following diseases:
   - **a.** Obesity
   - **b.** Diabetes mellitus
   - **c.** Chronic kidney disease
   - **d.** Metabolic syndrome

Future Therapeutic Directions

A. Infusion of recombinant ApoA-1 Milano without contamination of host protein is associated with significant reduction of atherosclerosis.

B. Conversion of α-HDL to pre-β-HDL by plasma selective delipidation can effectively remove lipid from arterial plaque.

C. Reconstituted infusible plasma-derived ApoA-I can enhance cholesterol efflux capacity—it is under trial.

Q95. Cardiac resynchronization therapy.

MJPRU/2015/MDIV (20)
TEERTHANKER MAHAVEER UNI, 2017 (10)
RAJIV GANDHI UNIVERSITY OF HEALTH SC, KARNATAKA, 2019 (10)

Write briefly about cardiac resynchronization therapy.

WBUHS, 2023 (10)

ANSWER

Introduction

It can be described as biventricular pacing or multisite ventricular pacing that involves simultaneous pacing of left as well as right ventricles in addition to conventional right ventricular endocardial leads, with or without right atrial lead. Coronary resynchronization therapy also involves another lead placement in coronary sinus to pace left ventricle.

Indications

A. It improves cardiac hemodynamics and symptoms.

B. It will prevent hospitalization.

C. It will improve mortality in patients with advanced heart failure with severe left ventricular dysfunction.

According to AHA guidelines:

A. Class I (indicated):
   - **a.** (With or without ICD)—patients are in sinus rhythm, LVEF of ≤35%, duration of QRS is ≥120 msec, NYHA functional class III or ambulatory IV heart failure symptom in spite of optimal medical therapy.
   - **b.** Patient is in sinus rhythm, LVEF ≤ 35%, LBBB with QRS duration of 150 msec, NYHA class II, III, or ambulatory IV heart failure symptom in spite of optimal medical therapy.

B. Class II (reasonable): CRT can be useful in following conditions—
   - **a.** Left ventricular ejection fraction of 35%, sinus rhythm, LBBB with QRS duration of 120–149 msec, NYHA class II, III, ambulatory IV heart failure symptom on guideline-directed optimal medical therapy
   - **b.** Left ventricular ejection fraction of 35%, sinus rhythm, non-LBBB pattern with QRS duration of at least 150 msec, and NYHA class III or ambulatory IV heart failure symptom on guideline-directed optimal medical therapy
   - **c.** Atrial fibrillation, LVEF of 35% on goal-directed medical therapy if:
      1. Patient requires ventricular pacing or otherwise meets CRT criteria, and,
      2. Atrioventricular nodal ablation or pharmacologic rate control will allow near 100% ventricular pacing with CRT.

d. On goal-directed medical therapy with LVEF of 35% and undergoing new or replacement device placement with anticipated requirement for significant (40%) ventricular pacing.

C. Class III (may be considered):

a. Left ventricular ejection fraction up to 30%, ischemic heart failure etiology, sinus rhythm, LBBB with QRS duration of at least 150 msec, NYHA class I symptoms on goal-directed medical therapy

b. An LVEF of ≤35%, sinus rhythm, non-LBBB pattern with QRS duration of 120–149 msec, NYHA class III or ambulatory class IV on guideline-directed optimal medical therapy.

c. An LVEF of 35%, sinus rhythm, non-LBBB pattern with QRS duration of at least 150 msec, and NYHA class ii symptoms on goal-directed medical therapy.

Contraindications to Cardiac Resynchronization Therapy

According to AHA guidelines:

A. Class III (no benefit):

a. New York Heart Association class I and II and non-LBBB pattern with duration of QRS of <150 msec.

b. Patients with comorbidities and/or frailty limit survival with good functional capacity to <1 year.

Role of Cardiac Resynchronization Therapy

A. Primary role of CRT is to improve systolic left ventricular dysfunction via improvement of efficiency of chambers that can lead to improvement of refractory heart failure.

B. Systolic and diastolic dimension of left ventricle will be decreased following prolonged CRT of at least 3 months.

C. There is also electrical remodeling.

D. In case of severe left ventricular disease CRT alone or in combination with ICD can improve the patients symptomatically.

Following factors are associated with improved outcome of CRT:

A. Women, because of lower left ventricular mass at the same duration of QRS as compared to men

B. Patients with nonischemic cardiomyopathy as there is chance of reversing of cardiac remodeling.

C. Patients with LBBB are more likely to improve function with CRT in comparison to non-LBBB, i.e., RBBB or IVCD.

D. Patients with wide QRS duration (150 msec) will improve more efficiently as compared to QRS duration of 120–149 msec.

E. Position of lead accounts for the response. Lead position in apical position as compared to mid and basal position is associated with improved outcome.

Following measures can be taken to prevent complications:

A. Preoperative antibiotic can be administered prior to implantation of ICD.

B. Chlorhexidine—alcohol is preferred for skin sepsis.

C. First choice of vein for insertion is cephalic or axillary veins.

D. Heparin bridging should be avoided in case of ICD as it will minimize the risk of hematoma and pocket infection.

E. Antibiotic eluting envelope in ICD to lower the risk of infection.

Devices for Implantation

It is an electronic device that senses intrinsic electrical rhythm and sends electrical signal as and when indicated. Permanent pacemaker involves insertion of leads in the endocardium (right atrium and right ventricle) or epicardium (left ventricle through the coronary sinus), these are ultimately connected to pacing generator placed subcutaneously in the infraclavicular region. In patient with heart failure CRT with biventricular pacing with or without ICD may be given.

Implantable cardioverter-defibrillator: It is the therapy of choice for prophylaxis in patient with risk of ventricular arrhythmias. The device offers tired therapy with programmable antitachycardia pacing schemes along with low-energy and high-energy shocks in the zones of multiple tachycardia.

Q96. Takayasu disease.

MGR/SEP2007/MDIV (5)

Current status of management of Takayasu arteritis.

AMU/2011/MDIV (20)

NTR UNIVERSITY OF HEALTH SC, VIJAYAWADA, ANDHRA, NOV 2020 (10)

ANSWER

Introduction

It is a rare systemic vasculitis of inflammatory origin involving large or medium-sized vessels—it is under the name of ophthalmologist Mikito Takayasu.

Etiology

Etiology is inflammatory—in this case several etiologic factors are proposed, these are mycobacterium tuberculosis, spirochetes, streptococcal infection, or circulating autoantibodies.

Antigen stimulates aortic tissue to express heat shock protein-65 leading to induction of MHC class I related chain A.

Natural killer cells and gamma delta T cells:

- **a.** Will infiltrate and recognize MHC class I related chain A present on the vascular smooth muscle cells and develop inflammation.
- **b.** Release proinflammatory cytokines leading to production of metalloproteinase that amplify inflammatory response as evidenced by stimulation of molecular expression on the vascular endothelial and smooth muscle cells and recruit more and more mononuclear cells.

T1 helper lymphocytes activate macrophages through interferon-γ leading to release of vascular endothelial growth factor resulting migration of smooth muscle cells and proliferation of intima.

Th17 after being induced by interleukin-23 activates infiltrating neutrophils and also aggravates vascular disease.

Cellular infiltrate consists of CD4+ and CD8+. Activated monocytes, macrophages, and T cells synthesize interleukin-6 which in turn:

- **a.** Activates B cells
- **b.** Enhances T cell cytotoxicity
- **c.** Enhances activity of natural killer cells
- **d.** Enhances proliferation of fibroblasts
- **e.** Increases acute phase protein synthesis

HLA-B*52 may be associated with Takayasu disease—it is highly prevalent in Asian population. It is also associated with aortic regurgitation and left ventricular wall abnormalities.

Other associated HLA alleles are HLA-B*39, HLA-DRB1*1502, and HLA-DRB1*0405 in Japanese patients.

Pathophysiology

This disease has a predilection for aorta and its branches. Lesions may be:

- **a.** Stenotic
- **b.** Occlusive
- **c.** Aneurysmal—it has areas of arterial narrowing.

Renal artery is involved in 24–68% of this disease, it is usually bilateral. It is associated with coexistent stenosis of perirenal aorta.

There may be associated congestive cardiac failure. If the pulmonary artery is involved, right branch is more affected than the left, patient may develop pneumonia, interstitial pulmonary fibrosis, and damages of the alveoli.

Other pathophysiological consequences are:

- **a.** Hypotensive ischemic retinopathy
- **b.** Myocarditis
- **c.** Pericarditis
- **d.** Cardiomyopathy
- **e.** Hypertensive encephalopathy
- **f.** Inflammatory bowel disease
- **g.** Carotid stenosis

Rarely, this arteritis is associated with the following conditions:

- **a.** Glomerulonephritis
- **b.** Polymyositis
- **c.** Rheumatoid arthritis
- **d.** Polymyalgia rheumatica
- **e.** Systemic lupus erythematosus
- **f.** Still disease
- **g.** Ankylosing spondylitis

Clinical Features

A. Constitutional symptoms:

- **a.** Fever
- **b.** Arthralgia
- **c.** Malaise
- **d.** Weight loss
- **e.** Headache

B. Cardiac and vascular features are:

- **a.** Carotid artery bruit
- **b.** Difference of blood pressure in the extremities
- **c.** Claudication
- **d.** Carotidynia or tenderness on the vessels
- **e.** Aortic regurgitation
- **f.** Pericarditis
- **g.** Hypertension
- **h.** Raynaud phenomenon
- **i.** Myocardial infarction
- **j.** Congestive cardiac failure

C. Neurological features:

 a. Visual disturbances—it is strongly associated with carotid artery disease

 b. Headache

 c. Transient ischemic attack

 d. Stroke

 e. Convulsions

D. Dermatological features:

 a. Pyoderma gangrenosum

 b. Erythema nodosum

 c. Ulcerated subcutaneous nodules

Classification Criteria

According to American College of Rheumatology:

A. Disease onset at 40 years or less

B. Claudication of the extremities

C. Decreased extremities of one or both brachial arteries

D. There is difference of at least 10 mm Hg in systolic blood pressure between the arms.

E. Bruit over the abdominal aorta or one or both subclavian arteries

F. Arteriographic demonstration of narrowing or occlusion of the entire aorta its primary branches or large arteries in the upper or lower extremities that is not due to arteriosclerosis, fibromuscular dysplasia or other causes.

Presence of three or more criteria has a sensitivity of >90%.

Other physical signs are:

A. Amaurosis fugax

B. Dilated cardiomyopathy

C. Myocardial infarction

D. Focal neurological deficit—which is consistent with cerebral infarction or TIA

E. Bruit in the carotid and abdominal arteries

F. Eclampsia

G. Subarachnoid hemorrhage—may be due to secondary hypertension

H. Pedal edema due to glomerulonephritis

I. Sensorineural hearing loss

J. Pulmonary hemorrhage

K. Ulcerative colitis

Evaluation

A. Laboratory studies:

 a. ESR: >50 mm/1st hour

 b. Leukocyte count: Elevated or near normal

 c. Moderate normocytic anemia

 d. Antibodies:

  1. Antinuclear antibodies

  2. Rheumatoid factor

  3. Antineutrophil cytoplasmic antibodies

  4. Anticardiolipin antibodies antiendothelial antibodies

  5. Antiaorta antibodies

 e. Vascular cell adhesion molecule-1

 f. Hypoalbuminemia

 g. Increased level of fibrinogen

 h. Increased α-2 globulin

 i. Increased γ-globulin

 j. Increased urinary protein consistent with nephrotic syndrome

 k. Human leukocyte antigens typing

Imaging

Ishikawa Criteria

A. Age younger than 40 years at the time of diagnosis or at onset of characteristic signs and symptoms of 1 month duration.

B. Two major criteria are:

 a. Lesion at right and left mid-subclavian artery with most severe occlusion in the mid portion of the artery from 1 cm proximal to the left and right respectively, of the vertebral orifices to a 3-cm distal point to the orifice which is determined by angiography.

C. Minor criteria are: Annuloaortic ectasia or presence of aortic regurgitation in angiography or echocardiography along with lesions involving any of the following vessels:

 a. Pulmonary artery

 b. Left mid-common carotid artery

 c. Descending aorta

 d. Abdominal aorta

 e. Distal brachiocephalic trunk

Ishikawa Clinical Classification

A. Group I: Uncomplicated disease with or without pulmonary artery involvement.

B. Group II: Mild/Moderate single complication together with uncomplicated disease.

C. Group III: Severe single complication together with uncomplicated disease.

D. Two or more complications together with uncomplicated disease.

Assessment of Disease Activity

New onset or worsening of two or more of the following features suggests active disease:

- **a.** Systemic features:
  - **1.** Fever
  - **2.** Arthralgia
- **b.** Elevated ESR
- **c.** Features of vascular ischemia or inflammation:
  - **1.** Claudication
  - **2.** Diminished or absent pulse
  - **3.** Bruit
  - **4.** Carotidynia
  - **5.** Asymmetrical blood pressure in either upper or lower limb or both.
- **d.** Typical features in angiography

Following biomarkers can establish the diagnosis:

- **a.** C-reactive protein
- **b.** Pentraxin-3
- **c.** Serum amyloid P

Angiography

Takayasu disease can be subdivided into following types based on angiographic involvement:

- **A.** Type I: Branches of the aortic arch
- **B.** Type IIa: Ascending aorta, aortic arch and its branches
- **C.** Type IIb: Type IIa region plus descending thoracic aorta
- **D.** Type III: Descending thoracic aorta, abdominal aorta, renal artery or any combination
- **E.** Type IV: Abdominal aorta, renal artery or both
- **F.** Type V: Entire aorta and its branches

Ultrasonography and CT Scan

It will give the detail of vascular wall, its lumen, blood flow through the vessels mainly through the carotid and subclavian arteries.

Magnetic Resonanace Angiography

It can delineate the lesion in any aortic branches and also in the smaller branches.

Positron Emission Tomography Scanning

It can detect the disease activity and the response to treatment.

Treatment

A. *Medical treatment*:

- **a.** Corticosteroid is the mainstay of treatment. Oral prednisolone 1 mg/kg of body weight to be given daily in single or in divided doses and to be tapered over weeks or months as the features subside. But in some cases long-term steroid is required.
- **b.** Interleukin-6 receptor inhibitor: As interleukin-6 is the major component of inflammatory process, human monoclonal antibody tocilizumab should be given as it will block the IL-6 receptor.
- **c.** B-cell depletion: Rituximab, chimeric IgG1 antibody will bind to CD20 present on the B cells and thus it will improve the clinical features of this disease.
- **d.** Cytotoxic drugs: In case of steroid-resistant cases or relapsing cases these drugs should be given and to be continued at least 1 year after remission and then should be tapered to discontinuation. The drugs are cyclophosphamide, methotrexate, and tacrolimus and mycophenolate mofetil.
- **e.** Anti-TNF agents: In case of active and relapsing Takayasu arteritis it can be given.
- **f.** Treatment of cardiovascular risk factors such as hypertension, diabetes mellitus, and dyslipidemia.

B. Surgical treatment:

- **a.** Indications of surgical repair:
  - **1.** Renovascular stenosis leading to hypertension
  - **2.** Aortic regurgitation
  - **3.** Claudication of the extremity induced by routine activity
  - **4.** Coronary artery stenosis leading to myocardial ischemia
  - **5.** Cerebral ischemia with or without critical stenosis in ≥3 cerebral vessels
  - **6.** Severe aortic coarctation
  - **7.** Thoracic or abdominal aneurysm
- **b.** Procedures:
  - **1.** Bypass graft surgery
  - **2.** Percutaneous balloon angioplasty
  - **3.** Angioplasty and stenting

Surgery may be unnecessary in case of aorta and splanchnic vessels due to presence of extensive collaterals.

But, critical stenosis should be intervened to prevent ischemia or stroke by graft of ascending aorta.

Renal artery can be treated by percutaneous transluminal angioplasty. Stent placement is required for:

a. Ostial lesion
b. Long segmental lesion
c. Incomplete relief of stenoses
d. Dissection

Pregnancy

Since Takayasu arteritis occurs in child-bearing age, hence issue of pregnancy is very important. Main maternal complication is hypertension. Fetal outcome depends upon:

a. The involvement of the vessels
b. Severity of maternal hypertension
c. Superimposed pre-eclampsia
d. Timing of adequate blood pressure control

Development of hypertension at the second stage of labor is a risk factor for cerebral hemorrhage. It can be overcome by shortening the second stage by low forceps delivery or vacuum extraction.

Q97. Sick sinus syndrome: diagnosis and management.

AMU/2011/MDI (10)
KERALA UNIVERSITY, 2017 (10)

ANSWER

Definition

It is also known as sinus node dysfunction characterized by SA node disorder due to impaired function of pace maker or transmission of impulses like:

a. Atrial tachyarrhythmias
b. Atrial bradyarrhythmias
c. Bradycardia alternating with tachyarrhythmia known as tachy-brady syndrome.

Etiology

Sinus node dysfunction can be classified into two categories:

A. Intrinsic pathology resulting from fibrosis of the nodal tissue:
   a. Age-related disorder of SA node
   b. Congenital disorder—results from several mutations in the ionic channel
   c. Arrhythmias
   d. Infiltrative disorder:
      1. Amyloidosis
      2. Sarcoidosis
      3. Hemochromatosis
      4. Collagen vascular disease
      5. Metastatic cancer
   e. Surgery:
      1. Damage of SA node or SA nodal artery from valve replacement
      2. Correction of congenital heart disease
      3. Cardiac transplantation
B. Extrinsic pathology affecting SA nodal function:
   a. Abnormally increased vagal tone:
      1. Carotid sinus hypersensitivity
      2. Vasovagal syncope
      3. Autonomic dysfunction
   b. Metabolic derangement:
      1. Hypothyroidism
      2. Hyperkalemia
      3. Hypokalemia
      4. Hypocalcemia
      5. Hypoxemia
      6. Hypothermia
   c. Obstructive sleep apnea may produce severe bradyarrhythmias due to severe hypoxia during the episode of apnea.
   d. Increased intracranial pressure (Cushing reflex)
   e. Pharmacologic agents and toxic agents:
      1. Lithium
      2. Sympathetic medications
      3. Digoxin

Pathophysiology

Sinoatrial node consists of collection of atrial myocytes which have been divided into two classically functional cells:

A. "P" cells or pace maker cells: These cells are responsible for intrinsic pace maker function.
B. "T" cells or transitional cells: These cells are responsible for propagation of impulse into the right atrium.

Dysfunction of any one of the cells responsible for development of different arrhythmias:

A. Abrupt and inappropriate: Severe sinus bradycardia
B. Sinus arrest or sinus pause: Here, there is ≥3 seconds of cessation of atrial activity characterized by the failure of SA node to generate action potential.

C. Sinoatrial exit block: it is characterized by failure of the "T" cells to transmit impulse into atrial musculature. There are three degrees of sinoatrial block:

a. First-degree SA block: It is usually subclinical and cannot be detected in electrocardiogram.

b. Second-degree SA block: It is again subdivided into two subtypes:

1. Second-degree type 1 SA block: Here, there is progressive shortening of PP interval followed by absence of next P wave.

2. Second-degree type 2 SA block: Here, there is drop of P wave without any preceding changes in the PP interval.

c. Third-degree SA block: It is characterized by complete failure of SA node to transmit impulse into atrial musculature which can be reflected in the ECG as absence of P wave. It is similar to sinus arrest.

D. Tachy-brady syndrome: It is characterized by bradyarrhythmias intervened by paroxysmal supraventricular arrhythmias mostly atrial fibrillation resulting from generation of abnormal automaticity of the atrial tissue. It is nearly 50% of sinus node disease.

E. Prolonged sinus pause occurring after cardioversion due to failure to resume sinus rhythm.

F. Atrial fibrillation with slow ventricular response in absence of AV nodal blocking agent occurring due to simultaneous degeneration of AV node. In these patients cardioversion results sinus pause due to associated sinus node disease.

G. Chronotropic incompetence—it is characterized by inappropriate bradycardia resulting inability to supply the metabolic demand.

History and Physical Examination

Natural history of sinus node dysfunction is slowly progressive, hence for many years the patient will be asymptomatic. But symptoms will develop due to hypoperfusion of the vital organ in the face of high oxygen demand.

A. Syncope results from:

a. Severe sinus bradycardia or sinus pause may produce hypoperfusion of the central nervous system.

b. Sudden termination of tachy-brady syndrome by cardioversion resulting sinus pause or making gross delay to return in sinus rhythm.

B. Abdominal pain results from gastrointestinal hypoperfusion.

C. Oliguria results from renal hypoperfusion.

D. Thromboembolism resulting cardioembolic stroke in case of atrial flutter or fibrillation—it carries worse prognosis.

E. Exercise intolerance and fatigue results from chronotropic incompetence.

F. Palpitation in the tachyarrhythmia phase of tachy-brady syndrome

G. Worsening of angina pectoris

H. Congestive cardiac failure

Evaluation

A. First step in the evaluation is to search for the reversible and correctable causes like electrolyte abnormalities, obstructive sleep apnea, offending drugs, and metabolic abnormalities.

B. Proper documentation of the correlation of the symptoms with bradycardia

C. To document symptomatic bradycardia, 12 leads ECG is not beneficial, hence 24 or 48 hours Holter monitoring or telemonitoring is useful to get symptomatic correlation with timing of bradycardia.

D. If Holter monitoring or telemonitoring fails to demonstrate this event, then external or implantable long event term monitor or loop recorder may be required.

E. In case of strong suspicion of sinus node dysfunction and failure to detect arrhythmias, electrophysiological study may be required.

F. Automatic modulation testing like prolonged sinus pause of >3 seconds after giving carotid sinus massage is suggestive of sinus node dysfunction.

G. Chronotropic incompetence can be tested by treadmill testing which can demonstrate symptoms like exertional symptoms and fatigue and patient will achieve 80% of maximum heart rate, but it is not validated.

Treatment

A. Treatment of reversible causes of sinus node dysfunction if identified.

B. After exclusion of reversible causes the definitive treatment is implantation of permanent pace maker if:

a. The patient has symptomatic bradycardia.

b. The patient demonstrates chronotropic incompetence.

c. Dysfunction of sinus node secondary to medication which is essential for another medical condition like requirement of β-blocker in case of atrial fibrillation in a case of tachy-brady syndrome but at the same time it will also suppress SA node that can lead to prolonged sinus pause along with syncope when tachycardia episode will cease.

d. Bradycardia of <40 beats/min but there is no documentation of symptoms with bradycardia.

C. Choice of pace maker: Dual chamber pace maker is of choice as there is chance of AV block along with sinus node dysfunction as it will reduce the incidence of atrial fibrillation and subsequent risk of thromboembolism as well as stroke will be minimized.

D. Anticoagulation is recommended as there is chance of thromboembolism in case of tachy-brady syndrome as there is atrial tachyarrhythmias.

E. As the risk of sudden death in sinus node dysfunction is very low, so there is not so much impact on the survival whether the patient is being treated with pace maker or not.

Q98. Ambulatory blood pressure monitoring.

MJPRU/2014/MDIV (10)
MJPRU/2015(S)/MDIV (10)
MJPRU/2015/MDIV (10)
KERALA UNIVERSITY, 2018 (10)

Home blood pressure monitoring guidelines.

DNB, 2022 (5)

Blood pressure variability and ambulatory blood pressure monitoring.

TEERTHANKER MAHAVEER UNI, 2017 (10)

Ambulatory blood pressure monitoring.

TEERTHANKER MAHAVEER UNI, 2019 (10)
AIIMS, 2023 (10)
SAMS (ODISHA), 2022 (10)

ANSWER

Indications of Ambulatory Blood Pressure Monitoring

A. Identification of white coat hypertension phenomena

B. Identification of masked hypertension phenomena

C. Identification of abnormal pattern of hypertension in 24 hours period

- **a.** Daytime hypertension
  - **1.** Siesta/Dipping/Postprandial hypotension
- **b.** Nocturnal hypertension
  - **1.** Status of dipping
  - **2.** Morning hypertension
  - **3.** Morning surge in blood pressure
  - **4.** Obstructive sleep apnea
  - **5.** Increased variability of blood pressure

D. Assessment of treatment

E. Assessment of hypertension in elderly

F. Assessment of hypertension in pregnancy

G. Assessment of hypertension in children and adolescent

H. Assessment of hypertension in high-risk patients

I. Identification of ambulatory hypotension

J. Identification of blood pressure in Parkinson disease

K. Endocrine hypertension

Threshold for Diagnosis of Hypertension based on Ambulatory Blood Pressure Monitoring

- **a.** 24-hour period: ≥130/80 mm Hg
- **b.** Daytime average: ≥135/85 mm Hg
- **c.** Night-time average: ≥120/70 mm Hg
- **d.** Clinic blood pressure: ≥140/90 mm Hg
- **e.** Home blood pressure: ≥135/85 mm Hg

Methods of Wearing Ambulatory Blood Pressure

Patient has to wear portable blood pressure device on the nondominant arm for 24–25 hours so that it will provide accurate information of blood pressure during day and night-time.

During fitting of portable device difference between the initial values and operator-measured value should not be >5 mm Hg. If the difference is very high cuff has to be removed followed by fitting again. At the time of inflation of cuff arm should be kept still, with cuff at the level of the heart, patient has to be calm and quiet.

After wearing the device the patient is asked to perform normal activities but he should be refrained from strenuous exercise.

The patient is asked to maintain the diary to take about his or her activities, time of drug ingestion, taking meals, bed time, and types of activities during daytime.

In clinical practice in the daytime, measurement should be taken at 15 minutes interval and during night at 30 minutes interval. But for all practical purpose, recording of blood pressure at equal interval throughout the day and night should be taken. Excessive time interval is not acceptable as it reduces the accuracy of measured blood pressure.

Data has to be downloaded in a computer and has to be analyzed. At least 70% of recorded blood pressure throughout the period should be satisfactory. Then blood pressure should be analyzed according to maintained diary where time of getting up from and going to bed has been written.

Importance of Dipping

Night to daytime blood pressure ratio means ratio between the average night-time and daytime blood pressure. Usually blood pressure drops at night—it is known as dipping. Though the dipping is normal in the population but night-time drop of blood pressure usually >10% of the values of daytime, i.e., ratio is <0.9. There are several categories of dipping:

- **a.** Absence of dipping: Rise in nocturnal blood pressure, i.e., ratio is >1.
- **b.** Mild dipping: 0.9–<1.0
- **c.** Dipping: 0.8–0.9
- **d.** Extreme dipping: <0.8

Following are the causes of absence of dipping:

- **a.** Obesity
- **b.** Salt sensitive subject
- **c.** Orthostatic hypotension
- **d.** Autonomic dysfunction
- **e.** Chronic kidney disease
- **f.** Old age
- **g.** Diabetic neuropathy
- **h.** Obstructive sleep apnea
- **i.** Excessive salt intake
- **j.** Sleep disturbance

Following additional information can be obtained from ABPM:

- **a.** Morning surge in blood pressure
- **b.** Variability in blood pressure
- **c.** Blood pressure
- **d.** Ambulatory arterial stiffness index

Prognostic importance of ABPM:

- **a.** Correlation with:
  1. Left ventricular hypertrophy
  2. Carotid-intima-media thickness
  3. Morbid and fatal events
- **b.** It can predict the risk of clinical outcome of cardiovascular events.
- **c.** Night to day ratio is a significant predictor of clinical cardiovascular outcomes. Cardiovascular incidences are more common in patients with nondipping of nocturnal blood pressure.

Q99. TNF-α blockers.

MUHS/NOV2014/MDI (10)

ANSWER

Following are the tumor necrosis factor-α with the indications of uses (Colored areas are the indication of disease):

Diseases	Adalimumab	Infliximab	Etanercept	Certolizumab	Golimumab
Rheumatoid arthritis					
Ankylosing spondylitis					
Psoriatic arthritis					
Plaque arthritis					
Adult Crohn disease					
Pediatric Crohn disease					
Ulcerative colitis					
Juvenile rheumatoid arthritis					
Hidradenitis suppurativa					
Uveitis					
Nonradiographic axial spondyloarthritis					

Structure and Mechanism of Actions of TNF-α

Anti-TNF agent	Structure	TNF-binding and action
Etanercept	Dimeric human recombinant fusion protein	• Binds with high affinity to TNF-α and TNF-β • It does not cause apoptosis of TNF-expressing cells
Infliximab	It is chimeric mouse-human monoclonal antibody	• It binds with high affinity to TNF-α but not TNF-β • It can bind also circulating or cell-bound molecules • It will be responsible for apoptosis of TNF-expressing cells
Adalimumab	Fully humanized IgG-1k monoclonal anti-TNF antibody	• It binds with high-affinity to TNF-α but not TNF-β • It can bind also circulating or cell-bound molecules • It will be responsible for apoptosis of TNF-expressing cells
Golimumab	Fully humanized IgG-1k monoclonal anti-TNF antibody	• It binds with high-affinity to TNF-α but not TNF-β • It can bind also circulating or cell-bound molecules • It will be responsible for apoptosis of TNF-expressing cells
Certolizumab	It lacks in Fc region	• Binds with high-affinity to TNF-α and TNF-β • It does not cause apoptosis of TNF-expressing cells

Adverse Effects

A. Common adverse effects are:

- **a.** Headache
- **b.** In case of subcutaneous route reaction at the injection sites
- **c.** In case of intravenous route infusion reaction
- **d.** Rashes
- **e.** Anemia
- **f.** Mild transaminitis
- **g.** Upper respiratory tract reaction
- **h.** Cough
- **i.** Sinusitis
- **j.** Diarrhea
- **k.** Abdominal pain
- **l.** Nausea

B. Serious reactions:

- **a.** Severe bacteria, fungal, and viral infection: These mainly occur where the patient is taking methotrexate and corticosteroids along with these drugs. There may be reactivation of latent pulmonary tuberculosis, hepatitis B and C infection. In case of latent tuberculosis, patient should receive antitubercular medications before starting TNF-α blockers.
- **b.** Malignancies: Risk of lymphoma is two to three times higher in elderly patients with RA. There is also high risk for developing nonmelanoma skin cancer in patients treating with these drugs.
- **c.** There is worsening of cardiac function in patients with rheumatoid arthritis receiving anti-TNF-α agents and NYHA class III and IV congestive cardiac failure.
- **d.** Drug-induced lupus: 50% patients can develop positive autoantibodies including ANA and DS-DNA. Clinical features are hemolytic anemia, thrombocytopenia, and leukopenia and skin rash.
- **e.** Demyelinating disorders: Following demyelinating diseases may occur in patients taking these agents:
  1. Multiple sclerosis
  2. Optic neuritis
  3. Myelitis
  4. Encephalitis
  5. Guillain–Barré syndrome
  6. Transverse myelitis
  7. Chronic inflammatory demyelinating polyneuropathy
- **f.** Skin infection:
  1. Lupus like rashes
  2. Erythema multiforme
  3. Cutaneous T cell lymphoma
  4. Hypersensitivity vasculitis
  5. New onset of psoriasis
  6. Granuloma annulare

g. Pregnancy and lactation: There is no controlled trial until now. There is class B pregnancy risk described by FDA.

Contraindications

A. Hypersensitivity reaction to the agent
B. Presence of sepsis
C. New York Heart Association class III and IV heart failure
D. Concomitant use of another biological immuno-suppressive agents

Q100. Stem cell therapy in cardiac diseases.
MUHS/NOV2014/MDI (10)

ANSWER

There are two types of stem cells used in the cardiovascular diseases:

A. Embryonic stem cells: It is derived during blastocyst stage from the inner mass of developing embryo. Characteristic features are:
   a. Proliferative properties
   b. Self-renewing properties
   c. Ability to differentiate into wide variety of cell types in cardiac myocytes
B. Adult stem cells:
   a. Bone marrow derived stem cells: Following subpopulation of stem cells are derived from the adult bone marrow—
      1. Hematopoietic stem cells
      2. Endothelial progenitor cells
      3. Mesenchymal stem cells

      In case of transfusion of unfractionated stem cells, the advantage is minimizing extensive ex vivo differentiation and isolation of stem cells, but the disadvantage is in case of unfractionated stem cells required therapeutically useful cells may be very small in amount. The alternate strategy is:
      1. Isolation and administration of endothelial progenitor cells that express CD133 on their surfaces and potentiate angiogenesis.
      2. Mesenchymal stem cells do not express CD133 or CD34, they can differentiate into adipocytes, bone, and cartilage and in certain special conditions to cardiac myocytes. Advantages of these cells are their low immunogenicity and its usefulness in case of nonavailability of autologous stem cells.
   b. Skeletal myoblast: These are the progenitor cells isolated from skeletal muscle biopsies and can differentiate into myotubes and after transplantation it will exhibit skeletal muscle phenotype and thereby can improve left ventricular systolic and diastolic dysfunction. But, these myocytes will not be coupled with cardiac myocytes electrically hence there is chance of developing arrhythmias.
   c. Resident cardiac stem cells: Recently, it has been demonstrated that a population of stem cells in the myocardium can be differentiated into cardiac myocytes which can be harvested from the cardiac biopsies. In case of myocardial infarction injection of these stem cells can improve cardiac systolic function.

Following are the methods of stem cell delivery:

A. Transvascular route: It is best suited for acute myocardial infarction with adequate reperfusion. If it is infused in the coronary arteries, it will remain in the injured myocardium as a result of activation of chemokines and adhesion molecules. Advantages of intracoronary infusion is direct infusion into the particular territory. Alternatively, it can be infused intravenously.
B. Direct injection into the left ventricular wall: This route is used when intracoronary route is not possible due to possible total occlusion of the coronary artery. There are three possible approaches of direct injection:
   a. Transendocardial approach: Here, needle of the catheter is directly advanced across the aortic valve to position it against the endocardial surface and the stem cells are directly injected into the left ventricle. By electrophysiological mapping scarred, ischemic, and viable myocardium can be differentiated.
   b. Transepicardial approach: In this method cells are injected during open heart surgery. The advantage is direct visualization of scarred, border zones, and infarcted areas.
   c. Delivery of the stem cells directly into myocardium through one of the cardiac veins: The disadvantage is—this process is very time-consuming as positioning the catheter is difficult.

Safety Concern

A. Arrhythmias: There is proarrhythmic effect with stem-cell transplantation. It may be due to injected stem cells that do not communicate with native cardiac myocytes electrically resulting slowed conduction leading to re-entrant arrhythmias. It has been recently suggested that skeletal myoblast is genetically engineered to express gap-junction protein named connexin-43 that will exhibit decreased arrhythmogenicity.

B. Restenosis, accelerated atherosclerosis, and coronary obstruction: According to recent reports that incidence of restenosis and atherosclerotic plaque progression have been increased after stem cell transplantation. If the stem cells are injected into the coronary circulation in large amount, they will adhere to each other producing aggregates thereby leading to occlusion of coronary vessels.

C. Abnormal cellular differentiation: As the stem cells can migrate to other tissues after being injected into the myocardium, it can be speculated that these cells can differentiate aberrantly leading to formation of tumor.

Tracking of Stem Cells

Major concern after delivery of stem cells is which cell will be remaining in the heart and which cells will end up in other organs. Within few hours after stem cell transplantation, it will not only be present in the heart but also in the lungs, kidney, spleen, and liver. Following methods are used to track the stem cells after injection:

a. MRI
b. Positron emission tomography
c. Scintigraphy

Evidences of Tissue Regeneration

Ultimate aim of stem-cell therapy is to regenerate cardiac tissue so that this tissue will contract other cardiac tissue in a synchronizing fashion to improve overall cardiac function in absence of proarrhythmic effect. Recently, it will also improve cardiac function independent of cardiac tissue regeneration. Locally injected stem cells will improve the left ventricular function by augmenting systolic function and through the release of paracrine mediators that can perform following functions:

a. Directly augment systolic function of the heart
b. Prevents apoptosis of ischemic myocardial cells
c. Promotes angiogenesis to limit the injury.
d. Promotes salvage of injured myocardium in absence of tissue regeneration.

These paracrine effects are useful in case of:

a. Acute myocardial ischemia
b. Hibernating myocardium

These paracrine effects are not beneficial in case of chronically infarcted myocardium with scar formation.

To promote regeneration of the cardiac tissue following factors needed to improve stem-cell transplantation:

a. Sufficient numbers of stem cells have to be delivered at the site of left ventricular dysfunction and to be present at that site.
b. New tissue administered should be electrically and mechanically coupled and well vascularized.

If autologous stem cells cannot be used to generate cardiac tissue, there is every chance of graft rejection.

Q101. Alteplase.

MUHS/NOV2014/MDIV (10)

ANSWER

Indications of this Thrombolytic Agent Produced by Recombinant DNA Technology

a. Acute myocardial infarction
b. Ischemic stroke
c. Pulmonary embolism
d. Occluded catheter

Mechanism of Actions

Alteplase acts as tissue plasminogen activator to break the plasminogen into proteolytic enzyme plasmin that breaks down fibrin and fibrinogen. Alteplase will be cleared by the liver primarily.

Administration

A. In case of acute ischemic stroke: 0.9 mg/kg is the total recommended dose. 10% of it is administered intravenously as a bolus over 1 minute and remaining 90% should be infused over 60 minutes. It should be transfused within 4.5 hours of onset of the disease.

B. In case of myocardial infarction: It is used in conjunction with heparin as well as aspirin.

   a. Intravenous bolus followed by 90 minutes of infusion: If weight is >67 kg—
      1. Bolus dose of 15 mg
      2. 30 minutes infusion of 50 mg
      3. 60 minutes infusion of 35 mg
   b. Intravenous infusion followed by 90 minutes of infusion if weight ≤ 67 kg:
      1. Bolus dose of 15 mg
      2. 30 minutes infusion of 0.75 mg/kg
      3. 60 minutes infusion of 0.5 mg/kg

- **c.** Intravenous infusion followed by 180 minutes of infusion if ≥65 kg:
  1. Bolus dose of 6–10 mg
  2. 60 minutes infusion of 50–54 mg
  3. 2 hours infusion at a rate of 20 mg/h

  Total dose should not exceed 100 mg.
- **d.** Intravenous infusion followed by 180 minutes of infusion < 65 mg:
  1. Bolus dose of 0.075 mg/kg
  2. In first hour at a rate of 0.675 mg/kg
  3. In next 2 hours at a rate of 0.25 mg/kg/h

  Total dose should not exceed 100 mg.

C. In case of pulmonary embolism: Intravenous infusion of 100 mg over 2 hours.

D. Clearance of catheter: 2 mg should be administered directly into the catheter at a concentration of 1 mg/mL. If the catheter remains occluded, second dose should be administered after 2 hours.

Adverse Effects

A. Fever

B. Bleeding: Risk is highest in following conditions—
- **a.** Recent intracranial hemorrhage
- **b.** Recent trauma
- **c.** Major surgery
- **d.** Uncontrolled hypertension
- **e.** Acute pericarditis
- **f.** Cerebrovascular disease
- **g.** Ophthalmic conditions
- **h.** Advanced age
- **i.** Concurrent anticoagulant or antiplatelet drugs
- **j.** Presence of any coagulopathy

C. Anaphylaxis

D. Angioedema

Contraindications

A. Intracranial hemorrhage

B. Internal bleeding

C. Subarachnoid hemorrhage

D. Stroke within last 3 months

E. Serious trauma in the head in last 3 months

F. Intracranial and intraspinal surgery in last 3 months

G. Conditions increasing the bleeding risk

H. Currently, severe uncontrolled hypertension

Q102. Stent in medicine.

MUHS/NOV2014/MDIV (10)

ANSWER

This question has been described in question number 62.

Q103. Ventricular tachycardia.

MUHS/NOV2014/MDIV (10)

Discuss the approach to a case of broad QRS tachycardia and its management.

MUHS/MAY2011/MDII (25)

Describe the anatomy and physiology of conduction system of the heart. Write in detail etiopathology, clinical features and management of ventricular tachycardia.

MUHS/MAY2009/MDI (25)

Ventricular tachycardia.

KERALA UNIVERSITY, 2021 (10)

Ventricular arrhythmias.

TEERTHANKER MAHAVEER UNI, 2019 (10)

SAMS (ODISHA), 2022 (10)

Wide complex tachycardia.

AIIMS, 2020 (10)

Write down the diagnostic approach of wide complex tachycardia. Describe the management of wide QRS complex tachycardia.

AIIMS (BBS), 2024 (10)

Discuss the electrophysiological mechanisms and diagnostic evaluation of ventricular arrhythmias.

WBUHS, 2024 (10)

Discuss the electrophysiological mechanisms and diagnostic evaluation of ventricular arrhythmias.

WBUHS, 2025 (10)

ANSWER

Definition

It is the most common form of wide complex tachycardia with rate of >100 beats/min arising from distal conduction system or ventricular myocardium or from both.

Types of Ventricular Tachycardia

It can be classified according to variation of morphology into following subtypes:

A. Monomorphic ventricular tachycardia: If the QRS complexes are identical from beat to beat if the tachycardia originates from same focus or circuit it is known as monomorphic ventricular tachycardia.

B. Polymorphic ventricular tachycardia: If the morphology of QRS complexes varies from beat to beat when it occurs from different foci in the ventricular myocardium it is known as polymorphic ventricular tachycardia. Torsades de pointes is a type of polymorphic ventricular tachycardia when it occurs in the setting of long QT interval or when there is waxing and waning of QRS amplitude in ECG.

It can be classified into following subtypes according to the duration:

A. Nonsustained ventricular tachycardia: It can be defined as when the beats of ventricular origin are >3 beats at a rate of >100 beats/min that lasts for <30 seconds.

B. Sustained ventricular tachycardia: It can be defined as when the beats of ventricular origin are >3 beats at a rate of >100 beats/min that lasts for >30 seconds or when there is hemodynamic instability occurring in <30 seconds.

There is another subtypes of ventricular tachycardia—it is known as bidirectional ventricular tachycardia—where there is beat to beat alteration in the QRS complexes in the frontal plane—it is associated with:

- **a.** Digitalis toxicity
- **b.** Catecholinergic ventricular tachycardia

Etiology

A. Ischemic heart disease

B. Congenital structural heart disease

C. Acquired and inherited cardiomyopathies

D. Infiltrative cardiomyopathy
- **a.** Sarcoidosis
- **b.** Amyloidosis
- **c.** Hemochromatosis

E. Electrolyte disturbances:
- **a.** Hypomagnesemia
- **b.** Hypocalcemia
- **c.** Hypokalemia

F. Drugs:
- **a.** Cocaine
- **b.** Methamphetamine
- **c.** Digitalis

G. Collagen diseases:
- **a.** Systemic lupus erythematosus
- **b.** Rheumatoid arthritis

H. Chagas disease

In case of younger people having age <35 years the causes are:

A. Myocarditis

B. Hypertrophic cardiomyopathy

C. Long QT syndrome

D. Right ventricular cardiomyopathy

E. Congenital coronary artery abnormalities

Clinical Features

Symptoms:

A. Palpitation, syncope, and lightheadedness—due to diminished cerebral perfusion or from structural heart disease

B. Chest pain from ischemia

C. Mental changes such as anxiety, agitation, and coma

D. Sensation of neck fullness from increased venous pressure

E. Dyspnea from
- **a.** Increased pulmonary venous pressure
- **b.** Contraction of left atrium against closed mitral valve

F. Patients may be asymptomatic.

G. Symptoms may be associated with triggered therapy.

H. Family history of sudden death

I. In case of athlete any risk of ventricular tachycardia should be determined.

J. Any history of sudden death in young following inherited arrhythmias should be evaluated:
- **a.** Short QT syndrome
- **b.** Long QT syndrome
- **c.** Brugada syndrome
- **d.** Arrhythmogenic right ventricular dysplasia
- **e.** Hypertrophic obstructive cardiomyopathy
- **f.** Catecholaminergic polymorphic ventricular tachycardia

Signs

A. Tachycardia
B. Cannon wave in the neck vein in case of sinus rhythm of atria
C. Tachypnea
D. Hypotension
E. Varying first sound due to AV asynchrony
F. Murmur of valvular heart disease or HOCM
G. S3 gallop
H. Crepitation in case of left ventricular heart failure

Investigations

A. In case of hemodynamically unstable patients advanced cardiac life support with electrical cardioversion to restore sinus rhythm, as the patients will be stabilized and ECG should be done.
B. If the patient is hemodynamically stabilized then ECG should be done along with measurement of serum electrolyte levels prior to cardioversion medically or direct current cardioversion.
C. ECG can be repeated after restoration of sinus rhythm or when VT is suspected in patient with syncope.
D. According to AHA 2017 following are the guidelines for the patient management with VT and to prevent sudden death:
   a. Assessment of risk of sudden death in patients with cardiomyopathies from HOCM, sarcoidosis, ARVD, or neuromuscular disease.
   b. Evaluation of genetic arrhythmia syndrome in patients of <40 years of age with unexplained sudden death, unexplained near drowning or recurrent syncope in absence of IHD or structural heart disease.
   c. Cardiac evaluation and genetic counseling and genetic testing as appropriated based on clinical findings in first-degree relatives of victims of sudden cardiac death having age of <40 years.
E. Screening of the first-degree relatives should be done if the patient is diagnosed as follows:
   a. Short and long QT syndrome
   b. Right ventricular dysplasia
   c. Hypertrophic obstructive cardiomyopathy
F. Familial screening should involve:
   a. Proper history
   b. ECG
   c. Echocardiography
   d. Treadmill testing

Laboratory Studies

A. Serum electrolytes such as potassium, ionized calcium, magnesium, and phosphate levels.
B. Serum level of digoxin, TCA
C. Toxicology screening—cocaine, methadone, and methamphetamine
D. Serum concentration of troponin T and I and other biomarkers if there is sign of ischemia. Persistent elevation of these cardiac enzymes suggests ongoing myocarditis.

Electrocardiography

A. Polymorphic VT: QRS complexes vary from beat to beat. The most common form is Torsade de Pointes, i.e., twisting the points. It may occur in case of sinus rhythm or following conditions those increase QT interval:
   a. Class 1A antiarrhythmic drugs
   b. Droperidol
   c. Hypomagnesemia

   Polymorphic VT can also be seen in case of myocarditis and ischemia.

   Typical Torsade de pointes can be seen in "long-short" sequence—longer RR interval leads to further prolongation of QT interval which is followed by early depolarization occurring during the time of repolarization.
B. Monomorphic VT: It is common in case of structural heart disease like scar which is common zone of slow conduction. It is rarely benign and rarely causes sudden death. Scar occurs in the following conditions:
   a. Prior infarct
   b. Primary cardiomyopathy
   c. Hypertrophy
   d. Surgical scar
   e. Degeneration of muscles

   Monomorphic VTs are named according to their sites of origin:
   a. Right ventricular outflow tract
   b. Left ventricular outflow tract
   c. Aortic root
   d. Left ventricular septum

   Re-entrant tachycardia occurs when electrical wavefront will travel through the slow conduction zone, i.e., damaged muscle protected by scar tissue thus allowing rest of the circuit to repolarize. In the scar-tissue wavefront breaks out to activate ventricle and again re-enters slow conduction zone.

ECG demonstrates:

a. Wide complex tachycardia—either VT or SVT with aberrant conduction. If there is difficulty in differentiating these two then it should be regarded as VT and should be treated accordingly.

b. AV dissociation—when it occurs, it is hallmark of VT. It may be due to the slower rate of depolarization atria from sinus node as compared to pathologic ventricular rate.

c. Retrograde conduction from the ventricle to atria through the AV node that can be demonstrated as wide QRS complexes with inverted "p" wave.

d. Fusion beat: It is the mixed morphology of normally conducted beat through the AV node/His-Purkinje system producing narrow QRS complex and simultaneous abnormal ventricular depolarization producing wide QRS complex.

e. Captured beat: Normally AV node is in refractory state due to depolarization as a result of retrograde conduction of rapid ventricular rate, but if the AV node is in nonrefractory state by chance, then normal atrial impulse will reach AV node and conduction will proceed normally through the His-Purkinje system to capture ventricle producing narrow QRS complex.

According to revised Brugada criteria:

a. Presence of initial R wave in lead aVR

b. Width of initial R or Q wave exceed 40 msec in aVR

c. Notching on the initial down stroke of a predominantly negative QRS complex in aVR

d. Ventricular activation velocity ration (Vi/Vt) is ≤ 1.

Echocardiography: It will demonstrate—

A. Left ventricular systolic function

B. Left ventricular wall motion abnormalities indicating prior scar

C. Findings suggestive of infiltrative diseases

Cardiac MRI: It can demonstrate—

A. Arrhythmogenic right ventricular dysplasia

Radionucleotide angiography: It can detect the cause of VT.

Assessment of Recurrent Syncope

A. Holter monitoring

B. Implantation of loop recorder having battery life

C. Provocative electrophysiological study

Genetic testing is required in following cases:

A. Long QT syndrome

B. Arrhythmogenic right ventricular dysplasia

C. Hypertrophic obstructive cardiomyopathy

D. Dilated cardiomyopathy

Myocardial Biopsy

It is usually done in case of suspected infiltrative diseases.

Treatment

A. *Unstable monomorphic VT* can be treated with synchronized direct cardioversion with starting energy dose of 100 Jules.

B. *Unstable polymorphic VT* immediate defibrillation, but due to difficulty in recognizing the QRS complexes synchronization of shock cannot occur.

C. *In stable patients with adequate organ perfusion and normal left ventricular function and no hemodynamic compromisation* treatment will depend upon:

a. Whether VT is monomorphic or polymorphic

b. Whether left ventricular function is normal or impaired, i.e., reduced ejection fraction.

D. *In stable patients with monomorphic VT and normal left ventricular function* sinus rhythm can be restored by intravenous procainamide, sotalol or amiodarone. In case of left ventricular failure intravenous lidocaine or amiodarone is preferred instead of procainamide as the later drug may exacerbate heart failure. But, amiodarone should not be the first choice in case of stable VT as its effect on myocardial function and refractoriness is gradual in onset. If the abode drug fails, then synchronized cardioversion of 50–200 Jules are the treatment of choice.

E. *Stable patients with polymorphic VT* terminates on its own but recurrence is common. Hence after return of sinus rhythm ECG should be done and analyzed to see whether QT interval is prolonged or not.

a. *Polymorphic VT with normal QT interval* should be treated in the line of monomorphic VT treatment.

b. *Polymorphic VT with QT prolongation* can be treated by magnesium sulfate, isoproterenol, pacing, or combination. Phenytoin and lidocaine can shorten the QT interval but due to QT prolongation effect procainamide and amiodarone are contraindicated.

F. In case of electrolyte imbalance correction of electrolyte abnormality should be done.

G. In case of digitalis toxicity administration of digitalis antibody is indicated.

H. After conversion to sinus rhythm it has to be determined that:

- **a.** Severity of heart disease
- **b.** Assessment of prognosis
- **c.** Formulation of best long-term treatment plan

So, options depend upon the severity of symptoms and types of structural heart disease and treatment includes:

- **a.** Antiarrhythmic medication: It includes lidocaine and amiodarone.
- **b.** Implantable cardioverter-defibrillator—It will terminate acutely ventricular arrhythmia and will give long-term management protocol in patients with VT.
- **c.** Catheter ablation: It is effective, but recurrent VT is not uncommon.

Cardioversion in Case of Acute VT

A. VT associated with unconsciousness with or without hypotension requires immediate 100–200 Jules biphasic cardioversion that will be administered according to ACLS guideline.

B. Reversible risk factors like hypokalemia should be addressed and drugs that are responsible for QT prolongation should be stopped.

C. In case of myocardial infarction VT should be corrected by intravenous lidocaine as the mechanism here is enhanced automaticity not the re-entry but this drug increases the risk of overall mortality. In Torsade de pointes intravenous magnesium sulfate is effective if QT interval is prolonged but in the baseline.

D. If above medical treatment fails the monophasic 100 Jules synchronized cardioversion to start with and can be increased if required.

E. In case of hemodynamic compromise with suspected VT or SVT with aberrant conduction, the patients should be treated like VT only.

F. In some cases of nonsustained VT, it can be treated medically or by catheter ablation.

Catheter Ablation

Endocardial or epicardial catheter placement for radiofrequency ablation is done to treat VT in following cases:

A. Left ventricular dysfunction in case of previous myocardial infarction

B. Cardiomyopathy

C. Bundle branch re-entry

D. Various forms of idiopathic VT

It can be used in conjunction with ICD in case of recurrent VT in order to reduce the frequency.

It can be used in case of idiopathic monomorphic VT that is resistant or intolerant to drug therapy or does not want to continue the drug therapy.

Current Recommendations

A. Patients with congestive heart failure with reduced ejection fraction should be managed with β-blocker, ACE inhibitors, or ARBs and mineralocorticoid receptor blocker to reduce the risk of sudden death.

B. In case of nonischemic cardiomyopathy, heart failure with reduced ejection fraction of ≤35%, ICD should be placed.

C. In case of IHD with monomorphic VT, medical therapy is required besides revascularization.

D. Catheter ablation is recommended in patients with:

- **a.** Previous myocardial infarction
- **b.** Storms of ventricular tachycardia. or
- **c.** Refractoriness to amiodarone
- **d.** Intolerant to antiarrhythmic therapy

Q104. Discuss physiology of cardiac conduction with special reference to AV node. Describe pathophysiology and management of supraventricular tachycardia.

MUHS/MAY2014/MDI (25)

Physiology of conduction in atrioventricular node.

MUHS/NOV2013/MDI (10)

ANSWER

Physiology of cardiac conduction has been described in question number 41.

Supraventricular tachycardia has been described in question number 9.

Q105. NT-ProBNP.

MUHS/MAY2014/MDIV (10)

SAMS (ODISHA), 2022 (10)

ANSWER

Introduction

NT-ProBNP acts as a significant indicator of heart failure and cardiac dysfunction.

Structure, Synthesis, and Secretion of NT-ProBNP

Brain natriuretic peptide is secreted from the left ventricular myocytes in response to stretching of these myocytes due to volume and pressure overload. Human gene encoding BNP is located in the chromosome 1. mRNA that encodes BNP consists of unstable repeat TATTTAT sequence. Under pathological conditions, unstable mRNA synthesizes pre-pro-BNP having 134 amino acid sequence which is then rapidly converted into pro-BNP by releasing 26 amino acid. This pro-BNP is split into inactive 76 amino acid residue, NT-ProBNP and 32 amino acid containing BNP by proNP convertase, corin or furin and are released into circulation.

Receptors of Natriuretic Peptides

There are three natriuretic peptide receptors for natriuretic peptide:

A. NPR-A: It is present in the vascular endothelium in large amount and also brain and kidney. It is the main effector of actions of ANP and BNP.

B. NPR-B

C. NPR-C

After activation of NPR-A and NPR-B, cyclic GMP with increased. BNP will bind to the NPR-A and work:

a. Against RAAS and sympathetic nervous system

b. To improve GFR

c. To improves filtration fraction

d. Diuretic effect

e. Vasodilatory effect

f. Natriuretic effect

Degradation of BNP and NT-ProBNP

A. NPR-C is responsible for receptor-mediated internalization and degradation to clear the natriuretic peptides from the extracellular fluid.

B. Neutral endopeptidase, dipeptidyl peptidase IV, and insulin degrading enzyme clear the BNP physiologically.

In 2015, sodium supranuclear complex having equal ratio of ARB valsartan and neprilysin inhibitor sacubitril have been approved by FDA for successful treatment of heart failure with reduced ejection fraction.

As Biomarker of Heart Failure

Heart failure can be divided into heart failure with normal or preserved ejection fraction and heart failure with reduced ejection fraction. According to AHA, NT-ProBNP acts as a biomarker for heart failure with cardiac dysfunction.

Level of NT-ProBNP in the Serum

A. In non-acute cases upper limit of normal of NT-ProBNP is 125 pg/mL and BNP is 35 pg/mL.

B. In acute cases upper limit of normal is 300 pg/mL and BNP level is 100 pg/mL.

If BNP level is <100 pg/mL—heart failure is unlikely.

If BNP level is 100–500 pg/mL—heart failure can be diagnosed based on clinical judgment.

If BNP level is >500 pg/mL—heart failure is possible and treatment should be started.

Diagnostic Role in Failing Heart

A. In case of acute IHD, BNP and NT-ProBNP level may reflect the severity of left ventricular dysfunction and it can guide the treatment benefit. It will be elevated for >12 weeks and is better diagnostic indicator than other markers.

B. In case of severe coronary artery disease the increased level of NT-ProBNP is strong predictor of cardiovascular event.

C. In case of atrial fibrillation, it will be elevated.

D. Left ventricular end-diastolic dysfunction and left ventricular volume are directly correlated with BNP level but inversely correlated with left ventricular ejection fraction in patients with dilated cardiomyopathy and hypertrophic cardiomyopathy.

E. Its level is significantly high in case of Takotsubo cardiomyopathy.

F. Ratios of early BNP/cTnT and BNP/CK-MB can differentiate Takotsubo cardiomyopathy from acute myocardial infarction.

Assessing the Severity and Prognosis of Heart Failure

It can assess the severity and prognosis of heart failure. This is the independent predictor of heart failure with reduced ejection fraction that can be determined by Doppler echocardiography. Reduced level will be correlated with clinical improvement of heart failure. Its level is also correlated with risk of death.

Therapeutic Role in Cardiac Dysfunction

Recombinant human natriuretic peptide with same amino acid sequence as that of BNP:

- **a.** It can dilate blood vessels.
- **b.** It effectively decreases preload and afterload.

Nesiritide is recombinant human natriuretic peptide is effective in case of heart failure by following mechanisms:

- **a.** Facilitates natriuresis.
- **b.** Facilitates diuresis.
- **c.** Inhibits RAAS.
- **d.** Increases cardiac output.
- **e.** Decreases wedge pressure in the pulmonary capillaries.
- **f.** Improves cardiac systolic and diastolic functions.

Q106. Discuss the management of heart disease in pregnancy.

MUHS/MAY2013/MDII (25)

What is pregnancy induced hypertension? Write about its pathophysiology, diagnosis and treatment and complications.

DNB, 2018 (1+2+2+3+2)

Effect of pregnancy on valvular heart diseases.

RAJIV GANDHI UNI OF HEALTH SC, KARNATAKA, 2016 (10)

Pregnancy and hypertension.

BHARATI VIDYAPEETH UNIVERSITY, SUMMER 2019 (10)

RAJASTHAN UNIVERSITY, 2019 (11)

Heart disease in pregnancy.

AIIMS, 2023 (10)

Hypertensive emergencies during pregnancy and their management.

AIIMS, 2023 (10)

Discuss hypertensive disorders in pregnancy. How will you manage them.

AIIMS (BBS), 2023 (10)

ANSWER

Specific Congenital Cardiovascular Diseases in Pregnancy

A. Atrial septal defect:

- **a.** Isolated ASD is well-tolerated in pregnancy.
- **b.** Paradoxical pulmonary embolism may occur.
- **c.** If ostium secundum is not corrected prior to pregnancy, it may produce complication.

B. Ventricular septal defect:

- **a.** Isolated VSD without pulmonary hypertension or correction of VSD prior to development of pulmonary hypertension is well-tolerated in pregnancy
- **b.** In case of VSD with pulmonary hypertension results in drop of blood pressure during or after delivery leads to reversal of shunt.

C. Patent ductus arteriosus:

- **a.** Patent ductus arteriosus in absence of pulmonary hypertension is usually well tolerated.
- **b.** Patent ductus arteriosus with PH results in drop of blood pressure during or after delivery leads to reversal of shunt.

D. Coarctation of aorta:

- **a.** During pregnancy it may be associated with following complications:
  1. Hypertension
  2. Congestive cardiac failure
  3. Aortic dissection
  4. Cerebral hemorrhage due to rupture of circle of Willis aneurysm

  Treatment:

  1. Control of hypertension to prevent cerebral hemorrhage
  2. β-blockers—it is the drug of choice. But excessive lowering of blood pressure should be prevented as to prevent compromisation of uteroplacental circulation.
  3. Prior to pregnancy coarctation of aorta associated its hypertension, heart failure and peak systolic gradient of >20 mm Hg has to be corrected.

E. Congenital bicuspid aortic stenosis should be corrected prior to pregnancy.

F. Pulmonary aortic stenosis:

- **a.** It is well tolerated during pregnancy.
- **b.** It should be corrected prior to pregnancy if the peak gradient is >60 mm Hg.

c. If there is right ventricular failure, percutaneous balloon valvotomy has to be done during pregnancy.

G. Epstein anomaly:
   a. Acyanotic patient can be tolerated in pregnancy.
   b. Cyanotic patients can precipitate heart failure, fetal immaturity, and fetal death.
   c. During labor and delivery, hemodynamic monitoring should be taken along with following measurement:
      1. Oxygen administration
      2. Rest
      3. Monitoring of blood gas

H. Tetralogy of Fallot:
   a. Patient can tolerate pregnancy if TOF has been treated in childhood and has:
      1. Little residual outflow gradient
      2. No pulmonary hypertension
      3. Preserved left ventricular function
   b. In case of partially corrected or uncorrected TOF pregnant patients and fetus can develop cyanosis as a consequence of right to left shunt due to:
      1. Increased blood volume
      2. Increased venous return
      3. Decreased systemic vascular resistance
      4. Fall in blood pressure during labor and delivery
   c. Following residual lesion may be present in case of partial correction:
      1. Right ventricular outflow tract obstruction
      2. Pulmonary regurgitation
      3. Right ventricular dysfunction

      There is risk of heart failure and arrhythmia.
   d. Poor prognostic signs are:
      1. Maternal hematocrit level of >60%
      2. Arterial saturation of oxygen below 80%
      3. Right ventricular hypertension
      4. Syncope

I. Eisenmenger syndrome:
   a. In case pregnant women mortality rate is 30–60%, chance of fetal loss is 50%. Hence, pregnancy should be discouraged.
   b. If pregnancy occurs, early abortion should be done. If the pregnancy is continued, in that case, following measures are to be taken:
      1. Continued administration of oxygen
      2. Physical activity should be restricted.
      3. Pulmonary vasodilators should be recommended.
      4. Since there is increased incidence of thromboembolism, anticoagulation is recommended in third trimester and up to 4 weeks of postpartum.
      5. Second stage of labor should be shortened by the use of forceps delivery.

Acquired Heart Diseases

A. Valvular heart diseases:
   a. Following types of valvular disease are associated with high-risk pregnancy and fetal risk:
      1. Symptomatic mitral stenosis
      2. Severe aortic stenosis
      3. New York Heart Association Class III/IV mitral regurgitation
      4. New York Heart Association class II/IV aortic regurgitation
      5. Valvular heart disease with pulmonary hypertension or left ventricular dysfunction.
      6. Mechanical prosthetic valves requiring anticoagulation.
      7. Hypertrophic cardiomyopathy
   b. Mitral stenosis: Increased blood volume in pregnancy will lead to increased pressure gradient across the mitral valve that leads to increased left atrial pressure and ensues the pulmonary edema resulting following symptoms:
      1. Dyspnea
      2. Orthopnea
      3. Paroxysmal nocturnal dyspnea
      4. Feature of atrial fibrillation in case of rapid ventricular rate

      These features are aggravated in case of moderate and severe mitral stenosis. These features are more aggravated during delivery or postpartum due to increased venous return.

      Treatment:

      It depends upon the following features:
      1. Severity of stenosis
      2. Symptoms
      3. Time of diagnosis

      Following treatments should be done:
      1. Prior to pregnancy severe stenosis with valvular area of <1 cm^2 or moderately severe mitral stenosis, percutaneous mitral balloon valvoplasty (PMVB) or repair of the valve if PMVB is not feasible.

2. In case of moderate stenosis symptoms assessment and exercise tolerance test (1.5 cm^2) should be done to decide requirement of any intervention needed prior to pregnancy.
3. If the valve is >1.5 cm^2, pregnancy can be well tolerated.
4. In case of pregnant woman, heart rate and the left atrial pressure should be kept low by β_1 blocker as it is the drug of choice in pregnancy, but β_2 blocker mediates uterine relaxation.
5. In case of atrial fibrillation digoxin can be given.
6. In case of deranged hemodynamic monitoring, electrical cardioversion can be administered safely in pregnancy.
7. Left atrial pressure can be managed by salt restriction and administration of diuretics.
8. In patients refractory to medical therapy PMBV or repair of mitral valve can be applied.
9. Cardiopulmonary bypass can be performed in pregnancy with normothermic perfusion with high volume of flow to the mother in lateral decubitus position of mother to minimize perfusion of placenta as there is chance of fetal demise.

B. Mitral regurgitation: The common causes are rheumatic heart disease and mitral valve prolapsed. This disease is usually well tolerated in pregnancy because:

a. Fall in systemic vascular resistance
b. Decrease in left ventricular afterload

But decompensation may occur in case of:

a. Associated hypertension
b. Atrial fibrillation

Treatment:

a. Asymptomatic patients should not be treated with any drug.
b. Decompensated heart failure patients can be treated with diuretics and digoxin.
c. Decompensated patients in peripartum period as a consequence of increased venous return as well as systemic vascular resistance can be treated by systemic vasodilator hydralazine. ACE-I and ARBs are contraindicated in pregnancy because of their teratogenic effects.

C. Aortic stenosis: It is commonly caused by congenital bicuspid aortic valve.

a. Mild to moderate aortic stenosis is well tolerated in pregnancy if left ventricular function is preserved.
b. In case of severe aortic stenosis with valvular area of <1 cm^2 and mean pressure gradient across the aortic valve is >40 mm Hg, there will be hemodynamic deterioration in pregnancy and it will precipitate heart failure and premature delivery. Patient develops dyspnea, chest pain, and syncope in 2nd trimester or early 3rd trimester of pregnancy.

Treatment:

a. In severe symptomatic aortic stenosis during pregnancy PABV should be done to reduce the chance of decompensation.

D. Aortic insufficiency: The common causes are—

a. Bicuspid aortic valve
b. Infective aortic endocarditis
c. Autoimmune disorders
d. Dilated annulus

It is well tolerated in pregnancy because of:

a. Reduced systemic vascular resistance
b. Rise in heart rate with shortened diastolic period

Symptomatic patients having decompensated heart failure are treated with:

a. Diuretics
b. Digoxin
c. Hydralazine to reduce the afterload

E. Hypertrophic cardiomyopathy: It has favorable outcome in pregnancy, but following symptoms may occur in women during pregnancy who were symptomatic prior to pregnancy:

a. Chest pain
b. Syncope
c. Worsening of dyspnea

During pregnancy following also may occur:

a. Supraventricular tachycardia
b. Atrial fibrillation
c. Hemodynamic deterioration
d. Ventricular arrhythmia
e. Fetal distress

Treatment:

a. Maintenance of adequate intravascular volume
b. Control of arrhythmias: β-blockers are the drug of choice.
c. Prophylactic implantable defibrillator can be advised prior to pregnancy in following cases:
   1. History of syncope
   2. Life-threatening arrhythmias
   3. Family history of sudden death

d. Vaginal delivery should be advised, β-adrenergic receptors, tocolytics, and prostaglandin have to be avoided.

e. Following should be avoided because all these reduce the intravascular volume:
   1. Blood loss
   2. Volume depletion
   3. Vasodilators
   4. Epidural anesthesia due to its vasodilatory effect
   5. Brisk diuresis immediately after postpartum as it will decrease intravascular volume.

F. Prosthetic valve: Bioprosthetic and homograft valves are safe for child as well as mother but there is an increased incidence of degeneration in younger people and is accelerated in pregnancy. Pregnancy should be discouraged because of this valve and anticoagulation requirement. Again, as pregnancy is thrombogenic state, there is also chance of thrombosis in case of nonuse of anticoagulation.

G. Hypertension:

a. Chronic hypertension: It can be defined as blood pressure of ≥140/90 mm Hg before 20 weeks of gestation and will persist beyond 42 days of postpartum period. It is associated with:
   1. Pre-eclampsia
   2. Eclampsia
   3. Fetal morbidity and mortality

   Treatment is to reduce the blood pressure to an optimum level to reduce the chance of:
   1. Cerebral hemorrhage
   2. Renal failure
   3. Left ventricular hypertrophy

b. Gestational hypertension: It is pregnancy-induced hypertension and will be resolved within 42 days of postpartum period. Outcome of gestational hypertension:
   1. Cardiovascular disease
   2. Future primary hypertension
   3. May be recovered by itself with good fetal and maternal outcomes.

c. Pre-eclampsia: It occurs in 10% of first pregnancy, 20–25% of chronic hypertension. It can be defined as:
   1. Blood pressure of ≥140/90 mm Hg
   2. >300 mg proteinuria in 24 hours urine collection, or
   3. In case chronic hypertension increases in proteinuria or loss of control of blood pressure.

   Symptoms are:
   1. Blurred vision
   2. Headache
   3. Dyspnea
   4. Abdominal pain
      Onset is in the 3rd trimester but will be recovered after delivery.
   5. In case of associated eclampsia grand mall seizures.

   Urgent delivery with rapid normalization of blood pressure is required in case of pre-eclampsia if it is associated with the following:
   1. Severe hypertension
   2. Hemolysis, elevated liver enzymes, low platelet count (HELLP) syndrome
   3. Abruption placenta
   4. Cerebral hemorrhage
   5. Pulmonary edema
   6. Renal failure

Pathophysiology of Pregnancy Induced Hypertension

A. Abnormal placentation: Normally trophoblast invades the maternal spiral arteries leading to dilatation and increased blood flow through the placenta. But if this invasion is insufficient, there will inadequate blood supply to the placenta resulting placental ischemia.

B. Endothelial dysfunction: Poor placental blood flow leads to increased release of antiangiogenic factors and proinflammatory cytokines into the maternal circulation that ultimately results severe endothelial dysfunction—this results in decreased production of potent vasodilator, nitric oxide resulting increased vascular resistance and hypertension. Again pro-inflammatory cytokines like interleukin-6, TNF-α produces placental hypoxia resulting endothelial activation, increased vascular permeability culminating worsening hypertension and end-organ damage

C. Imbalance between the vasoactive substances: Increased level of vasoconstrictors like thromboxane and endothelin and decreased level of vasodilators like nitric oxide results increase in the peripheral vascular resistance.

D. Dysregulated RAAS leads to fluid retention and increased blood pressure.

E. Placental ischemia leads to increased production of reactive oxygen species which results oxidative stress. Reactive oxygen species further damages endothelial cells and release of increased amount of inflammatory cytokines.

F. Normally immune status of the mother plays a crucial role in accepting the semi-allogenic fetus and placenta. If the immune response is abnormal against fetus and placenta—it will lead to endothelial dysfunction resulting hypertension.

G. During pregnancy, blood volume is increased to provide support the growing fetus. But, If the compensatory mechanism is affected, there is increased cardiac output and increased peripheral vascular resistance leading to development of hypertension.

Diagnosis of Pregnancy Induced Hypertension

A. Measurement of blood pressure:

a. According to hypertension criteria if systolic blood pressure is ≥140 mm Hg and diastolic blood pressure is ≥90 mm Hg in 2 separate occasions after 20 weeks' gestational period in previously normotensive woman.

b. Accurate position during blood pressure measurement—sitting upright position, proper size of cuff and after taking 5 minutes of rest.

B. Absence of proteinuria

C. Exclusion of other causes of hypertension

D. Monitoring of the symptoms like blurring of vision, headache, rapid gain of weight.

E. Laboratory tests:

a. Analysis of urine to exclude proteinuria

b. Blood tests:

1. Liver function test to detect liver involvement

2. Platelet count to detect thrombocytopenia—it suggests preeclampsia

3. Serum creatinine to exclude renal injury and chronic kidney disease.

Following drugs are given in case of hypertension in pregnancy:

Drug	Mechanism of action	Doses	Comments
Labetalol	α-β adrenergic blocker	20–80 mg intravenous infusion over 10–20 minutes, it can be given up to 300 mg	It is well tolerated, but should be avoided in asthma
Hydralazine	Vasodilator	5–10 mg intravenous infusion over 15–30 minutes	It is safe in pregnancy and lactation
Sodium nitroprusside	Arterial and venous dilator	0.5–5 μg/kg/min	Chance of fetal toxicity to thiocyanate
Long-term treatment of hypertension			
Methyldopa	Central α_2 agonist	250 mg thrice daily, it can be increased up to 4 g/day	It can be effective to control severe hypertension
Labetalol	α-β adrenergic blocker	200–2,400 mg/day in 2–3 divided doses	It is well tolerated, but should be avoided in asthma
Nifedipine	Calcium-channel blocker	Daily sustained release 120 mg/day	It can precipitate severe hypertension

Mechanism of action of the above drugs:

F. Hydralazine:

a. It will dilate the blood vessels

b. It will decrease the vascular resistance

c. It will relax the pre-capillary arteriole.

d. It will improve the placental circulation.

G. Labetalol:

a. It will dilate the blood vessels

b. It will reduce the peripheral vascular resistance.

c. It will maintain normal uteroplacental circulation.

For controlling seizures:

Magnesium sulphate: The loading dose is 6 mg intravenously to be given over 15–20 minutes followed by 2 g intravenously per hour. In absence of intravenous access 10 g intramuscularly followed by 5 g intramuscularly 4 hourly. Contraindication to magnesium sulphate:

a. Hypocalcaemia

b. Myasthenia gravis

c. Renal failure

d. Heart block

e. Cardiac ischemia

f. Myocarditis

Alternative drugs include:

- Phenytoin
- Diazepam
- Levetiracetam

In case of recurrent seizures: Additional 2–4 g magnesium sulphate intravenously over 5 minutes. If the seizures continues after 20 minutes or in spite of magnesium therapy, more than 2 seizures occur, 4 mg lorazepam has to be given over 3–5 minutes. Other alternative drugs include:

- Intravenous Sodium amobarbital 250 mg over 3 minutes.

- 10 mg loading dose of lorazepam intravenously over 2 minutes followed by 40 mg to be dissolved in 500 mL of normal saline for 1 day, this has to be followed by 20 mg in 500 mL normal saline in the 2nd day.
- 10 mg/kg Phenytoin in 30 minutes initially, after 2 hours 5 mg/kg over 5 minutes and this is followed by 300 mg intravenously over 10 minutes for 24 hours from the incidence of the last seizures.

During seizures, fetal monitoring should be done as during seizures, there is chance of maternal hypoxia and hypercapnia leading to bradycardia or tachycardia may occur.

H. Aortic dissection: It occurs in pregnant women in following conditions occurred in 3rd trimester and in peripartum period:

a. Systemic hypertension

b. Cocaine abuse

c. Coarctation of aorta

d. Turner syndrome

Management: Echocardiography can diagnose it and can be treated by β-blockers.

I. Coronary artery disease:

a. Myocardial infarction occurs in:

1. In older with in 3rd trimester with history of multiple pregnancies.

2. Following diseases may precipitate myocardial infarction:

- In situ coronary thrombosis
- Coronary dissection
- Coronary spasm

Treatment:

- Avoidance of thrombolytic agents
- Administration of β-blockers, low-dose aspirin, and nitrates
- Short-term administration of heparin is not associated with fetal and maternal side-effects.
- In case of anticipation of CABG or emergency angioplasty, coronary angiography can be performed.

J. Arrhythmias:

a. Atrial fibrillation:

According to AHA/ACC guidelines:

Class I:

1. A digoxin or a β-blocker or a nondihydropyridine calcium-channel antagonist is recommended to control ventricular rate in pregnant patient with atrial fibrillation.

2. Direct current cardioversion is recommended in pregnant patients who become hemodynamically unstable because of "atrial fibrillation".

3. Protection against thromboembolism is recommended throughout the pregnancy for all the patients with atrial fibrillation (except for those with lone atrial fibrillation and/or low thromboembolic risk). Therapy (anticoagulant or ASA) should be chosen according to the stage of pregnancy.

b. Supraventricular nodal re-entrant tachycardia: It is the most common in pregnant and nonpregnant women. In case of underlying heart disease, it can lead to hemodynamic deterioration. In this case adenosine can be administered safely in pregnant woman for diagnostic and therapeutic purpose.

c. Ventricular tachycardia: It is rare in pregnancy. It can be associated with:

1. Hyperemesis gravidarum

2. Thyrotoxicosis

All the antiarrhythmic drugs except amiodarone can be safely given in pregnancy.

K. Peripartum cardiomyopathy

L. Primary pulmonary hypertension:

a. It is associated with very high fetal as well as maternal mortality rate.

b. Other will die from right ventricular failure and fatal arrhythmia. Hence, pregnancy should be discouraged in these patients.

c. Symptoms become worsen in 2nd and 3rd trimester of pregnancy.

d. Anticoagulant may be recommended throughout gestation but must be in 3rd trimester.

Q107. ACLS guidelines for a patient with tachyarrhythmias and bradyarrhythmias.

BF/NOV2012/MD (20)

Recent trends in CPR.

MLB/MAY2009/MDIII (20)

Advanced cardiac life support.

VEER NARMAD SOUTH GUJARAT UNIVERSITY, 2022 (2.5)

ANSWER

According to the AHA 2020 guidelines:

Cardiopulmonary resuscitation for an adult

Step 1
Airway
- Tap or gently shake the victim to see if they are conscious
- Shout 'ARE YOU OK?' If no response, call out for help and attend to victim
- Tilt the head back by lifting the chin gently with one hand while pushing down on the forehead with your other hand. Do not close the victim's mouth completely

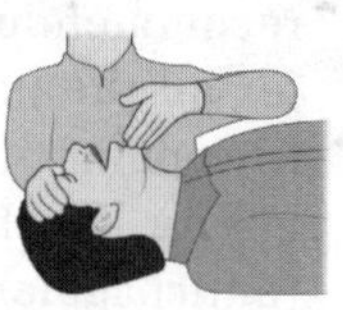
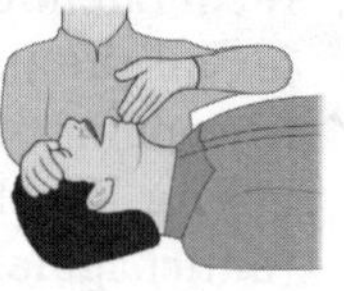
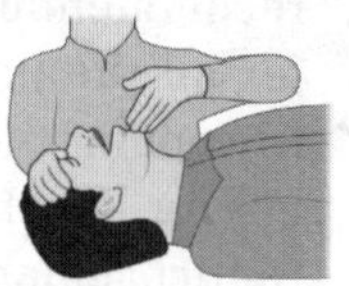
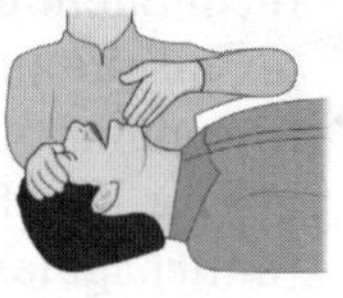

Step 2
Breathing
- Put your ear close to victim's mouth and nose for 3–5 seconds
- Look for the rise and fall of the chest
- Listen for breathing sounds
- Feel for breathing on your cheek

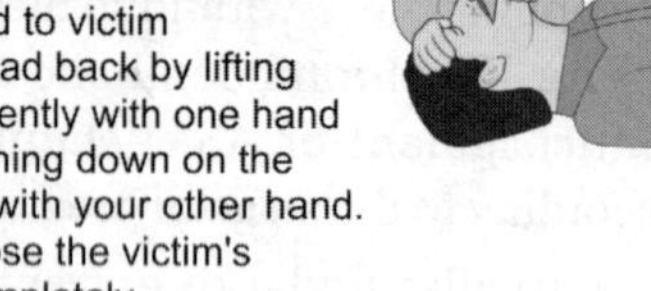

Step 3
If not breathing
- Pinch the nostrils shut, using your thumb and index finger
- Open your mouth wide and take a deep breath
- Place your mouth over the victim's mouth, making a tight seal
- Give 2 full breaths, pausing between them to take a breath
- Watch for the victim's chest to rise
- Check for pulse at side of neck for 5 to 10 seconds

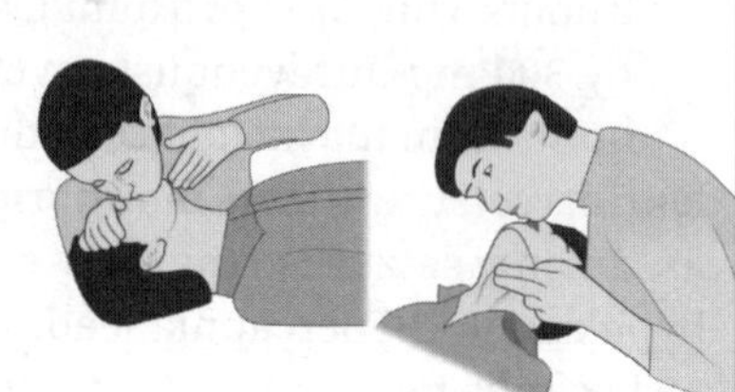

Step 4
If on pulse
- Locate notch at lower end of breastbone with two fingers. Place heel of other hand on breastbone next to fingers
- Remove hand from notch and put it on top of other hand keeping all fingers off chest
- Position shoulders over hands. Compress breastbone 1-1/2 to 2 inches. Do 15 compressions in 10 seconds following with 2 full breaths
- Do 4 cycles of 15 compressions and 2 breaths, checking pulse every minute

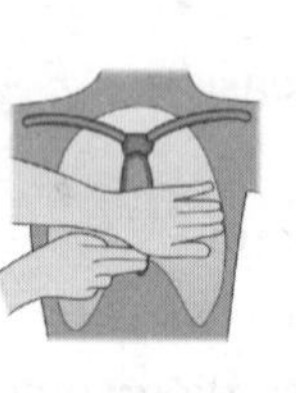
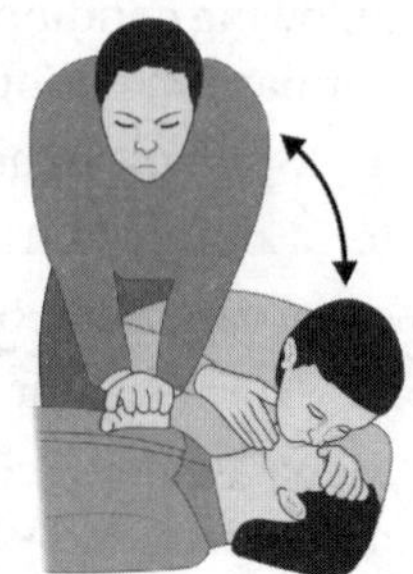

According to the AHA/ESC guidelines of bradyarrhythmias:

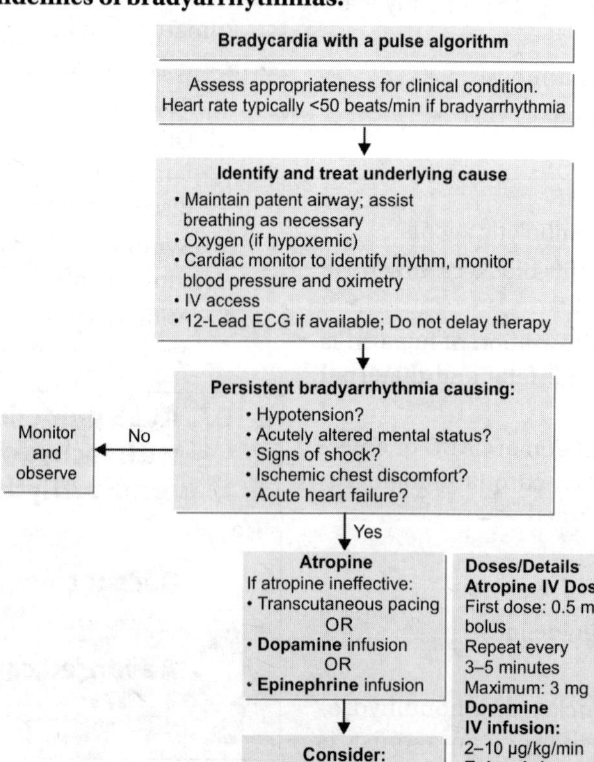

According to the AHA/ESC guideline of tachyarrhythmia:

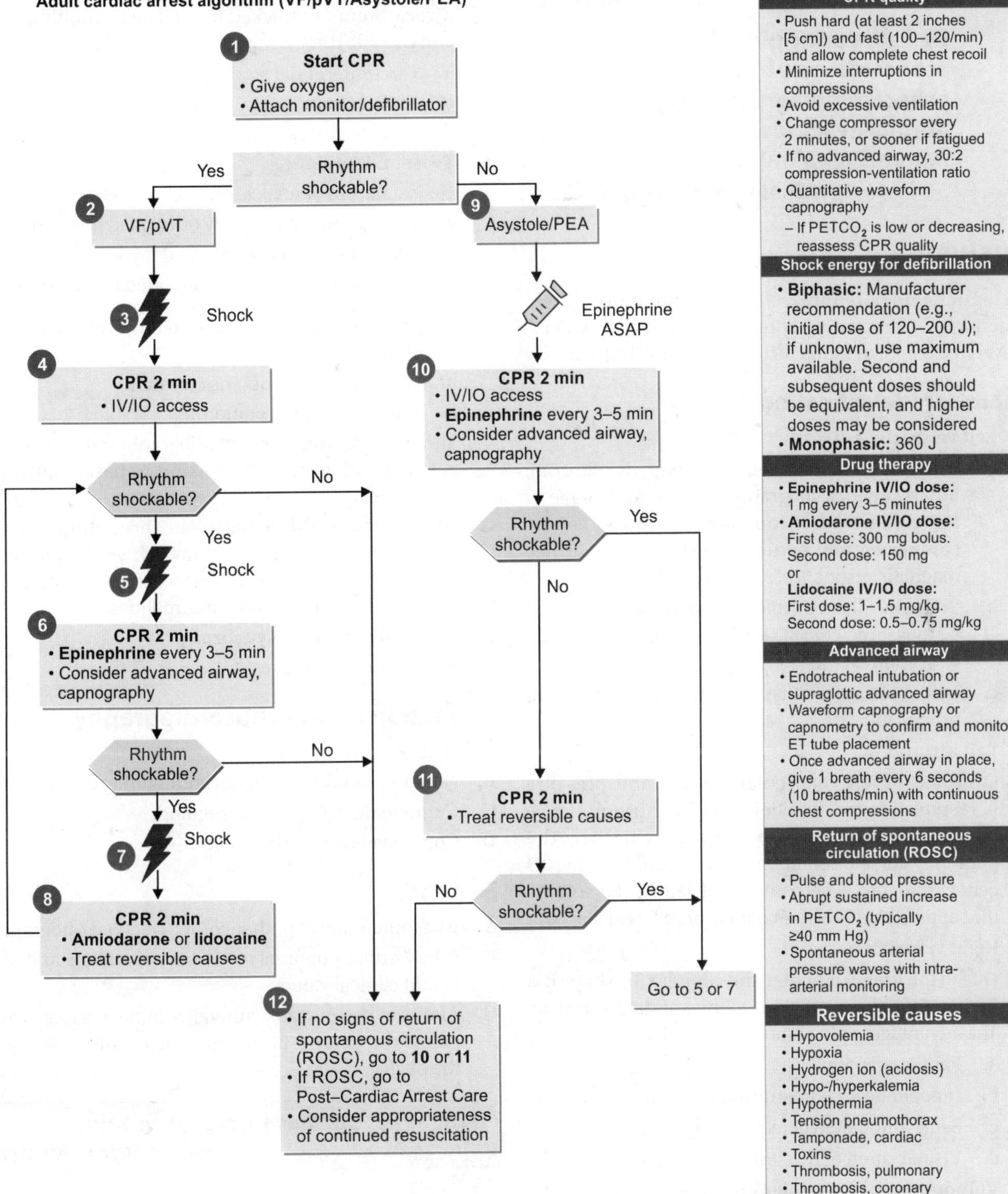

Q108. 3D Echocardiography.

BF/MAY2012/MDIV (10)

Describe principles of echocardiography. List echocardiographic findings in a normal heart. Mention the echo features of mitral regurgitation.

KERALA UNIVERSITY, 2022 (20)

ANSWER

For better understanding of human anatomy, three-dimentional echocardiography was introduced by Duke University School of Biomedical Engineering in 1990.

Chamber Identification

A. **Left ventricle:**
   a. In 2D echo the left ventricle shape is ellipsoid, but 3D echocardiography has the advantage of full-volume acquisition accurately and can be comparted and better correlated with cardiac magnetic resonance.
   b. Both end-diastolic and end-systolic volume can be measured with 3D echo and is more enhanced with contrast infusion.
   c. Left ventricular mass is better delineated with prognostic data.

B. **Left atrium:**

   Overload of left ventricular volume and pressure is responsible for remodeling of left atrium, hence left ventricular volume denotes whether the pathophysiologic condition is severe and chronic. 3D echocardiography determines left ventricular volume that approximates with that measured by cardiac MR.

C. **Right ventricle:**

   Due to the irregular border and complex 3D shape it is not possible to quantify the volume of right ventricle. The advantages of 3D echocardiography are:
   a. Fast acquisition
   b. Independent geometric assumption
   c. Semi-automated detection of border
   d. Visualization of dynamic right ventricular cast

D. **Volumetric color Doppler imaging:**
   a. It can assess the severity of valvular lesion with great reproducibility.
   b. In can directly visualize vena contracta area.
   c. It can visualize simultaneously the noncircumferential vena contracta area, nonspherical proximal isovelocity and multiple orifices.

E. **Speckle tracking echocardiography:**

   In 3D echocardiography speckles of whole myocardium are tracked in 3D space omnidirectally and provide three orthogonal strain values:
   a. Circumferential strain
   b. Radial strain
   c. Longitudinal strain

F. **Twist and torsion:**

   Helical nature of myocardium consists of:
   a. Right-handed obliquely orientated myocardium
   b. Circumferentially orientated myocardium
   c. Left handed obliquely orientated myocardium.

   So, from the apical point view, left ventricle contracts as spiral squeeze by:
   a. Apical counterclockwise rotation
   b. Basal clockwise rotation.

   Three-dimensional echocardiography can accurately calculate left ventricular torsion in basal and short axis planes.

G. **Wall motion abnormalities:** Three-dimensional echocardiography since all the left ventricular wall are visualized at a time, it can accurately estimate and quantify the wall motion abnormalities.

H. **Left ventricular dyssynchrony**

I. Valvular heart diseases

Limitation of 3D Echocardiography

A. Highly costly
B. Nonavailability of 3D echocardiography expertise
C. Cumbersome acquisition method
D. Complicated analysis software

Benefit

A. It has potentiality to enhance the 2D echocardiography.
B. It has strong potential to improve workflow and also to add clinical value.
C. After the use of transcatheter routinely intervention across the globe it produces a major role in sizing of the device.

Q109. Post-cardiac injury syndrome.

MGR/APR2016/MDII (7)

ANSWER

Definition

It is a heterogenous autoimmune-mediated condition involving pericardium, epicardium, and to some extent myocardium resulting from inflammation of pericardium resulting from the injury to pericardium.

Different Sub-titles of Postcardiac Injury Syndrome

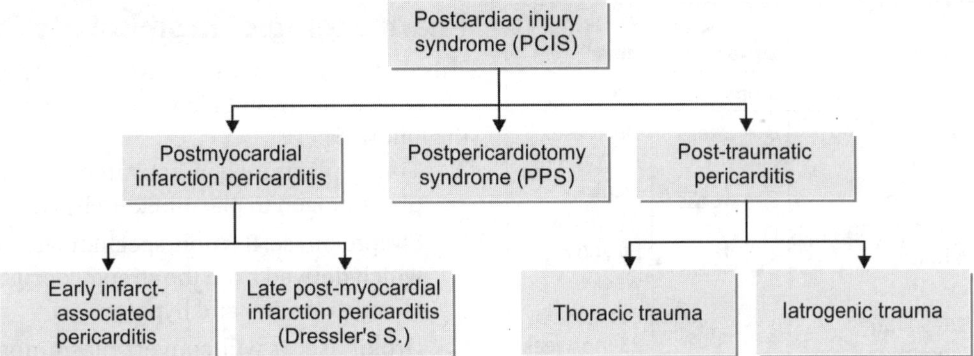

Postmyocardial Infarction Syndrome

It is of two types:

- **a.** Early infarct associated pericarditis: It occurs within 5 days of infarction. Major risk factor is delayed angioplasty and recurrence rate is low.
- **b.** Late infarct associated pericarditis or Dressler syndrome: It occurs 2–8 weeks after infarction with high level of recurrence.

Postpericardiotomy Syndrome

It is mainly the consequence of cardiac surgery, occurs after days to weeks after cardiac injury and pericardial effusion may develop.

Post-traumatic Pericarditis

It results from accidental blunt to sharp trauma or any iatrogenic trauma. Triggering factors are:

- **a.** Pace maker insertion
- **b.** Percutaneous coronary intervention
- **c.** Radiofrequency ablation
- **d.** Swan-Ganz catheterization

Etiopathogenesis

Damage to pericardial and pleural mesothelial cells and blood entering into the pericardial cavity are the triggering factors. There is positive correlation between the serum anti-mitochondrial antibody and incidence of postcardiac injury syndrome after cardiac injury. Systemic release of cardiac antigen as a result of cardiac injury activates innate immune system leading to initiation of adaptive immune response as evidenced by increase in antimitochondrial antibody titer as well as expansion of heart specific CD4 T cells, this cells recruit myelo-derived inflammatory cells to the heart. In the epicardium, pericardium, and myocardium inflammatory cells accumulate as compared to cardiac interstitium in spite of presence of cardiomyocytes specific autoimmune response—this suggests autoimmune pathogenesis of postcardiac injury syndrome.

Clinical Features

Symptoms

- **a.** Chest pain
- **b.** Low-grade fever
- **c.** Dyspnea

Signs

- **a.** Features of pericardial effusion
- **b.** Features of pleural effusion
- **c.** Pericardial friction rub on auscultation

Laboratory Investigations

- **a.** Leukocytosis
- **b.** Raised CRP
- **c.** ECG demonstrates:
  1. Widespread elevation of ST segment with concavity upward
  2. Depression of PR segment

Diagnostic Criteria

Any two of the following five criteria:

- **a.** Fever without alternative cause
- **b.** Pericarditic or pleuritic chest pain
- **c.** Pericardial or pleural rub
- **d.** Evidence of pericardial effusion
- **e.** Pleural effusion with elevated CRP

Treatment

Drug	Dose	Duration	Tapering dose
First line of therapy			
Aspirin Or Ibuprofen Or Indomethacin Plus Colchicine	750–1,000 mg 6 hourly Or 600–800 mg 6 hourly Or 25–50 mg 8 hourly Plus 0.6 mg 12 hourly	3–4 weeks Or 3–4 weeks Or 3–4 weeks Plus 3 months (1st episode) 6 months (recurrent)	Decrease by 250 mg/week Decrease by 200 mg/week Decrease by 25 mg/week Not to taper
Second line of therapy in refractory cases or contraindication to NSAIDs			
Prednisolone Plus Colchicine	0.2–0.5 mg/kg/day Plus 0.6 mg 12 hourly	2–4 weeks Plus 3–6 months	Gradual tapering by 0.2 mg/kg/week
Third line of therapy or pereicardiotomy			
Anakinra	1–2 mg/kg/day	Several months	Slow taper over 3 months
Azathioprine	1–3 mg/kg/day	Several months	Not to taper
IVIG	400–500 mg/kg/day	5 days	Not to taper

(NSAIDs: nonsteroidal anti-inflammatory drugs)

Follow-up

a. Inflammatory markers at 4 weeks after diagnosis
b. If the patient remains symptomatic or inflammatory marker remains elevated clinical follow-up should be done every 2 weeks.
c. If the patients become asymptomatic and inflammatory markers are normal, clinical follow-up should be done at every 3 months.

Q110. Discuss various strategies used to achieve reperfusion in coronary artery diseases.

KERALA UNIVERSITY, 2022 (20)

ANSWER

Pharmacologic Thrombolysis

This therapy involves administration of fibrinolytic agents to dissolve the thrombi in the coronary arteries. These are the following:

A. Tissue plasminogen activator: It will convert tissue plasminogen to plasmin thereby lysis of the clot.
B. Streptokinase: It is non-specific plasminogen activator which derived from the streptococcus. It can produce allergic reaction and hypotension.
C. Urokinase: It will convert plasminogen to plasmin directly thereby lysis of the clot.

Indications:

A. It should be most effective if it will be administered within 30 minutes to 1 hour of incidence.
B. If percutaneous intervention is not available.

Contraindications:

A. History of hemorrhagic stroke
B. Recent major surgery
C. Severe uncontrolled hypertension
D. Trauma

Percutaneous Coronary Intervention

It is a mechanical method of reperfusion by inserting a balloon catheter into the stenosed artery followed by placement of a stent in the affected position of the artery to keep the artery open.

A. Balloon angioplasty: In this method balloon is inflated at the affected site to compress the plaque against the wall of the artery.
B. Placement of a stent: In this method a mesh is deployed at the occluded site to make the vessel patent after balloon inflation. In case of drug eluting stent the drug is released to prevent the restenosis.

Indications of Percutaneous Coronary Intervention

A. In case of ST segment elevated myocardial infarction if it is performed within 90 to 120 minutes of the incident.
B. Lower risk of bleeding as compared to thrombolytic therapy.
C. This method requires specially trained personnel and well equipped catheterization laboratory.

Coronary Artery Bypass Graft

In this surgical procedure, a new route is being created around the blocked or narrowed artery by the graft taken from the saphenous vein or internal mammary artery.

Indications:

A. In case of complex coronary artery disease like left main coronary artery disease or multi-vessel disease.

B. In diabetic patient with high burden of atherosclerotic disease.

It will provide long term patency and relief from the symptoms.

Combination Therapies

In some cases combination of the above procedures are employed.

A. Facilitated PCI: If immediate PCI is not available, in that case initial thrombolytic therapy followed by PCI may be considered.

B. Rescue PCI: If the initial thrombolytic therapy is failed as evidenced by persistent chest pain or lack of resolution of ST segment in ECG.

Mechanical Circulatory Support

In case of cardiogenic shock to improve the cardiac hemodynamics intra-aortic balloon pumps or ventricular assisted device should be done while reperfusion strategies being implemented.

Adjunctive Pharmacotherapy

A. Antiplatelet agents: To prevent the formation of clot aspirin, P2Y12 inhibitors are given.

B. Anticoagulants: To prevent formation of thrombus heparin and bivalirudin are given.

C. Beta blockers, ACEI and statins are given to:

a. Manage the cardiac work load

b. Improve ventricular remodeling

c. Reduce the future cardiovascular events.

Q111. Discuss electrophysiological mechanisms and ECG features of supraventricular tachycardia.

WEST BENGAL HEALTH UNI, 2022 (10)

ANSWER

Electrophysiological mechanism of action potential of the heart initiate the propagation of the electrical impulse leading to contraction of the heart.

Pacemaker cells are:

A. Sinoatrial node is located in the right atrium and generates spontaneous electrical impulses as a result of spontaneous depolarization.

B. Atrioventricular node acts a gate keeper to delay the signals allowing the atrium to contract fully before the ventricles.

Following are the Key Phases of the Action Potential

Cardiomyocyte Action Potential: One Individual Cell

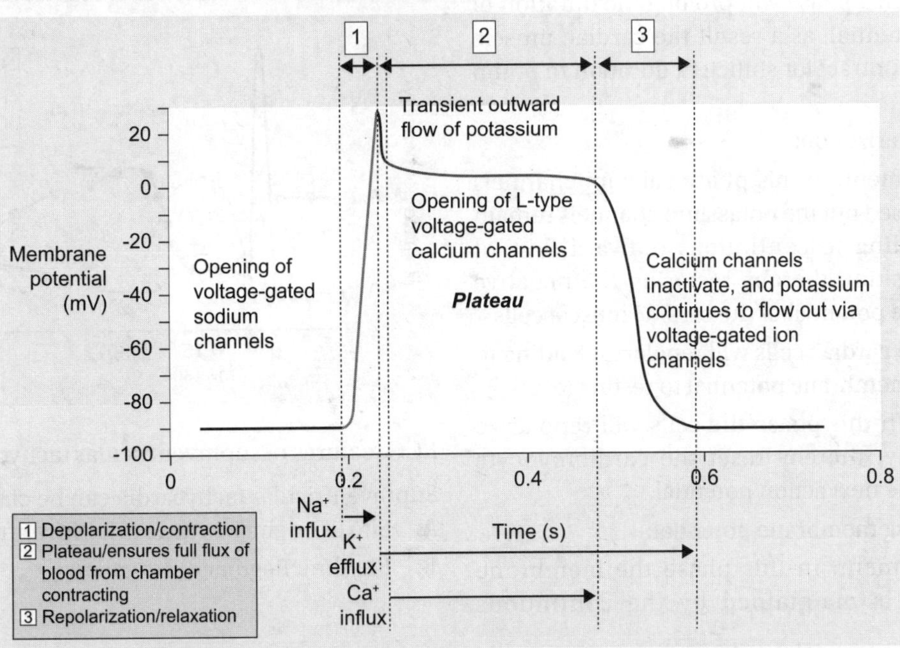

A. Phase 0: Rapid depolarization:

a. Ion movement: When the threshold voltage will be reached, there is rapid influx of sodium ion into cardiac muscle cells.

b. Effect: The potential of the cell membrane will be rapidly positive leading to initiation of depolarization of cardiomyocyte.

c. Role: There is rapid upstroke of the action potential and followed by rapid propagation of this potential along the atrial and ventricular muscle cells throughout the heart.

B. Phase 1: Early repolarization:

a. Ion movement: In this phase sodium channel will be closed and potassium channel opens leading to outward movement of potassium ion from the muscle cells.

b. Effect: There is partial repolarization of the membrane potential leading to slight dipping following rapid depolarization.

c. Key role: It is early and initial step toward repolarization, it prevents further rapid repolarization.

C. Phase 2: Plateau phase:

a. Ion movement: Calcium ions enter through the voltage gated L type calcium channels which balance the outward flow of the potassium ions through the potassium channels.

b. Effect: Here the membrane potential will be stable as a result of simultaneous inward flow of calcium and outward flow of potassium through the cardiac muscle cells.

c. Key role: This phase will prolong the duration of action potential, as a result the cardiac muscle cells will contract for sufficient duration to pump the blood.

D. Phase 3: Repolarization:

a. Ion movement: In this phase calcium channels will be closed but the potassium channels remain open leading to continuous outward flow of the potassium, thereby restoring the negative membrane potential of the cardiac muscle cells.

b. Effect: The cardiac cells will repolarize leading to return of membrane potential to resting level.

c. Ley role: In this phase the cells will repolarize completely, thereby reset the cardiomyocyte towards the next action potential.

E. Phase 4: Resting membrane potential:

a. Ion movement: In this phase the membrane potential is maintained by the continuous outward flow of potassium through the leak channels at the same time Na/K pumps act to maintain the correct ion gradient.

b. Effect: The membrane potential will be negative till the next depolarizing stimulus will act.

c. Key role: This phase ensures that this cardiac myocyte will be ready for the next depolarization stimulus.

Types of Channels

A. Fast response: These channels are present in the atrial and ventricular myosites and purkinje fibers. These cells have:

a. Rapid upstroke phase or phase 0 due to rapid influx of sodium ion

b. Distinct plateau phase or phase 2.

B. Slow response: These channels are found in sinoatrial and atrioventricular nodes. These cells rely on:

a. More influx of calcium ion during phase 0 leading to slow up stroke.

b. There is absence of well-defined plateau phase

c. There is absence of spontaneous depolarization in the phase 4.

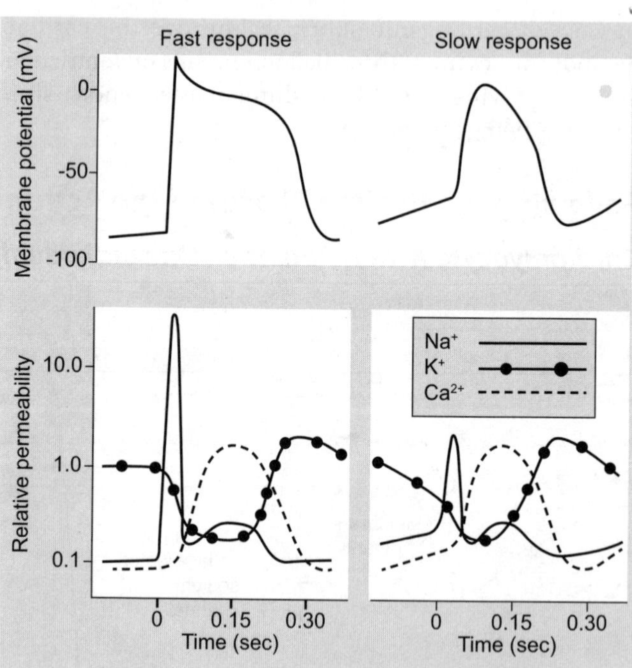

ECG features of supraventricular tachycardia:

Supraventricular tachycardia can be classified based on:

A. Site of origin, i.e., atria or atrioventricular node.

B. Rhythm: Regular or irregular.

Classifications Based on Site of Origin and Rhythm

A. Regular atrial tachycardia:
   a. Sinus tachycardia
   b. Atrial tachycardia
   c. Atrial flutter
   d. Inappropriate sinus tachycardia
   e. Sinus node reentrant tachycardia

B. Irregular atrial tachycardia:
   a. Atrial flutter with varying block
   b. Atrial fibrillation
   c. Multifocal atrial tachycardia

C. Atrioventricular regular tachycardia:
   a. AVRT
   b. AVNRT
   c. Automatic junctional tachycardia

ECG in Different Supraventricular Tachycardia

A. In sinus tachycardia:
   a. Heart rate is more than 100 beats/min
   b. Rhythm—regular.
   c. P, QRS, and T waves are normal.

B. Atrial tachycardia:
   a. Atrial rate more than 100 beats/min
   b. Morphology of P wave is abnormal due to its ectopic origin.
   c. Unifocal and identical P wave
   d. Baseline is isoelectric.
   e. QRS morphology is normal.

C. Atrial flutter with or without varying block:
   a. Narrow complex tachycardia
   b. Atrial rate is 300 beats/min
   c. Loss of isoelectric baseline.
   d. Inverted flutter wave in the form of "saw tooth" wave in II, III, and aVF.
   e. In V1 flutter wave is upright resembling P wave.
   f. Ventricular rate will depend upon the atrioventricular ratio—it may be 2:1, 3:1 or 4:1.

D. Atrial fibrillation:
   a. Irregularly irregular atrial rate.
   b. Fibrillary P wave in lead II and V1.
   c. Absent isoelectric baseline.
   d. Ventricular rate is variable.
   e. QRS complexes is less than 120 ms in absence of accessary pathway or aberrant conduction.
   f. Fibrillary wave amplitude is fine, i.e., less than 0.5 mm or coarse, i.e., more than 0.5 mm.

E. Multifocal atrial tachycardia:
   a. Heart rate is more than 100 beats/min
   b. Irregularly irregular rhythm i.e. varying RR, PP or PR intervals.
   c. Presence of at least three different morphologies in same leads.
   d. Baseline in between the P waves are isoelectric.
   e. Absence of single dominant pacemaker.
   f. Some of the P waves are non-conducted.

F. W-PW syndrome:
   a. PR interval is less than 120 ms.
   b. Slurring of the initial portion of QRS complex, i.e., delta wave.
   c. Duration of QRS complex is more than 110 ms.
   d. Discordant ST segment and T wave changes.
   e. Pseudoinfarction pattern in 70% of patients, i.e., R waves in V1–V3.

G. Automatic junctional tachycardia:
   a. Narrow QRS complexes
   b. Ventricular rate is 60 to 80 beats/min
   c. Presence of retrograde inverted P wave before, during or after QRS complexes in L-II, L-III, and aVF.
   d. As ventricular rate is more than atrial rate, there is dissociation between the atrial and ventricular rate.

H. AV nodal reentrant tachycardia:
   a. Heart rate 140–280 beats/min
   b. Narrow QRS complexes.
   c. P waves if present—demonstrate retrograde conduction with inversion of P waves in L-II, L-III, and aVF.
   d. May be rate related ST depression.

Q112. Describe through a flowchart the physiology of cholesterol transport. How will you assess major cardiovascular adverse events?

WEST BENGAL HEALTH UNI, 2022 (10)

ANSWER

Physiology of cholesterol transport:

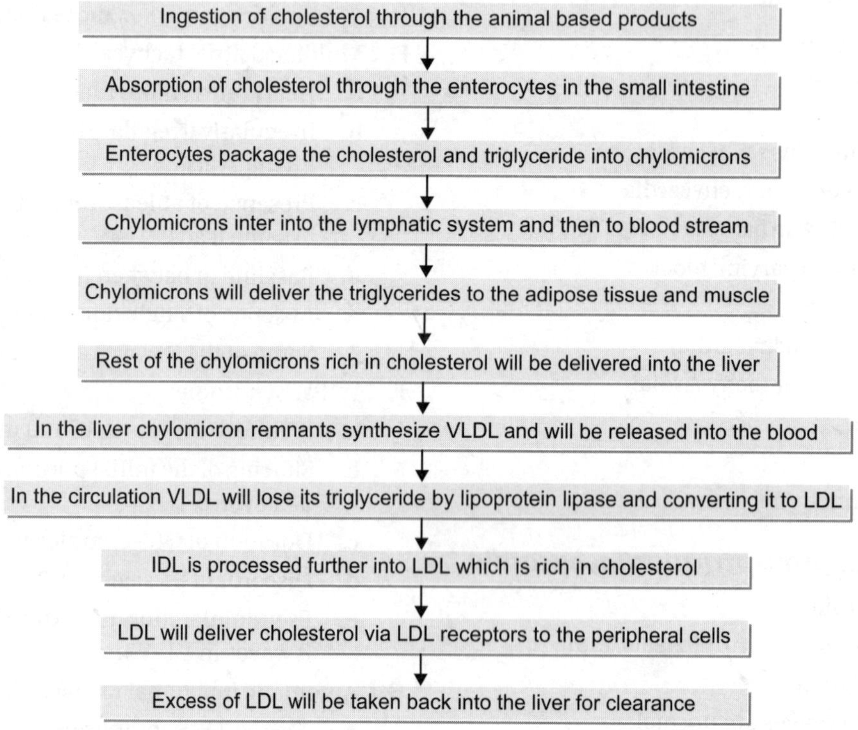

HDL pathway for cholesterol transport:

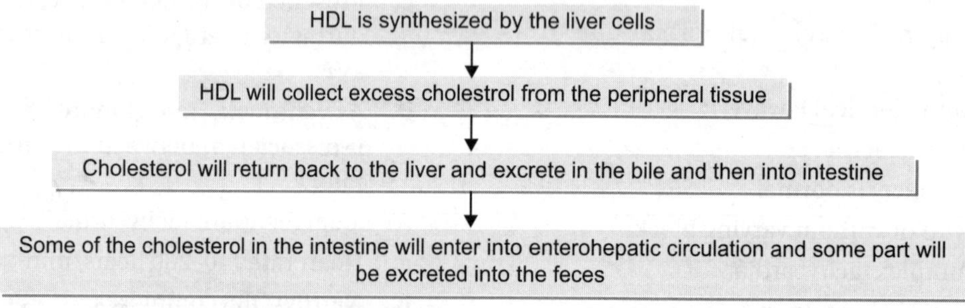

Assessment of Major Cardiovascular Events

Following are the cardiovascular events:

A. Heart failure due to ineffective pumping of the heart

B. Myocardial infarction due to damaged muscle tissue of the heart as a result of insufficient blood supply.

C. Cardiovascular death due to heart failure, arrhythmias

D. Unstable angina

Assessment:

A. Risk score assessment tools:

- **a.** Framingham risk score:
  - **1.** It will predict 10 years risk of coronary artery disease.
  - **2.** Risk factors:
    - Age
    - Total cholesterol
    - HDL cholesterol
    - Smoking status
    - Blood pressure
    - Diabetes
- **b.** Atherosclerotic cardiovascular disease (ASCVD) score:
  - **1.** It predicts risk of myocardial infarction, stroke and cardiovascular death.
  - **2.** Risk factors:

- Age
- Sex
- Race
- Total cholesterol
- Systolic and diastolic blood pressure
- Smoking status
- Diabetes
- Use and statin and antihypertensive drugs

c. Systemic coronary risk evaluation score:
   1. It predicts 10 years fatal risk of cardiovascular disease.
   2. Risk factors:
      - Age
      - Sex
      - Smoking status
      - Systolic blood pressure
      - Total cholesterol
   3. It focuses fatal events which is more relevant in our community.

d. $CHADS_2$ score and CHA_2DS_2-VASc score:
   1. It can predict score of stroke in patient with atrial fibrillation.
   2. Risk:
      - Congestive heart failure
      - Age ≥75 years (2 points)
      - Hypertension
      - Age 65–74 years (1 point)
      - Female
      - Diabetes
      - Stroke or transient ischemic event (2 points)
      - Vascular disease, i.e., prior history of myocardial infarction.

B. Clinical history:

a. Symptoms related to cardiovascular disease like chest pain, breathing difficulty, palpitations, fainting attack
b. Family history of premature cardiovascular risk
c. Physical examinations: Measurement of blood pressure, jugular venous pressure, heart sounds, signs of heart failure

C. Life style and behavioral factors:

a. Smoking
b. Dietary habit
c. Physical activity
d. Consumption of alcohol
e. Obesity

D. Laboratory examination:

a. Lipid profile
b. Total count
c. C-reactive protein
d. Blood sugar
e. HbA1c

E. Imaging and diagnostic testing:

a. Coronary artery calcium score: It will assess the extent of calcium plaques in the coronary artery which can predict the future cardiovascular risk.
b. Echocardiography: It can evaluate:
   1. Function of the heart, wall motion abnormality
   2. Structure of the heart
   3. Ejection fraction
c. Stress testing: It will detect ischemia during physical activity and pharmacologically induced tests.
d. Coronary angiography: It can detect the vascular blockage,

F. Biomarkers measurement:

a. Troponin: It is involved in contraction of cardiac muscles.
   1. It is highly sensitive marker in case of myocardial injury like myocardial infarction, acute coronary syndrome.
   2. Mild elevation of troponin may indicate future cardiovascular events.
b. B-type natriuretic peptide: It is released from the ventricular wall in response to either pressure or volume overload.
   1. It will be increased in heart failure.
   2. It can assess the severity of heart failure.
   3. It can differentiate heart failure from other causes of dyspnea.
c. C-reactive protein: It is produced by liver in response to infection.
   1. It is marker of systemic inflammation and increased in heater failure.
   2. It is associated with atherosclerosis.
   3. It can predict the risk of future cardiovascular events like myocardial infarction.
d. Lipoprotein A: It carries cholesterol in the blood.
   1. It is increased in case of myocardial infarction and atherosclerosis.

2. It is an independent risk factor.
3. In presence of positive family history of cardiovascular event of incase of high LDL level in the blood it will stratify the risk.

e. Fibrinogen: It is involved in the clotting and also act as acute phase reactant.
   1. Increased level of fibrinogen is associated with myocardial infarction or stroke.
   2. It will contribute to atherosclerosis and rupture of plaque.

f. Interleukin-6: It is proinflammatory cytokine which will play an important role in immune response.
   1. It is increased in systemic inflammation and associated with atherosclerosis progression.
   2. Its high level predict the outcome of cardiovascular events like myocardial infarction or stroke.

g. Myeloperoxidase: It is released from the activated neutrophil, and generates reactive oxygen species. Its high level is associated with:
   1. Oxidative stress and instable plaque in atherosclerosis.
   2. Increased cardiovascular events.

h. Growth differentiation factor-2: It is a stress related cytokine which linked to inflammation and tissue injury.
   1. Its increased level is associated with myocardial infarction, heart failure and other major cardiovascular events, acute coronary syndrome.
   2. It can predict the prognosis in patient with heart failure.

i. Soluble ST2: It is biomarker of cardiac stress.
   1. It is elevated in case of heart failure and predict worst outcome in case of major cardiovascular events.
   2. It will provide information regarding cardiac remodeling and fibrosis.

j. D-dimer: It is fibrin degradation production product and it is elevated during formation of active clot and breakdown of the clot.
   1. It is increased in pulmonary thrombo-embolism, and venous thromboembolism.
   2. It may also be increased in myocardial infarction and stroke.

k. Homocysteine: It is an amino acid if elevated is associated with endothelial dysfunction and fibrosis.
   1. Its high level is associated with myocardial infarction and stroke.
   2. Its high level contributes to vascular inflammation and also promotes clot formation.

Q113. Current status of diagnostic conclusion of non-invasive cardiac imaging.

SAURASHTRA UNIVERSITY RAJKOT, 2022 (20)

Cardiac imaging.

MAHARASHTRA UNI OF HEALTH SC, VIJAYAWADA, 2022 (10)

ANSWER

A. Diagnostic conclusion of non-invasive imaging:
   a. Cardiac function:
      1. Left ventricular ejection fraction
      2. Diastolic dysfunction by measuring mitral flow velocities, size of the left atrium and tissue Doppler imaging.
   b. Valvular diseases:
      1. Stenosis or regurgitation of valves
      2. Vegetations as seen in infective endocarditis or masses like mitral myxoma.
   c. Chamber size:
      1. Left ventricular hypertrophy
      2. Dilated left atrium
   d. Different types of congenital cardiac defect
   e. Pericardial diseases:
      1. Pericardial effusion
      2. Cardiac tamponade
   f. Pulmonary hypertension by measuring pulmonary artery pressure.
   g. Detection of aortic dissection or aortic aneurysm

B. Transesophageal echocardiography:
   a. Valvular heart disease
      1. Stenosis or regurgitation
      2. Vegetation in infective endocarditis
      3. Left atrial thrombus

- **b.** Congenital heart disease:
  - **1.** ASD
  - **2.** VSD
  - **3.** PDA
  - **4.** Patent foramen ovale
- **c.** Aortic pathology:
  - **1.** Aortic aneurysm
  - **2.** Aortic dissection
- **d.** Evaluation of the prosthetic valve:
  - **1.** Assessment of the structural integrity and function.
  - **2.** Detection of complication like dehiscence or thrombus formation.
- **e.** Pericardial effusion or pericardial tamponade
- **f.** Pulmonary vein assessment in patient who will undergo catheter ablation for atrial ablation.

C. 3D echocardiography:

- **a.** Valvular heart disease:
  - **1.** It helps in more precise evaluation of structural integrity and functional assessment of the cardiac valves,
  - **2.** In patients waiting for the valve replacement or repair, this will help to provide detail anatomical data as well as leaflet morphology and annular biometry.
- **b.** It will offer accurate visualization of the congenital defects like ASD, VSD, etc.
- **c.** It will detect accurately the ventricular volumes, ejection fraction, and assessment of global and regional wall motion.
- **d.** It can accurately identify any thrombus in the left atrial appendages in atrial fibrillation and helps in risk score assessment.
- **e.** It can detect accurately the position, site, size and attachment points of the thrombus in the cardiac chambers.

D. Speckle tracking echocardiography (staining): It will measure the deformation of the myocardium.

- **a.** It can detect the early dysfunction of the myocardium even before the gross decrease of ejection fraction in diabetes, cardiomyopathy, hypertension, chemotherapy induced cardiotoxicity.
- **b.** Global longitudinal strain: It is a measure of longitudinal contraction of the myocardium as compared to more traditional measure in case of heart failure, cardiomyopathies and ischemic heart disease.
  - **1.** Normal value is –18% to –20%.
  - **2.** Low value indicates impaired myocardial contractility in presence of normal ejection fraction.
- **c.** It can assess the impact of the valvular stenosis or regurgitation on the myocardium, can guide the timing of intervention of valvular defect.
- **d.** It can detect the regional wall motion abnormality, area if ischemic area in the myocardium in presence of nearly ejection fraction.
- **e.** It can monitor the early myocardial dysfunction in the patient receiving chemotherapy.
- **f.** It can assess the right ventricular function in patient with pulmonary hypertension.

Cardiac Magnetic Resonance Imaging

A. Comprehensive cardiac assessment:

- **a.** Anatomic visualization:
  - **1.** It will offer high resolution images of cardiac chambers, valves and surrounding structures.
  - **2.** It will demonstrate 3 dimensional imaging of cardiac chambers and cardiac masses.
- **b.** Functional evaluation:
  - **1.** It will evaluate ventricular volumes, ejection fraction and masses in the chambers.
  - **2.** It will evaluate wall motion abnormalities of free walls.

B. Characterization of tissues:

- **a.** It can evaluate myocardial fibrosis and scar tissue, that results from myocardial infarction, cardiomyopathies and myocarditis.
- **b.** By T1andT2 mapping it can detect diffuse fibrosis, myocardial edema and different infiltrative diseases like amyloidosis.
- **c.** By T2 mapping it can measure the deposition of iron in hemochromatosis and thalassemia after repeated blood transfusion.

C. Ischemic heart disease:

- **a.** By myocardial perfusion imaging it can evaluate myocardial blood flow during resting and stressful conditions and also the severity of coronary artery disease.
- **b.** In case of chronic coronary artery disease, it can detect the viable myocardium and also guide the decision regarding revascularization process.

D. Cardiomyopathies:

- **a.** It can evaluate and differentiate various types of cardiomyopathies based on pattern of fibrosis and hypertrophy.

b. By detailed tissue characterization it can evaluate constrictive physiology in the restrictive cardiomyopathies.

E. Valvular heart disease:
   a. It can evaluate the morphology, function, severity of regurgitation of valves with high accuracy.
   b. By using phase contrast imaging it can measure the blood flow across the valves thereby diagnose the severity of regurgitation and stenosis of the valves.

F. Congenital heart disease:
   a. It can evaluate the congenital septal defect, anomalous coronary arteries and abnormalities of the outflow tract.
   b. It also can monitor and evaluate the post-operative integrity and function of repaired congenital defects.

G. Pericardial diseases:
   a. It can evaluate inflammation, thickening, and accumulation of fluid in the pericardial spaces.
   b. It evaluates thickness of pericardium and ventricular interdependence in case of constrictive pericarditis.

H. Advanced cardiac MRI:
   a. Stress cardiac MRI: By physiological and pharmacological stress in can locate the sites of ischemia and sites of myocardial perfusion.
   b. 4D flow MRI: It will assess the blood flow dynamics in heart and great vessels which is very much essential in case of acquired and congenital heart diseases.
   c. Diffusion tensor imaging is emerging technique which can assess the architecture of myocardial fibers and deviation from any structural changes.

Cardiac Computerized Tomography

A. Coronary CT angiography: By this method it can demonstrate:
   a. Stenosis or blockage of the coronary arteries
   b. Anatomy of the coronary arteries
   c. Calcium deposits and calcium deposits.

B. Calcium scoring:
   a. It can assess and extent of coronary artery calcification.
   b. It can correlate with the future cardiovascular events.
   c. It can stratify the risk in asymptomatic patient.

C. It can assess and detect aorta, pulmonary arteries and cardiac masses.

Nuclear Cardiology

A. Single photon emission computerized tomography: By myocardial perfusion imaging:
   a. Can assess myocardial ischemia and viable myocardium.
   b. Can identify areas of reduced blood flow
   c. Can diagnose the coronary artery disease.

B. Positron emission tomography: It offers high spatial resolution as compared to SPECT it can evaluate:
   a. Myocardial perfusion
   b. Myocardial viability
   c. Inflammatory diseases like myocarditis, sarcoidosis.
   d. Metabolic activity of myocardium.

Emerging Techniques

A. Strain imaging (Speckle tracking): It can assess the myocardial deformation that can detect the systolic dysfunction prior to declining of ejection fraction.

B. Artificial intelligence and machine learning: It enable accurate interpretation of images.

Q114. ARNI.

MGR UNIVERSITY, TAMIL NADU, 2022 (10)

Neprilysin in heart failure.

TEERTHANKER MAHAVEER UNI, 2019 (10)
TEERTHANKER MAHAVEER UNI, 2020 (10)
SRI GURU RAMDAS UNI OF HEALTH SC, AMRITSAR, 2022 (10)

Angiotensin-Neprilysin in heart failure.

TEERTHANKER MAHAVEER UNI, 2020 (10)
DNB, 2021 (5)

ANSWER

Indications of ARNI

A. Heart failure with reduced ejection fraction in NYHA class III-IV. It will reduce the risk of cardiovascular death and hospitalization.

B. Heart failure following event of acute decompensated heart failure

Mechanism of Actions

A. Sacubitril (Neprilysin inhibitor):

- **a.** Neprilysin is responsible for breaking down several beneficial peptides like natriuretic peptide, bradykinin, and adrenomedullin. This naprilysin is inhibited by sacubitril leading to increase in the peptides that results in:
  1. Vasodilatation
  2. Natriuresis and diuresis
  3. Inhibition of cardiac fibrosis
  4. Decreased sympathetic tone leading to
     - Decreased heart rate
     - Decreased workload of the heart

B. Valsartan (angiotensin receptor II blocker): It blocks the angiotensin II type 1 thereby prevents the harmful effects angiotensin II like:

- **a.** Vasoconstriction leading to increase in the systolic blood pressure
- **b.** Increased secretion of aldosterone resulting in accumulation of sodium and water.
- **c.** Cardiac remodeling

Adverse Effects

A. Hypotension
B. Hyperkalemia
C. Renal impairment
D. Angioedema
E. Cough
F. Dizziness and fainting
G. Increase in serum creatinine

Contraindications

A. History of angioedema
B. Pregnancy
C. Severe renal impairment
D. Concurrent use of ACE inhibitors
E. Hyperkalemia
F. Severe hepatic impairment

Q115. Tropical endomyocardial fibrosis.

NTR UNIVERSITY OF HEALTH SC, VIJAYAWADA, ANDHRA, 2022 (10)

RAJIV GANDHI UNI OF HEALTH SC, KARNATAKA, 2016 (10)

NTR UNIVERSITY OF HEALTH SC, VIJAYAWADA, ANDHRA, 2018 (10)

ANSWER

Definition

It is characterized by fibrosis involving right and left ventricular endocardium leading to restriction of the ventricular contraction. Mostly occurring in tropical and subtropical regions.

Etiologies

A. Infections:

- **a.** *Plasmodium* species
- **b.** Microfilaria
- **c.** Schistosoma
- **d.** Helminths
- **e.** Arbovirus
- **f.** Toxoplasma

B. Environmental exposure:

- **a.** Cerium contaminated soil and food items

C. Immunologic mechanisms:

- **a.** Anti-myosin antibodies present in Dressler syndrome, post-cardiac transplant and rheumatic heart disease
- **b.** Deficiency of the key nutrients like magnesium and protein.

D. Genetic predisposition

Key Features in the Pathogenesis and Pathophysiology

A. Fibrosis: Dense fibrous tissue in the apices of the both ventricles extend to subendocardium involving chordae tendineae and papillary muscles.

B. Affected regions: Right ventricle is involved more commonly but, left ventricle may be involved.

C. Cardiac cavity: As the cavity of the heart is restricted, cavity is not filled adequately leading to diastolic dysfunction.

Clinical Presentation

A. Features of right sided heart failure like engorged neck vein, enlarged tender liver, ascites and peripheral edema. Giant v waves and rapid Y descent.

B. In case of left ventricular involvement fatigue, cachexia, orthopnea.

C. Thromboembolism: Due to risk of developing thrombi in the cardiac cavity there is chance of thromboembolism.

D. Features of valvular dysfunction like mitral regurgitation

E. Features of pulmonary hypertension, S3 and S4.

Diagnosis

A. Imaging: Echocardiography and cardiac MRI can demonstrate:

- **a.** Thickening of the left ventricular free walls
- **b.** Involvement of heart valves
- **c.** Fibrosis of the walls of ventricles
- **d.** Obliteration of the trabecular aspect of right ventricular cavity.

B. Cardiac hemodynamics:

- **a.** By cardiac catheterization, left ventricular tracing demonstrates dip and plateau pattern consistent with restrictive ventricular filling.
- **b.** Left ventricular end diastolic pressure
- **c.** Left ventricular angiography demonstrates obliteration of the apex of the involved ventricles.

C. Electron beam CT scanning: It will demonstrate:

- **a.** Obliteration of the apex of the inflow tract
- **b.** A band of low attenuation within the endocardium of the involved ventricles.

D. Cardiac MRI with gadolinium contrast demonstrates fibrosis of the endomyocardium.

E. Chest X-ray demonstrates:

- **a.** Mild to moderate cardiomegaly
- **b.** Enlargement of pulmonary artery
- **c.** Pulmonary vascular congestion

Treatment

A. Symptomatic relief by:

- **a.** Diuretic therapy
- **b.** ACE inhibitor
- **c.** Beta blocker

B. Antithrombotic therapy in patient with risk of thromboembolism.

C. In case of advanced heart failure surgery can increase the survival:

- **a.** Endocardectomy
- **b.** Valvular replacement

Q116. Give an overview of coronary circulation. Briefly describe how ECG can be used to localize the culprit vessel occlusion.

WEST BENGAL HEALTH UNI, 2021 (10)

ANSWER

Coronary circulation described in question number 39.

ST segment elevation	Affected myocardial area	Culprit coronary artery
V1 and V2	Septal wall	Proximal part of left anterior descending artery
V3 and V4	Anterior wall	Left anterior descending artery
V5 and V6	Apical wall	Distal left anterior descending artery
I and aVL	Lateral wall	Left circumflex artery
II, aVL, and III	Inferior wall	• 90% right coronary artery—90% • Left circumflex artery—10%
V7, V8, and V9	Posterior wall	• Right coronary artery • Left circumflex artery

Q117. What is cyanotic spell? Describe the mechanism of how squatting becomes beneficial in such a spell? Enumerate the conditions which may present with a cyanotic spell?

WEST BENGAL HEALTH UNI, 2021 (10)

ANSWER

Definition

Cyanotic spells or "Tet spell" can be defied as sudden bluish discoloration of the lips, skin and mucous membranes along with rapid breathing resulting from sudden reduction of the hemoglobin level I the blood commonly seen in the children with congenital cardiac defect.

Squatting is beneficial in cyanotic spell because of the following reasons:

A. Increase in the systemic vascular resistance. It will decrease the venous return to the heart from the lower half of the body. This resistance redirects the blood towards lung and thereby reduces the right to left heart shunt of the deoxygenated blood. The result is improved oxygenation of the blood.

B. Decreased right to left heart shunt: Squatting increases the systemic vascular resistance thereby reduces right to left heart shunt of deoxygenate blood and allowing large amount of blood to enter pulmonary circulation.

C. Increased return of oxygenated blood to the left side of the heart from the lung bed in presence of decreased right to left heart shunt leading to reduction of the cyanosis.

Causes of Cyanotic Spells

A. Causes related to congenital heart diseases:

- **a.** Tetralogy of Fallot: Here the defect is the decreased oxygenation along with increased demand during crying or exercise.
- **b.** Transposition of the great vessels: In this defect oxygenated blood goes to lung and deoxygenated blood goes to the body.
- **c.** Tricuspid atresia: In this defect due to abnormal development of tricuspid valve, deoxygenated blood cannot enter from right atrium to right ventricle leading to development of cyanosis due to insufficient oxygenation.
- **d.** Pulmonary atresia: Here due to abnormal pulmonary deoxygenated blood cannot go from right ventricle to lung bed leading to reduced oxygenation of the blood.
- **e.** Total anomalous pulmonary venous return: In this defect the pulmonary veins drain the oxygenated blood to the right atrium instead of left atrium resulting poorly oxygenated blood to the body.
- **f.** Epstein anomaly: In this defect malformed tricuspid vale leads to severe tricuspid regurgitation along with reduced flow of blood into the lungs resulting cyanosis.
- **g.** Double outlet right ventricle: Here both the aorta and pulmonary artery arise form right ventricle leading to distribution of oxygen poor blood throughout the body.

B. Non cardia causes of cyanosis in new born:

- **a.** Primary lung causes:
  1. Pneumonia
  2. Lobar emphysema
  3. Hypoplasia
  4. RDS
- **b.** Pulmonary hypertension
  1. Meconium aspiration
  2. Sepsis
  3. Pneumothorax
  4. Pneumonia
- **c.** Mechanical interference with lung function:
  1. Pneumothorax
  2. Congenital diaphragmatic hernia
  3. Chylothorax
  4. Pneumomediastenum

C. CNS causes:

- **a.** Seizures
- **b.** Encephalitis
- **c.** Severe hypermagnesemia
- **d.** Shock
- **e.** Severe hypoglycemia
- **f.** Congenital neuro-muscular condition
- **g.** Methemoglobinemia

Management of Cyanotic Spell

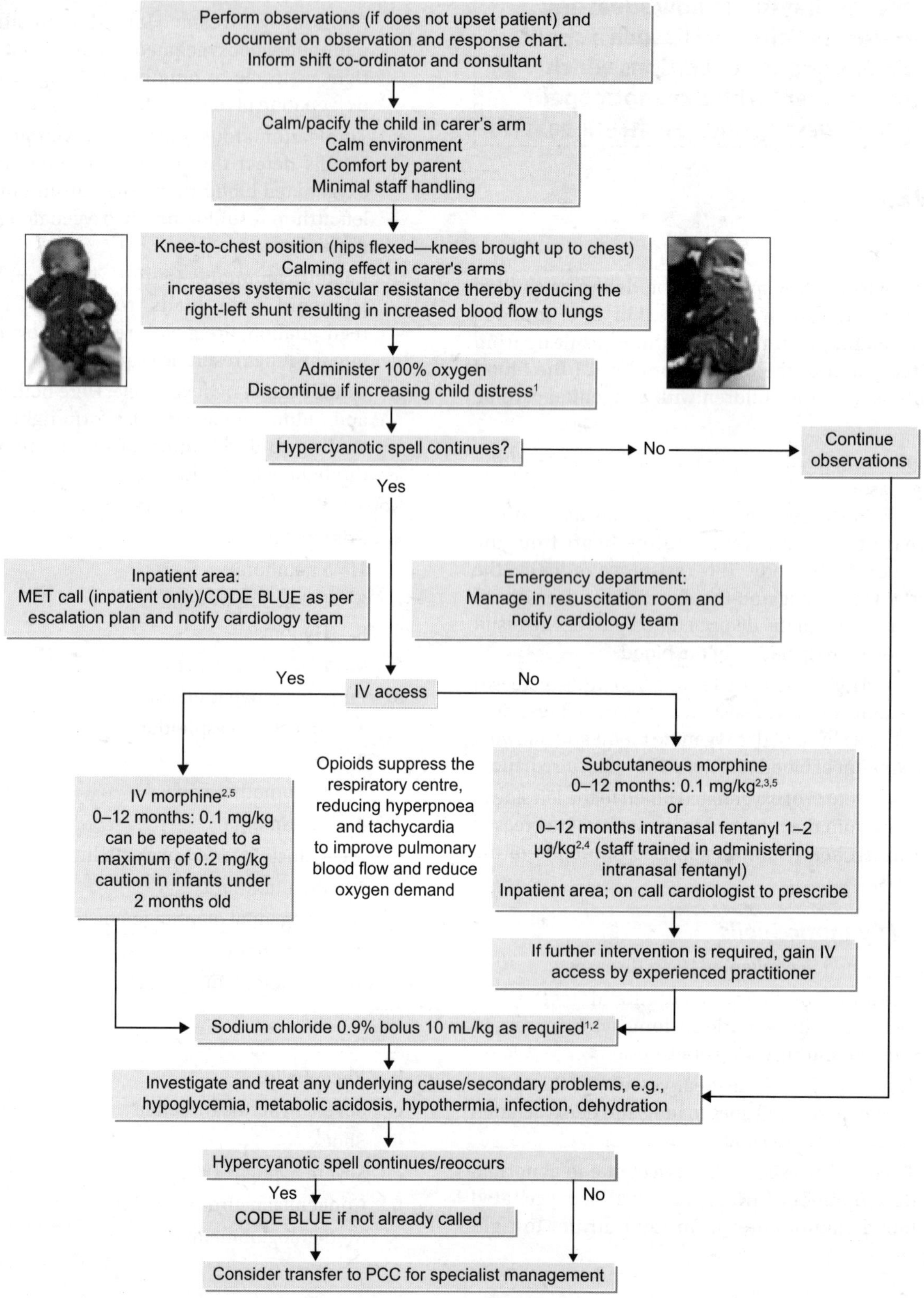

Q118. Ectopic pacemaker.
MGR UNIVERSITY, 2021, (10)

ANSWER

Ectopic pacemaker usually originates from within the heart which can generate impulses leading to development of different types of arrhythmias.

Following are the ectopic sites of origin of pacemaker:

A. Atria
B. Atrioventricular node
C. Ventricles

Causes of generation of ectopic pacemakers:

A. Reduced blood flow to the heart leading to ischemia.
B. Hypokalemia
C. Increased sympathetic tone in stress or any illness.
D. Stimulants like caffeine, nicotine
E. Cardiomyopathy
F. Myocardial infarction

Following are the clinical manifestations due to ectopic pace maker:

A. Atrial or ventricular premature contraction
B. Atrial flutter
C. Atrial fibrillation
D. Ventricular tachycardia
E. Ventricular fibrillation

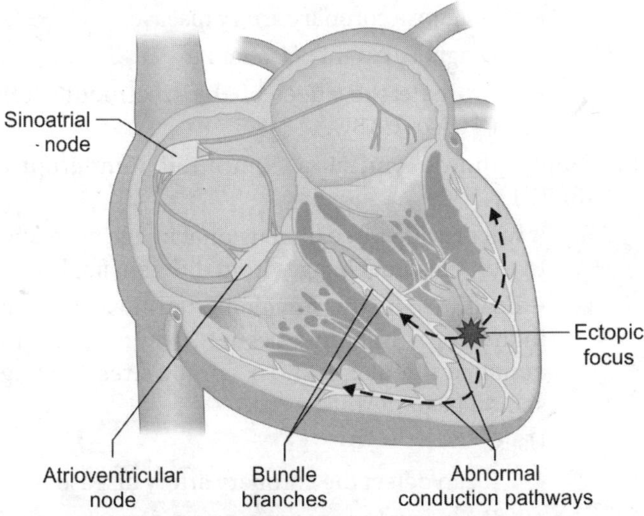

Q119. Purkinje fibers.
MGR UNIVERSITY, TAMIL NADU, 2021 (5)

ANSWER

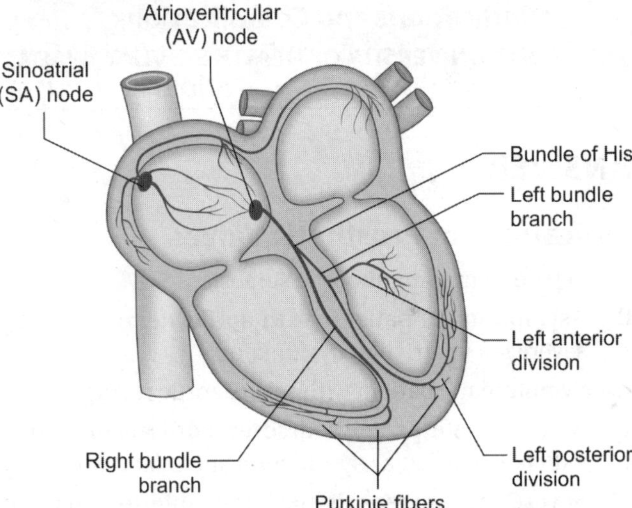

Purkinje fibers run along the inner wall of the both ventricles beneath the endocardium receiving impulses from the atrioventricular node and transmitting to the wall of the ventricles.

Branches: Two main branches—

A. Left bundle branch: It arises from the bundle of His and divides into two branches—
  a. Left anterior fascicle innervates the anterior and superior parts of the left ventricles.
  b. Left posterior fascicle innervates inferior and posterior parts of the left ventricle.

  This branch transmits impulses to throughout the left ventricle and helps to pump the blood out to the systemic circulation.

B. Right bundle branch arising from the bundle of His runs down the right side of interventricular septum and ensures the right ventricle to contract simultaneously with the left ventricle.

C. Terminal purkinje network: As the right and left bundle branches reach the ventricles, they will divide further into smaller numerous branches which will spread deep into the ventricular myocardium.

Functional Role of Purkinje Fibers

These branches ensure that electrical impulses generated from the SA node passing through the AV node then to bundle of his to purkinje fibers will be distributed uniformly throughout the ventricular myocardium.

This synchronous contraction of the both ventricle are responsible for pumping the blood simultaneously to pulmonary artery and aorta.

Q120. Prosthetic cardiac valves—Indications and Complications

NTR UNIVERSITY OF HEALTH SC, VIJAYAWADA, ANDHRA, 2021 (10)

ANSWER

Indications of Prosthetic Valves

A. Severe symptomatic aortic stenosis
B. Asymptomatic patients with aortic stenosis having severe left ventricular dysfunction.
C. Symptomatic patient with severe aortic regurgitation
D. Asymptomatic patient with severe aortic regurgitation with left ventricular dysfunction and dilatation.
E. Severe mitral stenosis not amenable to repair or balloon valvoplasty.
F. Evidence of recurrent embolic events despite prolonged anticoagulation.
G. Severe symptomatic mitral regurgitation.
H. Asymptomatic mitral regurgitation with left ventricular dilatation or reduced ejection fraction.
I. Infection with vegetation leading to destruction of the valve destruction or dysfunction.
J. Bicuspid aortic valve with severe dysfunction.
K. Dysfunction of previous prosthetic valves in the form of structural deterioration and thrombosis or paravalvular leak.

Complications of Prosthetic Valves

A. Thrombosis due to mechanical valves leading to obstruction of the valves resulting heart failure.
B. Thrombus from the valves after being dislodged will travel to the systemic arteries resulting stroke, ischemia of the limbs and other catastrophic events.
C. Anticoagulant related hemorrhage.
D. As the life span of the bioprosthetic valve is 10–15 years, after which the valve will tear or wear or calcified leading to valvular stenosis or regurgitation.
E. Infection of the prosthetic valves may occur within 2 months of surgery which should be hospital acquired or after 2 months of surgery which may come from blood borne infection.
F. There may be paravalvular leak due to improperly set valves or gradual loosening of the valves over time leading to heart failure or microangiopathic hemolytic anemia.
G. Mechanical destruction of the red blood cells leading to Microangiopathic hemolytic anemia.
H. Overgrowth of the tissue over the mechanical valve resulting pannus formation.
I. If the size of the prosthetic valve is relatively small as compared to body size there is suboptimal hemodynamic performance, as a result symptoms of heart failure will persists.
J. Rarely there may be mechanical failure of the mechanical valves like leaflet fracture. Tear or wear.

Q121. Nuclear cardiology.

VEER NARMAD SOUTH GUJARAT UNIVERSITY, 2021 (20)

Role of nuclear medicine in cardiology.

DNB, 2022 (5)

ANSWER

Nuclear cardiology involves nuclear imaging technique for evaluating the cardiac function and perfusion.

Following are the nuclear cardiology procedures:

A. Myocardial perfusion imaging:
   a. It will assess the blood flow to the cardiac muscles at rest as well as under stress.
   b. Procedure: Radiotracer Technetium 99 or thallium 201 is injected and picture will be taken by gamma camera. It will detect the area of reduced perfusion indicating blockage or damages in the coronary artery.
   c. Uses: It can:
      - Diagnose coronary artery disease
      - Diagnose extent of ischemia
      - Evaluate the effect of the treatment after PTCA or CABG.

B. Single photon emission computed tomography (SPECT):
   a. It will provide three dimensional image by taking two dimensional images from different angles.
   b. Procedures: It will provide better images of the infarcted or ischemic tissue. In some cases to enhance the diagnostic accuracy stress testing should be performed also.
   c. Uses:
      - It can detect the coronary artery disease
      - It can localize coronary artery disease
      - It can assess the myocardial viability.
      - It can predict the risk of heart attack.

C. Positron emission tomography:
   a. This highly sensitive technique evaluates viability, perfusion and perfusion of myocardium.

b. Procedure: The tracer used are rubidium 82 and fluorodeoxyglucose. It will provide clearer and high resolution images.
c. Uses:
   1. It can diagnose coronary artery disease.
   2. It can identify viable cardiac tissue for revascularization.
   3. It can assess the metabolic activity of the cardiac muscle cells.

D. Radionucleotide ventriculography:
   a. It can evaluate the pumping function of the heart by detecting the ejection fraction.
   b. Procedures: Here radiolabeled red blood cells are injected to detect the ejection fraction of the heart with each heartbeat.
   c. Uses: It can assess the function of ventricle in:
      1. Cardiomyopathy
      2. Heart failure
      3. Patient undergoing chemotherapy
      4. Patient undergoing radiotherapy.

Benefits of Nuclear Cardiology

A. Non-invasive assessment—it can detect the cardiac function without any invasive procedure.
B. Accurate diagnosis—it is highly sensitive in detecting:
   a. Coronary artery disease
   b. Viability of cardiac muscles
   c. Abnormalities in the perfusion.
C. Early detection prevents cardiac events: Functional perfusion—the procedures can assess performance of the heart by:
   a. Assessing the ejection fraction
   b. Assessing the perfusion of the heart.
D. It can guide the treatment decision by assessing the areas of reduced blood flow or infarcted area thereby provide decision regarding the PTCA or CABG.
E. It can assess the risk stratification based on perfusion defect, function of the heart.
F. Monitoring the treatment effectiveness: It can evaluate the effectiveness of treatment by—
   a. Stenting
   b. Bypass surgery
   c. Medical therapy
G. It will tailor the therapeutic plan
H. It can evaluate the heart failure or cardiomyopathy by assessing cardiac function.
I. It can predict the outcome based on extent of perfusion defect and function of the heart.
J. Radiation exposure is less—it makes safer.

Disadvantages of Nuclear Cardiology

A. In case of repeated exposure the radiation exposure will be increased.
B. The tests are highly expensive.
C. The tests are not available everywhere.
D. The tests take longer time to perform.
E. There may be allergic reaction to the radiotracers.
F. Certain conditions like obesity, breast tissue will interfere with the accuracy of the images.
G. If the patient is not cooperative, in that case this test is difficult to undertake.
H. The procedures requires highly skilled persons and very good interpreter is also necessary.

Q122. Primary angioplasty in acute myocardial infarction.

MAHARASHTRA UNIVERSITY OF HEALTH SCIENCE, 2020 (10)

Discuss indications for percutaneous coronary intervention and describe pre- and post-PTCA management of coronary artery disease.

TEERTHANKER MAHAVEER UNI, 2018 (10)

ANSWER

Key Indications of PTCA

A. Stable angina
B. Acute coronary syndrome:
   a. ST elevated myocardial infarction
   b. Non-ST-elevated myocardial infarction
C. Stress results demonstrating poor blood flow to the cardiac muscles.
D. Unstable angina
E. Angina due to narrowing of the left main stem coronary artery disease
F. In spite of post-coronary artery by-pass surgery there is refractory ischemia
G. Multivessel disease who is not a good candidate of CABG.

Pre-PTCA Assessment in Case of Coronary Artery Disease

A. Evaluation of the case of coronary artery disease:
   a. History and physical examination
   b. Diagnostic tests like:
      1. Electrocardiogram

2. Stress test
3. Echocardiogram
4. Coronary angiography to detect site and extent of coronary artery disease.

c. Medication taken by the patient:
   1. Antiplatelet drugs:
      - Aspirin should be prescribed before the procedure to reduce the risk of clot formation.
      - Clopidogrel or P2Y12 inhibitor may be given before or after the procedure to prevent formation of clot.
   2. Heparin should be given during the procedure to prevent clotting within the tubing.
   3. Statin should be used to stabilize the atherosclerotic plaque and to reduce the cardiovascular risk.

d. Pre-procedural anesthesia:
   1. Patient should be in fasting state for a period of 6 to 8 hours before the procedure it the procedure involves general anesthesia.
   2. The patient should be adequately hydrated if the contrast is used because it will protect the renal function.

e. Risk assessment:
   1. To prevent contrast induced nephropathy, adequate hydration is required because it will eliminate the contrast if it will be given.
   2. Prior to administration of the contrast, the patient should be enquired regarding the history of allergy to any contrast.
   3. Pre-procedural informed consent should be taken after explaining all the details of risk, benefits and possible complications of administering this contrast.

f. Education to the patient:
   1. The detail of the procedure and post-procedural care should be explained to the patient.
   2. Post-procedural care like monitoring of any symptom, any medicine to take and follow-up date.

g. Management of comorbidities:
   1. Hypertension: It should be kept in optimum level to minimize the symptom after or during the procedure.
   2. Diabetes mellitus: It should be controlled to prevent secondary infection.

Post-procedural follow-up:

A. Immediate care:
   a. Monitoring of vital signs like blood pressure, pulse, oxygen saturation.
   b. Site observation: Insertion site should be observed to seen any active bleeding, hematoma or inflammation.
   c. Continuous monitoring should be done to detect any ECG changes suggestive of arrhythmias.

B. Medications:
   a. Continuous therapy with clopidogrel or P2Y12 inhibitor should be administered to prevent stent thrombosis.
   b. Depending upon the stent used and the condition of the patient anticoagulant can be used.
   c. Statin should be continued for indefinite period.

C. To give relief from pain at the insertion site NSAIDs can be given.

D. Life style modification:
   a. Active heavy physical activity should be restricted for at least 24 to 48 hours and mild activity should be restricted.
   b. Following factors should be watched:
      - Balanced regular diet
      - Avoidance of smoking
      - Weight reduction to control.

E. Monitoring of complications like chest pain, severe bleeding, shortness of breath and advice should be given to inform at once any of these will start.

F. Follow-up care:
   a. Based on the risk factors and presence of any symptom, echocardiography, stress test should be advised.
   b. Follow-up visit to the clinic should be done to:
      1. Monitor the rate of recovery
      2. Assess the effectiveness of the procedure
      3. Adjust the medication if required.

G. Long term management:
   a. Patient should be instructed to take the medication prescribed till the next visit.
   b. Cardiac rehabilitation should be advised to aid in recovery.

Q123. Anatomy of conducting system of the heart. Enumerate the causes of bradycardia. Discuss the indications of permanent pacemaker implantation.

DNB 2018 (3+3+4)

ANSWER

Answers in Q41, Q90.

The Causes of Bradycardia

A. Intrinsic causes of bradycardia:
  a. Sick sinus syndrome due to dysfunction of the SA node of the conduction system.
  b. Heart block: It is due to delay or block in the conduction system from sinus node to atrioventricular node.
  c. Ischemic heart disease like myocardial infarction involving the conduction system of the heart.
  d. Myocarditis
  e. Congenital defect in the heart.

B. Extrinsic causes of bradycardia:
  a. Drugs:
    1. Beta blockers
    2. Calcium channel blockers
    3. Digoxin
  b. Electrolyte imbalance:
    1. Hyperkalemia
    2. Hypokalemia
    3. Hypercalcemia
  c. Hypothermia
  d. Hypothyroidism
  e. Increased vagal tone: Stimulation of parasympathetic nervous system by:
    1. Deep sleep
    2. Deep muscular relaxation
    3. Straining during defecation

C. Neurological causes:
  a. Increased intracranial pressure by:
    1. Brain tumor
    2. Intracranial hemorrhage
  b. Disorder of autonomic nervous system:
    1. Vasovagal syncope
    2. Autonomic failure

D. Systemic causes of bradycardia:
  a. Severe hypoxia depressing the cardiac activity
  b. Obstructive sleep apnea

E. Athlete

Q124. Classify oral anticoagulants. Describe their indications and contraindications.

DNB, 2018 (10)

Newer oral anticoagulants.

DNB, 2021 (5), DNB, 2019 (5)
BHARATI VIDYAPEETH UNIVERSITY, 2016 (10)
TEERTHANKER MAHAVEER UNI, 2017(10)

Target specific oral anticoagulant.

BHARATI VIDYAPEETH UNIVERSITY, 2019 (10)

Newer anticoagulants.

NTR UNIVERSITY OF HEALTH SC, VIJAYAWADA, ANDHRA, 2020 (10)

Enumerate the causes of non-valvular causes of atrial fibrillation. Discuss the role of various NOACs and bleeding risk assessment tools.

WEST BENGAL UNIVERSITY OF HEALTH SCIENCE, 2020 (10)

Novel oral anticoagulant.

SRI GURU RAMDAS UNI OF HEALTH SC, 2022 (10)

Oral anticoagulants.

RAJASTHAN UNIVERSITY, 2018 (10)
MANIPUR UNIVERSITY, 2018 (10)

ANSWER

Oral anticoagulant can be classified into following groups:

A. Vitamin K antagonists: It inhibits the synthesis of vitamin K dependent clotting factors like factors. Drug is warfarin.

B. Direct oral anticoagulants:
  a. Direct factor Xa inhibitors: It will directly inhibit the activated factor X, an essential component of coagulation cascade which is responsible for conversion of prothrombin to thrombin. The drugs are:
    1. Rivaroxaban
    2. Edoxaban
    3. Apixaban
  b. Direct thrombin inhibitors: This drug is responsible for inhibiting thrombin which converts fibrinogen to fibrin.
    1. Dabigatran

Indications for oral anticoagulants:

A. Vitamin K antagonists:
  a. Atrial fibrillation
  b. Prosthetic heart valves
  c. Deep vein thrombosis
  d. Pulmonary embolism
  e. Stroke prevention

B. Direct factor Xa inhibitors:
 a. Atrial fibrillation
 b. Deep vein thrombosis
 c. Pulmonary embolism
 d. Postoperative thrombo-prophylaxis
 e. Stroke prevention
C. Direct thrombin inhibitors:
 a. Atrial fibrillation
 b. Deep vein thrombosis
 c. Pulmonary embolism
 d. Stroke prevention

Contraindications for oral anticoagulants:
A. Active bleeding in case of:
 a. Active peptic ulcer disease
 b. Severe trauma
 c. Recent major surgery
 d. Uncontrolled hypertension
B. Severe impairment of liver leading to decreased production of clotting factors
C. Severe renal impairment with effective GFR of less than 15 mL/min leading to decreased rate of clearance of oral anticoagulants.
D. Pregnancy: These drugs cross the placenta leading development of fetal harm and increased of fetal hemorrhage.
E. Drug hypersensitivity.
F. Mechanical heart valves due to increased risk of thromboembolic events.
G. Recent hemorrhagic stroke
H. Severe uncontrolled hypertension with systolic blood pressure of more than 180 mm Hg and diastolic blood pressure of more than 110 mm Hg.
I. Recent surgery to spinal cord, brain, eyes those getting epidural anesthesia, having high risk of bleeding.
J. Thrombocytopenia
K. Endocarditis as there is increased risk of hemorrhagic complications.
L. Alcohol abuse as there may be already liver function impairment leading to increased risk of bleeding.

Different bleeding risk assessment tools:
A. HAS-BLED score:
 a. It can assess the bleeding risk in patient with atrial fibrillation who is on oral anticoagulant.
 b. Following factors are assessed:
  1. Hypertension
  2. Stroke
  3. History of bleeding
  4. Abnormal liver function test
  5. Abnormal renal function test
  6. Elderly
  7. Drugs
  8. Alcohol
  9. Labile INR
 C. It is simple and widely used
 D. Limitation is that this score overemphasizes the modifiable risk factors
B. ORBIT score:
 a. Following factors are assessed:
  1. Patient of more than 74 years of age
  2. Low hemoglobin
  3. Low hematocrit
  4. Insufficient renal function
  5. History of bleeding
  6. Treatment with platelets
 b. It is better for identifying the source of bleeding.
 c. Its use is limited in clinical practice.
C. ATRIA score:
 a. Factors assessed:
  1. Age ≥ 75 years
  2. Prior history of bleeding
  3. Hypertension
  4. Severely compromised renal function
 b. Here anemia is the key factor
 c. It is less specific.
D. ABC score:
 a. Factors used: clinical factors, hemoglobin, GDF-15 and troponin, age
 b. Its accuracy is improved due to use of biomarkers.
 c. Here laboratory testing is required.

Q125. Classify and enumerate the causes of cardiomyopathy. Write short notes on Takotsubo cardiomyopathy.

DNB, 2021 (1+4+5)

Brugada syndrome. Add a note on Takotsubo cardiomyopathy.

NTR UNIVERSITY OF HEALTH SC, VIJAYAWADA, ANDHRA, AUGUST 2020 (10)

Brugada syndrome discussed in Q144.

Takotsubo cardiomyopathy.

NTR UNIVERSITY OF HEALTH SC, VIJAYAWADA, ANDHRA, NOVEMBER 2022 (10)

SRI GURU RAMDAS UNI OF HEALTH SC, AMRITSAR, 2022 (10)

ANSWER

Notation	M **Morpho-functional Phenotype**	O **Organ/system Involvement**	G **Genetic inheritance Pattern**	E **Etiology**	S **Stage**

Characteristics	Proband's cardiomyopathy (CM) diagnosis (DCM, HCM, RCM, ARVC/D, LVNC)	Clinical history and evaluation
		- Organ involvement: Extracardiac organs/tissues
		- Multidisciplinary evaluation according per clinical needs or diagnostic hypothesis
			Genetic counseling with pedigree
			- Familial
			  - Inheritance AD, AR XL (R or D) or Matrilineal
			- Non-familial; Phenotypically sporadic
			  - Informative and non-informative families
			  - Consultant non-informed about family history
			Clinical family screening
			- Affected, asymptomatic relative unaware of the disease
			- Relatives with ECG and/or Echo abnormalities
			- Healthy family members with normal ECG and Echo
				Genetic testing in the proband
				- Positive
				  - Cascade genetic testing in relatives
				- Negative
				  - New tests novel genes
				  - Regular monitoring in relatives
					Functional status ACC/AHA, NYHA

Subscript	D Dilated H Hypertrophic R Restrictive R EMF Endomyocardial fibrosis LV = left ventricle RV = right ventricle RLV = biventricular A ARVC M = major m = minor c = category LV = left ventricle RV = right ventricle RLV = biventricular NC LVNC E Early, with type in parentheses NS Nonspecific phenotype NA Information nonavailable O Unaffected	H Heart LV = left ventricle RV = right ventricle RLV = biventricular M Muscle (skeletal) N Nervous C Cutaneous E Eye, Ocular A Auditory K Kidney G Gastrointestinal Li Liver Lu Lung S Skeletal O Absence of organ/system involvement e.g., in family members who are healthy mutation carriers; the mutation is specified in E and inheritance in G	N Family history negative U Family history unknown AD Autosomal dominant AR Autosomal recessive XLD X-linked dominant XLR X-linked recessive XL X-linked M Matrilineal O Family history not investigated Under inheritance still undetermined S Phenotypically sporadic (apparent or real)	G Genetic cause OC Obligate carrier ONC Obligate non-carrier DN De novo Neg Genetic test negative for the known familial mutation N Genetic defect not identified O No genetic test, any reason G-A-TTR Genetic amyloidosis G-HFE Hemochromatosis *Non-genetic etiologies:* M Myocarditis V Viral infection (add the virus identified in affected heart) AI Autoimmune/immunemediate; suspected (AI-S), proven (AI-P) A Amyloidosis (add type: A-K, A-L, A-SAA) I Infectious, non viral (add the infectious agent) T Toxicity (add cause/drug) Eo Hypereosinophilic heart disease O Other	ACC-AHA stage represented as letter A, B,C, D NA not applicable NU not used followed by NYHA class represented as roman numeral I, II, III, IV

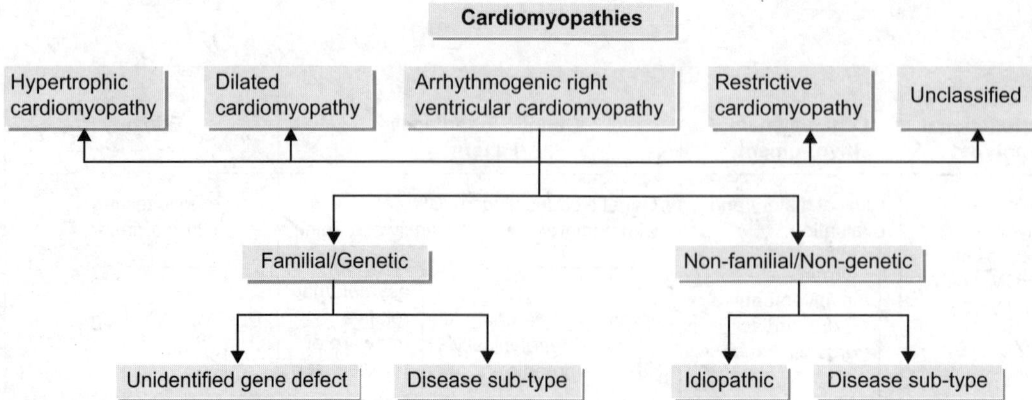

Takotsubo Cardiomyopathy

It is also known as stress induced cardiomyopathy or broken heart syndrome.

Pathophysiology

The exact mechanism is not clear, but it may be due to excessive release of catecholamine leading to myocardial stunning in absence of coronary obstruction resulting left ventricular apical ballooning seen in echocardiography or ventriculography. The stress may be due to:

A. Emotional stress

B. Physical stress like trauma or surgery

Other causes may be coronary artery spasm or microvascular dysfunction.

Estrogen has protective effects on the myocardium like vasodilation, protection against endothelial dysfunction and atherosclerosis. Hence in postmenopausal women suffer from this disease because of loss of protective effects.

Acute exacerbation of chronic inflammation may lead to emergence of this disease.

Risk Factors

A. Domestic abuse

B. Death of relatives

C. Accident

D. Major trauma

E. Natural calamities

F. Arguments

G. Financial loss

H. Diagnosis of acute medical illness

I. Stimulant drugs like cocaine or amphetamines

Clinical Features

A. Chest pain

B. Shortness of breath

C. Syncope

Following key features are required for the diagnosis of this disease:

A. Transient hypokinesia, akinesia or dyskinesia of the mid segment of left ventricles with or without the involvement of apex, abnormalities in the regional wall motion that extend beyond.

B. A stressful trigger may be single epicardial vascular distribution.

C. Absence of coronary artery disease or no evidence of acute plaque rupture.

D. Modest elevation of troponin or new ECG evidence of ST segment elevation with or without T wave inversion.

E. Absence of myocarditis or pheochromocytoma.

Diagnosis

A. ECG may demonstrate dynamic pattern of electrocardiographic changes like

- **a.** stage 1: ST segment elevation
- **b.** stage 2: Normalization of ST elevation
- **c.** stage 3: T wave inversion
- **d.** stage 4: Normalization of T wave or persistent inverted T wave.

B. Coronary angiography demonstrates no evidence of coronary obstruction.

C. Echocardiography demonstrated:

- **a.** Apical type—it is common:
  1. Systemic apical ballooning of left ventricle
  2. Depressed mid and apical segments
  3. Hyperkinesia of basal walls
- **b.** Apical variants:
  1. Mid-ventricular hypokinesia
  2. Basal type hypokinesia
  3. Focal type hypokinesia

D. Cardiac biomarkers demonstrated: Mildly elevated troponin.

E. Cardiac MRI demonstrates absence of myocardial scarring.

Management

A. Treatment of heart failure with ACEI, beta blockers or diuretics.
B. This disease will resolve within weeks and function of left ventricle will normalize.

Complications

A. Arrhythmias
B. Cardiogenic shock
C. Death
D. Recurrences of this disease.

Q126. Holiday heart syndrome.

DNB, 2022 (5)

ANSWER

Definition

It is characterized by evidence of arrhythmias following binge alcohol drinking in holiday or at the weekend.

Pathophysiology

A. Direct effect on the cardiac tissue: Alcohol has direct toxic depressant effect on the cardiac myocyte and also different cardiac channels.
B. Alcohol increases the atrial ectopy leading development of atrial fibrillation.
C. Alcohol due to its diuretic effect, produces dehydration along with hypokalemia and hypomagnesemia both of which may lead to enhanced arrhythmogenicity in the atria.
D. Ingestion of large quantity of alcohol activates the sympathetic nervous system resulting high levels of catecholamine levels in the blood which ultimately provoke arrhythmia.
E. Alcohol initiates inflammatory response in the heart leading to myocarditis which initiates and maintenance of arrhythmias.
F. Autonomic imbalance in case of alcohol drinking leads to increased sympathetic activation resulting arrhythmias.
G. Oxidative stress resulting from generation of reactive oxygen species damages the cardiac cells interfering the cardiac conduction.
H. Alcohol induced atrial remodeling will lead to chronic atrial fibrillation.
I. Alcohol induced vasodilatation will lead to decreased blood pressure and compensatory increased heart rate.

Clinical Features

A. Chest discomfort
B. Shortness of breath
C. Dizziness
D. Palpitation—transient or persistent.

Physical examination demonstrates:

A. Impaired mental status
B. Tachycardia
C. Hypotension
D. Pulse thread and irregular
E. Elevated jugular venous pressure
F. In case dilated cardiomyopathy there are signs of heart failure
G. Lower extremity edema
H. Tender hepatomegaly

Laboratory Tests

A. Hypomagnesemia
B. Hypokalemia
C. Complete blood count demonstrate—low red blood cells, white blood cells and platelet count.
D. Electrocardiogram and telemetry monitoring
E. Chest X-ray
F. Echocardiography

Management

A. Abstinence from alcohol
B. Heart rate is controlled by beta blockers and calcium channel blocker
C. Cardioversion may be required for rhythm control
D. Atrial fibrillation if lasts for more than 48 hours, anticoagulation should be given.

Complications

A. Life threatening arrhythmias
B. Persistent or chronic atrial fibrillation
C. Embolic stroke and systemic thromboembolism
D. Dilated cardiomyopathy
E. Congestive heart failure
F. Community acquired pneumonia
G. Death

Q127. Biosensors in hypertension.

DNB, 2022 (5)

ANSWER

Following biosensors are used in hypertension:

A. Wearable biosensors:
   a. Smart watches and wristbands: This optical sensors are used in:
      1. Measuring the blood pressure
      2. Analyzing the velocity of pulse waves
      3. Monitoring the variability of heart rate
   b. Skin patch biosensors: This flexible and adhesive biosensors are used in:
      1. Continuous tracking of blood pressure
      2. Integrating the vital signs like body temperature, heart rate and blood oxygen levels.

B. Implantable biosensors: This small implantable device is used for:
   a. Direct monitoring of blood pressure
   b. Communicating with the external devices for providing the data of blood pressure continuously without intervention of the patient.

C. Microfluidic biosensors: These will analyze the biomarkers in the body fluids like sweat and blood to detect any alteration in correlation with the change in the blood pressure. As, for example, serum sweat level will correlate with the blood pressure as it will be high in case of hypertension.

D. Electrochemical biosensors: It will detect a specific biomarker, i.e., nitric oxide that regulate the blood pressure and its alteration correlates with the hypertensive incident.

Advantages of the Biosensors

A. Biosensors continuously monitor the blood pressure round the clock to provide real time data so that proper timely intervention can be done.

B. Most of the biosensors are non-invasive or minimally invasive so that the patient does not feel discomfort with these biosensors.

C. The data from biosensors with be integrated with the digital platforms so that proper timely intervention plan can be made according to the pattern of changes.

D. The data of the biosensors can be provided to the healthcare providers through the telemedicine procedure so that treatment protocol can be made and remote monitoring of the patients are also done.

Disadvantages of the Biosensors

A. Calibration and accuracy:
   a. Wearable biosensors measure blood pressure through the measurement of the pulse velocity that may not be accurate as compared to the cuff based measurement of blood pressure.
   b. Sometimes temperature, skin contact or movement can affect the sensor accuracy.
   c. Wearable sensors should be regularly calibrated to maintain the accuracy as far as possible.

B. Cost of the biosensors:
   a. Biosensors that integrate with the telemedicine implantable devices or microfluidic are very much expensive and these have limited accessibility to the general populations.
   b. Again, maintenance of the device, replacement cost, software cost and its updates are highly expensive.

C. Limited long term reliable data and its impaction on the measurement of hypertension are not available, though these are very much popular. Again, many new biosensors are not validated in clinical trials and approved by the regulatory agencies.

D. Discomfort with wearing the biosensors:
   a. Many biosensors after wearing may produce skin irritation, allergic reaction with the skin.
   b. Sometimes the patient may feel discomfort wearing the bulky intrusive biosensors, again these require regular checking and changing.

E. Security concerns:
   a. Data collected from the biosensors will be transmitted to the cloud based system thereby the privacy of the collected data can be lost.
   b. The different platform and format used by different biodata lead to interoperability issue as a result, sharing the data between the devices are very much difficult.

F. Over acceptability on the technology:
   a. In some cases continuous monitoring of the patients may lead to false positivity, which may in turn lead to extra-alertness to that patient on the part of the healthcare providers as well as to the patient's party.
   b. Some contextual factors may not the recorded by the devices that may result in incomplete data collection:
      1. Psychological stress
      2. Adherence to the medications
      3. Life style factors

G. Batter life and power:

a. Battery life is a major hindrance in the wearable biosensors will require frequent recharge.

b. In some remote areas or during travel for long distance power supply wuill be a major hindrance.

H. Daily life activities interference:

a. Some biosensors may interfere with the physical activities or sleep.

b. In some cases biosensors may be a social stigma may not be aesthetically pleasant.

Clinical Applications

A. Biosensors can differentiate white coat hypertension from real hypertension by observing the real time data from the biosensors.

B. The data from biosensors can help the start the antihypertensive medication in a patient and also to monitor adjust the medications in the hypertensive patients.

C. It can also tract the healthcare providers to search for the cardiovascular risk factors in newly diagnosed hypertensive patient.

Q128. Subclinical atherosclerosis assessment in clinical practice.

DNB, 2022 (5)

How can you assess the subclinical atherosclerosis in clinical practice? Briefly discuss about the recent drugs used in heart failure.

WBUHS, 2025 (10)

ANSWER

Drugs in heart failure has been describe in the question of heart failure in question number 22 and 114.

Subclinical atherosclerosis is characterized by early stage of the disease where there is structural changes in the wall of arteries but there is no obvious clinical symptom. It can be assessed by the following methods:

A. Carotid intima-media thickness: It can be measured by the measuring the thickness of the inner 2 layers of the artery by ultrasound. Increased thickness is associated with the high risk of cardiovascular disease.

a. The measurement site is common carotid artery 1 cm proximal to its bifurcation.

Values:

a. Normal value is less than 0.6 cm.

b. Thickness between 0.6 and 1 cm—indicates early atherosclerosis—suggestive of intermediate cardiovascular risk.

c. If thickness is more than 1 cm—indicates advanced atherosclerosis.

Clinical importance:

a. It can diagnose subclinical atherosclerosis prior to appearance of symptom.

b. It can detect progress or regression of atherosclerosis in response to style changes or treatment of statin therapy.

B. Coronary artery calcium scoring: In this method, by the CT scan calcium can be quantified in the calcium plaques in the wall of the artery. A specialized software can measure the amount of calcium to provide total calcium score.

a. 0: Undetectable calcium

b. 1-99: Mild calcium build up—it is associated with low to moderate risk.

c. 100-399 indicates moderate amount of calcium—associated with moderate to high risk.

d. ≥ 400: Indicates high amount of calcium—it is associated with high risk.

Clinical importance:

a. It can stratify the risk.

b. High score is associated with high risk of cardiovascular diseases.

c. It can guide the static therapy. If the score is 0—no statin is needed, but if >100—indicates the initiation of statin therapy.

Limitations:

a. It cannot assess the non-calcified plaque.

b. There is risk of radiation exposure.

C. Ankle-brachial index: It can assess the peripheral vascular disease by comparing the ankle blood pressure with arm blood pressure by ultrasound or automated oscillometric device.

Ankle brachial index: Ankle blood pressure/arm blood pressure.

Value:

a. Normal value: 1-1.4—indicates no significant obstruction in the peripheral arteries.

b. Borderline value: 0.91-0.99—it indicates early peripheral artery disease.

c. Abnormal value: ≤0.90—it indicates significant reduction of blood flow through the peripheral arteries.

d. High value: ≥1.4—it indicates stiff or calcified non-compressible arteries seen in chronic kidney disease or diabetes. In this case toe-brachial index is required.

Clinical importance:

a. It can detect early peripheral artery disease and is associated with high risk of cardiovascular disease or strokes.

b. Low index is associated with increased independent cardiovascular risk.

D. Pulse wave velocity: It will measure the aortic wall stiffness by non-invasive method like tonometry. It can be calculated as:

Distance in meters/Transit time in seconds. Result is expressed in meter/second.

Value:

a. Normal value: 6–10 m/s

b. Increased value: Value more than 10 m/s indicates increased cardiovascular risk.

Clinical importance:

a. It indicates the increased stiffness of the arterial wall which is independent of cardiovascular risk.

b. It can detect the subclinical atherosclerosis before the clinical hypertension or cardiovascular disease will appear.

E. High resolution MRI: It can provide detailed imaging of the arterial wall:

a. Assess the plaque burden.

b. It can assess the composition of the plaque.

Clinical importance:

a. Early changes in the arterial wall prior to its calcification.

b. It will provide the comprehensive report regarding the vulnerability of the plaque.

But as it is operator dependent, it requires specialized training.

F. Flow mediated dilatation: It will measure the endothelial function in response to increased blood flow.

Clinical importance:

Method: Blood pressure cuff is inflated around the forearm for 5 minutes to occlude the blood flow. After dilatation there is surge in the flow of blood, it can evaluate the extent of dilatation. It can be calculated as:

(Post-occlusion diameter—Baseline diameter)/ Baseline diameter.

Values:

a. Normal value: It can dilate ≥ 10% in response to increased blood flow.

b. Impaired value: If the value is less than 7–10% indicates impaired endothelial function which may be associated with increased risk of cardiovascular disease.

Clinical importance:

a. It can detect early atherosclerosis which precedes the plaque formation.

b. It can monitor the early endothelial dysfunction especially in response to therapeutic intervention.

Q129. Targeted temperature management following cardiac arrest.

DNB, 2022 (5)

ANSWER

Targeted temperature, i.e., therapeutic hypothermia in the range of 32–36°C for a definite period is a therapeutic intervention after an episode of cardiac arrest in order to improve neurological recovery as well as to reduce the mortality.

Key aspect of targeted temperature management:

A. It is indicated in comatose patient after return to spontaneous circulation following an episode of cardiac arrest especially resulting from ventricular fibrillation or pulseless ventricular tachycardia.

B. Mechanism of action:

a. It will reduce the metabolic demand of the targeted tissue

b. It will slow the neurological damage

c. It will decrease the inflammatory response following global ischemia and reperfusion injury.

C. It has three phases:

a. Phase of induction: In this phase cooling has to be started by different cooling devices like
   - External cooling devices like cooling blankets, Ice
   - Internal cooling processes like intravascular cooling catheters and infusion of cold saline.

b. Phase of maintenance: Target temperature 32–36°C should be maintained for 24–36 hours.

c. Phase of rewarming: In this phase controlled rewarming at a rate of 0.25–0.5°C hourly to prevent electrolyte shift and hemodynamic instability.

D. Complications are the following:
  a. Arrhythmias
  b. Coagulopathies
  c. Infections
  d. Electrolyte imbalances

  So, monitoring of targeted temperature management is essential and in required management of the complications are essential.

E. Prognosis: This management improves the survival of the patient, but it will vary according to the characteristic of the patient and specific range of temperature used.

Q130. Pulsus alternans.

DNB, 2019 (4)

ANSWER

Pulsus Alternans

In this pulse there is alternate strong and weak beats suggesting alternate strong and weak force of cardiac pump.

Etiology

It suggests severe left ventricular systolic and diastolic dysfunction like:

A. Dilated cardiomyopathy
B. Coronary artery disease leading to left ventricular dysfunction
C. Severe aortic stenosis.
D. Heart failure

Clinical Implications

A. It is valuable sign of severe heart failure
B. It indicates poor prognosis.
C. It can be detected by measurement with blood pressure cuff or invasively by arterial catheter.

Q131. Etiology of atrioventricular block.

RAJIV GANDHI UNI OF HEALTH SC, KARNATAKA, 2016 (10)

Stoke-Adams attacks.

TEERTHANKER MAHAVEER UNI, 2017 (10)

ANSWER

Normally P wave is followed by QRS complex with fixed PR interval of 120 to 200 milliseconds. But in case of atrioventricular block the interval will be increased due to delay in conduction of electrical impulse from atria to ventricle.

Etiology of Atrioventricular Block

A. Congenital atrioventricular block:
  a. Congenital heart disease associated with congenital heart diseases:
    1. Transposition of great arteries
      - Atrioventricular canal defect
      - Left atrial isomerism
      - Tetralogy of Fallot
      - Heterotaxy syndrome
  b. Congenital atrioventricular defect not associated with congenital heart diseases:
    1. Immune mediated dysfunction of conduction system in the heart like SLE.
    2. Maternal viral infection

B. Acquired heart block:
  a. Myocardial ischemia/infarction
  b. Drugs:
    1. Digoxin
    2. Nondihydropyridine calcium channel blockers
    3. Beta blockers
    4. Class I and III antiarrhythmic drugs
    5. Lithium
    6. Donepezil
    7. Adenosine
  c. Electrolyte imbalance
  d. Endocrine disorders
  e. Toxins
  f. Age related degeneration of the conduction system
  g. Chronic idiopathic fibrosis like Lenegre disease, Lev disease.
  h. Vagal mediated block—it is nodal in origin.
  i. Myocarditis
  j. Lyme disease
  k. Infiltrative cardiomyopathies
  l. Rheumatic fever
  m. Infective endocarditis
  n. Aortic and mitral valve surgeries
  o. Trans-catheter aortic valve replacement

History and Physical Examinations

A. History related to the etiologies as described above.

B. Signs:

a. Mobitz type 1 second degree AV block is asymptomatic and it can be diagnosed by 12-lead ECG.

b. Symptoms are usually:

1. Dyspnea
2. Easy fatigability
3. Dizziness
4. Syncope

c. Physical examination in heart block:

1. Bradycardia
2. Irregular pulse
3. Hypotension
4. Presence of distended neck veins like giant "a" wave.

Classification of Atrioventricular Block

A. 1st degree AV block—it is characterized by the following features:

a. 1:1 association between P and QRS complex

b. Constant PR interval of more than 200 milliseconds.

c. Absence of any dropped beat

d. If the delay is more than 300 milliseconds then it is known as "marked" 1st degree atrioventricular block and P wave will be buried within preceding T wave.

B. Second degree AV block occurs due to intermittent AV conduction. It can be further classified into following 2 types:

a. Mobitz type 1 block—it is characterized by the following:

1. P wave exhibits constant rate of less than 100 beats/min.
2. Gradual prolongation of PR interval followed by a non-conducted P wave.
3. This is also known as Wenckebach phenomenon occurring at the site of AV node.

b. Mobitz type II block: It is characterized by the following:

1. P wave exhibits constant rate of less than 100 beats/min.
2. There is non-conducted of P wave at unpredictable interval.
3. Other P wave appear before and after non-conducted P wave and there is constant PR interval.
4. At least two consecutive P wave demonstration should be required to differentiate Wenckebach from type II block.

C. Second degree high grade block: It is characterized by:

a. Presence of ≥ 2 consecutive non-conducted P waves demonstrated at constant physiological rate.

b. Presence of AV conduction.

D. Third degree AV block or complete AV block:

a. Here there is block at the atrioventricular node resulting absence of any relation between P wave and QRS complexes. So atria and ventricles contract independently to other.

b. Atrial activity will, i.e., P wave will march through the QRS complexes at a faster rate than ventricles, so after 2 to 3 or more P waves followed by ventricular activity, i.e., QRS complex.

Diagnosis

A. 12 leads electrocardiogram demonstrating the above features.

B. Echocardiography will exclude or confirm the structural heart disease.

C. Cardiac MRI should be done to diagnose active or chronic myocarditis or infiltrative cardiomyopathies.

D. In case of sleep related AV block, this investigation is require to sleep apnea.

E. If the above non-invasive test fails to diagnose this disease, in that case electrophysiological study or implantable loop recorder.

F. Laboratory investigations:

a. Thyroid function test

b. Renal function test

c. Liver functional test

d. Serum electrolytes.

Treatment of Atrioventricular Block

A. Discontinue the any medication responsible for the block should be searched and if present should be stopped.

B. In patient with asymptomatic 1st degree and type 1 2nd degree heart block should not require any medication.

C. Patients with symptomatic high degree block type 2 2nd degree heart block and 3rd degree AV block has greater risk of progress towards asystole, ventricular tachycardia or sudden death, hence these patient require continuous cardiac monitoring.

D. For selecting the medications in high grade type 2nd degree heart block and 3rd degree heart block following parameters should be checked:
  - **a.** Hemodynamic stability
  - **b.** Assessment of systolic blood pressure
  - **c.** Severity and duration of the clinical symptoms
  - **d.** Level of heart block
  - **e.** Presence or absence of escape rhythm

E. In case of acute atrioventricular block:
  - **a.** In case of digoxin therapy, Lyme carditis or AV blocking drug overdose, specific reversal agents or targeted therapy can be administered.
  - **b.** In case of supra-Hisian AV block, intravenous atropine should be considered.
  - **c.** In case of symptomatic patient with 2nd degree AV block or 3rd degree AV block, dopamine or isoproterenol can be considered.
  - **d.** Symptomatic patient not responding to medical therapy or in cardiogenic shock, temporary transvenous pacemaker should be considered. But if the patient requires permanent pacemaker, it is not wise to give transvenous pacemaker initially as it may acquire infection.
  - **e.** If temporary pace maker is introduced it should be kept for shorter duration as it may produce:
    1. Infection
    2. Immobility
    3. Thromboembolism
    4. Cardiac perforation

F. Chronic management of AV block:
  - **a.** First degree, type 1 second degree or 2:1 AV block do not require pacemaker usually, hence they should be followed up, if the patient becomes symptomatic, he or she may require treatment.
  - **b.** Permanent pacemaker is the method of threating the following patients:
    1. Symptomatic 2nd degree AV block
    2. Symptomatic high grade 2nd degree AV block.
    3. Third degree AV block
  - **c.** Permanent pace maker along with defibrillator are required in 2nd or 3rd degree heart block associated with:
    1. Infiltrative cardiomyopathy
    2. Muscular dystrophy

d. Dual chamber pacemaker is recommended as compared to single chamber pacemaker according to the current guideline, but later one can be given in patient with atrial fibrillation or other comorbid conditions restricting the implantation of dual chamber pacemaker.

Prognosis

Prognosis depends upon:

A. Hypertension
B. Diabetes mellitus
C. Chronic kidney disease
D. Ischemic heart disease
E. Underlying heart disease

Q132. Electrocardiogram in non-cardiac diseases.

BHARATI VIDYAPEETH UNIVERSITY, WINTER 2016 (10)

ANSWER

A. Hyperkalemia:
  - **a.** Mild hyperkalemia (5.5 to 6.5 meq/L)
    1. Tall peaked T wave
    2. Short QT interval
    3. Flattening of P wave
  - **b.** Moderate hyperkalemia (6.5 to 7.5 meq/L)
    1. Disappearance of P wave
    2. Prolonged PR interval
    3. Depression of ST segment
    4. Continued peaks T wave
  - **c.** Severe hyperkalemia (more than 7.5 meq/L)
    1. More pronounced widened QRS complex
    2. Sine wave pattern—QRS complex combines with T wave
    3. Ventricular arrhythmias
    4. Asystole

B. Hypokalemia:
  - **a.** Prominent U wave in V2 to V4.
  - **b.** Flattened or inverted T wave
  - **c.** Depressed ST segment
  - **d.** Prolonged QT interval

- **e.** Increased risk of arrhythmias:
    1. Premature ventricular beats
    2. Ventricular tachycardia
    3. Ventricular fibrillation
    4. Torsades de pointes

C. Hypercalcemia:
- **a.** Shortened QT interval
- **b.** Shortened ST segment
- **c.** Tall T wave
- **d.** In severe cases J waves (Osborn waves)
- **e.** Sinus bradycardia
- **f.** Prolonged PR interval
- **g.** Wide QRS complex

D. Hypocalcemia:
- **a.** Prolonged QT interval
- **b.** T waves normal
- **c.** ST segment prolonged.
- **d.** Bradycardia
- **e.** Different types of arrhythmias

E. Pulmonary embolism:
- **a.** Sinus tachycardia
- **b.** S3Q3T3
- **c.** Right bundle branch BLOCK
- **d.** Right axis deviation
- **e.** Right atrial enlargement—P pulmonale
- **f.** Low voltage QRS complexes
- **g.** T wave inversion in V1 to V4.

F. Chronic obstructive pulmonary diseases:
- **a.** Low voltage QRS complexes in limb leads
- **b.** Right axis deviation
- **c.** P pulmonale
- **d.** Incomplete or complete right bundle branch block
- **e.** Poor R wave progression in precordial leads
- **f.** Right ventricular hypertrophy
- **g.** Multifocal atrial tachycardia
- **h.** Prolonged QTc interval
- **i.** Atrial arrhythmias

G. Stroke:
- **a.** Prolonged QT interval
- **b.** Flattened T wave in precordial leads
- **c.** Depression or elevation ST segments
- **d.** In subarachnoid hemorrhage prominent U waves
- **e.** In embolic stroke may be atrial fibrillation
- **f.** In cerebral hemorrhage ventricular arrhythmias
- **g.** Sinus tachycardia or sinus bradycardia as a consequence of autonomic dysregulation.
- **h.** In stroke of brainstem heart block
- **i.** In case of secondary hypertension left ventricular hypertrophy

H. Hyperthyroidism:
- **a.** Sinus tachycardia
- **b.** Atrial fibrillation
- **c.** Premature atrial contraction

I. Hypothyroidism:
- **a.** Bradycardia
- **b.** Low voltage QRS complexes
- **c.** Prolonged QT intervals
- **d.** Electrical alternans in case of pericardial effusion

J. Pheochromocytoma:
- **a.** Sinus tachycardia
- **b.** Ventricular tachycardia

K. Hypothermia:
- **a.** Sinus bradycardia
- **b.** PR interval prolonged
- **c.** QT interval prolonged
- **d.** QRS duration prolonged
- **e.** Presence of J wave in precordial leads

L. Sepsis or septic shock:
- **a.** Non-specific ST-T wave changes
- **b.** T inversion
- **c.** Sinus tachycardia

M. Renal failure:
- **a.** ST depression
- **b.** T wave inversion
- **c.** Low voltage QRS complexes

These changes will be resolved after dialysis.

N. Anemia:
- **a.** Sinus tachycardia
- **b.** Non-specific ST-T changes
- **c.** Features of myocardial ischemia

O. Liver disease: In cirrhotic cardiomyopathy
- **a.** QT interval prolonged
- **b.** Different types of arrhythmias

Q133. Biomarkers in heart disease.

BABA FARID UNI OF HEALTH SC, 2017 (10)

ANSWER

The answers are present in Q27, Q22, Q127.

Q134. High altitude systemic hypertension.
BABA FARID UNI OF HEALTH SC, 2017 (10)

ANSWER

High altitude systemic hypertension can be defined as development of hypertension in a person when he or she rises above 8,200 feet.

Mechanism of high altitude systemic hypertension:

A. Hypoxia induced vasoconstriction in the systemic and pulmonary vessels occurs with decrease in the partial pressure of oxygen in high altitudes. So there is redirection of the blood flow toward the lung which is better oxygenated.

B. Sympathetic nervous system will be activated to increase the heart rate and blood pressure for improving the oxygen delivery to the tissues. This hypertension will be sustained if the patient remains in that altitudes.

C. Hypoxia induced pulmonary vasoconstriction leads to pulmonary hypertension.

Renin-angiotensin-aldosterone system in response to hypoxia will be activated leading to fluid retention thereby increasing the blood pressure.

Following are the risk factors:

A. High altitude pulmonary edema
B. Pre-existing hypertension
C. Long stay in the high altitude
D. Genetic factors

Treatment:

A. Gradual ascent to the high altitudes to mitigate the risk of developing hypertension.

B. Pharmacotherapy ACEI, CCB or ARBs should be administered to treat hypertension.

C. Oxygen should be given to reduce hypoxia associated with generalized vasoconstriction that culminates hypertension.

Q135. Genetic advances in cardiomyopathy.
BABA FARID UNI OF HEALTH SC, 2017 (10)

Discuss genetic advances in cardiomyopathy.
WBUHS, 2024 (10)

ANSWER

Genetic advances in cardiomyopathies include knowing the etiology, diagnosis and therapies for that disease. These are the genetic following advances in cardiomyopathies:

A. Identification of the genes responsible for cardiomyopathies:

- **a.** In case of HOCM mutation of the following genes encoding the sarcomere proteins leading to defect in the contraction of the heart:
  1. MYH7 (Myosin heavy chain)
  2. MYBPC3 (Myosin binding protein C
  3. TNNT2 (Troponin 2)
- **b.** In case of dilated cardiomyopathy mutation of the following genes encoding cytoskeletal and nuclear envelope protein:
  1. LMNA—encodes lamin A/C
  2. TTN encoding titin

B. Next generation sequencing:

- **a.** It help in comprehensive screening of the multiple gene at a time.
- **b.** It can identify rare genetic variant
- **c.** It will provide better genotype to phenotype correlations like:
  - Mutation of *MYH7* genes is associated with risk of sudden cardiac death and more severe hypertrophy.
  - Mutation of gene *MYBPC3* is associated with more benign course in case of HOCM.

C. Gene therapy in case of cardiomyopathy is an ongoing research which includes:

- **a.** Use of CRISPR-Cas9 to edit and to correct mutation in the sarcomere genes.
- **b.** Replacement of *TTN* or *LMNA* genes can be done to correct the dilated cardiomyopathy.

D. Clinical implications of genetic advancement in cardiomyopathies:

- **a.** Through the family screening the family members at risk can be identified.
- **b.** Genetic advances helps us to personalize the therapy like selection of the patients for specific pharmacologic intervention.

E. Future implications:

- **a.** Pharmacogenetics: Specific genetic mutations can affect the responses to therapies based on this targeted therapies can be settled.
- **b.** Stem cell therapy can be started to regenerate the damaged myocardium.

Q136. Stokes–Adams attack.

TEERTHANKER MAHAVEER UNI, 2017 (10)

Conduction system of heart, Management of complete heart block.

SAMS (ODISHA), 2021 (10)

ANSWER

Conduction system of heart described in question number 41.

Stokes–Adams Syndrome

Definition

It can be defined as transient loss of consciousness due to dramatic drop of the cardiac output as a result of complete heart block producing reduced blood flow to the brain.

Etiology

A. Complete heart block
B. High grade type 2 second degree heart block
C. Sinus node dysfunction
D. Sick sinus syndrome
E. Paroxysmal ventricular tachycardia
F. Paroxysmal ventricular fibrillation
G. Drug induced bradyarrhythmias

Pathophysiology

Main pathophysiology is reduced stroke volume due to bradycardia or asystole resulting transient hypoperfusion of the brain. If the reduced cardiac output is 3 to 5 seconds there is transient unconsciousness whereas prolonged asystole for more than 10 to 15 seconds, there will be seizures.

Clinical Features

A. Transient and sudden loss of consciousness.
B. Due to decreased cardiac output, there will be pallor.
C. Prolonged asystole leads to occurrence of seizures.
D. During this episode of transient unconsciousness there may be extreme bradycardia or prolonged asystole.
E. But postsyncopal attack, the patient will regain consciousness with flushed face due to increased cardiac output.

Diagnosis

A. Electrocardiographic features:
- **a.** Extreme bradycardia
- **b.** Complete atrioventricular block with escape rhythm
- **c.** Intermittent high grade 2nd degree AV block
- **d.** May be presence of paroxysmal ventricular arrhythmias.

B. 24 hours Holter monitoring demonstrates different types of arrhythmias.
C. Electrophysiological study demonstrates the site of block in case of unexplained syncope.
D. Echocardiography demonstrates cause of this block.
E. To exclude metabolic cause:
- **a.** Serum electrolytes
- **b.** Thyroid function test

F. In case of drug toxicity serum level of the offending drug.

Treatment

A. Acute management:
- **a.** 0.5 mg atropine has to administer intravenously over 3 to 5 minutes to increase heart rate.
- **b.** Intravenous isoproterenol to increase the heart rate.
- **c.** In case of symptomatic patient transvenous pace maker.

B. Definite management:
- **a.** Implantation of permanent pacemaker as 1st line of treatment in case of complete AV block or severe arrhythmias.
- **b.** In case of ventricular arrhythmias implantable cardioverter defibrillator.

Q137. Calcium channel blockers.

BHARATI VIDYAPEETH UNIVERSITY, SUMMER 2016 (10)

MGR UNI, TAMIL NADU, 2017 (5)

ANSWER

Calcium channel blockers can be classified into two types based on the activity on the cardiac tissue or vascular tissue:

A. Dihydropyridine group: These drugs act on vascular smooth muscle cells of the vessels to produce vasodilatation. The drugs are:
- **a.** Amlodipine
- **b.** Nifedipine
- **c.** Felodipine

Indications for use:
- **a.** Hypertension

b. Chronic stable angina
c. Prinzmetal angina
d. Raynaud's phenomenon

B. Non-dihydropyridine group which act on the cardiac tissue leading to actions on cardiac conduction and contraction:
a. Verapamil—acts on cardiac smooth muscle cells
b. Diltiazem—acts both vascular and cardiac smooth muscle cells.

Indications for use:
a. Angina pectoris
b. Atrial flutter, atrial fibrillation
c. Supraventricular tachycardia
d. In some cases hypertension.

Mechanism of Actions

These drugs block the "L" type calcium channels in the cardiac and vascular smooth muscle cells by reducing the calcium ion intracellular level, thereby:

a. Dihydropyridine group of drugs decrease the peripheral vascular resistance leading to decrease in the systemic blood pressure
b. Non-dihydropyridine group of drugs decrease the heart rate, decrease the cardiac contractility and slower the atrioventricular nodal conduction.

Adverse Effects

A. Dihydropyridine group of drugs:
a. Peripheral edema
b. Headache, flushing
c. Reflex tachycardia

B. Non-dihydropyridine group of drugs:
a. Bradycardia
b. Atrioventricular block
c. Exacerbation of heart failure
d. Verapamil leads to constipation
e. Hypotension leading to dizziness

Contraindication to their Uses

A. Dihydropyridine:
a. Severe aortic stenosis
b. Severe hypotension
c. Cardiogenic shock

B. Non-dihydropyridine group of drugs:
a. Cardiac conduction disturbances
b. Sick sinus syndrome
c. Hypotension
d. Heart failure with reduced ejection fraction

Q138. Cardiomyopathies.

KERALA UNIVERSITY, APRIL 2018 (10)

ANSWER

Question 7, 35, 60, 135, 106.

Q139. Atrial flutter.

NTR UNIVERSITY OF HEALTH SC, VIJAYAWADA, ANDHRA, 2022 (10)A

ANSWER

Atrial flutter is a macro-reentrant tachycardia, can be typical or atypical based on its origin.

Etiology

It depends upon the presence of the reentrant mechanism to initiate tachycardia. Its electrical circuit has following circuits:

A. Areas of fast and slow velocities of conduction
B. Different refractory period
C. Functional core system.

Etiology

A. Structural heart disease
B. Hypertension
C. Chronic obstructive pulmonary disease
D. Past history of atrial fibrillation
E. Past history of cardiac surgery for congenital heart disease
F. Hyperthyroidism
G. Holiday heart syndrome

Pathophysiology

Typical flutter originates from right atrium at the level of tricuspid isthmus. Whereas, atypical flutter originates from right or left atrium, superior vena cava or terminal crest and it is non-isthmus dependent.

A. Reentrant mechanism: Atria is activated at a rate of 250–350 beats/min.
B. Ventricular response: As the electrical waves pass through the atrioventricular node—there will be delay due to long refractory period of this node, as a result ventricular response will be 150 beats/min. But this rate will vary according to the parasympathetic

response and as well as refractoriness of atrioventricular node.

C. Atrial-ventricular mismatch: Rapid atrial rate leads to reduced ventricular filling resulting insufficient contraction of the ventricle, thereby produce less cardiac output.

Clinical Features

A. Patient may be asymptomatic
B. Palpitation
C. Lightheadedness
D. Fatigue
E. Shortness of breath in presence of rapid ventricular conduction.
F. Decreased exercise tolerance

In case of rapid ventricular rate:
A. Hypotension
B. Syncope or near-syncope

On physical examination:
A. Irregularly regular pulse or regular pulse
B. Distended internal jugular vein
C. Abdominal distension
D. May be crackles in the both sides of the chest

Evaluation of atrial flutter:
Electrocardiogram:
A. Presence of flutter waves with absence of isoelectric line in between the FLUTTER waves
B. Atrial waves 300 beats/min, ventricular rate 150 beats/min or less, ratio being 2:1, 3:1 or 4:1.
C. In the inferior leads and V1: Flutter waves look like picket fence or saw tooth waves with negative P waves due to direction of vector.
D. R-R interval is regular.

Echocardiogram:
A. Status of atrium—dilated atrium due to chronic fibrosis.
B. Assessment of left ventricular ejection fraction.
C. Persistent tachycardia leads to tachycardia induced cardiomyopathy
D. Evaluation of thrombus in the ventricle as it is more frequently present.

Laboratory evaluation:
A. Thyroid function test
B. Complete blood count to evaluate anemia
C. Arterial blood gases to evaluate hypoxia
D. Evaluation of infection.
E. Pulmonary function test to evaluate ant persistent lung disease.

Treatment:
A. Rhythm control:
   a. It should be divided into two types—acute control and long term management.
      1. In acute setting and the patient is unstable—synchronized cardioversion to convert irregular to regular rhythm and stabilize the patient.
      2. In the stable patient following pharmacologic cardioversion should be administered:
         - Amiodarone
         - Class IA antiarrhythmic drugs: Quinidine, Disopyramide, and Procainamide
         - Class IC antiarrhythmic drugs: Propafenone and flecainide
         - Calcium channel blockers: Verapamil, diltiazem
         - Beta blockers: Metoprolol, Carvidolol and esmolol
B. Rate control:
   a. Beta blockers - Metoprolol to slow the ventricular rate by reducing the AV nodal conduction.
   b. Calcium channel blockers can be administered who cannot tolerate beta blockers.
   c. Digoxin It is less effective in acute control.
C. Administration of anticoagulant to prevent stroke as there is risk of thromboembolism. This should be done based on CHA_2DS_2-VASc score. If the age of the patient is more than 75 years, two extra points should be added.
D. Life style modification:
   a. Treatment and control the hypertension and lung disease if ant.

Q140. Clinical presentation in patients with VSD-PS physiology.
NTR UNIVERSITY OF HEALTH SC, VIJAYAWADA, ANDHRA, 2022 (10)

ANSWER

Following are the clinical manifestations in case of VSD-PS physiology:
A. Cyanosis: It occurs due to right to left heart shunt of deoxygenated blood into systemic circulation in presence of pulmonary stenosis.

B. Digital clubbing due to chronic hypoxemia

C. Weight loss due to increased metabolic demand along with low availability of oxygen.

D. Exercise intolerance due to decreased oxygen delivery to the tissues.

E. Secondary polycythemia due to increased red blood cell production due to chronic hypoxemia.

F. Presence of systolic thrill in the left 2nd intercostal space and left lower border of sternum.

G. Systolic murmur:

- **a.** Harsh systolic murmur is heard on the left lower border of sternum which is increased during inspiration having no radiation.
- **b.** Another localized harsh systolic murmur is heard in the left 2nd intercostal space.

Q141. Transcatheter aortic valve implantation.

GURU GOBIND SINGH, NEW DELHI, APRIL 2018 (10)

What is TAVI? Discuss the outline of management of a case of degenerative aortic stenosis

WEST BENGAL UNIVERSITY OF HEALTH SCIENCE, 2020 (10)

ANSWER

TAVI—it is known as trans-catheter aortic valve implantation, an invasive procedure for treating aortic stenosis

A. Indications:

- **a.** Severe symptomatic aortic stenosis
- **b.** The patient has high risk like extremes of age, other co-morbidities, frailty for aortic valve replacement surgically
- **c.** If the patient has contraindication for surgery like history of previous thoracic surgery, the patient is on radiotherapy.
- **d.** If the patient has history of bicuspid aortic valve disease
- **e.** If the patient has past history of bioprosthetic valve replacement which has been degenerated over time.

B. Disadvantages:

- **a.** Vascular complications like hematoma, bleeding, femoral artery damage
- **b.** There is risk of paravalvular leak
- **c.** After replacement of aortic valve, if there is involvement of left bundle branch leading to conduction disturbances, there may be need of pacemaker also.
- **d.** In case of younger patient the life span of the replaced valves may vary. Hence in these patients, use of this procedure may not be justified.

C. Contraindications:

- **a.** If the patient is of low risk.
- **b.** Following types of unsuitable anatomy:
  1. Heavily calcified annuli
  2. Small aortic annuli
  3. Abnormal size of iliofemoral vessels
- **c.** Presence of calcified bicuspid aortic valve.
- **d.** If the patient has significant coronary artery disease
- **e.** If the patient has severe aortic regurgitation.

D. Procedures:

- **a.** Preoperative evaluation:
  1. Imaging like echocardiography, CT angiography should be done to exclude bicuspid aortic valve, calcified aortic valve, and vascular access
  2. Patient should be evaluated by interventional cardiologist, radiologist, and cardiac surgeons.
- **b.** This operation should be performed under general anesthesia.
- **c.** Following vessels should be approached in this procedure:
  1. Femoral vessels
  2. Subclavian artery
  3. Direct approach to the aortic valve.
- **d.** Deployment of the aortic valve: Catheter with collapsed valve should be mounted over the balloon or self-expandable catheter and advanced to the point of aortic valve. The damaged valve should be either pushed aside or the new valve can be deployed within it by inflating the balloon.
- **e.** Post-procedural care: Immediately echocardiography should be done to confirm the valve replacement in proper position.
- **f.** The patient should be looked for any complications like
  1. Bleeding
  2. Stroke
  3. Any type of heart block
  4. Vascular injury

g. Recovery: In this procedure recovery should be fast.
h. Valve used are:
   1. Self-expanding CoreValve
   2. Balloon expandable Edward valve.

Management of a Case of Degenerative Aortic Stenosis

Assessment of the aortic stenosis:

A. Echocardiography, the gold standard procedure can assess the severity of the stenosis:
   a. Mild aortic stenosis: Valve area more than 1.5 cm^2 and transvalvular mean gradient is more than 20 mm Hg.
   b. Moderate aortic stenosis: Valve area more than 1.0 to 1.5 cm^2 and mean transvalvular gradient is 20 to 40 mm Hg.
   c. Severe aortic stenosis: Valve area less than 1.0 cm^2 and mean transvalvular gradient is more than 40 mm Hg.
B. Assessment of symptoms like chest pain, palpitation, syncope.
C. Evaluation of the following functional status:
   a. NYHA class.
   b. Society of Thoracic Surgeon Risk score using demography, clinical status, surgical variables, physiological parameters and functional status.

Medical management:

A. In case of asymptomatic patient:
   a. Regular monitoring of the aortic valve area by echocardiography by:
      1. Mild stenosis—every 3 to 5 years.
      2. Moderate stenosis—every 1 to 2 years.
      3. Severe stenosis—every 6 to 12 months.
   b Modification of the risk factors:
      1. Smoking cessation
      2. Control of hypertension
      3. Control of dyslipidemia
      4. Control of diabetes
   c. Symptomatic treatment:
      1. Medical therapy
      2. Use of diuretics to control heart failure by reducing preload.
      3. Beta blockers
      4. Angiotensin converting enzyme inhibitors

Definite Management

Surgical aortic valve replacement:

A. Standard management in case of mild to moderate risk
B. Bioprosthetic mechanical valve replacement.

Transcortical aortic valve replacement: It is done in case of—

A. In case of inoperability or high risk patient.
B. In case of elderly even if the risk is mild to moderate.

Choice of Procedure

A. In case of elderly of more than 75 years of age—surgical replacement, in case of younger patient—transcortical replacement.
B. If the surgical risk is very high, transcortical replacement is advisable.
C. Bioprosthetic valve is non-durable hence it is not usually done in younger patients.
D. Anatomy of the valve:
   a. Small annulus
   b. Severe calcification

Q142. Bradyarrhythmias.

TEERTHANKER MAHAVEER UNI, 2018 JUNE (5)

ANSWER

A. Bradyarrhythmia can be defined as heart rate below 60 beats/min. It can be classified into the following:
   a. Sinus node dysfunction:
      1. Sinus bradycardia: Heart rate is below 60 beats/min due to decreased automaticity of the sinus node.
      2. Sinus arrest: There is Failure of the sinus node to initiate impulse resulting pause in the rhythm of the heart.
      3. Sinoatrial exit block: Here the impulse is generated by the sinus node there is failure of the impulse to exit from the sinus node.
   b. Heart block:
      1. First degree heart block: Here PR interval is prolonged to more than 200 ms, but atrial impulse will be conducted to the ventricle.
      2. Second degree heart block:
         - Mobitz type 1 block: This is characterized by progressive increase in the PR interval

followed by drop of QRS complex. This occurs in the atrioventricular node.

- Mobitz type II block: Here the PR interval is fixed but there is non-conducted P wave. Here the block occurs below the atrioventricular node. There is increased incidence of complete heart block.

3. Complete heart block: Here no impulse is conducted to the ventricles leading to development of idioventricular rhythm.

Q143. Myocardial perfusion imaging.

TEERTHANKER MAHAVEER UNI, 2018 JUNE (10)

ANSWER

Myocardial perfusion imaging is a non-invasive imaging by which the flow of blood through the myocardium is evaluated.

Advantages of myocardial perfusion imaging:

A. PET scan is highly sensitive and specific in detecting the ischemic heart disease.

B. It can identify the patient at high risk so that early intervention can be applied.

C. It can evaluate the regional functional blood flow to detect the area of ischemia or scar.

D. It can assess the cardiovascular outcome and the survival of the patient.

E. It can determine which patient needs revascularization in the form of angioplasty.

Disadvantages of myocardial perfusion imaging:

A. Patient is exposed to radiation exposure in case of SPECT and PET thereby limiting the number of exposure in a patient.

B. The procedures are highly costly and some areas PET cannot be available.

C. The imaging may be susceptible to artefact from the body habitus especially breast or diaphragm which may interfere with the accurate evaluation.

Clinical implications of myocardial perfusion imaging:

A. It can detect the coronary artery disease by observing blood flow through the coronary artery.

B. In case of stable coronary artery disease it can assess the functional significance of lesions.

C. After the coronary artery intervention, it can detect further ischemia.

D. In case of heart failure it can evaluate the viable myocardium which can benefit from the revascularization procedure.

E. It can assess the cardiovascular risk in case of perioperative non-cardiovascular procedure.

Following are the myocardial imaging procedure:

A. Single photon emission computed tomography:

- **a.** In this procedure following radiopharmaceuticals are used:
  1. Technetium 99M based sestamibi or Tc99m tetraphosmin
  2. Thalium-201
- **b.** In this procedure either exercise or pharmacological stress is used to detect the myocardial perfusion under stress.
- **c.** Advantages:
  1. It is widely available and more affordable as compared to other procedure.
  2. It can assess severity of coronary artery disease and location of ischemia.
- **d.** Disadvantages:
  1. Its resolution is lower as compared to other procedure.
  2. There is chance of artefact.

B. Positron emission tomography:

- **a.** In this procedure following radiotracers are used:
  1. Rubidium-82 or N18 fluorodeoxyglucose
  2. Ammonia-13—it is used for perfusion imaging.
- **b.** It is more precise in detecting perfusion abnormalities as well as myocardial viability.
- **c.** Advantages:
  1. Its resolution is higher and more specific.
  2. Less chance of artefact
  3. It provides more information regarding the myocardial metabolism
  4. It is better in detecting the subclinical myocardial disease
- **d.** Disadvantages:
  1. It is more expensive
  2. It requires access to cyclotron in case of rubidium.

C. Magnetic resonance imaging:

- **a.** It is less commonly used for myocardial perfusion. Cardiac perfusion imaging in presence of stress can assess the blood flow through coronary artery.
- **b.** Advantages:
  1. It is noninvasive and absence of any radiation.
  2. It can give detailed picture of the perfusion.
  3. It can assess the myocardial scarring.

c. Disadvantages:
   1. Less widely available.
   2. In presence of pace makers or defibrillator it is not used.

D. CT angiography with myocardial perfusion imaging:
   a. It can assess the coronary arteries along with perfusion for understanding the coronary blood flow.
   b. Advantages:
      1. It will provide both functional and anatomical information of the coronary artery.
   c. Disadvantages:
      1. There is evidence of radiation exposure.
      2. It is limited to certain populations.

Q144. Brugada syndrome.

MAHARASHTRA UNI OF HEALTH SC, VIJAYAWADA, 2019 (10)

ANSWER

Definition

It is a congenital electrical disorder due to genetic mutation affecting the sodium channel in the cardiac muscle leading to abnormal ECG pattern and risk of sudden death.

Pathophysiology

The gene responsible mutation is *SCN5A* gene encoding alfa subunit of the sodium channel in the cardiac muscles. As a result of genetic mutation there is dysfunction of the sodium channel leading to reduced influx of sodium ion at the time of cardiac depolarization resulting imbalance between inward and outward current during early phase of depolarization in the right ventricular outflow tract—it leads to reentrant ventricular arrhythmias and ventricular fibrillation.

Here triggering factors are physiological and environmental factor like alcohol, sodium channel blockers and anesthetics.

Classifications

This disease has been classified according to the ECG pattern:

A. Type 1: It is characterized by coved type elevated ST segment of ≥2 mm and negative T wave at least one of the chest lead from V1 to V3 which may be spontaneous or drug induced and there is risk of arrhythmias.
B. Type 2: It is characterized by saddle type elevated ST segment followed by biphasic or positive T wave.
C. Type 3: It is similar to type 2 pattern but less than 1 mm elevated ST segment requiring drug challenge or additional criteria.

Clinical Features

A. Most of the patient is asymptomatic except it is diagnosed by ECG.
B. Symptoms:
   a. Syncope due to transient arrhythmias, here stress factors are fever, stress, and few medications.
   b. Agonal respiration at night due to ventricular arrhythmias.
   c. Sudden cardiac death as a result of ventricular fibrillation occuring at night or during rest.

Diagnosis

A. Proper history of syncope, nocturnal agonal respiration, family history of sudden death.
B. Pattern in the ECG
C. Administration of Provocative drugs like ajmaline, flecainide or procainamide will unmask the type 1 pattern.
D. Genetic testing to identify the SCN5A genetic mutation.

Treatment

A. Nonpharmacological management—avoidance of alcohol drugs those provoke arrhythmias.
B. Pharmacological management:
   a. Antipyretic for management of fever.
   b. Specific for this syndrome:
      1. Quinidine by inhibiting the outward current of potassium transiently thereby stabilizing the cardiac action potential.
      2. Isoproterenol is used in acute case to treat multiple arrhythmic event within a short period.
   c. Implantable cardioverter defibrillator: It will prevent sudden cardiac death in high risk patient.
   d. Application of radiofrequency in case of recurrent arrhythmic storms and targeting at the right ventricular outflow tract.

Q145. BROAD QRS tachycardia.

MAHARASHTRA UNIVERSITY OF HEALTH SC, VIJAYAWADA, 2019 (10)

ANSWER

It is characterized by heart rate of more than 110 beats/min and QRS complex duration of ≥ 120 milliseconds.

Classification

It is classified into following categories according to origin of electrical impulse:

A. Ventricular tachycardia resulting from origination of impulse in the ventricles.

B. Supraventricular tachycardia with aberration due to origination of electrical impulses from supraventricular area with pre-existing bundle branch block.

C. Pre-excitation due to involvement of accessary pathway.

Causes are the Following

A. Ventricular tachycardia:
- **a.** Dilated or hypertrophic cardiomyopathies
- **b.** Hyperkalemia
- **c.** Antiarrhythmic drugs like digoxin
- **d.** Ischemic heart disease
- **e.** Genetic disease:
  - **1.** Brugada syndrome
  - **2.** Long QT syndrome

B. Supraventricular tachycardia with aberration:
- **a.** AVNRT
- **b.** Atrial flutter
- **c.** Atrial fibrillation

C. Pre-excitation syndrome: Antidromic AVRT.

Clinical Features

A. Syncope

B. Dizziness

C. Palpitation

D. Pain chest—suggest ischemic heart disease

E. Dyspnea—suggest heart failure

F. Cardiac arrest due to ventricular fibrillation.

Diagnosis

A. Ventricular tachycardia:
- **a.** Duration of QRS complex—more than 140 milliseconds in case of right bundle branch block and less than 160 milliseconds in case of left bundle branch block.
- **b.** Capture beats or atrioventricular dissociation
- **c.** In the precordial leads concordance of QRS complexes which may be positive or negative.
- **d.** In V1-V2 R wave is more than 40 milliseconds.

B. Supraventricular tachycardia with aberrancy:
- **a.** Pre-existing bundle branch block
- **b.** P wave is normal PR interval is normal
- **c.** Rhythm is regular.

C. Pre-excitation syndrome:
- **a.** Broad QRS complexes
- **b.** Slurring in the upstroke of QRS complexes—delta wave
- **c.** In case of atrial fibrillation rhythm will be irregularly irregular.

Other Investigations

A. Echocardiography—to diagnose ischemic heart disease, dilated or right ventricular outflow tract obstruction.

B. Electrophysiological study: It is done for identification of arrhythmias.

C. Troponin—in case of myocardial infarction

D. Electrolytes: To detect electrolyte abnormalities

Treatment

A. In case of stable patient:
- **a.** Ventricular arrhythmias—amiodarone or procainamide or lidocaine, in case of Torsades de Pointes intravenous magnesium should be given.
- **b.** SVT with aberrancy:
  - **1.** For AVRT and AVNRT—adenosine
  - **2.** For reentrant tachycardia—calcium channel blockers or beta blockers
- **c.** For pre-excitation syndrome—amiodarone or procainamide

B. If the patient is unstable: The treatment of choice is synchronized cardioversion.
- **a.** In case of ventricular arrhythmias:
  - **1.** If the patient has been suffering from structural heart disease—ICD
  - **2.** For maintenance antiarrhythmic
  - **3.** Radiofrequency ablation of the abnormal tract
- **b.** In case of SVT with aberrancy: Radiofrequency ablation of the arrhythmogenicity tract.
- **c.** In case pre-excitation syndrome: Radiofrequency ablation of the accessary pathway.

Section 7 Pulmonology

Q1. Describe etiopathogenesis, pathology, and management of primary pulmonary hypertension.

PGI/NOV 2012 (10)

Pathophysiology, classification, diagnosis, and management of pulmonary hypertension.

DNBIII (A)/DEC2014 (10)

Primary pulmonary hypertension.

MGR/SEP2009/MDII (20)

Treatment of primary pulmonary hypertension.

GMC/2015/MDIV (10)

Pulmonary hypertension management.

AMU/2011/MDI (10) MUHS/MAY2014/MDIV (10)
BF/JUN2016/MDIV (10)

Discuss classification, pathophysiology, clinical features, investigations, and treatment of pulmonary hypertension.

MUHS/NOV2010/MDII (25)

Describe diagnosis and treatment of pulmonary artery hypertension.

MJPRU/2015(S)/MDIII (20)

Newer drugs in the treatment of pulmonary hypertension.

BF/OCT2011/MDIV (10)

Clinical features and management of pulmonary hypertension.

KUHS/MAY2014/MDII (10)

Describe etiology, clinical spectrum, differential diagnosis and management of pulmonary hypertension.

MLB/MAY2013/MDII (20)

Pathogenesis and management of pulmonary arterial hypertension.

DNB, 2022 (5)

Classify pulmonary hypertension.

DNB 2020 (5)

Discuss current classification, causes, investigations, and recent advances in the management of pulmonary arterial hypertension.

MAHARASHTRA UNI OF HEALTH SC, VIJAYAWADA, 2920 (25)

Pulmonary artery hypertension

SAURASHTRA UNIVERSITY, RAJKOT, 2020 (20)

Clinically classify pulmonary hypertension. How will you treat pulmonary arterial hypertension?

NTR UNI OF HEALTH SC, VIJAYAWADA, ANDHRA, 2020 (10)

Classify pulmonary hypertension. Write briefly about the new drugs used in the treatment of pulmonary hypertension.

WBUHS, 2020 (10)

ANSWER

Introduction

Normal pulmonary arterial pressure is 15–18 mm Hg at rest or 20–25 mm Hg during exercise.

Pulmonary hypertension is a group of diseases characterized by increased pulmonary vasculature resistance leading to right ventricular failure or premature death.

Hemodynamically, it is defined as increase in mean pulmonary arterial pressure to ≥25 mm Hg at rest or ≥30 mm Hg during exercise.

Etiology of Primary Pulmonary Hypertension

A. Idiopathic

B. Inherited pulmonary hypertension:

- **a.** ALK-1, CAV1, SMD
- **b.** BMPR2

C. Drugs- and toxin-induced

D. Unknown

E. Pulmonary veno-occlusive disease and/or pulmonary capillary hemangiomatosis

F. Chronic thromboembolic pulmonary hypertension

Pathophysiology of Pulmonary Arterial Hypertension

Following three mechanistic pathways are known to be perturbed in patients with pulmonary arterial hypertension (PAH):

a. Nitric oxide pathway: Nitric oxide is created in the endothelial cells by type III nitric oxide synthetase (eNOS), which induces guanylate synthetase to convert guanosine triphosphate to cyclic guanosine monophosphate (cGMP). cGMP activates cGMP kinase, which in turn opens cell membrane potassium channels which allow potassium to efflux, thus membrane depolarization and calcium channel inhibition.

b. Prostacyclin (PGI2) pathway: Production of PGI2 is catalyzed by prostacyclin synthetase in the endothelial cells. In pulmonary arterial smooth muscle cells (PASMCs), PGI2 stimulates adenylate cyclase thus increasing production from adenosine triphosphate (ATP) to cyclic adenosine monophosphate (cAMP) messenger that maintains PASMC relaxation and proliferation. Prostacyclin synthetase activity and prostacyclin levels are reduced in patients with PAH, which leads to a relative deficiency of its potent vasodilatory and antiproliferative effect. Moreover levels of the vasoconstrictor thromboxane A2 are increased.

c. Endothelin pathway: Here preproendothelin is converted to proendothelin then to endothelin 1 which acts on endothelin receptor B to produce:

1. Vasoconstriction
2. Smooth muscle cells proliferation

So, imbalance between vasoconstrictor substances (endothelin and thromboxane A2) and vasodilator substances (nitric oxide and prostacyclin) is responsible for development of pulmonary hypertension.

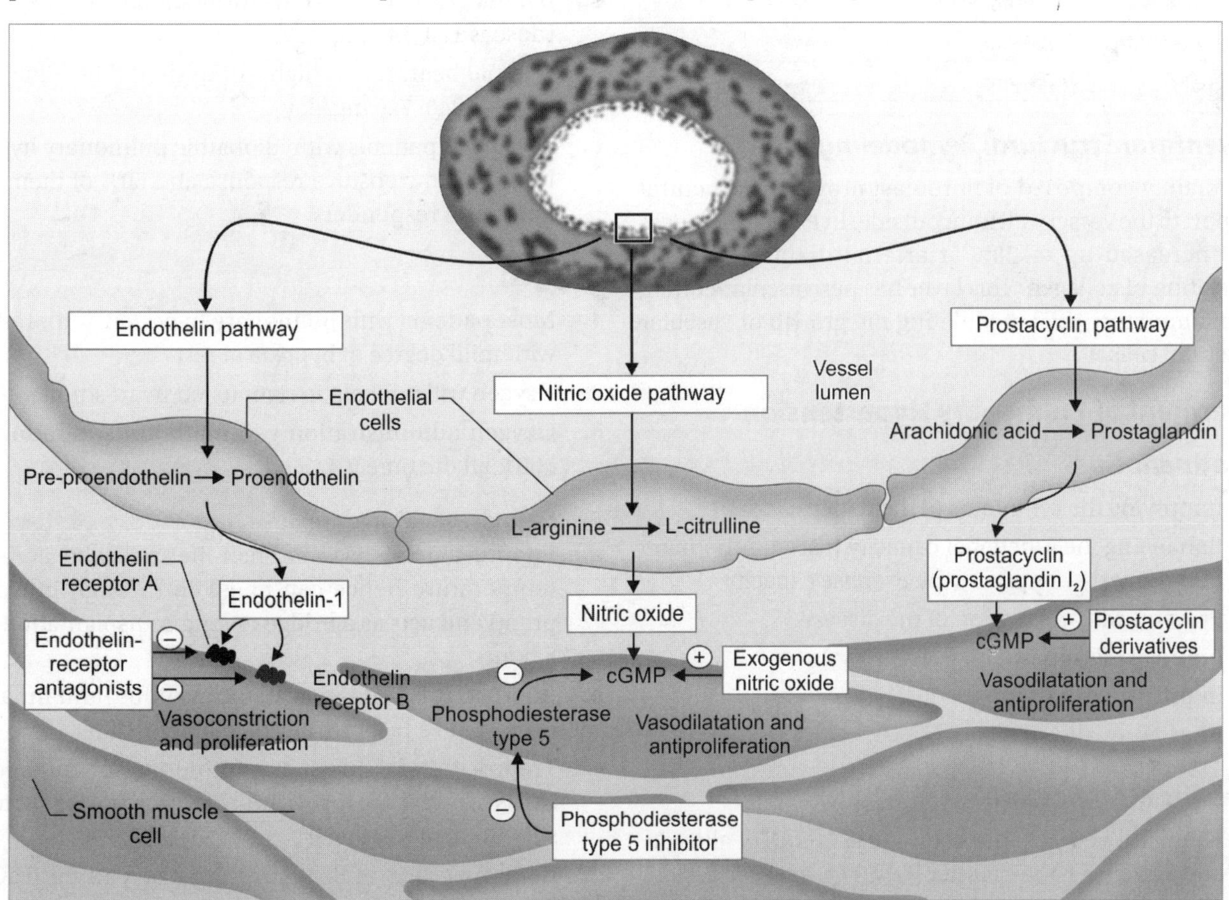

Pathology

Pathology of pulmonary vascular remodeling depends upon histological assessment of abnormal cellular components pulmonary vessel wall.

Intimal pathological remodeling according to stages of hypertension:

Type of cells	Smooth muscle cells		Extracellular matrix	Endothelial cells		
Lesion	Eccentric	Concentric	Fibrotic	Plexiform	Concentric	Dilatation
Normal pressure	Present	Absent	Absent	Absent	Absent	Absent
Mild/moderate PH	Present	Absent	Present	Absent	Absent	Absent
Severe PH	Present	Present	Present	Present	Present	Present

Plexiform lesion consists of network of vascular channels lined by endothelial cells and present in the branching points of muscular arteries. Distal to it there is formation of rosary of dilated channels, called angiomatoid lesion

Medial Pathological Remodeling According to Stages of Hypertension

Medial hypertrophy is present in very few pulmonary arteries and it is localized.

Type of cells	Smooth muscle cells	Extracellular matrix
Normal pressure	Present	Absent
Mild/moderate PH	Present	Present
Severe PH	Present	Present

Adventitial Structural Remodeling

It is mainly composed of fibroblast providing structural support to the vessel wall from outside. In PH the thickness will increased up to 28% of arterial diameter due to deposition of collagen. This layer has perivascular cuffing of inflammatory cells modulating the growth of vascular structural cells.

Treatment of Pulmonary Hypertension

Treatment Goal

a. Improving the symptoms of the patients
b. Enhancing the functional capacity (cardiopulmonary exercise test)—improves the exercise capacity
c. Prevents the progression of the disease
d. Improve the survival
e. Improve hemodynamics
f. Improve quality of life

Lifestyle Modification

a. Avoid use of oral contraceptives, extremes of altitude, and avoid over-the-counter (OTC) nasal decongestant as it produces tachycardia and vasoconstriction
b. Air travel is usually well tolerated
c. Aggressive treatment of anemia
d. Influenza and other vaccine administration
e. Avoidance of pregnancy

Pharmacotherapy

Calcium Channel Blocker

a. A minority of patient will benefit.
b. A positive response in acute vasoactivity test may demonstrate good response to long-term calcium channel blocker (CCB).
c. If initially heart rate is low—drug should be nifedipine (dose is 120–140 mg/day).
d. If initial heart rate is high—drug should be diltiazem (dose is 240–720 mg/day).
e. 10–15% of patients with idiopathic pulmonary hypertension show positive response and 50% of them are long-term responders.

Oxygen

1. Most patients with pulmonary hypertension present with mild degree of hypoxia at rest.
2. Oxygen will not help in right to left heart shunt.
3. Oxygen administration will maintain saturation of >90% all the time.

Prostanoids: The drugs are:

a. Epoprostenol: It has short half-life and stable at room temperature hence can be given through infusion pump and acts as a bridge to lung transplantation for 8 hours.
b. Iloprost: It is used in oral, intravenous, and inhaled route. Side effects are jaw pain and flushing.
c. Treprostinil: It is used as continuous subcutaneous infusion by microinfusion pump or small subcutaneous catheter.
d. Beraprost: It is orally active prostacyclin derivative but its effectiveness persists for 6 months.

Phosphodiesterase Type 5 Inhibitor

Pulmonary vasculature contains phosphodiesterase type 5, which is responsible for vasoconstriction. So, inhibitors of this enzyme are:

1. Sildenafil: Peak effect observed after 60 minutes. Approved doses are 20–80 mg three times per day.
2. Tadalafil: Peak effect observed after 90 minutes. Dose is once a day. Side effects are headache, flushing, and epistaxis.

Endothelin Receptor Antagonists

In patient with pulmonary hypertension, endothelin binds to endothelin receptor A and B and exerts its effect as vasoconstriction. So, the antagonists are the following:

1. Bosentan: It is orally active dual endothelin receptor A and B. It improves the exercise capacity but its hemodynamic and echocardiographic effects are variable. Dose is 62.5 mg twice daily and it can be increased up to 125 mg twice daily after 4 weeks. Side effect is elevated level of transaminases in 10% of patients hence monitoring of liver function test (LFT) is required.
2. Sitaxsentan
3. Ambrisentan

Balloon Atrial Septostomy

This is nothing but a creation of right to left heart shunt. It:

1. Decompresses right heart chambers
2. Decreases left ventricular preload
3. Improves cardiac output.
4. Improves systemic oxygen transport in spite of arterial desaturation.

Recommended technique is graded balloon atrial septostomy.

Pulmonary Endarterectomy

It is the treatment of choice in case of chronic thromboembolic pulmonary hypertension. By this procedure, there is dramatic fall in pulmonary vascular resistance with near normalization of pulmonary hemodynamics. But it requires good technical skillful hands.

Balloon Pulmonary Angioplasty

It markedly improves right ventricular end-diastolic and end-systolic volume index and improves the functional capacity.

Q2. Pathogenesis and management of pulmonary embolism (PE).

PGI/NOV 2012 (10)

A primigravida lady develops acute onset of breathlessness on the second day following delivery of a normal healthy baby. Discuss the possible causes and clinical approach to diagnosis and management.

DNBII/DEC2012 (10)

Discuss the risk factors, diagnosis, and management of acute PE in pregnancy.

DNBII/DEC2012 (10)

Diagnostic tests to rule in or rule out acute venous thromboembolism. Outline therapy for acute PE.

DNBIIIA/DEC2015 (10)

Discuss the etiopathogenesis, clinical features, management, and investigations of pulmonary thromboembolism.

MGR/APR2012/MDIII (15)

Discuss clinical features, diagnosis, and management of acute PE.

RGUHS/APR2001/MDII (25)

Clinical approach to diagnosis and management of pulmonary thromboembolism.

AMU/2011/MDIV (20)

Discuss clinical features of PE and management of massive pulmonary thromboembolism.

MUHS/MAY2013/MDI (25)

Discuss diagnosis and management of acute PE.

BF/MAY2012/MDIII (20)

Describe pathogenesis, risk factors, clinical manifestations, and management of pulmonary embolism.

DNB 2021 (10)

Clinical features, diagnosis, and treatment of pulmonary embolism.

DNB 2019 (10)

Pulmonary embolism: risk factors, clinical features, diagnosis, and management.

WBUHS, 2020 (10)

ANSWER

Introduction

Pulmonary embolism is the third most common cause of mortality after ischemic cardiac disease and cerebrovascular accident, most of the patients will die within few hours of incidence despite diagnostic advances.

Pathogenesis

Pulmonary embolism is acute chronic, most of PE develops from venous thromboembolism originating from veins of lower extremities. Virchow's triad are the main pathologic risk factors responsible for this condition, these are:

A. Hypercoagulability
B. Venous stasis
C. Vessel wall injury

Veins involved are:

A. Popliteal vein above the knee
B. Within the thigh femoral vein
C. Rarely pelvic vein.

Risk factors for this thromboembolic event are following:

Acquired risk factors:

A. Major risk factors are:
- **a.** Advanced age
- **b.** Prior thromboembolism
- **c.** Thrombophilia
- **d.** Major surgery
- **e.** Spinal cord injury

B. Moderate risk factors:
- **a.** Estrogen replacement therapy
- **b.** Smoking
- **c.** Family history of venous thromboembolism
- **d.** Obesity
- **e.** Pregnancy or postpartum period
- **f.** Malignancy
- **g.** Congestive heart failure
- **h.** Acute respiratory failure
- **i.** Chemotherapy

C. Weak risk factors:
- **a.** Bed rest of >3 days
- **b.** Age >40 years
- **c.** Extended immobility
- **d.** Air travel of >40 hours
- **e.** Obesity
- **f.** Varicose veins

D. Inherited risk factors are:
- **a.** Deficiencies of coagulation factors, protein C, and protein S
- **b.** Insufficiency of anticoagulant pathways, such as:
  1. Tissue factor pathway inhibitor
  2. Thrombomodulin and endothelin protein C inhibitor
- **c.** Elevated factor VIII
- **d.** Mutation of factor V. Blood group C to T variation at 10,034 position in fibrinogen gamma chain
- **e.** Hyperhomocysteinemia

Only blood group O is the protective factor for deep vein thrombosis (DVT).

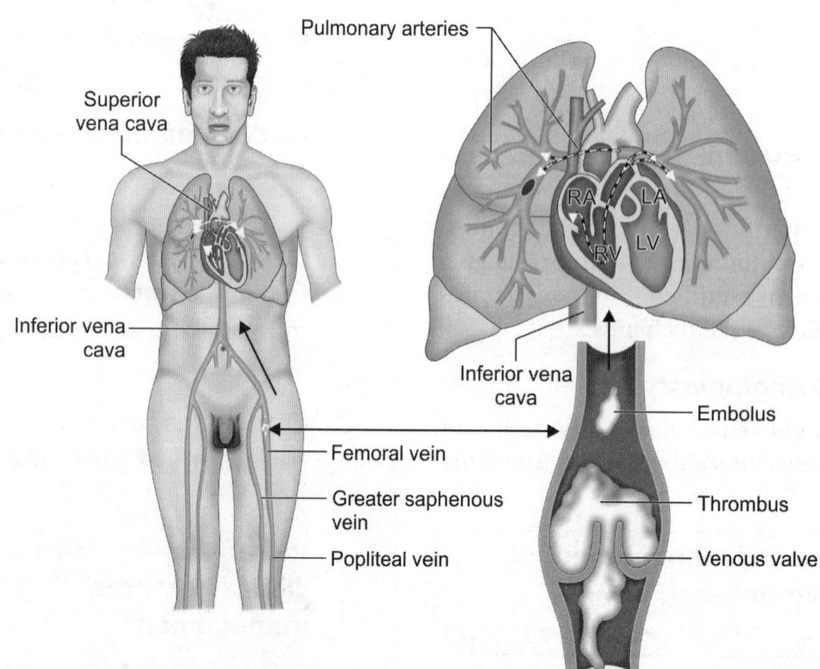

If the embolus is centrally in the pulmonary vessels and completely occlude the vessel, it is *acute embolism*. On the other hand if the embolus is contiguous and eccentric producing 50% obstruction with evidence of central recanalization, it is *chronic embolism*.

Pulmonary embolism may be central or peripheral.

Central PE includes:

- **a.** Pulmonary trunk
- **b.** Left and right pulmonary arteries
- **c.** Anterior trunk
- **d.** Right and left interlobar arteries

Peripheral PE includes:

- **a.** Segmental and subsegmental arteries of:
  1. Right upper lobe
  2. Right middle lobe
  3. Right lower lobe
  4. Left upper lobe
  5. Left lower lobe
  6. Lingula

In case of PE, following pathophysiological events occur:

A. If there is massive PE, it will lead to following circulatory compromise:

- **a.** Pulmonary hypertension
- **b.** Right ventricular dilatation with shifting of interventricular septum to the left
- **c.** Right-sided heart failure
- **d.** Low cardiac output ultimately producing cardiogenic shock
- **e.** Myocardial ischemia due to impaired coronary artery filling

B. Gas exchange abnormality:

- **a.** Low partial pressure of oxygen (PaO_2)
- **b.** Low arterial partial pressure of carbon dioxide ($PaCO_2$)
- **c.** Increased ventilation/perfusion (V/Q) mismatch
- **d.** Increased minute ventilation and increased dead space
- **e.** Peripheral vascular resistance due to release of humoral mediators, thromboxane A2, and serotonin from activated platelet from the unaffected lung

Clinical Features

A. Symptoms:

- **a.** Chest pain
- **b.** Breathlessness
- **c.** Fever
- **d.** Cough
- **e.** Hemoptysis
- **f.** Apprehension

B. Signs:

- **a.** Tachycardia
- **b.** Tachypnea
- **c.** Cyanosis
- **d.** Chest examination reveals:
  1. Crackles
  2. Pleural rub
  3. Accentuated pulmonary component of second heart sound
- **e.** Evidence of DVT in the peripheral leg veins

There is a scoring systems "Wells clinical prediction of pulmonary thromboembolism":

Clinical features	Points
Clinical symptoms related to DVT	3
Other diagnosis less likely than PE	3
Heart rate >100 beats/min	1.5
Immobilization or surgery within last 4 weeks	1.5
Previous history of deep venous thrombosis or pulmonary thromboembolism	1.5
Hemoptysis	1
Malignancy	1
Risk score interpretation	
High risk	>6
Moderate risk	2–6
Low risk	<2
Addition of D-Dimer will increase further the accuracy of prediction	

Following are the pulmonary syndrome:

A. Pulmonary infarction syndrome: It occurs due to peripheral pulmonary emboli. The hallmark are:

- **a.** Pleuritic chest pain
- **b.** Hemoptysis
- **c.** Radiological features: Classical wedge-shaped opacity with base toward the periphery

B. Isolated dyspnea syndrome:

- **a.** It is misdiagnosed as anxiety-related hyperventilation or asthma
- **b.** Patient will desaturate within few minutes while he is asked to walk or climbing upstairs

C. Syndrome-associated massive PE: Following features can be observed isolated or in combination:
   a. Sudden death: It occurs following straining over pain.
   b. Shock and/or prolonged syncope: It is feature of massive PE characterized by tachycardia, tachypnea, hypotension, sweating, and substernal chest pain.

D. Acute right heart failure: It is characterized by the following:
   a. Engorged pulsatile neck vein
   b. Prominent "a" wave in the venous pulse
   c. Right ventricular diastolic gallop
   d. Accentuated pulmonary component of second heart sound
   e. Enlarged and tender liver
   f. Pedal edema

E. Acute respiratory failure: It is characterized by:
   a. Dyspnea
   b. Excessive work of accessary muscles of respiration
   c. Tachycardia
   d. Tachycardia
   e. Cyanosis

F. Severe bronchospasm and pulmonary edema

G. Combination of B, C, D, and E. In this case following are the features:
   a. Shock
   b. Raised central venous pressure
   c. Hypotension
   d. Hypoxemic respiratory failure

Small often multiple pulmonary emboli produce following subtle features:
   a. Increasing unstable circulatory state
   b. Unexplained tachycardia and tachypnea
   c. Supraventricular tachycardia
   d. Postural hypotension
   e. Unexplained fever
   f. Syncope
   g. Icterus
   h. Rise in erythrocyte sedimentation rate (ESR)
   i. Unexplained fall in PO_2 or aggravation of already existing hypoxia.

Diagnosis

A. Chest radiograph: Following features may be seen:
   a. Focal oligemia
   b. Plate atelectasis
   c. Basal wedge-shaped shadow
   d. Pleural effusion

B. Electrocardiography:
   a. Normal in case of smaller PE
   b. Transient ST-T changes in 50% of cases
   c. S1Q3T3 with:
      1. Transient right bundle branch block
      2. Atrial fibrillation
   d. Severity of PE correlates with inversion of anterior lead T wave

C. D-dimer:

   It is product of breakdown of cross-linked fibrin and acts as sensitive marker of acute thrombosis. It is not specific for PE because fibrin is produced in following conditions:
   a. Infection
   b. Necrosis
   c. Inflammation
   d. Cancer

   D-dimer value of >500 μg/L cannot rule in this but value below this can rule it out

D. Biomarkers:

   Following biomarkers are associated with high mortality:
   a. Brain-natriuretic peptide
   b. N-terminal pro-brain natriuretic peptide
   c. Troponin

E. Lower limb venous compression ultrasonography:

   It is noninvasive test performed at bed side with sensitivity of 97% and specificity of 98% in case of proximal DVT. It is single most validated diagnostic test. It can detect femoropopliteal veins, ileac, renal veins, or inferior vena cava.

F. Arterial blood gases (ABGs):

   It may be present but not universal because, in 20% of patients with pulmonary thromboembolism have normal arterial oxygen pressure and normal alveolar-arterial oxygen gradient.

G. Echocardiography: It can be done as first-line test in case of suspected massive PE.

Findings are:

a. Presence and severity of right ventricular pressure overload indicates 30% obstruction in pulmonary artery
b. Increased right ventricular/left ventricular diameter ratio
c. Paradoxical septal wall motion abnormality
d. Dilatation of pulmonary artery
e. Evidence of tricuspid regurgitation

H. V/Q mismatch:

Perfusion scan is done by injection of macroaggregates of albumin labeled with technetium-99m. It is trapped in 0.1% pulmonary capillary. If this perfusion defect is large and/or segmental, it may clinch the diagnosis.

Ventilation scintigraphy with technetium-99m or xenon-133 will increase the specificity.

This is called normal ventilation but perfusion defect is highly predictive of pulmonary thromboembolism.

I. Helical CT pulmonary angiography:

It is the quickest and surest way to clinch the diagnosis and largely replaced V/Q mismatch test and invasive pulmonary angiography for following reasons:

a. In critically ill patients with right ventricular failure or shock it is most convenient, noninvasive, and quick method.
b. It is more frequent definite confirmation of pulmonary emboli.
c. CT angiography can detect pelvis and leg veins with same contrast injection.

Major limitations of helical CT pulmonary angiography are:

a. Inability to diagnose subsegmental branch emboli
b. Use of contrast material in case of renal failure
c. Patient is allergic to dye

J. Pulmonary angiography: It can detect subsegmental pulmonary emboli which may be missed by helical CT pulmonary angiography.

Prediction of Poor Prognosis in Pulmonary Embolism

A. Age >70 years
B. Hypotension
C. Shock
D. Oxygen saturation (SaO_2) < 90
E. Chronic obstructive pulmonary disease (COPD)
F. Cancer
G. Right ventricular thrombus
H. Respiratory rate > 20 mL/min
I. Raise BNP and pro-BNP
J. Elevated troponin I and T levels

Treatment

A. Unfractionated heparin or low-molecular-weight heparin (LMWH) can be given but later has following advantages over the former:

a. Easy to use
b. Longer half-life hence once or twice daily use is required
c. More predictable response
d. Standard dose is given
e. Low risk of heparin-induced thrombocytopenia
f. It will help the patient to get early discharge
g. It will act as a bridge till the change of LMWH to heparin

Dose:

a. Enoxaparin—1 mg/kg twice daily
b. Tinzaparin—175 units/kg once daily

B. Oral anticoagulant:

Warfarin is administered adjusted with international normalized ratio (INR) which has to be maintained to three to four times normal in case of PE or DVT. It will be affective after 4–5 days after administration.

But if warfarin is used only without heparin, it will paradoxically increases hypercoagulability due to lowering of protein C.

Duration of anticoagulant administration:

a. If the underlying precipitating factor is not available ideal duration is 3 months.
b. In patient with first episode of DVT or PE duration is 6–12 months.

Complications of warfarin in case of very high INR are:

a. Bleeding
b. Skin necrosis
c. Alopecia

Treatment of above complications:

a. Warfarin should be stopped.

b. Fresh frozen plasma can be given.

c. Low-dose oral vitamin K

If injection, vitamin K is given that will be resistant to warfarin for at least 7 days so it should be avoided.

C. Thrombolysis: It should be used in patient with PE having hemodynamic compromise.

a. Tissue plasminogen activator (TPA) acts on plasminogen to convert it to plasmin thereby dissolves the embolus; hence, it is also called medical embolectomy.

b. Streptokinase: It is used in poor countries as loading dose of 250,000 units over 30 minutes followed by 10,000 units in next 24 hours.

c. Alteplase: It is given as 100 mg given over 2 hours.

d. Tenecteplase: It is administered as 30–50 mg single bolus dose over 2 hours.

Only contraindication is uncontrolled bleeding.

D. Cardiopulmonary support:

a. In case of shock:

1. It can be treated with intravenous infusion of 1–2 mg isoproterenol in 500 mg of dextrose along with intravenous infusion of dextran:
   - To maintain central venous pressure to 12–14 mm Hg
   - To expand pulmonary vascular bed
   - To increase right ventricular stroke volume
2. In case of nonresponder dobutamine or dopamine may be given.

E. Oxygen should be administered at a rate of 6–8 L/min.

F. Surgical embolectomy: Large amount of thrombus can be removed by this method in following conditions:

a. Where thrombolysis is contraindicated.

b. Where there is risk of cardiovascular arrest and shock.

c. Who has severe right ventricular dysfunction

G. Catheter-directed modalities:

Several modalities are the following:

a. Ultrasound-assisted thrombolysis

b. Rheolytic embolectomy

c. Rotational embolectomy

d. Suction embolectomy

e. Thrombus fragmentation

Complications of these modalities are:

a. Pericardial hemorrhage due to perforation of pulmonary artery may also result cardiac tamponade.

b. Severe hemoptysis

c. Infection

d. Cardiac arrest

Q3. Physiology of sleep and pathophysiology of sleep apnea syndrome.

PGI/APRIL 2013 (10)

Obstructive sleep apnea (OSA) syndrome.

DNBII/JUNE2011 (10) MGR/APR2016/MDIV (7)

What is OSA syndrome? Risk factors for OSA syndrome and principles of its management.

DNBII/APR2016 (10)

Define OSA syndrome. Pathophysiology, diagnosis, and health complications of OSA.

DNBIIIA/JUN2016 (10)

Discuss the etiology, clinical features, and management of OSA.

MGR/OCT2003/MDI (15)

Diagnosis and management of OSA.

MJPRU/2015(S)/MDII (10)

Newer diagnostic modalities in treatment in sleep apnea.

BF/MAY2013/MDIV (10) BF/MAY2012/MDIV (10)

Discuss etiology, diagnosis, complication, and management of OSA.

ERA/MAY2012/MDII (25)

What is OSA? What are the health consequences? What are the side effects of cPAP?

DNB 2022 (5)

Diagnosis and treatment of OSA syndrome.

DNA 2019 (6)

Obstructive sleep apnea syndrome.

MGR UNI, TAMIL NADU, 2022 (10)

Diagnosis and management of sleep apneas.

NTR UNI OF HEALTH SC, VIJAYAWADA, ANDHRA, 2022 (10)

Obstructive sleep apnea.

KERALA UNIVERSITY, 2021 (10)

OSA

NTR UNI OF HEALTH SC, VIJAYAWADA, 2021 (10)

What is OSA? Briefly outline the clinical features and management strategies undertaken to tackle the problem.

WBUHS, 2023 (10)

Describe the pathophysiology and correlation with the clinical picture and the management of OSA syndrome.

WBUHS, 2025 (10)

ANSWER

Sleep is characterized by characteristic physiological changes, electroencephalogram (EEG) changes which can differentiate it from unconsciousness to unresponsiveness during anesthesia.

Physiology of Sleep

Wakefulness requires the activation of cortex supported by extensive subcortical network of pathways. Major neurotransmitters responsible for "ascending arousal system" are the following:

A. Excitatory norepinephrine released from locus ceruleus
B. Dopamine from ventral aqueductal gray matter
C. Serotonin released from midline raphe nuclei
D. Orexin from perifornical area—loss of these neurons is responsible for narcolepsy. It is characterized by excessive daytime sleepiness as well as fragmentation of sleep.
E. Acetylcholine from pedunculopontine tegmentum as well as laterodorsal tegmentum

But for initiation as well as maintenance of sleep requires inhibition of the activity of "ascending arousal system" through inhibitory neurons of ventrolateral preoptic (VLPO) area. It has been shown that there are adenosine receptors on this VLPO. Usually during wakefulness adenosine will be accumulated in the basal forebrain. During initiation of sleep adenosine acts as "sleep switch" and activates the receptors on VLPO. There are other molecules that take part in initiation and maintenance of sleep.

Now there are many inhibitor of VLPO activity.

A. Caffeine and theophylline antagonize the VLPO receptor activity and makes the person alert.
B. Monoaminergic arousal center also inhibits the activity of VLPO and produces the condition like "flip-flop" behavior where once the person at a given point of time may arise due to dominance of "arousal producing system" or sleep due to activity of VLPO.

Sleep has been divided into two forms:

A. Rapid eye movement (REM) sleep
B. Non-rapid eye movement (NREM) sleep

Sleep-wake cycle:

A. REM sleep occurs usually at 90 minutes cycle.
B. There are four to six cycles of REM and NREM sleep cycles in each night.
C. In late night, REM sleep becomes longer and NREM sleep becomes shorter.

Now the change over from REM sleep to NREM sleep is controlled by the following two systems:

A. Monoaminergic neurons
B. Certain subsets of cholinergic neurons present in the brainstem. It has inhibitory connection with two neurons present in the "ascending arousal system", these are:
  a. Serotonergic neurons in midline raphe nuclei
  b. Noradrenergic neuron in locus coeruleus

  So, during REM sleep cholinergic neurons become active and serotonergic and noradrenergic neurons will be silent and during NREM there will be opposite phenomenon.

Physiological Changes during Sleep

A. Respiratory system:
  a. During NREM sleep:
    1. Decrease in respiratory drive leading to decrease in minute and alveolar ventilation
    2. Mild hypoxia and mild hypercapnia but it will fail to augment respiratory drive

b. During REM sleep:
   1. Breathing will be irregular due to further increase of hypoxia and hypercapnia
   2. Loss of skeletal muscle tone also affect the respiratory muscles
   3. There will be ventilation—perfusion mismatch leading to arterial hypoxemia

B. Cardiovascular system:

a. Blood pressure, cardiac output, heart rate, and systemic vascular resistance decrease in NREM and tonic REM but increase during phasic REM sleep.

C. Central nervous system:

a. There is increase in cerebral blood flow to 50–100% above the resting level during tonic REM and even more in phasic REM sleep.

b. Cerebral metabolic rate, oxygen consumption, neuronal discharge, and autonomic sympathetic tone are reduced but parasympathetic tone is increased during NREM sleep but increased in phasic REM sleep.

D. Renal effect:

Glomerular filtration rate (GFR) and filtration fraction are reduced but antidiuretic hormone (ADH) secretion will increase leading to production of concentrated urine.

E. Endocrine system:

a. Melatonin release from pineal gland is under control of suprachiasmatic nuclei in pulse of 4–5 hours starting from dark onset, i.e., 9 PM, but this pulse is inhibited during bright light in the evening. It is best regarded as "opening the gate of sleep" not as hypnotic because during this period it is possible to maintain awake.

b. Prolactin level is low during day and high during sleep at night.

c. Growth hormone demonstrates also sleep-dependency.

d. Cortisol secretion decreases with sleep and increases in early morning and peaks after waking.

F. Temperature control:

a. Core body temperature decreases by 0.5°C and shivering threshold deceases.

b. Body temperature linked to circadian rhythm reaches nadir at nearly 3 AM.

Stages of Sleep

A. Stage 1: It is a transition from a state of wakefulness to state of drowsiness with closed eyes entering into stage 1 NREM sleep with rolling of eyes sometimes with hypnic jerks. It will stay only for 5–10 minutes but auditory stimuli can arouse the person.

B. Stage 2: In this stage body movement continues. It lasts for 10–20 minute in first two cycles but it will predominate in later cycles. This stage accounts for 50% of total sleep time.

C. Stage 3 and 4: These are the deep NREM sleep stage sometimes known as slow wave sleep stage. Auditory stimuli cannot arouse the person in this stage, but once awakened he will be disorientated and will react slowly.

Pathophysiology of Sleep Apnea

Obstructive sleep apnea can be defined as recurrent collapse of wall of pharynx during sleep leading to hypopnea or apnea despite full breathing efforts thus producing hypercapnia and hypoxia.

Upper airway is responsible for speech, swallowing, and passage of air and is composed of numerous muscles and soft tissue but no bony or rigid support. Moreover there is a collapsible portion extending from hard palate to larynx which is able to change during swallowing or speech momentarily during wakefulness but can collapse during sleep, it is more common in case of narrow airways.

General Factors

A. Sex: Males are much more susceptible to OSA as compared to females because of higher pharyngeal length and supraglottic resistance which may be due to obesity and deleterious effect of male sex hormones. In case of premenopausal women sex hormone will prevent OSA but after menopause there is increased prevalence of OSA due to decline in sex hormones.

B. Age: Pharyngeal resistance increases with increasing age of the patient which may be due to increased body weight.

C. Obesity: It has a strong relationship with the OSA because of the following:

a. Increases deposition of fat around the collapsed segment of pharyngeal wall compressing the upper airway. It also correlates with increased neck circumference.

- **b.** Obese patient has smaller lung volume and functional residual capacity (FRC) as compared to nonobese.

D. Genetics: It may be genetically correlated as sleep-related breathing disorders can be found in the relatives of patient of OSA.

E. Drugs:

- **a.** Ethanol increases incidence of OSA due to following:
  1. Reduction of muscle of upper airway
  2. Arousal response will be depressed
  3. Genioglossus muscle activity will be depressed during normal breathing as well as hypercapnia and hypoxia
  4. Depression of reticular activating system leading more pronounced depressant effect on upper airway muscle
- **b.** Chloral hydrate and anesthetics: Both will depress the reticular activating system which in turn depresses upper airway muscles.

Reduction of Upper Airway Caliber

There are number of factors which increase upper airway resistance and thus producing more negative intrapharyngeal pressure during inspiration in sleep. Factors responsible are:

A. Congenital:

- **a.** Micrognathia: This is due to closer position of base of the tongue to posterior pharyngeal wall which interferes with the function of genioglossus muscles
- **b.** Facial dysmorphism
- **c.** Adenoidotonsillar enlargement in children
- **d.** Mandibular abnormalities
- **e.** Choanal atresia

B. Acquired: Due to infiltration of the respiratory muscles with soft tissue:

- **a.** Myxedema
- **b.** Mucopolysaccharidoses
- **c.** Neoplastic tissue

C. Position of the head: It is very important in maintaining the patency of upper airway. Neck flexion is associated with increased resistance in the airway because of collapse mainly in obese, on the other hand neck extension is associated with resistance to collapse.

D. Opening of mouth: It increases the airway resistance due to dorsal movement of the ventrally attached dilator muscles leading to shortening of length of muscles.

E. Nose: It is the primary site of respiration both in sleep and wakefulness and it is responsible for >50% resistance in breathing due to the following factors:

1. Severe allergic rhinitis with deviated nasal septum
2. Unilateral nasal polyp in upper most nostril if the patient is in lateral recumbent position
3. Nasal packing to treat epistaxis
4. Topical anesthesia in the nose may increase the disordered breathing

Mechanical Factors

A. Posture: When the patient is in supine position:

- **a.** Cross-sectional area of the pharynx will be reduced as compared to sitting posture in snorers.
- **b.** Supraglottic resistance will be increased.
- **c.** Gravitational force acts on the pharyngeal muscles to narrow the airway.

B. Resistance in the upper airway: In case of OSA, patient has smaller upper airway as compared to non-OSA patient leading to higher inspiratory airflow resistance in the nasopharynx. During sleep there is resistance above the larynx. Inspiratory oropharyngeal resistance reaches high level between apneas and expiratory resistance shows significant increase as apnea approaches.

C. Collapsibility of upper airways: Upper airways extending from nasal choanae to epiglottis has no rigid support hence collapse easily in absence of force which maintains patency.

Abnormalities in Airway Muscle Function

Dilator muscles of upper airway mainly genioglossus distend the collapsible upper airway during inspiration. Breathing through the narrowed upper airways produces more negative and collapsing pressure which will be interacted by forceful contraction of dilator muscles to prevent airway obstruction. Drive of the dilator muscles are provoked by hypoxia and hypercapnia. So such coordination between the upper airway muscles and diaphragmatic muscle activity, defect response to the stimulus produce OSA.

Dilatation of alae nasi dilates anterior nares as a compensatory attempt to open the airway before lower of airway pressure due to contraction of intercostal and diaphragmatic muscle.

Genioglossus muscles prevent pharyngeal collapse by pulling the tongue forward.

Phasic inspiratory genioglossus muscle activity:

- **a.** Decreases during sleep in normal patient
- **b.** Almost absent during REM sleep

Phasic inspiratory genioglossus muscle activity:

- **a.** Increases from wakefulness to NREM sleep stage
- **b.** Increases between apneas in OSA patients
- **c.** Increases in older obese patients

Muscles attached to hyoid bones demonstrate phasic inspiratory activity and mechanical activity in response to hypercapnia. But neck flexion and mandibular abnormalities adversely affect the function of these muscles.

Tensor palatine muscle retracts the palate from the posterior pharyngeal wall to maintain the patency of pharyngeal cavity.

Correlation between upper airway muscle and diaphragmatic muscles:

Inspiratory drive activates and stabilizes upper airway muscles than diaphragmatic muscles thus counterbalances the force exerted by diaphragmatic and respiratory muscles. So any delay in upper airway muscle contraction relative to other respiratory muscles leads to narrowing of upper airway during sleep.

Upper Airway Reflexes

Upper airway reflexes are pressure sensitive, imbalance of which will lead imbalance between intrapharyngeal pressure and contraction of dilator muscles leading to OSA.

Feedback from the Lungs

Increased inflation of lung with increased rate of breathing at low lung volume will decrease the upper airway resistance. It will suggest that vagally-mediated reflexes at low lung volume can influence the caliber of upper airways.

Central Factors

These factors act at different levels from respiratory center to peripheral upper airway reflexes. Due to reduction of minute ventilation and reduced patency of upper airway during sleep produce hypoxia and hypercapnia. Difference in age and weight is responsible for difference in respiratory drive leading to resistance in pharyngeal muscles. Patient with OSA demonstrates increased and rapid ventilation and after apneas and doubling of tidal volume preceding apnea.

Periodicity of central drive: During hypoapneic period of breathing cycle due to low ventilatory drive timing and amplitude of inspiratory activity upper airway muscles favors upper airway occlusion. In between the upper airway occlusion phase there is increase in total pulmonary resistance.

Response to breath loading:

- **A.** Load detection threshold will be increased in patient with OSA during wakefulness.
- **B.** There is correlation between the degree of impairment of load detection and OSA severity.

Breath holding: Many chemical mechanical factors affect the duration of breath holding leading to development of some features of OSA.

Effects of oxygen supplementation: Administration of nocturnal oxygen can improve sleep disordered breathing, like 4 L/min can relieve bradycardia related to sleep apnea but fail to improve the day time sleepiness.

Arousal

Arousal of a patient with OSA can immediately relieve upper airway resistance and thus from OSA.

In normal individual, immediately after arousal there is fall in intrapharyngeal resistance leading to drop of end-tidal CO_2 tension as a result of hyperventilation. In case of no arousal there will be no hyperventilation which leads to increase in CO_2.

In patient with OSA, arousal usually coincides with increase in upper airway tone leading to relief from OSA. Upper airway mechanoreceptors are activated by airway occlusion leading to arousal. In REM sleep, cough and smooth muscle contraction in response to bronchopulmonary stimuli are blunted as it depends upon arousal. Also pulmonary stretch receptors in response to lung inflation do not cause arousal but can produce apnea in during NREM sleep.

Hypoxia is poorly related to arousal in patient with COPD and normal person, but *hypercapnia* activates upper airways receptor as well as receptor in the medulla and potentiates arousal.

Arousal response is responsible for shift of sleep from deeper to lighter stage, not complete awakening.

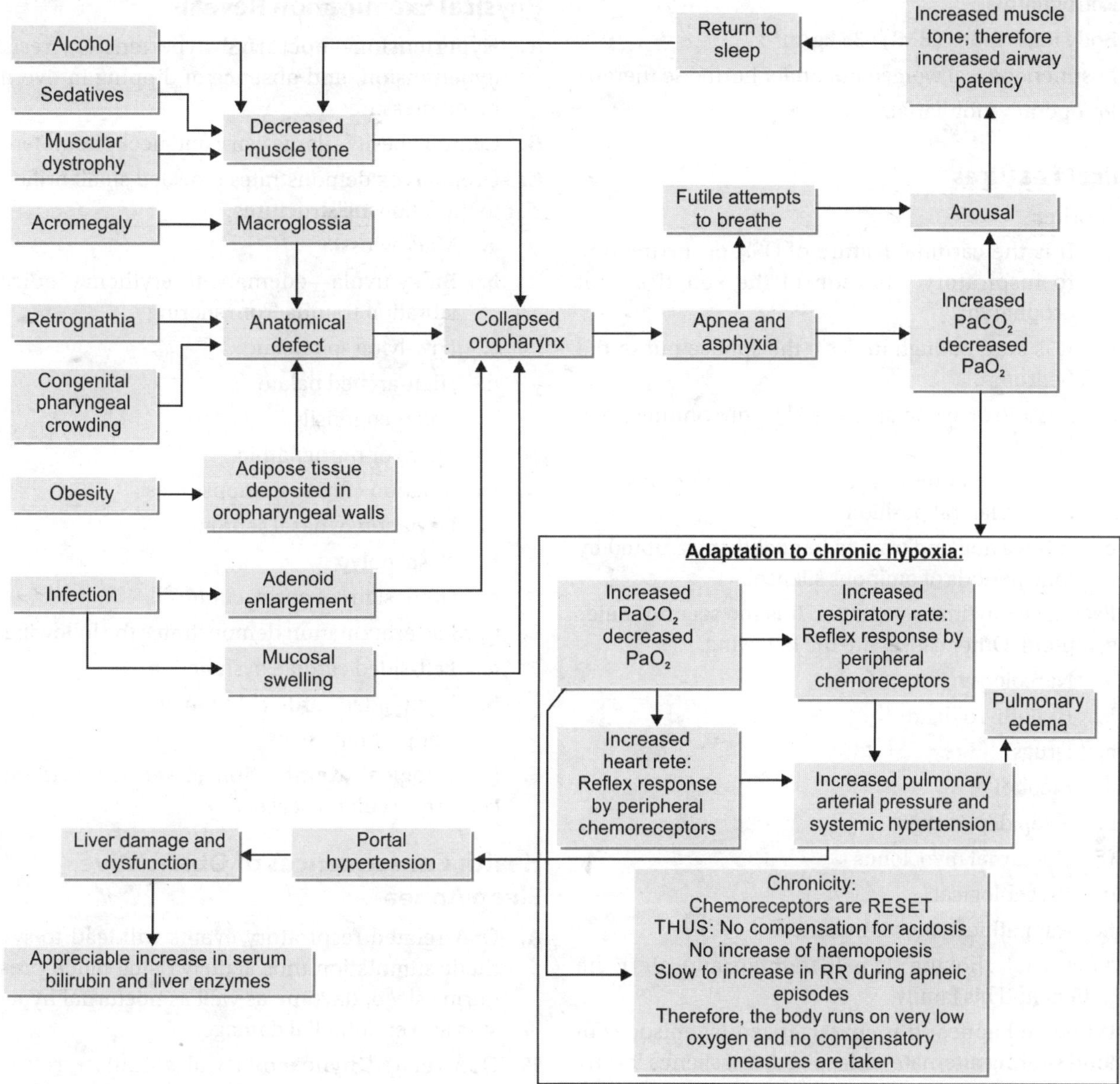

Definition of Obstructive Sleep Apnea Syndrome

It can be defined on the basis of daytime and nocturnal features and sleep study findings.

So, diagnosis requires:

A. Symptoms of nocturnal breathing disturbances such as snoring, gasping, snorting, or pause in breathing or evidence of daytime sleepiness or fatigue in spite of huge opportunities to get sleep which cannot be explained by any other medical problem.

B. According to sleep apnea study:

 a. More than and equal to five episodes of obstructive apnea or hypopnea per hour of sleep

 b. Or, in absence of any symptom, if apnea-hypopnea index (AHI) is >15 episodes/h.

Each episode of apnea or hypopnea represents the cessation of breathing for at least 10 seconds along with ≥3% reduction of SaO_2 with or without brain cortical arousal.

Predisposing Risk Factors for Obstructive Sleep Apnea Syndrome

A. Age: 40–70 years

B. Commercial motor vehicle driver

C. Male sex

D. Positive family history of OSA

E. Retrognathia
F. Body mass index (BMI) >35 kg/m^2
G. Postmenopausal women not under hormone therapy
H. Preoperative for bariatric surgery

Clinical Features

A. Snoring:
   a. It is the cardinal feature of OSA occurring due to inspiratory vibration of the soft tissue of oropharynx.
   b. It is loud enough to drive the spouse out of the bedroom.
   c. It is >50 db when measured by polysomnography (PSG).
   d. It is intermittent aggravated in supine position than in lateral position.
   e. It is waxing and waning in quality interrupted by long periods of ominous silence.
B. Excessive daytime sleepiness: It is the second major symptom. Other causes are the following:
   a. Narcolepsy
   b. Hypothyroidism
   c. Drugs
   d. Alcohol
   e. Sleep deprivation
   f. Nocturnal myoclonus
   g. Psychological
   h. Idiopathic hypersomnolence.
C. Nocturnal choking: It will frighten and alert the patient and his family.
D. Witnessed apnea: It is characterized by episodes of loud snoring alternate with episodes of silence lasting for 20–30 seconds. Apnea can be defined as cessation of breathing for >10 seconds, sometimes it may be longer to >60 seconds.
E. Other symptoms:
   a. Restlessness or nonrefreshing sleep
   b. Evidence of diaphoresis in the neck and chest
   c. Nocturia
   d. Morning headache
   e. Gastroesophageal reflux: It occurs due to increased intraabdominal pressure which is related to increased breathing effort during apneic episode.
   f. Mood disorders

Physical Examination Reveals

A. Hypertension—nocturnal hypertension, resistant hypertension, and absence of dipping in overnight blood pressure
B. Central obesity—large waist and neck circumference
C. Oropharynx demonstrates crowded small orifice due to the following structures:
   a. Macroglossia
   b. Bulky uvula—edema with erythema indicating vibration trauma from snoring
   c. Low-lying soft palate
   d. High-arched palate
   e. Enlarged tonsils
   f. Micro or retrognathia
D. Examination of nose demonstrates:
   a. Deviation of nasal septum
   b. Nasal polyp
   c. Other signs of obstruction
E. Cardiac examination demonstrates the following:
   a. Left-sided cardiac dysfunction
   b. Right-sided cardiac dysfunction
   c. Cor pulmonale
F. Neurological examination to see any evidence of cerebrovascular disease.

Health Consequences of Obstructive Sleep Apnea

A. OSA-related respiratory events will lead to sympathetic stimulation thus acutely rising blood pressure during sleep, daytime as well as nocturnal hypertension and endothelial damage.
B. OSA-related hypoxemia will stimulate release of reactive oxygen species and C-reactive protein (CRP) that leads:
   a. To exacerbation of lipolysis and insulin resistance
   b. To augmentation of prothrombotic and pro-inflammatory state
C. Inspiratory effort against occluded airway produces:
   a. Large swing in intrathoracic negative pressure
   b. Alteration of cardiac preload and afterload leading reduced cardiac function leading to surge in blood pressure of >40 mm Hg and tachycardia.
D. Hypertension may be due to activation of sympathetic nervous system, alteration of fluid balance, and

renin–angiotensin–aldosterone system. Following events will occur:

a. Blood pressure will raise the prehypertensive or hypertensive ranges
b. Increased incidence of nondipping pattern of overnight blood pressure
c. Increased incidence of resistant hypertension

E. Risk of cardiovascular diseases:

a. Coronary artery disease (CAD): It may occur directly or indirectly when associated with comorbidities such as obesity and hypertension. OSA may induce atherogenesis as there is evidence of CRP and increased endothelin levels. There is associated calcification of carotid artery atheroma or carotid artery wall thickness. OSA may induce acute nocturnal cardiac ischemia in patient with established CAD.
b. Heart failure with or without reduced ejection fraction
c. Atrial arrhythmia—bradyarrhythmia or tachyarrhythmias in patients with REM sleep
d. Ventricular arrhythmia

F. Risk of cerebrovascular diseases:

a. Increase risk of stroke in case OSA due to following factors:
   1. Reduction of cerebral blood flow
   2. Alteration of cerebral autoregulation
   3. Impaired endothelial function
   4. Impaired endothelial function
   5. Associated morbid factors:
      - Age
      - Sex
      - Smoking
      - Obesity
      - Use of alcohol

In patient with stroke and association with OSA there may be following unfavorable outcomes:

a. Impaired cognition
b. Delirium
c. Depression
d. Neurological worsening
e. Poor functional status

G. Psychiatric risk: There are significant neuropsychological impairments in patients with OSA. These are following:

a. Impairment of memory
b. Impairment of cognition
c. Impairment of attention
d. Depression
e. Impairment of general intellectual function

H. Metabolic risk:

a. Type 2 diabetes: There is associatioin with central obesity and OSA. It may be due to:
   1. Abnormality in glucose metabolism
   2. Increased insulin resistance

   Again, type 2 diabetes mellitus may itself produces OSA due to development of autonomic neuropathy.
b. Metabolic syndrome: It may occur in patient with other comorbidities such as obesity, hypertension, insulin resistance, and dyslipidemia. It may be due to severe stress imposed by OSA.

I. Sleepiness: Increased sleepiness may increase two- to threefold risk of occupational accidents or motor vehicle crashes. Even after treatment with continuous positive airway pressure (CPAP) there may be chance of residual sleepiness—its presence may be due to several factors:

a. Sleep time is insufficient
b. Treatment adherence is insufficient
c. Presence of other sleep disorders
d. Damage of brain affecting the area of alertness by prior hypoxia

J. In case of obese oral hypoglycemic agent (OHA) patients visceral adipose tissue will be increased releasing some amount of cytokines which aggravate sleepiness. So in this case also patients should be followed up to see:

a. Adherence to the treatment given
b. Presence of residual sleepiness
c. Whether sleep pattern is improved or not
d. Presence of any other disorders responsible for sleepiness

K. Motor vehicle accident: It occurs in these patients due to:

a. Lack of reaction of the sleepy driver to impending collision
b. Increased propensity to sleep in the early morning and late afternoon

   Incidence is 2–7 times higher as compared to normal population.

Diagnosis of Obstructive Sleep Apnea

A. Nocturnal oximetry: It is often used as "poor man's sleep study" in clinically suspected patient but it may miss OSA in a large number of patients.

B. Overnight PSG: Nocturnal laboratory-based dynamic PSG is the gold standard as it can measure throughout the night under monitoring of one technician:

- **a.** Recording of air flow and respiratory excursion
- **b.** SaO_2 of hemoglobin
- **c.** Position of the patient's body
- **d.** Electrocardiography
- **e.** Electroencephalography (optional)
- **f.** Electromyography (optional)
- **g.** Electrooculography (optional)
- **h.** Actigraphy (optional)

It can:

- **a.** Quantify the frequency and subtypes of abnormal movements of respiration dring sleep
- **b.** Change the oxygen dissociation curve
- **c.** Provide information regarding arousal and distribution of sleep stage
- **d.** Grade the OSA into mild, moderate, and severe
- **e.** Measure the limb movements by limb sensor

There are several variations in this study. If a patients is already diagnosed with OSA in the early part of night, in that case "split-night" study can be performed in the second half of the night to titrate with CPAP.

C. At home, PSG can be performed nowadays for:

- **a.** Reduced cost
- **b.** Light-weight machine
- **c.** Enhanced patient's convenience
- **d.** Better sleep in the family environment

Atypical report demonstrates:

- **a.** AHI scores
- **b.** Profile of SaO_2 overnight
- **c.** Respiration disturbance index—it includes:
  - **1.** Number of respiratory effort-related arousal
  - **2.** Number of apneas and hypopneas
- **d.** Sleep latency—it is the time measured from the light off to first sleep onset.
- **e.** Sleep efficiency—it can measures the percentage of time asleep relative to total time in the bed.
- **f.** Arousal index—it can measure number of cortical arousal per hour of sleep.
- **g.** Time of each stage of sleep
- **h.** Periodic limb movement index

Severity of OSA can be characterized according to the fragmentation of sleep which is associated with respiratory disturbances. Following are the relative metrics:

- **a.** Arousal index—it is the frequency of cortical microarousals per sleep-hour.
- **b.** Low sleep efficiency—sleep continuity is reduced.
- **c.** Time of stage N3 and REM sleep will be reduced.
- **d.** Increase in stage N1 sleep
- **e.** Abnormalities in cardiac rhythm
- **f.** Changes in the heart rate
- **g.** Surge in the blood pressure
- **h.** Detection of automatic arousal

Apnea-hypopnea index: It can deliniate number of apnea and hypopnea per hour of sleep.

Respiratory disturbance index: Number of apnea plus hypopnea plus respiratory effort-related arousal per hour of sleep.

OSAHS: AHI of 5–14 events/h
OSAHS: AHI of 15–29 events/h
OSAHS: AHI of ≥30 events/h

Treatment of Obstructive Sleep Apnea

Prior to treatment clinician should search for:

- **A.** Risk factors and comorbidities
- **B.** Lifestyle and behavioral factors

The aim of treatment should be the following:

- **A.** Reduction of weight
- **B.** Optimization of sleep time to 7–9 hours
- **C.** Regulation of sleep schedule having similar bedtime and similar wake time
- **D.** Avoidance of sleep in supine position
- **E.** Treatment of nasal allergies
- **F.** Increase in physical activities
- **G.** Elimination of alcohol intake within 3 hours of bedtime
- **H.** Minimal use of sedative medications
- **I.** Encouraging the patient not to drive in sedate condition

Methods of Treatment

A. CPAP is the standard method of therapy given through nasal mask or naso-oral mask to maintain the airway patent during sleep by holding the airway open. It should be done in laboratory by autotitrating device to know the optimum pressure setting with the aim:

- **a.** To reduce the number of apnea or hypopnea during sleep
- **b.** To improve the gas exchanges
- **c.** To reduce the number of arousals

Adherence to this method of CPAP can be improved by skilled heathcare team by following methods:

- **a.** Addressing the side effects of this method and the process of solution
- **b.** Giving motivational education to the patients

CPAP has beneficial effect on the following factors:

a. Reversion of desaturation
b. Blood pressure
c. Mood
d. Alertness of the patient
e. Quality of life
f. Sensitivity to insulin
g. Cardiovascular system
h. Ejection fraction of the heart
i. Recurrence of atrial fibrillation
j. Risk of mortality

Side effects are minor and these are the following:

a. Dry mouth
b. Conjunctivitis
c. Ocular irritation
d. Nasal congestion
e. Nasal abrasions and ulcers over the nasal bridge due to ill fitted mask
f. Rare and more dangerous complications are:
    1. Massive epistaxis
    2. Pneumothorax
    3. Pneumocephalus
    4. Increased intraocular pressure
    5. Rupture of tympanic membrane

B. Oral appliances: These will work by:

a. Advancing mandible
b. Repositioning of lower jaw to open the airway
c. Pulling the tongue forward

Two types of appliances:

a. Tongue repositioning appliances
b. Mandible repositioning appliances

Indication of oral appliances:

a. Mild obstructive sleep apnea hypopnea syndrome (OSAHS): Efficacy study demonstrate to reduce AHI by ≥50% in two-thirds of individual.
b. Who do not tolerate CPAP

Side effects are:

a. Pain in the temporomandibular joint
b. Movement of the teeth

C. Nasal expiratory positive airway device: It is single user device, it is inserted into the nares with adhesive tape.

It produces low inspiratory resistance on the other hand increased expiratory resistance so that upper airway will not collapse. It will improve following in case of mild OSAHS:

a. Sleep quality
b. Snoring
c. Daytime sleepiness

But there is problem with strict adherence.

D. Upper airway surgery:

Indications:

a. Snoring patient with mild OSAHS or
b. Cannot tolerate CPAP
a. Surgery is uvulopalato pharyngoplasty—here uvula, distal soft palate, tonsillar pillars, faucial muscles, and mucosa of pharynx are excised. Relapse rate is 50% of those who initially responded.

Contraindications:

a. Severe ISAHS
b. Obese patients with BMI of >30%.

Other method of surgeries are the following:

a. Bariatric surgery can improve obese patients with OSAHS and other obese-related health conditions
b. Stiffening of the soft palate by injection
c. Radiofrequency ablation
d. Laser-associated uvulopalatoplasty
e. Palatal implants
f. Tracheostomy
g. Septoplasty

E. Upper airway neurostimulation: Here pacemaker of neurostimulator is placed inferior to the clavicle. From here stimulator leads are tunneled via neck to stimulate unilateral hypoglossal nerve motor neurons innervating retractor and protrusor muscles of the tongue. From the pacemaker sensory leads are tunneled subcutaneously to stimulate intercostal muscles which can monitor respiration. Neurostimulator stimulate synchronously and continuously to protrude the tongue. After implantation stimulation titration should be done to adjust the stimulus frequency, intensity, and pulse width to such a tolerable levels so that restriction of inspiratory flow during sleep will be abolished.

a. Decrease the AHI
b. Improve the patient reported outcomes for at least 18 months such as quality of life and sleepiness
c. Mood
d. Improve oxygen desaturation index
e. Quality of life

Q4. Pathophysiology of acute respiratory distress syndrome (ARDS).
PGI APR 2013/MD1(10)

ARDS—definition, causes, and approach to management.
DNB/JUN2010 (10)

Define ARDS. Describe its clinical course and management.
DNBII/DEC2010 (10)

Define acute lung injury. Describe the etiology, pathophysiology, and management of acute lung.
DNBI/DEC2012 (10)

What are the common causes for ARDS? Pathophysiology and ventilator management in ARDS.
DNBIIIB/DEC2015 (10)

Acute lung injury.
MGR/MAR2009/MDII (6)

Discuss various mechanisms causing noncardiogenic pulmonary edema and management of ARDS.
MGR/FEB2005/MDI (15)

Define ARDS. Discuss etiology, diagnosis, and management of ARDS.
MJPRU/2015/MDIV (20)

ARDS definition.
MUHS/NOV2013/MDIV (10)

Ventilator strategies in adult respiratory distress syndrome.
MUHS/NOV2010/MDII (10)

Discuss recent trends in the management of ARDS.
BF/MAY2009/MDIV (20)

Pathology of acute lung injury.
MGR/APR2014/MDI (5)

Severe ARDS.
MGR/OCT2003/MDIII (5)

Noncardiogenic pulmonary edema.
BF/NOV2012/MDII (12)

Describe the etiology and management of resistance-expansion pulmonary edema.
BF/JUNE2016/MDIII (10)

Prone ventilation in acute respiratory distress syndrome.
DNB, 2022 (5)

Definition and causes of acute respiratory distress syndrome. What are the various strategies employed in mechanical ventilation in ARDS?
DNB 2020 (10)

Explain ventilation and perfusion. Discuss ARDS.
SAURASHTRA UN, 2022 (20)

A 40-year-old male with history of fever, cough and myalgia comes to OPD with sudden onset of breathlessness and SPO2 of 90%. Discuss the causes and management of the patient.
MGR UNI, TAMIL NADU, 2022 (10)

Ventilatory management in ARDS.
NTR UNI OF HEALTH SC, VIJAYAWADA, 2021 (10)

Acute respiratory distress syndrome.
MAHARASHTRA UNI OF HEALTH SC, VIJAYAWADA, 2020 (10)

ANSWER

Mechanical ventilation has been described in question number 19.

Ventilation and perfusion has been discussed in question number 34.

Definition

Acute respiratory distress syndrome or noncardiogenic edema is characterized by the following:

A. Previous history of perpetuating condition
B. Respiratory distress with hypoxemia refractory to supplemental oxygen therapy
C. Newly evolving bilateral pulmonary infiltrate
D. Pulmonary capillary wedge pressure is ≤18 mm Hg in spite of normal oncotic pressure.

Pathophysiology

The barriers in the lung to fluid and gases are:

A. Capillary endothelium

B. Interstitial area

C. Alveolar epithelium, which consists of:

  1. Flat alveolar type 1 cells
  2. Cuboidal alveolar type 2 cells

Both these types of cells:

- Produce tight barrier preventing the passage of solutes but allow the passage of gases, i.e., oxygen and carbon dioxide.
- Absorbs by vectorial transport excess fluid from alveoli through apical sodium channels and basolateral Na^+/K^+-ATPase pump.

3. Tight junctions

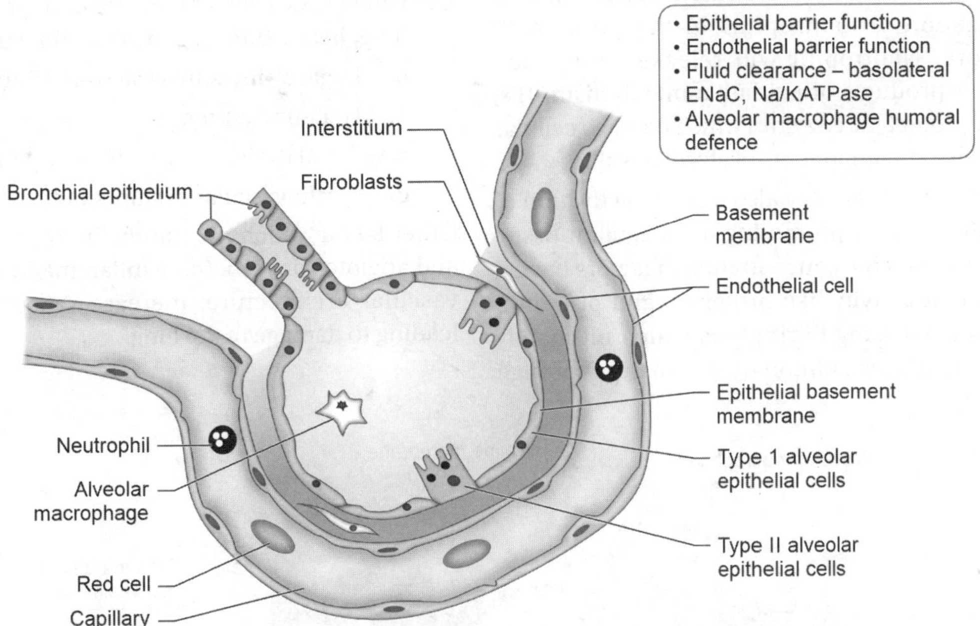

Again, type 2 cells produce surfactant which reduces surface tension of the alveoli preventing it from collapse.

Excess fluid in the interstitium can be removed by lymphatics.

According to recent molecular genetics a complex network of inflammatory cascade finely tuned by different modulators and regulators are responsible for development of ARDS as well as alteration of physiology in other organs.

Endotoxin released from focus of infection will perform three functions:

A. Cellular activation: Two types of cells are activated:

  a. Activated neutrophils release proteases, leukotrienes, such as interleukin 6 (IL-6) and IL-8, and reactive oxygen species

  b. Activated mononuclear cells release tumor necrosis factor-α (TNF-α), macrophage inflammatory protein 1 and 2, and neutrophil-activating peptide (NAP). TNF-α along with ILs recruit, activate, and promote adherence of neutrophils to vascular endothelium.

All the above factors damage the capillary endothelium and disturb pulmonary microcirculation leading to release of water from the capillary to interstitial spaces and alveoli producing pulmonary edema, pulmonary atelectasis, and pulmonary fibrosis. The effects are:

a. Fall in total lung capacity (TLC)

b. Reduction in FRC

c. Reduced pulmonary compliance

d. V/Q mismatch

e. Increased right-to-left heart shunt

f. Increase in minute ventilation and dead space

g. Low recoil pressure of lung at FRC will lead to smaller airway closure

h. Increasing noncompliant stiffening of lung

Pathologically, ARDS lungs are not homogeneously affected. There are four zones in the affected lung:

  1. Most dependent portion is not at all aerated but consolidated—it is "core" disease.

2. Zone above the most dependent zone is "collapse recruitable lung"—it can be recruited and aerated later.
3. Zone above it is inflammatory edema—weight of this zone responsible for producing "collapse recruitable lung".
4. Upper most zone is normal open lung.

B. Activation of complement pathway: After activation of this pathway, C5 will be released which will lead to aggregation of neutrophils in the pulmonary vasculature. Neutrophil will release superoxide radicals, byproducts of oxidative metabolism, ILs, and other proteolytic enzymes which damage cellular and noncellular components of alveolar wall.

C. This complement pathway also leads to activation of coagulation cascade promoting procoagulant tissue factors, decreases the concentration of factors having anticoagulant activity like protein C and protein S as well as decreasing fibrinolysis which ultimately obstruct and distort pulmonary vasculature through production of thrombin and fibrin. Thus pulmonary hypertension develops which:

a. Increase right ventricular overload leading to right ventricular failure.
b. Increased right ventricular diameter interventricular septum will shift to leftward reducing the left ventricular failing which in turn decreases cardiac output.

D. Direct toxic cellular injury of different organs, such as lung, heart, kidney, gastrointestinal tract, and brain.

a. In gastrointestinal tract—DVT and stress ulcers
b. Hepatic dysfunction
c. Renal dysfunction in 30–40% patients
d. Cardiovascular dysfunction

Other factors, such as endothelin-1, phospholipase A-2, and angiotensin-2 increase inflammation, destroy microvascular architecture, increase vascular permeability leading to damage of the lung.

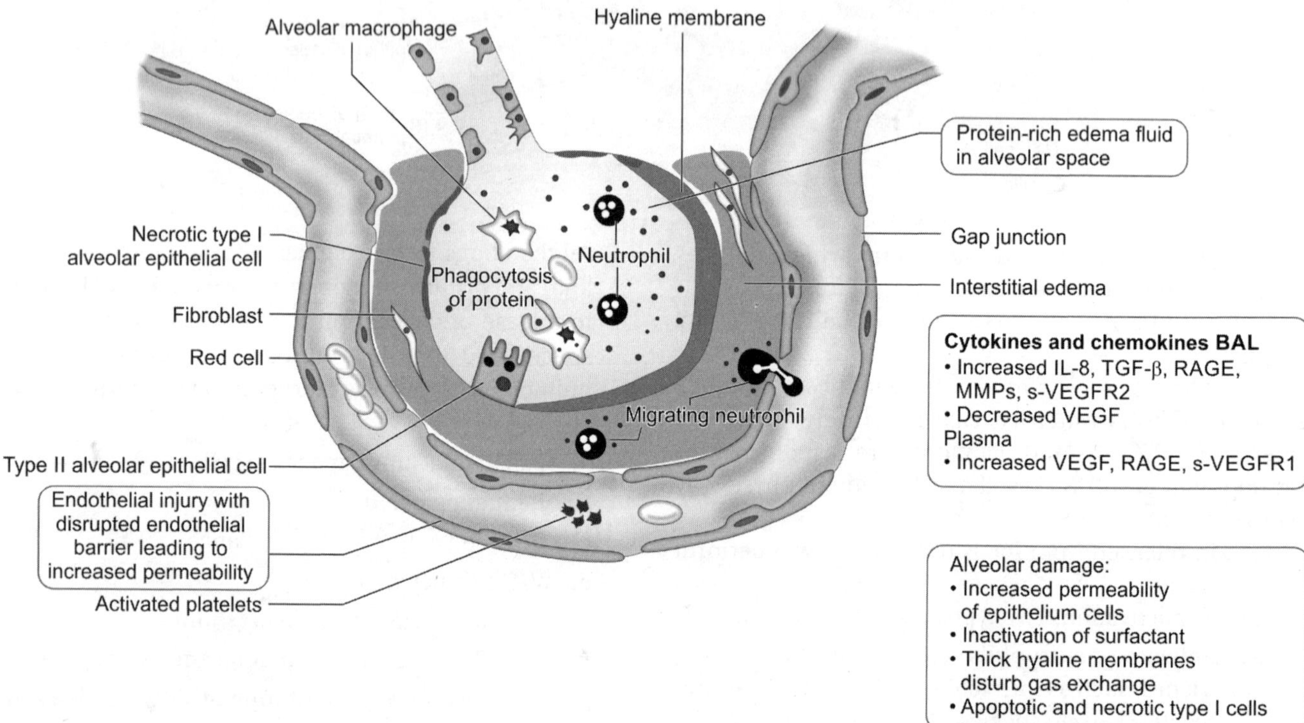

(BAL: bronchoalveolar lavage; IL: interleukin; MMPs: matrix metalloproteinases; RAGE: receptor for advanced glycation end products; S-VEFGR2: soluble vascular endothelial growth factor receptor 2; TGF: transforming growth factor; VEGF: vascular endothelial growth factor)

Arterial gas results in different stages of disease:

a. In early phase there is slight fall in PaO_2 and increased alveolar-arterial oxygen gradient as there is defect in diffusion only in this phase.
b. In late phase there is defect in diffusion and ventilation leading to hypoxia and hypercapnia.
c. In the fibroproliferative phase:
    1. Persistent hypoxemia

2. Lung compliance will be low
3. Dependent on ventilation

There are three phases of ARDS:

A. Exudative phase:
  a. Diffuse damage of type 1 pneumocytes and capillary endothelial cells
  b. Loss of tight junctional barriers to macromolecules and fluid
  c. In acute phase increased release of proinflammatory cytokines like IL-1, IL-8, TNF-α, and lipid mediators like leukotriene B leading to neutrophil recruitment into pulmonary interstitium and alveoli.
  d. Formation of hyaline membrane whorls in the alveoli by condensed plasma protein aggregates, cellular debris, and dysfunctional pulmonary surfactant that deposit in the alveoli and interstitium.
  e. Obliteration of pulmonary vasculature by microthrombi and fibrocellular proliferation.
  f. Pathophysiologic alterations are following:
    1. Collapse of dependent portion of the lung due to accumulation of fluid in the dependent portion of alveoli leading to:
      - Decreased compliance of lung
      - Presence of intrapulmonary shunting leading to hypoxemia
      - Increased work of breathing leading to dyspnea
    2. Reduction of pulmonary arterial blood flow in the ventilated portion of lung due to intravascular occlusion by microthrombi leading to increased dead space.
  g. This phase will last for 7 days.

B. Proliferative phase:
  a. During the initiation of lung repair alveolar exudates are organized.
  b. There is shift of neutrophil predominant to lymphocytes predominant infiltrate infiltrates.
  c. Proliferation of type II pneumocytes along the alveolar basement membrane during the process of repair.
  d. These new type II pneumocytes will synthesize new surfactant and will be transformed into type I pneumocytes.
  e. Reduced compliance of lung and gas exchange:
    1. Reduced vascular endothelial growth factor R1/2
    2. Neutrophil elastase and reactive oxygen species
  f. Duration of this phase is 7–21 days.

C. Fibroproliferative phase:
  a. Alveolar fluid and acute and chronic inflammatory infiltrate will be converted into extensive alveolar duct and interstitial fibrosis.
  b. Extensive disruption of acinar architecture will lead to emphysematous changes along with formation of bullae.
  c. Microscopic thromboembolic formation in the pulmonary vasculature leading to development of pulmonary hypertension.

Clinical Features

A. Dyspnea is the only symptom which will start after several hours to day before the respiratory consequences. But as the protein along with fluid will leak from vasculature into alveolar spaces and interstitium, dyspnea progressively worsens.

B. Restlessness

C. On examination:
  a. Tachycardia
  b. Tachypnea—in early phase it may be the only warning sign even in absence of normal chest X-ray and chest findings.
  c. Cyanosis may occur but may not be evidenced even in presence of hypoxemia.
  d. On auscultation there are crackles with occasional wheeze.

D. In case of worsening of respiratory failure, other organs may show features of dysfunction which may be due to widespread vascular endothelial changes.

Investigations

A. Chest X-ray:
  a. In early phase, it is normal at the onset but within short period interstitial and alveolar edema will develop.
  b. In established cases there is full blown pulmonary edema. To start with it is predominantly unilateral depending upon position of the patient but later on it will be bilateral.
  c. Both lungs are not symmetrically involved; one lung is involved more than the other.
  d. Cardiogenic pulmonary edema can be excluded by absence of Kerley lines, cardiomegaly, and vascular redistribution toward upper lobes.
  e. Infective changes can be differentiated by absence of consolidation.

B. ABGs:

a. In early phase, varying degrees of hypoxia without hypercapnia with respiratory alkalosis. As the interstitial and alveolar edema increases there will be true shunting of across the unventilated alveoli resulting more severe hypoxemia. Correction of hypoxemia is refract to oxygen therapy.

b. Hence to interpret PO_2 a standardized method in a patient receiving different concentration of supplemental oxygen ratio of PaO_2 to fraction of inspired oxygen (FiO_2) is used to categorize three types of ARDS:

1. Mild ARDS: PaO_2/FiO_2—>200 but ≤300

2. Moderate ARDS: PaO_2/FiO_2—100–200

3. Severe ARDS: PaO_2/FiO_2—<100

c. In later phase there is hypoxemia with hypercapnia with respiratory acidosis and metabolic acidosis.

d. Hypoxia refractory to administration of oxygen indicates:

1. V/Q mismatch

2. Increased right-to-left heart shunt

3. Increased dead space ventilation

C. Central venous balloon tipped catheterization through systemic vein to superior vena cava or through right atrium and right ventricle to pulmonary artery (Swan-Ganz catheter)—this catheter is usually advanced to smallest branch which can be totally occluded to prevent any forward flow of blood. This is called pulmonary artery occlusion pressure or pulmonary capillary wedge pressure. It can differentiate cardiogenic pulmonary edema from noncardiogenic pulmonary edema by following measure:

a. In case of cardiogenic edema: Due to back pressure of left atrium to pulmonary veins hydrostatic pressure in the pulmonary capillaries will be high.

b. In case of noncardiogenic edema left atrial pressure is normal—indicating that due to increased permeability of pulmonary capillaries there will be interstitial and alveolar edema.

D. Lung compliance: It will be decreased to 30 mL/cm of water.

E. Routine tests for measuring organ dysfunction:

a. Renal function

b. Liver function

c. Hematological parameters

F. Full bacteriological screening:

a. Blood culture

b. Tracheal aspirate

c. Urine culture

d. Bronchoalveolar lavage (BAL) culture

e. Culture of any other secretions

G. Bronchoscopy with study of bronchoalveolar fluid should be done in following conditions:

a. In case of bilateral pneumonia, it may be the cause of ARDS and it may mimic ARDS.

b. In case of alveolar hemorrhage, granulomatosis with polyangiitis, eosinophilic pneumonia, and disseminated malignancy of lung.

c. The organisms which cannot be found in endobronchial, tracheal aspirates, or in sputum.

Treatment

Mortality in ARDS is nearly 60%, of them most of the deaths are due to sepsis and multiorgan failure. Hence, close watch is required for these patients for:

a. Recognizing and treating the underlying medical or surgical disorders such as sepsis and pneumonia.

b. Minimizing of the unnecessary procedures and their complications.

c. Providing "bundle of care" approaches including prophylaxis against the following:

1. Prolonged mechanical ventilation

2. Gastrointestinal bleeding

3. Aspiration

4. Sedation

5. Venous thromboembolism

6. Infection of central venous catheter

d. Instantaneous recognition of nosocomial infection

e. Providing enteral nutrition

Treatment of Underlying Conditions

Etiology of ARDS should be searched and properly treated. Most of the etiologies of ADRS are mainly supportive except sepsis which should be recognized and promptly treated such as surgical drainage of abscess, urgent treatment of abdominal sepsis, or fulminant tropical conditions.

Respiratory Support

Respiratory support by mechanical ventilation is mainly supportive so that the lung will get sufficient time to recover from acute injury. To make this support effective following factors should be known:

a. Cardiorespiratory pathophysiology
b. The close interactions between heart and lungs
c. Importance of efficient oxygen transport
d. Complications and dangers of ventilatory support

Initiation of Ventilatory Support

Following are the indications of initiating ventilatory support:

A. Progressive hypoxemia refractory to oxygen inhalation
B. Marked unsustainable increase in work of breathing with respiratory rate >35–40 breaths/min an increase in minute volume to >12 L/min.

Noninvasive Ventilation

Patients with mild ARDS can be treated with:

A. CPAP: CPAP level are kept between 10 and 12 cmH_2O. Gas flow of >70 L/min is required to maintain the intrathoracic pressure at required CPAP level throughout respiratory cycle.
B. Bilevel positive airway pressure (BiPAP) ventilator with tight fitting mask: In this case expiratory positive airway pressure (EPAP) should be maintained at 7–10 cmH_2O and inspiratory positive airway pressure (IPAP) should be maintained at 15–18 cmH_2O. This setting is required for giving patient's comfort and maintaining SaO_2 of >90%.

Effect of Noninvasive Ventilation

a. Recruitment of collapsed alveoli
b. Increase in FRC
c. Increase in lung compliance
d. Reduction of work of breathing leading to unloading of respiratory muscles

Good response to noninvasive ventilation will start within 30 minutes of administration and it is characterized by following events:

a. Decrease in respiratory rate
b. SaO_2 will be improved
c. Patient's distress will be reduced

But endotracheal intubation with mechanical ventilation should be done in following cases:

a. Inability to maintain SaO_2 to >90%
b. Hemodynamic instability
c. Worsening of clinical condition

Following are the dangers in case of endotracheal intubation in ARDS:

a. Severe increase in hypoxia in an already hypoxic patients
b. Danger of gastric aspiration
c. Hemodynamic instability

Hence endotracheal intubation should be done by expert hand and patient should be under mild sedation with benzodiazepine or narcotic analgesic but in case of acute crisis succinylcholine can be administered.

Mechanical Ventilation

Principles of mechanical ventilation

There are two fundamental concepts in case of mechanical ventilation in patients with acquired immunodeficiency syndrome (AIDS):

a. Overdistention of the alveoli will be prevented by:
   1. Limiting the tidal volume
   2. Pause pressure
b. Positive end-expiratory pressure (PEEP) should so high that it prevents derecruitment of the alveoli at the end expiration.

Limitation of tidal volume

From different trial it has been shown that patients receiving lower tidal volume have lower mortality as compared to higher mortality in case of higher tidal volume.

Following are the protocol for ventilatory support in case of ARDS:

A. Setting of initial tidal volume to 8 mL/kg of predicted body weight and initial respiratory rate should be set to satisfy the patient's ventilatory requirement.
B. Then over next 1–3 hours tidal volume should be reduced to 7 mL/kg of predicted body weight and then to 6 mL/kg of predicted body weight with maintaining plateau pressure below 30 cmH_2O.

   Low tidal volume and limited plateau pressure to 30 cmH_2O will prevent:

   a. Undue over distension of alveoli—it will amplify already existed lung injury by following mechanisms:
      1. Increasing alveolar edema
      2. Increasing pulmonary cytokine production
   b. Increase in intra-alveolar and inspiratory pressure will increase the incidence of:
      1. Barotrauma
      2. Pneumothorax
      3. Pneumomediastinum
      4. Interstitial emphysema
      5. Subcutaneous emphysema
      6. Pulmonary hemorrhage

   c. Low tidal volume also decreases the production of IL-6, IL-1, and TNF-α which is also responsible for distant organ involvement along with aggravation of ARDS.

C. As tidal volume is decreased respiratory rate should be increased to maximum 35 breaths/min so that patient's minute ventilation can be maintained.

D. In that case hypercapnia is predictable and acceptable—$PaCO_2$ to above 40 mm Hg.

E. Now PEEP and FiO_2 have to be adjusted to maintain following oxygenation goal:
   a. PaO_2 of 60–80 mm Hg
   b. SaO_2 of 90–95%

   But PEEP should not be exceeded to >15–16 cmH_2O. In case of severe hypoxia, to counteract it FiO_2 can be increased to 100%. But over time FiO_2 should be decreased to 50–60% so as to maintain:
   a. PaO_2 near 60%
   b. SaO_2 close to 90%

F. In spite of these, if there is refractory hypoxemia IPAP to EPAP ratio of 1:2 to 1:1 is required.

Use of PEEP

It is the main stay of ventilation in ARDS. It acts by following mechanisms:
   a. Recruiting collapsed alveoli
   b. Restoration of FRC to normal
   c. Increase in lung compliance
   d. Redistribution of lung water within the alveolar spaces
   e. Improvement of V/Q mismatch
   f. Decrease the shunt and venous admixture
   g. It will deliver the oxygen in low concentration thus decreasing the chance of oxygen toxicity.
   h. It can prevent further lung injury if PEEP is properly adjusted by following mechanism:

      In the inspiratory phase of mechanical ventilation concertina effect of opening the alveoli—it is followed by during expiratory phase derecruitment well-nigh closure of alveoli—it leads to generation of shearing forces that worsen the lung injury further. So during mechanical ventilation "lung protection goal" has to be followed by adjusting the level of PEEP.

Level of PEEP varies individual to individual. PEEP is useful in patient having good proportion of recruitable lungs as compared to little proportion of recruitable lung where PEEP is of no use.

In the plotted pressure-volume curve there are two points—upper and lower inflection points. PEEP level has to be maintained little above the lower inflection point. But this curve relates to whole lung but it will not reflect the regional differences, i.e., some part is overdistended, some are collapsed or consolidated.

Positive end-expiratory pressure should be reduced to 5 cmH_2O if:
   a. There is no improvement in oxygenation as judged by PaO_2/FiO_2 ratio
   b. There is no increase in compliance

Ventilator modes

There are several modes of ventilation:

A. Volume control mode
B. Pressure control mode

Focus of all modes of ventilation:

A. Prevention of alveolar overdistension
B. Countering alveolar derecruitment
C. Avoidance of oxygen toxicity
D. Minimization of cardiovascular instability

Volume control mode is the most commonly adopted method for treating ARDS. But if pressure control mode is used following points have to be maintained:

A. PEEP of 6 mL/kg of predicted body weight
B. Peak pressure should not be >30 cmH_2O
C. Inspiration to expiration ratio is 1:2 or 1:1

High-frequency oscillating ventilation is generally accepted in case of children as it protects lung by giving very low tidal volume which is less than a dead space but at a high frequency.

Use of prone posture

In this prone position (face down) mechanical ventilation will improve exchanges of gases and thus reducing the mortality. Mechanism is not known but it helps in more even distribution of V/Q. Disadvantages of this prone position are the following:
   a. Great difficulty in nursing
   b. Chance of disconnection of the life-supporting lines
   c. Obstruction of the airway
   d. Facial-dependent edema
   e. Pressure sores leading to sepsis

Permissive hypercapnia

If the patient is under mechanical ventilation with the aim of lung protection goal, alveolar hypoventilation occurs with $PaCO_2$ of 60–70 mm Hg and respiratory acidosis but adverse effects such as arrhythmias and central nervous system (CNS) depression may occur. This hypercapnia is well tolerated by sedated patients. Permissive hypercapnia means slow rise at a rate of 10 mm Hg per hour, but if there is significant fall in pH then it will needs correction. In that case intravenous sodium bicarbonate has to be given temporarily to correct acidosis. But there is chance of fluid overload along with depletion of potassium in these patients who already has increased extravascular water content.

Open lung ventilation

In case of ARDS there are multiple areas of atelectasis at the bases due to reduced aeration of that part. Aim of open lung ventilation is to keep them open. This procedure is attempted in pressure-controlled ventilation with following parameters:

- **a.** Inspiration to expiration ratio of 1:1
- **b.** FiO_2—1
- **c.** PEEP to start with 15–20 cmH_2O in ARDS and lung will be opened with gradual increase by 2 cmH_2O of peak inspiratory pressure till it reaches 40–60 cmH_2O.

Successful recruitment of closed alveoli can be assumed by any of the following:

- **A.** Sudden sharp increase in PaO_2 to >450 mm Hg when the lungs open up fully.
- **B.** Proportional increase in tidal volume following peak expiratory pressure increase.

When the lung fully opens up, the adjustment of peak expiratory pressure with PEEP is required to maintain the lung open. The ideal pressure is 15–30 cmH_2O less than that required for opening peak pressure is able to maintain stable tidal volume. But open lung ventilation is not recommended as initial strategy of ventilation in ARDS patients.

Recruitment maneuvers

It is a method of brief application of high CPAP of 40 mm Hg for 40 seconds to open the collapsed alveoli. It may improve oxygenation but its use in undetermined. Adverse effects of this maneuver are:

- **a.** Hypotension
- **b.** Desaturation

These effects are self-limited and have no serious consequences.

Other measures are:

- **A.** Sedation:
  - **a.** It is invariably required for ARDS patients on mechanical ventilation to reduce their oxygen consumption and efficient ventilation.
  - **b.** Narcotics are required for relieving pain and suppression of respiratory drive.
  - **c.** Benzodiazepines are necessary for relieving anxiety.
  - **d.** Ideal dose, in case of mild or moderate ARDS, is the one which maintains efficient ventilatory support and makes the patient arouse easily, but in case of severe ARDS deep sedation is required.
- **B.** Paralytic agents: Use of paralytic agent will oxygenation through ventilatory support, but it has undesirable side effects. Hence, in case of severe ARDS having very low PaO_2/FiO_2 ratio.
- **C.** Fluid balance: Acute respiratory distress syndrome patient will not be overhydrated as it may worsen the pulmonary edema, so following precautions are necessary:
  - **a.** Left ventricular filling pressure to less than normal, i.e., pulmonary artery occlusive pressure of <4 mm Hg.
  - **b.** Central venous pressure to ≤4 mm Hg.

  Other fluid management strategies:
  - **a.** In patients with ARDS and hypoproteinemia, administration of furosemide and albumin to improve lung physiology. Since hypoproteinemia is a potential risk factor of ARDS, hence albumin administration improves the outcome of this ARDS.
- **D.** Circulatory support: Oxygen delivery to the tissue depends upon:
  - **a.** PaO_2
  - **b.** Cardiac output
  - **c.** Concentration of hemoglobin—it should be kept at 10 g/dL
  - **d.** Hematocrit level—it should be 35%

  Pressure support:
  - **a.** If the cardiac output is low—dobutamine
  - **b.** If the systolic pressure is below 90 mm Hg or systemic vascular resistance is low—dopamine or norepinephrine.

Support of other organ systems:

- **A.** Nutritional support:
  - **a.** 2,500 calories/day is required. But fluid restriction is vital as it may be detrimental to these patients.
  - **b.** Additional fluid can be removed by addition of loop diuretics if the renal function is good or ultrafiltration in case renal injury.
  - **c.** Feeding—it may be enteral, but in case of abdominal sepsis or ileus parenteral feeding is required.

B. Control of glucose: Blood glucose should be maintained in the range of 120–150 mg/dL.

C. DVT prophylaxis:

- **a.** Patient is always at risk of DVT and pulmonary thromboembolism, following are the risk factors:
  1. Prolonged immobility
  2. Trauma
  3. Sepsis
  4. Underlying illness
  5. Activation of coagulation pathways

  So, prophylaxis against DVT should be added.

D. Gastrointestinal bleeding: In patient on ventilatory support there is every chance of developing bleeding from stress ulcer. So, prophylaxis has to be added.

E. Role of corticosteroids: According to Society of Critical Care Medicine 1 mg/kg/day methylprednisolone may be given to moderate-to-severe ARDS with PaO_2/FiO_2 <200 and duration of disease is <14 days.

Q5. Write down the respiratory causes of dyspnea. How will you manage cardiac asthma?

MJPRU 2016/MDII (25)

ANSWER

Classification According to Severity of Dyspnea

Dyspnea can be defined as uncomfortable awareness of own respiratory effort. It can be classified into two types according to temporal factor:

A. Acute dyspnea:

This dyspnea can be defined as duration of dyspnea for 4–6 hours. This is tolerated badly. The most common causes are the following:

- **a.** Status asthmaticus
- **b.** Acute exacerbation of chronic bronchial asthma
- **c.** Pneumonia
- **d.** Acute pulmonary thromboembolism
- **e.** Pulmonary infarction
- **f.** Acute laryngotracheobronchitis

B. Chronic dyspnea:

It can be defined as duration of dyspnea for >1 month. Perception of this type is based on behavioral and physiologic response. The most common causes are the following:

- **a.** Alveolar causes:
  1. Bronchoalveolar carcinoma
  2. Chronic pneumonia
- **b.** Interstitial causes:
  1. Drugs (methotrexate)
  2. Radiation
  3. Lymphatic spread of malignancy
- **c.** Obstructive causes:
  1. Asthma
  2. Bronchitis
  3. Bronchiectasis
  4. Intrabronchial neoplasm
  5. Tracheomalacia
- **d.** Restrictive causes:
  1. Obesity
  2. Kyphoscoliosis
  3. Pneumothorax
  4. Pleural effusion
- **e.** Vascular causes:
  1. Idiopathic pulmonary hypertension
  2. Chronic pulmonary thromboembolism

Classifications According to Pathophysiology of Dyspnea

During breathing air enters through the nose from the atmosphere to the alveoli. In the alveoli oxygen and carbon dioxide transfer across the alveolar-capillary membrane. Carbon dioxide in bulk will be removed into atmosphere and blood will be oxygenated. This is a smooth process and is controlled through the following mechanisms:

A. Respiratory center controller:

It sends the efferent signal to muscles of ventilation and controls rate and depth of breathing. Following factors responsible for controlling the rate and depth of breathing:

- **a.** Hypoxia stimulates aortic and carotid bodies chemoreceptors from there afferent stimuli reach respiratory center.
- **b.** Hypercapnia: It diffuses into cerebrospinal fluid (CSF) and directly stimulates respiratory center.
- **c.** Stimuli from mechanoreceptors present in the trachea, larynx, large upper airways, skeletal, and respiratory muscles stimulates respiratory center.

- **d.** Stretch receptor present in the interstitium in the lung will be stimulated during interstitial lung disease (ILD) and interstitial pulmonary edema and send signals to respiratory center via vagus nerve.
- **e.** Drugs, like, aspirin directly stimulate respiratory center directly.
- **f.** Metabolic acidosis directly stimulates cerebral cortex.
- **g.** Patients with obstructive lung disease take breath slow and deep to minimize pleural pressure.
- **h.** Patients with restrictive lung diseases take shallow and rapid breath to minimize the work of breathing.

B. Ventilatory pump:

It is responsible for driving in and out the air of the respiratory system. It includes:

- **a.** Muscles involved in the ventilation
- **b.** Peripheral nerves supplying the respiratory muscles
- **c.** Pleura by producing negative pressure draw the chest cage outward and also the conducting airways which act as conduit for the flow of air from atmosphere to the alveoli and vice versa.

Following types of diseases responsible increase work of breathing:

- **a.** So any disease that produces reduced compliance of the lung or of the chest wall will obviously increases the work of breathing leading to breathlessness.
- **b.** Neurological disease, like, Guillain-Barré syndrome may produces weakness of the intercostal muscles and diaphragmatic muscle and increased work of breathing as these muscles require much more effort to create negative intrapleural pressure.

C. Impairment in gas exchange:

Impairment of gas exchange produces either hypoxia leading to hypoxic respiratory failure or hypercapnia leading to hypercapnic respiratory failure. There are following causes responsible for this type of impairment:

- **a.** V/Q mismatch which may occur in ARDS produces hypoxia but it can be relieved by oxygen supplementation.
- **b.** Intrapulmonary shunt which can occur in case atelectatic alveoli where there is no aeration, this is refractory to administration of oxygen.
- **c.** Thickened alveolar-capillary membrane reduces diffusion capacity of oxygen from alveoli to pulmonary capillary as occurs in case of ILDs. Here also high pressure oxygen may be of some help.

Management of Cardiac Asthma

It has been given in cardiology chapter Question Number 22.

Q6. Define hospital-acquired pneumonia. Discuss the etiology, diagnosis, and management of hospital-acquired pneumonia.

DNBII/DEC2012 (10)

Discuss the pathogenesis, clinical features, diagnosis, and treatment of nosocomial pneumonia.

MGR/SEP2007/MDIV (20)

Classify pneumonias. Discuss management of hospital-acquired pneumonia and its complications.

MUHS/MAY2013/MDII (25)

Discuss recent guidelines for prevention, diagnosis, and treatment for intensive care unit (ICU)-acquired pneumonia.

ERA/MAY2011/MDIV (10)

Treatment of health worker associated pneumonia.

MUHS/NOV2013/MDII (10)

Atypical pneumonia.

KUHS/MAY2014/MDII (10)

Etiology, clinical features, investigations, and treatment of atypical pneumonia.

DNB 2019 (10)

ANSWER

Definition

Hospital-acquired infections consist of three types:

A. Hospital-acquired pneumonia: It can be defined as pneumonias which are diagnosed 48 hours or more after admission.

B. Ventilator-associated pneumonias (VAPs): It can be defined as pneumonias which can be diagnosed 48 hours or more after endotracheal intubation and under ventilatory support.

C. Healthcare-associated pneumonias: It can be fined as pneumonias in a patient who will fill any one of the following criteria:

a. Patient has been admitted in an acute care unit of a hospital for ≥2 days within 90 days of diagnosis.

b. If the patient is residing in a nursing home or long-term care facility

c. If the patient receives antibiotic therapy or chemotherapy

d. If the patient received wound care within 30 days of current infection

e. If the patient attended hospital or hemodialysis units

Epidemiology

According to the Centers for Disease Control and Prevention (CDC) report:

A. Incidence of nosocomial pneumonia 0.9 per 1,000 ventilator days in case of medical ICU

B. Incidence of nosocomial pneumonia 2 per 1,000 ventilator days in case of medical ICU

Pathophysiology

Aspiration of Oropharyngeal Secretions

Source of Infected Secretions

A. In healthy adult, normal organisms that colonize the oropharyngeal mucosa are anaerobic organisms and harmless Neisseria pharyngitis. Whereas, in case ICU patients within 5–10 days gram-negative bacteria will colonize. So, aspiration of oropharyngeal secretions containing particulate matters and bacteria will retain in the lower respiratory tract.

B. Again, accumulated secretions in the larger as well as smaller airways

There are two sources of colonization:

A. Exogenous sources:

a. Hands

b. Clothing

c. Equipment of doctors, nurses, and heath cares

d. Unhealthy environment

e. Colonized instruments such as stethoscopes, humidifiers, respiratory equipment, and bronchoscope

f. Contaminated nebulizers

B. Endogenous sources:

a. Contamination and colonization in the oropharynx, proximal trachea, gastrointestinal tract, and endotracheal and tracheostomy tube.

During tracheal intubation or tracheostomy:

a. There is aspiration of oropharyngeal pathogens and inability of intrinsic respiratory defense to work against the pathogens leading to nosocomial pneumonias.

b. Pathogens will grow on the inner surface of the tube and aspirated or translocated into the lower respiratory tract.

After endotracheal intubation it will be lined by a biofilm of exopolysaccharide matrix within which bacteria will grow and cannot be eradicated by antibiotics and host immune response. But during tracheal aspiration, mechanical ventilation and bronchoscopy this infected biofilm will be dislodged into lower respiratory tract leading to nosocomial pneumonia. In case of severely ill patients this colonization is perpetuated.

Other invasive diagnostic and therapeutic procedures also promote aspiration and transfer of infected oropharyngeal contents into lower respiratory tract.

Usually upper respiratory tract will be colonized first but *Pseudomonas aeruginosa* will infect only the lower tract.

In case of healthy individual, fibronectin will cover the oropharyngeal epithelium and thus prevents colonization of gram-negative bacteria, but in case of critically ill patients this protective layer will be lost leading to adhesion and followed by colonization of bacteria with the oropharyngeal epithelial cells. Receptors will also be increased in the upper and lower respiratory tract in these patients.

Risk factors are the following:

a. Increasing age

b. Smoking

c. Obesity

d. Prolonged ventilation

e. Malnutrition

f. Major surgery

g. Underlying serious diseases

Gastric Colonization

Gastric acid will kill the bacteria swallowed from saliva. But if the gastric acidity is suppressed by antacids, histamine type 2 blocker or proton pump inhibitor, bacteria will survive, multiply, and colonize in the gastrointestinal tract. In following conditions, gastric aspirates containing gram-negative bacteria will enter into lower respiratory tract leading to aspiration pneumonia:

a. Sedate patients
b. Unconscious patients
c. Following large amount of vomiting
d. Obtunded patients

So, stress ulcer treatment with sucralfate will no significantly increase the gastric pH and thus decreases the incidence of nosocomial pneumonia.

Hematogenous Spread Producing Pneumonia

A. Catheter-related sepsis and other sources of sepsis
B. Infected emboli from septic thrombophlebitis.

Inhalation Pneumonia

Contaminated respiratory equipment in the form of infected aerosols having particle size of 3–5 micron will deposit in the terminal bronchioles and alveoli leading to nosocomial pneumonia.

Iatrogenic Causes

During suction of the tracheobronchial tree through the tracheostomy or endotracheal tube, lack of aseptic precaution will produce pneumonia.

Factors Responsible for Nosocomial Pneumonias

A. Host factors:
  a. Overwhelming infections like:
    1. Severe sepsis
    2. Burns
    3. After major surgery
    4. Prolonged shock
    5. Severe trauma
  b. Background factors:
    1. Advancing age
    2. Diabetes mellitus
    3. Renal dysfunction
    4. Hepatic dysfunction
    5. Malnutrition
    6. Underlying malignancy
    7. Cardiac dysfunction
  c. Total parenteral nutrition
B. Therapeutic interventions:
  a. Endotracheal intubation
  b. Tracheostomy
  c. Nasogastric tube
  d. Use of invasive procedures
  e. Use of immunosuppressive or chemotherapy therapy
  f. Prolonged use of antibiotics
  g. Colonization of gram-negative bacteria in the gastrointestinal tract
C. Environmental factors:
  a. Overcrowding
  b. Increased prevalence of multidrug resistant (MDR) organisms
  c. Contaminated hands of ICU personnel
  d. Unclean environment

Clinical Features

A. Fulminant infections of respiratory tract due to gram-negative pathogens such as *Pseudomonas aeruginosa* and *Acinetobacter* producing respiratory failure
B. Fever, purulent sputum
C. Respiratory failure producing persistent hypoxia in spite of high FiO_2, peak expiratory flow (PEF) rate
D. Feature of septic shock like hypotension, multiorgan failure requiring dialysis

Clinical Diagnosis of Nosocomial Pneumonia

A. Chest X-ray demonstrating new or progressive alveolar infiltrate
B. Fever
C. Leukocytosis of >12,000/cc or leukopenia of <4,000/cc
D. Appearance of purulent sputum or in case of VAP purulent tracheal secretions

Presence of abnormal radiographic infiltrate plus at least two out of three clinical criteria is highly sensitive but less specific. But when all three criteria plus fresh alveolar infiltrate are present it is less sensitive but more specific.

Microbiology

Following factors are responsible for nosocomial pneumonia depends upon several factors:

a. Patients and healthcare workers in ICUs
b. Gravity of underlying illness
c. Duration of mechanical ventilation
d. Invasive or noninvasive methods used to collect the material for examinations
e. Previous antibiotic therapy

Each ICU has own pattern of distribution of bacteria for development of nosocomial pneumonia. Organisms in these units are usually *Acinetobacter*, *Klebsiella*, and

Pseudomonas aeruginosa. They may be MDR—usually to carbapenem and colistin. Other bacteria are methicillin-resistant staphylococci.

Diagnosis

Bacteriological examinations such as Gram stain, culture, and sensitivity of lower respiratory secretions collected invasively or noninvasively are helpful for the diagnosis and will direct the antibiotic treatment. Negative culture will make the diagnosis of nosocomial pneumonia unlikely. Quantitative culture method having cutoff point of 10^6 colony-forming unit/mL will increase the specificity of diagnosis of nosocomial pneumonia.

A. Noninvasive methods:
- **a.** Examination of sputum in patient with artificial airway
- **b.** Examination of aspirates collected by suction through the endotracheal tube or tracheostomy

B. Invasive methods:
- **a.** Collection of samples for lower respiratory tract in the area of radiographic infiltrate by protected specimen brush
- **b.** Bronchoalveolar lavage—10^3–10^5 colony-forming unit/mL is considered as positive
- **c.** Blinded invasive procedures, like:
  1. Blinded bronchial brushing samples
  2. Mini-BAL
  3. Blinded sampling with protected specimen brush

In well-developed countries, bronchoscopic diagnostic procedures are required in following situations:
- **a.** Specificity of the diagnosis will be improved
- **b.** Use of unnecessary use of antibiotics
- **c.** Where smears and cultures will be negative

In case of underdeveloped countries, noninvasive method of diagnoses are used.

Antibiotic Therapy

Selection of antibiotic therapy will depend upon the following:

A. Awareness and knowledge of core organisms prevalent along with their culture and sensitivity to different antibiotics in ICU

B. Time of onset of VAP

C. Presence of risk factors for multidrug-resistant (MDR) pathogens and its clinical back ground

D. Any history regarding the antibiotic administered prior to onset of pneumonia

Clinical Background

A. Risk factors for MDR-resistant organisms:
- **a.** Current hospitalization of 5 days or more
- **b.** Antibiotic therapy within past 90 days
- **c.** Immunosuppressed patients
- **d.** Multiple invasive procedures
- **e.** Comorbid states
- **f.** Marked severity of critical illness
- **g.** High frequency of organisms resistant to multiple drugs

B. Following features of severe nosocomial pneumonia:
- **a.** Rapid radiographic progression
- **b.** Respiratory failure with increasing hypoxia
- **c.** Severe sepsis with hypotension with or without multiorgan failure
- **d.** Acute kidney injury requiring hemodialysis

Principles of Antibiotic Therapy

Empiric antibiotic therapy in case of nosocomial pneumonia with no risk factor:

A. *Streptococcus pneumoniae* and *Haemophilus influenzae*: Ceftriaxone or amoxicillin plus clavulanic acid

B. Enterobacteriaceae: Piperacillin plus tazobactam

Empiric antibiotic therapy in case of nosocomial pneumonia in presence of risk factor:

A. Enterobacteriaceae, *Pseudomonas aeruginosa, Acinetobacter baumannii,* and other gram-negative bacilli: Cefepime or piperacillin plus tazobactam or carbapenem

Here the antibiotic choice depends upon:

A. Prevalence and culture of the organisms in that unit

B. Severity of the disease

If MDR pathogen is suspected, in that case combination of two or more antibiotics should be used to wide cover of the organisms. In that case following combinations should be started:
- **a.** Piperacillin-tazobactam plus vancomycin/teicoplanin
- **b.** Carbapenem plus vancomycin/teicoplanin

In case of MDR *Pseudomonas* or *Acinetobacter* colistin should be added with carbapenem to enhance the maximum synergistic activity.

If methicillin-resistant *Staphylococcus aureus* (MRSA) is suspected then vancomycin has to be added with above antibiotics.

In case of aspiration of oropharyngeal content or gastric content, the clindamycin or metronidazole has to be added.

Once reports of culture sensitivity are obtained then in the organism is showing resistant to any antibiotic then that antibiotic has to be omitted and another antibiotic sensitive to that pathogen has to be added.

Duration of Therapy

A. If there is sharp improvement of the clinical condition within 3–4 days after starting the therapy, and SaO_2 improves along with the declining of inflammatory marker level, in that case antibiotics should be withdrawn after 7–10 days.

B. In following case antibiotic should be continued for several weeks:

- **a.** In case of breakdown of lung tissue forming one or more abscesses
- **b.** In presence of empyema
- **c.** Persistent intra-abdominal sepsis

Q7. Discuss the etiology, management, and complications of community-acquired pneumonia (CAP).

DNBII/JUN2013/ (10)

Discuss the infective agents in community-acquired and nosocomial pneumonia. Outline the outline the management in both types.

DNBIIB/DEC2014 (10)

Enumerate the etiologic agents of CAP. How will you assess the severity of CAP? Outline the management of CAP in a 50-year-old male patient.

DNBII/APR2016 (2)

CAP.

MGR/OCT2015/MDIII (7)

KUHS/MAY2013/MDII (10)

Treatment of CAP.

MGR/APR2013/MDIII (7)

Discuss the definition, risk factors, clinical features, and treatment of pneumonia.

MGR/MAR2002/MDI (25)

Describe the etiology, clinical features, diagnosis, treatment, and complications of severe CAP.

MGR/SEP2006/MDIII (15)

Discuss epidemiology, pathophysiology, clinical feature, and management of CAP.

GMC/2016/MDII (20)

Discuss the pathophysiology of lobar pneumonia in relation to clinical signs.

KUHS/MAY2014/MDI (10)

Lobar pneumonia.

MGR/APR2013/MDI (5)

Empirical antibiotic treatment in case of community acquired pneumonia.

DNB 2020 (6)

Classify pneumonia syndrome and pathological stages of consolidation.

DR YSR UNI OF HEALTH SC, VIJAYAWADA, ANDHRA, 2022 (10)

Draw bronchopulmonary segments. Write about etiology and pathology of lobar pneumonia.

DR YSR UNI OF HEALTH SC, VIJAYAWADA, ANDHRA, 2022 (10)

Community acquired pneumonia.

MGR UNIVERSITY, TAMIL NADU, 2020 (10)

ANSWER

Definition

Pneumonia can be defined as infection as well as consolidation of lung parenchyma caused by bacteria and viruses. There are four types of pneumonia:

A. CAP

B. Hospital-acquired pneumonia

C. VAP

D. Healthcare-associated pneumonia: It means CAP that is caused by MDR pathogens associated with hospital-acquired pneumonia.

Etiology

A. Bacteria:

- **a.** Typical bacterial pathogens:
  - **1.** *Streptococcus pneumoniae*—it is less common after increasing use of pneumococcal vaccine.

2. *Staphylococcus aureus*
3. *Haemophilus influenzae*
4. *Klebsiella pneumoniae*
5. *Pseudomonas aeruginosa*

b. Atypical bacterial pathogens:
1. *Mycoplasma pneumoniae*
2. *Chlamydia pneumoniae*
3. *Legionella pneumophila*

c. Anaerobic bacteria:
1. Oral anaerobes
2. Anaerobes

B. Viruses:
a. Influenza
b. Parainfluenza
c. Adenoviruses
d. Metapneumoviruses
e. Respiratory syncytial viruses (RSVs)
f. Varicella-zoster
g. Measles

Epidemiology

Over all attack rate in adult is 5.16–12 cases per 1,000 persons per year. In case of CAP due to influenza virus attack and mortality rate are in winter but in tropical countries incidence can be increased in rainy season. Epidemiology of pneumonia has been changed in Asian countries recently due to following reasons:

a. Changes in the type of population at risk
b. Changes in antimicrobial agents in case of microbes
c. Identification of new microbes as an etiological agent
d. Widespread use of *Haemophilus influenzae*, pneumococcal, and influenza in the West.

Epidemiological Risk Factors

A. CAP occurs at any age but most vulnerable groups are extremes of age—children of <5 years and adult of >65 years of age. In elderly, associated morbidities are:
a. Congestive cardiac heart failure
b. Chronic obstructive lung disease
c. Diabetes
d. Chronic renal failure

B. Alcoholism: It will hamper the mechanisms of the respiratory tract by following mechanisms:
a. It facilitates colonization of bacteria in the respiratory tract.
b. It hinders mucociliary transport.
c. It impairs swallowing and cough reflexes thus facilitating aspiration.
d. It impairs the function of alveolar macrophage, neutrophil, lymphocyte, and monocyte.

C. Poor nutrition: Impaired nutrition is responsible for following abnormal functions:
a. It impairs cellular immunity.
b. It impairs function of macrophages.
c. It will decrease the level of immunoglobulin A2 (IgA2).

Thus, it increases the frequency of mortality of pneumonia in children of developing countries.

D. Immunosuppression: It will increase the propensity to develop pneumonia.

E. Smoking: It will impair respiratory mechanism by following methods:
a. It adversely affects mucociliary transport.
b. It will affect humoral and cellular immune responses.
c. It increases adherence of *Streptococcus pneumoniae* and *Haemophilus influenzae*.

F. Poverty: Increased risk of pneumonia due to following related factors:
a. Poor nutrition
b. Poverty
c. Overcrowding
d. Poor hygiene
e. Inhospital living conditions

G. Aspiration:
a. Aspiration of gastric contents leads to chemical inflammation leading to:
1. Hemorrhagic bronchitis
2. Well-marked bronchospasm
3. Alveolar hemorrhage
4. Damage of surfactant leading to atelectasis

b. Aspiration of gastric content in patients on proton pump inhibitor leads to pneumonia
c. Aspiration of oropharyngeal contents leads to:
1. Anaerobic organism-related pneumonia—anaerobic streptococci and *Bacteroides* species.
2. Gram-negative organisms

Following are the risk factors for different etiological agents:

Agents	Risk factors
Pneumococcal pneumonia	• Dementia • Seizures • Heart failure • Alcoholism • Cerebrovascular disease • COPD • Tobacco smoking • Gag reflexes
MRSA pneumonia	• Skin colonization • Infection with community-acquired MRSA
Enterobacteriaceae	• Hospitalized patient • Patient received antibiotic therapy • Comorbidities such as alcohol, heart failure, or renal insufficiency
Pseudomonas aeruginosa	• Bronchiectasis • Cystic fibrosis • Severe chronic obstructive lung disease
Legionella pneumophila	• Male sex • Diabetes • Hematogenic malignancy • Severe renal disease • Cancer • Human immunodeficiency virus (HIV) infection • Smoking • Recent hotel stay • Ship cruise

Pathogenesis

Bacteria enter the lower respiratory tract by four mechanisms:

A. Bacteria in the form of small droplets enter into tracheobronchial tree.

B. Aspiration of gastric and oropharyngeal contents through larynx to tracheobronchial tree. This occurs mainly in deep sleep, especially in elderly or during seizures, unconsciousness. It is the most common pathway.

C. Less commonly *Staphylococcus aureus* spreads from distal primary sources like tricuspid endocarditis or from direct introduction into the veins through bloodstream to lung.

D. Direct contagious extension of infection from infected mediastinal or pleural space.

Host Defense Factors

Following defense factors protect the human being from infection of the lung parenchyma:

A. Hair and turbinates in the nasal cavity capture large inhaled particles prior to their entry into lower respiratory tract.

B. Airway lining present in the branching of tracheobronchial tree traps the microbes from where the mucus and local antibacterial factors kills followed by clearing them.

C. Two reflexes—gag and cough reflexes are the protective reflexes against the aspiration of oropharyngeal contents.

D. Normal flora present in the oropharyngeal mucosa prevents pathogenic bacteria from binding to the mucosal surface thus decreasing the risk of pneumonia.

After Entry into Lower Respiratory Tract

A. When the pathogens reach the lower respiratory tract by overcoming the host defense alveolar macrophages assisted by surfactant protein A and D produced by surfactant kill and clear the pathogens by their opsonizing properties and antibacterial as well as antiviral activities.

B. When the macrophages engulf killed or living pathogens they will be eliminated by mucociliary elevator or by lymphatics completely. But when the amount of pathogens overwhelms the capacity of macrophages to kill then the clinical pneumonia ensues.

C. Then in response to survived pathogens series of inflammatory response starts. Macrophages release proinflammatory cytokines such as IL-1 and TNF resulting fever.

D. Released chemokines, IL-8, and colony-stimulating factor attract neutrophils at the site of infection producing sputum and in the peripheral blood leading to leukocytosis.

E. Inflammatory mediators released by neutrophils as well as alveolar macrophages produce leak at the alveolar-capillary membrane which to start with as localized leak then can spread to the surrounding area. Sometimes red blood cells (RBCs) will also pass through the leak and thus produces rusty sputum or hemoptysis. This alveolar-capillary leak produces crackles on auscultation and hypoxemia detected in blood gas analysis. This hypoxemia will be aggravated by hypoxemic pulmonary vasoconstriction.

F. Systemic inflammatory response syndrome increases the respiratory drive leading to tachypnea and respiratory alkalosis.

G. There will be decreased compliance leading to dyspnea of the lung due to following factors:

- **a.** Increased capillary leak
- **b.** Increased respiratory drive
- **c.** Respiratory alkalosis
- **d.** Increased secretion in the alveoli
- **e.** Bronchospasm due to infection

H. If reduced lung volume and compliance along with intrapulmonary shunting of blood are enormously severe this will lead to respiratory failure and death.

Pathology

A. Earliest phage is presence of edema due to accumulation of proteinaceous exudate with pathogens in the alveoli—this phase is not clinically evident.

B. Next phase is red hepatization phase: In this phase cellular and intra-alveolar exudate are composed of leaked erythrocytes, influxed neutrophil required for host defense, and occasionally bacteria.

C. Gray hepatization: In this phase cellular and intra-alveolar exudates are composed of lysed and degraded erythrocytes, no new erythrocyte, large number of neutrophils, abundant accumulated fibrin, but no bacteria. This phase corresponds to:

- **a.** Improved gas exchange
- **b.** Containment of infection

D. Phase of resolution: In this phase alveolar exudate is composed of largely reappeared macrophages and debris of neutrophils, but no bacteria and fibrin.

This is classically seen in case of lobar pneumonia due to pneumococcus but not in other etiologies.

Pathologically pneumonia can be divided into three types:

A. Lobar pneumonia: It involves entire lobes but not limited by segmental boundaries and appears as dense consolidation. Here the spread of infection is due to:

- **a.** Alveolus to alveolus
- **b.** Acinus-to-acinus through the pores of Kohn

Classical example of pneumonia is pneumococcal pneumonia.

B. Bronchopneumonia: Here distal airways are inflamed along with involvement of alveoli. So it appears as patchy distribution depending on which airways are involved. Examples are staphylococcal pneumonia or pneumonia due to other gram-negative bacilli.

C. Interstitial pneumonia: It is characterized by presence of infiltrate in the interstitial space not involving alveolar space, but in severe cases interstitial infiltrate may spread into alveolar spaces. Classical example is viral pneumonia.

Clinical Features

A. Symptoms:

- **a.** Fever may be with shaking chill.
- **b.** Cough: It may be nonproductive in case of viral or mycoplasma pneumonia. But in case of bacterial pneumonia, it is mucoid, purulent, or blood-tinged sputum or rusty sputum.
- **c.** Hemoptysis in case of community-associated MRSA (CA-MRSA) involvement.
- **d.** If the patient is unable, speak full sentence—suggest breathlessness.
- **e.** If parenchymal involvement extends to pleura—pleuritic chest pain.
- **f.** 20% patients may develop nausea, vomiting, and diarrhea.
- **g.** Other features are fatigue, myalgia, headache, and headache.

B. Physical examinations:

- **a.** General survey:
  1. Tachypnea
  2. Tachycardia
  3. May be cyanosis
  4. High temperature
- **b.** Systemic examination:
  1. On inspection, movement on the affected side will be diminished.
  2. On palpation:
     - Movement diminished
     - Trachea central
     - Presence of vocal fremitus
  3. Percussion note will be woody dull indicating consolidation or fibrosis or atelectasis but centrally positioned trachea excludes last two diagnoses.
  4. On auscultation:
     - Breath sound bronchial
     - Vocal resonance increased
     - In case of resolution phase there may be presence of crackles
     - Presence of pleural rub in presence of pleural pain

Specific Features in Different Types of Pneumonia

A. In case of pneumococcal pneumonia:
- **a.** It usually follows viral upper respiratory infection
- **b.** Onset is abrupt with high fever and shaking chills
- **c.** Cough is productive, purulent, or rusty sputum

B. In case of mycoplasma pneumonia:
- **a.** Young adults are mainly affected
- **b.** Onset is insidious
- **c.** Fever is not high, chills are often absent
- **d.** Cough is prominent symptoms but nonproductive

C. In case of staphylococcal or gram-negative bacillary pneumonia:
- **a.** Patient has underlying medical problem or patient is receiving antibiotics
- **b.** It may be due to secondary complication of influenza infection
- **c.** It is blood-borne disseminated infection

D. In case of pneumonia due to anaerobic organism:
- **a.** It occurs due to aspiration of oropharyngeal contents in patient having poor dentition, gingivitis, periodontal abscess, and impaired consciousness
- **b.** Onset is gradual
- **c.** Odor of the sputum is foul, suggest anaerobic infection
- **d.** As a result of extensive necrosis there may be formation of anaerobic abscess

E. In case of *Legionella* pneumophila infection:
- **a.** It is localized outbreak
- **b.** Patient impaired respiratory defense is affected
- **c.** Associated involvement of other systems such as gastrointestinal, hepatic, renal, and CNS involvement

Diagnostic Procedures

A. Chest radiography can demonstrate the distribution, extent of the disease, and can give the clue to the nature of etiology.
- **a.** Lobar distribution in streptococcal pneumoniae or *Klebsiella pneumoniae*
- **b.** Patchy localized or extensive distribution in staphylococcal pneumonia
- **c.** Pneumatocele suggests staphylococcal pneumonia
- **d.** Interstitial infiltrates in mycoplasma and viral pneumonia
- **e.** In case of *Legionella* infection lesion will be patchy or consolidated unilobar distribution
- **f.** Aspiration of oropharyngeal content in the dependent region of the lung like:
  1. Lower lobe in case of up-right patients
  2. In case of supine patient:
     - Posterior segment of upper lobe
     - Superior segment of lower lobe

In strongly suspicious patient having CAP but normal chest X-ray, empiric antibiotic therapy should be started and then after 48 hours repeat chest X-ray has to be done to see whether it is really present or not. Radiological improvement to treatment is lags behind the clinical improvement like in case of pneumococcal pneumonia it takes 6 weeks to clear and in case of staphylococcal or *Legionella* pneumonia it takes much longer. Age is the main predictor of speed resolution. In elderly patient, resolution takes longer time. It lesion will persist in spite of treatment or it will increase or it will recur then one has think about obstruction of bronchus or endobronchial tumor or foreign body.

B. Gram stain and culture of sputum: First point in case of staining is that sample must be suitable for culture, i.e., sputum sample must have <10 squamous epithelial cells and ≥25 neutrophils per high-power field. But there are few practical problem regarding collection of sputum, these are:
- **a.** Usually lower respiratory tract secretion is contaminated with upper respiratory tract commensal organisms; in that case in the laboratory the sample has to be diluted with sterile saline so that only bacteria will be present in the sample to get growth in the culture.
- **b.** Single dose of antibiotic can hinder the growth of the pathogen in the culture medium.
- **c.** Routine culture of sputum is not useful for three different causes of pneumonia; these are *Legionella*, *Chlamydophila*, and *Mycoplasma*.

  In case of intensive care admitted patient, deep suction aspirate or BAL collected via bronchoscopy or non-bronchoscopically or sample by needle aspiration of lung can be sent. In case of *Legionella*, special culture medium is available.

C. Blood culture: At least two samples for culture has to be taken from two different sites. Results of properly collected blood from hospitalized patients of CAP even prior to antibiotic therapy are 5–14%. Most commonly isolated pathogen is *Streptococcus pneumoniae*. Because of the low yield of pathogen it is not considered as real-time investigation in this patient. But in following types of patient blood should be sent for culture:

a. Neutropenia secondary to pneumonia
b. Asplenia
c. Complement deficiencies
d. Chronic liver disease
e. Severe community-acquired pneumonia

D. Urine antigen test: Two commercially available tests in urine are:

a. Pneumococcal polysaccharide capsular antigen can be detected in urine even in the patient who is in antibiotic therapy with sensitivity and specificity of 70% and >90%, respectively and it will be detectable 7–14 days after pneumococcal bacteremia.
b. *Legionella* serogroup type 1 antigen is detected in urine in patient with sensitivity and specificity of 70% and 99%, respectively.

E. Sputum and blood antigen test: In case of pneumococcal pneumonia, polysaccharide antigen of pneumoniae can be diagnosed by countercurrent immunoelectrophoresis and latex agglutination. Other pathogens detected by immunodetection in the sputum are *Legionella pneumophila, Pneumocystis carinii* and *Chlamydia pneumoniae.* In suspected case of *Legionella* following specific tests should include:

a. *Legionella* antigen in urine
b. Direct antibody test is positive with antibody titer being 1:256
c. Isolation of the *Legionella* in culture or fourfold rise in antibody titer

F. Polymerase chain reaction (PCR): It can detect deoxyribonucleic acid (DNA) or ribonucleic acid (RNA) of the pathogens. PCR of nasopharyngeal swab is the standard test for nucleic acid detection of:

a. *Legionella pneumophila*
b. *Chlamydia pneumoniae*
c. *Mycoplasma pneumoniae*
d. Mycobacteria
e. Influenza
f. Coronaviruses

In patient with pneumococcal pneumonia, whole blood PCR can diagnose bacterial load and is associated with septic shock and even death.

G. Biomarkers: Two important biomarkers are:

a. Acute phase reactant is CRP in presence of inflammation can identify:
   1. Worsening of the disease
   2. Treatment failure
b. Procalcitonin—it is helpful in following conditions:
   1. Distinguish bacterial from viral infection
   2. It can determine need for antibacterial therapy.
   3. It can help to take decision regarding the discontinuation of treatment.
   4. In presence of specific history and physical examination, it can help for antibiotic stewardship.

H. ABGs:

a. In early case: Hypoxemia, hypercapnia, and respiratory alkalosis
b. In late case: Hypoxemia, hypercapnia, and respiratory acidosis

I. Hematological findings:

a. Leukocytosis with neutrophilia—bacterial pneumonia
b. In case of overwhelming sepsis there will be leukopenia
c. In case of viral infection normal leukocyte count with lymphocytosis
d. Presence of cold agglutinins—mycoplasma pneumonia
e. Liver and renal function tests, hyponatremia due to syndrome of inappropriate secretion of antidiuretic hormone (SIADH)—can be found in *Legionella* infection.

Treatment

Estimation of Severity of Pneumonia

Confusion, uremia, respiratory rate, blood pressure, and age > 65 years (CURB-65): It includes following variables:

A. Confusion
B. Urea > 7 mmol/L
C. Respiratory rate > 30 breaths/min
D. Blood pressure—systolic <90 mm Hg or diastolic <60 mm Hg
E. Age > 65 years

Group 1: 0–1—low mortality, domiciliary treatment
Group 2: 2–3—9.2% mortality, hospitalized treatment
Group 3: ≥3—22% mortality, admission in ICU

According to American Thoracic Society Guidelines

Any one major or two minor criteria suggests severe CAP:

A. Major criteria:
  - **a.** Septic shock
  - **b.** Need for mechanical ventilation

B. Minor criteria:
  - **a.** PaO_2/FiO_2 <250 kPa
  - **b.** Multilobar shadowing on chest radiography
  - **c.** Systolic blood pressure of <90 mm Hg

Following factors require hospitalization: If any one of CURB criteria is fulfilled and any one of more of the following:

- **a.** Hypothermia or hyperpyrexia
- **b.** Pulse >120 beats/min
- **c.** Multilobar involvement or presence of cavitation or moderate pleural effusion or metastatic complications
- **d.** Anemia, thrombocytopenia, or marked leukopenia
- **e.** PaO_2/FiO_2 < 250 kPa or PaO_2 <60 mm Hg or arterial pH <7.3
- **f.** Presence of significant comorbid disease, like:
  1. Moderately severe COPD
  2. Congestive heart failure
  3. Immunodeficiency states
  4. Cardiac disease
  5. Immunosuppression from any disease
- **g.** Management in home is impossible because:
  1. Poor compliance
  2. Altered mentation

Choice of antibiotics is influenced by following factors:

- **a.** Presence of coexisting illness
- **b.** Any history of recent treatment with antibiotics
- **c.** Residence in nursing home
- **d.** How much severity of illness at the initial presentation.

Category of patient	Common organisms	Other organisms	Initial therapies
Outdoor patients having no cardiopulmonary disease or any risk factor	*Streptococcus pneumoniae* *Mycoplasma pneumoniae* Respiratory viruses *Haemophilus influenzae*	*Legionella pneumophila* Endemic fungi *Mycobacterium tuberculosis*	Azithromycin Or Clarithromycin 500 mg twice daily Or Doxycycline 100 mg twice daily
Outdoor patient having cardiopulmonary disease or any other risk factor	*Streptococcus pneumoniae* *Mycoplasma pneumoniae* Respiratory viruses *Haemophilus influenzae* Aerobic gram-negative bacilli Anaerobes *Chlamydia pneumoniae*	*Legionella pneumophila* Endemic fungi *Mycobacterium tuberculosis*	Oral quinolones like levofloxacin 750 mg daily Or β-lactam along with macrolide like azithromycin 500 mg twice daily Or Third-generation cephalosporin like cefuroxime 500 mg twice daily
Hospitalized patients	*Streptococcus pneumoniae* *Mycoplasma pneumoniae* Respiratory viruses *Haemophilus influenzae* Aerobic gram-negative bacilli Anaerobes *Chlamydia pneumoniae* *Legionella pneumophila*	*Mycobacterium* catarrhalis *Mycobacterium tuberculosis* Endemic fungi	Co-amoxiclav 1.2 g 8 hourly intravenously Or Ceftriaxone 2 g twice daily intravenously + Azithromycin orally 500 mg twice daily
Severely ill patients	*Streptococcus pneumoniae* *Mycoplasma pneumoniae* Respiratory viruses *Haemophilus influenzae* Aerobic gram-negative bacilli Anaerobes Chlamydia pneumoniae *Legionella pneumophila*		Amoxicillin 500 mg orally twice daily + Piperacillin-tazobactam 4.5 g thrice daily Or Meropenem 1 g thrice daily intravenously + Vancomycin 500 mg four times daily (if suspected MRSA) + Macrolide

In Case of Pseudomonas Infection

Piperacillin-tazobactam 4.5 g intravenously 6 hourly or 1–2 g cefepime twice daily or imipenem 500 mg 6 hourly or 1 g meropenem 8 hourly intravenously + levofloxacin 750 mg intravenously four times daily.

In Case of MRSA

Linezolid 600 mg or 15 mg/kg vancomycin intravenously initially with adjusted doses + 300 mg clindamycin.

Duration of Treatment

A. In case of uncomplicated pneumonias due to streptococcal pneumoniae, *Haemophilus influenzae* and *Mycobacterium catarrhalis* treatment should be continued for 7–10 days.

B. In case of pneumonias due to *Mycoplasma pneumoniae* and *Legionella pneumophila* treatment duration is 2–3 weeks.

C. In case of nonbacteremic staphylococcal pneumonia treatment duration will be 2 weeks.

D. In case of staphylococcal pneumonia with complicated empyema treatment duration will be 4–6 weeks.

Supportive Treatment

A. If the patient is in respiratory distress with PaO_2 of <90 mm Hg, 2–4 L/min oxygen inhalation.

B. If PaO_2 is <60 mm Hg with rising $PaCO_2$, respiratory acidosis, with copious respiratory secretion mechanical ventilatory support is essential.

C. If the patient is unable to cough but has copious secretion—endotracheal intubation for proper aspiration of secretion.

D. If the patient is hypotensive due to shock, inotropic agents such as dopamine and dobutamine and vasopressors like norepinephrine have to be administered.

E. Pleural pain can be treated by nonsedative analgesic.

F. Physiotherapy should be avoided in case of severely ill patients but it can assist in expectoration.

Q8. Risk factors, prevention, diagnosis, and management of VAP.

DNBIIA/DEC2015 (10)

VAP.

MGR/APR2015/MDII (7)

PGI/APR2013/MDIII (10)

AMU/2011/MDII (10)

Prevention strategies of VAP.

MGR/OCT2011/MDIV (7)

Discuss etiology, epidemiology, clinical manifestation, diagnosis, and treatment of case of VAP.

BF/MAY2010/MDII (30)

Etiological causes, clinical presentation, and management of VAP.

DNBI/DEC2010 (10)

Define VAPs. Enumerate the microbes causing it and outline the treatment approach.

DNBIV/JUN2010 (10)

Ventilator associated pneumonia.

DR YSR UNI OF HEALTH SC, VIJAYAWADA, ANDHRA, 2022 (10)

ANSWER

Definition

It can be defined as pneumonia developed after 48 hours of endotracheal intubation and patient under ventilatory support.

Etiology

Agents are subdivided into MDR and non-MDR bacterial pathogens.

A. MDR bacterial pathogens:
- **a.** MRSA
- **b.** *Pseudomonas aeruginosa*
- **c.** *Legionella pneumophila*
- **d.** *Acinetobacter*
- **e.** Antibiotic-resistant Enterobacteriaceae
- **f.** *Burkholderia cepacia*
- **g.** *Aspergillus* species

B. Non-MDR bacteria:
- **a.** *Streptococcus pneumoniae*
- **b.** *Haemophilus influenzae*
- **c.** Methicillin-sensitive *Staphylococcus aureus*
- **d.** Antibiotic-sensitive Enterobacteriaceae:
  1. *Enterobacter* species
  2. *Proteus* species
  3. *Escherichia coli*
  4. *Klebsiella pneumoniae*
  5. *Serratia marcescens*

Pathogenesis

Frequency of diagnosis depends upon the duration of mechanical ventilation having highest hazards ratio in first 5 days. Following five factors are very important in the pathogenesis:

- **a.** Microorganisms colonization in the oropharynx:
  1. Normal flora elimination
  2. During the time of intubation aspiration of large volume oropharyngeal secretion
  3. Gastroesophageal reflux
  4. Overgrowth of bacteria in the stomach cavity
- **b.** Aspiration of the organisms from oropharynx to lower respiratory tract.
- **c.** Altered normal host defense mechanisms—glycocalyx biofilm formed on the surface of endotracheal tube by pathogenic bacteria protects the bacteria from antibiotics. Later on these bacteria will be dislodged during suction and either fragments of it containing bacteria will embolize distal airways or reinoculate in the trachea.
- **d.** Microaspiration around the endotracheal tube:
  1. Endotracheal intubation
  2. Pooling of secretion above the endotracheal tube
  3. Ventilation duration will be prolonged
  4. Abnormal swallowing function
- **e.** Alteration of oropharyngeal flora due to following risk factors:
  1. Antibiotic selection pressure
  2. Antibiotic exposure
  3. Cross infection from other colonized patients
  4. Malnutrition
  5. Contaminated equipment

Clinical Features

Symptoms and signs are similar to that of community-acquired pneumonia.

There is presence of new or changing radiographic infiltrate will be demonstrated in chest X-ray.

Diagnosis

New guideline of ventilator-associated conditions:

- **A.** Possible VAP: After third day of ventilation and within 2 days of worsening of oxygenation, any one of the following criteria should be met:
  - **a.** Purulent tracheobronchial secretion demonstrating >25 neutrophils as well as <10 squamous epithelial cells per low power field.
  - **b.** Culture of sputum/endobronchial aspirates or BAL fluid or lung tissue or protected specimen brushing is positive.
- **B.** Probable VAP: After third day of ventilation and within 2 days of worsening of oxygenation, any one of the following criteria should be met:
  - **a.** Purulent secretion from one or more specimen of respiratory tract and any one of the following:
    1. More than 10^5 colony-forming unit/mL in endotracheal aspirate.
    2. More than 10^4 colony-forming unit/mL in BAL fluid
    3. More than 10^4 colony-forming unit/mL in lung tissue
    4. More than 10^3 colony-forming unit/mL in protected specimen brushing
  - **b.** One of the following without the need for purulent respiratory secretions:
    - **a.** Pleural fluid aspirated following paracentesis or ICD is culture positive
    - **b.** Histopathology of lung tissue is positive
    - **c.** Serology positive for common viral infections such as RSV, adenovirus, and influenza virus.

Treatment

Important risk factors for MDR-resistant bacteria:

- **A.** 5 or more days of hospitalization
- **B.** Evidence of antibiotic therapy in past 90 days
- **C.** Markedly severe critical illness
- **D.** Patients are immunocompromised
- **E.** Patients have multiple comorbidities
- **F.** Evidence of high frequency of antibiotic-resistant organisms
- **G.** History of multiple invasive procedures

Empiric therapy for MDR-resistant organisms and no risk factor:

- **A.** *Streptococcus pneumoniae* or *Haemophilus influenzae*:
  - **a.** Ceftriaxone 2 g twice daily or,
  - **b.** Amoxicillin + clavulanic acid or,
  - **c.** Levofloxacin 750 mg four times daily or,
  - **d.** Cefepime 2 g intravenously 8 hourly
- **B.** Enterobacteriaceae—piperacillin-tazobactam 4.5 g 6 hourly

Empiric therapy for MDR-resistant organisms and presence of risk factors:

- **A.** Enterobacteriaceae, *Pseudomonas aeruginosa* or *Acinetobacter baumannii* and other gram-negative bacilli:

One from this column	One from this column
Piperacillin-tazobactam—4.5 g 6 hourly **or,**	Amikacin 15–20 mg/kg intravenously 24 hourly
Cefepime 2 g intravenously 8 hourly **or,**	Ciprofloxacin 500 mg intravenously 8 hourly
Imipenem 500 mg intravenously 6 hourly **or,**	Levofloxacin 750 mg intravenously 24 hourly
Meropenem 1 g intravenously 8 hourly **or,**	Colistin 5 mg/kg intravenously as loading dose
Ceftazidime 2 g 8 hourly	Then 2.5 mg × [1.5 × CrCl + 30] intravenously 12 hourly

But in case of risk factors for MRSA:

A. Linezolid—600 mg intravenously 12 hourly

B. Adjusted dose of vancomycin

Specific Treatment

A. After diagnosis of etiological agents in patient with MDR risk factors a single most appropriate antibiotic should be used. In minority of cases two or three drug combination are used.

B. In case of negative tracheal aspirate or presence of below threshold result of culture antibiotic should be discontinued and alternative diagnosis should be searched. So if the site of infection is changed the spectrum of pathogens is also changed, in that case 7–8 days course of therapy will be sufficient.

C. For covering wide spectrum of gram-negative and gram-positive organisms:

- **a.** Combination of piperacillin-tazobactam + vancomycin/teicoplanin

  Or

- **b.** Carbapenem + vancomycin/teicoplanin

D. In case of *Pseudomonas* or *Acinetobacter*:

- **a.** Combination of piperacillin-tazobactam + vancomycin/teicoplanin

  Or

- **b.** Carbapenem + vancomycin/teicoplanin

  Or

- **c.** Colistin intravenously

Duration of Treatment

A. In case of absence of any risk factor treatment duration is 7–10 days.

B. In case of presence of risk factor duration of treatment is 15 days.

Treatment Failure

A. VAP due to MRSA with high minimum inhibitory concentration (MIC) is associated with 40% failure when treated with standard dose of vancomycin, but there is risk of renal toxicity. In that case linezolid will be preferred as it is renal-friendly and in case of high MIC isolates of MRSA.

B. In case of *Pseudomonas aeruginosa* there is high chance of development of β-lactam resistance during therapy.

C. Recurrent VAP is also possible during therapy development of biofilm present on the endotracheal tube helps reintroduction of same microorganism in the secretion.

D. Other causes of treatment failure are:

- **a.** Development of new superinfection
- **b.** Presence of extrapulmonary infection
- **c.** Occurrence of drug toxicity

Complications

A. Prolongation of mechanical ventilation leading to increased stay in ICU

B. Necrotizing pneumonia leads to:

- **a.** Pulmonary hemorrhage
- **b.** Bronchiectasis
- **c.** Parenchymal scarring leading to recurrent pneumonia

C. High catabolic risk due to loss of muscles and general debilitation from VAP.

Prevention

Most important preventive interventions are:

- **a.** Avoidance of ventilation
- **b.** Minimization of duration of ventilation, but aggressive extubation can result in
  1. Reintubation
  2. Increased risk of aspiration
  3. Risk of VAP
- **c.** Successful noninvasive ventilation can prevent mechanical ventilation.
- **d.** Daily holding of sedation
- **e.** Formal weaning protocol
- **f.** Short course of prophylactic antibiotic therapy can reduce the risk of early onset VAP in comatose patients as it may be caused by non-MDR pathogens. Whereas, prolonged course of antibiotic therapy is associated with VAP due to lethal MDR pathogens.
- **g.** Minimization of microaspiration around the endotracheal tube—it can be done by:
  1. Elevating the head end of the bed between 30 and 60° above horizontal

2. Use of special endotracheal tube to remove the pooled secretion successfully
3. Careful transport of the patient outside the ICU for investigation

h. Avoidance of overgrowth of bowel flora by use of agents which will raise the gastric pH in liver transplant recipients, and undergoing major intra-abdominal procedures.

Pathogenesis	Methods of prevention
Normal flora elimination	Short course of antibiotic
Gastroesophageal reflux	Prokinetic drugs Postpyloric enteric feeding Avoidance of gastric residuals
Bacterial overgrowth	Decontamination of gastrointestinal tract with rifaximin Not to use prophylactic agents that will not elevate gastric pH
Aspiration of oropharyngeal content during intubation	Short course of antibiotic in patient in coma
Aspiration of large volume of oropharyngeal content	Endotracheal intubation Small bowel decompression Avoid sedation Rapid sequence intubation
Cross infection from other colonized patients	Proper washing of hands with alcohol based rub Isolation of the patients Education regarding control of infection Reusable equipment cleaning
Endotracheal intubation	Use of noninvasive ventilation
Long duration of ventilation	Weaning protocols Daily awakening from sedation
Pooled secretion above the endotracheal tube	Elevation of head, Continuous aspiration of the oropharyngeal contents From subglottic areas by separate endotracheal tube Avoidance of reintubation Sedation must be minimized
Abnormal swallowing function	Rapid percutaneous tracheostomy
Lower respiratory tract defense of host is altered	Strong glycemic control Lower hemoglobin transfusion

Q9. Allergic bronchopulmonary aspergillosis (ABPA).

KUHS/MAY2013/MDII (10)
DNBIII/JUN2011 (10)
MGR/OCT2015/MDIII (7)

Bronchopulmonary aspergillosis.

MGR/APR2016/MDI (5) BF/MAY2009/MDIII (10)

Discuss pathophysiology, clinical features, and management of ABPA.

BF/NOV2013/MDI (10)

Allergic bronchopulmonary aspergillosis.

MGR UNI, TAMIL NADU, 2022 (10)
SAURASHTRA UNIVERSITY, RAJKOT, 2020 (20)

ANSWER

Definition

It is progressive disease due to hypersensitive host response to intermittent or continuous exposure of bronchi to hyphae of *Aspergillus fumigatus* leading to eosinophilic infiltration in the periphery of lung, bronchial plugging with mucus containing fungal hyphae and bronchial wall inflammation thus producing bronchiectasis.

Pathogenesis

Spores of *Aspergillus* are inhaled and will be deposited in the proximal bronchial wall

↓

Under proper humidity and temperature, spores turn into hyphae and colonize bronchial wall

↓

In patients with bronchial asthma and cystic fibrosis, impaired ciliary function help in colonization

↓

These fungal hyphae further impair ciliary function mediated by gliotoxin and other toxins produced by *Aspergillus fumigatus* leading to more and more colonization of hyphae.

Adhesion of *Aspergillus* to the bronchial wall is also important for colonization in susceptible individuals. It also adheres to subepithelial fibronectin and other components which are exposed after bronchial wall tissue damage.

After colonization of the fungus immunological response started issuing through the antigen from colonizing fungus within the airway leading to following types of immune response:

A. Type I immunogenic response: This type of reaction is due to degranulation of mast cells leading to release of histamines, leukotrienes, and different cytokines. This is associated with increased level of nonspecific and *Aspergillus*-specific IgE.

B. Type III immunologic response: This is characterized by polyclonal antibody response to *Aspergillus* antigen leading to increase in the level of both total and *Aspergillus* antigen-specific IgA and IgG, as a result there is local deposition of immune complexes leading to inflammatory response and thus damages bronchial wall.

C. Type IV immunologic response: Here *Aspergillus* antigen is presented to T cells leading to TH2-CD4-T cell response. TH2 cells being activated release large amount of cytokines IL-4, IL-5, and IL-13.

All the above immunologic responses attract large number of eosinophils and produce submucosal inflammation containing neutrophilic infiltration which ultimately leads to granuloma formation. As a result following things will occur:

- **a.** Airways obstruction
- **b.** Mucus plugging of small bronchial cavity
- **c.** Damage of bronchial wall tissue.

Protease derived from *Aspergillus fumigatus* is responsible for:

- **a.** Bronchial wall tissue injury
- **b.** Triggering of hypersensitivity
- **c.** Release of proinflammatory cytokines

In case of bronchial asthma this ABPA can occur in following cases:

- **a.** Genetic predisposition
- **b.** T cell antigen responsiveness
- **c.** Specific human leukocyte antigen DR subtype among six subtypes.

Pathology

There are three specific features which are:

A. Lung parenchyma is infiltrated with eosinophil which leads to fleeting types of radiological shadows.

B. Mucus plugs obstruct the bronchi lead to atelectasis of segments of the lung, lobe, or sometimes whole lobe. Composition of mucus plug are:

- **a.** Curschmann's spirals
- **b.** Fungal hyphae
- **c.** Charcot Leyden crystal—it is eosinophilic degradation product

C. Eosinophilic infiltration and granuloma formation of walls of proximal bronchi mainly in upper lobe leading to:

- **a.** Thickening of bronchial wall
- **b.** Fibrosis of bronchial wall
- **c.** Bronchiectasis

Clinical Features

It occurs mainly in adult patients suffering from preexisting asthma, but can occur in infant or children.

There are following types of presentation in ABPA:

A. Asymptomatic in patient of preexisting asthma in the form of accidental finding of radiological infiltrate.

B. Classical presentation may be in the form of fever, cough with expectoration, and sputum containing brownish or brownish-black viscid pellets of sputum which contains hyphae of *Aspergillus*.

C. Acute exacerbation of bronchial asthma.

D. Recurrent episodes of ABPA leading to evidence of bronchiectasis due to severe bacterial broncho-pulmonary infection.

There are five stages of the disease:

- **a.** Stage I—acute stage: It is characterized by following:
  1. Symptoms of acute asthma
  2. Presence of peripheral eosinophilia
  3. All the immunological features of ABPA-S are present
  4. Fleeting type of pulmonary infiltrate
  5. Patient will respond to steroids and antifungal antibiotics
- **b.** Stage II—stage of remission: It is characterized by the following:
  1. Resolution of symptoms and pulmonary infiltrate
  2. Significant attenuation of immunological responses
  3. Lowering of peripheral eosinophilia
- **c.** Stage III—stage of exacerbation: It is characterized by the following:
  1. Exacerbation or worsening of clinical features
  2. Recurrence of pulmonary infiltrate
  3. Recurrence of immunological responses
  4. Recurrence of pulmonary eosinophilia

d. Stage IV—stage of corticosteroid dependent asthma: Here:
   1. Elevation of immunological features will be persistent
e. Stage V—fibrosis mainly involving upper lobe: It is characterized by the following:
   1. Refractory to steroid
   2. Evidence of fibrotic lung disease
   3. Evidence of both restrictive and obstructive lung diseases in lung function test
   4. Presence of bronchiectasis—evidence of infection

There are two patterns of ABPA:

A. ABPA-S: Seropositive ABPA without any radiological evidence of bronchiectasis.
B. ABPA-B: Here there is radiological evidence of bronchiectasis.

Diagnosis

Criteria for diagnosis of ABPA:

A. History of asthma:
   a. Pulmonary eosinophilia
   b. Acute exacerbation of asthma
   c. Unexplained bronchiectasis or upper lobe fibrosis or atelectasis of bronchopulmonary segment or upper lobe
B. *Aspergillus* skin test using standardized extract of *Aspergillus fumigatus* antigen: Positive test is characterized by appearance of wheal and flare of 3 mm within15 minutes of administration—it will detect *Aspergillus*-specific IgE, but it is not specific for ABPA as in 25% of asthma patients this test may be positive.
C. Serum IgE and IgG levels: Total IgE level will be >1,000 IU/L—it is due to nonspecific rise in IgE. But IgE specific to *Aspergillus* will also be raised, its absence of rise will make this diagnosis more unlikely. In case of remission its level will be decreased below 1,000 IU/L. IgG to *Aspergillus* will also be raised.
D. Serum precipitin antibodies to *Aspergillus* antigen: It will be raised in 70% of patients. It is less sensitive as compared to skin prick test but more specific.
E. Presence of *Aspergillus* hyphae in the sputum: It is confirmatory but its absence cannot rule out the ABPA because it is not always found in the sputum.
F. Radiological changes in chest X-ray:
   Transient pulmonary changes:
   a. Transient pulmonary infiltrate with eosinophilic pneumonia: It is characterized by the following:
      1. Typical segmental distribution and fleeting in character
      2. Well-marked peripheral eosinophilia
      3. Sometimes there is perihilar infiltrate
      4. Perihilar hilar adenopathy
   b. Plugging of bronchi by mucus plug producing atelectasis: It is segmental or lobar or may be whole lung. Atelectatic lung will reopen after coughing mucus plug or removal of plug by bronchoscopy.

   Permanent pulmonary changes:
   a. Tram-line shadows extending outward from hilum—it represents dilated bronchi with thickened walls. Presence of upper lobe fibrosis.
   b. Gloved finger like shadow due to dilated bronchi filled up with mucus. After expectoration of mucus bronchi remains dilated with thickened walls.
G. CT scan of chest:
   a. Bronchiectasis of upper lobe classically central in character
   b. In advanced cases there is wide-spread bronchiectasis
   c. Transient pulmonary infiltrate—if it is perihilar it resembles tumor masses
   d. Areas of distal atelectasis and mucus plug in the bronchi that may not be evident in chest X-ray

Treatment

A. Corticosteroids: It is the mainstay of treatment as:
   a. It will prevent increasing lung damage
   b. It will prevent recurrence
   c. Relief of symptoms
   d. It will reduce the airway obstruction
   e. It will reduce serum IgE level
   f. It will reduce peripheral eosinophilia
   g. It will reduce pulmonary infiltrate

   Dose is: In stage I and II—0.5 mg/kg daily for 2–3 weeks followed by tapering of the dose 5–10 mg every 2–3 weeks to reach the maintenance dose of 5–7.5 mg daily.

   Monitoring of the disease: Serum IgE level should be monitored with in few months followed by periodic intervals as if it will rise significantly it will indicate acute exacerbation and initiate reintroduction of steroid therapy.

   In case of very occasional exacerbations the patient will receive steroids during exacerbations only whereas long-term exacerbations are required in following cases:
   a. Very frequent exacerbations of ABPA
   b. There is progressive damage of lung.

B. Inhaled β2 agonists: It together with corticosteroids will relieve airways obstruction.

C. Itraconazole: This antifungal drug acts by following mechanisms:

- **a.** It will reduce colonization of fungal hyphae.
- **b.** It will reduce the steroid dose.
- **c.** It will reduce the pulmonary infiltrate.
- **d.** It will reduce the IgE level.
- **e.** It will improve the exercise tolerance and lung function.

Dose is 200 mg twice daily for 16 weeks.

Adverse effects:

- **a.** Adrenal insufficiency by:
  - **1.** Direct depression of adrenal gland
  - **2.** Reducing the clearance of steroids
- **b.** Hepatotoxicity

D. Omalizumab: This monoclonal antibody can reduce the disease activity and has steroid sparing effect. Dose is 375 mg subcutaneously every 2 weeks.

E. In patient with ABPA with bronchiectasis it requires airway clearance treatment.

F. In case of bronchiectasis, antibiotics can be added to prevent secondary bacterial infection.

Complications

- **A.** Bronchiectasis
- **B.** Severe airways obstruction
- **C.** Pulmonary fibrosis
- **D.** Aspergilloma
- **E.** Lobar atelectasis or whole lung atelectasis
- **F.** *Aspergillus* sinusitis
- **G.** Mildly invasive aspergillosis

Q10. Discuss idiopathic pulmonary fibrosis (IPF) and its management.

DNBIII/JUN2010 (10)

Interstitial pulmonary fibrosis.

MUHS/MAY2011/MDII (10)

Fibrosing alveolitis.

SNMC/MAY2013/MDIII (10)

Idiopathic pulmonary fibrosis.

MAHARASHTRA UNI OF HEALTH SC, VIJAYAWADA (10)

NTR UNI OF HEALTH SC, VIJAYAWADA, SEPTEM, ANDHRA, 2020 (10)

ANSWER

Definition

Idiopathic pulmonary fibrosis is also known as cryptogenic fibrosing alveolitis or usual interstitial pneumonia. It can be defined as chronic progressive fibrosing interstitial pneumonia occurring in elderly associated with radiologic and/or histological pattern of usual interstitial pneumonia.

Pathophysiology

Idiopathic pulmonary fibrosis is an epithelial-fibroblastic disease where homeostasis of alveolar epithelial cells is disrupted by endogenous or environmental stimuli leading to diffuse activation of epithelial cells associated with aberrant repair. The inciting events are smoke, environmental pollutants and dust, viral infections, chronic aspiration, and gastroesophageal reflux.

Inciting events first injure type I alveolar epithelial cells. During repair process type II alveolar epithelial cells will proliferate and later on differentiate into type I cells to complete the process of repair. But most important in this process is the intactness of basement membrane which will be disrupted in this disease.

Alveolar epithelial cells release a large number of prefibrotic cytokines and growth factors such as platelet-derived growth factor, tumor growth factor-α, and transforming growth factor-β—these are responsible for proliferation and migration of fibroblast leading to increased accumulation of extracellular matrix followed by generation of fibrosis.

There are genetic mutations of several biological pathways responsible for injury to lung followed by repair and production of repair in the peripheral airways.

- **a.** Mutation of genes encoding surfactant protein A2 and C increase stress of endoplasmic reticulum in alveolar type II cells which leads to susceptibility to chronic injury of lung.
- **b.** Multimeric enzyme systems of telomerase RNA component and telomerase reverse transcriptase repairs shortened telomeres. Mutation of the genes affecting these produce abnormalities in telomerase function thus decrease the replication of progenitor cells and impairs wound healing.
- **c.** Overexpression of *MUC5B* gene that is involved in mucin production in the peripheral bronchial pathways—it will increase the susceptibility to interstitial pulmonary fibrosis.

These above mechanisms are not present in all the patients with IPF but these mechanisms will increase the hope of invention of new therapies.

Clinical Features

History

A. Dyspnea—it is insidious and progressive
B. Dry cough
C. Weight loss
D. Associated symptoms are low-grade fever, fatigue, arthralgia, or myalgia. Duration of symptoms between assumption and establishment of diagnosis may be several years.
E. In 5% patients there is presenting symptom.
F. Other histories like occupational history like exposure to asbestos, silica, heavy metal contaminating patient's ventilatory system, social, recreational and environmental history, drug history like intake of bleomycin, amiodarone, etc.
G. History of OSA syndrome

Physical Signs

A. Digital clubbing
B. Pedal edema
C. Pulmonary dry crackles

Complications

A. Respiratory infection
B. Pulmonary hypertension
C. Acute exacerbation of pulmonary fibrosis
D. Thromboembolic disease
E. Lung cancer
F. Acute coronary syndrome
G. Adverse effects of medicine

Investigations

A. Laboratory studies:
- **a.** In 30% of patients, high titer of antinuclear antibodies (ANAs) or rheumatoid factor.
- **b.** Raised CRP
- **c.** Increased ESR
- **d.** Hemoglobin will be raised due to chronic hypoxemia producing secondary polycythemia.
- **e.** To distinguish it from other ILDs following tests are useful:
    1. Matrix metalloproteinase-7
    2. Surfactant protein-D
    3. Chemokine ligand-18
    4. Kreb von den Lungen-6

B. Imaging studies:
- **a.** Chest X-ray: Typical findings are:
    1. Peripheral reticular opacities (curvilinear densities)
    2. Honeycombing (coarse reticular pattern)
    3. Loss of lower lobe volume
- **b.** High-resolution computed tomography (HRCT): It is more sensitive and more specific for the diagnosis. The positive findings are:
    1. Peripheral, patchy, reticular, subpleural, and bibasilar opacities
    2. Interlobar septal thickening
    3. Intralobar line
    4. In the areas of severe reticular markings there is evidence of traction bronchiectasis.
    5. Less than 5 mm round translucencies known as honeycombing in the subpleural areas—it suggests irreversible fibrosis.
    6. Ground-glass opacities may be present but is less extensive.

C. Pulmonary function tests (PFTs):
- **a.** Reduction of tidal volume, vital capacity (VC), TLC, FRC, and forced vital capacity (FVC)
- **b.** Due to decreased lung compliance pressure/volume curve will be shifted to the right.
- **c.** Restrictive ventilatory defect
- **d.** Reduced diffusion capacity of carbon monoxide.

D. 6-minute walk testing:

Desaturation below 88% during this walk test suggestive of high mortality. If it is associated with progressive decline of diffusing capacity of the lung for carbon monoxide (DL_{CO}) is less than 15% or more—is strong predictor of high mortality.

E. Bronchoalveolar lavage:
- **a.** Increased number of neutrophils present in 90% and lymphocytes in 40–60% of patients of IPF.
- **b.** Proper analysis of this fluid can exclude other diseases such as infection, malignancy, eosinophilic pneumonia, and alveolar proteinosis.

F. Surgical lung biopsy:

Histological findings are the following:
- **a.** Heterogeneous, variegated appearances, inflammation, fibrosis, and honeycombing with alternating areas of healthy lung.
- **b.** Areas of fibrosis characterized by deposition of fibroblasts and myofibroblast in linear fashion in

the midst of pale-staining matrix. It is present in subpleural or paraseptal areas.

c. Honeycombing—it is characterized by cystic dilatation of bronchioles lined by ciliated columnar in the areas of scarred lung tissue.
d. Absence of granuloma—its presence indicates other disorder.

Treatment

Currently, there is no effective drug which can prevent or reverse the progression of fibrosis of lung. But now there are two drugs which can reduce but not reverse or stop the progression of disease and it can be measured by proper lung function test. These drugs are:

A. Pirfenidone: It will inhibit the number of prefibrotic cytokines like tumor growth factor-β.
B. Nintedanib: It is tyrosine kinase inhibitor and it blocks and reduces the signal of fibrogenic growth factors such as platelet-derived growth factor, vascular endothelial growth factor, and fibroblast growth factor.

Though IPF is chronic fibrotic disease, but due to intercurrent problem there may be acute exacerbation of this disease. Following are the criteria of acute exacerbation of IPF:

a. Previous or concurrent diagnosis of IPF
b. Worsening of hypoxemia from a known baseline ABG level
c. Unexplained worsening or development of dyspnea within 30 days
d. Endotracheal aspiration or BAL shows no evidence of infection
e. HRCT demonstrates ground-glass abnormality or consolidation superimposed on background of honeycomb or reticular pattern—which is consistent with interstitial pattern.
f. Exclusion of other causes such as PE, left-sided heart failure, and other causes of lung injury.

In this case corticosteroid like methylprednisolone 2 mg/kg for 2 weeks followed by slow tapering along with proper antibiotics.

Q11. Describe pathophysiology, clinical presentation, and management of high-altitude pulmonary edema (HAPE).

DNBIV/JUN2012 (10)

HAPE.

MJPRU/2015/MDIII (6)

ANSWER

Barometric pressure at the sea level is 760 mm Hg.
Partial pressure of inspired oxygen at sea level is 150 mm Hg.
Partial pressure of carbon dioxide at normal ventilation is 40 mm Hg.
Alveolar oxygen partial pressure = Pressure in the inspired oxygen – Partial pressure of carbon dioxide
= 150 – 40
= 110 mm Hg

Normal alveolar-arterial pressure gradient is 10–15 mm Hg in case of healthy individual, hence arterial partial pressure gradient is:
Alveolar oxygen partial pressure - 10 mm Hg = 100 mm Hg
As any person ascends gradually, barometric pressure will decline gradually thus pressure of inspired oxygen, alveolar oxygen partial pressure, and arterial PaO_2 also will be reduced gradually.

Epidemiology

Most of the individual resolve mountain sickness within few days but few individuals who lives at sea level may develop lethal complications like HAPE or high altitude cerebral edema. Its frequency depends upon:

a. Rate of ascent
b. Altitude reached
c. Duration of rest at lower level of altitude which is essential for acclimatization. If a person reaches 4,000–5,000 ft in the span of 3 days his chance of developing complication is less than who climbs this height in a single day.

Risk Factors

High-altitude pulmonary edema develops within 2–4 days after arrival and does not occur after 4 days because adaptation in that altitude will render the pulmonary vessels less susceptible to hypoxia. Risk factors for HAPE are:

a. Rapid rate of ascent
b. History of HAPE
c. Too cold temperature in the environment
d. Respiratory tract infection
e. Abnormalities in cardiopulmonary circulation producing pulmonary hypertension, so in these cases echocardiography is required when HAPE will be developed at <300 m altitude:
    1. Large patent pulmonary ovale—it is four times more common in HAPE susceptible individual.
    2. Primary pulmonary hypertension

3. Mitral stenosis
4. Unilateral absence of pulmonary artery

Pathogenesis

Main pathogenesis is the hypoxic vasoconstriction leading to pulmonary hypertension (pulmonary capillary pressure of >18 mm Hg) which is uneven throughout the lungs.

Where vasoconstriction is severe alveoli will be protected from pulmonary edema.

Where vasoconstriction is less severe pulmonary edema will be developed due to following reasons:

a. Increased intracapillary pressure
b. Damage of capillary wall due to increased blood flow
c. Sheer stress damages capillary wall
d. Increased permeability of capillary endothelium due to release of kinin and cytokines.

Following are the causes of hypoxic pulmonary vasoconstriction:

A. Endothelial dysfunction leading to decreased release of nitric oxide usually plays a role in hypoxic pulmonary vasoconstriction which is supported by alleviating the following after administration of phosphodiesterase-5 inhibitor:
   a. Reduced exercise tolerance
   b. Altitude-induced pulmonary hypertension
   c. Hypoxemia
B. Triggered sympathetic drive:
   a. Produces pulmonary vasoconstriction
   b. Extravasation of fluid from pulmonary capillaries to alveoli
C. Exercise and cold produces pulmonary vasoconstriction
D. Inflammation may be an etiological factor as there is evidence of raised ESR and peripheral leukocytosis
E. Impaired transepithelial clearance of sodium and water from the alveoli

Again some patients with severe vasoconstriction at high altitudes will not develop pulmonary edema.

Clinical Features

Symptoms usually occur in those persons who will ascend high altitudes at rapid pace without any acclimatization.

A. Symptoms are:
   a. Rapidly progressive dyspnea
   b. Cough—it starts as dry cough then it becomes productive and frothy occasionally blood tinged.
   c. Central cyanosis
B. Signs are:
   a. Tachypnea
   b. Tachycardia
   c. Raised jugular venous pressure
   d. Pedal edema
   e. Later hypotension
   f. On palpation:
      1. Right ventricular heave
      2. Palpable pulmonary second heart sound
   g. On auscultation: Loud pulmonary second heart sound
C. Death may occur due to:
   a. Gross pulmonary edema
   b. Severe hypoxemia
   c. Coma

Investigations

A. Chest X-ray demonstrates patchy or localized opacities in both lungs. But there is absence of Karley's B line or Bat's wing appearance.
B. Electrocardiography demonstrates right ventricular strain or right ventricular hypertrophy.
C. Blood gas analysis demonstrates hypoxemia with respiratory alkalosis but if the patient is taking acetazolamide there will be metabolic acidosis.
D. Comet-tail scoring in ultrasound can evaluate extravascular lung water at high altitude. It can detect HAPE whether it is clinical or subclinical.

Treatment

A. Problem has to be recognized in the incipient stage. Breathlessness and dry cough should be treated.
B. Patient should be taken to lower altitude.
C. In the meantime oxygen should be administered through mask with reservoir bag to maintain the FiO_2 to >90%.
D. Drugs administered are:
   a. Sustained release nifedipine 30 mg orally once or twice daily for treatment.
   b. Tadalafil 10 mg 12 hourly orally is given for treatment.
E. Intravenous furosemide has to be given to reduce edema.
F. Provision of well-equipped portable hyperbaric chamber for mountaineering.
G. Inhaled nitric oxide and EPAP is also useful but it is not available in this settings.

Prevention

A. Gradual ascent by providing sufficient time for acclimatization.

B. Sustained release nifedipine 30 mg once or twice daily in patient with past history of HAPE or who wants to ascent rapidly.

C. Salmeterol 125 µg has to be inhaled 12 hourly as preventive treatment.

D. Tadalafil 10 mg twice daily.

E. Dexamethasone 8 mg twice daily. It will:
   - **a.** Increase the availability of endothelial nitric oxide
   - **b.** Alter excessive sympathetic activity

Q12. Describe the role of inflammatory mediators in bronchial asthma. Discuss the management of acute severe asthma.

DNBI/JUN2013 (10)

Define atopy. Outline the pathophysiology of bronchial asthma. Pulmonary function abnormalities in bronchial asthma.

DNBI/APR2016 (10)

Management of acute severe asthma.

MGR/OCT2003/MDI (5) PGI/NOV2013/MDIII (10)

Newer drugs in the management of bronchial asthma.

MGR/OCT2003/MDIII (5)

Discuss the recent concepts in the pathogenesis of bronchial asthma. Outline the management of acute severe asthma. Add a note on newer anti-asthmatic drugs.

MGR/SEP2002/MDIII (25)

Discuss the recent advances in management of bronchial asthma.

AMU/2011/MDII (20)

Discuss the newer concepts in pathophysiology, types and treatment of bronchial asthma.

BF/NOV2012/MDIV (20)

Acute life-threatening asthma.

MC/2015/MDIII (10)

Discuss pathogenesis, newer diagnostic modalities and recent guidelines in the treatment of bronchial asthma.

WBUHS 2022 (10)

GINA criteria for bronchial asthma and the treatment of bronchial asthma.

DR YSR UNI OF HEALTH SC, VIJAYAWADA, ANDHRA, 2022 (10)

How will you assess and monitor asthma severity? Discuss detail about the management of asthma.

TEERTHANKER MAHAVEER UNI, 2020 (10)

Outline the role of airway inflammation and inflammatory mediators in triggers of bronchial asthma.

WBUHS, 2024 (10)

Enlist the causes of acute pulmonary edema. Outline the assessment of severity and management of ARDS.

WBUHS, 2024 (10)

ANSWER

Definition

Asthma can be defined as reversible narrowing of the airways leading to reduction of airflow producing respiratory discomfort and wheezing.

Predisposing Factors

A. Atopy: It is a major risk factor. Atopy is genetically determined due to production of IgE antibody. In case of previously sensitized individual, asthma may be exacerbated by repeat exposure to various allergens. Patient having atopic asthma may suffer from allergic rhinitis in 80% of cases and also atopic dermatitis. Nearly 50% patients suffer from atopy but only few of them will suffer from asthma. So genetic or other environmental factors may predispose to development of asthma in these atopic individuals. Allergen in case of allergic rhinitis has protease activity. These allergens are derived from house dust mites, cat, dog fur, and cockroaches in the inner cities pollens, grass and rodents in case of laboratory workers.

B. Genetic predisposition: Asthma occurs in the first-degree relatives of asthma patients and higher incidence of concordance if monozygotic twin as compared to dizygotic twins. Genetic screening, classical linkage analysis as well as single nucleotide polymorphisms of candidate genes suggest that:

a. Asthma is polygenic

b. Small effects of single gene may not replicate in different populations. So interactions between different genes are important.

Following genes or genetic regions are responsible for atopic asthma:

a. 5q region near major locus for controlling IgE levels, increased release of T-helper cell-2, IL-4, IL-5, IL-9, and IL-13, corticoid receptor, genetic coding of β2 receptor, and granulocyte-macrophage colony-stimulating factor.

b. Chromosome 11q is responsible for atopy, positive skin test, and serum IgE levels

c. Chromosome 12q controls the β-subunit of nuclear factor-γ (NF-γ) and interferon

d. Chromosome 5q31-33 region is cytokine-cluster gene

e. Chromosome 6 controls release of eosinophil

f. Chromosome 16 controls serum IgE levels

g. Other genes include:

1. ADAM-33
2. DPP-10
3. ORMDL3

h. Few genetic regions also influence the therapy:

1. Arg-Gly-16 variant in the β2 receptor is associated with reduced response to β2 agonist
2. In the promoter region of 5-lipoxygenase repetition of Spl recognition will affect the response to antileukotrienes.

Environmental Factors

A. Infections: Rhinovirus infection can trigger acute exacerbations but there is association of RSV and asthma in infancy. Again, Mycoplasma and Chlamydophila are implicated in severe asthma. But their role in absence of other factors in the development of asthma is controversial. According to one theory, viral infection in childhood is causally associated with late-asthma. Again according to "hygiene hypothesis" in childhood lack of microbes and their byproducts like endotoxin will preserves T-helper cell-2 at birth, but in case of exposure there is shift toward protective T-helper cell-1 immune response that mediates allergic reaction.

B. Diet: According to observational studies diet containing following low level of antioxidants is associated with asthma:

a. Vitamin A

b. Vitamin C

c. Magnesium

d. Selenium

e. Omega-3 fatty acids

Following high level of antioxidants are associated with asthma:

a. Omega-6 fatty acids

b. Sodium

Obese female is important risk factor for asthma.

C. Air pollution:

a. Outdoor pollutants:

1. Sulfur dioxide
2. Ozone
3. Diesel particulate matters
4. Nitrogen dioxide

b. Indoor pollutants:

1. Nitrogen oxide from cooking stoves
2. Passive cigarette smoking

D. Allergen from followings:

a. Most common triggering allergens are *Dermatophagoides* species

b. Cats

c. Domestic pets

d. Cockroaches

e. Ragweed

f. Grass and tree pollen: It is responsible for allergic rhinitis but in thunderstorm particles released from disruption of pollen grains produces asthma—it is called thunderstorm asthma.

E. Drugs:

a. Beta-adrenergic blocking agents

b. Selective β2 blockers

c. Angiotensin-converting enzyme inhibitors (ACEIs)

F. Occupational exposure:

a. At workspace:

1. Small animal allergens in laboratory workers

2. Fungal amylase in wheat flour in bakers
3. Aerosols of cleaning liquid in cleaners

b. Other chemicals are toluene diisocyanate, trimellitic anhydride, etc.

G. Obesity: It is more common in obese people of >30 kg/m^2.

H. Physical factors: Cold air and hyperventilation

I. Other factors:

a. Lower maternal age
b. Prematurity
c. Low-birth-weight
d. Breastfeeding

Pathogenesis of Bronchial Asthma

There are several complex and inter-related events which act serially leading to airway hyperresponsiveness and airflow obstruction, these events are:

a. Cellular infiltration
b. Injury to epithelial cells
c. Release of cytokines
d. Remodeling of airways

In case of cellular infiltration many cells are involved, no key cell is predominant.

A. Mast cells: Different allergens, exercise, and hyperventilation activate mast cells through the IgE-dependent mechanism and release following mediators:

a. Histamine
b. Prostaglandin D2
c. Cysteinyl-cytokines
d. Chemokines
e. Growth factors

B. Macrophages cells: These are derived from monocytes, activated via low affinity IgE receptors by allergen and serves following two opposite functions and hence their role in asthma is uncertain:

a. Inflammatory response through the release of certain cytokines
b. Release of antimediators like IL-10

C. Dendritic cells: This antigen-presenting cell is present in the airway epithelium. These cells process the already taken up allergens into peptides and present these peptides to uncommitted T lymphocytes in the local lymph nodes for production of antigen specific T cells. Immature dendritic cells in the respiratory tract with the help of IL-12 and TNF-α promote differentiation of Th2 cell. In asthmatic patients, cytokine thymic stromal lymphopoietin (TSLP) from airway epithelial cells direct dendritic cells to release chemokines which attract Th2 cells into the respiratory airways.

D. Eosinophils: In response to allergen eosinophils are recruited and adhered to the vascular endothelial cells through interaction between adhesion molecules, eosinophils degranulate to release toxic proteins like major basic protein and eosinophilic cationic protein which along with other eosinophilic products increase the airway hyperresponsiveness and damage the airway epithelium, as a result barrier function will be disrupted thus allowing the inhaled material into deeper part of the mucosa. This damaged epithelium will amplify the inflammatory response through the production of cytokines and chemokines and perpetuate edema through vasodilatation mediated by leukotrienes, prostaglandins, and nitric oxide. Eosinophils are also responsible for remodeling of airway epithelium and exacerbation of asthma through the release of growth factors.

E. Neutrophils: In case of severe asthma, acute exacerbation of asthma increased number of activated neutrophils are present but in case of mild or moderate asthma neutrophil may be predominant, these patients are resistant to anti-inflammatory effect of steroid.

F. Lymphocytes: These cells play an essential role in the production of inflammatory response through:

a. The release of specific types of cytokines
b. Recruitment and survival of eosinophils
c. Maintenance of mast cell population in the airways.

In normal person Th1 cells are predominant, but in asthmatic patient Th2 cells are predominate and perform several functions:

a. Chemoattraction, growth, and degranulation of eosinophils, through the release of IL-5
b. Increased synthesis of IgE and airway remodeling through the release of IL-13
c. Different types of proinflammatory effect, increased synthesis of IgE, and promoting differentiation to Th2 cells from native T cells by released IL-4
d. Neutrophil recruitment by IL-17

Other types of lymphocytes:

a. CD4+ NK T lymphocytes also express IL-4.
b. Regulatory T cells determine the expression of other T lymphocytes. E.g., few subsets of these regulatory cells express transcription factor

FOXP3 in asthma patients and it lead to increased differentiation to Th2 cells.

c. Innate T cells having no T cell receptors release Th2 cytokines that is regulated by epithelial cytokines IL-33 and IL-25.

G. Structural cells: These are airway epithelial cells, fibroblasts, smooth muscle cells that are the sources of inflammatory mediators, and these are the major sources in chronic inflammation of the airways.

H. Inflammatory mediators: Multiple inflammatory mediators such as histamine, prostaglandin D2, and cysteinyl-leukotrienes released from mast cells perform following different functions:

1. Contraction of airway smooth muscles
2. Increases microvascular leakage
3. Increases secretion from the mucosa
4. Attract other inflammatory cells

I. Cytokines: These are the following:

a. Th2 cytokine are IL-4, IL-5, IL-9, and IL-13 produce allergic inflammation.

b. Proinflammatory cytokines are TNF-α and IL-1β—it amplifies inflammatory response.

c. Epithelial cells secrete TSLP—it increases the chemokines which attract Th2 cells.

d. Anti-inflammatory cytokines are IL-10 and IL-12—it is deficient in asthma patients.

J. Chemokines: These will attract inflammatory cells of bronchial pathways.

a. Eotaxin (CC11) from epithelial cells specifically attracts eosinophils via CCR3.

b. CCL17 and CCL22 from epithelial cells attract Th2 cells via CCR4.

K. Increased oxidative stress: Macrophages, neutrophils, and eosinophils produce reactive oxygen species and it can evidenced by:

a. Increased concentration of 8-isoprostone in expired air.

b. Increased concentration of ethane, product of lipid oxidation in expired air.

It is related to the following:

a. It can information regarding disease severity.

b. It will amplify inflammatory response.

c. It may reduce response to corticosteroids.

L. Nitric oxide: It is produced by nitric oxide synthetase in the airway epithelial cells and mast cells. As it is related to eosinophilic inflammation, fractional exhaled nitric oxide is increased in the diagnosis of asthma.

M. Transcription factors: Following are the transcription factors:

a. NF-κβ

b. Activated protein-1

These will orchestrate expression of multiple inflammatory genes.

c. NF of activated T cells

d. GATA-3

These express Th2 cytokine in Th2 and IL-C2 cells.

Effect of Common Provocative Stimuli

A. Inhaled allergen:

a. It is processed by dendritic cells leading to release of cytokine mediators.

b. If the asthmatic patient possesses IgE antibody to a specific antigen then this antibody will bind to specific receptors on the mast cell surface and basophils in the blood. But if the antigen is inhaled then this antigen binds and crosslinks to IgE antibody present on the surface of the mast cells residing in the bronchial lumen, as a result mast cells will be activated to release the different mediator performing following functions:

1. Bronchoconstriction
2. Increased epithelial permeability
3. Antigen is allowed to access a large number of mast cells containing IgE antibody residing within the epithelium leading to same sequence of actions.

c. Major mediators in allergic asthma are:

1. Histamine: It serves following actions:
   - Contraction of bronchial smooth muscles
   - Increased vascular permeability
   - Formation of airway edema
   - Stimulation of irritant receptors triggering vagus nerve stimulation resulting further bronchoconstriction.
2. Leukotrienes: It is called slow reacting substance of anaphylaxis formed in the mast cells after antigenic exposure. It is synthetized from arachidonic acid by lipoxygenase enzyme to leukotriene C4, D4, and E4. LTC4 and LTD4 are potent bronchoconstrictors. This arachidonic acid also produces prostaglandins by cyclooxygenase enzyme. Hence, if asthmatic patient will take nonsteroidal anti-inflammatory drugs (NSAIDs) it will inhibit the cyclooxygenase pathway leading

to shifting of the whole pathway toward lipoxygenase pathway thus exacerbation of asthma will take place.

B. Inhaled irritants: Inhaled irritants stimulate irritant receptors present on the wall of the larynx, trachea, and large bronchi, from here travels through the afferent pathway to CNS, after processing it passes through the efferent vagus nerve to bronchial smooth muscles to produce bronchial constriction. It also stimulates IgE antibody containing mast cells residing in the bronchial tree to release different mediators that serve different functions.

C. Respiratory tract infection: Mechanism of bronchoconstriction by respiratory tract infection is not clear but following factors may be responsible:

- **a.** Epithelial injury caused by release of mediator of inflammation
- **b.** Stimulation of irritant receptors
- **c.** Nonspecific bronchial hyperresponsiveness

D. Exercise: It will produce bronchoconstriction in patients with hyperresponsiveness in following ways: During exercise with increased minute ventilation cold and dry air will flow through the airways. This air will be warmed and humidified by water that evaporates from the airway epithelium, as a result the airway becomes cool stimulating bronchial smooth muscles leading to bronchial constriction by following mechanisms:

- **a.** Alteration in ionic movement after drying the mucosa
- **b.** Release of mediators
- **c.** Hyperemia of bronchial mucosa following warming
- **d.** Stimulation of irritant receptors.

Effect of Inflammation

A. Airway epithelium:

Different triggering factors will damage the airway epithelium which contributes airway hyperresponsiveness in the following ways:

- **a.** Loss of barrier function which allows penetration of allergens
- **b.** Loss of enzymes like neural endopeptidase that degrades proinflammatory mediators
- **c.** Loss of epithelial-derived relaxant factor
- **d.** Exposure of sensory nerves leading to its irritant effect

B. Fibrosis: There is deposition of type III and V collagen along with eosinophilic infiltration below the basement membrane through the release of transforming growth factor-β leading to subepithelial fibrosis and thickening of the basement membrane. There is also alteration phenotype of airway epithelial cells, so in severe cases there will be fibrosis of wall of the airway leading to irreversible narrowing of the bronchial wall.

C. Vascular response:

- **a.** Increased blood flow through the airway that contributes to narrowing
- **b.** Increased number of blood vessels in the asthmatic airways in response to growth factors
- **c.** Microvascular leakage from postcapillary venules leading to edema in the airway and exudation of plasma

D. Mucus hypersecretion:

- **a.** Increased mucus secretion leading to formation of viscid mucus plug occluding the small airways
- **b.** Hyperplasia of submucosal glands that confined to large airways
- **c.** Increased number of epithelial goblet cells

E. Smooth muscles of the airways:

- **a.** Inflammatory mediators modulate the ion channels that alter the resting membrane potential of the smooth muscle cells leading to alteration of excitability of the cells.
- **b.** Various growth factors like platelet-derived growth factor or endothelin-1 released from inflammatory or epithelial cells stimulate airway smooth muscle cells leading to hyperplasia and hypertrophy of these cells.
- **c.** These cells also release cytokines and chemokines in asthmatic patients.

F. Neural regulation:

- **a.** Acetylcholine released from the cholinergic nerve endings acts on muscarinic receptors leading to bronchoconstriction.
- **b.** Inflammatory neuropeptides activate sensory nerves leading to reflex cholinergic bronchoconstriction.
- **c.** Inflammatory peptides irritate sensory nerve endings present in the airway epithelium and become hyperalgesic.
- **d.** Neurotrophins released from mast cells and airway epithelial cells proliferates and sensitize the airway sensory nerves.
- **e.** Nerves in the airway release substance P which is responsible for inflammatory effect.

Pathophysiology

Pathological changes such as contraction of smooth muscle cells, inflammatory edema of mucous, and submucosal glands, and excessive viscid mucus secretion are present in different levels of tracheobronchial tree from trachea to peripheral airways of <2 mm in diameter. As a result there is difficulty in airflow during inspiration and expiration.

A. During inspiratory phase of respiratory cycle, lumen of intrathoracic airways will be larger due to increased negative intrapleural pressure so air will enter into the lung normally.

B. During expiratory phase of respiratory cycle, pleural pressure will be relatively positive which will be transmitted to the intrathoracic airways which lead to decrease in their diameter. So in case of asthmatic patients, there is greater difficulty in expiration which will be exacerbated more in case of forced expiration as the pleural pressure will be much more positive.

During the Attack

a. Decrease in expiratory flow rate

b. Decrease in FVC

c. Decrease in forced expiratory volume in 1 second—it is more pronounced (FEV_1)

d. Ratio of FEV_1/FVC

e. Decreased mid-expiratory flow rate between 25% and 75% of VC

f. Increased in residual volume (RV): It may increase to 200% of the predictive value, which may be due to premature closure of the small airways due to small muscle contraction, presence of mucus plug, and inflammatory edema of the bronchial wall.

g. Increased FRC due to air trapping

h. There is dynamic hyperinflation: Prolong expiration time is required as airways are obstructed and the patient will not get sufficient time to exhale fully of the previous breath before the next breath will resume in patient with rapid respiratory rate. Another hypothesis is due to persistent activity of inspiratory muscles. Patient cannot exhale fully; as a result throughout the expiration lung volume will be maintained at a higher level than expected. But the disadvantage is due to reduced compliance of respiratory system there is increased work of breathing. Mechanical disadvantage is diaphragm is lower and flatter.

Between the Attack

a. Normalization of FVC and FEV_1

b. Improvement of maximal mid-expiratory flow rate

c. Mild increase in RV

In case of chronic asthmatic patient in between the attack there will abnormal FEV_1 and FVC.

Arterial Blood Gases in Asthma

a. Hypoxemia due to V/Q mismatch. In asthmatic patient, airway resistance is unevenly distributed, as a result in some part of lung resistance is increased and in some part it is less, so more air will go to less involved areas. On the other hand, perfusion is preserved in poorly ventilated regions; so low V/Q ratio in the affected areas is responsible for hypoxemia. Since the affected areas are large as compared to less involved areas hence areas of increased V/Q ratio of less involved areas cannot compensate for V/Q ratio of more affected areas, hence hypoxemia occurs.

b. Hypocapnia occurs in acute attack due to hyperventilation due to stimulation of irritant receptors present on the airways, lung, and chest wall. But in case prolonged attack there will be worsening of airway obstruction and respiratory muscle fatigue producing hypercapnia.

Clinical Features

Symptoms

Four most common symptoms are cough, dyspnea, chest tightness, and wheezing. All symptoms are variable. But most important is identification of precipitating factors described above.

Patients may complaint of unexplained cough (cough variant asthma) occasionally with thick tenacious mucus plug which may be difficult to expectorate.

Again, some asthmatic patients may precipitate asthma after ingestion of aspirin due to overproduction of leukotrienes.

Some patients have also associated nasal polyp—it is called triad asthma or Samter's syndrome or aspirin-induced respiratory disease.

Signs

There is tachypnea, tachycardia, and hyperinflation of the chest.

On auscultation, diminished vesicular breath sound with prolonged expiration and rhonchi.

Presence of rhonchi occurs in case of chronic obstructive lung disease, partial bronchial obstruction due to foreign body, congestive cardiac failure. Again, all the asthmatic patient may not produce wheeze. In case of severe asthma there will be no wheeze—it is called silent chest. Severe attack not responding to initial treatment with bronchodilators is called status asthmaticus. Severity of asthma can be assessed by:

- **a.** Frequency of exacerbation
- **b.** Presence of nocturnal symptoms
- **c.** Variability of pulmonary function
- **d.** Magnitude of abnormality

Diagnosis

A. PFT:

- **a.** Reduced FEV_1, FVC, and PEF rate
- **b.** Reversibility is demonstrated by giving inhalation of short-acting β_2 agonist (SABA) like albuterol 400 μg or 2–4 weeks trial of 30–40 mg oral corticosteroids daily—it shows >12% and 200 mL increase in FEV_1.
- **c.** PEF rate: Its usefulness are the following:
  1. Diurnal variation of air flow obstruction can be measured by twice daily measurement.
  2. Monitoring the course of the disease
  3. It will alert the patient for adjusting the medication regimen.
- **i.** Flow volume curve will demonstrate decreased mid-expiratory flow rate between 25 and 75% of VC.
- **d.** Whole body plethysmography will demonstrate increase in RV, FRC, and TLC.
- **e.** Gas diffusion as measured by carbon monoxide transfer is nearly normal.

B. Air responsiveness: Histamine or methacholine challenge test to demonstrate the required concentration of these mediators can reduce the FEV_1 by 20%. This is only done following cases:

- **a.** When there is doubt in diagnosis in spite of normal PFT
- **b.** Diagnosis of chronic cough

In case of history of exercise-induced asthma exercise should be done to show the evidence of postexercise bronchoconstriction.

C. Hematological investigation:

- **a.** Blood count—eosinophilia
- **b.** IgE—total and allergen specific antibody

D. Sputum examination: It may show presence of eosinophil in the sputum smear.

E. Chest X-ray:

- **a.** It is usually normal but in case of severe patient there will be hyperinflation.
- **b.** There may be evidence of pneumothorax.
- **c.** Presence of lung shadow indicates pneumonia eosinophilic infiltrate.
- **d.** Flattening of diaphragm suggestive of severe asthma.

F. HRCT: It demonstrates:

- **a.** Areas of bronchiectasis in case of severe asthma
- **b.** Thickening of bronchial wall, but these are not diagnostic of asthma

G. Skin test: It is positive in case of inhalant allergens such as house dust, mite, cat fur, and grass pollen but it is negative in case of intrinsic asthma. But it is not useful test as many patients with allergic sensitivities do not suffer from asthma; again many asthma patients have no allergic background.

H. Fraction of exhaled nitric oxide: Airway epithelial cells synthesize and release nitric oxide, its concentration will be increased in the exhaled gas in case of inflammation of the airway in presence of eosinophils due to increased level of enzyme inducible nitric oxide synthetase. It is useful in following cases:

- **a.** Eosinophilic airway inflammation
- **b.** It is the marker of active inflammatory response.
- **c.** It can guide the response to corticosteroid therapy.
- **d.** It can titrate the gradual reduction in the dose of corticosteroids.

Treatment

A. Bronchodilator therapy: There are three classes of bronchodilator drugs:

- **a.** β_2 agonists:
  1. It acts on β_2 receptors to increase cAMP by activating adenylate cyclase. cAMP activates protein kinase A, it will phosphorylates several regulatory protein to produce bronchodilatation.
  2. It will also increase cAMP level in the mast cells and thus inhibits the release of chemical mediators which also produce bronchoconstriction.
  3. It will reverse and prevent the contraction of bronchial muscles.

4. It will reduce the exudation of plasma.
5. It will inhibit the sensory nerve activation.
6. It will downregulate the number of β_2 receptors on inflammatory cells.

It has no effect on inflammatory cells and airway hyperresponsiveness.

Types of β_2 agonists:

1. SABA:
   - Albuterol and terbutaline. Duration of action is 3–6 hours.
   - It acts as rapid symptom reliever as its onset of action is very rapid.
   - It prevents exercise-induced asthma if it is taken prior to exercise.
   - It is user in high dose through nebulizer or metered dose inhaler.
2. Long-acting β_2 agonist (LABA):
   - Salmeterol and formoterol. Duration of action is 12 hours.
   - Indacaterol, olodaterol, and vilanterol. Duration of action is 24 hours.
   - It should not be given without inhaled corticosteroids (ICS) as they cannot control inflammation.
   - Along with ICS it will improve the exacerbation and dose of steroids can be decreased.

Side effects:

1. Muscle tremor and palpitation mainly in elderly
2. Small fall in plasma potassium as a result of increased uptake by skeletal muscles
3. Development of tolerance by mast cell receptor but no decrease in bronchodilator response in smooth muscle cells

Safety:

1. Due to increased use of SABA for rescue there is increased incidence of death in asthma patients
2. If ICS is not used along with LABA there is little increase in death as LABA fails to suppress the underlying inflammation.

b. Anticholinergic: These are muscarinic receptor antagonists.
   1. It will prevent the cholinergic nerve-induced stimulation bronchial smooth muscles hence it is less potent than β_2 receptor agonists.
   2. It will also decrease the mucus secretion.

Types:

1. Short-acting drug is ipratropium bromide—it is available as aerosol for inhalation.
2. Long-acting drug is tiotropium bromide and glycopyrronium bromide. It is given in those patients who are not controlled by maximum dose of ICS plus LABA.

These drugs are given through nebulizer in case of severe asthma but after giving β_2 agonists.

c. Methylxanthines:
   1. Theophylline will inhibit the enzyme phosphodiesterase. As this enzyme is responsible for degradation of cAMP, inhibition of this enzyme will automatically increases the level of cAMP in the mast cells and bronchial smooth muscle cells. But the level of this drug responsible for degradation of the enzyme will be higher as compared to actual level of the drug achieved, hence whether this mechanism is responsible in not known.
   2. It activates key nuclear enzyme histone deacetylase 2 (HDAC2) and thus switching off the inflammatory genes already activated which reduce the insensitivity of corticosteroid in case of severe asthma.

Clinical uses:

1. Orally theophylline is used once or twice daily to maintain serum concentration of 5–10 mg/L.
2. It may be used as additional bronchodilator in case of severe asthma when plasma concentration of 10–20 mg/L is required.

Side effects:

Side effects are related to its serum concentration but rarely seen if it is <10 mg/L.

1. Due to phosphodiesterase inhibition nausea, vomiting and headache, diuresis, and palpitation
2. In high concentration cardiac arrhythmias, seizures, and death due to its A1-receptor antagonistic action
3. CYP450 enzyme in the liver will metabolize theophylline, hence allopurinol or erythromycin elevate the blood level of theophylline by blocking this enzyme.

B. Controller therapies:

a. ICS:
   1. Mode of action:
      - It reduces number of eosinophils in the sputum and the airways.

- It reduces mast cell number in the bronchial wall mucosa.

2. Molecular mechanism of action: It will switch off transcription of multiple-activated genes encoding different inflammatory proteins such as cytokines, inflammatory enzymes, and adhesion molecules, TNF-α, inducible form of nitric oxide synthetase, and inducible form of cyclooxygenase by following mechanisms:
   - Inhibition of transcription factor NF-$\kappa\beta$
   - Recruitment of HDAC2 to the inflammatory gene complex
   - Activation of anti-inflammatory genes like mitogen-activated protein kinase phosphatase-1
   - Increased expression of β_2 receptors
3. Clinical use:
   - It is effective once daily in case of mildly symptomatic patient
   - Exercise-induced asthma
   - Nocturnal exacerbation
   - Prevent severe exacerbation
   - Early treatment will prevent irreversible changes that occur in chronic asthma
   - It is used in persistent asthma.
4. Side effects:
   - Oropharyngeal candidiasis
   - Hoarseness of voice
   - At high-dose suppression of plasma and urinary cortisol concentrations

b. Systemic corticosteroids:

1. It can be given as 30–45 mg orally once daily for 5–10 days to treat acute exacerbation of asthma without any tapering of dose.
2. In 1% of patient maintenance dose is required.
3. Systemic side effects are diabetes, hypertension, truncal obesity, osteoporosis, depression, proximal myopathy, depression, etc. In some patients regular bone density measurement is also required.

c. Cromones:

Drugs are cromolyn sodium and nedocromil sodium.

1. Mechanism of actions: It blocks exercise, allergen, and sulfur dioxide-induced asthma by flowing mechanisms:
   - It inhibits mast cells.
   - It inhibits sensory nerve activation.

These are effective in childhood asthma. It has little benefit in long-term control of asthma.

d. Antileukotrienes:

Mast cells and eosinophils release cysteinyl-leukotrienes through activation of cys-LT_1 receptors, which produces:

1. Potent bronchoconstriction
2. Microvascular leakage
3. Eosinophilic inflammation

It is less effective to control asthma as compared to ICS and less effect on inflammation of airways, only it can be used as add-on therapy who are not controlled by low doses of ICS. It is less effective than LABA.

Drugs are:

1. Montelukast
2. Zafirlukast

These two drugs are responsible for antagonizing the action of leukotrienes blocking the receptors.

3. Zileuton: It inhibits the lipoxygenase enzyme and thus reduces leukotriene production.

e. Anti-IgE antibodies:

Omalizumab blocks the binding of IgE on the receptors on the mast cells thus inhibits IgE-mediated reactions. It prevents acute exacerbation in severe asthmatic patients. It is given in highly selected patients containing high level of IgE antibodies and not controlled by maximal dose of inhaler therapy.

It is given subcutaneously every 2–4 weeks.

f. Anti-IL-5 antibodies:

1. Antibodies blocking IL-5: Mepolizumab and reslizumab
2. Antibodies blocking its receptor: Benralizumab

Mode of actions:

1. It will reduce the blood and tissue eosinophils.
2. It will reduce the exacerbation in asthmatic patients containing large number of eosinophils in the sputum in spite of therapy with ICS.

g. Immunotherapy:

Injection of pollen, house dust, and mites are not very effective to control asthma. It may cause anaphylaxis but it can be reduced by sublingual dose.

h. Bronchial thermoplasty:

In this method thermal energy can ablate the airway smooth muscle thus it reduce the smooth muscle mass acute exacerbation and can control asthma. It can be given in highly selected patients who are not controlled by maximum inhaler therapy.

i. Alternative therapy:

Nonpharmacologic treatment includes:

1. Acupuncture
2. Hypnotherapy
3. Yoga
4. Breathing control
5. Speleotherapy
6. Chiropraxis

But these treatments are less efficacious and cannot be recommended.

Stepwise therapy in case of asthma according to severity and ability to control asthma:

				Oral corticosteroid
		LABA	LABA	LABA
	Low-dose ICS	Low-dose ICS	High-dose ICS	High-dose ICS
SABS as required for relief of symptoms				
Mild intermittent asthma	**Mild persistent asthma**	**Moderate persistent asthma**	**Severe persistent asthma**	**Very severe persistent asthma**

Clinical Features of Acute Severe Asthma

A. Symptoms:
   a. Increase in chest tightness
   b. Respiratory distress
   c. Wheezing
   d. Inability to complete the full sentences

   Above symptoms are not relieved by inhaler.

B. Signs:
   a. Cyanosis
   b. Tachycardia
   c. Tachypnea
   d. Increased action of accessary muscles of respiration
   e. Pulsus paradoxus
   f. Chest examination:
      1. Hyperinflation of the chest
      2. Diminished vesicular breath sound with prolonged expiration
      3. Rhonchi may be heard or chest may be silent

C. PFT demonstrates:
   a. Hypoxemia
   b. Hypocapnia

Treatment of Acute Severe Asthma

A. Administration of oxygen by face mask to maintain the SaO_2 to 90%

B. Administration of high dose of SABA through nebulizer or metered dose inhaler with spacer

C. In severely ill patients with impending respiratory failure: Intravenous β_2 agonists

D. If there is no satisfactory response, anticholinergic agents has to be added or can be given as added drug.

E. In case of patients refractory to inhale therapies, slow infusion of aminophylline to be given with constant monitoring of the blood level if the patients are already on oral theophylline.

F. Magnesium sulfate can be given intravenously or by nebulization while the patients are on β_2 agonists, but is usually not recommended.

G. In case of impending respiratory failure with normal or mildly elevated PCO_2 prophylactic intubation can be given.

H. In case of respiratory failure intubation has to be given under halothane anesthesia, but sedative never be given because it will depress ventilation.

I. Antibiotics should not be administered if there is no sign of pneumonia.

Q13. What is pneumothorax? What are its types? Describe the clinical features and management of tension pneumothorax.

DNBIIB/DEC2013 (10)

Causes and management of recurrent spontaneous pneumothorax.

MGR/APR2012/MDIV (7)

What is spontaneous pneumothorax and what are the causes of this condition? Write about the clinical features and radiological findings of this condition. What are the pathological types and management of spontaneous pneumothorax?

MUHS/NOV2014/MDII (25)

Define pneumothorax. Enumerate the types of pneumothorax. Clinical features and management of tension pneumothorax.

DNB 2018 (10)

ANSWER

Definition

Accumulation of air in between the visceral and parietal pleura is called pneumothorax.

Types

A. Spontaneous pneumothorax: This type of pneumothorax occurs in absence of any antecedent trauma to thorax.It is of two types:
 a. Primary spontaneous pneumothorax: There is no definite abnormality of the lung adjacent to pleura. The most common cause is rupture of subpleural apical air-pocket or blebs mainly occurs in smokers suggestive of subclinical lung disease. Half of the patients have recurrences.
 b. Secondary spontaneous pneumothorax: There is presence of abnormality of lung adjacent to pleura mainly chronic obstructive lung disease and this is life-threatening as lung reserve is limited in these patients.
B. Traumatic pneumothorax: It occurs from penetrating and nonpenetrating trauma to thorax. It may be gunshot or penetrating knife wound or introduction of air via needle into pleural space.
C. Tension pneumothorax: This occurs in case of mechanical ventilation to tracheobronchial tree.

Spontaneous Pneumothorax

Primary spontaneous pneumothorax occurs in young male between 20 and 40 years of age and common in India.

Risk Factors

A. Smoking is most important risk factor. Incidence is seven times greater in smokers who smoke 1–12 cigarettes per day, 21 times greater in those who smoke 13–21 cigarettes per day.
B. Family history of homocystinuria
C. Marfan syndrome
D. Thoracic endometriosis
E. Birt–Hogg–Dubé syndrome: It is autosomal dominant, characterized by benign skin tumors, renal cancer, and associated with increased incidence of this pneumothorax.

Pathophysiology

Spontaneous pneumothorax occurs due to rupture of subpleural bleb or small bullae. Bleb is small air-filled spaces present in between visceral pleura and lung substance where small bulla is the air-filled spaces present within the lung substance. It occurs in 75% of cases. These blebs develop due to rupture of few alveolar walls as a result of nonspecific infection which is more common in smokers. This air passes along the interstitial spaces to subpleural area. In few cases in the periphery of lung alveolar wall will be damaged producing peripherally placed bullae.

This pneumothorax occurs at lung apex in tall individual as there is high transpulmonary pressure at the apex. Primary pneumothorax is independent of change of intrathoracic pressure.

According to recent concept, increased porosity of the lung is identified by fluorescein-enhanced autofluorescence technique. From this porous area air will enter into the pleural space to produce spontaneous pneumothorax.

Clinical Features

A. Most of the patients are clinically silent. Few patients present with acute onset of chest pain or dyspnea or both.
B. Dry cough
C. On physical examination:
 a. Diminished movement on the affected side
 b. Bulging of the same side of the chest
 c. Shifting of mediastinum to opposite side
 d. On percussion the affected side is tympanic
 e. On the affected side breath sound and vocal resonance is absent

Diagnosis

A. Chest X-ray: In full expiration it is sensitive in picking up small pneumothorax. Features are:
   a. Hypertranslucent area in the affected part of the thorax.
   b. Shifting of mediastinum to opposite side if the size of pneumothorax is sufficiently large.
   c. 10% patients demonstrate small amount of pleural effusion.

B. CT scan of chest: It can diagnose:
   a. Cyst or small bullae not seen in chest X-ray
   b. In case of female, diffuse cystic lung disease
   c. It can differentiate large bulla from localized pneumothorax
   d. Confirmation of suspected localized pneumothorax
   e. To detect persistent air leak in case of recurrent pneumothorax

Volume of pneumothorax can be quantified by volume of hemithorax occupied by pneumo part of the thorax by Light's index:

Percentage of pneumothorax = 100 – [(Diameter of collapsed lung)^3/(Diameter of hemithorax)^3] × 100

Management

Small pneumothorax of <3 cm with minimal symptoms and stable cardiopulmonary system will be absorbed spontaneously but slowly provided pleural space will be closed. Pressure of gas present in the pneumothorax is higher than the combined partial pressure of those gases in capillary and venous blood.

For example, pressure of gases in pleural cavity is little below the atmospheric pressure, i.e., 756 mm Hg. Partial pressure of gases in mixed venous blood is 706 mm Hg. (PO_2 40 + PCO_2 46 + PN_2 573 + PH_2O 47) mm Hg. So this pressure is 50 mm Hg below that is present in pleural space producing a pressure gradient for diffusion of gas from pleural space to mixed venous blood, thus there is continuous diffusion of gases leading to slow reduction of size of pneumothorax till complete resorption of gases.

High level of oxygen has to be administered at the same time to enhance the process of absorption of gases. Because following administration of oxygen most of the nitrogen in the arterial blood will be replaced by oxygen thus lowering the PN_2 in the mixed venous blood and increasing the rate of absorption of nitrogen considerably.

Again after administration of pure oxygen PO_2 of the arterial blood though will be increased considerably but most of the oxygen will be extracted by tissue thus pressure of oxygen in capillary and venous blood will be lowered to a considerable extent. So pressure gradient of oxygen between pleural space and mixed venous blood remains large. So net result of oxygen inhalation favors both oxygen and nitrogen absorption.

If the pneumothorax is symptomatic, i.e., >4 cm, it should be withdrawn from the pleural space by simple needle. If aspiration is not successful, in that case intercostal drainage is necessary with 10–14 Fr needle. Gentle suction is needed to avoid reexpansion edema. If the lung is expanded or there is no further bubbling in the water sealed bottle, then the tube has to be clamped for another 24 hours and repeat chest X-ray has to be done to confirm that there is no further air leak.

Patient should be under observation to see whether the expansion of the lung will be complete or not and if it is again gradually increasing.

If there is persistent leak for >3 days in spite of chest tube drainage then surgical therapy has to be done.

Surgical Treatment

A. If there is persistent leak, i.e., edge of the tear in the pleura and adjacent lung remains open for free egress of air from the lung into pleural space which may be due to:
   a. Fibrotic thickened pleura in that area
   b. Pleural adhesion holding the edge of the tear

B. Recurrence of unilateral pneumothorax

C. Following the occurrence of contralateral pneumothorax

D. Occurrence of bilateral synchronous pneumothorax

E. If patient's job demands the further recurrence

Methods of Surgery

Video-assisted thoracoscopic surgery—stapling of blebs and small bullae by use of:
   a. Endostapler
   b. Laser ablation
   c. Electrocoagulation

This is followed by pleurodesis by following methods:
   a. Mechanically by pleural abrasion
   b. Partial pleurectomy
   c. Chemically by talc insufflation

Recurrence rate following this method is very low.

Recurrence:
   a. Risk of recurrence of primary pneumothorax is 30%, mostly in the first year.
   b. Risk of contralateral pneumothorax is 10–15% after primary case.
   c. Recurrence rate is higher in smoker and tall thin person.

Tension Pneumothorax

Etiology of tension pneumothorax:

- **A.** Central venous catheterization
- **B.** Lung biopsy
- **C.** Percutaneous tracheostomy
- **D.** Barotrauma due to positive pressure ventilation
- **E.** Thoracocentesis
- **F.** Insertion of pacemaker
- **G.** Bronchoscopy
- **H.** Cardiopulmonary resuscitation
- **I.** Intercostal nerve block

Pathophysiology

It is direct complication of disruption of dynamics of pleural cavities. Pressure in the pleural cavity is negative as compared to positive atmospheric pressure. The tendency of the inward recoil of the lungs is counteracted by the outward recoil of the chest wall cavity and pressure gradient in the pleural cavity. Pressure in the pleural cavity compresses the lung thereby reducing the ventilation as well as oxygenation.

In case of tension pneumothorax, the mediastinum will be pushed to the contralateral side. It will compresses the superior vena cava leading to reduction of the venous return and thereby reducing the cardiac output which aggravates the hypoxemic states due to increased pulmonary vascular resistance.

Circulatory collapse leads to acidosis resulting cardiac arrest if the disease cannot be managed timely.

History and clinical examination:

- **A.** To detect the etiology history of trauma should be searched.
- **B.** Sudden shortness of breath,
- **C.** Pleuritic chest pain radiating to back and shoulder.
- **D.** Clinical signs:
  - **a.** Tachycardia
  - **b.** Tachypnea
  - **c.** Retraction of chest wall
  - **d.** Cyanosis—central
  - **e.** Distension of jugular vein
  - **f.** Reduced tactile fremitus on the ipsilateral side
  - **g.** Trachea shifted to the opposite side.
  - **h.** In some cases subcutaneous emphysema

Evaluation

- **A.** X-ray chest demonstrates one or more of the following:
  - **a.** A thin line representing the edge of the visceral pleura
  - **b.** Effacement of the lung markings distal to that line
  - **c.** Complete collapse of the ipsilateral lung
  - **d.** Shifting of the mediastinum away from the side of tension pneumothorax
  - **e.** Subcutaneous emphysema
  - **f.** Deviation of the trachea away from the side of affection.
  - **g.** Flattening of the hemidiaphragm on the affected side.
- **B.** Ultrasound of the chest demonstrates:
  - **a.** Absence of lung sliding
  - **b.** Presence of lung point

Management

Management depends upon the hemodynamic stability of the patient. Airway, breathing, and circulation should be maintained if the suffering from the chest trauma.

- **A.** Administration of 100% oxygen:
  - **a.** Decreases the size of pneumothorax by decreasing the partial pressure of the nitrogen in the alveoli.
  - **b.** Creates a diffusion gradient for nitrogen thereby accelerating the resolution of pneumothorax.
- **B.** Positive pressure ventilation should be avoided initially as it increase the size of tension pneumothorax, but after giving the chest tube drainage it can be given.
- **C.** If the patient is hemodynamically unstable, immediate decompression by introduction of needle with angiocatheter at 2nd intercostal space in the midclavicular line above the rib, so collapsed lung will be re-expand.
- **D.** Removal of the introduced needle when:
  - **a.** Lung is fully expanded.
  - **b.** There is no air-leak.
  - **c.** Clinical improvement of the lung.
- **E.** Surgical intervention is required when:
  - **a.** Bilateral pneumothoraces
  - **b.** Pulmonary decompression sickness
  - **c.** If the air-leaks are not resolved within 7 days.
- **F.** Pleurodesis as it decreases the recurrence. It can be done by:
  - **a.** Mechanical processes:
    1. Abrasive scratchpads
    2. Dry gauze
    3. Stripping of parietal pleura
  - **b.** Chemical processes by administration of:
    1. Talc
    2. Minocycline
    3. Doxycycline
    4. Tetracycline

Q14. Classification, etiology, diagnosis, and treatment of lung abscess.
DNBIIIA/JUN2015 (10)

ANSWER

Definition

Lung abscess can be defied as single or multiple discrete areas of necrosis of parenchyma.

Classification

A. Primary lung abscess: It occurs due to aspiration caused by anaerobic bacteria in absence of pulmonary or systemic condition.
B. Secondary lung abscess: It occurs in the setting of underlying conditions:
   a. Postobstructive process: Presence of foreign body or tumor in the bronchus
   b. Systemic process: HIV infection and immuno-compromising condition

Primary Lung Abscess

Major risk factor for primary abscess is aspiration, following patients are very susceptible to aspiration:
   a. Altered mental status
   b. Drug over dose
   c. Alcoholism
   d. Seizures
   e. Bulbar dysfunction
   f. Prior cerebrovascular or cardiovascular disease
   g. Neuromuscular disease
   h. Esophageal dysmotility
   i. Esophageal stricture or tumor

In patients suffered from gingivitis or periodontal disease following bacteria are colonized:
   a. Anaerobic bacteria:
      1. *Peptostreptococci*
      2. *Prevotella*
      3. *Bacteroides*
      4. *Streptococcus milleri*
   b. Microaerophilic streptococci

Pathogenesis

Susceptible patient carry overwhelming burden of aspirated material and fail to clear the bacterial load along with further damage of lung parenchymal tissue by gastric acid, as a result pneumonitis will develop initially. Then over 7–14 days, there will be parenchymal necrosis flowed by cavitation—but this progress depends upon host-pathogen interaction. Later on extensive necrosis occurs due to polymicrobial infection.

Secondary Lung Abscess

Its pathogenesis depends upon the predisposing factors.
A. In case of partial bronchial obstruction oropharyngeal contents are failed to be cleared from the lung, as a result there is parenchymal necrosis by pathogens leading to abscess formation.
B. In case of systemic disease, immunosuppression in case of organ transplantation there is impairment of host defense mechanisms leading to increased susceptibility to secondary infection by polymicrobes and opportunistic pathogens thus lung abscess formation.

The organisms are:
   a. *Staphylococcus aureus*
   b. Gram-negative rods:
      1. *Pseudomonas aeruginosa*
      2. Enterobacteriaceae
      3. *Aspergillus*
      4. *Cryptococcus*
      5. *Nocardia*
      6. *Legionella pneumophila*
      7. *Pneumocystis carinii*

Other process of secondary lung abscess formation:
A. Bacteremic spread from distant infection:
   a. *Staphylococcus aureus* in case of tricuspid valve endocarditis
   b. Infection starting from pharynx to neck and carotid sheath due to Fusobacterium necrophorum in Lemierre's syndrome.
B. Bacteremic spread from anywhere in the body from any cause produces seeding in the body like infected central venous catheter, intravenous drug users, and heroin injection.
C. Endemic infection with or without immuno-suppression—different types of *Mycobacterium* like *avium, tuberculosis, kansasii, Histoplasma capsulatum, Blastomyces, Paragonimus westermani,* and *Strongyloides stercoralis.*

Pathogenesis

Abscess starts with an area of large consolidation or small areas of consolidation which later on coalesces to form large consolidation. In the consolidated areas necrosis starts which later on produces suppuration.

This area later on communicates with bronchus to produce profuse foul-smelling expectoration. Since this abscess communicates with bronchus, there will be air-fluid level. Real abscess cavity contains necrotic tissue as pus which is lined by inflammatory infiltrate and it is surrounded by fibrotic capsule if the abscess cavity is chronic or in acute cases it is surrounded by consolidated lung tissue.

Fate of the Abscess

a. In acute case, it is healed completely with or without fibrosis.
b. If the abscess is close to pleura, it will produce empyema.
c. It the abscess cavity opens into pleural cavity, it will produce pyopneumothorax.
d. Abscess cavity ruptures into pleural cavity bronchopleural fistula can occur.
e. Metastatic spread of infection can produce cerebral abscess.
f. Thin-walled sterile cavity may be formed whose inner lining will be epithelized or fibrous tissue.

Site of Abscess in the Lung

a. Posterior segment of upper lobe
b. Apical segment of lower lobe
c. Posterior segment of lower lobe

Right lung is mostly affected because right main bronchus is less angulated. Location of secondary abscess depends upon the underlying cause.

Clinical Features

A. In the formative phase:
   a. Fever with chill and rigor
   b. Severe prostrations
   c. Lassitude
   d. Dry cough
   e. Chest pain, if there is pleural involvement
B. If the abscess cavity communicates with bronchus:
   a. Coughing out large amount of foul smelling sputum
   b. Fever becomes low grade
   c. Systemic toxicity will be reduced
C. On physical examination:
   a. Tachypnea
   b. Tachycardia
   c. Diminished movement of the affected part of the chest
   d. Dull or impaired percussion note because of surrounding consolidation
   e. Breath sound is diminished in the affected areas, sometimes there is cavernous or amphoric breath sound depending upon the size of bronchus communicating with the cavity.
   f. Sometimes there may be crepitations
   g. In chronic lung abscess, clubbing may be present
   h. Absence of gag-reflex
D. If there is frequent small aspiration into lung tissue, this will produce multiple microabscesses which later on coalesce to form large abscess. These patients present with the following:
   a. Insidious onset of low-grade fever
   b. Dry cough to start with which becomes productive later on with foul-smelling sputum
   c. As areas of necrosis are increased clinical features become more pronounced
   d. In these patients lung abscess is diagnosed very late and is established by imaging studies or HRCT.

Complications

a. Empyema
b. Pyopneumothorax
c. Bronchopleural fistula
d. Overwhelming sepsis
e. Multiorgan failure in immunocompromised patients
f. Secondary amyloidosis in case chronic lung abscess in rare cases

Diagnosis

A. Chest X-ray:
   a. In early case there are multiple infiltrates, which later on coalesce to form cavity in different lobe as described above and after a week cavitation may be seen.
   b. In chronic lung abscess, shape of the cavity will be irregular surrounded by ring-shaped consolidated lung.
   c. When it opens into communicating bronchus there will be air-fluid level.
   d. Evidence of associated empyema
   e. Evidence of associated pyopneumothorax
B. CT scan of chest:
   a. It can define the abscess better.
   b. It can provide earlier definition of cavitation.

c. It can yield additional information regarding the underlying cause of abscess.
d. It can produce distinction between pleural infection and peripheral lung abscess as empyema requires urgent pleural drainage or CT-guided percutaneous needle aspiration.

C. Microbiology:
   a. Pus should be collected in a specialized technique like transtracheal aspiration or BAL with protected brushes for collection as it will avoid contamination from the oral cavity. But risks of the above procedures are:
      1. Spillage of content of the abscess into other lung
      2. Production of pneumothorax
      3. Development of bronchopleural fistula

      In case of immunosuppressed patient these procedures are particularly important as these patients are very fragile, at high risk of infection and infection with polymicrobes.
   b. Sputum can be collected which may show polymicrobial infection, but may not reflect the anaerobic organisms.

Treatment

A. In case of primary lung abscess:
   a. Clindamycin 600 mg three times daily intravenously till the disappearance of fever or clinical improvement then 300 mg orally four times daily

      Or,
   b. B-lactam or β-lactamase combination intravenously till the patient is stable then oral amoxicillin-clavulanate

      During the course of antibiotics, imaging at regular interval and total therapy is 3–4 weeks or as long as 14 weeks.

      Metronidazole can be used for anaerobic organism but it is not effective for microaerophilic streptococci or other mixed flora of oral cavity.

      If the patients fail to improve, additional studies are required to know the underlying condition, if any.

B. In case of secondary lung abscess:

   Choice of antibiotic depends upon:
   a. Nature of pathogen
   b. Immune status of the host
   c. Treatment of underlying condition which led to lung abscess

10–20% patients fail to respond as evidenced by continued fever and progressive increase in size of the abscess cavity. If the size of the cavity is >6–8 cm in diameter, it is less likely respond to antibiotic therapy, in that case following two surgical procedure are undertaken:
   a. Surgical resection of the abscess cavity
   b. CT-guided percutaneous drainage of abscess if the patient is poor surgical candidate

Possible complications of percutaneous drainage:
   a. Bacterial contamination of pleural space
   b. Pneumothorax
   c. Hemothorax

Q15. Bronchopulmonary segments and its significance.

MGR/OCT2012/MDI (5)
MGR/OCT2011/MDI (5)
MGR/MAR2009/MDI (5)
MGR/SEP2010/MDI (5)
MGR/SEP2007/MDI (5)
RGUHS/MDI (10)
BF/MAY2009/MDI (8)

Respiratory unit.

MGR UNI, TAMIL NADU, 2022 (5)

Bronchopulmonary segment.

MGR UNI, TAMIL NADU, 2021 (5)

ANSWER

Definition

Bronchopulmonary segment can be defined as one segmental bronchi along with structurally and functionally independent unit of lung lobe. This is basically anatomic, functional as well as surgical units of lungs. Kramer and Glass in 1932 coined this phrase "bronchopulmonary segment".

Characteristics of Bronchopulmonary Segments

A. It is the largest subdivision of lobe of a lung.
B. It is pyramidal in shape with apex toward root of hilum.
C. Each bronchopulmonary segment is independent unit of lung.

D. Each bronchopulmonary segment has separate branch of pulmonary artery, segmental bronchus, and autonomic nerves and lymphatic vessels.

E. Segmental vein runs through connective tissue in between the bronchopulmonary segments.

F. Bronchopulmonary segment and bronchovascular segment are not same as there is no vein here.

G. Infection in any bronchopulmonary segment is restricted to that segment, but tuberculosis and bronchogenic carcinoma will spread to other segments.

Name of the bronchopulmonary segments (according to American Thoracic Society of Great Britain):

Right lung bronchopulmonary segments

Upper lobe	Apical
	Anterior
	Posterior
Middle lobe	Medial
	Lateral
Lower lobe	Superior
	Medial basal
	Anterior basal
	Lateral basal
	Posterior basal

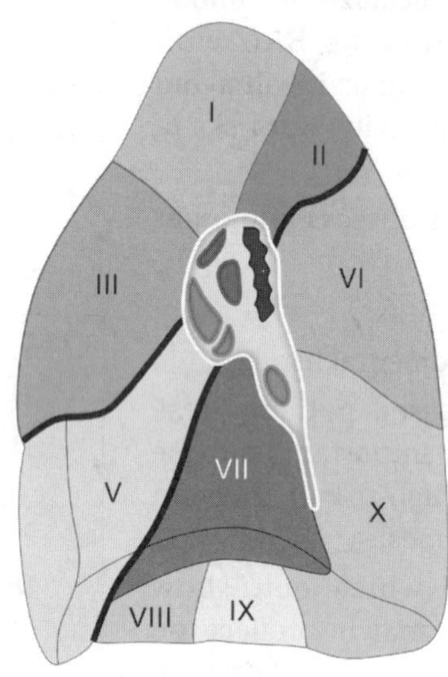

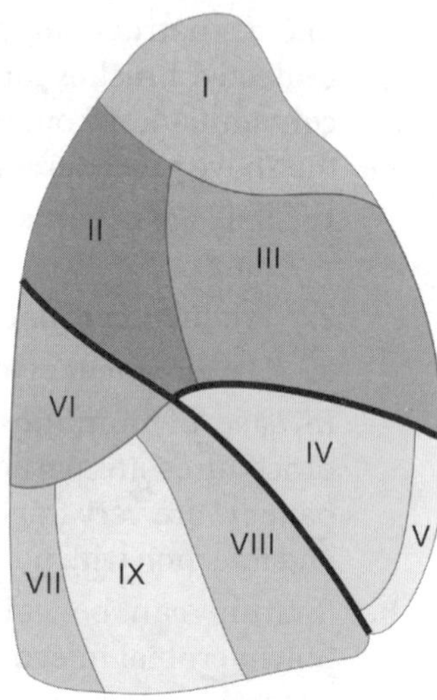

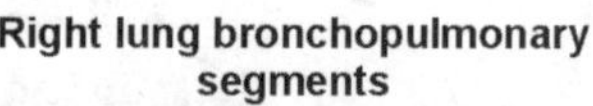
Right lung bronchopulmonary segments

Upper lobe	Apical
	Anterior
	Posterior
Middle lobe	Medial
	Lateral
Lower lobe	Superior
	Medial basal
	Anterior basal
	Lateral basal
	Posterior basal

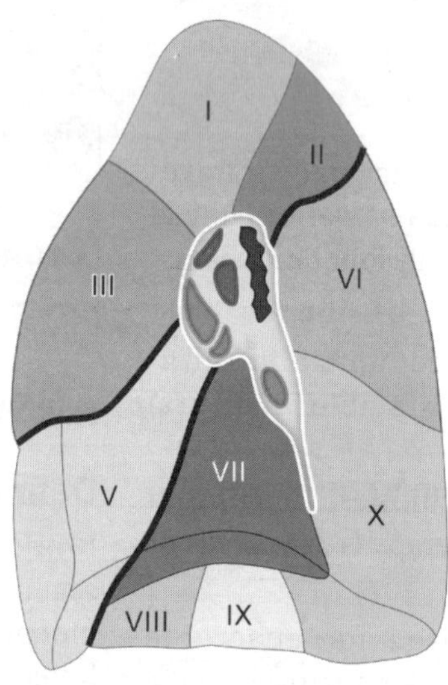

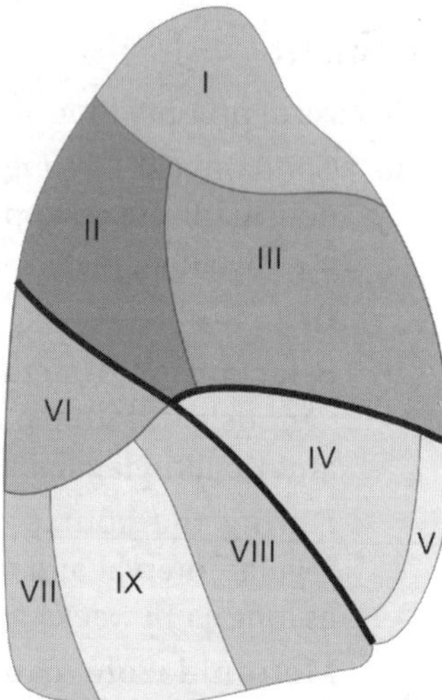

Clinical Importance of Bronchopulmonary Segment

A. Double lesion sign: It is characterized by collapse of multiple lobes or segments in certain combinations—it will rule out malignancy.

Exceptions are:

- **a.** Primary malignancy or metastasis
- **b.** Multicentric neoplasms
- **c.** Extension of lesions through fissures

B. Silhouette sign: It is characterized by localized parenchymal lesion, i.e., intrathoracic lesion having similar radiologic density in contiguity of heart, aorta, or diaphragm which obliterates the border due to loss of radiologic contrast.

- **a.** Right cardiac border—right middle lobe
- **b.** Left cardiac border—Lingula
- **c.** Aortic knuckle—left upper lobe and anterior right upper lobe

d. Right aortic border—middle lobe and anterior right upper lobe
e. Hemi diaphragm—basal segment of lower lobe from medial to lateral, anterior basal, medial basal, and posterior basal segments.

C. In case of tuberculosis: Apical and posterior segments of upper lobe are involved because of high V/Q ratios with elevated alveolar PO_2 as compared to other zones.
D. Sequestration of lung: Posterior basal segment of lower is involved, left more than the right.
E. Cancerous lesion: It usually involves anterior segment of right upper lobe.
F. Lung abscess: Posterior segment of right upper lobe or superior or posterior basal segments of lower lobe of right lung are involved because:
   a. Right bronchus is more vertical
   b. Aspirated secretion will gravitate into these lobes in supine position
G. Aspiration pneumonia will occur in apical segments of both lower lobes or posterior segment of right upper lobe
H. Bronchiectasis mostly occurs in left lower lobe because the bronchus is longer and narrower in this lobe.

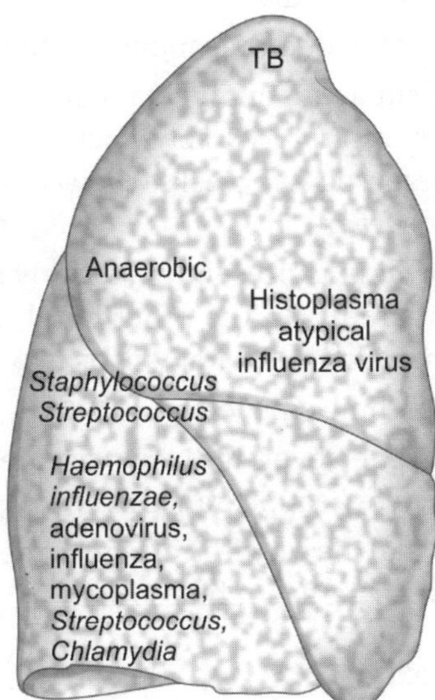

Surgical Importance

Postural drainage and percussion: Patient should be positioned in such a way retained secretion in the bronchopulmonary tree can be drained out of the lungs by gravity by rhythmic percussion on the chest wall. Position of the patient is such that each bronchopulmonary segment should be vertical so that liquid inside the bronchus will be drained into main stem bronchi and lastly out of the lung.

A. Apical segment of both upper lobes: High long sitting with 30–45° backward on reclined sitting.
B. Anterior segments of both upper lobes: Patient should be in supine position in flat bed with pillow under the head and knee.
C. Posterior segments of left upper lobe: Thorax is elevated for 30° with raising the head-end of the bed by 30°, patient will be turned one quarter from prone position to right side and pillow will be under left shoulder.
D. Posterior segment of right upper lobe: Thorax is elevated for 30° with raising the head-end of the bed by 30°, patient will be turned one quarter from prone position to left side and pillow will be under right shoulder.
E. Superior segment of both lower lobes: Patient should be prone flat with pillow under the hips and knees but nothing under the head.
F. Lateral basal segment of right lower lobe: Patient should lie on left side with leg end elevated by 30° and the patient will flex the upper leg over a pillow support.
G. Lateral basal segment of left lower lobe: Patient should lie on right side with leg end elevated by 30° and the patient will flex the upper leg over a pillow support.

Q16. Describe etiology, clinical features, diagnosis, and treatment of empyema thoracis.

MGR/APR2003/MDIII (25)

ANSWER

Definition

It can be defined as accumulation of pus within the pleural space. If the pus is localized in the pleural space, it is called intrapleural abscess.

Causes

A. Pulmonary infection:
   a. Bacterial causes
   b. Tubercular infection
   c. Pneumonia due to other microorganism
   d. Fungal infection
   e. Lung abscess
   f. Infected bronchiectasis

- **g.** Infection distal to obstruction in the bronchus which may be due to:
  - **1.** Lung cancer
  - **2.** Foreign body
- **B.** Esophageal perforation
- **C.** Subdiaphragmatic abscess
- **D.** Postoperative complication after cardiothoracic surgery
- **E.** Blunt or perforating trauma to the chest
- **F.** Hepatic abscess:
  - **a.** Amebic abscess
  - **b.** Pyemic abscess
- **G.** Primary pleural involvement—bacteremic or pyemic abscess

Predisposing Factors

- **A.** Alcoholism in 30% cases
- **B.** Immunocompromised state
- **C.** Diabetes
- **D.** Underlying chronic lung disease
- **E.** Neurologic disorder causing aspiration

Bacteriology

- **A.** Gram-positive cocci like *Streptococcus pneumoniae* and other streptococcal species
- **B.** *Haemophilus influenzae*
- **C.** *Staphylococci*
- **D.** *Mycobacterium tuberculosis*
- **E.** Anaerobic organisms from aspiration pneumonia
- **F.** *Legionella monocytogenes*
- **G.** *Pseudomonas aeruginosa*
- **H.** *Klebsiella pneumoniae*
- **I.** *Acinetobacter*
- **J.** Enterobacteria

Pathogenesis

- **A.** In the first stage, there is presence of sterile exudative collection in the pleural cavity with few leukocytes.
- **B.** Within few days it enters into the intermediate stage where fluid will be more turbid, containing marked leukocytes and many bacteria. In this stage, fibrous septa will be formed that loculate the pleural fluid into different compartments.
- **C.** In the final stage, pus becomes localized and collections walled off from the rest of the pleural space producing intrapleural abscess.

In case of pleuropulmonary infection becomes chronic. Ultimately fibrous tissue encircles the lung by laying down the fibrous tissue in peels thus making the lung functionless.

If the localized empyema is present anteriorly within the thoracic cavity it points empyema necessitates. The area of "point" is a bulge which produces impulse during coughing and it pulsates during palpation. Ultimately the bulge may open producing a sinus through which the pus seen coming out.

Types of empyema:

- **A.** Total empyema
- **B.** Encysted empyema
- **C.** Interlobar empyema
- **D.** Diaphragmatic empyema

Clinical Features

- **A.** In case of acute empyema:
  - **a.** Patient will present with fever with chill and rigor, tachycardia and tachypnea, intercostal tenderness on palpation, leukocytosis if the pleural effusion is large, or there is presence of underlying pneumonia.
  - **b.** If the pleural fluid is not drained there will be overwhelming sepsis, hypotension, shock, and multiorgan failure.
  - **c.** In case of pneumonia induced ARDS
- **B.** In case of subacute empyema, patient may recover from lower respiratory tract infection and fever may subside for few days to weeks followed by appearance of low grade fever.
- **C.** If the empyema is present posteriorly signs of fluid will be apparent. On the other hand, if the fluid is present anteriorly or laterally signs may be absent.
- **D.** In case of chronic empyema:
  - **a.** Low grade fever followed by afebrile period followed by reappearance of fever.
  - **b.** There may be no clinical sign if the collection is present in paravertebral space.

Imaging Studies

- **A.** X-ray chest:

  Convex border of the ill-defined homogeneous opacity in the pleural space which points toward walled-off.
- **B.** CT scan of chest reveals:
  - **a.** Thickened visceral and parietal pleura
  - **b.** Multiloculated pleural effusion with multiple fibrin strands in 80% cases. But it can be observed

in case of untreated or inadequately treated pleural effusion.

c. There may be air-fluid level in following conditions:
   1. In case of bronchopleural fistula
   2. Empyema caused by anaerobic organisms
   3. After paracentesis

d. It can resemble lung abscess, but it can be differentiated from lung abscess by following features:
   1. Compression of the adjacent lung
   2. Thickened visceral and parietal pleurae that are separated by fluid
   3. Formation of blunt angle with the chest wall
   4. Within the opacity there is absence of vessel markings. In case abscess wall will be smooth, occasionally irregular and thickened as in case of staphylococcal abscess.

C. Pleural fluid examination: Presence of pus in the aspirate confirms empyema, foul odor in the fluid occurs in anaerobic infection. During aspiration fluid should be collected from more than one location, because one may demonstrate clear fluid which may be due to inability of the organism to cross to the fibrin partition to enter into that cavity.

In case of complicated pleural effusion and empyema:

a. Low pH (7.1)
b. Low glucose (<40 mg/dL)
c. Raised lactate dehydrogenase (LDH) (>1,000 IU/L)
d. Elevated white blood cell count
e. Presence of elevated amylase points toward pancreatic etiology.
f. Culture of the fluid will be positive in untreated cases and negative in treated cases.
   1. Gram-positive culture: Community-acquired pneumonia
   2. Gram-negative culture:
      - Nosocomial pneumonia
      - Elderly or immunosuppressed patients having community-acquired pneumonia
   3. Anaerobic culture positive in case of:
      - Aspiration pneumonia
      - Lung abscess
   4. If culture is negative: Possibility of tubercular infection

D. Bronchoscopy:

It is useful in following conditions:

a. It can determine the nature of obstruction—tumor or foreign body
b. For study of the microbiological study of pleural fluid
c. It can determine the exact location of bronchopleural fistula
d. For aspiration of bronchial secretion in patients with excessive secretions

Management

A. Antibiotic therapy:

Empirical antibiotic therapy has to be started after taking the fluid for examination. Antibiotic should cover gram positive, gram negative, and anaerobic organisms. So combination of amoxicillin with piperacillin tazobactam along with clindamycin or metronidazole (in anaerobic infection) should be started intravenously. Instillation of antibiotic should not be done into the pleural cavity for following reasons:

a. Introduction of fresh infection
b. In case of inflammation of pleura concentration of antibiotics will be above the MIC

Duration of antibiotic administration is 4–6 weeks

B. Drainage of pleural fluid:

a. Indication:
   1. In case of localized frank pus in the pleural cavity
   2. In case of acute empyema if the quantity of fluid is >1.5 L and patient is in sepsis
   3. If the refilling of plural cavity after more than two paracentesis
   4. If there is bronchopleural fistula
   5. Following the assessment of pleural fluid by Light's criteria
   6. If the pH of pleural fluid is <7.2
   7. Presence of pus.

b. Drainage of fluid

It should be done by inserting the needle in the most dependent portion of the empyema under CT guidance.

c. Duration of drainage:

It should be continued till the closing of abscess cavity and there is no fluid to be drained. It may take several months.

C. Administration of fibrinolytic agents:

The aim is to break down the fibrin strands for complete drainage of pleural fluid. Successful fibrinolysis can reduce the need for surgery.

Instillation of 200,000–250,000 IU streptokinase or 30,000–100,000 IU urokinase into the pleural space daily for 5–6 days or in can be continued for 10–12 days. Contraindications of this therapy are:

a. Bronchopleural fistula where liquefied pleural fluid will be flooded into the lungs
b. Sepsis with deranged coagulation profile
c. Patients with coagulation disorders

D. Combination of fibrinolytic agents with deoxyribonuclease:

Deoxyribonuclease (DNAase) is introduced with the aim that it will reduce the viscosity and fibrinolytic agents will break down the fibrin strands so that proper drainage of fluid can be done. This combination can be called as "rescue therapy". Indications are:

a. Ongoing signs of infection
b. Poorly draining of loculated empyema
c. Failed antibiotic therapy and conventional drainage
d. Who needs surgical debridement

E. Surgical therapy:

Indication:

a. Failed medical treatment
b. Failure of closing of tube drainage to close the empyema cavity
c. Incorrect drainage procedure
d. Multiple loculations within the empyema cavity
e. Persistent underlying cause of empyema like bronchogenic carcinoma and foreign body
f. Persistent bronchopleural fistula
g. Persistent esophagotracheobronchial fistula
h. Persistent of empyema cavity

Different procedures:

a. Resection of ribs with insertion of large bore drainage tube at proper site of collection
b. Video-assisted thoracoscopic approach to break the loculations within the empyema for proper drainage through large bore tube
c. Thoracoscopic approach to break the loculations and decortication of lung surface and followed by drainage through large bore tube
d. Open thoracotomy for full decortication of lung followed by breaking down the loculi in the empyema cavity and then toileting the pleural cavity.

Q17. Interstitial lung disease.

MLB/MAY2013/MDII (20)
SNMC/MAY2013/MDI (10)

Write about the management of ILD.

ERA/NOV2012(S)/MDIII (25)

Diagnosis and management of ILD.

BF/MAY2013/MDII (10)

Write pathogenesis, causes, evaluation, and treatment of patient of ILD.

MUHS/MAY2012/MDII (25)

Discuss the management and recent advances in the management of ILD.

MUHS/MAY2014/MDIV (25)

Classification, pulmonary function testing, and treatment of ILD.

DNBIIIA/JUNE2015 (10)

Differentiate between obstructive and restrictive lung disease. Write down the classification of interstitial lung disease.

DNB 2021 (10)

Describe the functional anatomy of lungs, the physiology of breathing and respiratory function abnormalities in obstructive versus restrictive lung diseases.

DNB 2020 (10)

Classify interstitial lung disease, pathogenesis, diagnosis and management of non-specific interstitial pneumonia.

DR YSR UNI OF HEALTH SC, VIJAYAWADA, ANDHRA, 2022 (10)

Diagnosis and management of interstitial lung disease.

KERALA UNIVERSITY, 2020 (8)

Describe the pathogenesis, etiology, evaluation, and treatment of chronic interstitial lung disease.

NTR UNI OF HEALTH SC, VIJAYAWADA, SEPTEM, ANDHRA, 2020 (10)

ANSWER

Functional anatomy of the lungs will be answered in question number 15, 25, and 34.

Features	Obstructive lung disease	Restrictive lung disease
Definition	Narrowed bronchi leading to decreased airflow	Decreased compliance and expansion of lung
Total lung capacity	Increased or normal	Decreased and normal
Forced expiratory volume in 1 second	Markedly decreased	Decreased
Forced vital capacity	Decreased or normal	Decreased
FEV1/FVC	Decreased to less than 70%	Increased more than 80%
Residual volume	Increased	Decreased
Pattern of air flow	Obstructive pattern of airflow scooped flow-volume curve	Narrowed flow volume loop
Symptoms	Wheeze, diminished vesicular breath sound with prolonged expiration	Respiratory distress, Shallow breathing
Response to bronchodilators	Improves	No improvement

Definition

Interstitial lung disease can be defined as a group of disorders that affect following parts of the lung:

- **a.** Interstitium of the lung
- **b.** Air spaces with their epithelial linings
- **c.** Peripheral airways
- **d.** Bronchopulmonary vessels with their endothelial linings

Classification

Interstitial lung disease:

A. Idiopathic interstitial pneumonia:

- **a.** IPF
- **b.** Idiopathic nonspecific interstitial pneumonia
- **c.** Respiratory bronchiolitis—ILD
- **d.** Desquamative interstitial pneumonia
- **e.** Cryptogenic organizing pneumonia (COP)
- **f.** Acute interstitial pneumonia
- **g.** Idiopathic lymphoid interstitial pneumonia
- **h.** Idiopathic pleuroparenchymal fibroelastosis
- **i.** Unclassifiable idiopathic interstitial pneumonia

B. Autoimmune ILDs:

- **a.** Rheumatoid arthritis
- **b.** Interstitial pneumonia with autoimmune features
- **c.** Systemic lupus erythematosus (SLE)
- **d.** Sjögren's syndrome
- **e.** Polymyositis and dermatomyositis
- **f.** Mixed connective tissue diseases
- **g.** Systemic sclerosis
- **h.** Other connective tissue diseases

C. Hypersensitivity pneumonitis (HP)

D. Sarcoidosis

E. Others:

- **a.** Lymphangioleiomyomatosis (LAM)
- **b.** Langerhans' cell histiocytosis
- **c.** Drug-associated ILD
- **d.** Vasculitis or granulomatosis associated ILD
- **e.** ILDs related to other occupational disorders

Classification of idiopathic interstitial pneumonia according to the American Thoracic Society:

Histopathological pattern	Clinical diagnosis
Usual interstitial pneumonia	Idiopathic pulmonary fibrosis
Organizing pneumonia	Cryptogenic organizing pneumonia
Respiratory bronchiolitis	Respiratory bronchiolitis-associated ILD
Nonspecific interstitial pneumonia	Nonspecific interstitial pneumonia
Diffuse alveolar hemorrhage	Acute interstitial pneumonia
Desquamative interstitial pneumonia	Desquamative interstitial pneumonia
Lymphocytic interstitial pneumonia	Lymphocytic interstitial pneumonia

Diagnosis of Interstitial Pneumonia

A. Age:

- **a.** Less than 60 years old—idiopathic interstitial pneumonia and nonspecific interstitial pneumonia
- **b.** More than 60 years old but rare under 50 years of age—IPF
- **c.** Between the age of 20 and 40 years—sarcoidosis, Langerhans cell granulomatosis, LAM, and connected tissue disease-associated ILD

B. Sex:

- **a.** Females—LAM and connected tissue disease-associated ILD

b. Males—Langerhans cell granulomatosis, rheumatoid arthritis-associated ILD, IPF, and occupation- or exposure-related ILDs

C. Duration of symptoms:

a. Acute presentation of days to weeks—unusual in ILD but common in heart failure, pneumonia, or acute exacerbation of COPD. But eosinophilic pneumonia, granulomatosis with polyangiitis, acute interstitial pneumonia, and HP can present acutely.

b. Chronic presentation of months to years—IPF

c. Subacute presentation of weeks to months—sarcoidosis, connective tissue disease-associated ILDS, drug-induced ILD, and COP

D. Respiratory symptoms:

a. Dyspnea—it is a cardinal symptom in IPF, present during undue exertion like climbing upstairs but will be absent at rest. But it is relentlessly progressive over months and years and ultimately present at rest but relieved with oxygen.

b. Many patients are asymptomatic despite abnormal chest X-ray of CT chest findings.

c. Cough:

1. Dry cough with no diurnal variation—IPF
2. Cough due to prominent airway involvement—sarcoidosis and HP
3. Cough with hemoptysis—IPF with diffuse alveolar hemorrhage (DAH), LAM, pulmonary infection due to traction bronchiectasis, or on immunosuppressive therapy

d. Fatigue—ILD

e. Pleuritic chest pain—possibility of pneumothorax

f. Wheeze in ILD due to sarcoidosis or extrinsic pneumonitis

g. Associated joint pain and fever—collagen vascular disease or sarcoidosis

E. Past medical history:

a. History of connective tissue diseases such as joint deformity and Raynaud's phenomenon

b. History of malignancy may be associated with dermatomyositis with COP and sarcoid-like reaction

c. History of allergic rhinitis or asthma—suggests granulomatous with polyangiitis

F. Family history:

a. Idiopathic interstitial pneumonia in close relatives is strong risk factor

b. Nonspecific interstitial pneumonia

c. Desquamative interstitial pneumonia

d. Genetic factors for IPF is:

1. Promoter variant of mucin gene (MUC5B)
2. Genetic determinants influencing telomere length like telomerase reverse transcriptase gene

G. Social history:

a. Smoking—respiratory bronchiolitis, desquamative interstitial pneumonia relate ILD, and two-thirds of IPF.

b. Occupational and environmental exposure like exposure to asbestos and silica

H. History of medications:

a. Drugs for treating the inflammatory and granulomatous lung disease—azathioprine, methotrexate, rituximab, TNF-α blocking agents

b. Nitrofurantoin

c. Amiodarone

d. Bleomycin

Physical examination:

A. Crackles—dry Velcro-like crackles are heard at the base during the end part of inspiration. At early stage it can be heard when the patient is asked to lean forward with deep breathing. It will not change with coughing—it is pathognomonic of IPF.

B. Crackles are less common in granulomatous ILD-like sarcoidosis.

C. Associated wheeze is found in sarcoidosis, HP, eosinophilic pneumonia, and granulomatous polyangiitis.

D. Clubbing—present in IPF and rare in sarcoidosis, collagen vascular disease with ILD.

E. Evidence of pulmonary hypertension as evidenced by palpable pulmonary 2nd sound, right ventricular hypertrophy, and engorged pulsatile neck vein—indicates grave prognosis

F. Other extrapulmonary features are:

a. Raynaud's phenomenon and sclerodactyly—sarcoidosis

b. Erythema nodosum—sarcoidosis

c. Subcutaneous nodule—rheumatoid arthritis

d. Café-au-lait spot—tuberous sclerosis associated with LAM

Laboratory Studies

A. Radiology:

a. Chest X-ray: Following features can be found:

1. Enlarged hilar lymph nodes, presence of central nodular opacities in mid to upper zones—sarcoidosis

2. Presence of basilar reticular pattern and small cystic spaces in a patient not suffering from heart failure—IPF

Chest X-ray diagnosis is seldom confident. It cannot determine the disease activity and it cannot provide any information whether is it reversible or not.

B. Chest CT scan:

a. It is the standard care for initial evaluation.

b. It can spare the patient with the risk of lung biopsy because:

1. Classical history in an elderly and typical HRCT pattern can negate the biopsy.

c. It can detect the extent of disease.

d. It can provide the information of advanced disease like honeycombing.

e. It can provide the information of coexisting disease like emphysema cancer.

f. HRCT can demonstrate that which lobe or segment is required for lung biopsy.

g. Ground-glass pattern in HRCT can increase the survival by treatment as compared to reticular pattern.

h. It can demonstrate cavity or infiltrate which points toward tuberculosis.

i. Septal carcinoma can be picked by HRCT as compared to chest X-ray.

j. For diagnosing usual interstitial pneumonia following three radiological features are necessary:

1. Honeycombing

2. Reticular abnormalities

3. Basal and subpleural predominance

Findings in HRCT in different ILDS:

a. IPF:

1. Subpleural reticulation with posterior basal predominance

2. Honeycombing with traction bronchiectasis

b. Nonspecific interstitial pneumonia:

1. Diffuse subpleural symmetric reticular and ground-glass opacities

2. Volume contraction and traction bronchiectasis of lower lung zones

c. Smoking-related ILD:

1. Central bronchial wall thickening

2. Peripheral bronchial wall thickening

3. Centrilobular nodules

4. Ground-glass opacities

d. Cryptogenic organizing pneumonia:

1. Patchy migratory subpleural consolidation

2. Occasional ground-glass opacities

e. Acute interstitial pneumonia:

1. Patchy bilateral ground-glass opacities

2. Dependent region of air-space consolidation

f. Acute exacerbation of Idiopathic interstitial pneumonias:

1. Bilateral ground-glass opacities with air space consolidation

g. Collagen vascular disease:

1. Like nonspecific interstitial pneumonia and idiopathic interstitial fibrosis

h. Lipoid interstitial pneumonia:

1. Ground-glass appearances

2. Septal thickening

3. Cysts

4. Diffuse or lower lung distribution

i. Organizing pneumonia:

1. Peribronchial or subpleural consolidation

C. Lung biopsy:

a. Fiberoptic bronchoscopy: Its usefulness:

1. It can diagnose specifically ILD

2. Serial lavage fluid examination can reveal vasculitis associated with ILD

3. Cellular examination reveals:

- Chronic eosinophilic pneumonia if eosinophil count in peripheral blood is 25%
- Lipoid pneumonia if there is presence of fat globules in macrophages

4. Transbronchial lymph node biopsy can diagnose granulomatous lung disease in sarcoidosis or hypersensitivity pneumonia

b. Surgical lung biopsy:

It can be done in video-assisted approach as it will reduce the operation time length.

Evidences of histopathological features:

a. UIP:

1. Heterogeneous areas of young connective tissues

2. Scarring
3. Honeycombing
4. Normal lung

b. Nonspecific interstitial pneumonia:
1. Inflammation followed by alveolar septal thickening
2. Spatially or temporarily homogenous

c. Desquamative interstitial pneumonia:
1. Accumulation of macrophages within the alveolar spaces
2. Mild interstitial thickening
3. Homogenous involvement

d. Acute interstitial pneumonia:
1. Acute edema
2. Hyaline membrane
3. Inflammation of interstitium
4. Organization of airspaces

e. Lipoid interstitial pneumonia:
1. Diffuse infiltration of alveoli by lymphocytes
2. Infrequent lymphoid hyperplasia

f. Organization pneumonia:
1. Intraluminal organizing fibrosis in bronchioles alveolar ducts and alveoli

D. PFTs:

a. Restricted type of PFTs as evidenced by the following:
1. Reduced TLC
2. Reduced symmetrical reduced FEV_1
3. FVC

b. Reduced diffusion capacity to carbon monoxide—this test is less specific for ILD.

c. Reduced FEV_1/FVC ratio may be an associated defect in case of sarcoidosis, hypersensitivity pneumonia, and LAM.

Pulmonary function test is rarely diagnostic but it can diagnose the extent of the disease. Serial FVC and T_{LCO} measurement are correlated with the mortality of this disease. 10% and 20% decline in FVC and T_{LCO} from the baseline are associated with 2.4-fold increase in mortality.

E. 6-minute walk test: Desaturation below 88% during this walk test suggestive of high mortality. If it is associated with progressive decline of DLCO is less than 15% or more is strong predictor of high mortality. Desaturation to 88% from the baseline either during or end of the walk is powerful predictor of mortality of ILD.

F. Hematological abnormalities:

a. Eosinophilia—suggests HP

b. Serology to be tested according to past history of connective tissue diseases

Treatment

Currently there is no effective drug which can prevent or reverse the progression of fibrosis of lung. Steroid will much more harm than good. Triple therapy with steroid, azathioprine, and N-acetylcysteine is recently proved to worse. But now there are two drugs which can reduce but not reverse or stop the progression of disease and it can be measured by proper lung function test. These drugs are:

A. Pirfenidone: It will inhibit the number of prefibrotic cytokines like tumor growth factor-β, stimulate collagen synthesis, and blocks proliferation of fibroblast. It will slow the annual decline of FVC by 50%. Dose is 1,800 mg per day. But due to its adverse effect like gastric distress its dose should be increased gradually and to be taken after food. Other adverse effects are abnormal liver function and photosensitivity reaction.

B. Nintedanib: It is tyrosine kinase inhibitor and it blocks and reduces the signal of fibrogenic growth factors like platelet-derived growth factor, vascular endothelial growth factor, and fibroblast growth factor—these receptors are involved in the development of fibrosis. Dose is 150 mg twice daily and it shows 50% decline in speed of reduction of FVC.

Though IPF is chronic fibrotic disease, but due to intercurrent problem there may be acute exacerbation of this disease. Following are the criteria of acute exacerbation of IPF:

a. Previous or concurrent diagnosis of IPF

b. Worsening of hypoxemia from a known baseline ABG level

c. Unexplained worsening or development of dyspnea within 30 days

d. Endotracheal aspiration or BAL shows no evidence of infection

e. HRCT demonstrates ground-glass abnormality or consolidation superimposed on background of honeycomb or reticular pattern, which is consistent with interstitial pattern.

f. Exclusion of other causes such as PE, left-sided heart failure, and other causes of lung injury.

In this case corticosteroid like methylprednisolone 2 mg/kg for 2 weeks followed by slow tapering along with proper antibiotics.

General Measures

a. Administration of oxygen by bag mask

b. Cough usually cannot respond to antitussive

c. In case of gastroesophageal reflux disease (GERD), proton pump inhibitors should be administered to prevent reflux of acid, bile reflux, and pepsin as these may be responsible for progression of fibrosis.

d. Sleep apnea—it may coexist with ILD hence these patient may benefit from positive air-way pressure.

e. Pulmonary rehabilitation

Lung Transplantation

It is the only option in younger patient with advanced fibrosis. Survival rate is 75% at 1 year to 50% in 5 years.

Complications

A. Acute exacerbation of ILD:

It can be defined as acute worsening of respiratory distress with decline of lung function without any identifiable cause. Following are the diagnostic criteria:

a. Previous or concurrent diagnosis of interstitial pulmonary fibrosis

b. Unexplained worsening of respiratory distress within the past 30 days

c. HRCT demonstrates new bilateral ground-glass opacities along with exclusion of alternating cause of pulmonary infection.

Incidence is 1–20%. It is the major cause of mortality in patient with IPF and it is the most common cause of death. Autopsy findings in these patients are:

a. Background of UIP

b. Pattern of DAH

c. Concurrent organizing pneumonia may be present.

Management:

a. Hospitalization with supplementation of oxygen

b. Noninvasive ventilation to be given as it may eliminate the need for mechanical ventilation.

c. Large pulse of steroid like 500 mg of methylprednisolone to be given intravenously for 3 days

d. Other agents are tacrolimus, cyclophosphamide pulses, cyclosporine, polymyxin-B-immobilized fiber cartridge, and thrombomodulin.

e. Newer antifibrotics

B. Opportunistic infection: In our country tuberculosis is the most frequent complication.

C. Bronchial carcinoma: 10% death is due to this disease arising from diffuse areas of scarring. These are:

a. Localized adenocarcinoma

b. Alveolar cell carcinoma

It can be treated by chemotherapy and surgical resection.

D. Heart failure and ischemic heart disease: It occurs from pulmonary hypertension and right heart failure. It occurs in elderly. There may be left ventricular dysfunction.

E. PE: It produces 3–7% of death in IPF.

F. Pneumothorax: It can complicate ILD. Prolonged intercostal drainage is required

Q18. Describe principles of oxygen therapy in chronic obstructive lung disease.

ERA/MAY2012/MDII (10)

Discuss cor pulmonale and its management.

ERA/MAY2011/MDIII (10)

COPD with type II respiratory failure.

SNMC/MAY2013/MDIV (10)

Discuss recent trends in COPD management.

ALLD/MAY2007/MDII (10)

Discuss clinical feature, diagnostic criteria, and management of COPD.

AMU/2011/MDIII (20)

Discuss the evolving trends in the management of COPD.

MGR/MAR2007/MDIV (15)

Types of emphysema.

MGR/MAY2011/MDI (5)

Systemic manifestation of COPD.

DNBIIIA/DEC2014 (10)

Structural lesion in chronic bronchitis.

MGR/OCT2012/MDI (5)

A 40-year-old male, who has been suffering from chronic cough and copious purulent expectoration for 4 years presented with anasarca. Discuss the approach to history, clinical examination, differential diagnosis, laboratory evaluation, and treatment.

MJPRU/2015(S)/MDII (20)

Alpha-1 antitrypsin deficiency and its clinical manifestations.

BF/JUN2016/MDII (10)

Smoking cessation.

BF/MAY2009/MDIV (10)

Pulmonary rehabilitation.

KUHS/NOV2013(S)/MDII (10)

Pathophysiology of emphysema.

MGR UNI, TAMIL NADU, 2022 (5)

GOLD criteria of COPD and management of COPD.

NTR UNI OF HEALTH SC, VIJAYAWADA, ANDHRA, 2022 (10)

Contemporary diagnosis and recent advances in the management of chronic obstructive lung disease.

MGR UNI, TAMIL NADU, 2021 (15)

Discuss the newer therapies in chronic obstructive pulmonary lung disease.

NTR UNI OF HEALTH SC, VIJAYAWADA, SEPTEM, ANDHRA, 2020 (10)

Cor pulmonale.

RAJIV GANDHI UNI OF HEALTH SC, KARNATAKA, 2020 (10)

Discuss pulmonary function test. Write in brief about asthma-COPD overlap syndrome.

WBUHS, 2023 (10)

Discuss the etiopathology, risk factors and guidelines in the management of chronic obstructive lung disease.

WBUHS, 2024 (10)

ANSWER

Pulmonary function test has been described in question number 25.

Introduction

Chronic obstructive pulmonary disease is a preventable, treatable but progressive and not fully reversible respiratory disease of disturbances in air flow which may be due to involvement of airways or lung parenchyma or both. Mainly two disorders are commonly involved; these are chronic bronchitis and emphysema.

Chronic Bronchitis

It can be defined as chronic cough with production of sputum for at least 3 months per year for 2 or more consecutive years. Chronic bronchitis can be subclassified into three types:

- **A.** Simple bronchitis—it can be characterized by hypersecretion of mucus.
- **B.** Mucopurulent bronchitis—it can be characterized by production of mucopurulent sputum.
- **C.** Chronic obstructive bronchitis—it can be characterized by hypersecretion of mucus along with obstruction of airways.

Chronic bronchitis usually will be precipitated by respiratory tract infection and it is responsible for recurrent worsening of symptoms.

Emphysema

It can be defined as permanent abnormal enlargement of airspaces distal to terminal bronchioles along with disruption of alveolar walls but without fibrosis which may not limit airflow.

COPD

According to the ATS and European Respiratory Society, COPD can be defined as preventable and treatable disease characterized by not fully reversible airflow limitation, but this limitation is progressive and occurs due to inflammatory response to noxious agents such as smoke and gases.

Pathogenesis

Comorbidities:

- **A.** Osteoporosis
- **B.** Anemia
- **C.** Weight loss
- **D.** Skeletal muscle dysfunction
- **E.** Lean muscle mass loss

F. Sleep disorder

G. Psychological problems such as depression and anxiety

H. Associated with diabetes mellitus, ischemic cardiac disease, and peptic ulcer disease

Smoking

Smoking affects at the following level of respiratory system:

A. Bronchi: Smoking affects both structure and function of the mucous secreting apparatus in the bronchial wall.

a. There is hyperplasia and hypertrophy of the mucous secreting glands leading to increased secretion of mucus, as a result airway wall will be thickened.

b. Airway lumen will be narrowed due to:

1. Increase in number and size of the gland
2. Increased secretion of mucus
3. Influx of inflammatory cells such as neutrophils, macrophäges, and cytotoxic T lymphocytes
4. Release of various inflammatory mediators such as leukotriene B4, IL-8, and TNF-α, will amplify inflammatory process further in the bronchial airways and lung parenchyma
5. Reactive oxygen species in the cigarette smoke and released from inflammatory cells also involves in this process.
6. Neutrophil elastase produced by neutrophils also stimulates secretion of mucus which overwhelm the activity of secretory leuko-protease inhibitor produced by airway epithelial cells and mucus secreting cells.
7. As a result of long-term exposure to smoke there will be structural changes in the cilia lining in the bronchial lumen which will impair mucociliary clearance from the lumen.
8. Pipe and cigar smoking are also responsible for development of chronic bronchitis but risk are less as smoke of pipe and smoke are not inhaled extensively.

B. Small airways involving bronchioles of <2 mm in diameter are predominantly affected. As a result of smoking there will be narrowing of bronchiole, inflammation of the wall of the bronchiole, and residual fibrosis all of which predispose to airway narrowing and it is mainly responsible for obstruction of airway in COPD.

C. Pulmonary parenchyma:

a. There is destruction of connective tissue matrix ofthe walls of the alveoli by proteolytic enzymes released by inflammatory cells as in case of emphysema. This is explained by protease-antiprotease hypothesis. Elastase, a serine protease, most important proteolytic enzyme released from neutrophils within the lungs, also known as neutrophil elastase is responsible for destruction of structural protein of alveoli elastin which will lead to destruction of alveoli. Inhibitor of neutrophil elastase known as α1 antitrypsin is normally present in the lung. Balance between the elastase and its inhibitor will prevent the destruction of the alveolar walls. But in smoking, there is increased release of neutrophil in the alveolar wall which will increase the synthesis of elastase thus there is shift the balance toward the destruction of the elastin of the alveolar wall.

b. There is oxidant stress due to release of oxidants from cigarette smoke damages the alveolar epithelium and other structural components of lung such as elastin and collagen.

c. Matrix metalloproteinases produced by alveolar macrophages and neutrophils will also capable of breaking down the alveolar wall structure which is normally inhibited by tissue inhibitor matrix metalloproteinases. But in case smoking there is increased influx of neutrophils as well as macrophages, as a result there is increased burden of matrix metalloproteinases in the alveolar walls which overwhelm the activity of their inhibitors leading to enhanced destruction of alveolar walls.

C. Environmental and indoor pollution:

a. Air pollution does not initiate COPD but exacerbate the preexisting disease.

b. Occupational exposure to pollutants in case of miners or organic antigen in case of agricultural workers is responsible for chronic bronchitis.

c. Indoor cooking involving biomass fuels produces COPD.

D. Infection:

Different types of viral and bacterial infections will not initiate the disease but may be responsible for worsening of symptoms, bacterial infection is responsible for superinfection in case of preexisting viral infection. Childhood respiratory tract infection affects the growth and function of the lung and enhances the development of COPD in adulthood, hence in case smoker development of COPD is not uniform.

E. Genetic factors:

   a. One important hereditary factor responsible for development of emphysema is α1 antitrypsin, a glycoprotein, a serine protease inhibitor (PI). It is produced in the liver and released in the circulation; this enzyme is encoded by SERPINA1 gene. Among >100 different alleles of this enzyme each person has two gens, one from paternal and the other from maternal. Normal allele is M allele having two genes MM. In case of normal MM phenotype, the blood level of the inhibitor enzyme is 200 mg/dL.

      In case of variant alleles, known as Z, sequence of amino acids in the inhibitor will be altered which in turn impairs the secretion from the liver, site of synthesis. So this abnormal PI will remain in the globules in the liver resulting liver disease but small amount will circulate in the blood. In case of ZZ phenotype, blood level of this inhibitor is only 15% of the normal or 30 mg/dL. On the other hand, heterozygotes having MZ phenotype intermediate level of this enzyme, i.e., 50–60% is present. So ZZ phenotype is responsible for premature development of emphysema in third or fourth decade if patient is smoker. In these ZZ phenotype patients, there is absence or very low level of α_1-antitrypsin which allow elastin to destroy the alveolar walls in unchecked fashion leading to development of emphysema.

   b. There is hyperresponsiveness of bronchial smooth muscles and mucous glands to smoke, which leads to bronchoconstriction declining pulmonary function.

   c. Pulmonary tuberculosis is associated with obstruction of the airways during active phase and also several years after treatment due to inflammation followed by fibrosis, the degree of obstruction varies with the length of the treatment and extent of the disease. This airway obstruction is the result of immunological response to mycobacterial antigen.

   d. In chronic severe asthma, airway obstruction is irreversible due to remodeling of airways along with thickening and fibrosis.

Pathology

Pathology of chronic bronchitis includes:

A. Mucus secreting glands: There is hyperplasia and hypertrophy of mucus secreting glands which can be assessed by comparing the thickness of mucus secreting glands with the total thickness of wall of the airway and the ratio is known as Reid index—it is increased in chronic bronchitis.

B. Goblet cells are abundant throughout the airways and more in the proximally, in chronic bronchitis their number is also increased and more in the periphery.

C. The glands secrete mucus, but in chronic bronchitis its amount and character are increased.

D. Large bronchial wall demonstrates evidence of inflammation, cellular infiltration, and variable fibrosis.

E. Diameter of the smaller airways is narrowed due to inflammation of the bronchial smooth muscles, variable degree of fibrosis, hyperplasia of goblet cells, and increased amount of mucus. Airway resistance varies inversely to the thickness of the bronchial lumen. So, as diameter of the bronchial lumen decreases airway resistance increases.

F. Inflammation of mucosa and submucosa leads to excessive mucus secretion.

G. There is infiltration of mucosa, submucosa and mucous gland and bronchial wall with neutrophil and macrophages and activated CD8 suppressor cells which increases during acute exacerbation. There is loss ciliary epithelium in the airway.

Pathology of emphysema includes:

A. In case of emphysema there is destruction of alveolar wall leading to enlargement of terminal airspaces. It can be described as acinar unit—it can be described as an unit supplied by single terminal bronchiole. Emphysema is of three types:

   a. Centriacinar or centrilobular emphysema: Here there is predominant involvement of proximal part of the acinus and respiratory bronchiole. Here the affected area is irregular sparing the alveolar tissue between the dilated respiratory bronchiole at the center of acinus. It is found in smoker.

   b. Panacinar emphysema: Here there is uniform involvement of acinus involving respiratory bronchiole, alveolar duct, and alveolar sac beyond the terminal bronchiole. It is found in case of α1 antitrypsin deficiency. Lower zones are involved than upper zones.

   c. Periacinar or paraseptal emphysema: Here enlarged airspaces are present at the periphery against fixed structure like lung fissure, pleura, or septum.

B. Macroscopically airspace is visible when it is enlarged >1 mm. Bulla—it is formed by rupture of many adjacent walls of alveoli resulting formation of airspace of >1 cm in diameter. Large bullae are formed by coalescence of small bullae and it may occupy large part of the lobe.

C. Vascular changes:
   a. There is thickening of intima, increased number of smooth muscle along with infiltration of macrophages, and CD8 suppressor T lymphocytes in the media
   b. With the progression of the disease more and more thickening of intima and media along with deposition of collagen
   c. Hypoxia and hypercapnia will be the triggering factor for vasoconstriction

Pathophysiology of Chronic Obstructive Pulmonary Disease

Pathophysiology is dependent upon the complex interaction of centrally conducting airways of >2 mm, peripherally conducting airways of <2 mm in diameter, lung parenchyma, respiratory muscles, diaphragmatic muscle, and chest wall mechanics. So, abnormalities of any one of the above will culminate gas exchange abnormalities leading to breathlessness, cough, respiratory failure, and death.

Functional Abnormalities in Case of Chronic Bronchitis

A. In case large airways increased number and size of the gland and increased formation of mucus produce excessive cough and sputum that do not correlate with degree of airway obstruction. But if there is associated mild airflow obstruction, it suggests associated emphysema.

B. If there is associated hyperactivity of airway smooth muscles, it leads to constriction of airway smooth muscles which is responsible for reversible airflow obstruction which is known as asthma-COPD overlap syndrome.

C. Airway cross-sectional area and resistance will be increased by the following:
   a. Intraluminal secretions
   b. Bronchospasm
   c. Wall edema
   d. Infiltration of inflammatory cells
   e. Enlargement of mucus secreting gland and goblet cells
   f. Varying level of fibrosis.

   In case of mild affection of peripheral airways there is 10–20% of airway resistance.

D. Following abnormalities in expiratory flow rates are seen:
   a. FEV_1—decreased
   b. FEV_1/FVC—decreased
   c. Maximal mid-expiratory flow rates—decreased
   d. No improvement in these flow rates after use of inhaled bronchodilator. But in case of asthma-COPD syndrome these flow rates will be improved.

E. Abnormalities in lung volumes in PFT:
   a. TLC: It is normal as there is neither alteration of elastic recoil of lung nor respiratory muscle strength.
   b. FRC remains normal as both chest wall and lung recoil are unaltered. But if there is tachypnea and expiration is prolonged the patient will get sufficient time to reach normal resting end-expiratory point during expiration.
   c. RV will be increased when more peripheral airways are involved as there is chance of air trapping by occlusion of small airways.

Functional Abnormalities in Case of Emphysema

A. As the primary problem in emphysema is elastic recoil of lung, so there is decrease in driving pressure during expiration to expel the air from the alveoli leading to air trapping.

B. Indirect effect on collapsibility of the airways. Normally walls of the airways are pulled outward from the adjacent lung tissue by supporting structures thus prevent collapse of airways. But in case of emphysema as there is absence of radial traction of the airways due to loss of supporting structure, so the airway will collapse and it will be enhanced by strong expiratory pressure during forced expiration.

C. Alteration of compliance curve: It relates transpulmonary pressure to gaseous volumes within the lung. As emphysematous lung resists expansion less as compared to normal, the curve will be shifted upward and to the left—so at any given transpulmonary pressure lung volume will be increased.

D. Alteration in the volume:
   a. Total lung volume—increased because of loss of elastic recoil of the lung will give smaller force to oppose the action of inspiratory musculature.
   b. FRC—if it is increased, there is gross imbalance between the inward recoil of lung and outward recoil of chest wall shifting the force in favor of chest wall.

c. RV—increased because poorly supported airways are very susceptible to closure during forced expiration.

Mechanisms of abnormal gas exchange:

A. In obstructive lung disease, pathological changes in the airways are not uniformly distributed. In case of chronic bronchitis, some airways become plugged with secretions and some airways remain normal, so ventilation is not distributed differentially. So areas of the lung supplied by diseased airways are underventilated as compared to normal areas. But blood will flow in the areas of underventilated lung producing V/Q mismatch and low V/Q ratio resulting hypoxemia without hypercapnia.

B. In some obstructive lung disease there is impairment of carbon dioxide, the possible mechanisms are as follows:

- **a.** Increased work of breathing
- **b.** V/Q mismatch producing high V/Q in some areas producing dead space and in some areas low V/Q ratio due to shunt. When shunt areas are increased then there will be carbon dioxide gas retention.
- **c.** Abnormalities in the central ventilatory drive
- **d.** Fatigue in the respiratory muscles will lead to acute retention of carbon dioxide in patient with respiratory failure.

C. In case of obstructive lung disease diaphragmatic muscles are flattened, so the contraction is less effective and less efficient. Again, when FRC is increased then the diaphragm will be flattened and muscle of diaphragm is already shortened even prior to inspiration. So flattened diaphragm is itself is a mechanical disadvantage.

Pulmonary Hypertension

Primary cause of pulmonary hypertension in COPD is chronic hypoxia, but other causes are hypercapnia, polycythemia, and reduction of the pulmonary vascular bed.

A. Hypoxia produces intense vasoconstriction of pulmonary arteriole, it may be reversible after correction of hypoxia but vascular remodeling will not be fully reversed.

B. Hypercapnia also produces vasoconstriction by changes in the pH arterial blood due to increased PCO_2.

C. In case of chronic hypoxia, there is secondary rise in hematocrit leading to secondary polycythemia which increases the blood viscosity thus increases pulmonary hypertension.

D. In case of emphysema, there is loss of pulmonary vascular bed due to loss of alveoli, thus large amount of pulmonary vascular bed will be lost which leads to increased arterial pressure.

As a result increased work load in the right ventricle making it hypertrophied and eventually fails.

Clinical Features

A. History:

- **a.** Proper history regarding smoking has to be taken in absence of genetic, environmental or occupational predisposition, because smoking of <10–15 packs per year is unlikely to produce chronic obstructive lung disease.
- **b.** History regarding outdoor or indoor pollution like dust or biofuels is needed.

B. Symptoms:

- **a.** Dyspnea
- **b.** Cough with expectoration—many of the patients may start with cough with expectoration preceding the development of dyspnea.
- **c.** Wheeze
- **d.** Chest discomfort: It usually occurs during the time exacerbations mainly due to increased workload of breathing.
- **e.** Pleuritic chest pain: It may occur due to:
  1. Pulmonary infarction
  2. Pneumonia
  3. Pneumothorax
- **f.** Hemoptysis occurs due to:
  1. Acute pulmonary infarction
  2. Bronchogenic carcinoma
- **g.** Weight loss and muscle wasting occur due to poor nutrition and in some patients chronic symptoms are punctuated by period of exacerbations which is characterized by worsening of symptoms precipitated by viral and bacterial infections and may require alteration of medications. Other factors responsible for acute deterioration of breathlessness are:
- **a.** New strain of bacteria colonized in the tracheobronchial tree
- **b.** Air pollutants
- **c.** Sudden bronchospasm in patients having pre-existing asthma
- **d.** Heart failure
- **e.** Unknown cause

Dyspnea is graded according to Modified Research Council Dyspnea Scale:

Category	Degree of dyspnea	Effect
0	None	Not being troubled by shortness of breath except with strenuous exercise
1	Slight	Being trouble by shortness of breath when hurrying on the travel or walking up to a slight hill
2	Moderate	Walks slower than people of same age on the travel because of shortness of breath
3	Moderately severe	Patient has to stop because of shortness of breath when walking at own pace on the travel
4	Severe	Stops for breath after about 100 yards or after few minutes on the travel
5	Very severe	Too breathless to leave the house or breathless when dressing or undressing

Oxygen cost diagram is more sensitive in diagnosing dyspnea. Here patients mark the point beyond which he or she becomes breathless on a 10 cm line. It starts with zero and from there up to a point where the patient becomes breathless will be marked and that score is the degree of breathlessness.

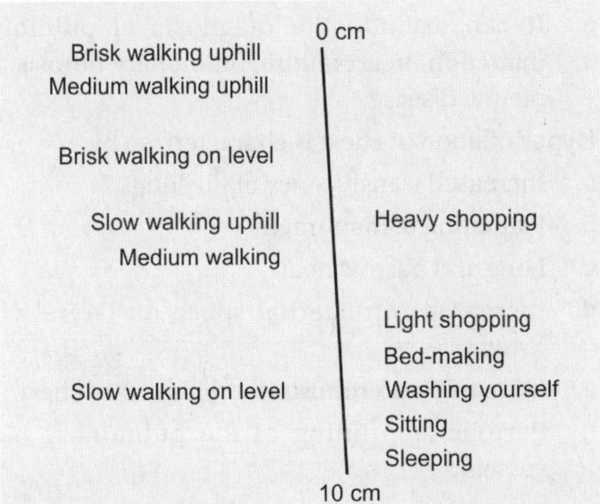

Physical Findings

A. General examination:

a. Tachypnea

b. Forced expiration time is >5 seconds

c. Increased work of accessary muscles of respiration

d. In case of severe COPD:

1. Pursed lips in emphysema
2. Cyanosis in case chronic bronchitis
3. Clubbing is usually not present. Its presence indicates bronchiectasis and bronchogenic carcinoma
4. Drowsiness or even comatose due to carbon dioxide retention
5. Flapping tremor
6. Seizures and papilledema due to carbon dioxide retention
7. Patient's position is "tripod"—it is characterized by leaning forward on his straight arms allowing fixation of both clavicles and proper and maximum use of accessary muscles.

B. Respiratory system examination:

a. Barrel-shaped chest due to overinflated lung—it can be characterized by:

1. Increased anteroposterior diameter
2. Kyphosis
3. Elevation of sternum
4. Ribs are horizontally placed
5. Prominent sternal angle
6. Wide subcostal angle
7. Reduction of space in between suprasternal notch and cricoid cartilage

b. Indrawing of intercostal spaces and suprasternal notch during inspiratory phase—as a result of strong contraction of intercostal muscles due to increased negative intrapleural pressure.

c. Flattening of diaphragm tugs lower costal margin inward during inspiration.

d. On palpation:

1. Poor expansion of chest
2. Apical impulse may not be palpated

e. On percussion:

1. Hyper-resonant note is found
2. Absence of hepatic and cardiac dullness
3. In case of advanced COPD, total loss of cardiac dullness

f. On auscultation:

1. Diminished breath sound with prolonged expiration
2. Wheeze is polyphonic
3. Presence of crackles at both bases during early inspiration

4. In case of advanced COPD—breath sound will be further diminished, wheeze is not heard. But during forced expiration wheeze may be heard.

C. Cardiovascular system:

A. General features related to cardiovascular system:
   a. Tachycardia
   b. High pulse pressure
   c. High volume pulse
   d. Pulsus paradoxus due to marked swinging of intrapleural pressure during inspiration and expiration
   e. Neck vein is pulsatile and engorged

B. Proper cardiovascular system:
   a. Faint or absent apical impulse
   b. In case of cor pulmonale:
      1. Right ventricular heave indicating right ventricular hypertrophy
      2. Palpable pulmonary 2nd heart sound

   On auscultation:
      1. Right ventricular gallop—3rd heart sound
      2. Loud 2nd heart sound
      3. Systolic murmur of tricuspid incompetence increased during inspiration
      4. There may be blowing diastolic murmur, called Graham Steel murmur due to dilated pulmonary artery with pulmonary incompetence—it is best heard in 2nd and 3rd intercostal space in the 2nd intercostal space.

   In case of right heart failure:
      1. Tender hepatomegaly which can be palpated due to flattening of diaphragm

Chronic Obstructive Pulmonary Disease Phenotypes

A. Blue bloater: It occurs in severe chronic bronchitis. In this case face becomes puffy, sometimes cyanosed, not unduly tachypneic

B. Pink puffer: Here the patient is emphysematous, tachypneic, with all accessary muscles of respiration being hyperactive, plethoric face with pursed lips.

Investigations of Chronic Obstructive Pulmonary Disease

A. Hematological investigations:
   a. Complete blood count to detect leukocytosis in case of suspected infection
   b. Packed cell volume (PCV): It detects polycythemia. It occurs when PaO_2 is <55 mm Hg. Polycythemia is diagnosed when:
      1. PCV is > 47% in women and >52% in men
      2. Hemoglobin is >16 g/dL in women and >18 g/dL in men
   c. Full biochemical study
   d. Blood gas analysis suggesting presence or absence of hypoxemia and hypercapnia
   e. Electrocardiogram (ECG) manifestation of cor pulmonale:
      1. Peaked P in lead II and avF
      2. Clockwise rotation
      3. Tall R in V1
      4. Right bundle branch block pattern

B. Chest X-ray:
   a. It can exclude the diagnosis of pulmonary infarction, heart failure, pulmonary fibrosis, and pleural disease.

   Hyperinflation of chest is characterized by:
   a. Increased translucency of the lungs
   b. Flattening of diaphragm
   c. Long and narrow heart
   d. Increased retrosternal space on lateral chest X-ray
   e. Increased anteroposterior diameter of chest
   f. Peripheral pruning of the pulmonary blood vessels
   g. Paucity of vascular markings—it results from destruction of septa of alveoli along with enlargement of alveolar spaces—it is known as arterial deficiency pattern of emphysema.
   h. In case of α1 antitrypsin deficiency arterial deficiency pattern are seen in the lower lobe.
   i. In case of pulmonary hypertension:
      1. Enlargement of proximal pulmonary artery
      2. Pronounced tapering of the distal blood vessels
      3. Cardiomegaly indicating right ventricular hypertrophy
   j. Presence of bullae—it is radiolucent space of 1 cm or more in diameter surrounded by thin outline

C. HRCT:

It can characterize the extent and distribution of emphysema whether it is panacinar, centrilobular or septal.

D. Assessment of lung function: It is of vital importance because:

a. When clinically diagnosis may be missed COPD

b. Objective diagnosis of COPD by this basic test

c. Degree of COPD can be assessed by spirometry

Spirometry

A. Gold spirometric classification of degree of COPD:

Grade	Types	Features
I	Mild COPD	$FEV_1/FVC < 70$ $FEV_1 \geq 80\%$ of predicted
II	Moderate COPD	$FEV_1/FVC < 70$ $FEV_1 \geq 50\%$ and <80% of predicted
III	Severe COPD	$FEV_1/FVC < 70$ $FEV_1 \geq 30\%$ and <50% of predicted
IV	Very severe COPD	$FEV_1/FVC < 70$ FEV_1 <30% of predicted

FEV_1 and FVC are influenced by:

a. Speed of inspiration

b. Presence and duration of end-inspiratory pause prior to forced expiration

If forced expiratory maneuver is preceded by slow inspiration and long inspiratory pause then forced expiratory flow will be lower.

Severity of symptoms, comorbidities, and risk of exacerbations assess the risk of COPD.

Revised GOLD assessment of COPD:

GOLD: Severity of airflow limitation (it is based on post-bronchodilator FEV_1)		
Stage	**Severity**	**FEV_1 (% predicted)**
In case of patients with FEV_1/FVC		
GOLD 1	Mild	≥80
GOLD 2	Moderate	50–79
GOLD 3	Severe	30–49
GOLD 4	Very severe	<30
GOLD: Assessment of symptoms and risk of exacerbations		
	Assessment of symptoms	
Exacerbations/ Hospitalizations	mMRC 0–1, CAT <10	mMRC ≥ 2; CAT ≥ 10
0–1: Exacerbations without hospitalizations	A	B
≥2 exacerbations or ≥1 hospitalization	C	D

mMRC: modified Medical Research Council dyspnea scale, refer to http://www.catestonline.org

Global Initiative for Chronic Obstructive Lung Disease (GOLD) guidelines (www.goldgopd.org)

Source: www.goldcopd.org

CAT–COPD assessment test http://www.catestonline.org

A. Group A:

a. Low risk

b. Less symptoms

c. 0–1 exacerbation per year and prior hospitalization

d. CAT score <10

e. mMRC grade: 0–1

B. Group B:

a. Low risk

b. More symptoms

c. 0–1 exacerbation per year but no prior hospitalization for exacerbation

d. CAT ≥ 10

e. mMRC grade: ≥ 2

C. Group C:

a. High risk

b. Less symptoms

c. ≥2 exacerbations per year or ≥1 hospitalization for exacerbations

d. CAT < 10

e. mMRC grade: <2

D. Group D:

a. High risk

b. More symptoms

c. ≥2 exacerbations per year or ≥1 hospitalization for exacerbations

d. CAT ≥ 10

e. mMRC grade: ≥2

Testing of Reversibility Obstruction of Airways

It will differentiate asthma from COPD because asthma is completely reversible but COPD in poorly reversible. In this test, forced expiratory maneuver can be measured after four to five puffs of bronchodilators. Absolute change in FEV_1 of >200 mL or increase in FEV_1 by 12% or more has been considered as significant as per GOLD guidelines. Whereas according to the British Society Guidelines FEV_1 of >200 mL or increase in FEV_1 by 15% or more. But if there is no reversibility with bronchodilators then corticosteroids can be tried to demonstrate the reversibility of the bronchoconstriction.

Static Lung Volume

a. TLC—increased

b. FRC—increased

c. RV—increased

d. Ratio of RV/TLC—increased

All the above volumes are increased due to air trapping and hyperinflation of lung.

Flow-volume Loops

Expiratory flow rate at different lung volumes is reduced because of limitation of airflow in COPD.
Inspiratory capacity:

- **a.** It reflects changes in hyperinflation and it is simple to measure.
- **b.** It reflects the FRC, so if there is any change in FRC there will be opposite change in inspiratory capacity (IC).
- **c.** It is good predictor of maximal tidal volume during exercise.
- **d.** It will evaluate the progress as well as status of COPD.

Carbon Monoxide Transfer

- **A.** Carbon monoxide transfer factor is reduced in emphysema—it occurs due to:
  - **a.** Reduction of surface volume
  - **b.** Inequality of V/Q ratio
- **B.** In case of chronic bronchitis: diffusion capacity will be normal.

Complications of Chronic Obstructive Pulmonary Disease

- **A.** Recurrent infection
- **B.** Pneumothorax
- **C.** Atelectasis of lung
- **D.** Lung cancer
- **E.** Thromboembolic diseases
- **F.** Systemic complications

Treatment of Chronic Obstructive Pulmonary Disease

Objective of management of COPD:

- **A.** Prevention of progression of disease: Key element is cessation of smoking, but other elements are occupational pollutants, indoor pollution, combustion of biofuels, and environmental pollution—these has to be mitigated or completely abolished. Smoking of cigarettes can be replaced by nicotine replacement therapy (NRT) or/and use of bupropion.
  - **a.** NRT can be given in the form chewing gum or skin patch or as nasal spray or inhaler. Side effects may occur who use to take <10 cigarettes per day. It has to be avoided in case of patients with peptic ulcer disease, ischemic heart disease, and pregnant and breastfeed women.
  - **b.** Bupropion is given as 150 mg twice daily for 6–8 weeks. Side effects are headache and seizures; hence, it is avoided in case of epileptics.
  - **c.** Varenicline:
    1. New alternative to NRT
    2. It is partial acetylcholine receptor agonist
    3. It is 12 weeks course
    4. Adverse effects are nausea and high suicidal attempts
- **B.** Relief of symptoms: Breathlessness, cough, and poor tolerance to exercise can be relieved by bronchodilators and corticosteroids.

Management of COPD based on GOLD assessment of symptoms and risk of exacerbations:

Category	Symptoms	Risk	Suggested treatment
All			
A	Less symptomatic: Mild or infrequent symptoms or CAT <10	Low risk No or 1 exacerbation in the past year but absence of hospitalization	SABA or combination of SABA and anticholinergic Alternative drugs are LABA
B	More symptomatic: Moderate-to-severe symptoms or CAT ≥ 10	Low risk No or 1 exacerbation in the past year in absence of hospitalization	**First choice:** LABA or LAMA based on symptoms SABA for control of symptoms **For persistent symptoms:** Regular treatment with LAMA + LABA
C	Less symptomatic: Mild or infrequent symptoms or CAT <10	High risk ≥2 exacerbations per year associated with ≥1 hospitalizations	**First choice:** Regular treatment with LAMA SABA is for control and relief of symptom **For acute exacerbations:** Regular treatment with LAMA + LABA Or LABA + ICS

Continued

Continued

Category	Symptoms	Risk	Suggested treatment
D	More symptomatic: Moderate-to-severe symptoms or CAT ≥ 10	High risk ≥2 exacerbations per year along with one or more hospitalizations	**First choice:** LABA + LAMA or LABA + ICS in case of asthma-COPD overlap syndrome SABA is used to control symptoms LAMA only in case of contraindication for LABA **For further exacerbations:** Regular treatment with LABA + LAMA + ICS Or LABA + ICS (in asthma-COPD overlap)

(ICS: inhaled corticosteroids; LABA: long-acting bronchodilator; LAMA: long-acting muscarinic agents; SABA: short-acting bronchodilator)

Simplified form of Management According to mMRC Criteria

a. Severe or very severe COPD: LABA + LAMA + ICS

b. Moderately severe disease: LABA + LAMA

But in case of frequent exacerbations: LABA + LAMA + ICS

c. Mild symptoms: SABA on SOS basis

But in case of frequent breathlessness: LABA on long-term basis

d. Mild-to-moderate COPD with frequent exacerbations: ICS + LABA or, ICS + LAMA

C. Pulmonary rehabilitation:

Following have to be excluded prior to rehabilitation:

a. Ischemic heart disease

b. Arrhythmias

c. Arthritis

After exclusion of the above cases following are the indications:

a. Poor exercise tolerance due to well-marked dyspnea—class III/IV severe chronic obstructive lung disease

b. In patient with grade II chronic obstructive lung disease having dyspnea with reduced effort tolerance

c. History of frequent visit to emergency department or frequent hospitalization

d. Patients requiring psychological help as well as adjustment

Following features of pulmonary rehabilitation:

a. Exercise training—it is characterized by graded exercise under supervision like lower limb exercise through cycling and walking, but during this time, if required, administration of oxygen.

b. Breathing exercise and training:

1. Diaphragmatic breathing
2. Pursed lip breathing characterized by slow complete expiration followed by slow complete inspiration
3. Rhythmic breathing during activity
4. Allowing for full respiration
5. Yoga breathing exercise
6. Conservation and reduction in energy requirement through using proper use of body mechanics

c. To alleviate anxiety and depression psychological counseling

d. Education for maintaining proper healthy and disciplined lifestyle

e. Nutritional guidance:

1. In case of patients with weight loss or loss of body muscle mass there is increased chance of mortality. So proper nutrition is required.
2. In case of overweight patient balanced diet is required to lose weight.

D. Oxygen therapy:

Indications for continuation of oxygen therapy COPD patients:

a. Stable COPD on medical therapy having PaO_2 of <55 mm Hg with SaO_2 of <90%

b. $PaCO_2$ of <55 mm Hg along with packed cell volume of >55%

c. Right heart dysfunction showing P pulmonale in ECG and peripheral edema

Objective of oxygen therapy is:

a. To maintain PaO_2 of >60 mm Hg

b. At night flow of oxygen should be increased to maintain saturation of 90%

c. To relieve dyspnea during activity and during rest
d. To reduce pulmonary hypertension
e. To improve cognition
f. To improve the quality of life

Nocturnal hypoxemia is dangerous because it can induce:

a. Dangerous arrhythmia
b. Pulmonary hypertension
c. Poor cognition during the day
d. Daytime hypersomnolence

Hence, oxygen flow at night should be increased.

But in case of patients with severe hypoxemia and severe hypercapnia uncontrolled oxygen therapy can relieve hypoxemia but at the cost of hypercapnia, as a result the patient will become increasing drowsy or comatose, hence controlled oxygen therapy with venture mask or nasal prongs at a rate of 1–2 L/min.

E. Control of hypercapnia:

End-stage COPD increases hypercapnia which may lead to drowsiness or coma. It usually increases at night, so it will be difficult for the patient to arouse in the morning. Drowsy state will lead to poor cough reflex which in turn leads to retention of sputum in the throat that may aspirate and imbibe infection. So, in this case, noninvasive ventilation at night using BiPAP and CPAP machine can prevent this worsening of $PaCO_2$.

F. Treatment of right heart failure:

a. Controlled oxygen therapy by noninvasive ventilation, but in case of severe hypercapnia ventilatory support may be required.
b. Restriction of salt and water
c. Aldactone at 50–100 mg/day to excrete salt and water but serum level of potassium should be checked as this drug may produce severe hyperkalemia.
d. Measures to be taken to reduce lung hyperinflation as it may help to pulmonary hypertension.
e. In patient with cor pulmonale right heart failure cannot be corrected by high dose of diuretics unless hypercapnia will be corrected to 45–55 mm Hg.
f. Prophylactic treatment of pulmonary thromboembolism
g. Treatment of complications

G. Interventional therapy in case of stable COPD:

a. Bullectomy: In patients with large one or more bullae surgical removal of bullae can relive dyspnea at rest and on effort.
b. Reduction of lung volume: In case of upper lobe emphysema surgical removal of lung volume can improve exercise tolerance and improve survival.

Indications of lung volume reduction surgery:

1. Severe emphysema restricted to upper lobe and low exercise capacity in spite of optimal medical treatment
2. Upper lobe involvement with good exercise capacity
3. Reduced exercise capacity in absence of lower lobe disease

Contraindication of lung volume reduction surgery:

1. FEV_1 is <20% predicted with either homogeneous emphysema or diffusion capacity of carbon monoxide of <20% predicted.
2. Low exercise capacity but no lower lobe disease.

c. Bronchoscopic intervention:

In patients with severe asthma, appropriate placement of valves and coils bronchoscopically can reduce end-expiratory volume and improve exercise tolerance after 6–12 months post-surgically.

d. Transplantation of lung:

Indications of transplantation:

1. BODE index ≥ 7. BODE index includes following parameters:
   - BMI
   - Degree of airflow obstruction
   - Dyspnea exercise capacity
   - FEV_1
2. $FEV_1 \geq$ 15–20% predicted
3. During last 1 year three or more severe exacerbations
4. One severe exacerbation includes hypercapnic respiratory failure
5. Moderate-to-severe pulmonary hypertension

Contraindications to lung transplantation:

1. History of malignancy in past 2 years
2. Persistence of substance addiction in last 6 months of surgery
3. Persistent hepatitis B or C or HIV infection
4. Other organ system dysfunction

Survival rate of lung transplantation:

1. 1 year survival rate is 90%
2. 2 years survival rate is 65–90%
3. 5 years survival rate is 41–50%

H. Future hope:
- **a.** Endobronchial instillation of biological sealants
- **b.** Thermal airway ablation
- **c.** Placement of airway stents
- **d.** Mepolizumab—monoclonal antibody against IL-5 which is used in eosinophilic asthma indicating the role of allergy in case of COPD.

Q19. Mechanical ventilator and its indications, advantages and complications.

DNBIII/JUN2010 (10)

What are the types of mechanical ventilators? Describe the indications and complications of mechanical ventilation.

DNBII/JUN2012 (10)

Describe the indications and complications of mechanical ventilation.

DNBIII/DEC2011 (10)

Mechanical ventilatory support.

MJPRU/2015/MDI (10)

Enumerate clinical conditions requiring mechanical ventilation. Mention the types of invasive and noninvasive ventilatory support. Discuss general considerations of management of ventilated patient.

MGR/OCT2013/MDIV (15)

Continuous positive airway pressure.

MGR/OCT2015/MDIV (7)

ANSWER

Indications of Mechanical Ventilation

A. Established acute respiratory failure:
- **a.** Primary ventilatory failure where both the lungs are normal:
  1. Poisonings depressing CNS
  2. Head injury or increased intracranial tension producing altered consciousness
  3. Neuromuscular disorders such as poliomyelitis, myasthenia gravis, and infective polyneuritis
  4. Neurotoxic snake bite
  5. Severe tetanus
- **b.** In patient with deep coma due to:
  1. Depressed respiratory center
  2. Obstructed airway by mucus plug
  3. Patchy atelectasis
  4. Worsening of hypoxia and hypercapnia
- **c.** Acute pulmonary diseases producing inability to maintain PaO_2 of >55 mm Hg
  1. Fulminant pneumonia
  2. Acute lung injury
- **d.** Acute fulminant pulmonary edema producing choking of alveoli
- **e.** Massive PE
- **f.** Acute exacerbation of COPD which is unresponsive to therapy
- **g.** Massive atelectasis
- **h.** Acute severe asthma not responsive to conventional therapy
- **i.** Severe fatigue of respiratory muscles

B. Incipient respiratory failure:
- **a.** Increased ventilatory demand which cannot be met by normal respiration as a result there will be respiratory muscle fatigue like in acute severe asthma. These patients are unable to sustain ventilatory rate to >35–40/min or minute ventilation of >10–12 L/min.
- **b.** Obese patients undergoing upper abdominal surgery because there is splinting of dome of diaphragm and at the sometime there is loss of basal lung volume.
- **c.** Progressive worsening of acute parenchymal lung disease along with progressive impairment of PFT.
- **d.** Respiratory muscle fatigue in poor risk surgical patients due to old age, chronic lung disease, and debility and electrolyte imbalance.

C. Low output states associated with:
- **a.** Cardiogenic shock
- **b.** Septic shock with multiorgan failure

D. Purposeful hyperventilation:
- **a.** In case of head injury to decrease intracranial tension
- **b.** In case of massive cerebrovascular accident to reduce cerebral edema after cardiopulmonary resuscitation

Advantages of Mechanical Ventilation

A. Major advantages of volume-targeted ventilatory support:

- **a.** It is easy application
- **b.** Provision of fixed tidal volume in the face of changes in the resistance of the airways or changes in pulmonary compliance

B. Major advantages of pressure-cycled or pressure-targeted ventilation:

- **a.** Gas is delivered at fixed preset pressure

Complications of Mechanical Ventilation

A. Alveolar hyperventilation producing $PaCO_2$ of <25 mm Hg which in turn is responsible for:

- **a.** Respiratory alkalosis
- **b.** Tetany
- **c.** Decreased cerebral blood flow
- **d.** Shifting of potassium ion from extracellular fluid to intracellular fluid causing arrhythmias
- **e.** Difficulties in weaning

B. Atelectasis:

- **a.** Segmental or lobar or massive atelectasis producing rise in static compliance and endotracheal tube may be slipped into right main bronchus thus producing collapse of part or whole left lung.
- **b.** Diffuse airspace atelectasis producing collapse of many scattered alveoli of both lungs and static tidal volume of 10 mL/kg. It is suspected when there is fall in compliance of lung and increase in alveolar-arterial oxygen gradient but normal chest X-ray.
- **c.** Different areas showing uneven compliances leading to uneven distribution of inspired gas as well as difficulty in mechanical ventilation.
- **d.** Nosocomial infection
- **e.** Auto-positive end-expiratory pressure or auto-PEEP can be characterized by unintentional PEEP occurring at the time of delivery of new inspiratory breath before the end of expiration. It occurs in:
  1. COPD where there is air trapping due to prolonged expiration through the narrowed airways
  2. Age > 60 years
  3. Use of small-sized endotracheal tube
  4. Mechanical ventilation is ≥10 L/min
  5. In case COPD increase in tidal volume
  6. Increase in compliance
  7. Increased respiratory rate leads to increased air trapping
  8. Reduced expiratory flow rate with decreased with shorter expiratory time
- **f.** Hypotension:
  1. High inflation pressure
  2. Use of PEEP
  3. In patients with overinflated lungs in patients with emphysema

  All of which reduce venous return and filling of heart leading to fall in blood pressure.
- **g.** Barotrauma, volume trauma, or biotrauma:
  - Barotrauma occurs in high inflation pressures or high tidal volume when PEEP is being used.

    It will take the form of:

    Tension pneumothorax—it can lead to cardiorespiratory failure and death

    Interstitial emphysema:

    Surgical emphysema of soft tissues in the neck

    Mediastinal emphysema:
  - Volutrauma: It will be produced by high tidal volume producing damage of alveoli.
  - Biotrauma: Overstretched alveoli along with high tidal volume produce cytokines that will injure the lung and other organs—it is known as biotrauma.
- **h.** Clashing with the machine: It occurs due to following causes:
  1. Alveolar hypoventilation
  2. Obstructed endotracheal tube or tracheostomy tube due to bronchospasm or mucus plug
  3. Atelectasis, pneumonia, and pneumothorax
  4. Shock from any cause, electrolyte imbalance, and blood loss
  5. Strong respiratory drive as a result of altered mechanics in presence of diseased lungs producing mismatch with the machine
- **i.** Gastrointestinal complications:
  1. Gastric dilatation
  2. Paralytic ileus
  3. Gastrointestinal bleeding
- **j.** Water retention producing some degree of pulmonary edema

Types of Ventilator used in Case of Intermittent Positive-pressure Ventilation

Two types of ventilators:

A. Pressure limited ventilation:

There are two types of pressure-limited ventilators:

a. Pressure support ventilation: This form is patient-triggered, pressure-limited, and flow-cycled. In this case ventilator will sense when patient starts his breath, at once the ventilator assists the patients by providing a sufficient amount of positive pressure into the airway. The level of pressure support will be reached very rapidly and that will be maintained throughout the most part of inspiration. But when the inspiratory airflow will fall below the specified level of target, i.e., 25% of PEF ventilator stops assisting patient's inspiration. But this volume of each breath will vary according to the following:

1. Patient's pattern of breathing
2. Mechanical properties of the lung
3. Preset level of inspiratory pressure support

But the disadvantage of this ventilator is when the patient stops spontaneous breathing there will be no backup from the machine side, hence this machine is used in case of conscious patients because this patient can determine the timing and depth of breathing.

b. Pressure-controlled ventilation: In this machine target level of pressure is set by the clinicians, hence initiation of breath and duration of inspiration and expiration are set in the ventilator by the clinicians. But change in airway resistance of change in lung compliance of the patient can alter the volume of the gas when the specified target will be reached. It is used primary in case of ARDS where there is problem with oxygenation due to decreased lung compliance.

B. Volume-cycle ventilation:

a. Volume-cycled ventilation: In this mode, a constant volume of air will be given during inspiration by the machine followed by passive expiration is allowed. Here constant tidal volume is provided. The advantage of this mode is the pressure required to deliver the targeted amount of air will vary according to changes in the compliance of lung and airway resistance in the lung. But in case of conscious patient this mode is uncomfortable because it dictates the patient to initiate the inspiration. Hence, it is mostly used in comatose and anesthetized patient because this patient cannot initiate the inspiration by his own.

b. Assist-control ventilation: In this mode ventilator will be sensed when the patient initiates inspiration, then the ventilator will deliver a specified volume of air as already set by the machine. So, respiratory rate will be determined by the patient but tidal volume is by the machine. So, if the respiratory rate falls below a specified level, then this machine will take the backup and deliver a minimal number of breaths. As for example, the respiratory rate is set up in the machine as 12 breaths/min, now if the patient's breath falls below that specified rate and 5 seconds is lapsed from the patient's previous breath, then machine will start automatically.

c. Intermittent mandatory ventilation: In this mode the machine will deliver already specified number of breaths per minute and specified amount of tidal volume of air containing inspired oxygen, but in between the breaths delivered by the machine the patient starts breathing spontaneously from oxygen source. Since the patient's breath is not controlled by machine hence tidal volume will be determined by the patient.

d. Synchronized intermittent mandatory ventilation: In this mode machine-delivered breaths coincide with and assist with the patient's own breath. Hence, this mode allows the patient's respiratory muscles to exercise between the assisted breaths and useful for preparing the patient for weaning. But tachypneic patient tries to exhale during ventilator-assisted breath in inspiratory cycle, so airway pressure exceeds the inspiratory pressure limit and thus ventilator-assisted breath will be aborted which lead to drop in minute volume below the level already set by the operator.

Basic Initial Ventilator Set Up

A. Tidal volume: It is set up in between 5 and 10 mL/kg of body weight. Its selection is governed by:

a. Nature of the disease
b. Appropriate minute ventilation equipment
c. Pulmonary compliance
d. Airway resistance
e. Airway pressure

f. PaO_2
g. $PaCO_2$

Low tidal volume results:

a. Hypoxemia
b. Atelectasis
c. Hypoventilation

High tidal volume results:

a. Respiratory alkalosis
b. Reduced venous return leading to decreased cardiac output
c. Barotrauma, volutrauma, and biotrauma

In case of normal lung in case of neuromuscular disease, coma, poisoning, and CNS disease tidal volume is set at 10 mL/kg

In case of stiff lung in ARDS, tidal volume to start with will be at 10 mL/kg followed by reduction to 5–7 mL/kg.

B. Respiratory rate: It is generally set at 10–14 breaths/min.

In case of stiff lung, it will be 20–25 breaths/min and lower rate is found in case of COPD. High respiratory rate can lead to:

a. Respiratory alkalosis
b. Auto-PEEP
c. Barotrauma

Low respiratory rate will lead to:

a. Hypoxemia
b. Hypoventilation

C. Minute ventilation: It is set at 5–10 mL/min and is controlled by:

a. Respiratory mechanics
b. Nature of the disease

D. Inspiration:expiration ratio: It is set at 1:3 to provide sufficient time for expiration.

E. Oxygen concentration: FiO_2 is to start with 1.0, but after 15–20 minutes it will be reduced in such a way that PaO_2 can be maintained at ≥60 mm Hg and SpO_2 will be ≥90%.

F. Inspiratory flow rate: It is set at 40–60 mL/min in case of volume-targeted ventilation, but in case of high inspiratory demand it can be increased to 60–100 mL/min.

Q20. ABG in respiratory diseases

MGR/APR2014/MDI (5)

Arterial blood gas analysis.

MGR UNIVERSITY, TAMIL NADU, 2020 (10)

ANSWER

Arterial blood gas is a common diagnostic tool for the evaluation of partial pressure of the gases and acid-base content. Analysis of blood can be done from the blood obtained from the artery, vein or capillary, but ABGs can assess properly PaO_2 and carbon dioxide.

Components of the ABG

A. pH: It measures the acid-base balance in the blood (normal is 7.35–7.45)

B. PaO_2: It is the PaO_2 in the arterial blood (normal is 75–100 mm Hg)

C. $PaCO_2$: It is the partial pressure of carbon dioxide in the blood (normal is 35–45 mm Hg)

D. HCO_3: It is the calculated concentration of bicarbonate in the blood (normal is 22–26 mEq/L)

E. Base excess/deficit: It is the calculated base excess or deficit in the arterial blood (normal is –4 to +2)

F. SaO_2: It is the calculated arterial SaO_2 (95–100%)

There are six steps for analysis of ABGs:

A. In the first step: pH has to be measured to detect any acid base imbalance.

a. If pH is >7.45, it indicates:
   1. Primary metabolic alkalosis
   2. Primary respiratory alkalosis
   3. Both respiratory and metabolic alkalosis

b. If pH is <7.35, it indicates:
   1. Primary metabolic acidosis
   2. Primary respiratory acidosis
   3. Both respiratory and metabolic acidosis

c. If pH is within normal range, it indicates:
   1. Normal acid-base status
   2. Mixed disturbances but balanced

B. Second step is to look for arterial PCO_2:

a. If PCO_2 is >45 mm Hg, it indicates respiratory acidosis.
b. If PCO_2 is <35 mm Hg, it indicates respiratory alkalosis.

C. In the third step, it has to be determined that whether change is respiratory or metabolic. So relation between direction of change of pH and PCO_2 has to be solved in the following manner:

Respiratory acidosis	pH low	PCO_2 high
Metabolic acidosis	pH low	PCO_2 low
Respiratory alkalosis	pH high	PCO_2 low
Metabolic alkalosis	pH High	PCO_2 high

D. In the fourth step, it is to be ascertained that whether there is appropriate compensation for primary disturbance.

Primary disturbance	Compensatory response	Expected magnitude of response
Metabolic acidosis	Low PCO_2	$PCO_2 - 1.5 \times (HCO_3^-) + 8 \pm 2$
Metabolic alkalosis	High PCO_2	PCO_2 increases 6 mm Hg for each 10 mEq/L increase in HCO_3^-
Acute respiratory acidosis	Increased HCO_3^-	HCO_3^- increases 1 mEq/L for each 10 mm Hg increase in PCO_2
Chronic respiratory acidosis (3–5 days)		HCO_3^- increases 3.5 mEq/L for each 10 mm Hg increase in PCO_2
Acute respiratory alkalosis	Decreased HCO_3^-	HCO_3^- decreases by 2 mEq/L for each 10 mm Hg decrease in PCO_2
Chronic respiratory alkalosis	Decreased HCO_3^-	HCO_3^- decreases by 5 mEq/L for each 10 mm Hg decrease in PCO_2

E. In the fifth step there is calculation of anion gap: It can be measured by following equation:

Anion gap = [Na+] – {[Cl-] + [HCO_3^-]} -12 ± 2.

Normal anion gap is 12 mEq/L. In case of hypoalbuminemia normal anion gap will be 2.5 mEq/L lower for each 1 g/dL decrease in serum albumin.

F. In the sixth step, if there is increased anion gap then the ratio of change in anion gap to change in HCO_3^- has to be ascertained.

a. If the ration is between 1 and 2, it indicates uncomplicated metabolic acidosis.

b. If the ratio falls outside this range, it indicates another metabolic disorder is present.

1. If the ratio is <1, it indicates presence of concurrent nonanion gap metabolic acidosis.
2. If the ratio is >2, it indicates the presence of concurrent metabolic alkalosis.

Q21. Development of lung.
MGR/OCT2013/MDI (5)

ANSWER

Stages of Development of Lung

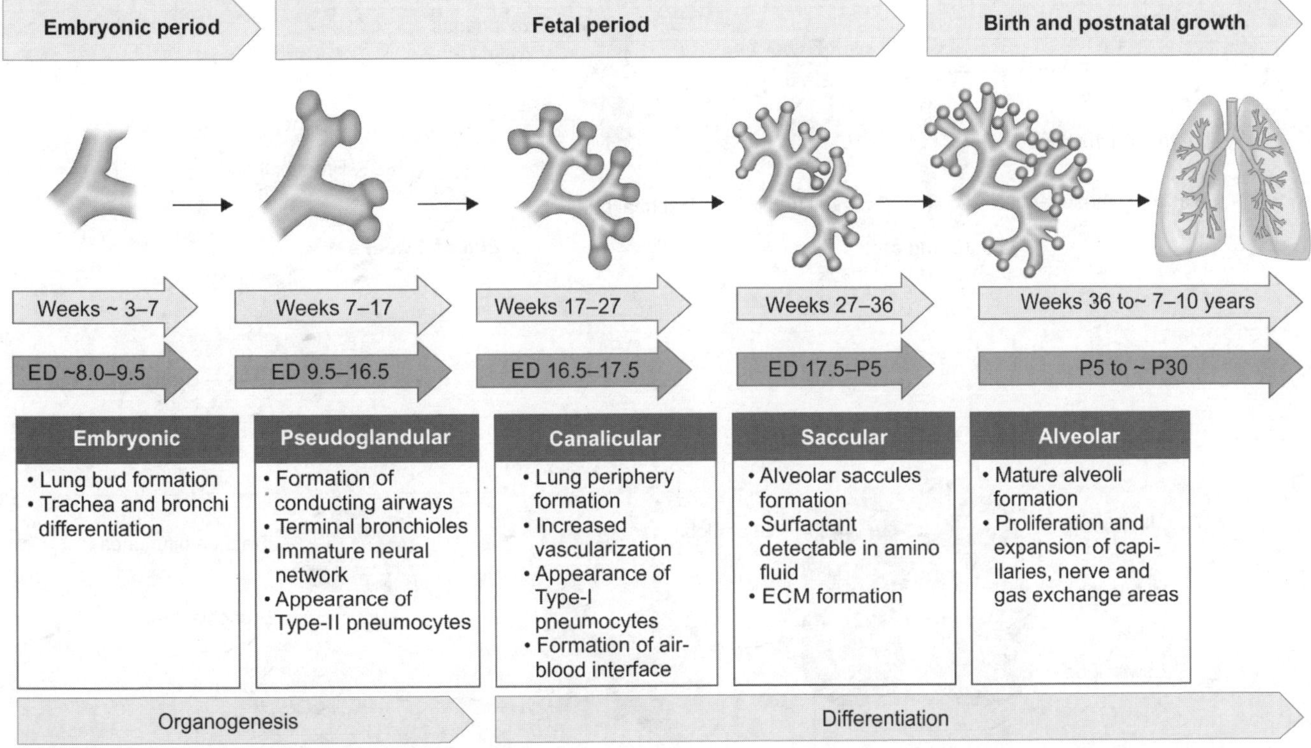

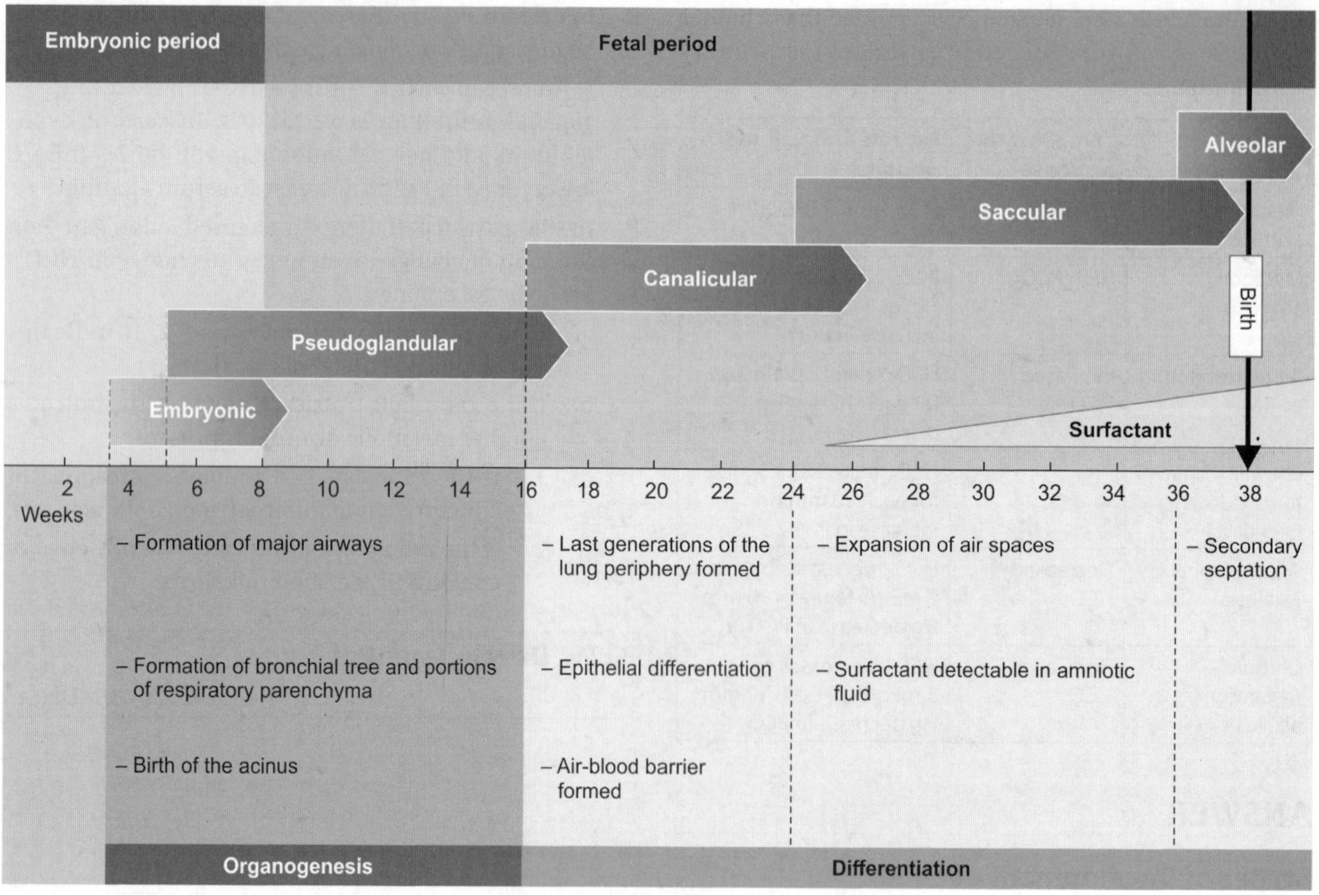

Embryonic period
Fetal period
Alveolar
Saccular
Canalicular
Birth
Pseudoglandular
Embryonic
Surfactant
2
4
6
8
10
12
14
16
18
20
22
24
26
28
30
32
34
36
38
Weeks
– Formation of major airways
– Formation of bronchial tree and portions of respiratory parenchyma
– Birth of the acinus
– Last generations of the lung periphery formed
– Epithelial differentiation
– Air-blood barrier formed
– Expansion of air spaces
– Surfactant detectable in amniotic fluid
– Secondary septation
Organogenesis
Differentiation

Pharynx
Laryngotracheal tube
Splanchnic mesoderm
Beginning of 4th week
Tracheal buds
Esophagus
Trachea
Tracheal buds
Trachea
Bronchial bud
End of 4 weeks
Bronchial buds
Trachea bifurcates
Bronchial buds
Bronchial buds develop
Upper lobe
Middle lobe
Lower lobe
Upper lobe
Lower lobe
8 weeks

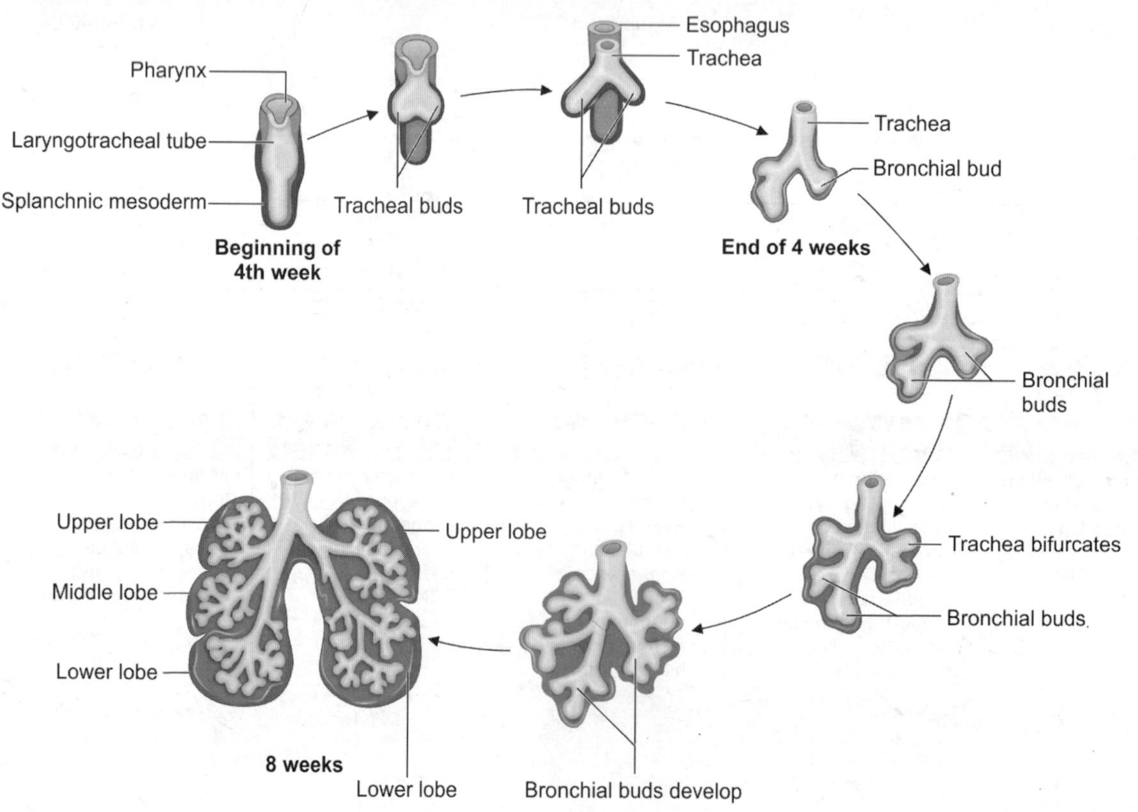

Q22. Describe the lung problem in environmental disorders.

DNB/DEC2014 (10)

ANSWER

Introduction

Environmental and occupational lung diseases are very difficult to distinguish; again in some cases both will interact together such as smoking and genetic factors to produce lung disease. Again, for the management of the patients, environmental or occupational etiologies are essential, such as in case of HP and occupational asthma, triggering environmental agents are required as their avoidance can give relief to the patients from those diseases.

History and Assessment of Exposure

Most important is the patient's history as it will reveal the etiology.

A. Enquiry about the specific work practices like
   - **a.** Presence of visible dust
   - **b.** Chemical odors
   - **c.** Specific contaminants involved
   - **d.** Use of respiratory protective equipment
   - **e.** Size of the work spaces
   - **f.** Presence or absence of ventilation at work spaces
   - **g.** Alternate source of exposure to toxic agents
      1. Hobbies
      2. Characteristic of houses
      3. Exposure to secondary smoke
      4. Proximity to industrial areas

Short-term as well as long-term exposure to potentially toxic agents recently or distant past is also considered.

Occupational exposure	Nature of respiratory diseases	Investigations
Inorganic dusts		
Asbestos required in mining, repair of ship, construction	Fibrosis (asbestosis) Pleural disease Cancer Pleural mesothelioma	Chest X-ray shows irregular or linear opacities in lower lung. Ground-glass appearances in the lung parenchyma HRCT shows subpleural curvilinear lines of 5–10 mm in length parallel to pleural surface PFT: Restrictive pattern of lung disease. Decreased static lung volume, low diffusion capacity, and mild obstruction to airflow in case of peribronchiolar fibrosis
Silica used in mining, stone cutting, quarrying and sandblasting	Fibrosis (silicosis) Progressive massive fibrosis Tuberculosis Chronic obstructive lung disease Lung cancer	Chest X-ray shows intense miliary infiltration and consolidation. HRCT shows crazy paving pattern In long-term cases chest X-ray shows small round opacities in upper lobes which in absence of further exposure coalesces to form nonsegmental conglomerates of irregular masses of >1 cm in diameter (complicated silicosis) which ultimately progresses to progressive massive fibrosis Calcification in hilar nodes showing "egg-shell" appearances
Coal exposure in mining	Coal worker's pneumoconiosis Progressive massive fibrosis Chronic obstructive lung disease	Chest X-ray shows small-rounded opacities not associated with impairment in PFT In complicated case, nodules are >1 cm in diameter in upper lobe of lung
Beryllium used in processing of alloys	Chronic granulomatous disease Lung cancer Acute pneumonitis (rare)	Chest X-ray shows nodular and septal opacities PFT shows restrictive or obstructive ventilatory defect and decreased diffusion capacity Assay for specific cell-mediated immune response like lymphocyte proliferation testing in nuclear workers, tuberculin testing in healthcare persons
Aluminum, cobalt, titanium, nickel, tungsten carbide	Wide spectrum from acute pneumonitis to lung cancer Giant interstitial pneumonitis	

Continued

Continued

Occupational exposure	Nature of respiratory diseases	Investigations
	Organic dust	
Cotton dust used in milling, processing	Byssinosis producing asthma-like syndrome Chronic bronchitis Chronic obstructive lung disease	PFT shows significant drop in FEV_1 over the course of work shift on Monday In case of long-standing exposure, PFT demonstrates obstructive pattern of lung disease
Grain dust used in dock workers, milling and bakers	Chronic obstructive lung disease Chronic bronchitis Asthma	PFT shows reduced FEV_1, FEV_1/FVC ratio
Other agricultural dust like vegetable products, fungal spores, animal dander, bird's feces, animal feces	Hypersensitivity pneumonitis like farmer's lung Bronchial asthma Chronic bronchitis	PFT shows reduced FEV_1, FEV_1/FVC ratio Specific IgG precipitating antibody titer for agent responsible for developing hypersensitivity pneumonitis (pigeon antigen)
Toxic chemicals	Bronchial asthma Chronic obstructive lung disease Chronic bronchitis Pneumoconiosis Lung cancer Hypersensitivity pneumonitis	
	Environmental agents	
Uranium, radon, secondhand tobacco, tobacco smoke, biomass, polycyclic aromatic hydrocarbons, welding fumes, wood finishing	10% cases of lung cancer Chronic bronchitis Bronchial asthma Lung fibrosis	

For rating respiratory impairment following tests are performed:

A. PFT for static lung volume and diffusion capacity

B. Cardiopulmonary testing for assessing maximal consumption of oxygen

C. Methacholine challenge test for assessing airway hyper-reactivity in case of normal spirometry

General Environmental Exposure

Outdoor Air Pollution

Standard of each toxic outdoor pollutant is regularly updated by Environmental Protection Agency (EPA) in the following website: http://www.epa.gov/criteria-air-pollutants/naaqs-table%20

Two types of outdoor environmental pollutants:

A. Stationary sources: Power plants and industrial complexes

B. Mobile sources like motor vehicles

Some pollutants may be changed after chemical reactions like:

A. Sulfur dioxide and other particulate matter emitted from coal-fired power plant will react with air to produce acid sulfates and aerosols which transport for long distance in atmosphere.

B. Nitrogen oxides and other volatile compounds, the product of automobile exhaust, will form ozone after reacting with sunlight.

Symptoms are breathlessness, cough, production of sputum, and chest pain. In case of long-standing exposure, the symptoms will exacerbate. High level of exposure is associated with increased mortality and morbidity. Fine particulate matter is responsible for cardiovascular morbidity and mortality. These particles generate oxidative stress leading to injury and inflammation in the lung parenchyma and bronchial wall generating autonomic and systemic inflammatory response and this will induce endothelial cell dysfunction.

Increased traffic congestion involving motor vehicles in absence of pollution control will lead to high level of outdoor pollution.

Indoor Exposure

These are secondhand tobacco smoke, wood smoke, radon gas, and biological mass. Children of smoker parents may suffer from bronchial asthma, chronic bronchitis, and reduced level of pulmonary functions measured from spirometry from childhood.

A. Radon gas is a risk factor for lung cancer, because the active ingredient of radon, radon-222, and immediate precursor radium-226 originating from decay of uranium-238 are responsible for this. Amount of radon gas origination depends upon the amount of radium present in the earth. If smokers are present in home, the radon particles will be attached with the smoke particles, hence the problem is potentially greater.

B. Bioaerosols containing antigenic material of fungi, dust mites, dander of pets, and cockroaches are potential risk factors for developing asthma.

C. Indoor chemical agents such as formaldehyde, perfumes, pesticides, and nitrogen oxides are responsible for "tight building syndrome" or "building-associated illness"; here small particulate matters are responsible for respiratory illness which can be relieved by avoidance of exposure.

D. Household air pollutions such as crop residues and charcoal are responsible for more than 4% of disability in the form of bronchial asthma, lung cancer in women, and lower respiratory tract infection in children and cardiovascular diseases in men.

E. Kerosene is used as fuel during cooking mainly in rural areas of developing countries inside the home having poor ventilation. As a result, the women and children are constantly exposed to high level of smokes which may lead to different types of pulmonary diseases.

Household air pollutant is also responsible for outdoor pollution.

Q23. Describe etiology, clinical features, and management of HP.

DNBIIIB/DEC2013 (10)

ANSWER

Definition

Hypersensitivity pneumonitis is a group of immunologically-mediated disorders characterized by inflammatory response to alveoli, bronchiole, and interstitium due to repeated triggering by antigen containing organic dust.

Etiology

Agents	Exposure	Antigens
Plant proteins		
Farmer's lung	Moldy hay	*Thermoactinomyces vulgaris* *Saccharopolyspora rectivirgula*
Baggasosis	Moldy pressed sugarcane	*Thermoactinomyces vulgaris* *Thermoactinomyces sacchari*
Malt worker's lung	Contaminated barley	*Aspergillus clavatus*
Mushroom worker's lung	Moldy compost and mushroom	*Saccharomyces rectivirgula* *Thermoactinomyces vulgaris*
Compost lung	Compost	*Thermoactinomyces vulgaris* *Aspergillus* species
Wood pulp worker's lung	Contaminated wood pulp or dust	*Alternaria* species
Tobacco worker's lung	Mold on tobacco	*Aspergillus* species
Summer type hypersensitivity pneumonitis in Japan	Contaminated house furnishings	*Trichosporon cutaneum*
Animal proteins		
Bird-fancier's disease	Pigeons, parrots, chicken, geese, and ducks	Avian droppings, feathers, and serum. Antigens are glycoprotein with IgA activity
Insect proteins		
Miller's lung	Contaminated grain	*Sitophilus granarius*
Chemical		
Chemical worker's lung	Spray paint, glues, and polyurethanes	Diisocyanate and trimellitic anhydride
Epoxy resin lung	Heated epoxy resin	Phthalic anhydride
Thatched roof lung	Dried leaves and grasses	
Air conditioner lung	Contaminated air conditioner	
Others		
Coffee worker's lung	Coffee bean dust	

Pathophysiology

A. Genetic susceptibility:

a. Major histocompatibility complex (MHC) is responsible for immunologic mechanism for HP. DR and DQ of Class II MHC are associated with increased risk of developing HP.

b. Patients with polymorphism of transporter-associated antigen processing genes may also be susceptible to HP.

c. Promoter variants in tissue inhibitor of metalloproteinase-3 (TMP) may possess protective effect in an unknown mechanism.

B. Though many patients may precipitate HP following viral infection, pesticides exposure has been considered as an important risk factor.

C. Paradoxical effect of smoking: Usually HP is less frequent in smokers as compared to nonsmoker because smoker will produce low level of specific antigen during their exposure to environmental antigen. But if HP develops, it will produce chronic course with recurrent exacerbations and poor survival.

D. Tolerance to specific factor: Few people will develop mild lymphocytic alveolitis or will be asymptomatic when exposed to environmental antigen and ultimately become tolerant to that antigen and it is mediated by specific subsets of CD4+ T lymphocytes which is responsible for maintaining balance between tissue damage and tissue protection effect of immune response.

E. Immunopathology: HP develops in patients in response to inhaled antigen through the development of following types of response:

a. Type III immunologic response: It is characterized by formation of antigen-antibody complexes triggered by complement system as evidenced by increased level C1q, C3, and C5a in the BAL fluid, increased blood level of IgG mostly, and also IgM and IgA. These antigen-antibody complexes release proinflammatory cytokines such as ILs and TNF-α leading to inflammatory changes in the lung. It is responsible for acute form of HP.

b. Type IV immunological response: It is characterized by release of neutrophils initially followed by release of activated lymphocytes, CD8 lymphocytes and thus ratio of CD4:CD8 will be reduced. Histologically it will form granuloma. In case of subacute or chronic form of HP, antigen reacts with CD4+ cells to release various effector subsets of which granuloma formation requires different mediators Th1 like cytokines, TNF-α, interferon-α, and toll-like receptor-9-mediated dendritic cell response.

c. In genetically predisposed patients repeated antigenic exposure ultimately activates proliferation of fibroblast leading to pulmonary fibrosis.

d. Nonantigenic factors such as organic dusts, mycotoxins, endotoxins, and histamine-releasing substances directly activate alveolar cells.

e. Some proteins having immunogenic adjuvants activate macrophages and complement system leading to HP.

Histopathology

Main histopathological features are:

A. Presence of poorly defined small scattered granuloma

B. Presence of mononuclear and lymphocytic infiltrate in the alveoli and interstitial tissue

C. Inflammation of bronchioles

D. Presence of granuloma. Within the granuloma presence of intense expression of cathepsin K in the epithelioid cells and macrophages.

E. In case of chronic HP evidence of architectural distortion with presence of fibrosis involving upper lobes

Above features are uniformly distributed all over the lung but discordant findings may be observed.

Clinical Features

A. Acute HP will develop within 4–12 hours of exposure, peak within 6–24 hours, and subside within 2–4 days without treatment after cessation of exposure and the features are characterized by:

a. Constitutional symptoms such as fever, chills, myalgia, and prostrations

b. Respiratory features such as cough, breathlessness, and chest discomfort. Physical findings are tachypnea, cyanosis, tachycardia, and basal crackles

c. There may be wheezing due to bronchial hyperresponsiveness and normal chest X-ray

B. In subacute and chronic form there may not be any relation between antigenic exposure and clinical presentation. The features are:

a. Dyspnea

b. Cough which will be increased progressively with or without expectoration

c. Easy fatigability
d. Malaise
e. Digital clubbing
f. In case of chronic progressive pulmonary fibrosis there may be chronic hypoxemic respiratory failure and cor pulmonale.

Investigations

A. Chest X-ray:
 a. Normal chest X-ray cannot exclude HP
 b. Diffuse ground-glass shadow and reticulonodular infiltrate
 c. In case of chronic HP:
  1. Bilateral upper lobe fibrosis
  2. Upward retraction of hila
  3. Loss of lung volume in the upper and middle lobes of the lung
  4. Reticulonodular opacities

B. High-resolution computerized tomography:
 a. Centrilobular nodules of 2–4 mm in diameter are distributed in the middle and lower lobes closely related to bronchioles.
 b. Ground-glass opacities indicate alveolitis due to ongoing antigenic exposure.
 c. Consolidation may be observed rarely which will resolve spontaneously.
 d. Expiratory air trapping: It will produce mosaic appearances of the involved lung field. The affected areas look like dark and lucent as compared to the surrounding areas.
 e. Fibrosis: In case of chronic form it is characterized by loss of lung volume, traction bronchiectasis, and linear reticular opacities all leading to honeycombing affecting upper and middle lobes.
 f. Emphysema: In farmer's, lung emphysema is predominant than fibrosis, involves upper lobes more due to bronchiolitis-induced obstruction of distal airways.

C. Bronchoalveolar lavage studies: It will demonstrate marked increase in T lymphocytes with CD8 predominance which is unusual in nonspecific interstitial pneumonia, usual interstitial pneumonia, and sarcoidosis.

Diagnostic criteria as proposed by hypersensitivity pneumonitis study group are as follows:

A. Exposure to already known antigen
B. Recurrent respiratory symptoms
C. Precipitin antibodies
D. Inspiratory crackles
E. Symptoms will start within 4–8 hours of antigenic exposure
F. Loss of weight

Management

A. Mainstay of the treatment is the avoidance of exposure like
 a. Use of dust mask with filters, adequately improved storage facilities and mechanization of farming processes
 b. Avoidance of pigeon dust and droppings
 c. Removal of pet birds from the home is of immense importance

B. Corticosteroids:
 a. Though acute episode sometimes resolves spontaneously without treatment but corticosteroid can be given as a short course and it can show significant improvement in the physiological parameters, mainly diffusion capacity within 2 months.
 b. In subacute case, prednisolone can be administered at a dose of 0.5 mg/kg over 3–4 weeks followed by gradual tapering of the dose and it should be stopped after 4–6 months.
 c. In case of progressive and chronic disease, same dose of steroid has to be started followed by gradual tapering over 4–6 months till 10 mg/day maintenance dose will be reached. In few cases there may be relapse after withdrawal of the drug if the antigenic nature is completely unknown.

C. In case of chronic progressive cases cyclophosphamide or azathioprine can be added to steroid.

Q24. Define noninvasive ventilation. Mention indications and contraindications for its use. What are the advantages and disadvantages?

DNBIIIB/DEC2013 (10)

Noninvasive ventilation.

DNB, 2020 (5)

Noninvasive ventilation uses in pulmonary diseases.

KERALA UNI, 2022 (10)

Noninvasive ventilation in acute and chronic respiratory failure.

NTR UNI OF HEALTH SC, VIJAYAWADA, ANDHRA, 2022 (10)

Noninvasive ventilation.

NTR UNI OF HEALTH SC, VIJAYAWADA, ANDHRA, 2021 (10)

Noninvasive ventilation.

WBUHS, 2020 (10)

ANSWER

Definition

Noninvasive ventilation can be defined as delivery of mechanical ventilation to the lungs by technique that does not require any invasive process.

The goals of noninvasive intubation:

A. Overcome auto-PEEP
B. Giving rest to respiratory muscles
C. Provide relief from respiratory distress
D. Avoidance of endotracheal intubation
E. Avoidance of complications
F. Provision of respiratory failure to be resolved and improvement of gas exchange

Types of noninvasive ventilation:

A. Negative-pressure ventilation:
- **a.** It is the main process of noninvasive ventilation during early 1900s.
- **b.** It was extensively used during polio epidemics.
- **c.** "Iron lung", i.e., tank ventilator was used at that time.

It applies negative pressure uniformly around the patient's body resulting drop of pressure around the thorax. This negative pressure will be transmitted into the pleural space and alveoli, as result a pressure gradient will be developed between the lungs and the mouth cavity. So the gas will flow inward into the lung. In this process head of the patient is exposed into the room.

It works in the following way:
- **a.** It will prevent the respiratory muscle to work and prevent muscle fatigue.
- **b.** It will augment tidal volume.
- **c.** It will overcome intrinsic PEEP.
- **d.** It will reduce the afterload thus enhancing the cardiac function.
- **e.** It will revise microatelectasis and thus improve the lung compliance.
- **f.** It will reduce the production of carbon dioxide.
- **g.** It will stent the airway.

In case of hypoxemic respiratory failure:
- **a.** It will increase the FiO_2
- **b.** PEEP—it will perform:
  1. Increment V/Q relationship
  2. Decrease in the shunt
  3. Increase in FRC
  4. Recruitment of alveoli
  5. Decrease in work in breathing as well as respiratory rate

In case of hypercapnic respiratory failure:
1. It will reduce the airway resistance.
2. It will improve ventilation and $PaCO_2$.
3. It will off-set auto-PEEP.

Advantages of noninvasive ventilation:
- **a.** It is noninvasive so it will reduce the need for nasogastric tube.
- **b.** It will improve lung mechanics.
- **c.** It will reduce resistive work that will be imposed by invasive ventilation.
- **d.** Ventilation is done with low pressure.
- **e.** It will correct the gas exchange.
- **f.** It will correct mental status.
- **g.** It can be applied intermittently.
- **h.** It can be terminated any time.
- **i.** This procedure need not require any sedation.
- **j.** It will obviously avoid complications of invasive ventilation like gastrointestinal bleeding, deep venous thrombosis, respiratory infection, and sepsis.
- **k.** It will avoid the complications of endotracheal intubation like trauma during the process and aspiration of nasopharyngeal contents.
- **l.** It will decrease mortality related to respiratory failure.

Disadvantages of noninvasive ventilation:
- **a.** System:
  1. Slow correction of abnormalities in gaseous exchange
  2. Time commitment
  3. It will produce gastric distension
- **b.** Interface between instrument and lung:
  1. Necrosis of the skin
  2. Skin rash
  3. Leak
  4. Irritation of eye and ear
  5. Pressure in the sinus

- **c.** Airway:
  - **1.** Aspiration in the lung
  - **2.** Limitation in respiratory clearance

Contraindications of noninvasive ventilation:

- **a.** Cardiopulmonary arrest
- **b.** Inability to protect airway from secretions
- **c.** Hemodynamic instability
- **d.** Mental changes such as seizures and encephalopathy
- **e.** Multiorgan failure
- **f.** Facial deformity
- **g.** Gastrointestinal bleeding
- **h.** Intractable vomiting
- **i.** Tumor in the head and neck or extrinsic compression of the airway
- **j.** History of recent neurosurgery
- **k.** Untreated pneumothorax

Following patients are selected for noninvasive ventilation:

- **a.** Chronic obstructive lung disease with respiratory failure
- **b.** Asthma
- **c.** OSA syndrome
- **d.** ARDS
- **e.** Cor pulmonale
- **f.** Restrictive lung disease
- **g.** Neuromuscular disease
- **h.** Postextubated patients

Procedure for noninvasive ventilation:

- **A.** Step 1: Firstly one has to diagnose the cause of respiratory failure and whether it is correctable by noninvasive ventilation or not.
- **B.** Step 2: Clinical presentation and ABG analysis
- **C.** Step 3: Exclusion of the situations where this ventilation is unsafe.
- **D.** Successful application:
  - **a.** Choice of ventilator and interface
  - **b.** Choice of settings
  - **c.** Reassess the patient and readjust the machine
  - **d.** Assessment of success, failure, and weaning from ventilation

Modes of ventilation:

- **a.** CPAP
- **b.** BiPAP, i.e., noninvasive ventilation with pressure support ventilation
- **c.** Average volume assured pressure support
- **d.** Adaptive servo ventilation
- **e.** High flow nasal cannula

Q25. Describe various ventilatory functions. Discuss flow-volume curves in obstructive and restrictive lung disease.

DNBIVA/DEC2013 (10)

Describe PFT and their interpretation in relation to various pulmonary diseases.

DNBIV/JUN2010 (10)

Interpretation of lung function tests.

MGR/APR2013/MDI (5)

PFTs.

MGR/MAR2008/MDI (4)
MUHS/MAY2010/MDI (10)
KUHS/MAY2014/MDI (10)

Compare and contrast the spirometry in obstructive versus restrictive lung disease.

BF/MAY2013/MDIII (10)

Respiratory function tests and their relevance.

PGI/APR2014/MDI (10)

Describe the functional anatomy of lungs. Discuss various lung function tests.

MUHS/NOV2014/MDI (25)

Describe various ventilatory functions. What are the normal flow-volume curve and how to differentiate between obstructive and restrictive lung disease?

DNBIII DEC2010 (10)

How would you differentiate obstructive and restrictive lung disease? Give an account of management of ILD.

MJPRU/2016/MDII (25)

Pulmonary function test.

MGR UNI, TAMIL NADU, 2022 (5)

Describe various pulmonary function tests in health and disease.

MAHARASHTRA UNI OF HEALTH SC, VIJAYAWADA, 2022 (25)

Describe noninvasive procedures in respiratory diseases.

MAHARASHTRA UNI OF HEALTH SC, VIJAYAWADA, 2022 (10)

How will you diagnose common respiratory abnormalities using different parameters in a lung function test.

WBUHS, 2021 (10)

Pulmonary function test in health and disease.

SAURASHTRA UNIVERSITY, RAJKOT, 2020 (20)

Pulmonary function test.

NTR UNI OF HEALTH SC, VIJAYAWADA, SEPTEM, ANDHRA, 2020 (10)

NTR UNI OF HEALTH SC, VIJAYAWADA, SEPTEM, ANDHRA, 2020 (10)

ANSWER

Introduction

Pulmonary function test is a most important and valuable investigation for managing a patient with suspected or previously diagnosed pulmonary disease as they monitor the treatment response and further investigation, if required.

Indications of Pulmonary Function Tests

A. For evaluation of clinical or radiological features relating to respiratory diseases:
   - **a.** Cough
   - **b.** Wheeze
   - **c.** Breathlessness
   - **d.** Crackles
   - **e.** Abnormal chest X-ray

B. Monitoring the patients with already existing respiratory diseases for response to treatment or progression of the disease:
   - **a.** Bronchial asthma
   - **b.** COPD
   - **c.** Interstitial pulmonary fibrosis
   - **d.** Pulmonary vascular disease

C. In patient with systemic diseases having respiratory complications:
   - **a.** Neuromuscular diseases
   - **b.** Connective tissue disorders

D. Evaluation of patients prior to following operations:
   - **a.** Cardiothoracic surgery
   - **b.** Abdominal surgery
   - **c.** Resection of lung

E. Surveillance following transplantation of lung for:
   - **a.** Infection
   - **b.** Obliterative bronchiolitis
   - **c.** Acute rejection

F. Evaluation for risk factors leading to lung diseases:
   - **a.** Occupational exposure
   - **b.** Environmental exposure
   - **c.** Radiations
   - **d.** Toxins
   - **e.** Medications

Contraindications of Pulmonary Function Tests

A. Myocardial infarction occurred in last month
B. Thoracic or abdominal aneurysm
C. Recent pneumothorax
D. Recent eye surgery
E. Unstable angina
F. Recent thoracoabdominal surgery

Categorization of Pulmonary Function Test

Mechanical Ventilatory Function of Lung or Chest Wall

A. Bedside PFT
   - **a.** Sabrasez breath holding test: The patient is asked to take full but not too deep breath and then hold it as long as possible.
     1. More than 25 seconds—normal cardiopulmonary reserve
     2. 15–25 seconds—limited cardiopulmonary reserve
     3. Less than 15 seconds—very poor cardiopulmonary reserve

     25–30 seconds: 3,500 mL VC
     20–25 seconds: 3,000 mL VC
     15–20 seconds: 2,500 mL VC
     10–15 seconds: 2,000 mL VC
     5–10 seconds: 1,500 mL VC

b. Schneider's match blowing test: It will measure maximum breathing capacity. Here the patient is asked to blow the matchsticks kept at 15 cm distance in the same level with mouth opened, head static and chin supported. During the time there will be no air movement in the room.
   1. Patient cannot blow the match:
      - Maximum breathing capacity is <60 L/min
      - FEV_1 < 1.6 L/min
   2. Patient is able to blow out the match:
      - Maximum breathing capacity is >60 L/min
      - FEV_1 > 1.6 L/min

c. Cough test: Patient is asked to take deep breath followed by cough. Following is noticed:
   1. Strength of cough
   2. Ability to cough
   3. Effectiveness of cough

   Cough is inadequate if:
   1. FVC is <20 mL/kg
   2. FEV_1 is <15 mL/kg
   3. PEF rate < 200 mL/min

d. Forced expiratory time

e. De-Bono whistle blowing test

B. Static lung volume

a. Tidal volume: This is the amount (500 mL) of air entering the nose or mouth in each breath.

b. Expiratory reserve volume (ERV): This is the amount of air (1.5 L) that can be exhaled during maximum forced expiration that starts at the end of tidal expiration.

c. Inspiratory reserve volume (IRV): This is the amount of air (2.5 L) that can be inhaled during maximum forced expiration that starts at the end of tidal inspiration.

d. VC: This is the volume of air (4.5 L) that can be exhaled during maximum forced expiration after taking maximum forced inspiration. It is the summation of tidal volume plus IRV plus ERV.

e. IC: This is the amount of air (3 L) that can be inhaled with maximum effort after tidal expiration. It is tidal volume plus IRV.

f. RV: This is the amount of air (1.5 L) that will remain after forced expiration.

g. FRC: This is the amount of air (3 L) that will be present in the lung at the end of tidal expiration. It is ERV plus RV. Functions of FRC:
   1. Partial inflation of lung is helpful for preventing atelectasis.
   2. It will minimize the work of breathing.
   3. It buffers for maintaining the steady arterial PO_2.
   4. It will store oxygen.

h. TLC: This is the amount of air (5–6 L) that is inhaled after maximal inspiratory effort. It is RV plus ERV plus tidal volume plus IRV.

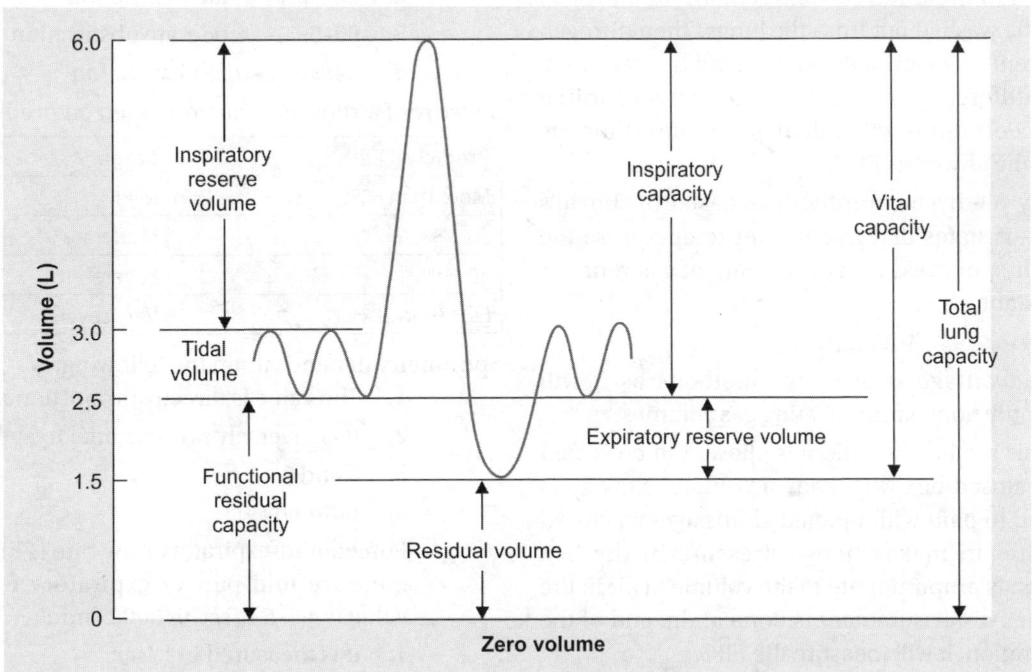

In case of restrictive and obstructive lung diseases following will be volume of lung:

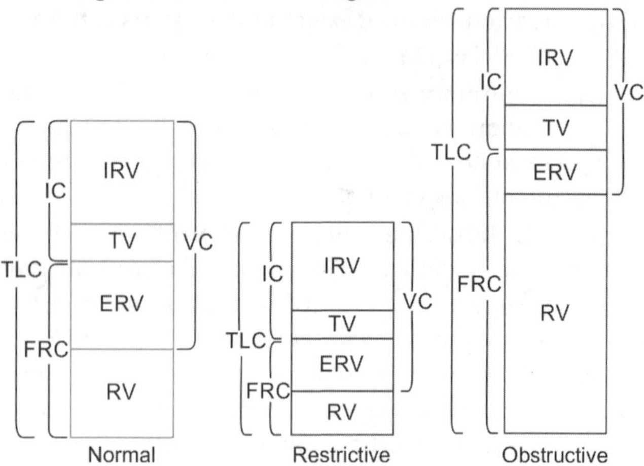

C. Dynamic lung volume:

It can be measured by following technique:

a. Inert gas like helium gas dilution technique: Patient is asked to breathe 10–15% helium which commences at any point of end-tidal respiration. Breathing is continued until steady lower helium concentration will be reached. Now concentration of helium in the spirometer and in the lung will be same. Helium will be diluted by gas which is present in the lungs. As for example, if 50 mL of helium is introduced and concentration of helium is 1%, volume of the lung will be 5 L.

b. Nitrogen washout technique: The patient is asked to breathe 100% oxygen, all the nitrogen will be washed out from the lungs. Then nitrogen content of the exhaled volume will be measured. So, difference in the final exhaled and initial concentrations will calculate the intrathoracic volume as well as FRC.

c. Body plethysmography: It is based on Boyle's law—it states that at constant temperature the product of pressure and volume of gas remains constant.

$$P_1V_1 = P_2V_2$$

Its advantage is over two methods as it will quantify noncommunicating gas volumes.

In this method, a patient is allowed to be seated in a closed box with known volume. Now he is asked to pant with opened glottis against closed shutter to make change pressure in the box which is proportionate to the volume of air in the chest. As measurement is done at the end of the expiration, it will measure the FRC.

d. FVC: The amount of air exhaled after taking maximal inspiration as long as and as quickly as possible. It indirectly reflects the property of airway resistance. Interpretations of percentage predicted are the following:

1. 80–120%—normal
2. 70–79%—mild reduction
3. 50–69%—moderate reduction
4. <50%—severe reduction

e. FEV_1: The volume of air exhaled in first second is FEV_1. Normally FEV_1 is 80% of FVC. When forced expiratory volume can be charted against time—FEV_1. It will measure severity of the airway. Normal is 3–4.5 L.

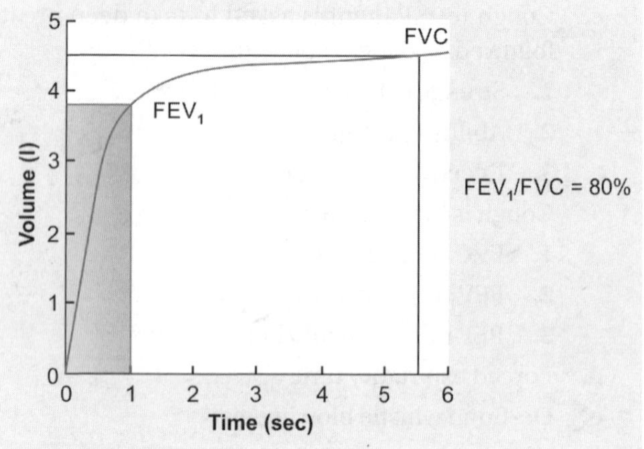

f. FEV_1/FVC: Its interpretation:

1. >75%—normal
2. 60–75%—mild obstruction
3. 50–59%—moderate obstruction
4. <49%—severe obstruction

Severity of airflow obstruction based on predicted FEV_1:

Predicted FEV_1	Stage
More than 80%	Mild
50–79%	Moderate
30–49%	Severe
Less than 29%	Very severe

Spirometry depends upon the following:

1. The value is directly proportional to height
2. It is inversely proportional to age
3. Gender
4. Ethnicity

g. Forced mid-expiratory flow rate (FEF_{25-75}): It will measure mid-part of expiratory flow. Normal value is 4.5–5 L/sec or 300 L/min.

1. It is measured in L/sec.

2. It will reflect effort independent expiration.
3. It will measure the status of smaller airways.
4. It is highly variable.
5. It will depend highly on FVC.

Interpretation:

1. >60%—normal
2. 40–60%—mild obstruction
3. 20–40%—moderate obstruction
4. <20%—severe obstruction

h. PEF rate: It is the maximum flow rate measured during a FVC maneuver in initial 0.1 second. The patient is asked to take deep inspiration and then to expire forcefully and as quickly as he or she can and thus maximum airflow can be measured. Forced expiratory flow is between 200 and 1,200 mL of FVC. It reflects larger airway function. Normal value:

1. 450–700 L/min in males
2. 300–500 L/min in females

Its significance: Value of <200 L/min signifies

1. Impaired coughing
2. Postoperative complication

i. Maximum volume ventilation: It is the maximum volume of air that can be breathed in and out of the lungs in 1 minute by maximum effort.

a. It will measure the speed and efficiency of filling and emptying of the lungs during increased respiratory effort.
b. It is 30–40 times the normal baseline value of FEV_1. Value is 150–175 L/min
c. It is decreased in:
   1. COPD
   2. Upper airway obstruction
   3. Poor strength of respiratory muscles
   4. Low value correlates with reduced exercise capacity
   5. Value below 40–45 L/min is contraindication to pneumonectomy

D. Bronchodilator response of airways in the lung:

Pre- and post-bronchodilator spirometry demonstrates:

a. There is increase either in FEV_1 or FVC of 12% of the baseline value.
b. Increase in baseline value of FVC or FEV_1 of more than 200 mL will correlate with the reversibility of obstruction.
c. Reduction of RV or FRC in absence of any change in FVC or FEV_1 suggests symptomatic relief.
d. Negative response may not suggest that bronchodilator is of no benefit.
e. Increase in FVC or FEV_1 after use of bronchodilator in spite of normal spirometry indicates occult limitation of air flow.

E. Bronchoprovocation test:

Here methacholine or histamine is used to provoke the bronchoconstriction. Positive test is characterized by:

a. Fall in 15–20% in FEV_1 after inhalation of these bronchoconstrictor agents.
b. It can identify occult asthma.
c. Bronchoconstriction test may be positive in following cases:
   1. Allergic rhinitis
   2. COPD
   3. Upper respiratory tract infection
   4. Nasal allergy with absence of asthma

Spirometry can detect the following:

a. It can detect obstructive lesion in the major airways
b. Characterization of lesion:
   1. Location whether it is intrathoracic or extrathoracic
   2. Whether it is fixed or variable

So the lesions are:

a. Variable intrathoracic lesion: Intratracheal tumor and tracheomalacia

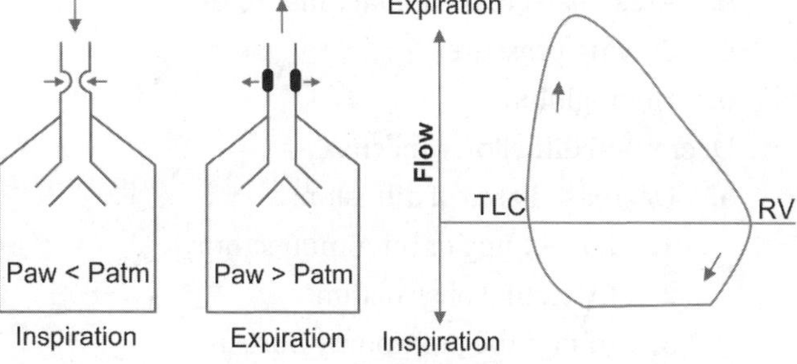

Variable extrathoracic

b. Fixed intrathoracic or extrathoracic lesion: Tracheal stenosis, intratracheal mass, and surgical stenosis

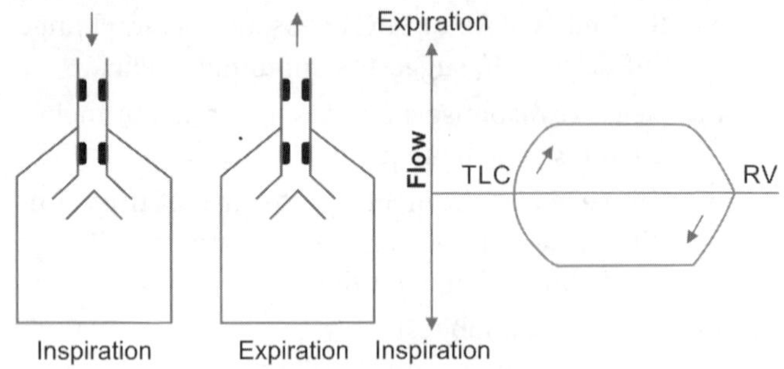

Fixed (Intra-or extrathoracic)

c. Variable extrathoracic lesion: Tumor, paralysis of vocal cord, and goiter

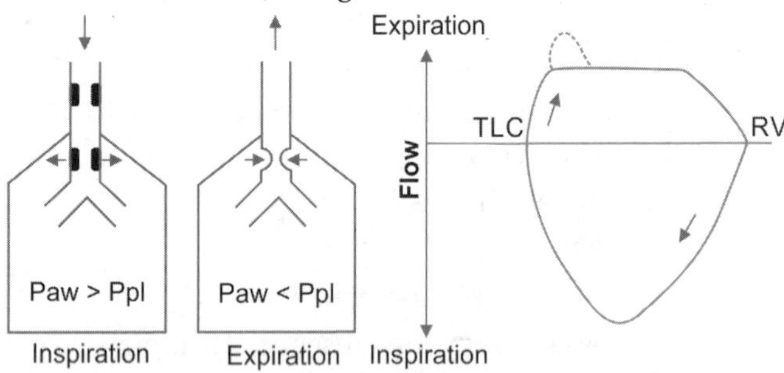

Variable intrathoracic

F. Diffusion capacity: It will estimate the transfer of oxygen in the alveolar air into the RBC. Here the subject is asked to exhale up to RV and then inhale maximally the test gas 0.3% carbon dioxide with dilution of 10% helium gas. Rate of disappearance of carbon monoxide during breath-hold time of 10 seconds is estimated by infrared analyzer. Factors that affect the diffusion capacity:
   a. Thickness of the membrane
   b. Area of alveolar capillary membrane
   c. Driving pressure
   d. Hemoglobin

   Decreased diffusion capacity:
   a. Decreased area of diffusion:
      1. Lobectomy or pneumonectomy
      2. Bronchial obstruction
      3. Interstitial pulmonary fibrosis
      4. Recurrent PE
      5. Pulmonary hypertension
      6. Pulmonary vasculitis
   b. Increased thickness of alveolar-capillary membrane:
      1. Pulmonary vascular disease
      2. Interstitial pulmonary fibrosis
      3. Chronic heart failure
   c. Decrease in driving pressure:
      1. Pressure of carbon monoxide
      2. Smoking
   d. Hemoglobin:
      1. Anemia
      2. Hemoglobinopathy

   Increased diffusion capacity:
   a. Polycythemia
   b. Left to right shunt
   c. Exercise
   d. Obesity
   e. Pulmonary hemorrhage
   f. Asthma

G. 4- and 6-minute walk test:
   a. It can detect hidden diffusion defect.
   b. SaO_2 has to be measured at rest, after 6 minutes' walk.
   c. In case of healthy subject, 500–600 meters is usually covered.
   d. Measurements to be taken at the end of 6 minutes' walk:
      1. Distance walked in meters
      2. SpO_2
      3. Maximum heart rate
      4. Borg scale assessment to measure dyspnea and fatigue of leg

      Desaturation occurs in following circumstances:
      1. Shunt
      2. Diffusion defect
      3. V/Q defect

      Criteria for supplementation of oxygen:
      1. $SaO_2 < 88\%$ or PO_2 55 mm Hg
      2. Pulmonary hypertension or polycythemia or PO_2 59 mm Hg

H. Maximal inspiratory pressure (Pi-max) and maximal expiratory pressure (Pe max):
   a. It can measure the strength of respiratory muscles.
   b. It can demonstrate the pressure the patient can generate during inspiration (Pi) and during expiration (Pe).
   c. Normal value:
      1. During inspiration: –60 cm of water
      2. During expiration: +120 cm of water

I. Airway resistance:

   a. It can measure the pressure difference between alveoli and mouth per unit airflow by plethysmography. Normal resistance is 2.5 cm of water/L/sec.

J. Compliance of lung:

   a. It can measure the change in volume per unit change of pressure.

   b. Patient is asked breathe out 500 mL at a time from TLC and esophageal pressure will be measured through balloon catheter placed in the esophagus. During this time glottis must be opened and lung will be allowed to become stabilized for few seconds. At every expiration of 500 mL of air, readings of esophageal pressure have to be take and plotted as pressure-volume curve.

   c. Normal value is 200 mL/cm of water.

   d. Low compliance is seen in:

      1. Interstitial pulmonary fibrosis

      2. Pulmonary edema

      3. Adult respiratory distress syndrome

      4. Diffuse bilateral inflammatory disease

   e. Compliance of lung is increased in emphysema

Flow-volume Loops or Curves

It relates the lung volume during maximal inspiration after maximal exhalation (except RV) and maximal expiration (TLC) after complete inspiration. Its advantage is that it can demonstrate whether the airflow is appropriate for that particular lung volume. Air flow is slower at low lung volume because of decreased elastic recoil of the lung at lower lung volume. In case of pulmonary fibrosis due to lower lung volume air flow will be decreased.

A. Flow volume loops in normal conditions:

   a. Inspiratory loop is symmetrical and convex.

   b. Expiratory limb is linear.

   c. Airflow at the mid-point of inspiratory capacity and expiratory capacity are measured and compared.

   d. Maximal inspiratory flow (MIF) at 50% of FVC is greater than maximal expiratory flow (MEF) at 50% of FVC due to dynamic compression of airway during exhalation.

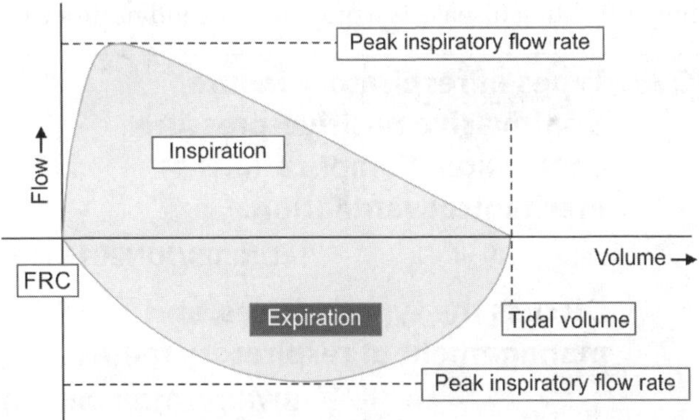

B. Flow volume loops in obstructive airway disease:

   a. Although air flow is diminished expiration will be prolonged, so MEF < MIF

   b. Low peak inspiratory flow

   c. Low PEF

   d. Expiratory flow curve fails to reach "zero" point

   e. "Scooped out" expiratory flow pattern

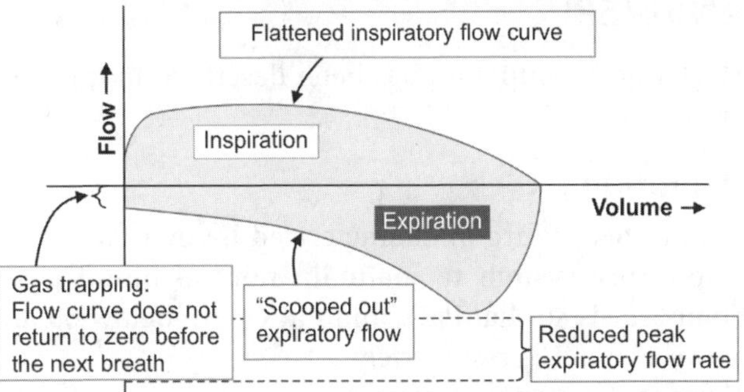

C. Flow-volume loop in case of restrictive lung disease:

   a. It will show diminished size of normal lung volume due to reduced volume of the lung.

   b. Characteristic low lung volume

   c. Rapid decrease in inspiratory flow

   d. Expiratory flow will be rapid having high expiratory flow rate

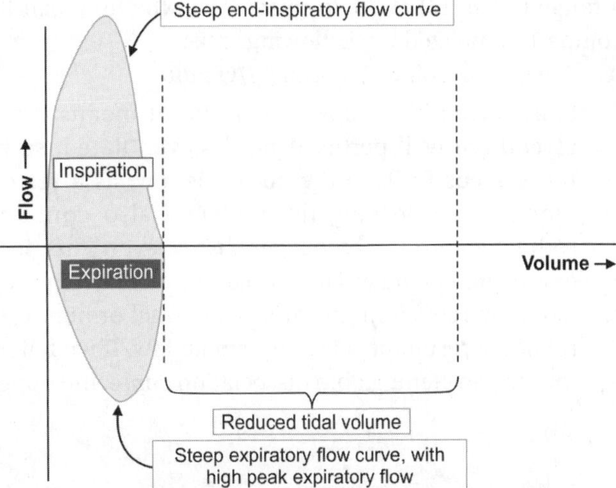

Interstitial lung disease is written in question number 17.

Q26. Types of respiratory failure. Noninvasive positive-pressure ventilation. Complications of mechanical ventilation.

DNBIIB/JUN2015 (10)

Discuss the types, causes, and management of respiratory failure.

BF/NOV2012/MDII (30)

Noninvasive ventilation.

BF/MAY2010/MDIV (10)

Describe acute respiratory failure and mechanical ventilatory support.

SAURASHTRA UNI, RAJKOT, 2021 (20)

ANSWER

Mechanical ventilation has been described in question number 19.

Definition

Respiratory failure in characterized by inability of the respiratory system to maintain normal blood gases homeostasis so that PaO_2 and $PaCO_2$ are below 60 and above 50 mm Hg, respectively.

There are four types of failure:

A. Type 1 or hypoxic respiratory failure where PaO_2 is <60 mm Hg due to failure of oxygenation.

Pathophysiology of hypoxic respiratory failure: Normal V_A, i.e., the difference between minute ventilation and dead space is 4–5 L and normal perfusion quotient is 5 L, so the V/Q ratio is 0.8–1 in case of normal lung in spite of differential ratio in different parts of the lung having a range of 0.8–1.2 L. So, in this context the lung can be compartmentalized into following areas:

A. Areas of alveoli with normal V/Q ratio

B. Some alveoli have low V/Q ratio—it means these alveoli are well perfused but less ventilated, so in these areas PaO_2 in the alveoli is low; as a result, bloodstream leaving these alveoli also contains reduced amount of oxygen. Now even this less oxygenated blood will mix with the blood having SaO_2 of nearly 100% from the areas of normal or high V/Q ratio, the resultant SaO_2 will remain low. If we follow the oxygen-hemoglobin dissociation curve, the upper part of the curve is plateau shaped; hence after full saturation of hemoglobin with oxygen there will no further increase in oxygen concentration of oxygen. On the other hand, PaO_2 in the alveoli may be very high.

C. Some alveoli have high V/Q ratio, i.e., these alveoli are very well ventilated but less perfused, so in these areas, PaO_2 is high but partial pressure of carbon dioxide will be low.

D. Some alveoli are ventilated but not perfused; here the V/Q ratio will reach infinity. So, here the alveoli will create increased physiological dead space.

E. Some alveoli are atelectatic, so in these areas the blood will pass without being oxygenated creating a type of shunt and this is most important cause of refractory acute hypoxemic respiratory failure. A small amount of shunt (5%) can be seen in the normal lung like:

a. Bronchial venous blood directly drains into left atrium through pulmonary veins

b. Small amount of venous blood from coronary veins drains into left ventricle Thebesian veins.

But in case of atelectatic lung it will reach up to 35–50%. As this percentage increases there will be more and more hypoxemia.

So, severity of hypoxemic respiratory failure will depend upon the proportion of above V/Q mismatching, but if the shunt proportion is high, prognosis will be grave.

In resting patient, diffusion abnormality is not responsible for hypoxemia, but regional variation in pulmonary compliance results in low V/Q ratio.

The causes are:

a. Alveolar flooding or pulmonary edema:

1. Cardiogenic pulmonary edema:

- Elevated pulmonary microvascular pressure like heart failure
- Intravascular volume overload like ARDS (low pressure pulmonary edema) and this cannot be explained by fluid overload as well as shunt physiology requiring PEEP. The clinical causes of heart failure:

  Gastric aspiration

  Near drowning

  Acute pancreatitis

  Multiple blood transfusion

  Aspiration pneumonia

B. Type II or hypercapnic respiratory failure or ventilatory failure where the partial pressure of carbon dioxide is <50 mm Hg and PaO_2 is < 60 mm Hg in arterial blood due to inability of the lung to eliminate carbon dioxide.

Pathophysiology of ventilatory failure:

Normally carbon dioxide produced in the tissues is removed by ventilation through lungs. Tension of alveolar carbon dioxide (P_ACO_2) and $PaCO_2$ is usually maintained at around 40 mm Hg by adjusting V_A (difference between minute ventilation V_E and physiological dead space ventilation V_D) and VCO_2. So any change in VCO_2 will lead to change in V_A, so the relationship between V_A, VCO_2, and P_ACO_2 can be calculated as:

$P_ACO_2 = PaCO_2 = (VCO_2/V_A) \times \text{Constant } (0.86)$

Or, $P_ACO_2 = PaCO_2 = VCO_2/(V_E - V_D)$ = Volume of carbon dioxide/(Minute ventilation – Dead space). From this equation it can be explained that rise in arterial PaO_2 due to ventilatory failure occurs due to either fall in V_A, which may be due to fall in minute ventilation, or increase in dead space or increase in tissue production of carbon dioxide without any increase in V_A.

The causes are as follows:

a. Impairment of CNS to breathe
   1. Injury to brainstem
   2. Overdose of sedative drugs
   3. Severe hypothyroidism
   4. Sleep-induced apnea
   5. Vocal cord paralysis

b. Impairment of strength and failure of neuromuscular junction in the respiratory system:
   1. Impaired neuromuscular transmission:
      - Myasthenia gravis
      - Amyotrophic lateral sclerosis
      - Guillain–Barré syndrome
      - Poliomyelitis
      - Tetanus
      - Botulism
   2. Myopathy
   3. Fatigue
   4. Electrolyte derangement like
      - Hypokalemia
      - Hyperkalemia
      - Hypomagnesemia
      - Prolonged ventilator dependence
      - Phrenic nerve disorder

c. Increased load on the respiratory system:
   1. Resistive loads like bronchospasm in case of bronchial asthma or in acute crisis in chronic bronchitis and emphysema—here minute ventilation will be decreased at the cost of increased dead space.
   2. Tracheal or subglottic stenosis
   3. In children epiglottitis
   4. Reduced lung compliance:
      - Alveolar edema
      - Intrinsic PEEP or auto-PEEP
   5. Reduced compliance of chest wall:
      - Pleural effusion
      - Pneumothorax
      - Abdominal distension
      - Kyphoscoliosis
      - Flail chest
   6. Due to increased requirement of minute ventilation:
      - Pulmonary embolus will produce acute rise in dead space
      - Sepsis
      - Increased fraction of dead space

C. Type III or perioperative respiratory failure:

It occurs due to:

a. Perioperative atelectasis because after general anesthesia there is collapse of dependent lung due to decrease in FRC thus increasing closing lung volume

b. Cardiothoracic surgery

c. Major upper abdominal surgery which may splint the diaphragm and upper abdominal mechanics are deranged.

As a result small lung due to atelectasis of dependent lung with high diaphragm produces hypercapnia.

D. Type IV respiratory failure:

It occurs in case of shock. Due to low cardiac output there is hypoperfusion of respiratory muscles. Respiratory muscles utilize only oxygen from 5% of cardiac output. But in shock patients may develop respiratory distress, lactic acidosis, and anemia.

Clinical Features of Acute Respiratory Failure

A. Hypoxemia is the basic feature of hypoxemic respiratory failure and it can be detected by pulse oximeter even before the development of cyanosis. Well marked hypoxemia coexists prior to cyanosis because it is only clinically evident when capillary concentration of reduced hemoglobin exceeds 5 g/dL. Patient with hemoglobin of <7 g/dL may die due to severe hypoxemic failure prior to development of cyanosis. Again in anemia hyperdynamic circulation prevents the development of cyanosis. Other features are restlessness, confusional state, anxiety, and restlessness.

B. Compensatory mechanisms due to hypoxia are:

- **a.** Tachycardia
- **b.** Hypertension

Both are due to sympathetic stimulation.

- **c.** Tachypnea due to stimulation of chemoreceptors present in the carotid body and aorta. But in case of CNS depression or weakness of respiratory muscles tachypnea is not evident.
- **d.** In case of elderly, diabetic neuropathy with CNS depression above features may not be evident.
- **e.** In case of severe hypoxemic failure:
  1. Severe bradycardia
  2. Hypotension
  3. Lactic acidosis
  4. Arrhythmias
  5. Circulatory failure
  6. Death
- **f.** Myocardium has no reserve for oxygen, so in case of hypoxemia cardiac muscles suffer from hypoxia resulting in depression of cardiac function and produce bradycardia, hypotension, increased ectopic activity, and different types of tachyarrhythmias.

C. Hypercapnia:

- **a.** Due to depressant effect on cardiovascular system producing:
  1. Cutaneous flushing
  2. Warmth
  3. Sweating
  4. Bounding pulse
- **b.** Depressant effect of CNS:
  1. Confusion
  2. Behavioral disturbances
  3. Inversion of sleep rhythm
  4. Progressively increasing drowsiness leading to coma also known as carbon dioxide narcosis when partial pressure of carbon dioxide will reach 80–100 mm Hg. Coma occurs when it will reach >100 mm Hg.
  5. Flapping tremor
  6. Plantars are usually flexor but they may be extensor
  7. High level of arterial carbon dioxide may produce headache, seizures, and papilledema all of which may simulate intracranial tumor
  8. Sympathetic nervous system stimulation may produce tachycardia and hypertension, but these features depend upon the balance between depressant effect on cardiovascular system and stimulant effect on sympathetic nervous system.

D. Dyspnea: Some patients may be aware of dyspnea, but many patients with respiratory failure are not dyspneic. Again many dyspneic patients may not suffer from respiratory failure.

Complications of Acute Respiratory Failure

A. Most important complication is nosocomial infection which is present who are on artificial airway or mechanical ventilation.

B. Complications of mechanical ventilation

C. Fluid-electrolyte imbalances

D. Acid-base imbalance

E. Segmental or lobar atelectasis in patients with hyper-secretion of mucus

F. Paralytic ileus

G. Gastric dilatation—it may be responsible for aspiration of oropharyngeal contents.

Management of Acute Respiratory Failure

A. Maintenance of airway patent: Airways are plugged with retained respiratory secretions, mucus plugs, food particles and thus obstruct lumen of the airway, which may be responsible for V/Q mismatch; in some cases areas of atelectasis may be responsible for shunt thus creating severe hypoxemia. So this secretions have to be liquefied by following mechanisms:

- **a.** Liquefaction of secretion: Drying of secretion can be done by following mechanisms:
  1. Administration of intravenous fluid to hydrate the patient.

2. Humidification of inspired gas is utmost important in case of patients on endotracheal tube or tracheostomy tube, because in absence of humidification the respiratory secretions become inspissated and block the larger airways and endotracheal tube producing disastrous consequences.
3. Use of normal saline: In patients of asthma on ventilatory support, instillation of normal saline drop by drop through the tracheostomy or endotracheal tube to liquefy the inspissated secretions.
4. Though acetylcysteine is a good liquefactant, a very small amount instillation may produce severe bronchospasm and will increase the volume of secretion in the tracheobronchial tree.

B. Promotion of cough: In case of patient with respiratory failure, cough should not be suppressed and always promoted. It is due to major surgery like abdominal or open heart surgery, where analgesic should be used to give relief from pain but its dose should not be like that which will produce respiratory depression.

C. Physiotherapy of chest should be required along with tracheal stimulation as in critically ill patient proper physiotherapy may spell the difference between the survival and death.

D. Removal of secretion by suction:

- **a.** In case of critically ill patient, if the patient is unable to spit or cough out the accumulated secretion in the mouth and upper respiratory tract, regular and frequent suction of the secretion is required to prevent aspiration into the lung parenchyma.
- **b.** Accumulated secretion around larynx is suctioned by laryngoscope.

The above suctions also induce cough which are added help. But this suction should not traumatize the pharyngeal and laryngeal mucosa as it induces bleeding and mucosal sloughing further worsening the airway.

E. Endotracheal intubation: If the above processes fail to clear the airway or by giving oropharyngeal or nasopharyngeal airway, then endotracheal intubation is required to clear the trachea and larger airways. Common indications of endotracheal intubation are as follows:

- **a.** In case of comatose patient, the inability of the patient to clear the airway of secretions
- **b.** Very poor cough reflex
- **c.** Very critically ill patients
- **d.** Paralysis of palate and pharynx
- **e.** Four common conditions in case of critically ill patients:
  1. Administration of respiratory depressant as poisons
  2. Cerebrovascular accidents
  3. Any cause producing coma
  4. Following major surgery

F. Maintenance of adequate ventilation:

In case of apneic patients or in patients on feeble respiration following process of ventilations can be applied:

- **a.** Mouth-to-mouth breathing
- **b.** Mask fitted to Ambu bag fed with 100% oxygen
- **c.** Endotracheal intubation

G. Use of respiratory stimulants:

- **a.** Its use in case of critically ill patients is limited because this drug in addition to stimulate respiratory center also acts as analeptic and awaken the patients so ventilation may be impossible.
- **b.** Good physiotherapy during analeptic phase will mobilize the secretions from the respiratory tract so that it will be coughed up or can be suctioned.
- **c.** Adverse effects are:
  1. Vomiting
  2. In large dose, it will produce twitching or seizures
- **d.** Valid use of stimulant:
  1. It will tide over the critical period during the transfer to ICU.
  2. In case of hopelessly crippled COPD, this stimulant can be used as conservative measure.
- **e.** Respiratory stimulant having least side effect is doxapram; dose is 1–3 mg/min up to 600 mg.

H. Treatment of cause of acute respiratory failure:

- **a.** Treatment of infections
- **b.** Removal of air in case of tension pneumothorax
- **c.** Urgent removal of foreign body present in the trachea or large bronchus
- **d.** Tapping of fluid from unilateral massive pleural effusion

e. With the help of bronchoscopic suction along with proper physiotherapy expansion of atelectatic lobe can be enhanced.

f. Myasthenia gravis can be treated by prostigmine or antivenom in case of snake bite.

g. Administration of naloxone in case of narcotic poisoning.

h. In case of acute severe asthma β2-agonists, oral or intravenous corticosteroids can be given.

Q27. Neural circuit responsible for cough reflex. Enumerate the causes of cough. Clinical histories and findings which would help to localize the cause of cough in a given individual.

DNBI/APR2016 (10)

Cough reflex.

MGR/MAY2011/MD (5)

ANSWER

Cough is a protective reflex responsible for:

a. Clearing the respiratory tract of respiratory secretions

b. Protecting the lungs from aspiration of oropharyngeal contents

Two types of cough:

a. Voluntary cough

b. Involuntary cough which can arise from stimulation of rapidly activating irritant receptors that present in the larynx and tracheobronchial tree, pleura, esophagus, stomach, and external auditory meatus.

A. Sensory nerve endings or primary adapting receptors are stimulated by following stimuli:

a. Chemical stimuli such as capsaicin and smoke

b. Mechanical stimuli such as dust, tumor within the airway, extrinsic mechanical pressure on the airway, or interstitial pulmonary fibrosis producing distortion of the airways

c. Mucosal inflammation like tracheobronchitis

B. Another type of receptors known as "slowly adapting stretch receptors" terminates inspiration after the lung will reach an adequate level of inflation and starts expiration.

C. Another type of fibers, C fibers, is present in the mucosa of respiratory tract and wall of the alveoli that are sensitive to chemical like capsaicin and bradykinin.

Cationic ion channel known as transient receptor potential vanilloid 1 is present in C fibers and rapidly adapting receptors—these are sensitive to chemical capsaicin.

Sensory impulses from the above receptors travel via vagus and superior laryngeal, trigeminal, and phrenic nerves to tractus solitarius in the brainstem identified as "cough center".

a. Vagus nerve carries impulses from larynx, trachea, bronchi, pleura, esophagus and stomach and external auditory meatus via auricular branch.

b. Glossopharyngeal nerve carries impulses from pharynx.

c. Trigeminal nerve carries impulses from nose and paranasal sinuses.

d. Phrenic nerve carries impulses from pericardium and diaphragm.

From the cough center efferent impulses through the cranial and phrenic nerves to muscles of respiration and diaphragm and accessory muscles of respiration thus complete the reflex arc.

To start with there is rapid inspiration followed by sequentially closure of glottis due to adduction of vocal cords, contraction of ribcage muscles of expiration, abdominal muscles leading rise in pleural and intrapulmonary pressures up to 200 mm Hg. Now with sudden release of laryngeal contraction and opening of glottis rapid expiratory flows are generated that will exceed normal "envelope" of MEF. The associated bronchial smooth muscle contraction and dynamic compression of the airways will narrow the bronchial lumen and maximize the expiratory airflow. This kinetic energy present in the expiratory flow is sufficient to dislodge the mucus present in the bronchial lumen and it is directly proportional to square of the velocity of expiratory flow. Sound is produced by vibration of tracheobronchial walls and secretions present in the lumen.

The propulsion of secretions by effective cough depends upon lung volume.

a. In healthy adult at high lung volume, "equal pressure points" are present in the large airways, hence propulsive force is large.

b. In case of critically patients at low lung volume "equal pressure points" are located near the alveoli, so propulsive forces is feeble toward mouth.

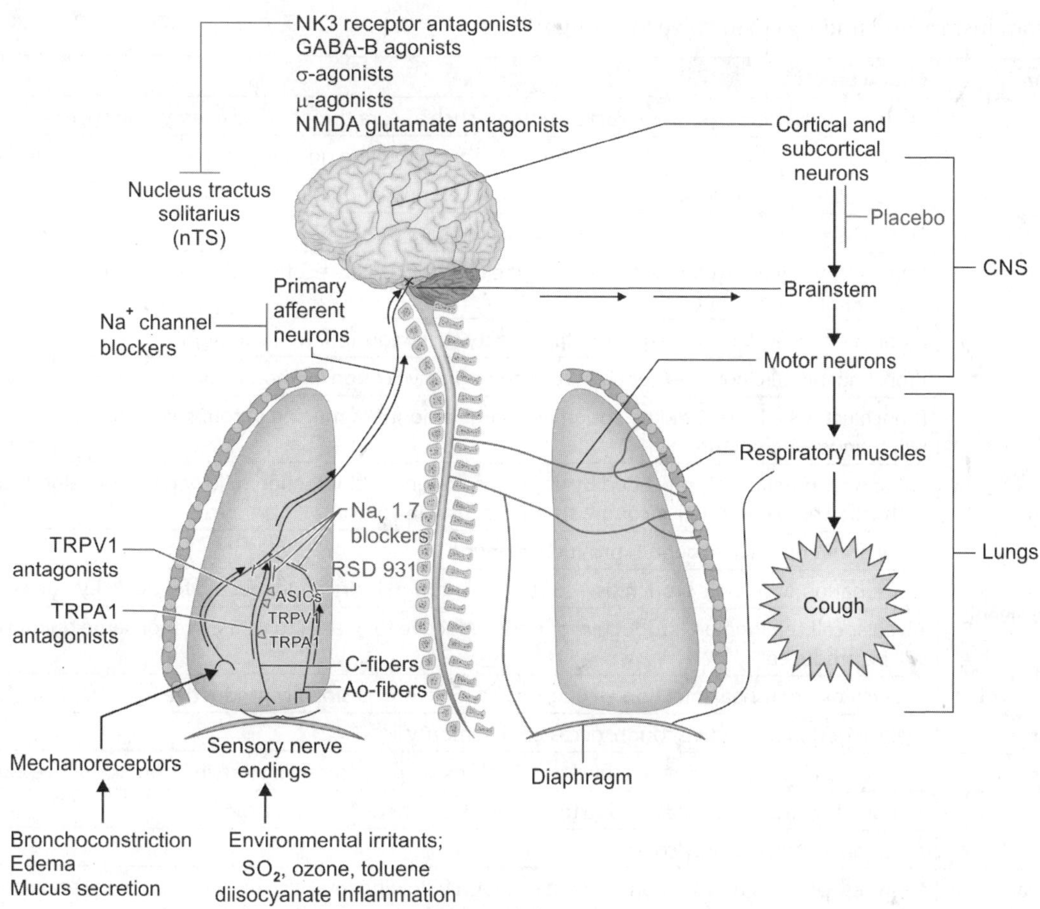

Causes of Cough

A. Acute cough: It usually starts suddenly and will be resolved within 3–4 weeks.

- **a.** Acute upper respiratory tract infection
- **b.** Acute asthma
- **c.** Acute sinusitis
- **d.** Acute rhinitis
- **e.** Acute exacerbation of COPDs
- **f.** Pulmonary infarction
- **g.** Acute pleurisy

B. Chronic cough:

- **a.** Smoking
- **b.** Occupational lung diseases:
  - **1.** Asbestosis
  - **2.** Pneumoconiosis
  - **3.** Silicosis
  - **4.** Byssinosis
- **c.** Chronic pulmonary infection:
  - **1.** Tuberculosis
  - **2.** Lung abscess
  - **3.** Bronchiectasis
  - **4.** Bronchitis
  - **5.** Fungal infection
- **d.** Granulomatous lung disease: Sarcoidosis
- **e.** Tumors of lung:
  - **1.** Bronchoalveolar carcinoma
  - **2.** Bronchogenic carcinoma
  - **3.** Other tumors of lung
- **f.** Interstitial lung diseases:
  - **1.** Interstitial lung disease
  - **2.** Infiltrative disorders of the lung
- **g.** Aspiration of foreign body
- **h.** Pleural pathology:
  - **1.** Chronic pleural effusion
  - **2.** Mesothelioma
- **h.** Cardiovascular causes:
  - **1.** Mitral stenosis
  - **2.** Congestive cardiac failure
  - **3.** Pulmonary infarction
- **i.** Gastrointestinal causes:
  - **1.** Gastroesophageal reflux
  - **2.** Large diaphragmatic hernia
- **j.** Unexplained cough

Evaluation from history and findings to localize the cough:

Causes of cough	Characteristics
Pharynx	Pharyngitis: Upper respiratory tract symptoms such as sore throat, nasal allergy, and sneezing
Larynx	Laryngitis, whooping cough, laryngeal tumor—harsh barking quality, persistent, and associated with stridor
	Left-sided vocal cord paralysis—bovine cough, i.e., inefficient low pitched with hoarseness of voice
Trachea	Tracheitis—dry painful cough, running nose, and sore throat
Bronchus and alveoli	Bronchitis—dry or productive on most of the days for >3 consecutive months and for >2 years, worse in the morning, sputum is mucoid
	Asthma—repeated cough expectorating scanty sticky sputum, worse at night
	Bronchogenic carcinoma—productive or nonproductive cough for months or years with occasional hemoptysis
	Bronchiectasis—long-standing cough with large amount of mucoid or foul-smelling sputum, the amount will change with posture
	Lobar pneumonia—it is preceded by upper respiratory tract infection followed by dry painful cough to start with followed by productive cough, sputum is rusty in color
	Bronchopneumonia—cough is productive or dry
	Exacerbation of chronic bronchitis—to start with cough is dry, then mucoid followed by purulent sputum
	Alveolar cell carcinoma—productive or nonproductive for weeks to years, later on large quantity of sputum will be produced
	Tuberculosis or fungal infection—cough is productive, occasionally productive
Benign tumor	Inefficient nonproductive cough, occasional hemoptysis
Interstitial tissue	Interstitial lung disease due to infiltration or fibrosis—persistently distressing nonproductive cough
Mediastinum	Tumor—breathlessness, cough due to compression on trachea and bronchi
	Aortic aneurysm—brassy cough
Gastrointestinal causes	Gastroesophageal reflux—nonproductive cough following intake of heavy meals or in recumbent position, this is associated with heart burn and belching, acid regurgitation
	Neuromuscular disease of upper esophagus—associated with eating or drinking
Foreign body intake	In the upper airway—cough is associated with stridor and asphyxia
	In the lower airway—nonproductive cough with wheeze
Cardiovascular causes	Left ventricular failure—cough aggravated in supine position and relieved in recumbent position. Expectoration of pink frothy sputum
	Pulmonary infarction—sudden cough with hemoptysis, pleural effusion, cyanosis, and shock
	Congestive cardiac failure—chronic cough with expectoration and pedal edema
Drugs	Angiotensin-converting enzyme inhibitor—nonproductive cough usually occurs in women, it occurs after commencement or years after use
Debility and weakness	Inefficient and inadequate cough

Timing of cough:

A. Morning cough—smoker

B. Nocturnal cough—postnasal drip, congestive cardiac failure, and left ventricular failure

Type of cough	Causes
Dry hacking cough	Allergy, infection, anxiety neurosis, tumor, and interstitial lung disease
Chronic productive cough	Lung abscess, bronchiectasis, chronic bronchitis, tuberculosis, and bacterial pneumonia
Barking cough	Epiglottic disease
Stridor	Tracheal obstruction
Associated with eating or drinking	Upper esophageal muscular disease
Inadequate cough	Debility and weakness
Wheezing	Asthma, allergy, and COPD

Following information can be obtained from the sputum:

A. Amount of sputum:

a. Large amount of sputum:

1. Bronchiectasis
2. Lung abscess
3. Bronchoalveolar carcinoma

b. Scanty amount of sputum:

1. Bronchial asthma
2. Early phase of pneumonia

B. Character of the sputum:

a. Clear watery frothy serous sputum:

1. Acute pulmonary edema
2. Bronchoalveolar carcinoma

b. Clear, gray/white frothy mucoid sputum:

1. Chronic asthma
2. Tumors
3. Tuberculosis
4. COPD

c. Yellow sputum: Staphylococcal pneumonia

d. Rusty sputum: Acute lobar pneumonia

e. Pink frothy sputum: Left ventricular failure

f. Black-colored sputum: Town dweller

g. Blood-tinged sputum: Streptococcal pneumonia

h. Bloody sputum: pulmonary emboli, tuberculosis, bronchiectasis, and bleeding disorders

C. Viscosity of sputum:

a. Highly viscous:

1. Early stage of lobar pneumonia
2. Bronchial asthma
3. Chronic bronchitis

b. Small bronchial cast-like twig: Bronchopulmonary aspergillosis associated with asthma

D. Odor:

a. Lung abscess

b. Infective bronchiectasis

c. Anaerobic organisms

Q28. Trace the pathway of cough reflex. What are the causes of hemoptysis? Outline evaluation of a patient with hemoptysis.

DNBIB/JUN2016 (10)

Describe causes, evaluation, and treatment of patients with massive hemoptysis.

DNBI/DEC2011 (10)

ANSWER

Pathway of cough reflex in Question Number 27.

Causes of Hemoptysis

Main causes	Diseases
Infective or inflammatory	Bronchitis and bronchiectasis
Infection in the lung parenchyma	Tuberculosis, pneumonia, and lung abscess
Fungal disorders	Aspergillosis, fungal ball in the tuberculous cavity, cystic residue of sarcoidosis, bronchiectatic area
Noninfective inflammatory	Goodpasture syndrome and Wegener granulomatosis
Tumor	Tracheal tumor, laryngeal tumor, bronchial adenoma, and bronchogenic carcinoma
Vascular disorder	Pulmonary infarction, arteriovenous malformation, aortic aneurysm penetrating into tracheobronchial tree
Cardiac cause	Mitral stenosis and left ventricular failure
Hematological	Blood dyscrasia
Drugs	Anticoagulant
Trauma	Foreign body
Liver	Amebic liver abscess perforating into right pleural cavity producing anchovy sauce-like pus

Approach to a Patient with Hemoptysis

A. Onset:

a. Sudden onset: Pulmonary thromboembolism, bronchiectasis, rupture of aortic aneurysm into bronchial tree, and acute bleeding disorders.

b. Chronic onset: Bronchogenic carcinoma, tuberculous cavity, bronchial adenoma, and bleeding disorders

c. When hemoptysis is the only symptom: Aspergilloma and *Echinococcus*

B. Amount of blood: 400 mL of blood/day or 100–150 mL per vomit is called as massive hemoptysis.

a. Large amount at a time: Pulmonary tuberculosis, bronchogenic carcinoma, bronchiectasis, and rupture of aortic aneurysm into bronchus

b. Small amount of blood at a time: Immunological cause, chronic bronchitis, pneumococcal and *Klebsiella pneumoniae*, and trauma to chest

c. Streak of blood: Pharyngitis, chronic bronchitis, and bleeding disorders

C. Age of onset:
  a. Childhood: Nasal polyp, foreign body, trauma to chest, arteriovenous fistula, and bronchiectasis due to Kartagener syndrome
  b. Middle age: Chronic bronchitis, immunological causes, left ventricular failure, and trauma to chest.
  c. Elderly: Bronchogenic carcinoma, chronic bronchitis, post-primary tuberculosis, left ventricular failure, and post-lung biopsy

D. Associated symptoms:
  a. Cough with mucoid sputum, low grade fever, and night sweat: Pulmonary tuberculosis
  b. Early morning cough, mucoid sputum, chest pain, and recurrent respiratory distress: Chronic bronchitis
  c. Cough with:
    1. Red currant jelly sputum: *Klebsiella pneumoniae*
    2. Rusty sputum in patient with alcoholism and diabetes: Lobar pneumonia
    3. In winter season having history of influenza, yellow-colored sputum: Staphylococcal pneumonia
    4. Red-colored foul-smelling sputum: Lung abscess
    5. Blood mixed with necrotic lung tissue: Gangrene of the lung
  d. Old debilitated elderly bed-ridden patient with history of aspiration of gastric contents: Lung abscess
  e. History of cough with respiratory distress in immunocompromised patients

Physical examinations also to be performed for:

A. Anemia, jaundice, cyanosis, clubbing, decubitus, edema, blood pressure, pulse, lymphadenopathy, nails, facial swelling, facial examination, bleeding in other sites, activity of other accessory respiratory muscles, upper and lower limb, and rashes in the body.

B. Thorough examinations of chest and heart are required to diagnose the cause of hemoptysis.

Investigations

A. Hematological examination has to be done to see complete blood count, peripheral blood picture

B. Biochemical examination for LFT, urea, and creatinine

C. Urine analysis for RBC cast, RBC in urine, and granular cast

D. Sputum for Gram stain, acid-fast stain, culture, and PCR

E. Electrocardiography to diagnose the cardiac cause of hemoptysis

F. Chest X-ray:
  a. Upper lobe pulmonary infiltrate—pulmonary tuberculosis
  b. Consolidation of lower lobe—pneumococcal pneumonia
  c. Wedge-shaped opacity with apex toward hilum and base toward periphery—pulmonary infarction
  d. Visible dilated bronchi with persistent consolidation—bronchiectasis
  e. Consolidation and cavitation with air-fluid level in posterior segment of right upper lobe—lung abscess
  f. Mass, visible collapse, and peripheral or apical mass—bronchogenic carcinoma to be proved by fine-needle aspiration cytology (FNAC)
  g. Double right border of heart and left atrial enlargement—mitral stenosis

G. Bronchoscopy to be done to diagnose foreign body, bronchial adenoma, bronchogenic carcinoma

H. Special test are the following:
  a. Mantoux test—tuberculosis
  b. Serological test: Antineutrophil cytoplasmic antibody (ANCA), peripheral (p-ANCA) to diagnose collagen vascular disease
  c. Combined immunofluorescence with specific immunoassay for antibodies to PR3 and MPO increases the sensitivity to Wegener granulomatosis and microscopic polyangiitis
  d. Anti-GBM antibodies—Goodpasture syndrome
  e. Computerized tomography pulmonary angiogram for pulmonary infarction
  f. CECT with FNAC—bronchogenic carcinoma
  g. Positron emission tomography (PET)—to detect local and systemic spread of bronchogenic carcinoma
  h. Aortography—aortic aneurysm
  i. MR angiography—to delineate aneurysm
  j. Mediastinoscopy with biopsy of the nodes: Pulmonary tuberculosis and bronchogenic carcinoma

k. Echocardiography to detect heart cause
l. CT scan to differentiate lung abscess from empyema

Q29. Lymphatic drainage of the lung.

MGR/OCT2014/MDI (5)
MGR/APR2013/MD (5)

ANSWER

Pulmonary lymph nodes are divided into two main groups:

A. Intrapulmonary lymph nodes: These are present beneath the visceral pleura.
B. Bronchopulmonary lymph nodes: These will be subdivided into two groups:
   a. Lobar lymph nodes
   b. Hilar lymph nodes

Pulmonary lymphatics can be subdivided into two groups:

A. Interstitial-venous lymphatics (interstitial lymphatics):
   a. Subpleural lymphatics
   b. Lymphatics present in the interlobular connective tissue
   c. Lymphatics related to pulmonary vein
B. Bronchoarterial lymphatics (parenchymal lymphatics):
   a. Lymphatics related to bronchus
      1. Submucosal lymphatics
      2. Lymphatics in the bronchial adventitia
   b. Lymphatics related to pulmonary artery

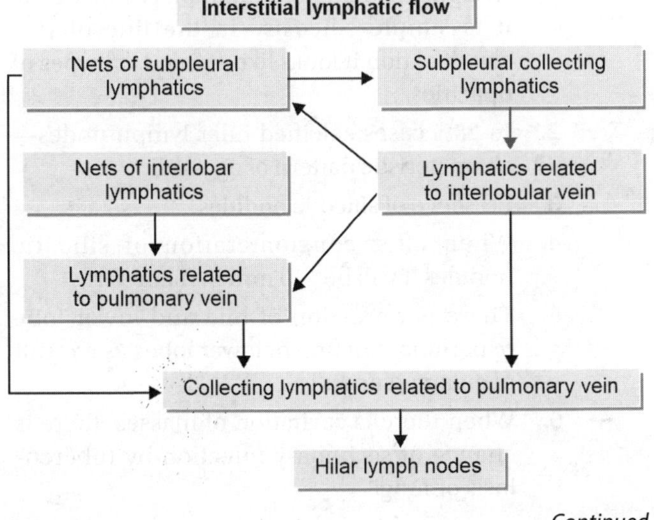

Continued

Continued

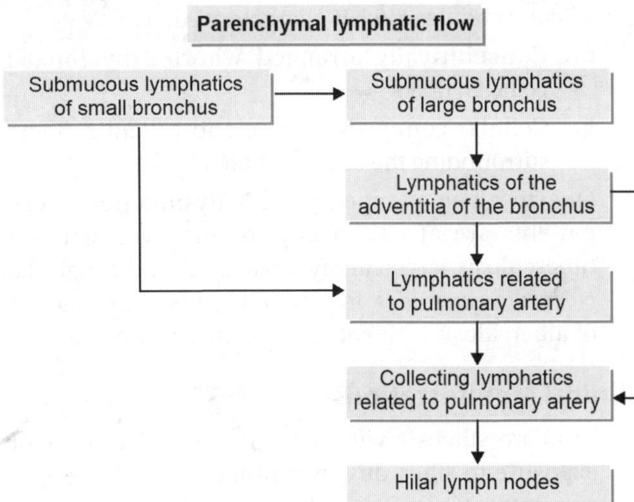

Q30. Silicosis of lung.

MGR/OCT2013/MDI (5)

ANSWER

Introduction

It is an occupational lung disease producing irreversible fibrosis due to inhalation, retention, and reaction to free silica in dose-response fashion after many years of exposure.

Persons Affected

People affected are usually working in the mines, ceramics, foundries, potteries, stone crushing, and slate pencil industries. People are engaged with drilling, mining, quarrying, tunneling, abrasive blasting, etc.

Forms of silica present in two forms:

A. Crystalline silica: Quartz (most common type), cristobalite, and tridymite. Last two are formed when quartz are exposed to high temperature.
B. Amorphous silica

Pathogenesis

Silica dust will react with aqueous media to form free oxygen radical which thereby injure alveolar macrophages in the lung parenchyma leading to release of inflammatory cytokines such as ILs and TNF-β. End result is inflammation of pulmonary parenchyma leading to necrosis.

Pathology

A. In case of heavily exposed persons to sandblasting in closed spaces or tunneling through the rock, silicosis may appear within 10 months of exposure—it is acute silicosis.

B. The hallmark of chronic form is the development of silicotic nodule which is characterized by:

a. Concentrically arranged whorled hyalinized collagen fibers

b. Cellular connective tissue and reticulin fibers surrounding the collagen fibers

C. Due to alveolar macrophages dysfunction these patients are at risk of developing mycobacterial tuberculosis, atypical mycobacteria, and fungi like *Nocardia asteroides*. In case of increased prevalence of tuberculosis incidence in silicotic workers is 20%.

Clinical Manifestations

A. In acute silicosis within 10 months to 2 years of exposure to silica dust symptoms are fever, cough, respiratory distress, weight loss, and pleuritic pain. If it progresses it will progress to progressive massive fibrosis; in that case it demonstrates crackles on auscultation.

B. Chronic silicosis occurs after 15–20 years of exposure to low level of silica dust. It is of two types:

a. Simple silicosis

b. Complicated silicosis

Usually patient is asymptomatic, but symptoms such as chronic cough and respiratory distress occur when radiographic changes are more marked. Sputum production is increased due to silica-induced chronic bronchitis aggravated by smoking. On physical examination, there is crackles and wheeze on auscultation.

If the disease progresses to massive fibrosis, there will be increasing dyspnea, cough, along with decreased breath sounds while ausculting the upper lobes.

In Acute Silicosis

Radiological Manifestations

a. Chest X-ray demonstrates in the lower zones. There is ground-glass opacity which may coalesce over times to form "mass-like" opacities involving mid zone and upper zones bilaterally but not necessarily symmetrical.

b. HRCT chest: It will demonstrate:

1. Bilateral centrilobular nodular opacities
2. Ground-glass opacities
3. Areas of consolidation
4. Absence of crazy pavement appearance seen in the alveolar proteinosis is not seen here

Bronchoalveolar Lavage

It is performed to exclude infection, eosinophilic pneumonia, and alveolar hemorrhage.

Histopathology

A. In the alveoli:

a. Proteinaceous fluid

b. Type II pneumocytes

c. Desquamated pneumocytes

d. Macrophages

e. Silica particles

B. Interstitium demonstrates the presence of inflammatory cells

C. Little or absence of fibrosis

Prognosis

A. Death will result from respiratory failure and cor pulmonale.

B. Survival is not >4 years.

Treatment

A. Avoidance of further exposure completely

B. Whole lung lavage will give symptomatic relief and slow the progression of disease

C. Corticosteroids

D. Lung transplantation

In Case of Chronic Silicosis

Radiological Investigation

a. Chest X-ray:

1. Rounded opacities in the upper lobes without any impaired pulmonary function—it is simple silicosis—in the line of ILO classification it looks like "q" and "r" types of opacities.
2. In 20% cases calcified hilar lymph nodes—characteristic pattern of eggshell.
3. Presence of silicotic nodules.
4. When after conglomeration of silicotic nodules it will be >10 mm in diameter.
5. There is retraction of hila and lower lobe hyperinflammation of lower lobes as a result of enlarged nodules.
6. When there is cavitation of masses, there is chance of secondary infection by tuberculosis or fungi.

b. HRCT chest:
   1. Centrilobular, symmetrical silicotic nodules having sharp margins.
   2. Coalescence of silicotic nodules lead to formation of nonsegmental conglomerates of irregular masses having diameter of >1 cm—called complicated silicosis.
   3. When these masses enlarge to great extent, it is known as progressive massive fibrosis.

Pulmonary Function Test

a. Decreased diffusion capacity to carbon monoxide
b. Decreased FVC
c. FEV_1/FVC reduced
d. Hypoxemia

Fluorodeoxyglucose (FDG)-PET Studies

a. It can distinguish between malignancy and silicotic nodules.
b. In case of PMF this scan may be positive.

Bronchoalveolar Lavage

It is helpful in differentiating it from malignancy and infection.

Complications

A. Pulmonary tuberculosis
B. Nocardia infection
C. Chronic necrotizing aspergillosis
D. Lung cancer
E. Collagen diseases such as production of autoantibodies against ANA, rheumatoid factor, systemic sclerosis, and rheumatoid arthritis
F. Chronic kidney disease
G. Chronic bronchitis
H. Accelerated silicosis: There is rapid development within 10 years of very high exposure to silica. Patient is asymptomatic, only radiological abnormal findings are present. But there may be cough, dyspnea, and crackles on auscultation.

Treatment

A. No specific treatment
B. General measures are:
   a. Management of airway obstruction
   b. Treatment of infection
   c. Treatment of respiratory failure and pneumothorax
   d. Treatment of coexisting tuberculosis, if present

Q31. Control of ventilation.

MGR/APR2012/MDI (5)

Ventilation and its related disorders.

BF/MAY2010/MDI (9)

Alveolar hypoventilation.

KUHS/MAY2013/MDII (10)

ANSWER

Arterial level of carbon dioxide is maintained between 37 and 43 mm Hg. But tissue will produce carbon dioxide continuously which will be eliminated by respiratory system. The relation between carbon dioxide production (VCO_2) and arterial partial pressure of CO_2 is described in following equation:

$$PaCO_2 = k \times (VCO_2/VA),$$

where VA = Fresh gas alveolar ventilation which can be calculate as minute ventilation × (1-Vd/Vt), where Vd/Vt is dead space fraction representing the amount of air that will remain within the conducting airways at the end of complete expiration. So, any change in ventilation will also reflect the changes in $PaCO_2$, VCO_2, minute ventilation, and dead space.

Main function of the lung is to maintain normal PaO_2 and $PaCO_2$ through the proper exchange of oxygen and carbon dioxide by the process of ventilation and this process has three elements:

A. Sensory system which sends sensory inputs to brainstem regulatory center. It consists of three types of receptors:
   a. Central chemoreceptors: It is situated beneath the floor of fourth ventricle and bathed in the extracellular fluid of brain in close relation of medullary respiratory center. As the composition of the extracellular fluid depends upon the local blood supply, local metabolism as well as CSF, it is influenced by pH of the blood and fluid. But among all most important is CSF which is separated from the blood vessels by blood-brain barrier; it is highly permeable to CO_2 but impermeable to H^+ and HCO_3 ions. If PCO_2 rises, CO_2 will enter into the CSF and reacts with water to form H^+ ions thereby stimulating chemoreceptors to increase ventilation and leading to reduction of H^+ ion and CO_2 concentration in CSF. For a given increase in PCO_2 pH of CSF changes much greater as compared to that in the blood because of much lowering buffering capacity of CSF. If for a prolonged period pH of CSF is lowered, then to compensate it HCO_3

will diffuse into CSF and restore the pH. This restoration of pH is much faster as compared to that in the blood because pH of blood takes time to restore for >2 days by renal compensation.

b. Peripheral chemoreceptors: There are two types of receptors:

1. Carotid bodies present at the bifurcation of common carotid artery and composed of two types of cells:
   - Type 1 cells will store dopamine and are present in close to nerve endings to carotid sinus nerve.
   - Type II cells is rich in blood supply.

   These receptors are sensed by changes in pH, PO_2, and PCO_2 in the blood and release the neurotransmitters that stimulate the afferent nerve endings in the carotid body which in turn sends impulse to CNS through the carotid body. Because of high blood supply carotid bodies respond to arterial PO_2 changes, i.e., fall in PO_2 or increase in PCO_2. So stimulation of carotid bodies by hypoxemia, hypercapnia and lowered pH increases ventilation.
2. Aortic bodies are present in the above and below the aortic arch.

c. Lung receptors:

1. Pulmonary stretch receptors: These slowly adapting stretch receptors are present in the airways, smooth muscles being stimulated during inflation of lung and remaining stimulated throughout the inflation procedure. The impulses from the receptors reach the medullary center through the vagus nerve which in turn inhibits the activity of inspiratory muscles. Just opposite procedure is observed during deflation. This will result in "self-regulating negative feedback," also known as "Hering-Breuer initiation reflex". As a result of stimulation of this reflex respiratory rate will be decreased due to increase in expiratory time.
2. Irritant receptors: These rapidly acting pulmonary stretch receptors are present between the airways epithelial cells and stimulated by cold air, dust, or other noxious agents. The impulses travel via myelinated fibers of vagus nerve to produce bronchoconstriction and hyperpnea.
3. J receptors: These receptors are present in the alveolar walls close to the capillaries. Afferent impulses from these receptors travel via slowly conducting unmyelinated fibers of vagus nerve to central medullary center leading to rapid and shallow breathing as seen in case of left ventricular failure and ILDs.
4. Bronchial C receptors: These are present very close to bronchial circulation and its stimulation results in:
   - Rapid shallow breathing
   - Bronchoconstriction
   - Increased secretion of mucus

B. Central controlling mechanism involving brainstem which receives sensory inputs from peripheral sensory system and sends efferent signals to effector system. In the brainstem there are three groups of loosely arranged neurons—these are the following:

a. Medullary respiratory center: It is present in the reticular formation in the mid-brain in the floor of fourth ventricle and divided into two groups:

1. Dorsal group controls inspiration
2. Ventral group controls expiration

It has its own intrinsic rhythm, sends repetitive nervous impulses to respiratory muscles and diaphragm and it will maintain this basic rhythm even in absence of sensory afferent stimuli. This intrinsic rhythmicity of medullary respiratory center is characterized by a latent period followed by progressive increase in discharge of action potentials to the respiratory muscles along with progressive increase in the strength of contraction of inspiratory muscles. After this action potential from the center to inspiratory muscles will be turned off, as result process of expiration begins—it is passive relaxation of chest wall to a position of equilibrium at the level of FRC. But active relaxation begins when ventral group of neurons will begin the discharge.

b. Apneustic center: This center is present in the lower pons. It will stimulate dorsal group of neurons present in the medullary center to release progressively increasing action potentials to the inspiratory muscles. Transection above this level will produce apneustic breathing characterized by prolonged respiratory effort being interrupted by transient respiratory efforts.

c. Pneumotaxic center: This center is present in the upper pons. It is able to regulate the rate and depth of respiration by inhibiting the action potentials from the ventral group of neurons of medullary respiratory center to inspiratory muscles and thereby it act as a fine tune of the inspiratory medullary center.

d. Cortex: It will override the brainstem center and control voluntary ventilation. So in case of hyperventilation there is substantial reduction of $PaCO_2$, but voluntary hypoventilation is not strong enough because of lowered PO_2 and $PaCO_2$.

Centers in the cerebrum are influenced by limbic system of brain and hypothalamus through the effect of fear, rage, and emotion.

C. Effector system is mainly respiratory muscles and diaphragm controlling ventilation.

Other receptors are:

a. Receptors of nose and upper airways: In response to mechanical and chemical stimuli, receptors from nose, nasopharynx, larynx, and trachea produce sneezing, coughing, bronchospasm, and laryngeal spasm.
b. Receptors present in the intercostal muscles and diaphragm: Receptors present in the muscle spindles are stimulated as a result of stretch of the muscles and control the strength of contraction of respiratory muscles. Excessive stimulation of these receptors leads to uncomfortable awareness of own respiratory effort.
c. Arterial baroreceptors: Increased blood pressure causes sudden reflex hypoventilation through the stimulation of carotid and aortic baroreceptors.
d. Receptors from muscles and joints stimulate ventilation during early phase of exercise.

In case of excess respiratory muscle strength in healthy person:

In healthy person, neural input delivered to respiratory muscles will contract with adequate amount of strength to overcome the elastic loads generated in the chest wall and resistive loads provided by lung parenchyma and airways and respiration will continue indefinitely.

In case of increased load or decreased strength of respiratory muscles:

A. Increased load:
   a. Chest wall disease like kyphoscoliosis, obesity, and ascites
   b. Sleep disordered bleeding
   c. Parenchymal lung and airway disease like ILD, atelectasis, obstruction of airways, and PE
B. Decreased strength:
   a. Impaired neuromuscular transmission such as amyotrophic lateral sclerosis, phrenic nerve injury, myasthenia gravis, and lesions in the spinal cord
   b. Decreased strength of muscles such as myopathy, malnutrition, and fatigue
   c. Diminished drive like sleep disordered breathing, stroke, hypothyroidism, narcotics or sedative drug use, and alveolar hypoventilation

The result is diminished minute hypoventilation resulting in hypercapnia.

In case of increased respiratory drive with acceptable strength:

If there is excessive respiratory drive coupled with normal muscle strength in absence of any lung or chest wall disease, the result is alveolar hyperventilation leading to hypocapnia.

Clinical Features

All the features are nonspecific, which are as follows:

A. Dyspnea during daily activities and decreased exercise tolerance. In case of COPD there is excessive sputum production whereas ILD cough without mucus production.
B. Orthopnea occurs due to reduced force of respiratory muscles.
C. Again, in case of amyotrophic lateral sclerosis or muscular dystrophy there is weakness of extremities or bulbar symptoms prior to sleep disturbances.
D. Poor quality of sleep with snoring
E. Anxiety
F. Daytime somnolence
G. Early morning headache
H. Neuromuscular disease producing impaired cough. With the progress of neuromuscular weakness respiratory muscles and diaphragm will be in mechanical disadvantage mainly in supine position as the abdominal contents will move upward.

Clinical course of chronic hypoventilation in case of neuromuscular or chest wall disease:

A. In asymptomatic stage—normal daytime PaO_2 and $PaCO_2$, it is followed by nocturnal hypoventilation. It occurs during both REM and NREM sleep.
B. Finally when there is fall in VC daytime hypercapnia will develop. But the progress will depend upon the progress of respiratory muscle weakness. So, the hallmark of alveolar ventilation syndrome is increase in alveolar PCO_2 and arterial PCO_2 resulting in respiratory acidosis with compensatory rise in concentration of plasma bicarbonate.
C. Again, there is obligatory fall in alveolar pressure of oxygen resulting in hypoxemia. If hypoxemia

is severe it will lead to cyanosis and secondary erythrocytosis.

D. Combination of hypoxemia and hypercapnia produces pulmonary vasoconstriction leading to pulmonary hypertension, right ventricular hypertrophy, and right heart failure.

Diagnosis

Following two are suggestive of hypoventilation:

A. Elevated plasma bicarbonate
B. Absence of volume depletion

Arterial blood gases demonstrate in chronic hypoventilation

A. Elevated arterial PCO_2
B. Normal pH

Evaluation of etiologies of lung disease or chest wall abnormalities can be done by physical examination, proper investigations, and PFTs.

Obstruction sleep apnea syndrome which may lead to hypoventilation can be diagnosed by following tests:

A. Berlin questionnaires—these are validated.
B. Epworth Sleepiness Scale (ESS)—it measures daytime sleepiness, but score of ≥10 in any patient requires further investigations.
C. STOP-Bang questionnaires—these are not validated. These are used in case of preoperative anesthesia to assess the future risk of developing OSA; hence, they are validated in surgical clinics.

If there is no abnormality in ventilatory function and there is no increase in minute ventilation in response to hypercapnia, then there is defect in respiratory drive. It will be more marked during sleep and PSG reveals central apnea or hypopnea. In that case brain imaging can detect the structural defect in the brain.

Patients with respiratory muscle weakness can be assessed by the following measurements:

A. Maximal inspiratory and inspiratory pressure
B. FVC

These patients may also suffer from central sleep apnea or hypopnea or OSA resulting hypoxemia. So, in this group of patient night-time oximetry and capnometry during PSG will characterize the sleep disturbances.

Treatment

A. Nocturnal noninvasive positive-pressure ventilation (NIPPV): It is successfully used in following cases:
   a. Central apnea
   b. OSA
   c. Neuromuscular disorders
   d. Chest wall disorders
   e. Daytime hypercapnia

   According to the Advanced Life Support (ALS) guidelines, NIPPV is used in patients with nocturnal hypoventilation along with any one of the following criteria:
   a. $PaCO_2 \geq 45$ mm Hg
   b. Nocturnal oximetry demonstrates SaO_2 of ≤88% for 5 consecutive minutes
   c. Maximal inspiratory pressure <60 mm Hg
   d. FVC is <50% predicted
   e. Sniff nasal pressure < 40 cm of water

   But now NIPPV is used in all patients with neuromuscular or chest wall disorders demonstrating nocturnal hypercapnia but no daytime hypercapnia.
B. In some institution, pressure or volume preset modes mechanical ventilatory support is given in these patients.
C. Pharmacological therapy:
   a. Correction of metabolic alkalosis because plasma bicarbonate will elevated out of proportion of amount of chronic respiratory acidosis.
   b. Moist oxygen inhalation for correction of hypoxemia, polycythemia, and pulmonary hypertension, but in some cases it may worsen hypercapnia.
   c. In case of cervical spinal cord disorders affecting phrenic nerve, diaphragm or phrenic nerve pacing. But prior to this procedure nerve conduction studies should be performed to demonstrate to ensure that phrenic nerve bilaterally are sound.

Q32. Surfactant.

MGR/APR2014/MDI (5)

Surfactant.

MGR UNI, TAMIL NADU, 2022 (5)

ANSWER

Surfactant is produced by type II alveolar epithelial cells that show lamellar bodies on electron microscopy. These bodies after being extruded in to the alveolar liquid are spread as thin layer at the liquid-air interface. Component of the surfactant responsible for lowering of surface tension is dipalmitoylphosphatidylcholine (DPPC). This chemical is synthesized in the lung from the fatty acids extracted from the blood or synthesized in the lung. It is produced in the fetal life. In absence of this surfactant, newborn baby will develop severe respiratory distress which if not recognized or untreated may die.

Actions:

A. It prevents and stabilizes the alveoli.

B. Low-surface tension within the alveoli increases the lung compliance and at the same time will reduce the work of breathing.

C. This surfactant at the corner of the alveoli forces to draw the fluid accumulated in the interstitium and outside the capillaries thus preventing pulmonary edema.

This molecule has hydrophobic bond at one end and hydrophilic bond at other end. After alignment on the wall of the alveoli intermolecular repulsive forces will counter the attracting forces present between the liquid surface molecules thus preventing increase in the surface tension which is more marked in alveoli with smaller volumes. If the film of surfactant gets compressed, reduction in surface tension will be much more because crowded DPPC molecules will repel each other to a great extent.

Among the four surfactant proteins, surfactant proteins B and C are hydrophobic proteins, composed of 2–4% of surfactant mass. These lower the surface tension at the alveolar air fluid interface during expiration and prevent atelectasis.

Surfactant protein A is hydrophilic lectin; it regulates inflammation of lung.

Surfactant D produced by type II alveolar epithelial cells and Clara cells are responsible for removal of pathogen by binding with it.

Q33. Microscopic structure of the lung.

MGR/APR2012/MDI (5)

Describe with a schematic diagram of alveolo-capillary membrane. How will you assess functions of pulmonary interstitium?

WBUHS 2022 (10)

ANSWER

Function of pulmonary interstitium has been described in question number 25.

Lung is composed of respiratory bronchioles along with alveoli present in the wall of the bronchiole in respiratory zone of the lung. Histological section of airways demonstrates:

A. Airways: It is composed of the following layers:

a. Mucosa:

1. It is composed of pseudostratified columnar epithelial cells. These cells are several layer thick due to columnar shape and position of nuclei at variable positions in the cells. Cilia present on the surface of the mucosa propel tracheobronchial secretions along with the inhaled particle toward pharynx and thus protect the deeper airways. The ultrastructural features of the cilia are as follows:
   - Central pair of microtubules
   - Outer ring of nine double microtubules. It has following substructure:

     Small side arm known as dynein arms containing ATP dynein in the outer double microtubules. These are responsible for normal functioning of cilia.

2. In between the ciliated epithelial cells, there are mucin secreting epithelial cells, known as goblet cells, prevalent in proximal airways and decrease peripherally and absent in terminal bronchioles, produce and release large glycoprotein mucin which binds with water and other molecules and expands to form viscus mucous gel. There are two forms of mucin:
   - MUC5AC: It is produced by goblet cells and is most abundant.
   - MUC5B: It is produced by submucosal glands.

In between the epithelial cells, there are tight junctions that prevent entry of inhaled particles and to the deeper level in the airway.

3. Basal cells: These are present deep in the mucosa. These will transform, differentiate, and replenish into ciliated epithelial cells and goblet cells.
4. Club cells: These are interspersed in between ciliated epithelial cells. These act as progenitor cells for ciliated epithelial cells and serve following protective functions:
   - Synthesis of immune molecules
   - Produce some amount of mucus and surfactant proteins
   - Metabolism of inhaled chemicals
5. Kulchitsky cells or pulmonary neuroendocrine cells:
   - These are present in airway epithelium.
   - They produce serotonin, dopamine and norepinephrine and products of polypeptide as they are a part of amine uptake and decarboxylation.
   - They sense the composition of inspired gas and thus controls the regional V/Q.

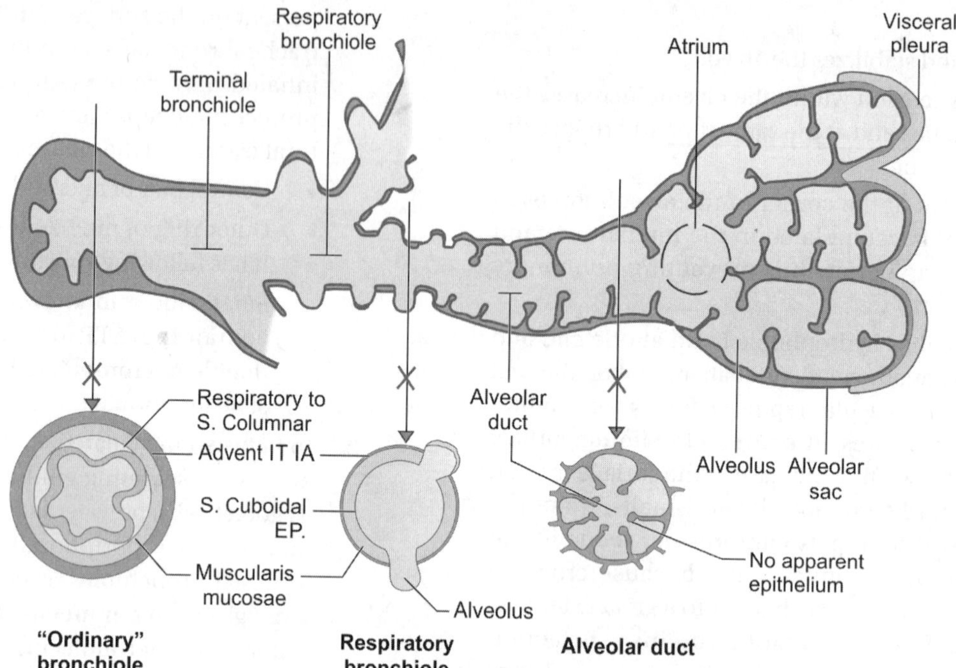

b. Submucosa: It is composed of two following structures:
   1. Bronchial mucous gland: It is present in between the band of smooth muscles.

      Base of the gland is composed of following cells:
      - Mucous cells
      - Serous cells

      Mucin secreted by this gland is composed of:
      - Mostly water
      - Mucins—mainly MUC5B
      - Immunomodulators
      - Electrolytes
      - Lipids
      - Cellular debris
   2. Smooth muscles
   3. Loose connective tissue
   4. Nerves
   5. Lymphatic vessels

c. Basement membrane in between the mucosa and submucosa

d. Fibrocartilaginous layer: It contains cartilage rings and supports the other airways.

e. Peribronchial tissue containing lymphatics and nerves within the fat

There are following changes seen from proximally to distally through the tracheobronchial tree:

a. Epithelial cells become progressively thinner ultimately to cuboidal cells at the level of terminal bronchiole.

b. The number of the goblet cells will be decreased gradually and ultimately disappear in the terminal bronchiole.

c. Club cells in the small airways are responsible for mucin production.

d. Mucous glands are present in trachea, large and medium size bronchi, gradually decrease in number distally and ultimately are absent from the level of bronchioles.

e. There is change in the configuration of smooth muscles at different levels of the tracheobronchial tree:
   1. In the trachea and large bronchi, smooth muscles are arranged spirally or in bands
   2. In smaller bronchi and bronchiole, smooth muscles encircle as a continuous layer
   3. In the distal tracheobronchial tree, smooth muscles occupy nearly total thickness of airway wall.

f. Cartilage: There are changes in the configuration of cartilage:
   1. In the trachea, it is horseshoe shaped having free of cartilage in the posterior aspect.
   2. In the bronchial wall, cartilage plate becomes smaller and distally less numerous.
   3. In the bronchiole, it is absent.

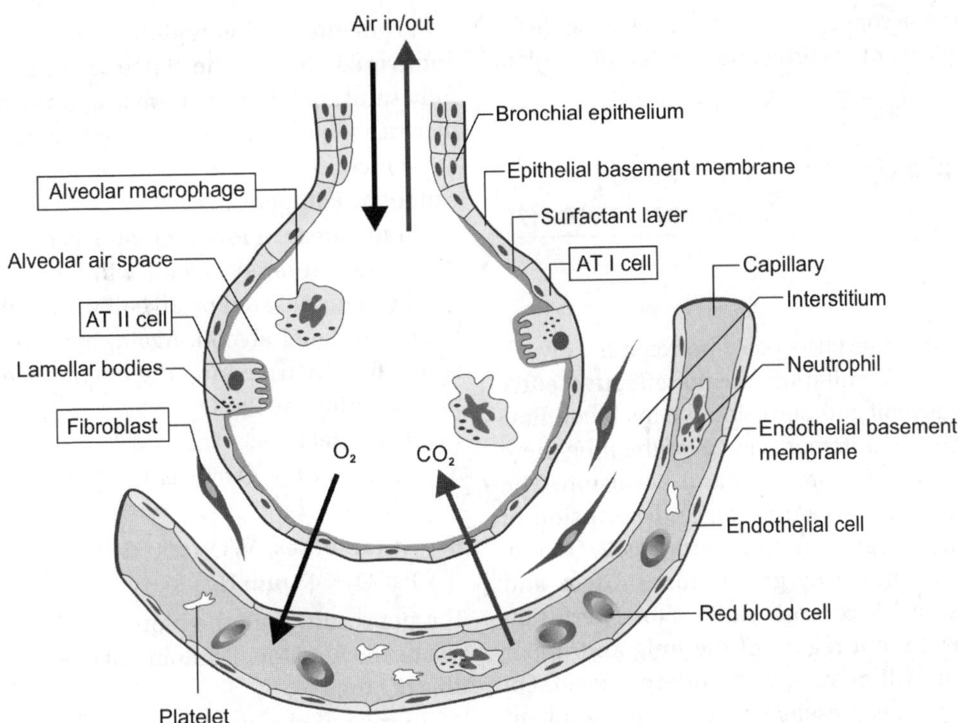

Wall of the alveoli are covered with two different types of epithelial cells:

A. Type I cells: These are less in number but their cytoplasmic extensions cover >95% of alveolar surface area and acting as barrier to prevent movement of fluid into the alveolar lumen. They have few cytoplasmic organelles and thus important for ion and fluid balance in the lung.

B. Type II cells: These are cuboidal in shape abundant in number, but due to their short cytoplasmic projection they cover only 5% of alveolar surface. They have many cytoplasmic organelles such as mitochondria, Golgi bodies, and endoplasmic reticulum for their following synthetic functions:

a. Surfactant production: Inclusion bodies known as lamellar bodies, packaged form of surfactant will be released into alveolar lumen. It is composed of protein, carbohydrate, and fat. It acts as detergent, responsible for reducing the surface tension of the alveoli.

b. Repair of alveolar epithelial surface: After damage of type I cells, type II cells become hyperplastic. Some hyperplastic type II cells will undergo apoptosis and rest of the cells will differentiate into type I cells.

c. Transport of ion and fluid by controlling trans-epithelial transport of sodium and chloride.

Along the wall of the alveolar wall pulmonary capillaries run as intercommunicating vessels. Junctions between endothelial cells of the capillaries allow small molecular weight proteins.

In between the capillary endothelial cells and alveolar epithelial cells there is basement membrane in some areas and in other areas there is presence of interstitial spaces—its major components are:

a. Collagen

b. Proteoglycans

c. Elastin

d. Nerve endings

e. Macromolecules that are involved in the interaction between cell-to-cell and cell-to-matrix

f. Fibroblast-like cells

g. Lymphocytes

h. Cells which appear as transitional state in between blood monocytes and alveolar macrophages

Within the alveolar lumen, alveolar epithelial cells are covered by:

a. Thin layer of fluid immediately adjacent to epithelial cells

b. Surface layer of surfactant produced by type II cell

c. Alveolar macrophages—these are responsible for phagocytosis of bacteria and inhaled particulate matter.

Q34. Ventilation/perfusion quotient.

MGR/APR2015/MDII (7)

ANSWER

In the lung, gas exchange takes place between the alveoli and the capillaries. Ventilation means effective entry and exit of air in alveoli and perfusion means blood flow into the capillaries. In different regions of the lung there are variable degrees of ventilation and perfusion. The collective changes in the ventilation and perfusion of different pulmonary regions are measured as V/Q ratio. Blood flow is determined by gravitational forces and hydrostatic pressure; hence larger share of total perfusion occurs in the dependent region of the lung and upper pulmonary region will be relatively underperfused. On the other hand, there is presence of ventilation gradient in lung; thus upper lung region is overventilated and dependent region will be underventilated. So the ration = is increased in apical region resulting in high PaO_2 and low $PaCO_2$ and decreased in basal regions of lung resulting in low PaO_2.

In a single alveolus:

A. If there is ventilation but there is no perfusion, in that case V/Q ratio will be infinity and that alveolus acts as dead space.

B. On the other hand if there is no ventilation but perfusion is maintained, in that case V/Q will be zero, i.e., there is presence of shunt and hemoglobin remains desaturated while leaving the capillary.

In case of alveolar-capillary unit:

A. If V/Q is infinity, i.e., ventilation but without perfusion (dead space), PAO_2 will be very high as that of air whereas $PACO_2$ will be zero as there is no perfusion and CO_2 will not enter into the alveoli. So in the dead space of lung no exchange of gas takes place between alveoli and blood.

B. If V/Q is zero, i.e., no ventilation but perfusion, in that case blood leaves the capillary as mixed venous blood (PaO_2 = 40 mm Hg but $PaCO_2$ = 46 mm Hg). So this unit acts as shunt.

In the region of high V/Q ratio, blood is fully oxygenated, i.e., hemoglobin is fully saturated but it cannot compensate the region with low V/Q ratio where hemoglobin may not be fully saturated. So net result is the hemoglobin will not be fully saturated.

From the oxyhemoglobin dissociation curve it is confirmed that in the flat upper part hemoglobin is fully saturated, here administration of oxygen only can increase the alveolar oxygen content but never boost the oxygen content of the blood. So areas of low V/Q ratio cannot be compensated.

In the areas of low V/Q ratio, capillary blood leaving the hypoventilated alveoli will have high $PaCO_2$ and can be compensated by alveoli with high V/Q ratio, i.e., hyperventilated alveoli. Again, hyperventilation will be stimulated by triggering the chemoreceptors by $PaCO_2$ thus lowering the $PaCO_2$.

In the normal lung:

A. At the apex: V/Q ratio is 3.3. PaO_2 = 132 mm Hg. $PaCO_2$ = 28 mm Hg.

B. At the bases: V/Q ratio is 0.63, PaO_2 = 90 mm Hg, $PaCO_2$ = 43 mm Hg.

The net result of all the blood coming from whole lung will be the function of amount of blood coming from each area of lung.

In case of chronic obstructive lung disease, appearance of increased amount of dead space leads to high V/Q ratio.

Q35. Enumerate the causes of pulmonary infiltrate with eosinophilia. Clinical manifestations of eosinophilic granulomatosis with polyangiitis.

DNBIIIA/JUN2016 (10)

Wegener granulomatosis.

MGR/APR2015/MDI (5)

Pulmonary infiltrate with eosinophilia and eosinophilic pneumonia.

DNB, 2022 (5)

ANSWER

Definition

Eosinophilic pneumonia can be characterized by presence of infiltrate predominantly containing eosinophils in the alveoli as consolidation which is accompanied by peripheral eosinophilia. Pathologically it can be characterized by:

a. Macroscopically solid airless gray lung tissue

b. Microscopically:

  1. Alveoli filled with eosinophils, monocytes, and macrophages

2. Eosinophilic extension into interstitial tissue and bronchial walls
3. Perivascular inflammation but without actual infiltration of vessel wall

Classification

A. Parasitic causes of eosinophilia
B. Drugs: NSAIDs
C. Pollen
D. Contact with nickel
E. Sensitization to ivy
F. Brucella infection
G. Spanish toxic oil syndrome
H. ABPA
I. Pulmonary vasculitis: Eosinophilic granulomatosis with polyangiitis or Churg–Strauss syndrome
J. Hypereosinophilic syndrome:
K. Unknown causes:
   a. Intrinsic or extrinsic asthma
   b. Acute eosinophilic pneumonia
   c. Cryptogenic chronic eosinophilic pneumonia

Eosinophilic Granulomatosis with Polyangiitis

Definition

It is characterized by the following:
   a. Eosinophil rich granulomatous inflammation involving respiratory tract
   b. Small- and medium-vessel necrotizing vasculitis
   c. Asthma
   d. Peripheral eosinophilia

Epidemiology

A. Globally incidence is 2.5 cases/year per 100,000 adults.
B. All the ages are involved but age involved is 15–70 years with mean age of 38 years.
C. It is more common in male as compared to females.

Pathophysiology

It is idiopathic but now-a-days develops secondary to number of agents i.e. there is association with use of leukotriene receptor antagonists. ICS will control asthma but masks vasculitis but withdrawal of steroids will unmask active vasculitis. Administration of leukotriene antagonist improves asthma control allowing the steroid to be tapered or stopped and thus unmasking the vasculitis. Other drugs responsible for this disease are mesalazine, freebase cocaine, and propylthiouracil.

Clinical Features

There are three phases:
A. Prodromal phase: In this phase there is allergic rhinitis and asthma
B. Eosinophilic phase: This phase of infiltrative disease like gastroenteritis or eosinophilic pneumonia.
C. Vasculitis phase: In this phase there is systemic small-to-medium vessel vasculitis along with granulomatous inflammation.

All the three phases may not be evident in all patients and in any patient these phases may not be evident in the above orders.
   a. Asthma: It is the cardinal feature, present in 98% of patients, may precede vasculitis by 3–10 years, but sometimes it will coincide with the appearance of vasculitis. Patients with persistent and chronic asthma are on steroid and mask the features of vasculitis.
   b. Paranasal sinusitis: It occurs in 60% of patients. There may be allergic rhinitis or necrotizing vascular lesions in the upper airways.
   c. Pulmonary manifestations: It occurs in 39% of patients. The features are:
      1. Transient peripheral pulmonary infiltrate
      2. Alveolar capillaritis producing hemoptysis
      3. Eosinophilic pleural effusion
      4. Rarely cavitation or consolidation
   d. Dermatologic manifestations:
      1. Palpable purpura
      2. Urticarial rash
      3. Livedo reticularis
      4. Digital ischemia
      5. Necrotic bullae
      6. Nodules
   e. Rheumatological features: Arthralgia, arthritis is rare.
   f. Renal manifestations: Pauci-immune glomerulonephritis
   g. Gastrointestinal manifestations:
      1. Abdominal pain
      2. Bloody diarrhea
      3. Abdominal crises as in Henoch–Schönlein purpura
   h. Peripheral nervous system: Mononeuritis multiplex
   i. Cardiac manifestations:
      1. Myocarditis
      2. Pericarditis
      3. Myocardial infarction

Investigations

A. Hematological features:
   a. Peripheral eosinophilia
   b. Mild anemia
   c. Raised ESR
   d. Increased CRP
   e. Increased IgE
   f. In 40% of patients, ANCA will be positive. Pattern of staining is positive for perinuclear ANCA.
B. Blood biochemistry:
   a. Serum creatinine
C. Urine for microscopy for proteinuria, microscopic hematuria, and cast
D. Radiology:
   a. Chest X-ray: It will demonstrate the following features:
      1. Bilateral transient infiltrate
      2. Localized nodular or patchy opacities that may cavitate
      3. Extensive air space consolidation signifies intra-alveolar hemorrhage
      4. Pleural effusion
E. Electromyography
F. Nerve conduction studies
G. Echocardiography
H. Holter monitoring
I. Upper gastrointestinal endoscopy to detect gastrointestinal bleeding
J. Biopsy from the different sites: It can confirm the diagnosis but not essential for the diagnosis. Depending on the involvement of the organ biopsy can be taken from lung, kidney, skin, nerves, or muscle. The following possible findings are:
   a. Small necrotizing granuloma—characterized by eosinophilic center surrounded by giant cells and macrophages
   b. Small arteries and venules involved in vasculitis
   c. In kidney, there are evidences of focal and segmental glomerulonephritis

Treatment

A. Steroid: It is the drug of choice. Dose is 1 mg/kg/day.
B. Life-threatening involvement of lung can be treated by 1 g methylprednisolone intravenously daily for 3 consecutive days followed by oral steroid.
C. Immunosuppressant can be given if there is presence of vasculitis.

Prognosis

A. 5 years survival rate is 25%.
B. Administration of steroid can improve the rate of survival to 70%.
C. Death in this case occurs due to the following:
   a. Myocarditis due to coronary arteritis
   b. Myocardial infarction due to coronary arteritis
   c. Alveolar hemorrhage
   d. Renal failure
   e. Gastrointestinal bleeding
   f. Status asthmaticus

Eosinophilic Pneumonia

Definition

It can be defined as heterogeneous group of the disorders of lung characterized by peripheral eosinophils, i.e., eosinophil count more than 500/cc along with presence of increased number of eosinophils in the bronchoalveolar lavage fluid or eosinophilic infiltration in the pulmonary parenchyma.

Etiology

A. Idiopathic
B. Drugs:
   a. Ampicillin
   b. Phenytoin
   c. Nitrofurantoin
   d. Iodides
C. Environmental triggers
D. Allergic bronchopulmonary aspergillosis
E. Hypereosinophilic syndrome
F. Smoking
G. Parasitic infection:
   a. Ascariasis
   b. Hook worms
   c. Strongyloides
   d. Toxocara

Pathophysiology

Normal eosinophil count is 0–500/cc. Main function of eosinophils are:

A. Host defense
B. Modulation of inflammation
C. Destruction of tissue.
D. Kill parasites, cancer cells, and respiratory epithelial cells.

In eosinophilic lung diseases, there is presence of eosinophils in the lung parenchyma and airways.

Three grades of eosinophilia:

A. Mild eosinophilia—500 to less than 1,500/cc.
B. Moderate eosinophilia—1,500–5,000/cc
C. Severe eosinophilia—more than 500/cc.

The following substances released from the eosinophils and activated macrophages contribute to lung damage:

A. Release of toxic granules—damage of epithelial cells and nerves.
B. Release of leukotriene and platelet activating factors—recruitment of inflammatory cells and contraction of smooth muscle cells.
C. Release of cytokines—damage of tissue along with remodeling.

Clinical Features

A. Common features are cough, fever, night sweat, and respiratory distress.
B. Acute eosinophilic pneumonia develops within 2 weeks, there may be pleuritic chest pain, and there may be feature of acute lung injury or acute respiratory distress syndrome.
C. The course is slowly progressive in case of chronic eosinophilic pneumonia. Presentation may be weight loss, progression of respiratory distress.

Evaluation

A. Idiopathic acute eosinophilic pneumonia: It is diagnosis of exclusion. The features are the following:
   a. Eosinophil count in the bronchoalveolar lavage fluid is more than 25%.
   b. Moderately elevated IgE
   c. Marked leukocytosis
   d. Restrictive ventilator defect with reduced DLCO in the pulmonary function test.
   e. Nonspecific chest X-ray with subtle ground glass appearance.
   f. Small to moderate bilateral pleural effusion
   g. Fluid analysis demonstrates high pH and marked eosinophilia.
   h. CT scan can confirm the diagnosis.
B. Chronic eosinophilic pneumonia: It is based on clinical, BAL fluid, and radiographics features:
   a. Marked eosinophilia in the bronchoalveolar lavage fluid—more than 40% of white blood cells.
   b. Moderate leukocytosis with peripheral blood eosinophilia
   c. Elevated ESR
   d. In half of the patient IgE levels are elevated.
   e. Moderate normochromic and normocytic anemia along with thrombocytosis
   f. Bilateral infiltrates in the mid and upper zones of the lung.

Treatment

A. Intravenous or oral systemic glucocorticoids are administered as soon as possible to get rapid improvement within 24 to 48 hours as there is chance of acute respiratory failure in absence of glucocorticoids. After resolution of respiratory failure the steroid should be continued for further 2 to 4 weeks. There is complete resolution of symptoms after 1 to 2 months.
B. In case of chronic eosinophilic pneumonia, oral steroids should be given for 2 to 3 weeks after resolution of symptoms. Treatment should be continued for at least 3 months and optimally for 6 to 9 months. After discontinuation of oral steroids, inhaled corticosteroid should be initiated.

Q36. Hyaline membrane disease.

MGR/MAR2009/MDIV (6)

MGR/OCT2013/MDIV (7)

Hyaline membrane disease.

MGR UNIVERSITY, TAMIL NADU, 2020 (10)

ANSWER

Introduction

It is also called infant respiratory distress syndrome in which the baby requires much more oxygen to breathe. It is the most common problem in the premature babies; it will worsen within 48–72 hours after birth but improves with treatment. 90% of patients will survive.

Pathophysiology

Surfactant is composed of four apoproteins and six phospholipids. DPPC is the principal phospholipid. Phosphatidylglycerol is 4–15% of phospholipids. It is important for maturity of lung and normal lung function. It starts producing in the fetus from 24 to 28 weeks of gestation and it starts appearing in amniotic fluid from 28 to 32 weeks of gestation. By 35 weeks adequate amount of surfactant will be produced. Surfactant will keep the alveoli open during expiration by reducing the surface tension of the alveolar wall. In absence of adequate amount of surfactant alveoli collapse, as it collapses the damaged cells will accumulate in the airways producing a membrane like structure called hyaline membrane. It is composed of proteins, cellular debris, and exudates. So the breath of the baby becomes harder and harder. As a result diffusion of gases will enormously affect producing hypoxemia and hypercapnia and respiratory acidosis. Progresses of this disease can be determined by following factors:

A. Age of the baby
B. Severity of the disease
C. Presence or absence of infection
D. Presence of patent ductus arteriosus (PDA)

Risk Factors for Hyaline Membrane Disease

A. Caucasian baby
B. Male babies
C. History of previous baby having hyaline membrane disease
D. Cesarean section
E. Perinatal infection
F. Cold stress as it will decrease the surfactant production
G. Asphyxia immediately before, during, and after birth
H. History of multiple births
I. Baby with PDA
J. Diabetic mother

Clinical Features

A. Cyanosis
B. Tachypnea
C. Flaring of nostrils
D. Difficulty in breathing at birth
E. Grunting sounds during breathing
F. Retraction of chest
G. Respiratory distress syndrome decreases with the following:
  a. Use of antenatal steroid
  b. Prolonged rupture of membrane
  c. Maternal narcotic addiction
  d. Pregnancy-induced hypertension
  e. Chronic maternal hypertension
H. Secondary deficiency of surfactant in case of infant in following cases:
  a. Intrapartum asphyxia
  b. Pulmonary hemorrhage
  c. Meconium aspiration pneumonia
  d. Oxygen toxicity due to barotrauma
  e. Congenital diaphragmatic hernia
  f. Pulmonary infections

Complications of Hyaline Membrane Disease

A. Leaking of air from the lung into the following structures:
  a. Pneumomediastinum
  b. Pneumopericardium
  c. Pneumothorax
B. Pulmonary interstitial emphysema
C. Bronchopulmonary dysplasia
D. Pulmonary hemorrhage
E. Septicemia
F. Apnea
G. Bradycardia
H. Retinopathy of prematurity
I. Failure to thrive
J. Necrotizing enterocolitis
K. Intraventricular hemorrhage
L. Periventricular leukomalacia
M. Hematologic problems such as anemia and polycythemia
N. Metabolic complications such as hypoglycemia and hypothermia

Diagnosis

A. Fetal lung maturity test: It can be estimated by estimation of lecithin to sphingomyelin ratio.
B. Testing the presence of phosphatidylglycerol in the amniotic fluid during amniocentesis.
C. Blood gases demonstrate:
  a. Metabolic and respiratory acidosis
  b. Hypoxia from right to left shunting through the pulmonary vessels.
D. Chest X-ray demonstrates:
  a. Bilateral diffuse reticular granular or ground-glass shadowing
  b. Poor expansion of lung
  c. Prominent bronchioles in the background of collapsed alveoli
  d. Cardiomegaly due to prenatal asphyxia, maternal diabetes, poor expansion of lung, or PDA
E. Echocardiography: It will demonstrate:
  a. Presence of PDA
  b. Pulmonary hypertension

F. Pulmonary function testing:

- **a.** Decrease in lung compliance
- **b.** Airway resistance may be normal or increased

Treatment

A. Nasal CPAP in case of spontaneously breathing premature infants immediately after delivery as it will prevent immediate intubation as well as replacement of surfactant to decrease bronchopulmonary dysplasia.

B. Corticosteroids: One course of steroid will reduce the incidence of respiratory distress syndrome and neonatal death. It should be given in case of premature delivery of the baby. If the mother does not deliver the baby within 1 week then another course of steroid is given.

C. Surfactant: It will reduce the mortality by 50%. Early administration of surfactant followed by removal of nasal catheter will decrease the need for mechanical ventilation and decrease the pulmonary leakage. Dose is 50–200 mg/kg. Bolus administration of surfactant after adequate recruitment of lung with administration of 3–4 cm PEEP will distribute the surfactant homogeneously throughout the lung. Most of the neonates require two doses but as many as four doses can be administered at 6–12-hour interval. If the neonate improves after single dose, respiratory distress is unlikely, but if the neonate fails to improve after full course then following factors should be excluded:

- **a.** Infections like pneumonia
- **b.** PDA
- **c.** Complications of ventilation

Q37. Radiological presentation and clinical classification of bronchogenic carcinoma.

MGR/OCT2012/MDIV (7)

Small cell lung cancer (SCLC).

MGR/MAR2008/MDI (5)

Molecular genetics in lung carcinoma.

MGR/MAR2007/MDI (5)

Staging of lung cancer.

MUHS/MAY2011/MDIII (10)

Discuss cytological basis, tumor, node, and metastasis (TNM) staging, clinical features, laboratory findings, and management of lung cancer.

MGR/OCT2011/MDII (25)

Write targeted therapy in lung cancer.

WBUHS, 2020 (10)

ANSWER

Molecular Genetics in Case of Lung Carcinoma

All cancer cells usually acquire six hallmark capabilities, these are as following:

- **A.** Self-sufficiency in growth signals
- **B.** Insensitivity to antigrowth signals
- **C.** Evading apoptosis
- **D.** Limitless replicative potential
- **E.** Sustained angiogenesis
- **F.** Tissue invasion and metastasis

These orders of hallmark capabilities vary from tumor to tumor. Cancer arises from increased accumulation of gain-of-function of oncogenes and at the same time loss-of-function of tumor-suppressor genes.

In case of lung cancer the cell of origin is not known, but according to evidence:

- **a.** Alveolar epithelial cells or type II epithelial cells give rise to lung adenocarcinoma.
- **b.** In case of small cell lung carcinoma neuroendocrine cell is the cell of origin.

According to stem cell theory:

In a tumor, small subsets of cells are known as stem cells which are responsible for the full malignant behavior of the tumor, large bulk of the cells are the off-springs of the stem cells. Again, most of the cells clonally related to stem cells cannot regenerate to malignancy phenotype. This theory proves that even total cancer therapy fails to eradicate the stem cells from the body in spite of complete clinical response; hence disease recurs and it may be more resistant to targeted therapy.

Lung cancer cells harbor multiple chromosomal abnormalities like:

- **a.** Deletion
- **b.** Insertion
- **c.** Mutation
- **d.** Amplification
- **e.** Translocations

Earliest sets of oncogenes found to be aberrant was MYC family of transcription; these are:

- **a.** MYC
- **b.** MYCN
- **c.** MYCL

Among them MYC is frequently activated by amplification and transcriptional dysregulation of gene in case of small cell and non-small cell carcinoma and there is no MYC-specific drug till date.

Adenocarcinoma has been extensively studied for genomic gains and losses and somatic mutations. Among the different kinds of aberrations "driver mutations" involve major class where mutations occur in genes encoding signaling proteins which are responsible for initiation and maintenance of tumor cells.

One set of mutation involves epidermal growth factor receptor (EGFR) belonging to ERBB or HER family of proto-oncogenes that involves:

- **a.** ERBB1 or EGFR
- **b.** ERBB2 or HER2
- **c.** ERBB3 or HER3
- **d.** ERBB4 or HER4

These genes will encode cell surface receptors which consist of two domains, these are:

- **a.** An extracellular ligand binding
- **b.** An intracellular tyrosine kinase domain

When ligand binds to receptor, it will activate dimerization and autophosphorylation of tyrosine kinase that initiate cascade of intracellular events leading to:

- **a.** Increased cellular proliferation
- **b.** Angiogenesis
- **c.** Local and distant metastasis
- **d.** Decreased apoptosis

Lung adenocarcinoma arises as a result of expression of mutant EGFR. It is also sensitive to EGFR-tyrosine kinase inhibitors.

Other examples of driver mutations in case of lung adenocarcinoma are:

- **a.** GTPase KRAS
- **b.** Serine-threonine kinase BRAF
- **c.** Lipid kinase PIK3CA

Recently, a new subset of lung adenocarcinoma has been identified due to aberrant activation of tyrosine kinase ALK, ROS1, NTRK, and RET in presence of chromosomal rearrangement.

In case of lung cancer, most of the driver mutations are exclusive—it suggests acquisition of any one of these mutation is sufficient for genesis of tumor.

Recently three possible targets are found for squamous cell carcinoma of lung, these are:

- **a.** FGFE1 amplification
- **b.** DDR2 mutation
- **c.** PIK3CA mutations or PTEN loss

Following suppressor genes are inactivated during the process of tumorigenesis:

- **a.** TP53
- **b.** RB1
- **c.** RASSF1A
- **d.** LKB1
- **e.** CDKN2A/B
- **f.** FHIT

90% of small cell lung carcinoma harbor mutation of RB1 and TP53.

Cytological Basis of Lung Cancer

Main diagnosis of lung cancer is based on morphological and cytological features which are correlated with clinical as well as radiological features.

Immunohistochemistry is used:

A. To verify any neuroendocrine differentiation within the tumor with the help of following markers:

- **a.** Neuron-specific enolase (NSE)
- **b.** CD56
- **c.** NCAM
- **d.** Synaptophysin
- **e.** Chromogranin
- **f.** Leu7

B. To differentiate primary from metastatic adenocarcinoma.

Thyroid transfer factor-1 (TTF1) is present in both thyroid and pulmonary tumor. It is positive in 70% lung adenocarcinoma and if primary thyroid tumor has been excluded, then it can be accepted as reliable marker of primary lung cancer. But negative TTF1 cannot exclude the possibility of lung as primary.

Napsin-A (Nap-A), aspartic protease, is important in the maturation of surfactant B7 and it expressed in the cytoplasm of type II pneumocytes. It is present in >90% of adenocarcinoma.

Both TTF-1 ND Nap-A can differentiate:

A. Primary adenocarcinoma where both are positive

B. Primary lung squamous cell carcinoma where both are negative

C. Small cell lung carcinoma where TTF-1 is positive but Nap-A negative

Again cytokeratin 7 (CK-7) and cytokeratin 20 (CK-20) are used for narrowing the diagnosis:

A. Squamous cell carcinoma, non-small cell carcinoma, small cell lung carcinoma, and mesothelioma are positive for CK-7 but negative for CK-20

B. Squamous cell carcinoma is negative for CK-20 and CK-7

P63 is a useful marker for non-small cell carcinoma with squamous differentiation

Mesothelioma is difficult to differentiate from adenocarcinoma by morphology and immunohistochemistry. But CK-5/6, calretinin, and Wilms tumor gene-1 are positive for mesothelioma.

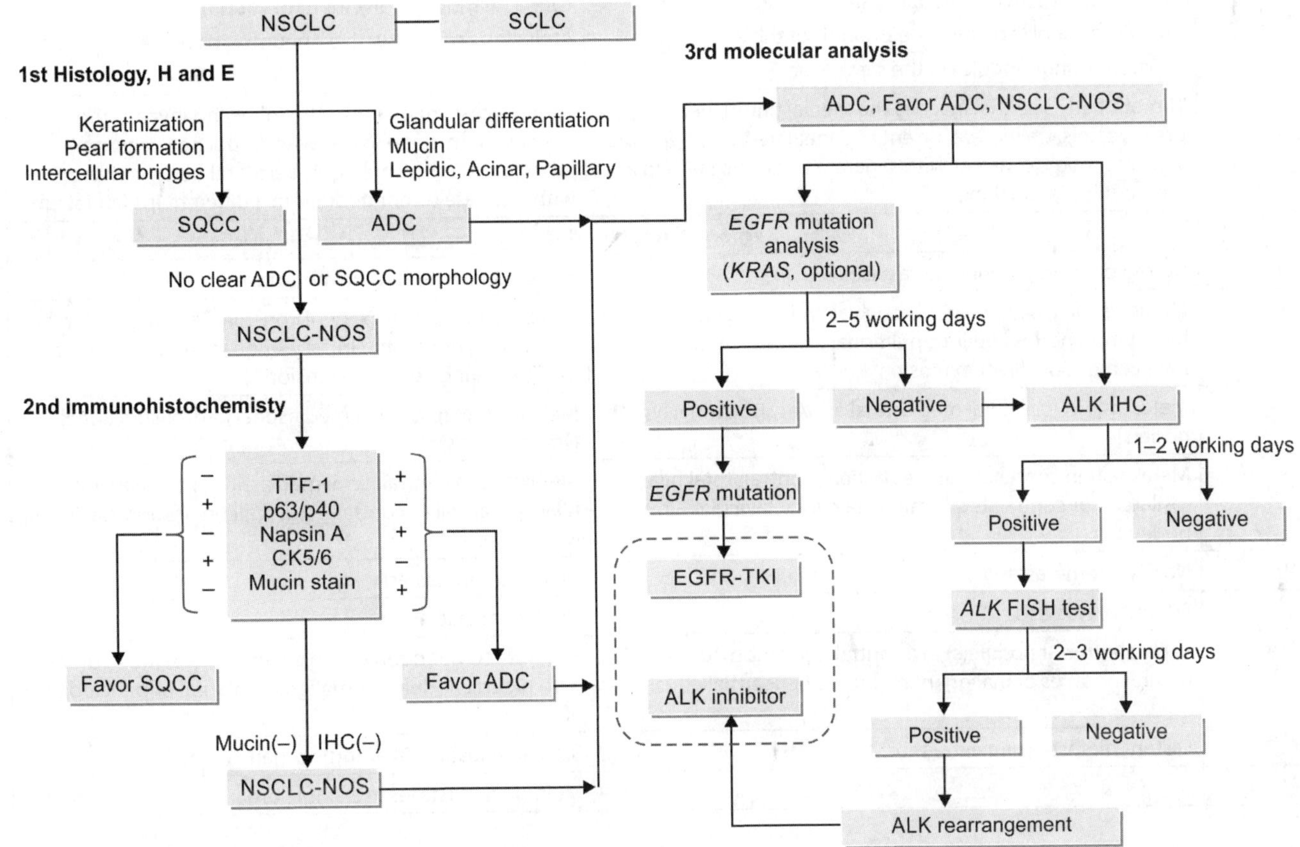

TNM Staging of Nonsmall Cell Lung Cancer

Primary tumor		
Primary tumor (T)	TNM staging (7th edition)	TNM staging (8th edition)
T1	Tumor ≤ 3 cm in diameter, surrounded by lung or visceral pleura, without invasion more proximal than lobar bronchus	T1 tumor ≤ 3 cm in diameter surrounds by lung and visceral pleura without evidence of main bronchus
T1a	Tumor ≤ 2 cm in diameter	Tumor < 1 cm
T1b	Tumor > 2 cm, but ≤ 3 cm in diameter	Tumor ≥ 1 cm but ≤ 2 cm
T1c	NA	Tumor > 2 cm but ≤ 3 cm
T2	Tumor > 3 cm but ≤ 7 cm or tumor with any of the following features: Involves bronchus ≥ 2 cm distal to pleura Invades visceral pleura Associated with atelectasis or obstructive pneumonitis that extends to the hilar region but does not involve the entire lung	T2 tumor > 3 cm but ≤ 5 cm or tumor with any of the following features that does not involve the entire lung Involves bronchus ≥ 2 cm distal to pleura Invades visceral pleura Associated with atelectasis or obstructive pneumonitis that extends to the hilar region

Continued

Continued

T2a	Tumor > 3 cm but ≤ 5 cm	Tumor > 3 cm but ≤ 4 cm
T2b	Tumor >5 cm but ≤ 7 cm	Tumor >4 cm but ≤ 5 cm
T3	Tumor > 7 cm or any of the following: Directly invades any of the following: Diaphragm, chest wall, phrenic nerve, mediastinal pleura, parietal pericardium, and main bronchus < 2 cm from the carina (without involvement of carina) Atelectasis or obstructive pneumonitis of the entire lung Separate tumor nodules in the same lobe	Tumor > 5 cm but ≤ 7 cm or any of the following: Directly invades any of the following: Diaphragm, chest wall, phrenic nerve, mediastinal pleura, parietal pericardium, and main bronchus < 2 cm from the carina (without involvement of carina) Atelectasis or obstructive pneumonitis of the entire lung
T4	Tumor of any size that invades the mediastinum, heart, great vessels, trachea, recurrent laryngeal nerve, esophagus, vertebral body, carina or with separate tumor nodules in a different ipsilateral lobe	Tumor size 7 cm or any of the following invades the mediastinum, heart, great vessels, trachea, recurrent laryngeal nerve, esophagus, vertebral body, carina or with separate tumor nodules in a different ipsilateral lobe
Regional lymph nodes		
N0	No regional lymph node metastases	No regional lymph node metastases
N1	Metastasis in ipsilateral peribronchial and/or ipsilateral hilar lymph nodes and intrapulmonary nodes, including involvement by direct extension	Metastasis in ipsilateral peribronchial and/or ipsilateral hilar lymph nodes and intrapulmonary nodes, including involvement by direct extension
N2	Metastasis in ipsilateral mediastinal and/or subcarinal lymph node(s)	Metastasis in ipsilateral mediastinal and/or subcarinal lymph node(s)
N3	Metastasis in contralateral mediastinal, contralateral hilar, ipsilateral or contralateral scalene or supraclavicular lymph node(s)	Metastasis in contralateral mediastinal, contralateral hilar, ipsilateral or contralateral scalene or supraclavicular lymph node(s)
M0	No distant metastasis	No distant metastasis
M1	Distant metastasis	Distant metastasis
M1a	Separate tumor nodule(s) in a contralateral lobe, tumor with pleural nodules or malignant pleural or pericardial effusion	Separate tumor nodule(s) in a contralateral lobe, tumor with pleural nodules or malignant pleural or pericardial effusion
M1b	Distant metastasis (in extra thoracic organs)	Single metastasis in a single organ
M1c		Multiple metastases in a single organ or in several organs

Staging of Small Cell Lung Cancer

According to the American Joint Committee on Cancer: SCLC has been divided into two stages:

A. Limited stage: It is confined to ipsilateral hemithorax and it will be encompassed within tolerable radiation port. Hence, contralateral supraclavicular nodes, involvement of recurrent laryngeal nerve, and superior vena caval obstruction are all part of limited disease.

B. Extensive disease: It is characterized by overt metastases demonstrated by both physical and imaging system. Hence, cardiac tamponade, bilateral pulmonary parenchymal involvement, and malignant pleural effusion are described as extensive diseases.

Physiologic Staging

In patients with lung cancer other than smoking, cardiovascular disease and COPD are the comorbid conditions.

To improve preoperative conditions following conditions have to be addressed:

A. Correctable conditions such as anemia, arrhythmias, fluid and electrolyte imbalance, and infections

B. Smoking

C. FEV_1 if >2 L or >80% of predicted value—patient can tolerate pneumonectomy

D. If FEV_1 is >1.5 L but <2 L then patient can tolerate lobectomy

E. If FEV_1 is borderline, then cardiopulmonary exercise testing is performed

F. If the maximum oxygen consumption is <15 mL/kg/min then patient is at risk of postoperative complication.

Clinical Features

Patient's presenting features depend upon the following:

A. Primary lesion:
   a. Adenocarcinoma is within the lung parenchyma and peripherally situated; hence there may be delay in local intrathoracic symptoms.
   b. In case of squamous cell carcinoma, it is confined to the thorax for longer time; hence intrathoracic spread and local lung related symptoms are more common.
   c. In case of small cell carcinoma, it arise from central airways and spread is fast and quickly metastasize; hence presenting symptoms may be locally or distant related.

B. Local tumor growth
C. Invasion of adjacent structures
D. Obstruction of the adjacent structures
E. Growth at distant metastatic sites
F. Paraneoplastic syndrome

So the symptoms are as follows:

A. Cough: Dry cough may occur due to:
   a. Tumor in the central airways producing narrowing of the bronchial lumen
   b. Involvement of major central airways, carina, main bronchi, and lobar bronchi
   c. Impairment of mucociliary clearance
   d. Development of pneumonia distal to airway obstruction
   e. Complete bronchial obstruction producing atelectasis of the involved lobe produces cough along with respiratory distress.

   Type of cough or change in character of cough mainly in smokers.

   Ulcerating or obstructing lesions present in the large bronchus—dry brassy cough accompanied by noisy breathing, stridor along with wheeze.

   Productive cough having yellow-colored sputum:
   a. Due to infection.
   b. Excessive bronchorrhea seen in:
      1. Invasive adenocarcinoma
      2. Bronchoalveolar carcinoma

B. Hemoptysis: It occurs in 5–10% of patients, is rarely profuse, and sometimes there may be streak of blood on the sputum mainly in the mornings.

C. Dyspnea: Dyspnea, productive cough are present in 25% of patients. It may occur in:
   a. Progressive obstruction in a major bronchus
   b. Increasing obstructive emphysema of a lobe in case of involvement of lobar bronchus.

   It may be associated with monophonic inspiratory wheeze (Chevalier sign)

   There are other causes of dyspnea:
   a. Pneumonia distal to obstructive lesion
   b. Lobar atelectasis
   c. Pleural effusion
   d. Extensive involvement of lung parenchyma
   e. Left vocal cord paralysis
   f. Extensive pressure on large airways due to extensive mediastinal involvement

D. Chest pain:
   a. Dull aching or ill-defined intermittent or continuous pain results from tumor involvement of the chest wall, mediastinum, pleura, and vertebral body.
   b. Pleural pricking aggravated during respiration in case of pleural involvement.
   c. In case of superior sulcus tumor, i.e., Pancoast tumor arising in the apex of the lung produces shoulder pain with radiation along the arm.

E. Wheeze: It is a symptom of central airways obstruction. There is fixed monophonic wheeze which can be differentiated from bronchial asthma or chronic bronchitis that produces polyphonic wheeze.

F. Systemic features:
   a. Fever of low grade
   b. Weight loss
   c. Lassitude
   d. Anorexia

In case of intrathoracic spread:

A. Involvement of left recurrent laryngeal nerve producing hoarseness
B. Involvement of sympathetic trunk produces Horner's syndrome characterized by partial ptosis on the affected side, small pupil, absence of sweating on the ipsilateral half of the face, and loss of ciliospinal reflex.
C. Superior vena caval syndrome due to occlusion of superior vena cava by:
   a. Tumor
   b. Thrombus due to slow flowing of blood
   c. Extrinsic pressure or infiltration of the venous wall by infiltration of the wall or by pressure
   d. It occurs in small cell carcinoma
   e. It is characterized by:
      1. Puffiness of face
      2. Plethoric face with congested conjunctiva
      3. Engorged poorly pulsatile jugular vein

4. Presence of collaterals visible in the upper part of the chest

f. Malignant mediastinal lymphadenopathy due to spreading of tumor cells by:
   1. Lymphatics
   2. Blood
   3. Direct extension

g. Dysphagia due:
   1. Pressure of the malignant nodes
   2. Direct invasion of the tumor

h. Pericardial involvement producing features of pericardial effusion, cardiac tamponade, and arrhythmias.

i. Involvement of chest wall or vertebrae producing chest pain, back pain occurs due to:
   1. Direct extension of tumor
   2. Blood borne spread

Superior sulcus tumor at the vault of the pleura and the apex of the lung produces shoulder pain radiating down the arm toward the finger. It may be associated with erosions involving:

a. Posterior portion of 1st and 2nd ribs
b. 7th cervical, 1st and 2nd dorsal vertebrae

There may be involvement of sympathetic trunk producing Horner's syndrome.

Distant Extrathoracic Manifestations

It occurs in 50% of squamous cell carcinoma, 80% of adenocarcinoma and large cell carcinoma, and 90% of small cell carcinoma. Features may occur according to organ involvement. Features are as follows:

A. Brain metastasis present with:
   a. Headache
   b. Nausea
   c. Vomiting
   d. Seizures
   e. Neurological deficit

B. Bone metastases may present with:
   a. Pain
   b. Pathological fractures
   c. Features of cord compression
   d. Epidural metastasis

C. Features of bone marrow involvement are:
   a. Leukoerythroblastosis
   b. Cytopenias

D. Liver metastasis presents with:
   a. Hepatomegaly with normal LFT
   b. Right upper quadrant pain
   c. Anorexia
   d. Weight loss
   e. Jaundice in case of biliary obstruction by enlarged metastatic glands at the porta hepatis upon bile duct

E. Adrenal metastasis in case of small cell carcinoma rarely produces adrenal insufficiency

Paraneoplastic Syndrome

A. Hypercalcemia: It occurs in case of squamous cell carcinoma due to:
   a. Multiple bony metastases
   b. Parathyroid hormone-related protein
   c. Calcitriol
   d. Cytokines

   Clinical features are nausea, vomiting, lethargy, dehydration, constipation, polyuria, confusion, drowsiness, and coma. Cardiovascular effects are shortened QT interval, heart block, ventricular arrhythmias, and ultimately cardiac arrest.

B. SIADH: It occurs in 10% of SCLC patients due to:
   a. Inappropriate secretion of ADH
   b. Increased secretion of atrial natriuretic peptide (ANP)

   Diagnostic criteria are:
   a. Hyponatremia—serum sodium is <135 mEq/L
   b. Plasma osmolality < 280 mOsmol/kg
   c. Inappropriately concentrated urine i.e. > 100 mOsmol/kg of water
   d. Urine sodium > 20 mEq/L
   e. Clinical euvolemia
   f. Normal function of adrenal, thyroid, and renal function

   Clinical features are:
   a. Vomiting
   b. Drowsiness
   c. Confusion
   d. Coma
   e. Seizures

C. Ectopic corticotropin hormone syndrome occurs due to SCLC tumor. It is observed in:
   a. Carcinoid tumor of lung
   b. Neuroblastoma
   c. Thymic tumor
   d. Medullary thyroid carcinoma

Features suggestive of ectopic corticotropin production are:

a. Marked elevation of urinary cortisol, i.e., >500 μg/24 hours
b. Plasma corticotropin >200 pg/mL

D. Dermatomyositis polymyositis

E. Clubbing and hypertrophic pulmonary osteoarthropathy: It is characterized by:

a. Periostitis
b. Painful arthropathy
c. Marked finger clubbing

Features are:

a. Pain, tenderness, and swelling over the affected bones
b. Radiologically distal ends of radius, ulna, tibia, and fibula

F. Hyperthyroidism

G. Gynecomastia

H. Pigmentation due to α- and β-melanocyte stimulation

I. Hyperglycemia or hypoglycemia

J. Growth hormone excess

K. Galactorrhea

L. Neurologic syndrome:

a. Peripheral neuropathy—painful, sensory, or sensory motor neuropathy
b. Lambert–Eaton syndrome
c. Myasthenic syndrome
d. Cerebellar degeneration
e. Encephalomyelopathy
f. Cerebellar degeneration

Paraneoplastic syndrome is immune mediated, hence a number of autoantibodies are identified, and these are:

A. Antinuclear neuronal antibody I (ANNA I) associated with SCLC

B. Antinuclear neuronal antibody II (ANNA II) associated with SCLC

C. CRMP-5 associated with SCLC and thymoma

D. Anti-Purkinje antibody (anti-Yo) associated with ovarian cancer and breast cancer

Lambert–Eaton myasthenic syndrome due to impaired release of acetylcholine at the motor nerve endings due to antibodies against P/Q type presynaptic voltage-gated calcium channels—It is characterized by:

a. Weakness of the muscles
b. Depressed tendon reflexes
c. Autonomic disturbances

This disease is associated with allotypes Gm2 and HLA-B8.

Diagnosis

Tissue diagnosis:

A. Tissue diagnosis is the preferred method of diagnosis in case of lung cancer. A core biopsy is preferred to adequate tissue diagnosis and it can be obtained in the following ways:

a. Bronchial biopsy
b. Transbronchial biopsy
c. Fiberoptic bronchoscopy FNAC
d. Percutaneous biopsy under image guidance
e. Endobronchial ultrasound

B. Depending upon the location of lymph node it can be sampled by:

a. Transesophageal endoscopic ultrasound-guided biopsy
b. Endoscopic biliary ultrasound
c. Blind biopsy

C. In case of clinically palpable lymph node or skin metastasis, biopsy can be taken directly from the sites.

a. Lymph nodes
b. The soft tissue mass
c. Lytic bone lesions
d. Pleura
e. Bone marrow
f. Liver
g. Adequate cell block from suspected malignant pleural effusion, if required; repeated thoracentesis is required.

Diagnosis of yield depends upon following factors:

a. Type of tumor
b. Location of tumor
c. Size of the tumor
d. Technical aspect of the procedure like experience of bronchoscopist and pathologist

Bronchoscopic examination is necessary in case of centrally located lesions like:

a. Squamous carcinoma
b. SCLC
c. Endobronchial tumor-like carcinoid tumor

Transthoracic biopsy is required for:

a. Adenocarcinoma of lung
b. Large cell carcinoma

Bronchial specimen includes:

a. Bronchial wash
b. Bronchial brush
c. Bronchoalveolar lavage
d. Transbronchial FNA
e. Core biopsy

More tissue is required for:

- **a.** More accurate histological classification
- **b.** Mutation analysis
- **c.** Investigational purpose

Sensitivity of bronchoscopic and tissue biopsy is 85–90%. Sensitivity is highest for larger lesions and peripheral lesions. Core biopsy specimen is superior to other specimen.

Sputum cytology:

It is inexpensive and noninvasive but its value in diagnosis is of low yield due to poor preservation of cells and less capability of obtaining the good specimen. The yield is higher in case of centrally located lesion like SCLC and squamous cell carcinoma. The chance or more positivity is more in case of repeated sampling.

Bronchoscopy: By this method:

- **a.** A tumor arising within lobar bronchus can be removed by lobectomy
- **b.** If the tumor extends into the main bronchus and the tumor is >1 cm away from the carina—pneumonectomy
- **c.** Spreading of tumor to mediastinal structures in the form of widening and fixity of the carina, subcarinal nodes involvement, inwards pressure on the lateral bronchial and tracheal wall by enlarged paratracheal glands—suggests unresectability.

Positron emission tomography:

It can detect distant metastasis for extrathoracic as well as intrathoracic staging. Specificity is 88% and sensitivity is 94%.

False-positive results can occur in following cases:

- **a.** Tuberculosis
- **b.** Fungal infection
- **c.** Sarcoidosis
- **d.** Inflammatory disorders
- **e.** Rheumatoid nodules

False-negative results are obtained in following cases:

- **a.** Alveolar cell carcinoma
- **b.** Carcinoids
- **c.** Tumor of <1 cm in size

Treatment

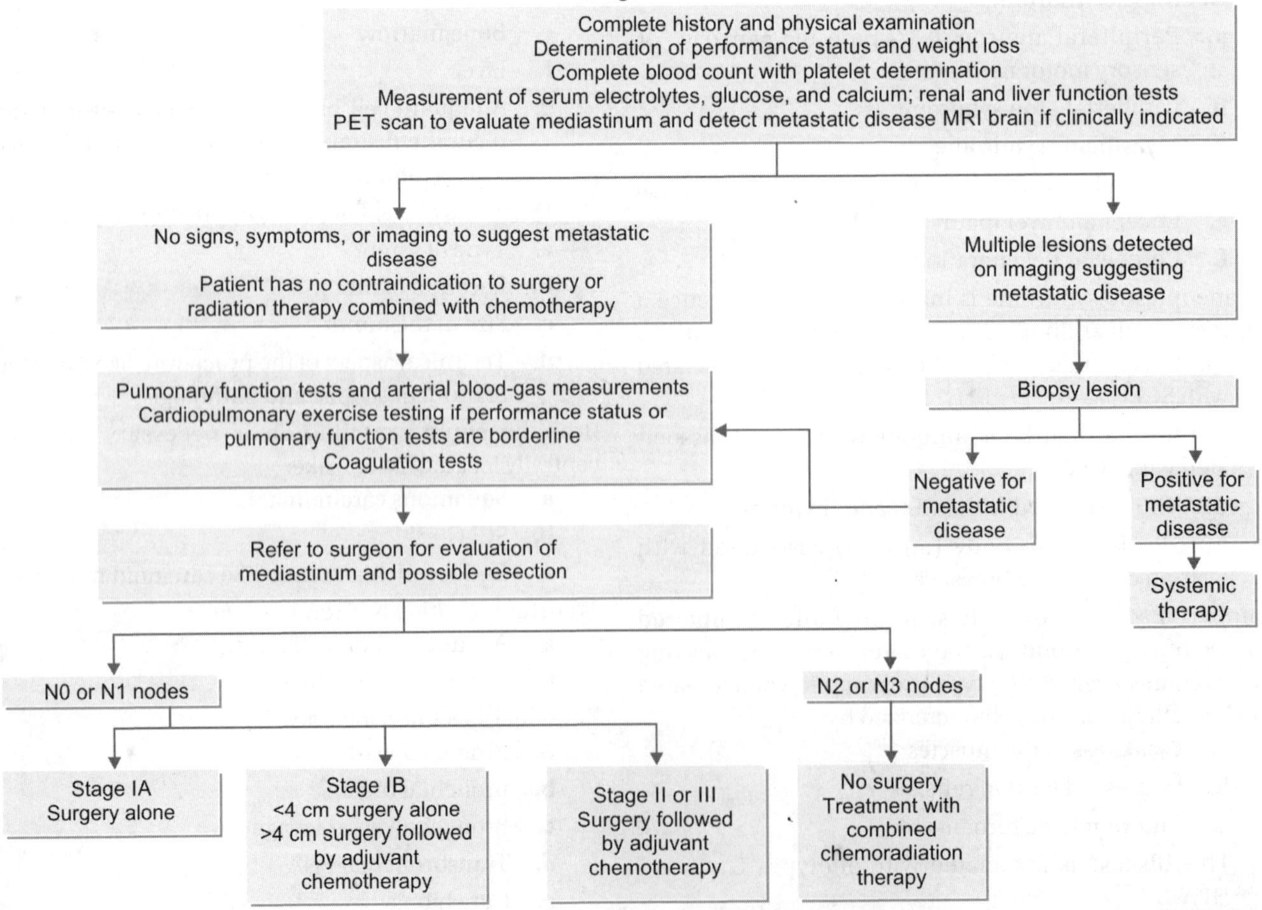

Continued

Continued

Management of small-cell lung cancer

Complete history and physical examination
Determination of performance status and weight loss
Complete blood count with platelet determination
Measurement of serum electrolytes, glucose, and calcium; renal and liver function tests
PET scan to evaluate for metastatic disease
MRI of brain

- No signs, symptoms, or imaging to suggest metastatic disease
  - Patient has no contraindication to combined chemotherapy and radiation therapy → Combined modality treatment with platinum-based therapy and etoposide and radiation therapy
  - Patient has contraindication to combined chemotherapy and radiation therapy → Sequential treatment with chemotherapy and radiation therapy
- Metastatic disease suspected on imaging or laboratory work → Biopsy most distant site of disease
  - Negative for metastatic disease → (back to: Patient has contraindication to combined chemotherapy and radiation therapy)
  - Positive for metastatic disease → Chemotherapy alone and/or radiation therapy for palliation of symptoms

Note: Regardless of disease stage, patients who have a good response to initial therapy should be considered for prophylactic cranial irradiation after therapy is completed.

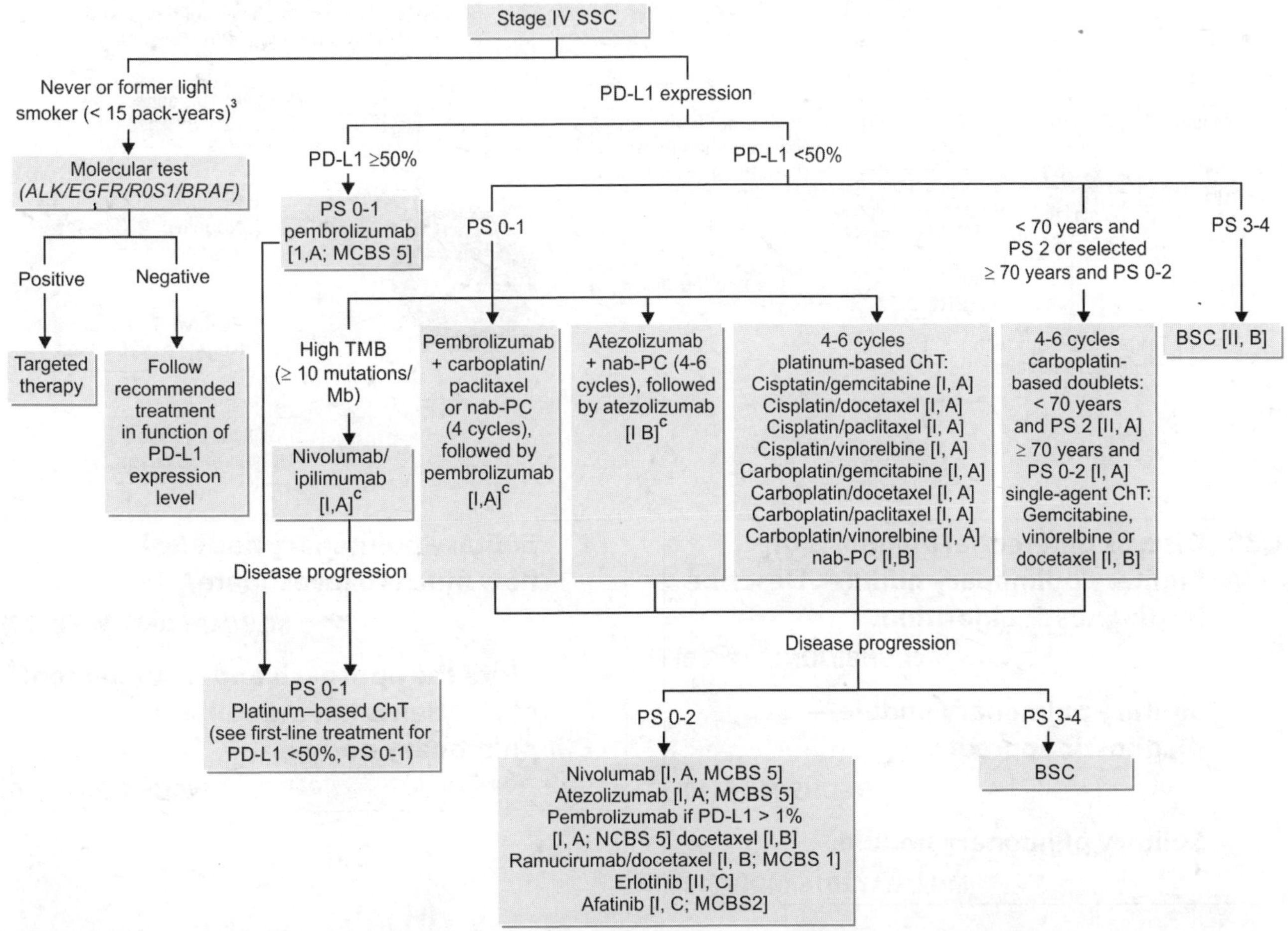

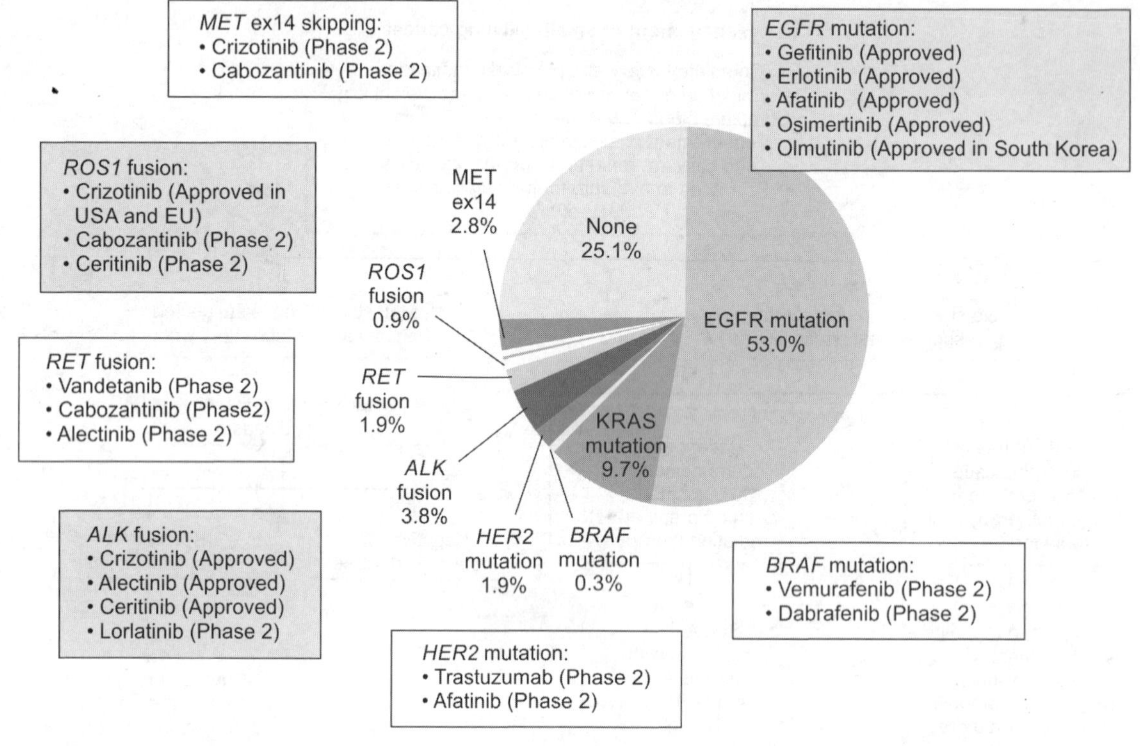

Common mutations in lung Ca driving targeted therapy

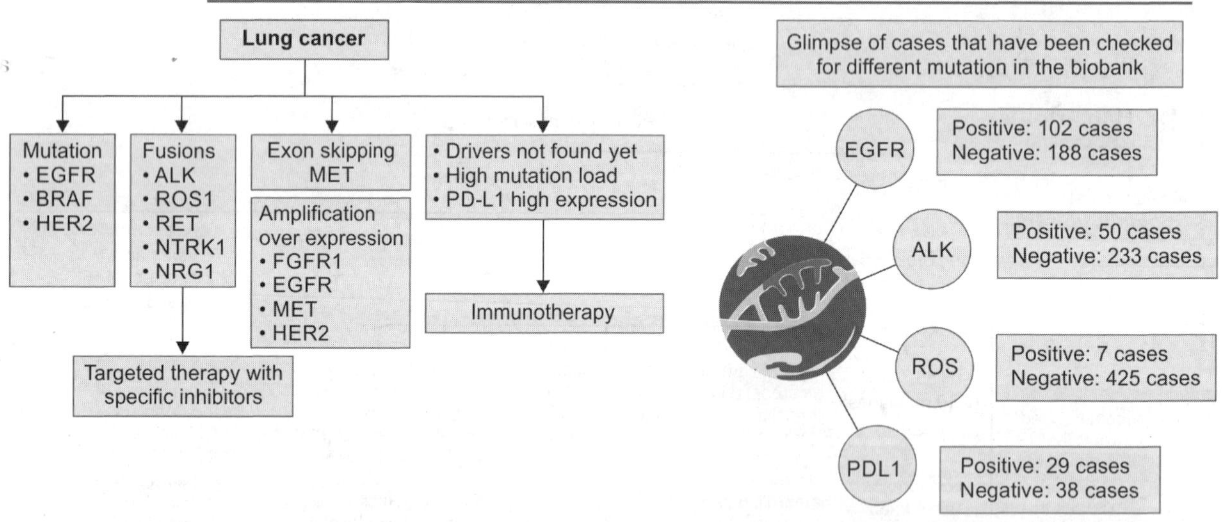

Q38. Discuss differential diagnosis of "solitary pulmonary nodule". Describe its diagnostic algorithm.

DNBI/JUN2012 (10)

Solitary pulmonary nodule—diagnostic approach.

RGUHS/MDII (10)

Solitary pulmonary nodule.

MUZ/MAY2016/MDIV (10)

Solitary pulmonary nodule: How and how much to investigate?

MLB/MAY2009/MDIII (30)

Write the approach and management of a patients having solitary pulmonary nodule.

WBUHS, 2024 (10)

ANSWER

Definition

Solitary pulmonary nodule can be defined as round well-marginated opacification having 3 cm in diameter present in the pulmonary parenchyma.

Differential Diagnosis of Pulmonary Nodule

Causes	Conditions
Congenital	Bronchogenic cyst, sequestration, and bronchial atresia with mucoid impaction
Benign causes	Arteriovenous malformation and hamartoma
Malignant causes	Small cell carcinoma, non-small cell carcinoma, lymphoma, and single metastasis from breast, colon, and kidney
Inflammatory infectious	Abscess, pneumonia, septic embolus, and granuloma
Noninfectious inflammatory	Rheumatoid nodule, amyloidosis, Wegener granulomatosis, subpleural nodule, focal scarring, and infarction

Approach to Diagnosis

Clinical history:

A. Age:
- **a.** Children:
  - **1.** Hamartoma
  - **2.** Bronchogenic cyst
  - **3.** Pneumonia
  - **4.** Lung abscess
- **b.** Young adult:
  - **1.** Pneumonia
  - **2.** Lung abscess
  - **3.** Bronchogenic carcinoma
  - **4.** Lymphoma
  - **5.** Granulomatous disease
  - **6.** Collagen vascular disease
- **c.** Elderly:
  - **1.** Bronchogenic carcinoma
  - **2.** Lymphoma
  - **3.** Metastasis
  - **4.** Amyloidosis

B. Sex:
- **a.** Male: Small cell carcinoma
- **b.** Female:
  - **1.** Adenocarcinoma of lung
  - **2.** Collagen vascular disease

C. History of hemoptysis:
- **a.** Lung abscess
- **b.** Bronchogenic carcinoma
- **c.** Lobar pneumonia

D. History of cough:
- **a.** Bronchogenic carcinoma
- **b.** Round pneumonia
- **c.** Pulmonary infarction
- **d.** Collagen vascular disease
- **e.** Tubercular granuloma

E. Sputum:
- **a.** Blood streak sputum—bronchogenic carcinoma
- **b.** Rusty sputum—round pneumonia
- **c.** Foul sputum—lung abscess
- **d.** Mucoid sputum—pulmonary infarction
- **e.** Impacted mucus—bronchial atresia

F. History of fever:
- **a.** Round pneumonia
- **b.** Lung abscess
- **c.** Pulmonary infarction
- **d.** Bronchogenic carcinoma
- **e.** Active collagen vascular disease

G. History of exposure to asbestos, uranium, radon, and silica

H. Family history of:
- **a.** Bronchogenic carcinoma in first-degree relative
- **b.** Collagen vascular disease
- **c.** Lymphoma

I. Surgical history regarding the operation of nodule in the lung

Physical examination:

A. General survey:
- **a.** Anemia:
  - **1.** Collagen vascular disease
  - **2.** Bronchogenic carcinoma
  - **3.** Granulomatous disease
- **b.** Cyanosis:
  - **1.** Pneumonia
  - **2.** Pulmonary infarction
- **c.** Raised temperature:
  - **1.** Round pneumonia
  - **2.** Lung abscess
  - **3.** Pulmonary infarction due to septic embolus
  - **4.** Active collagen vascular disease

d. Tachycardia:
   1. Pulmonary infarction due to septic embolus
   2. Round pneumonia
   3. Lung abscess
   4. Active collagen vascular disease

B. Respiratory system examination:
   a. Presence of bronchial breath sound:
      1. Round pneumonia
      2. Lung abscess
   b. Crepitation:
      1. Pulmonary infarction due to septic embolus
      2. Round pneumonia
      3. Lung abscess
      4. Active collagen vascular disease

Investigations:

A. Hematology:
   a. Anemia:
      1. Bronchogenic carcinoma
      2. Active collagen vascular disease
      3. Tubercular granuloma
      4. Lung abscess
   b. Leukocytosis:
      1. Round pneumonia
      2. Lung abscess
      3. Bronchogenic carcinoma
   c. Raised ESR:
      1. Active collagen vascular disease
      2. Lung abscess
      3. Round pneumonia
      4. Bronchogenic carcinoma
   d. Leukopenia: Active collagen vascular disease

B. Radiological features: Following features have to be noted:
   a. Size of the nodule: Increase in size suggests lung cancer. But small size of the nodule cannot rule out cancer.
   b. Margin of the nodule: There may be overlap between benign and malignant nodule regarding margin and contour of the nodule.
      1. Benign
      2. Pulmonary metastasis
   c. Spiculated margin: It may occur due to growth of the malignant cells along the interstitium of lung. It occurs in other cases:
      1. Focal atelectasis
      2. Progressive massive fibrosis
      3. Lipoid pneumonia
      4. Tuberculoma
   d. Lobulated margin due to differential growth of the nodule: Lung carcinoma
   e. Halo sign around the nodule:
      1. Adenocarcinoma in situ
      2. Pulmonary metastasis
      3. Kaposi sarcoma
   f. Reverse halo sign:
      1. COP
      2. Lung cancer after radiofrequency ablation
   g. Attenuation of fat:
      1. Hamartomas
      2. Lipoid pneumonia
      3. Metastasis from liposarcoma
      4. Pulmonary neoplasm
   h. Calcification within the nodule: There are eight types of calcifications which are:
      1. Central dense nidus (benign)—granulomatous disease
      2. Laminated (benign)—granulomatous disease
      3. Popcorn (benign)—hamartoma
      4. Diffuse solid (benign)—granulomatous disease
      5. Punctate—lung cancer
      6. Dendriform—lung cancer
      7. Reticular—lung cancer
      8. Amorphous—lung cancer
   i. Cavitation within the nodule:
      1. Pulmonary infarction
      2. Lung abscess
      3. Infectious granuloma
      4. Vasculitis
      5. Primary malignancies or secondaries
   j. Wall thickness:
      1. More than 15 mm—suggest malignancies
      2. 5 mm—suggests benign
      3. Between 5 and 15 mm suggests benign or malignant

   Calcification may also be seen in primary central lung carcinoid, bronchogenic carcinoma, metastasis, and mucinous adenocarcinoma.

   k. Bubbly lucencies found in:
      1. Sarcoidosis
      2. Organizing pneumonia
      3. Adenocarcinoma

l. Air bronchogram sign: Air-filled bronchi surrounded by airless lung tissue suggesting patency of the proximal airway and evacuation of air from alveoli by absorption atelectasis:
   1. Malignant nodule from lymphoma
   2. Infection

Treatment of Lung Nodule

Fleischner Society Guidelines of Treatment

A. Solid nodule:

a. Less than 6 mm in low risk patient—no treatment is required and do not need follow-up. In high risk patient, the optional treatment is repeat CT scan after 1 year.

b. If diameter is between 6 and 8 mm, regardless of risk in patient repeat CT scan chest should be done after 1 year and again after 18–24 months.

c. If the size of the nodule is more than 8 mm, repeat CT scan should be done after 3 months with PET scan or tissue biopsy. In case of very high risk patient, tissue biopsy is very essential for the diagnosis.

B. Ground glass nodule:

a. If the diameter of the nodule is less than 6 mm, no follow-up.

b. If the diameter is more than 6 mm, repeat CT scan should be done every 6–12 months followed by every 2 years for total 5 years.

c. If the nodule partly solid—reaction should be considered.

C. For partly solid nodule:

a. Less than 6 mm size—routine follow-up.

b. If size more than 6 mm—repeated CT scan at 3 and 6 months.

1. If the nodule gradually increases in size, and solid part is more than 6 mm, the patient should be considered as high risk, in that case resection should be considered.
2. CT scan should be followed up yearly for next 5 years, size is unchanged and solid component is less than 6 mm.

According to American College of Physician:

A. If the size of the nodule is stable for next 2 years, no more testing is required.

B. Solid nodule having size of less than 8 mm has been divided into two groups: With risk or without risk of malignancy.

a. If the size is less than 4 mm and no risk of malignancy, optimal follow-up is required.

b. If the size of the nodule is 4–6 mm, in that case CT scan should be done at 12 months.

c. If the size is 6–8 mm, follow-up is required at 6–12 months then again at 18–24 months.

d. If there is risk of malignancy and the size is less than 4 mm, then repeat CT scan is required at 12 months.

e. In patient having risk factor for malignancy and the size is 4–6 mm, follow-up CT scan should be done at 6 to 12 months and again at 18–24 months.

f. In patient having risk factor for malignancy and the size is 6 to 8 mm, follow-up CT scan should be done at 3–6 months and again at 9–12 months and again at 24 months.

C. If the size of the solid nodule is 8–30 mm, these patient should be subdivided into low, moderate and high pretest probability groups.

a. In case low pretest probability group, low dose CT scan should be done at 3–6 months, 6–12 months, and lastly 18–24 months.

b. In case of moderate pretest probability group, serial CT scan or PET CT scan should be done.

c. In case of high pretest probability group, surgical section or biopsy should be performed from that nodule.

D. In patient with part solid nodule—repeat CT scan should be done at 3 months.

a. If the solid component is less than 5 mm, then yearly CT scan is recommended for next 3 years.

b. If the solid component is more than 5 mm, then excision biopsy or surgical resection is required.

E. In patient with non-solid nodule of

a. Less than 5 mm in size—no further evaluation is required.

b. More than 5 mm in size, annual CT scan is should be performed at 3 years.

c. More than 1 cm in size—repeat imaging should be done at 3 months then, biopsy or surgical resection should be warranted.

F. In patient with ground-glass nodule of

a. Less than 5 mm in size, repeat CT scan is required at 2–3 years,

b. More than 5 mm in size, repeat CT scan should be performed at 3 months, if the nodule persists, subsequent CT scan is performed up to 3 years. Even after 3 years the nodule persist, surgical excision is required.

Q39. Massive pleural effusion.

MLB/MAY2009/MDII (20)

Discuss the etiology, pathophysiology, clinical features, and management of pleural effusion.

MGR/MAR2009/MDIV (20)

Malignant pleural effusion.

MJPRU/2015(S) (10)

MJPRU/2013/MDII (10)

Enumerate the causes of recurrent pleural effusion.

DNB 2018 (2)

ANSWER

Introduction

Pleural membrane is doubled layered covering inner surface of chest wall and outer wall of the whole lung separated by thin layer of fluid of 10–30 mL, called plasma infiltrate—it is formed at a rate of 0.3–0.5 mL/kg/day and protein content of 0.9–1.2 g/dL. Pleural membrane is lined by single layer of mesothelial cells having a surface area of 2,000 cc in standard 70 kg man. It helps in smooth expansion of lung in the thoracic cage.

Accumulated fluid in the pleural cavity is called pleural effusion.

Pathophysiology of Development of Pleural Effusion

Visceral and parietal layers play in homeostasis of fluid homeostasis. Both production and absorption of pleural fluid is 0.2 mL/kg/h; it means that total volume of fluid will be turn over within an hour and parietal pleura takes part in this process. But the exception is left heart failure where the fluid will come from visceral pleura. Pleural fluid will also be absorbed by the lymphatics present in the parietal pleura. The reabsorption power in these lymphatics will be increased up to 20 times if the production of fluid in the pleural cavity is abnormally increased. So in the healthy person both production and absorption of fluid are in equilibrium. In the pleural cavity, it is formed by the interaction of three mechanisms, these are:

A. Hydrostatic pressure of blood and pleural fluid

B. Oncotic pressure of protein in the blood and pleural fluid

C. Capillary permeability

If the hydrostatic pressure is increased and plasma oncotic pressure is decreased in the blood as compared to pleural fluid, the fluid will enter across the blood vessels into the pleural cavity. This is called transudate.

On the other hand, if the capillary permeability is increased the fluid along with plasma albumin will cross into pleural cavity. This is called transudate.

In both cases lymphatic channels will fail to absorb the fluid from the cavity.

Causes of Pleural Effusion

Causes	Type of effusion
Congestive cardiac failure	Transudate
Liver disease and cirrhosis	Transudate
Nephrotic syndrome	Transudate
Myxedema	Transudate
PE	Transudate
Sarcoidosis	Transudate
Cancers like: Lung Breast cancer Pleural mesothelioma	Exudate
Infection in the pleural space	Community-acquired or nosocomial infection
PE	Exudate
Gastrointestinal diseases like: Pancreatitis Esophageal perforation Intra-abdominal abscesses	Exudate
Rheumatic disease like: SLE Rheumatoid arthritis Systemic sclerosis Wegener granulomatosis Sjögren's syndrome Amyloidosis	Exudate
Meigs syndrome	Exudate
Radiation	Exudate
Lymphangiomyomatosis	Transudate
Langerhans cell granulomatosis	Exudate
Hemothorax	Exudate
Chylothorax	Exudate
Drugs: Amiodarone, methotrexate, ergot alkaloids, beta-blockers, phenytoin	

Clinical Features

Symptoms

Clinical features depend upon the following features:

a. Rate of accumulation of pleural fluid
b. Amount of fluid
c. Underlying cause

A. Most common symptom is pleural pain as the pleural inflammation, stabbing, or pricking in nature arising from parietal pleura as there is no nociceptive fiber present on the visceral pleura. It will start at the site of pleural effusion and linked with respiratory cycle. But it will decrease as the effusion starts increasing. But the pain is diffuse when the pathological process involves the parietal pleura as in empyema, pleural mesothelioma, pleural metastasis, and mediastinal pleura.

B. Next common symptom is respiratory distress and it depends upon size of effusion. In case of massive pleural effusion lung in the involved side will collapse; thus lung volume will be diminished leading to dyspnea.

C. Dry cough due to compression of lung by effusion.

D. Trepopnea: It means development of respiratory distress when the patient lies down on the side of pleural effusion.

Other symptoms and signs to diagnose the etiology of pleural effusion:

Symptoms	Suggested etiology
Ascites	Cirrhosis
Orthopnea	Heart failure and pericarditis
Lymphadenopathy	Tuberculosis and malignancy
Peripheral edema	Heart failure and cirrhosis
Unilateral edema	Pulmonary infarction
Weight loss	Tuberculosis and malignancy
Hepatosplenomegaly	Cirrhosis, malignancy, and tuberculosis
Distended neck veins	Heart failure and pericarditis
S3 gallop	Heart failure
Hemoptysis	Malignancy and tuberculosis, and PE
Fever	Tuberculosis, parapneumonic effusion, and malignancy

Signs

A. General examination reveals:

a. Anemia—malignancy and tuberculosis
b. Jaundice—cirrhosis
c. Cyanosis—cardiac failure
d. Tachypnea
e. Tachycardia
f. Clubbing—tuberculosis, empyema, bronchogenic carcinoma, and cirrhosis
g. Lymphadenopathy

B. Respiratory system examination:

a. On inspection:
1. Fullness on the affected side of the chest
2. Movement of the affected part is diminished

b. On palpation:
1. Trachea will be shifted toward opposite side
2. Movement of the affected part will be diminished
3. Apical impulse will be shifted to opposite side
4. Intercostal tenderness with raised temperature—empyema

c. On percussion
1. On the affected part percussion will be stony dull
2. Just above the level of pleural effusion—woody dull
3. Above the level of second part or apical area—percussion is resonant
4. On the non-affected side: Percussion note is hyperresonant due to compensatory emphysema.

d. On auscultation:
1. Breath sound is absent on the areas of pleural effusion
2. In the upper part breath sound is vesicular
3. Just above the level—bronchial breath sound due to collapsed lung and patent bronchus
4. On the non-affected side—breath sound is normal

Clinical clue to the diagnosis:

Disease	Symptoms
Congestive cardiac failure	Hypoxia, peripheral edema, and pulmonary edema
Bacterial pneumonia	Cough with expectoration, fever, and pulmonary infiltrate
Malignancy	History of cancer, mass, and features of superior vena caval obstruction
Abdominal causes	Abdominal pain, chills, fever, nausea, and vomiting
Cirrhosis	History of alcohol abuse, ascites, and signs of hepatocellular failure

Continued

Continued

Disease	Symptoms
Meigs syndrome	History of ovarian tumor
Pancreatitis	Abdominal pain, nausea, vomiting, and raised amylase and lipase
Chylothorax	Chest mass, chyle in the pleural fluid
Nephrotic syndrome	Pedal edema and proteinuria
Rheumatoid arthritis	Swell and tender joints and deformed joints

Light Criteria

Pleural effusion is exudative if at least one of the following criteria is positive:

A. Protein concentration in the pleural fluid divided by protein concentration in the blood is >0.5

B. Lactate dehydrogenase concentration in the pleural fluid is >200 IU or greater than two-thirds of upper limit of LDH in the blood.

C. Lactate dehydrogenase in the pleural fluid divided by that of the serum is >0.6

But if the two above criteria are combined then it makes Light's criteria more sensitive and specific.

Diagnosis

A. Chest X-ray (PA view):

- **a.** Homogeneous opacity on the affected side having upper concave border form Ellis S-shaped curve with highest point toward axilla.
- **b.** Mediastinum will be shifted toward opposite side in case of large effusion.
- **c.** In case of mild effusion: Blunting of the costophrenic angle.
- **d.** There is evidence of tenting of diaphragm indicating pleural fibrosis.
- **e.** Walled off pleural effusion present on the anterior and lateral pleural surface can be seen. But loculated effusion behind the heart, along the mediastinum and subpulmonic effusion may not be diagnosed.

B. Ultrasonography:

- **a.** Its sensitivity is 100%.
- **b.** It can be diagnosed in critically ill patient in whom it can differentiate basal consolidation, atelectasis basal pleural thickening from pleural effusion.

C. HRCT:

- **a.** It can diagnose pleural or pulmonary pathologies.

D. Aspiration of pleural fluid:

Bilateral pleural effusion usually needs diagnostic or therapeutic tap. In case of unilateral pleural effusion it is tapped for diagnosis of the etiology or in case of massive effusion to relieve the patient from respiratory distress and to prevent cardiac or respiratory decompensation.

It is generally safe but one has to stop aspiration when there is appearance of cough. There are complications of aspiration, these are as following:

- **a.** Vasovagal syncope
- **b.** Bleeding due to injury to vessels
- **c.** Pneumothorax

If the large quantities of fluid are aspirated there is cough due to re-expansion of pulmonary edema and the whole procedure has to be stopped.

E. Pleural fluid analysis:

Physical characteristics for diagnosis of pleural effusion:

Characteristics	Diagnosis
Anchovy brown fluid	Ruptured amebic liver abscess
Black fluid	*Aspergillus* infection
Milky fluid	Chylothorax or pseudochylothorax
Putrid smell	Anaerobic empyema
Bile staining	Chylothorax due to biliary fistula
Urine	Urinothorax
Presence of food particles	Esophageal perforation

Tests recommended for any diagnosis of pleural effusion	
Lactate dehydrogenase	To diagnose transudate or exudate
Microscopy and culture	Aerobic or anaerobic, blood culture may be indicated
Recommended tests for specific diagnosis of pleural effusion	
pH	Pleural fluid acidosis is found in pleural infection, tuberculosis, malignant pleural effusion, and rheumatoid arthritis, more acidosis in malignant pleural effusion decreases the survival and lower chance of survival from pleurodesis
Glucose	In rheumatoid disease, empyema, tuberculosis, and malignancy
Acid-fast bacilli, culture and Sensitivity of *Mycobacterium tuberculosis*, PCR using 16S-rRNA	Suspected tuberculous pleurisy

Continued

Continued

Triglyceride and cholesterol	Chylothorax, in pseudochylothorax raised cholesterol and low triglyceride level
Amylase	Acute pancreatitis, esophageal perforation, and tuberculosis
Hematocrit	<0.5 × peripheral blood hematocrit suggests hemothorax, <1% indicates PE, trauma, and malignancy
NT-proBNP	Systolic and diastolic heart failure
Tumor markers	Carcinoembryonic antigen, CA-125, 15.3, cytokeratin 19 fragment, and mesothelin testing

Differential blood count:

A. Raised neutrophil count in parapneumonic pleural effusion, empyema, and PE.

B. Predominant increased lymphocyte count is found in tuberculosis, congestive heart failure, malignant pleural effusion, and long-standing pleural effusion.

Q40. Describe the extent of different parts of pleura, its nerve supply, blood supply, and its recesses.

MGR/MAR2007/MD (5)

Parietal pleura.

MGR UNI, TAMIL NADU, 2021 (5)

ANSWER

Pleura is a serous membrane which folds on itself to form two layers in between which there is a cavity called pleural cavity containing few mL of serous fluid. So, two layers of pleura are visceral and parietal pleura.

A. Visceral pleura:

- **a.** It adheres to as well as covers the lobes and roots of both lung.
- **b.** It dips into the fissures in between the lobes called parietal pleura.
- **c.** Pulmonary ligament extending from hilum to diaphragm consists of two apposed layers of visceral pleura which is ultimately continuous with the parietal pleura.

B. Parietal pleura:

- **a.** It lines the inner wall of chest cavity or outer wall of pleural cavity.
- **b.** It has been subdivided into four parts according to the structures it covers:
  1. Diaphragmatic pleura: It covers and closely adheres to superior surface of diaphragm.
  2. Mediastinal pleura:
     - It covers all the structures in the mediastinum
     - It is continuous with the visceral pleura which covers the root of the lung
     - It covers and is closely adherent to the pericardium
  3. Costal pleura:
     - It will cover inner surface of thoracic wall
     - It is loosely attached to inner thoracic wall by endothoracic fascia which covers inner surfaces of deepest layer of muscles in the thoracic wall
  4. Cervical pleura:
     - It is also called cupola.
     - It will cover the apex of the lung loosely projecting into the neck superior to 1st rib.
     - Endothoracic fascia associated with this pleura is known as suprapleural membrane, also known as Sibson's fascia—it is tent-like thickened structure.

Pleural Recesses

Inferiorly lung does not fill the pleural cavity completely, so in few places parietal pleura appose each other producing pleural recesses—these are usually filled by the lung during deep inspiration. Clinically these recesses are important as there may be collection of fluid in certain diseases which can be drained easily. There are two recesses:

A. Costodiaphragmatic recesses:

- **a.** In this area, costal pleura will reflect back onto the diaphragm to form diaphragmatic pleura.
- **b.** It is clinically more important.
- **c.** These are deeper during expiration and shallower during inspiration.

B. Costomediastinal recesses:

- **a.** It is present behind the sternum where costal pleura will fold on itself to become mediastinal pleura.
- **b.** It is more conspicuous on the left side around the left heart

Pleural Reflections

A. Sternal line of pleural reflection: It is sharp, abrupt, and anteriorly present where costal pleura is continuous with mediastinal pleura.

B. Vertebral line of pleural reflection: It is gradual and rounder the posterior counterpart of sternal line where costal pleura is continuous with mediastinal pleura.

C. Costal line of pleural reflection: It is sharp area where costal pleura becomes continuous with diaphragmatic pleura.

Blood Supply of Visceral Pleura

A. Arterial supply: Branches of bronchial and pulmonary veins
B. Venous drainage: Pulmonary vein

Blood supply of parietal pleura:

A. Cervical pleura: Intercostal vessels
B. Costal pleura: Intercostal vessels
C. Diaphragmatic pleura:
    a. Outer part: Intercostal vessels
    b. Inner part: Pericardiophrenic vessels
D. Mediastinal pleura: Pericardiophrenic vessels

Nerve Supply of Pleura

A. Visceral pleura: No nerve supply
B. Parietal pleura:
    a. Cervical pleura: Intercostal vessels
    b. Costal pleura: Intercostal vessels
    c. Diaphragmatic pleura:
        1. Outer part: Intercostal vessels
        2. Inner part: Pericardiophrenic vessels
    d. Mediastinal pleura: Pericardiophrenic vessels

Q41. Bronchial thermoplasty.

AMU/2011/MDI (10)

ANSWER

Introduction

Bronchial thermoplasty is an innovative method of treatment of asthma by preventing the hyperresponsiveness of smooth muscles of the airways by delivering radiofrequency energy in a specific amount through a dedicated catheter.

Asthma is produced as a result of interaction of airway hyperresponsiveness and variable obstruction to airway.

Indications

A. Severe persistent asthma in adult requiring maintenance ICS like >1,000 μg/day beclomethasone as well as LABA like ≥100 μg/day salmeterol, may be the receiver of leukotrienes modifier, ≥10 mg/day oral steroids.

Contraindications

A. Presence of implantable electronic device
B. Known hypersensitivity to the drugs which is used during bronchoscopy
C. Severe comorbidity increasing the risk of the procedure

Technique

It is done through bronchoscopy in three separate procedures with intervening period of 3 weeks in between the procedures because

a. It will reduce the bronchial wall edema
b. It will minimize the risk of acute exacerbation of asthma
c. It will reduce the length of the procedure

All the accessible airways are treated excepting right middle lobe as it may induce right middle lobe syndrome.

Proper oxygenation via nasal cannula with appropriate monitoring of vital signs like blood pressure, pulse oximetry should be continued during the procedure.

Under conscious sedation delivery of radiofrequency energy through bronchoscope can be done through oral or nasal approach, but later approach is preferable because of less gagging and less amount of secretions. But patient should receive preprocedural steroids and bronchodilators.

After properly examining the airways Alair catheter has to be introduced through the working channel of bronchoscope under direct vision. At the tip of the catheter there are four electrode baskets present containing heating and temperature sensing elements to get feedback control.

After reaching the proper site to be treated four electrode arrays have to be expanded to make the four wires in firm contact with the wall of the airway circumferentially. Energy is delivered by the bronchoscopist through footswitch and controller controls the temperature through feedback system to maintain the temperature 65°C for 10 seconds.

Right and lower lobes are treated by separated procedure and both upper lobes are treated in third procedure. Each procedure requires 50–75 activations to cover the targeted airway.

Postprocedural Care

Patient should be under observation for 3–4 hours after each procedure. Postprocedural follow-up includes following:

a. FEV_1
b. Vital signs
c. Gag reflex

Complications

A. Recurrent atelectasis of lung secondary to fibrin plug
B. Inflammatory reaction with microvascular alteration following high thermal stimulation leading to release of inflammatory mediators
C. Lung abscess

Q42. Oxygen dissociation curve.

RGUHS/MDI (10)

Hemoglobin with altered oxygen affinity.

DNB 2020 (5)

ANSWER

Introduction

Oxygen dissociation curve represents graphically the affinity of hemoglobin after hemoglobin, i.e., the relationship between SaO_2 of hemoglobin and PaO_2.

Only 2–3% of oxygen will be dissolved in plasma rest will be attached with the hemoglobin molecules depending upon the PaO_2, higher the partial pressure greater will be the binding with hemoglobin—this combination is called oxyhemoglobin. When hemoglobin is 100% saturated then each gram of hemoglobin contains 1.39 mL of oxygen, but blood contains normally some inactive hemoglobin, hence only 1.34 mL of oxygen combines with hemoglobin.

Relations between Saturation of Hemoglobin and Partial Pressure of Oxygen

Normal PaO_2 is 80–100 mm Hg, whereas saturation of hemoglobin is 93–97% with average of 97%.

This curve is "S" shaped—its flat upper portion represents loading of oxygen onto hemoglobin in the lungs. PaO_2 entering the lungs exceeds the oxygen concentration in the blood in the venous blood that returns to the lungs. As result, hemoglobin binds easily to the hemoglobin. Hence, this flat portion of the curve is protected for generation of patient's oxygen status. As for example, if the patient's PaO_2 drops to 70 mm Hg from 96 mm Hg, patient's saturation of hemoglobin will drop to 92% from 97%. Again, by giving supplemental oxygen PaO_2 can increase to >100% but hemoglobin saturation will never be >100%.

In the lower steep portion of the curve below the knee, PaO_2 is between 40 and 60 mm Hg because large amount of oxygen will be released into the tissues due to increased oxygen demand. In this, portion of the curve moderate changes in PaO_2 will lead to large amount of change in saturation of hemoglobin. So, at this point supplemental oxygen can enormously increase saturation of hemoglobin.

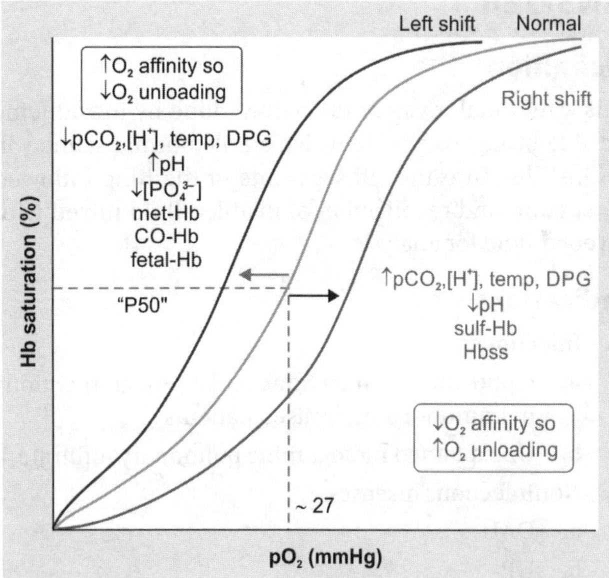

Factor Affecting the Oxygen Dissociation Curve

A. pH: Acidic pH will shift the curve to the right whereas, alkaline pH will shift the curve to left. Deoxygenated hemoglobin will bind to hydrogen ion more avidly as compared to oxyhemoglobin thus reducing the blood pH and also lowering the affinity hemoglobin for oxygen—this is known as Bohr effect.
B. Temperature: Rise in temperature will shift the curve to right, whereas fall in temperature will shift the curve to the left.

So, higher PO_2 is required for binding of hemoglobin with a given amount of oxygen and index used is known as p50 for this shift. Higher the p50 lower the affinity of hemoglobin for oxygen.

C. Concentration of 2,3-diphosphoglycerate (DPG): It is present in RBCs in large amount. It is produced by glycolysis via Embden-Meyerhof pathway. This highly charged anion will bind to beta chain of deoxyhemoglobin. So, when amount of 2,3-DPG will be increased in the RBC, curve will be shifting to the right and thus release more oxygen in to blood.
D. Carbon dioxide level: If PCO_2 increases, pH of the blood will be decreased thus shifting the curve to right.
E. Fetal hemoglobin shifts the curve to the left.
F. Sickle cell hemoglobin will shift the curve to the right.
G. Sulfhemoglobin will shift the curve to the right.

Q43. Bronchoalveolar lavage.

MJPRU/2015/MDII (10)

ANSWER

Definition

It is a minimal invasive procedure done by introducing flexible bronchoscope in which sterile normal saline will be instilled into the subsegments of the lung followed by suction and recollection of instilled fluid mixed with alveolar fluid for analysis.

Indications

A. Infections:

- **a.** Opportunistic infections and atypical infections in immunocompromised patients
- **b.** Unexplained radiographic pulmonary infiltrate

B. Noninfectious diseases:

- **a.** DAH
- **b.** HP
- **c.** ILDs
- **d.** Pulmonary alveolar proteinosis
- **e.** Eosinophilic pneumonia
- **f.** Chronic asbestosis
- **g.** Chronic berylliosis

C. Neoplastic lung diseases

Procedures

Prior to collection of alveolar fluid adult flexible bronchoscope with 3–6 mm tip is introduced into tracheobronchial tree and wedge in the bronchiole for inspection of airways so that it will minimize the introduction of bronchial wall debris and RBCs into the distal airways and alter the composition of the lavage fluid.

Now 20–40 mL of sterile normal saline at room temperature is injected via handled syringe into the bronchoscope. This is done for three to five times till total up to 300 mL of sterile fluid is injected. Returned yield sample of 30% total instilled amount will be considered as adequate return—only 10–20 mL is ultimately required for cellular and infectious workup.

A. In case of localized disease as evidenced by chest X-ray or HRCT of chest, bronchoscope can be introduced into specific subsegment to visualize the distal airways in the center of the real image.

B. In case of diffuse image as evidenced by HRCT of chest, most common location of collection of fluid is middle lobe or lingula. In the supine position during bronchoscopy, anteriorly projected locations of these areas allow maximal collection of fluid. In case of nonaccessibility, superior or anterior segments of either lobes are of choice. This process allows to collect fluid from at least 1 million of alveoli.

Collection and Analysis

Collected fluid is pooled, mixed, and its volume has to be recorded. Sample should be sent in ice if the transportation is >1 hour as fluid is only viable for 4 hours in the room temperature.

- **a.** It should be analyzed for red and white blood cells.
- **b.** Esterase staining is required for differentiating immature macrophages from large lymphocytes.
- **c.** Irons, inorganic dusts, malignant cells, microorganisms, and other types of staining are required.

This fluid is not valid for diagnosis if fluid demonstrates following features:

- **a.** <2 million of total cells
- **b.** <10 alveolar macrophages per high-power field
- **c.** Large number of RBCs in the fluid due to trauma
- **d.** Presence of degenerative changes in the fluid

In case of nonsmokers, average number of cells in the fluid is 100–150,000/mL. In case of smoker, it will be increased up to fourfold, most of them are neutrophils and macrophages.

Contraindications

A. Myocardial infarction within last 4 weeks

B. Unstable angina

C. Uncontrolled arrhythmias

D. Refractory hypoxemia

E. Hemodynamic instability

Following cell line cutoff will support the diagnosis:

A. Increase neutrophils of >5%:

- **a.** ARDS
- **b.** IPF
- **c.** Connective tissue disorders
- **d.** Infections

B. Eosinophilia: >25% suggests:

- **a.** Acute eosinophilic pneumonia
- **b.** Chronic eosinophilic pneumonia
- **c.** Churg–Strauss syndrome

C. Lymphocytosis of >50%—HP

D. When lymphocyte count is ≥15%, then CD4 and CD8 cells ratio will be assessed.
   a. Elevated CD4:CD8 ratio suggests
      1. Chronic HP
      2. Berylliosis
      3. Sarcoidosis
      4. Asbestosis
      5. Crohn's disease
      6. Connective tissue disorders
   b. Normal ratio suggests:
      1. Tuberculosis
      2. Malignancies
   c. Low ratio suggests:
      1. Acute HP
      2. Drug-induced pulmonary disease
      3. Silicosis
      4. HIV infection
      5. COP

E. Progressive blackening of aliquots of bloody fluid suggests DAH

F. Hemosiderin-laden macrophages are also seen

G. This fluid also detects:
   a. *Cytomegalovirus* or herpes simplex in the intranuclear or intracytoplasmic inclusion
   b. *Mycobacterium tuberculosis*
   c. Fungi

Complications

A. Hypoxemia

B. Post-bronchoalveolar lavage fluid

C. Bronchospasm

D. Pneumothorax rarely

Q44. Muscles of respiration.

MGR/MAY2011/MDI (5)

ANSWER

There are two sets of muscle usually responsible for respiration like during inspiration and expiration.

During inspiration primary muscle is diaphragmatic muscle, other muscles being external intercostal and internal intercostal muscles during quiet respiration. Other muscles such as scalene and parasternal intercostal muscles also come into play during inspiration.

Accessory muscles of respiration, namely sternocleidomastoid and trapezius muscles, do not usually play their game during quiet respiration but start playing when functions of diaphragmatic muscles are impaired or in case of significantly increased ventilation.

Diaphragm at its lateral aspect is in contact with inner part of lower ribcage—this area is known as zone of apposition. Here, the diaphragmatic muscle fibers are arranged vertically. So, at the time of contraction there is shortening of these vertically orientated muscle fibers, thus diminishing the zone of apposition and more medial dome of diaphragm will descend. So, downward descent of the diaphragm will increase the intra-abdominal pressure and pushes the abdominal content downward and abdominal wall outward. At the same time diaphragmatic contraction lifts the lower ribs and expands the lower chest downward and another muscle, external intercostal muscle which is present in between the ribs will contract to rotate the lower ribcage outward like "bucket handle" movement.

Upper chest wall moves outward anteroposteriorly like "pump handle" movement by the contraction of scalene muscles and parasternal intercostal muscles along with external intercostal muscles.

So, the effect is expansion of chest anteroposteriorly and above downward with reduction of intrathoracic pressure; as a result air will flow into the lungs. But during forceful inspiration, accessory muscles of respiration will enter in the game to assist the primary inspiratory muscles.

Efficacy of diaphragmatic contraction depends upon its initial shape and length of diaphragmatic muscles. Usually, in case of any muscle if the initial length is short, in that case strength of contraction will be diminished, but diaphragm is the only exception where the length of the muscles of diaphragm if longer prior to contraction as in case of emphysema, its strength of contraction will be diminished during inspiration. So, diaphragm will be flattened, area of apposition will be diminished and less downward and outward movement of the lower ribcage during inspiration will be evident.

In the extreme cases, diaphragm will be flattened horizontally and there will be absence of zone of apposition and no effective downward drawing of lower ribcage during inspiration as in case of severe chronic obstructive lung disease.

Diaphragm is supplied by phrenic nerve from 3rd, 4th, and 5th cervical segments. In case of phrenic nerve paralysis, diaphragm is drawn upward during inspiration due to increased negative intrapleural pressure and moves downward during expiration due to increased intrapleural pressure. This is called paradoxical movement of the diaphragm which can be proved by "sniff test".

On the other hand, expiration is a passive process where chest wall as well as lungs will come into their resting position. But when patient coughs or expel the air forcefully, expiratory muscles like abdominal muscles like internal and external obliques, transverse abdominis, and chest muscle like internal intercostal muscle will come into play.

Q45. Mediastinum.

MGR/MAR2010/MDI(5)

Anatomy of mediastinum and mediastinal compression syndrome.

MUHS/MAY2010/MDI (10)

Discuss the clinical approach to a patient presenting with mediastinal mass.

BF/NOV2013/MDII (10)

Mediastinum.

MGR UNIVERSITY, TAMIL NADU, 2020 (5)

ANSWER

Introduction

Mediastinum is the vertical region within the chest between the two pleural cavities bounded by:

- **a.** Superiorly by thoracic inlet
- **b.** Inferiorly by diaphragm
- **c.** Posteriorly by vertebral column
- **d.** Laterally by mediastinal pleural reflections

Anatomy of Mediastinum

Mediastinum is divided into three divisions such as anterior, middle, and posterior parts based on lateral view of chest X-ray.

Anterior compartment is bounded by:

- **a.** Anteriorly by inner surface of sternum
- **b.** Posteriorly by anterior surface of pericardium, great vessels, and anterior surface of trachea
- **c.** Superiorly by thoracic inlet
- **d.** Inferiorly by diaphragm

Contents of the anterior mediastinum are:

- **a.** Thymus gland
- **b.** Pericardial fat
- **c.** Lymph glands
- **d.** Connective tissue

Middle mediastinum or visceral compartment is bounded by:

- **a.** Anteriorly by posterior limit of anterior mediastinum
- **b.** Posteriorly by:
  - **1.** Posterior surface of great vessels
  - **2.** Posterior surface of trachea and its division into two main bronchi
  - **3.** Posterior pericardial surface
- **c.** Superiorly by thoracic inlet
- **d.** Inferiorly by diaphragm

Contents of the middle mediastinum:

- **a.** Pericardium
- **b.** Heart
- **c.** Aorta
- **d.** Great vessel
- **e.** Superior vena cava along with the large veins draining into this vein
- **f.** Pulmonary vessels
- **g.** Trachea along with two major bronchi
- **h.** Phrenic nerves
- **i.** Lymph glands

Posterior mediastinum is bounded by:

- **a.** Anteriorly by posterior aspect of middle mediastinum
- **b.** Posteriorly by anterior aspect of vertebral bodies and paravertebral sulci
- **c.** Superiorly by thoracic inlet
- **d.** Inferiorly by diaphragm

Contents of posterior mediastinum:

- **a.** Descending aorta
- **b.** Esophagus
- **c.** Sympathetic trunk on each side of vertebral column
- **d.** Azygos and hemiazygos veins
- **e.** Thoracic duct
- **f.** Intercostal nerves

Following are the mediastinal masses:

A. Masses in the anterior mediastinum:

- **a.** Thymoma
- **b.** Thymic carcinoma
- **c.** Thymic hyperplasia
- **d.** Thymic lymphoma
- **e.** Thymic cyst

f. Thymic carcinoid
g. Germinal cell tumors
   1. Teratoma
   2. Seminoma
h. Intrathoracic goiter
i. Aortic aneurysm
j. Parathyroid adenoma

B. Masses in the middle mediastinum:
a. Lymphoma
b. Metastatic enlargement of lymph nodes
c. Benign mediastinal lymphadenopathy
d. Bronchogenic cyst
e. Enterogenous cyst

C. Masses in the posterior mediastinum:
a. Neurofibroma
b. Schwannomas
c. Esophageal carcinoma
d. Hiatus hernia
e. Achalasia cardia
f. Pott's disease with paravertebral cold abscess
g. Descending aortic aneurysm
h. Enterogenous cyst
i. Nerve sheath tumor
j. Extramedullary hematopoiesis

Approach to a Case of Mediastinal Mass

A. Asymptomatic presentation: One-third of the patients are asymptomatic and can be diagnosed by routine chest X-ray. 15% are malignant.

B. Compression of the neighboring structures: Symptoms of compression, though more common in case of malignant tumor, can occur in case of large benign tumor. The following structures are compressed:
a. Pressure on the superior vena cava producing superior vena caval syndrome which can be characterized by:
   1. Progressively engorged but nonpulsatile jugular vein
   2. Signs of venous engorgement:
      - Slight puffiness of the face mainly around the eyes
      - Chemosis of the conjunctiva in the early morning
      - Flushed face due to facial congestion on bending or during stooping to take something or tying the shoelace.
b. Compression of the trachea producing stridor
c. Compression of bronchus producing monophonic wheeze
d. Compression of the bronchus producing atelectasis of the lobe
e. Pressure on the esophagus producing dysphagia
f. Compression of left recurrent laryngeal nerve produces abductor paralysis of left vocal cord leading to hoarseness of voice
g. Cardiac compression or pericardial invasion will lead to palpitation, chest pain, and rhythmic disturbances.
h. Pressure of sympathetic trunk by malignant tumor leads to Horner's syndrome
i. Compression of intercostal nerves while emerging from vertebral foramina leads to intercostal neuralgia
j. Intraspinal mass produces pressure on the spinal cord leading to neurological deficits
k. Presence of bone erosion involving ribs and vertebrae produces pain and tenderness on the bone
l. Presence of unequal pulses or absent pulses in both upper limbs associated with mediastinal mass due to aortic aneurysm

Other systemic features:

A. Malignant masses spread to outside the mediastinum like:
a. Pleural effusion due to pleural involvement
b. Lymphadenopathy in neck and axilla
c. Hepatosplenomegaly

B. Specific features depend upon nature of mass:
a. Thymoma produces features of myasthenia gravis
b. Germ cell tumor produces gynecomastia
c. Mediastinal lymphoma produces Pel–Ebstein fever.

C. Nonspecific features are low-grade fever, lassitude, and weight loss.

D. Paraneoplastic syndrome:

Diseases	Features
Thymoma	Myasthenia gravis
	Red cell hypoplasia
	Acquired hypogammaglobulinemia
Thymic carcinoid	SIADH
	Cushing's syndrome

Continued

Continued

Diseases	Features
Intrathoracic goiter	Hyperthyroidism
	Hypothyroidism
Pheochromocytoma	Hypertension
Germ cell tumor	Klinefelter's syndrome
	Gynecomastia
Sarcoidosis	Hypercalcemia
Tumor of autonomic ganglion	Horner's syndrome
	Hypertension
	Diarrhea

Investigations of Mediastinal Masses

Nature of investigation	Features
Proper clinical history and examination	
Chest X-ray	Pericardial cyst or aortic aneurysm
HRCT	More accurate delineation of features present in X-ray
CT scan	For CT-guided FNAC from suspected tumor
Magnetic resonance imaging	It will determine invasion of vascular and neural tumor
	It will detect the infiltration of the tissue by malignant tumor
	T1 and T2 images clearly delineate mediastinal masses from the surrounding tissues—it is more useful in case of broncho-genic carcinoma and inflammatory masses
	Infiltration of the brachial plexus as well as vertebral foramina near the thoracic inlet
Ultrasound examination of scrotum	It can diagnose suspected germ cell tumor
Positron emission tomography-CT	In suspected lymphoma
	It can help to identify the suspected lesion from where biopsy can be taken
	It can monitor response to treatment
Radionuclide studies	^{131}I can diagnose substernal goiter
	^{131}I-metaiodobenzylguanidine uptake can diagnose pheochromocytoma
	Gallium scan—distinguish between lymphoma from thymoma
	Gallium can be picked up by bronchogenic carcinoma or inflammatory mass
	Tc-99m sestamibi diagnose parathyroid adenoma

Continued

Continued

Nature of investigation	Features
Biochemical markers	Alpha-fetoprotein (AFP), β-human chorionic gonadotropin (β-hCG), and carcinoembryonic antigen (CEA)—anterior mediastinal masses
	Serum level of β-hCG and AFP will rise in case of nonseminomatous malignant germ cell tumor
	Estimation of metanephrines and normetanephrines in blood and urine in case of suspected pheochromocytoma
	Raised level of epinephrine and norepinephrine in case of paraganglioma and neuroblastoma
Biopsy procedures	CT-guided Trucut biopsy is preferred to FNAC
	Endobronchial biopsy
	Surgical biopsy: In case of substernal lesions, anterior mediastinoscopy followed by biopsy (Chamberlain's procedure) Cervical mediastinoscopy in case of middle mediastinum for sampling of paratracheal and subcarinal glands Video-assisted thoracoscopic surgery under general anesthesia can visualize structures within the thorax along with biopsy from these structures

Q46. Respiratory acidosis.

MGR/SEO2010/MDI (5)

ANSWER

Definition

Acute rise in PCO_2 and hydrogen ion with fall in pH indicates acute respiratory acidosis. In this, there is rise in concentration of carbonic acids. In this type of acidosis, there is compensatory rise in serum bicarbonate which increases 1 mmol/L for each 10 mm Hg increase in $PaCO_2$ due to cellular buffering mechanism.

But after number of hours or days kidneys try to retain bicarbonate, thereby returning the value of pH value toward normal but not entirely normal—this is known as chronic respiratory acidosis. In this type of acidosis (>24 hours), there is increase in serum bicarbonate by 4 mmol/L for each 10 mm Hg increase in $PaCO_2$ by renal adaptation. But serum bicarbonate will not rise above 30 mmol/L.

Causes of Respiratory Acidosis

A. Central respiratory depression:
   a. Drugs such as sedatives and anesthetics
   b. Stroke
   c. Infection
B. Airway involvement:
   a. Bronchial asthma
   b. Respiratory tract obstruction
C. Lung parenchymal diseases:
   a. Chronic bronchitis
   b. Emphysema
   c. Pneumoconiosis
   d. Adult respiratory distress syndrome
   e. Barotrauma
D. Neuromuscular diseases:
   a. Myasthenia gravis
   b. Poliomyelitis
   c. Muscular dystrophies
   d. Myopathy
   e. Kyphoscoliosis
E. Miscellaneous:
   a. Obesity hypoventilation syndrome
   b. Hypoventilation
   c. Maladjusted mechanical ventilation where there is acute rise in PCO_2 due to fever and sepsis.

Clinical Features

Clinical features depend upon:
   a. Severity and duration of respiratory acidosis
   b. Underlying cause
   c. Presence of hypoxemia

Rapid rise in $PaCO_2$ may produce:
   a. Dyspnea
   b. Confusion
   c. Psychosis
   d. Hallucination
   e. May progress to coma

In case of chronic hypercapnia:
   a. Sleep disturbances
   b. Daytime somnolence
   c. Loss of memory
   d. Impairment of coordination
   e. Motor disturbances like:
      1. Asterixis
      2. Myoclonic jerk
      3. Tremor
   d. Features of raised intracranial tension:
      1. Headache
      2. Papilledema
      3. Abnormal reflexes
   e. Focal vasoconstriction produces focal muscle weakness

Diagnosis

A. Detailed history of drugs, alcohol, and physical examination of the patients
B. PFTs like:
   a. Spirometry
   b. Diffusion capacity of carbon monoxide
   c. Static lung volume
C. ABG analysis for $PaCO_2$, pH, bicarbonate, and PaO_2
D. Measurement of hematocrit
E. Assessment of upper airway, pleura, chest wall, and neuromuscular junction

Treatment

Management of respiratory acidosis depends upon:
   a. Severity of respiratory acidosis
   b. Onset of acidosis

The measurements are as follows:
   a. Reversion of underlying cause
   b. Restoration of adequate alveolar ventilation
   c. Tracheal intubation with assisted mechanical ventilation
   d. Administration of moist oxygen in case of severe obstructive pulmonary disease and chronic carbon dioxide retention

Rapid correction of respiratory acidosis should be avoided because of following probable complications:
   a. Cardiac arrhythmias
   b. Reduced cerebral perfusion
   c. Seizures

In case of chronic respiratory acidosis, $PaCO_2$ should be reduced gradually with the following aims:
   a. Restoration of $PaCO_2$ to baseline level
   b. Enhancement of renal excretion of bicarbonate by providing sufficient potassium and chloride
   c. Measurements for improvement of lung function

Q47. Drug-induced lung diseases.

MGR/OCT2003/MDI (5)

ANSWER

Almost all the drugs which are effective therapeutically may also produce adverse effects in the lung.

Mechanisms of Drug-related Injury

A. Contraction of bronchial smooth muscles, bronchospasm, and dyspnea

B. Production of increased endothelial permeability leading to development of pulmonary edema

C. By the drug metabolites, drug plus heptane producing inflammation of lung parenchyma, airways, and pleura

D. Enhanced fibrogenesis leading to:

- **a.** Pulmonary fibrosis
- **b.** Pulmonary hypertension
- **c.** Bronchiolitis obliterans
- **d.** Veno-occlusive disease

E. Due to drug-induced capillaritis or use of anticoagulants severe bleeding occurs within the lung parenchyma or within the pleura

Nature and Sites of Drug-induced Lung Injury

A. Parenchymal injury:

- **a.** HP, drugs involved are:
  1. Gold and methotrexate produce acute pneumonitis
  2. Nitrofurantoin and sirolimus produce chronic toxicity
- **b.** Eosinophilic pneumonia, drugs responsible are:
  1. Antiepileptic such as carbamazepine and phenytoin
  2. NSAIDs
  3. Minocycline
  4. Antidepressants
- **c.** Diffuse alveolar damage, drugs responsible are:
  1. Antineoplastic drugs in multidrug chemotherapeutic regimes such as busulfan, bleomycin, mitomycin C, chlorambucil, and melphalan
  2. Newer nitrosourea like etoposide
  3. Tyrosine kinase inhibitors such as imatinib and gefitinib
  4. Granulocyte monocyte colony-stimulating factors
- **d.** Granulomatous inflammation, drugs responsible are:
  1. Interferon α and β
  2. Methotrexate
  3. Sirolimus
  4. Etanercept
- **e.** Organizing pneumonia, drugs responsible are:
  1. Statins
  2. Methotrexate
  3. Interferon α and β
- **f.** DAH, drugs responsible are:
  1. Anticoagulants such as abciximab, fibrinolytic agents, sirolimus, and clopidogrel
  2. Drug-induced capillaritis by hydralazine and penicillamine
  3. Thrombocytopenia by abciximab
- **g.** Pulmonary fibrosis, drugs responsible are:
  1. Bleomycin
  2. Busulfan
  3. Lomustine
  4. Carmustine
- **h.** Pulmonary edema, drugs responsible are:
  1. Antimitotic drugs like gemcitabine
  2. IL-2
  3. Salicylates

B. Effect on the airways:

- **a.** Acute bronchospasm, drugs responsible are:
  1. Aspirin
  2. NSAIDs
  3. Beta blockers
- **b.** Upper airway obstruction, drugs responsible are:
  1. ACEIs
  2. Anaphylaxis from any drugs
- **c.** Bronchiolitis obliterans, drugs responsible are:
  1. Penicillamine
- **d.** Cough, drugs responsible are:
  1. ACEI
  2. Angiotensin II receptor antagonists

C. Pleural injury:

- **a.** Pleural effusion due to:
  1. Antiepileptic such as carbamazepine and phenytoin
  2. NSAIDs

3. Minocycline
4. Antidepressants

b. Pleural thickening and fibrosis:
1. Methysergide
2. Ergot compounds

D. Injury to pulmonary circulation:
a. Pulmonary hypertension by anorectic drugs like aminorex
b. Pulmonary veno-occlusive disease by cytotoxic drugs, radiation therapy, or marrow transplant
c. Obstruction of pulmonary circulation by acrylate glue

E. Drug-induced SLE: Drugs are:
1. Isoniazid
2. Hydralazine
3. Procainamide
4. Interferon
5. TNF-α

F. Neuromuscular disorders: Drugs are:
1. Aminoglycosides
2. Muscle relaxants
3. Neuroleptics
4. Corticosteroids
5. Opiates

Diagnosis

Following are the features which help in the diagnosis:

A. Increase in cough, respiratory distress in patient on >200 mg/day of drugs for >6–12 weeks
B. Exclusion of other lung diseases
C. Presence of ground-glass appearance or reticular shadow in HRCT or chest X-ray
D. Exclusion of heart failure and absence of radiological improvement following use of diuretic
E. After withdrawal of drugs, there is clinical and radiological improvement.

Gold standard is lung biopsy but it is rarely necessary.

Q48. Extracorporeal membrane oxygenation (ECMO).

MJPRU/2015/MDIV (10)

ANSWER

Definition

It is a form of cardiopulmonary life support where the blood is drained out of the vascular system and after circulation outside the body through the oxygenator by mechanical pump is returned into the circulation. Outside the body hemoglobin will be fully saturated with oxygen and carbon dioxide will be removed from the body.

Indications of Extracorporeal Membrane Oxygenation

A. Cardiac support:
a. Patients with low cardiac output of <2 L/min/m^2 with severe hypotension leading to diminished tissue perfusion in spite of full dose of ionotropic support and use of aortic balloon pump.
b. Refractory cardiogenic shock from any cause
c. Severe cardiomyopathy
d. After cardiac surgery inability to wean from cardiopulmonary bypass
e. Bridge to cardiopulmonary transplant
f. As bridge to long-term ventricular assist device
g. Post-transplant graft failure

B. Respiratory support:
a. Severe respiratory failure from ARDS
b. Management of advanced respiratory disease
c. As a bridge to heart-lung transplant

Technique

A. Veno-venous ECMO:
a. In case of use of single cannula, blood is withdrawn by the cannula from superior vena cava or right atrium and after being fully oxygenated blood is returned to right atrium.
b. In case of use of double cannula, blood is withdrawn from feral vein by a cannula and will be returned after being fully oxygenated into internal jugular vein or femoral vein through the other cannula.

B. Veno-arterial ECMO: The main aim is to bypass both lungs and heart. So by using one cannula, blood is withdrawn from the superior vena cava and after being fully oxygenated blood is returned into either carotid, femoral, or axillary artery.

Complications

A. Bleeding: This most frequent complication occurs at following sites:
a. At the site of insertion of cannula
b. At the site of operative site
c. Internal site:
1. Intracerebral
2. Intraperitoneal

3. Retroperitoneal
4. Intra-abdominal

Bleeding occurs due to:

a. Heparinization
b. Platelet dysfunction
c. Hemodilution of clotting factors

B. Systemic thromboembolism: It occurs due to development of thrombus within the extracorporeal circuit.

C. Neurological complications:

a. Seizures
b. Cerebral hemorrhage
c. Cerebral infarction

D. Hypertension: It is very dangerous as it is risk factor for stroke or intracerebral bleeding.

E. Sepsis with multiorgan failure

F. Mechanical complication due to formation of clot in the circuit

G. Complications related to veno-arterial ECMO:

A. When both femoral and femoral arteries are used, cardiac thrombosis is a possible complication due to retrograde flow into the ascending aorta.

B. Since whole oxygenated blood will return to femoral artery leading to preferential perfusion of oxygen in the lower limbs and abdomen, there will be cerebral hypoxia and decreased coronary perfusion.

Conclusion

Extracorporeal membrane oxygenation is the efficient life support in case of refractory respiratory and cardiac failure; 75% ARDS patients require ECMO now. It is also demonstrating good results when using in case of ARDS in case H1N1 infection. But it should be remembered that it is only the supportive therapy, not the modifier of the natural history of the parent disease.

Q49. Discuss "lung as an endocrine organ."

MUHS/MAY2011/MDIV (25)

ANSWER

Lungs are involved in the synthesis, storage, release, activation, and inactivation of hormones.

A. Synthesis and release of hormones from the lungs:

a. Histamines and other mediators of anaphylaxis: In case of type 1 hypersensitivity reaction or anaphylaxis, the mediators of anaphylaxis such as histamine, prostaglandin, and bradykinin are released from the mast cells present in the lung, polymorphs and other cells also contribute. Release of these mediators is inhibited by:

1. Alpha-adrenergic blockade
2. Beta-adrenergic stimulation
3. Atropine
4. Methylxanthines
5. Prostaglandin E

Release of mediators is enhanced by:

1. Cholinergic stimulation
2. Alpha-adrenergic stimulation
3. Beta-adrenergic inhibition

Release of mediators is influenced by alteration of intracellular level of cAMP.

b. Prostaglandins: These compounds are synthesized and released from the lung in normal conditions, but synthesis and release are catalyzed by:

1. Anaphylaxis
2. Mechanical ventilation at large volumes
3. Respiratory alkalosis
4. PE
5. Pulmonary edema

Effect of prostaglandin release depends upon the type of released prostaglandins.

1. Prostaglandin E2 (PGE2)—vasodilator and bronchodilator which is responsible for hypotension due to hyperventilation and PE.
2. Placental growth factor (PGF): It is vasoconstrictor and bronchoconstrictor and exacerbates the bronchial asthma.

c. Vasoactive polypeptide: Lungs contains kallikrein such as enzymes and large amount of kininogens which will break down to kinins; one of them is bradykinin responsible for anaphylaxis. These kinins dilate systemic and pulmonary blood vessels.

B. Pulmonary metabolism of vasoactive hormones:

a. Biogenic amines:

1. Lung will eliminate serotonin from the circulation through its uptake and inactivation.
2. Lungs play little role in metabolism of histamine as compared to liver and kidney
3. In case of catecholamine, 30–40% of norepinephrine is metabolized by the lungs but epinephrine is unaffected.

b. Prostaglandins: A specific enzyme in the lung oxidizes prostaglandin molecules at 15-carbon atom position to form 15-hydroxyprostaglandin dehydrogenase. The metabolism of prostaglandin in the lungs is selective such as PGE and PGF are metabolized whereas PGA will be nearly unaffected and there will be little loss of its activity.

c. Polypeptides and proteins:
   1. Proteolytic enzymes: Lungs are enriched with an enzyme, Trasylol, which inhibits several kinds of proteolytic enzymes, kallikreins. The significance of its metabolism in the lungs is not known.
   2. Bradykinin: It is effectively removed by the lungs though kininase is widely distributed in many tissues in the body. Its destruction is accomplished by:
      - Either removal of C-terminal residue by kininase-I
      - Or, removal of C-terminal dipeptide by kininase II

   But destruction of bradykinin is selective process; hence substances closely related to bradykinin like eledoisin, physalaemin, and substance P are not metabolized in the lungs.
   3. Angiotensin: Only this hormone is activated in the lung more effectively than blood. Here angiotensin I is converted into angiotensin II by splitting the C-terminal dipeptide leaving 8-residue peptide, which is angiotensin II.

Similarities between the metabolism of bradykinin and prostaglandin are as follows:

A. Activation of angiotensin I and inactivation of bradykinin are accomplished by removal of C-terminal dipeptide.
B. In the plasma membrane of pulmonary capillary endothelial cells, both the enzymatic processes will take place.
C. Angiotensin I and bradykinin will disappear completely during first circulation through the lungs.
D. Peptides from certain snake venom will potentiate the action of bradykinin but inhibit the action of angiotensin I.

   4. Other peptides: Hormones of posterior pituitary are not metabolized in the lung.

C. Hormones that influence respiratory function:

Many humoral substances influence the structure and functions of the lung.

a. Smooth muscle of bronchi and pulmonary vessels:
   1. Bronchoconstriction done by:
      - Catecholamine
      - Prostaglandins
      - Vasoactive intestinal peptide
      - Vasoactive lung peptide
   2. Bronchodilatation done by:
      - Histamine
      - $PGF_{2\alpha}$
   3. Vasodilatation done by:
      - PGF
      - Vasoactive intestinal peptide
      - Vasoactive lung peptide
   4. Vasoconstriction done by:
      - Norepinephrine
      - $PGF_{2\alpha}$

b. Ventilation:
   1. Vasoactive intestinal peptide in case of cirrhosis fails to be inactivated, so the active hormones will be responsible for hyperventilation, vasodilatation, and increased cardiac output.
   2. Number of bronchoactive amines by their direct effect on maintaining the caliber of alveolar duct and bronchi will influence the ventilation.
   3. High blood level of prostacyclin is responsible for hyperventilation in late pregnancy.

c. Maturation of lung and surfactant secretion:
   1. Glucocorticoids and ACTH accelerate the functional maturation of lung as well as induce premature production of alveolar surfactant as manifested by sudden increase in osmophilic inclusion bodies which is precursor of surfactant.

Q50. Approach and management of pulmonary sarcoidosis.

BF/NOV2013/MDII (10)

ANSWER

Definition

Sarcoidosis is characterized by presence of noncaseating epithelioid granuloma in different organs in the body as a result of immune response to unknown antigen; lung is the main involved organ.

Epidemiology

This disease is world-wise in distribution, women are mostly affected than men, age group being 20–40 years and second peak after the age of 50 years. Clinical presentation varies according to geographical location and ethnicity like:

- **a.** Erythema nodosum and Lofgren's syndrome are common in Scandinavian countries.
- **b.** Cardiac involvement is common in Japanese people.
- **c.** Disease is more severe with increased mortality in African–Americans and Africans.
- **d.** Skin lesions such as lupus pernio, nodules, and plaques are common in South Africa.
- **e.** Increased mortality due to progressive pulmonary fibrosis is more common in UK.

This disease is very uncommon in Southeast Asia except Japan, but rarely seen in Hong Kong and rare in Korea.

Etiology

Interaction between unknown antigen and genetic, host and environmental factors comes into play in development of sarcoidosis.

- **A.** Antigenic protein products of microorganisms produce immune response leading to formation of noncaseating granuloma.
- **B.** Several potential autoantigens such as vimentin, ATP synthetase, and Lysyl transfer RNA-induced host-antigen reaction producing autoantibodies stimulate the T-helper lymphocytes in the lung and blood leading to granuloma formation.
- **C.** There is link between environment and sarcoidosis as evidenced by presence of seasonal clustering of disease in winter and early spring.
- **D.** In some transplanted patients sarcoidosis may develop in recipient after transplantation due to transfer of transmissible agents.
- **E.** Other organisms may be regarded as etiologies such as chlamydia and lymphocytic DNA viruses such as Epstein–Barr virus, cytomegalovirus, HTLV1, and *Propionibacterium acnes* DNA.
- **F.** Inorganic dust like silica.

Genetic factors:

- **A.** Human leukocyte antigens:
  - **a.** HLA-DR3 has association with HLA-DR1 and HLA-DR4 has protection against sarcoidosis.
  - **b.** HLA-DRB1 0301 or HLA-DQB1 0201 is associated with mild sarcoidosis
  - **c.** There is association of acute sarcoidosis and HLA-B8, class 1 antigen.
  - **d.** Several HLA class II genes act independently or are converted to develop sarcoidosis.
- **B.** Non-HLA candidate antigens: These genes are responsible for:
  - **a.** Processing of antigen
  - **b.** Presentation of antigen
  - **c.** Activation of macrophages and T cells
  - **d.** Cell recruitment

  Candidate protein genes are:
  - **a.** Angiotensin-converting enzymes
  - **b.** CC chemokine receptor—CCR5 acts as receptor for macrophage inflammatory proteins as well as monocyte chemotactic protein 2
  - **c.** Clara cell 10-kDa protein
  - **d.** Heart shock protein
  - **e.** IL-1, IL-4R, IL-18, and interferon-α
  - **f.** Vascular endothelial growth factor

Pathogenesis

Initial event in sarcoidosis is alveolitis and critical cells responsible are macrophages and T lymphocytes. Alveolar macrophages process the antigens leading to recruitment of helper T lymphocytes CD4+ cells into the lung; as a result there will be decrease in T4 lymphocytes in the blood. There is also local proliferation of T cells in the lung. Many proinflammatory cytokines and chemokines such as IL-2, IL-12, interferon-γ, and TNF-α are responsible for:

- **a.** Recruitment and activation of inflammatory cells
- **b.** Perpetuation of inflammatory response
- **c.** Initiation of granuloma formation

Two active chemokines are also responsible for recruitment of neutrophils in active sarcoidosis; they are:

- **a.** IP-10
- **b.** RANTFS

There is also development of cell-mediated immunity in these patients as a result of depletion of T lymphocytes in the peripheral blood as evidenced by negative tuberculin test and decreased response to viral and fungal antigens. So the patient will be susceptible to opportunistic infection.

On the other hand, T lymphocytes activate B-lymphocytes to produce different immunoglobulins leading to development of polyclonal hyperglobulinemia, production of various antibodies against various viral antigens, formation of immune complexes, and formation of erythema nodosum, uveitis.

Alveolar macrophages derived from mononuclear cells and also from local proliferation are responsible for two functions—being antigen-presenting as well as antigen processing-cells produce proinflammatory cytokines which are responsible for proliferation and activation of T4 cells and macrophages.

- **a.** Inflammatory response is Th1 type in sarcoidosis and it is associated with cytokines like IL-2, interferon-γ, and TNF-α.
- **b.** Macrophages produce IL-12 and thus it will intensify Th1 response and induce TNF-α production by T and natural killer cells.
- **c.** Both macrophages and lymphocytes will produce IL-18 and it will increase INF-γ by T and natural killer cells.

Hence in active sarcoidosis, both IL-12 and IL-18 are present in high concentration in blood.

Pathology

Characteristic histological finding in sarcoidosis is formation of granuloma. As a result of influence and stimulation of cytokines, alveolar macrophages will be differentiated into epithelioid cells and then to giant cells which are surrounded by CD8 T lymphocytes, mononuclear cells, and B lymphocytes which will be encased by fibrous tissue formed from fibroblast proliferation. Th1 cells when switch to Th2 cells will produce IL-4 which in association with fibroblastic growth factor, platelet-derived growth factor, insulin-like growth factor-binding protein, and granulocyte-macrophage colony-stimulating factor stimulate fibroblast to lay down fibrous tissue.

In the lung, granulomas are distributed in perivascular and peribronchial regions. These granulomas later on persist or resolve or coalesce to destroy lung tissue leading to fibrosis mainly involving upper lobe.

In addition to granuloma, intrathoracic lymph nodes and alveolitis may occur. Alveolitis is composed of macrophages and lymphocytes.

Granuloma secrete following factors:

- **A.** Epithelioid cells in the granuloma secrete angiotensin-converting enzyme (ACE) thus increasing the serum level of ACE—though it is nonspecific marker it can give the estimation of burden of granuloma and sarcoid activity.
- **B.** Vitamin D3 is secreted in large amount which in turn increases the absorption of calcium leading to hypercalcemia. Among the two allele variants of vitamin D receptor, gene B allele is associated with sarcoidosis.

Clinical Presentation

- **A.** Nearly two-thirds of patients are usually asymptomatic and accidentally diagnosed when bilateral hilar lymphadenopathy is detected in routine chest X-ray.
- **B.** In other patients, there may be cough and exertional dyspnea because in 90% cases lung and intrathoracic lymph nodes are involved. To start with dyspnea is with exertion, but as the disease progresses it will be present at rest also. Dyspnea may be due to the following factors:
  - **a.** Obstruction to the airways
  - **b.** Restrictive lung disease
  - **c.** Both obstructive and restrictive lung disease
  - **d.** Compression of large airways by enlarged mediastinal lymph nodes

  Cough to start with is dry but if there is progressive fibrosis and bronchiectasis it will be productive; in that case expectoration may be mucoid or yellow.
- **C.** Hemoptysis
- **D.** Wheezing in case of endobronchial involvement due to airway obstruction which can be relieved by bronchodilators.
- **E.** Vague chest pain
- **F.** Constitutional symptoms are lassitude, fever, malaise, weight loss, and arthralgia which may be seen in 20% of patients and can occur with any one organ involvement.

Physical Findings

- **A.** Rhonchi in case of airways obstruction
- **B.** Crackle is usually absent but in 20% patients it may be present.

Extrapulmonary Manifestations

- **A.** Lofgren's syndrome—it is characterized by high fever, erythema nodosum, hilar lymphadenopathy, and polyarthritis associated with uveitis.
- **B.** Cutaneous sarcoid:
  - **a.** Lupus pernio: Present in the face as dull red or reddish-brown lesion plaques on the nose, skin below the eyes, and cheeks.
  - **b.** Erythema nodosum: Painful reddish nodules involving the lower limbs.
  - **c.** Sarcoid nodules may be formed in the scar tissue.

C. Ocular sarcoid:
   a. Uveitis
   b. Conjunctivitis
   c. Chorioretinitis
   d. Optic neuritis

D. Lymph nodes: These nodes are nontender, mobile, and discrete
   a. Hilar region
   b. Abdomen

E. Liver and spleen:
   a. Multiple hypoechoic lesions in the spleen
   b. Granulomatous hepatitis
   c. Chronic cholestasis
   d. Hepatomegaly or hepatosplenomegaly

F. Neurosarcoid:
   a. Headache
   b. Mental confusion
   c. Seizures
   d. Cranial nerve involvement producing optic neuritis and facial palsy
   e. Sarcoid granuloma deposition in the hypothalamus or pituitary gland
   f. Aseptic meningitis
   g. Transverse myelitis due to deposition of sarcoid granuloma in the spinal cord
   h. Obstructive hydrocephalus due to obstruction in the third ventricle

G. Sarcoid involvement in the heart:
   a. Dilated or congestive cardiomyopathy
   b. Left ventricular failure or congestive cardiac failure
   c. Bundle branch block or complete heart block
   d. Different arrhythmias

H. Hypercalcemia due to increased conversion of 1-hydroxy vitamin D3 to 1,25-dihydroxy vitamin D3 which increases absorption of calcium. As a result, following may occur:
   a. Nephrocalcinosis
   b. Renal stones

I. Kidney: Noncaseating granulomatous renal disease producing renal dysfunction.

J. Upper respiratory tract:
   a. Epistaxis
   b. Sinusitis
   c. Nasal congestion
   d. Destruction of nasal septum producing saddle nose deformity
   e. Laryngeal stridor due to laryngeal sarcoid and hoarseness of voice

K. Salivary gland: Parotid, submandibular, and lacrimal gland involvement leading to dry eyes and xerostomia.

L. Muscle and joint:
   a. Muscle weakness and pain in the muscles resembling polymyositis
   b. Punched-out lesions in the metacarpophalangeal and interphalangeal joints
   c. Lytic bony lesions in the spine and long bones

M. Hematogenous involvement:
   a. Granulomatous lesion in the bone marrow
   b. Hypersplenism
   c. Peripheral lymphopenia

Investigations

A. Chest X-ray: It is abnormal in 90% of patients. It is used as grading system of sarcoidosis:
   a. Stage 0: Normal chest radiograph in 5–10% of patients.
   b. Stage I: Bilateral hilar lymphadenopathy in 40% patients, it is associated with right paratracheal, subcarinal, or pretracheal lymph adenopathy.
   c. Stage II:
      1. Hilar adenopathy with or without mediastinal adenopathy associated with pulmonary infiltrates in perivascular or peribronchial reticulonodular involving upper and mid-zones
      2. Discrete pulmonary nodules
      3. Fluffy alveolar infiltrate looking like small areas of consolidation
      4. Miliary pattern of shadow
   d. Stage III: Pulmonary infiltrate consisting of reticulonodular or alveolar shadows in upper and mid-zones of lungs without hilar or mediastinal lymphadenopathy.
   e. Stage IV:
      1. There is extensive fibrosis with traction bronchiectasis
      2. Pulling of hila
      3. Presence of small and large bulla and honeycombing appearances involving upper lobe, lingual, and right middle lobe.

B. HRCT:

a. It can detect adenopathy and pulmonary infiltrates which cannot be diagnosed by chest X-ray.

b. It can delineate exact nature and distribution of infiltrate.

c. Distribution of infiltrate is peribronchial, perivascular, or may be along the lung fissures.

d. Honeycombing and ground-glass opacities which cannot be seen in chest X-ray.

It is useful in case of the following:

a. Evaluation of suspected sarcoidosis in patients presenting with extrapulmonary sarcoid.

b. Prior to intake of biopsy from enlarged mediastinal nodes

c. For evaluation of uncommon X-ray appearances in sarcoidosis

d. For evaluation of bronchiectasis, fibrocystic disease, and mycetoma.

C. PET scan:

It cannot differentiate sarcoid from malignancy. Following are the mediastinal masses, but along with MRI it can evaluate cardiac sarcoidosis

D. Lung function test:

It may demonstrate obstructive or restrictive pattern or both.

In case of restrictive defect, following pattern can be seen:

a. Fall in carbon monoxide diffusion—it is the earliest feature

b. Decrease in total lung volume

c. Later fall in VC

d. Fall in RV

e. Fall in FRC

Obstructive pattern can be demonstrated as follows:

a. Decreased FEV_1

b. Reduced FVC

c. Reduced FEV_1/FVC ratio

d. Reduced expiratory flow rate

In case of combined defect, following features are seen:

a. Reduced carbon monoxide diffusion

b. Reduced FVC

c. Reduced lung volume

d. Significantly reduced expiratory flow rates

e. Reduced FEV_1/FVC ratio

In case of extensive fibrosis of lung, there is hypoxemia.

E. Fiberoptic bronchoscopy with transbronchial biopsy

Here, diagnostic yield is 60–90%. Four to six biopsies are usually taken.

F. Endoscopic bronchial ultrasound-guided transneedle bronchial biopsy:

Its advantages are:

a. High diagnostic yield

b. Reduction of injury to mediastinal vessels

c. Superior to standard transbronchial needle biopsy

G. Bronchoalveolar lavage fluid:

CD4:CD8 ratio of 3:5 is diagnostic of sarcoidosis.

H. Mediastinoscopy with biopsy: It can be used when all the above invasive procedures will fail.

I. Video-assisted thoracoscopic biopsy:

It is done in case of necrotizing sarcoid granulomatosis biopsy from solid lesion in the lung.

J. Other sites from where biopsy can be taken:

a. Skin

b. Peripheral lymph nodes

c. Conjunctiva

d. Minor salivary glands

e. Liver

K. Blood biochemistry:

a. T4 cell will be decreased.

b. CD4 level decreased and CD8 level increased

c. Increased level of ACE

d. Increased level of vitamin D3

e. Serum calcium level increased

Progression of the Disease

Natural course of this disease is variable.

A. Clinical and radiographic features of two-thirds patients will be resolved within 1–2 years.

B. In some patients, radiographic changes will persist with or without symptoms.

C. 10% patients will progress continuously clinically and radiologically with or without extrapulmonary manifestations and ultimately becomes debilitated.

D. Following factors are associated with worse prognosis:

a. Age of onset >40 years

b. Progressive pulmonary fibrosis

c. Chronic uveitis

d. African descent

e. Hypercalcemia

f. Presence of lupus pernio affecting the face

Treatment

Indications of Steroid Therapy

A. Severe form—Lofgren's syndrome
B. Persistent hypercalcemia
C. Chronic pulmonary sarcoidosis associated with deterioration of lung function
D. Renal dysfunction
E. Hepatic dysfunction
F. Neurosarcoidosis
G. Cardiosarcoidosis
H. Sarcoid myopathy
I. Disfiguring lupus pernio in the face
J. Splenomegaly with multiple hypoechoic lesion in the spleen
K. Uveitis not responding to topical steroid therapy or showing frequent relapse

Corticosteroids	30–40 mg/day. But in case of extrapulmonary sarcoid 60 mg/day	Dose has to be tapered slowly every 3–4 weeks to reach a maintenance dose of 5–10 mg/day Treatment has to be continued for at least 12 months. If it is stopped before this period it may relapse In some patients, it may be continued for 2–3 years to make the disease under control
	In case of life-threatening sarcoidosis with eye involvement	Intravenous methylprednisolone 0.5–1 g/day for 3–4 days followed by 60 mg/day prednisolone orally which has to be tapered slowly

Refractory to Steroid Therapy

Immunosuppressive therapy should be given in following cases:

A. Patients unresponsive to steroids
B. There is frequent relapse
C. There are untoward side effects of steroids

Prior to start of immunosuppressive therapy, the following baseline investigations should be done:

- **a.** Liver function test
- **b.** Complete blood count
- **c.** Serum creatinine

Following drugs are given:

Hydroxychloroquine	It is given in neurosarcoidosis and dermal sarcoid
Methotrexate	Steroid-resistant cases. Dose is 5–7.5 mg weekly and can be increased by 2.5 mg/week till the total dose of 10–15 mg weekly Folic acid should be taken daily at 5 mg except the date on which methotrexate has to be taken 10 mg steroid can be given simultaneously with methotrexate therapy
Leflunomide	In case steroid-resistant case, 20 mg/day
Azathioprine	In steroid-resistant cases, 50 mg/day for 2 weeks and it can be increased up to 100 mg/day
Mycophenolate mofetil	In neurosarcoidosis, ocular sarcoid hepatitis and steroid-resistant pulmonary sarcoid
Anti-TNF: Drugs are the following: Infliximab Adalimumab Etanercept	Infliximab: 3–5 mg/kg at 0, 2, 6, and 12 weeks Adalimumab: 40 mg every week or every other week subcutaneously in case of pulmonary sarcoid

Symptomatic Therapy

A. Embolization of culprit vessels in case of hemoptysis
B. In hypoxemic respiratory failure, continuous oxygen support at 1–2 L/min in PaO_2 is <55 mm Hg in resting state.
C. Prostacyclin epoprostenol can be used in case of long-term treatment in pulmonary hypertension. In some cases, oral drugs such as sildenafil or bosentan can be given.
D. In case of sarcoid-induced arrhythmias:

- **a.** Antiarrhythmic drugs
- **b.** Defibrillator
- **c.** Automatic implantable cardioverter

E. In case of congestive cardiomyopathy:

- **a.** Loop diuretics
- **b.** Afterload reducing agents
- **c.** Spironolactone
- **d.** Digoxin
- **e.** Beta-blocker can be used judiciously

F. Lung transplantation:

In case of advanced pulmonary sarcoidosis, it is the ultimate choice. Mortality of the patient awaiting for transplant is very high.

Indications of lung transplantation are:

a. FVC is <50% of predicted value
b. DLCO is <50% of predicted value
c. Declining of pulmonary function in spite of full medical therapy

Following are the risk factors in patients awaiting for transplantation:

a. Pulmonary hypertension
b. African–American race
c. Right atrial pressure of >15 mm Hg
d. Increased quantity of supplemental oxygen.

Q51. Extensively drug-resistant (XDR) tuberculosis.

MJPRU/2015/MDIV (10)

Bedaquiline

DNB 2020 (5)

X-DR TB.

MGR UNIVERSITY, 2021 (10)

ANSWER

Definition

Pre-extensive drug-resistant tuberculosis: This is characterized by tuberculosis resistant to isoniazid, rifampicin along with any one fluoroquinolone.

Extensive drug-resistant tuberculosis: This tuberculosis is characterized by resistance to isoniazid, rifampicin, fluoroquinolone, and any one of the second-line injectable class of drugs such as amikacin, kanamycin, and capreomycin.

Types of Extensive Drug-resistant Tuberculosis

A. Drug resistant among the new cases (primary cases): This patient is characterized by evidence of drug resistance in patients who have not been treated for tubercular disease or who received treatment for tuberculosis for <1 month.
B. Drug resistance among the previously treated patients (secondary cases): This can be defined as drug resistance in such patients who have already antitubercular drugs for >1 month.

Pathogenesis

Extensive drug resistance occurs in following cases:

A. If patients took the drugs irregularly
B. If physicians prescribed drug is incorrect dose and incorrect drugs.

Resistance to antitubercular drug mainly occurs due to spontaneous mutation of chromosomes at a rate of 10^6 to 10^8 bacterial replication which corresponds to average expected frequency of spontaneous mutation of chromosomes. This mutation results unlinked resistance, hence, probability of resistance to all three drugs is in order of 10^{18} to 10^{20}. A large tubercular cavity contains nearly 1 million of bacteria; hence, the chance of resistance is not at all possible if all the three drugs are used in combination. That is why short course therapy is of choice nowadays.

Genetic basis:

Antitubercular drug	Genes involved in resistance
Isoniazid	*KatG*
	inhA
Rifampicin	*rpoB*
Streptomycin	*RpsL*
	rrs
Ethambutol	*EmbAB*
Pyrazinamide	*pcnA*
Fluoroquinolones	*gyrA*

Drug-resistant strains can be prevented by taking the following measures:

a. Adherence to principles of sound treatment
b. Administration of at least two bactericidal drugs to which bacteria are susceptible.
c. Fixed dose combination use
d. Supervision of treatment with patient support
e. Verification that patient has successfully completed the course.

Transmission of drug-resistant strain can be prevented by the following mechanisms:

a. Control of infection through the respiratory tract
b. Early detection of people with active tuberculosis
c. Immediate treatment with effective drugs

Clinical Features of XDR Tuberculosis

Patients are clinically indistinguishable from drug sensitive tubercular patients. A cardinal rule to suspect drug-resistant tuberculosis is the following:

A. Past history of treatment for tuberculosis
B. Contact with patients with proven MDR-tuberculosis
C. HIV-positive patients with suspicion of developing XDR-tuberculosis

Diagnosis of XDR-TB

A. X-pert MTB or XDR
B. Hain genotype Line Probe Assay
C. Genotype test

Treatment of XDR-tuberculosis

Principles of Treatment

A. Regimen should be planned according to history, drug susceptibility tests, genetic test, Hain LPA assay, and Gene-Xpert test.

B. The right number of drugs has to be added.

C. Selection of right number of drugs from different groups of drugs: At least five drugs have to added in the intensive phase, these are:

- **a.** Pyrazinamide
- **b.** One drug from group A
- **c.** One drug from group B
- **d.** Two drugs from group C
- **e.** If the minimum number of drugs cannot be incorporated, then one from group D and one from group D3 may be added to make the total number to five.
- **f.** In some case, high dose of isoniazid—10–15 mg/kg can be added to strengthen the treatment.

D. Treatment should be given for right duration. According to WHO, total duration of treatment should be 22–24 months, among which 5 months will be intense phase where injectable agent should be given and it should be discontinued after 4 months of culture conversion.

E. Right dose with highest end of the range should be used to compensate the inherent weakness of the drugs, otherwise underdosing may produce treatment failure or overdosing produces toxicity.

F. Drugs should be given daily not intermittently

G. Close monitoring of the drug toxicity

H. Whenever possible early surgery is required because in case of more resistant strain threshold for surgery will be low.

I. Proper address of other comorbid conditions like malnutrition, poverty, diabetes, biomass exposure, etc.

Outcome of XDR-TB

A. Mortality is 30%.

B. In case of HIV-positive patient mortality will be higher.

Bedaquiline

This new drug is mycobacterial ATP synthetase inhibitor. Recommended dose is 400 mg for 2 weeks followed by 200 mg thrice weekly for 22 weeks. Now WHO recommends to use this drug for only 6 months.

Adverse effects: It can produce QT prolongation; hence, ECG monitoring is essential. It is used cautiously in case of elderly and HIV-positive patients. It is advised not to use in case of pregnant women and children.

Delamanid

It is nitro-dihydroimidazooxazole derivative. It will inhibit synthesis of mycolic acid.
Recommended dose is:

- **a.** 50 mg twice daily for 24 weeks in case of 20–35 kg
- **b.** 100 mg twice daily in case of >35 kg of body weight

Side effects: It prolongs the QTc interval. Hence, it is contraindicated where the QTc interval is >500 ms.

Patients with XDR-TB have poor prognosis because only end-of-life treatment can be given to these patients because nearly all the treatment options have been exhausted.

Aggressive treatment with five effective drugs under strict observation, bactericidal monitoring, and intensive support from the patient can avert death.

If the patient has sufficient pulmonary reserve having localized disease to one lung, lobectomy or wedge resection can be performed.

XDR-TB may be complicated by medical as well as social factors, hence:

- **a.** This patient should be admitted in specialized center.
- **b.** Patient should require adequate support from the community.
- **c.** Treatment should be given as ambulatory basis.

WHO classification of drugs of MDR-TB:

Steps	Drug group	Options
Add later generation fluoroquinolones	Levofloxacin	A
	Moxifloxacin	
	Gatifloxacin	
Add one second-line injectable drug	Amikacin	B
	Capreomycin	
	Kanamycin	
	(Streptomycin)	
Add two or more second-line drugs	Ethionamide/ Protionamide	C
	Cycloserine/Terizidone	
	Linezolid	
	Clofazimine	
Add pyrazinamide and any other first-line drug to strengthen the regimen	Pyrazinamide	D1
	Ethambutol	
	High dose isoniazid	

Continued

Continued

Steps	Drug group	Options
Add bedaquiline or delamanid	Bedaquiline	D2
	Delamanid	
Add any of the three drugs if the regimen cannot be composed otherwise	Para-aminosalicylic acid	D3
	Imipenem-cilastatin	
	Meropenem	
	Amoxicillin-clavulanate	

Q52. Discuss the etiology, pathophysiology, clinical features, and management of cystic lung disease.

MGR/APR2016/MDII (15)

ANSWER

Cyst can be defined as round circumscribed area which is surrounded by thin wall of fibrous and epithelial tissue of variable thickness. Lung cyst is formed by various mechanisms:

- **a.** Airway obstruction with distal dilatation of airspaces
- **b.** Necrosis of the walls of alveoli
- **c.** Lung parenchymal destruction by proteases

Cyst usually contains air, but in few occasions, it may contain liquid or solid material.

Causes of Cystic Diseases of Lung

- **A.** Pulmonary Langerhans cell histiocytosis
- **B.** Lymphangioleiomyomatosis
- **C.** Lymphocytic interstitial pneumonia
- **D.** Follicular bronchiolitis
- **E.** Light chain deposition disease
- **F.** Amyloidosis
- **G.** Pneumocystosis
- **H.** Paracoccidioidomycosis
- **I.** Constrictive bronchiolitis
- **J.** Desquamative interstitial pneumonia
- **K.** Hypersensitivity pneumonitis

Pulmonary Langerhans Cells Histiocytosis

Definition

This disease is characterized by accumulation of proliferation of mononuclear cells along with infiltration of Langerhans cell in the interstitium and small bronchiole of the lungs.

Pathogenesis

- **A.** Presence of immune complexes in the blood and also bound to the tissues
- **B.** Nonspecific increase of IgG in the BAL fluid
- **C.** Abnormalities in the T cell function

In case of smoker, glycoproteins present in the smoke being immunostimulant together with other regulatory glycoprotein peptides perform a role in the pathogenesis.

According to one hypothesis, Bombesin secreted by neuroendocrine cells is increased in the lungs in case of smokers. It will activate monocytes which in turn stimulate epithelial cells and fibroblasts and at the same time stimulate macrophages to produce cytokines. These cytokines stimulate as well as activate Langerhans cells present in the lung.

Relation with malignancy:
Few subsets of these patients associated with BRAF V600 mutation are prone to develop:

- **a.** Lymphoma
- **b.** Bronchogenic carcinoma
- **c.** Pulmonary carcinoid tumor
- **d.** Mediastinal ganglioneuroma

Pathology

The characteristics of the disease are:

- **A.** Infiltrate containing eosinophils, lymphocytes, and plasma cells
- **B.** Granuloma
- **C.** Langerhans cells are characterized by abundant acidophilic cytoplasm in the mononuclear cells having irregular, elongated nuclei with prominent grooves and folds.
- **D.** During healing, there is fibrosis leading to honeycombing of the lung marked in the upper lobes.

Clinical Features

- **A.** 10–25% are asymptomatic; presence of nodular lesions in the upper and mid-zones of both lungs can be diagnosed.
- **B.** Two most important symptoms are cough and respiratory distress during exertion.
- **C.** Appearance of recurrent spontaneous pneumothorax
- **D.** Constitutional symptoms are low-grade fever, fatigue, and weight loss.
- **E.** Extrapulmonary manifestations are:
  - **a.** Bone pain, pathological fractures in case of bone involvement
  - **b.** Diabetes insipidus in case of CNS involvement

c. Maculopapular erythematous lesions, crusted seborrheic lesion if skin is involved
d. Pulmonary arteriopathy
e. Veno-occlusive disease

F. Physical findings:
a. Clubbing is uncommon
b. On auscultation rhonchi in some patients, crackles in upper lobe in some cases and in some cases both are present.

G. With progression of the disease there is increasing fibrosis leading to:
a. Hypoxemic respiratory failure
b. Pulmonary hypertension
c. Cor pulmonale
d. Congestive cardiac failure

Investigations

A. Chest X-ray demonstrates:
a. Micronodular lesions, occasionally miliary lesions in the mid and upper zones of both the lungs
b. Superimposed cystic ring shadows due to cavitation of the nodular lesions
c. Coalescing of small cystic lesion resulting in large bullae formation

B. HRCT thorax: It will demonstrate:
a. Nodules in upper and mid-zones
b. Progression of nodular lesion toward cavitation
c. Increasing fibrosis leading to honeycombing appearance
d. Ground-glass appearance
e. Large cysts and bullae

C. PET-scan:
a. In early disease, there is increased uptake associated with nodular lesion
b. In late stage, there is negative PET-scan associated with fibrosis and honeycombing.

D. Lung function test demonstrates both restrictive and obstructive patterns as evidenced by:
a. Decrease in the ratio of FEV_1/FVC
b. Decreased DLCO
c. Standard 6-minute walk test will show low SaO_2.

E. Bronchoalveolar lavage fluid:
a. >5% Langerhans cells suggest this disease
b. <4% Langerhans cells are found in:
1. ILD
2. Bronchiolitis
3. Bronchoalveolar carcinoma

F. Lung biopsy:
a. Transbronchial lung biopsy is 10–40% positive
b. Open lung biopsy is the procedure of choice.

Treatment

A. Prednisolone 40 mg/day for 4 weeks; then its dose will be gradually reduced by 5 mg every 3–4 weeks to maintenance dose of not >10 mg/day.

B. In case of rapidly progressive disease not controlled by steroids, cytotoxic drugs such as cyclophosphamide, methotrexate, or chlorambucil may be tried.

C. Cladribine, cytotoxic drug that is toxic to monocytes and lymphocytes is used in progressive disease.

D. In case of BRAF V600 mutation can be treated by targeted therapy vemurafenib, a BRAF inhibitor.

E. Pulmonary hypertension can partially respond to conventional therapy.

F. Bone lesion can be treated by radiotherapy.

G. Pneumothorax can be treated by:
a. Chest tube drainage
b. In case of recurrence pleurodesis

H. In case of rapidly progressive disease, bone marrow transplantation

I. Advanced disease with respiratory failure, the treatment is lung transplantation.

Lymphangioleiomyomatosis

Definition

This disease occurring in mainly women of child-bearing age is characterized by infiltration of the lung by unusual form of smooth muscle cells, called LAM cells leading to cyst formation along with destruction of lung tissue.

Pathogenesis

Hamartin (TSC-1) on chromosome 9 tuberin (TSC-2) on chromosome 16 is responsible for controlling cell growth and survival through the rapamycin-signaling pathway. Mutation of these two genes results in activation of mTOR kinase and S6 kinase leading to:
a. Increased synthesis of protein
b. Proliferation of cells
c. Migration of cells
d. Invasion of the tissue

Mutation and heterogenicity of TSC-2 genes are responsible for sporadic disease. These LAM cells have the capability to metastasize; hence it can involve transplanted lung leading to its recurrence.

LAM cells have estrogen and progesterone receptors—these show female sex hormones, mainly estrogen that has propensity for evolution of this disease.

Pathology

Microscopically there are:

- **a.** Proliferation of LAM cells in the airways leading to obstruction of the airways
- **b.** Proliferation within the lymphatic vessels leading to lymphatic obstruction
- **c.** Proliferation within the vessels leading to obstruction or rupture of the vessels leading to alveolar hemorrhage

LAM cell is a type of smooth muscle cell expressing actin, desmin, and vimentin on their surface. These cells stain with HMB-45. Estrogen receptor present on the LAM cell is associated with antiapoptotic protein Bcl-2.

Clinical Features

- **A.** Progressive breathlessness
- **B.** Associated wheeze
- **C.** Hemoptysis may occur
- **D.** Pleuritic chest pain due to unilateral or bilateral recurrent pneumothorax
- **E.** Unilateral or bilateral chylous pleural effusion may be recurrent and associated with chyloptysis.
- **F.** Extrapulmonary manifestations are:
  - **a.** Angiomyolipoma
  - **b.** Abdominal lymphadenopathy
  - **c.** Abdominal LAM
  - **d.** Chylous ascites
  - **e.** Tuberous sclerosis

Investigations

- **A.** Chest X-ray:
  - **a.** Reticular shadowing with thin-walled cyst
  - **b.** Septal Kerley B line
  - **c.** Small cysts may coalesce to form large cyst.
  - **d.** Pneumothorax
  - **e.** Pleural effusion—chylous
- **B.** HRCT thorax: Following features are described:
  - **a.** Evenly distributed thin-walled cysts of 2–20 mm in both the lungs with normal intervening parenchyma. They may coalesce to form large cyst of 5–10 cm.
  - **b.** Presence of ground-glass densities representing recent pulmonary hemorrhage
  - **c.** Hilar lymphadenopathy
  - **d.** Retrocrural lymphadenopathy
- **C.** HRCT of abdomen:
  - **a.** Angiomyolipoma indicated by presence of fat of >10 Hounsfield density.
  - **b.** Lymphadenopathy along the course of axial lymphatics—it may be retrocrural, retroperitoneal, or pelvic.
- **D.** Lung function test:
  - **a.** In early stage, it is normal.
  - **b.** As the disease progresses:
    1. Both obstructive and restrictive pattern are seen.
    2. Reduced DLCO
    3. Hypoxemia
    4. Worsening of hypercapnia

Treatment

- **A.** Hormone therapy with:
  - **a.** Drug for oxygen blockade
  - **b.** Oophorectomy was recommended in earlier days producing depletion of estrogen.
- **B.** Sirolimus: There are two different complexes which involve mTOR-1 and mTOR-2. Sirolimus partially inhibits mTOR-1 but some degree of inhibition also in case of mTOR. Dose is 2 mg/day, but after getting the stability of the lung disease dose can be reduced to 1 mg/day.

  Adverse effects are: mucosal ulcers, infection, hyperlipidemia, amenorrhea, impairment of renal function, hypertension, and thrombocytopenia.
- **C.** Everolimus: This drug is not approved for sporadic LAM, dose is 2.5 mg/day increasing to 10 mg/day.
- **D.** Inhibitors of autophagy:

  By this mechanism, cells maintain energy hemostasis and recycle proteins

  Hydroxychloroquine blocks the autophagy and induces death of the cells. This inhibition of autophagy will induce the effect of sirolimus on LAM.
- **E.** Treatment of airways obstruction:
  - **a.** By bronchodilators in the form of inhaled or nebulization of β2 agonist
  - **b.** Oxygen therapy in case of increasing dyspnea with hypoxemic respiratory failure
- **F.** Pneumothorax:
  - **a.** Chest drainage
  - **b.** In case of recurrence pleurodesis
  - **c.** Lung transplantation

G. Chylous effusion:
   a. Octreotide to reduce the lymph production which can be done by reducing the splanchnic blood flow.
   b. Low fat diet to reduce the lymph production
   c. In case of symptomatic patient, drainage of effusion
   d. Surgical measures:
      1. Pleurodesis
      2. Pleurectomy
      3. Ligation of thoracic duct
      4. Pleuroperitoneal shunt

Birt–Hogg–Dubé Syndrome

It is an autosomal dominant disease characterized by renal neoplasm, pulmonary cysts, and follicle tumor seen in fourth or fifth decade of life, sex ratio being equal.

Pathogenesis

Mutation of FLCN present in the chromosome 17p leading to mTOR-signaling abnormality. Another possible pathway is abnormal expression of TGF-β or neoplasia protein.

Pathology

A. Intraparenchymal air-filled cyst surrounded by normal lung tissue
B. Abnormal proliferation and infiltration of cells

Clinical Features

A. Pulmonary manifestation
B. Dermatological manifestation
C. Renal manifestation: Cyst to tumor

HRCT Thorax

It demonstrates multiple thin-walled lentiform or round well-defined cyst having size of 2–78 mm, basilar, subpleural, or medial in distribution.

Pulmonary function is normal.

Till date there is no treatment for pulmonary cyst.

Lymphocytic Interstitial Pneumonia

It is benign lymphoproliferative disease characterized by lymphocytic and plasmacytic infiltrate producing lymphoid aggregates affecting the alveoli and interlobar septa affecting mainly women of fifth or sixth decade.

Associated diseases are many connective tissue diseases, Epstein–Barr infection, and acquired immunodeficiencies.

Clinical Features

Clinical features are cough, fatigue, dyspnea, and chest pain.

Lung function test: Restrictive pattern

Investigations

A. Chest X-ray:
   a. Thin-walled cyst having different shapes of 30 mm in diameter
   b. Diffusely distributed but mainly in lower lobe along the peribronchovascular bundle.
B. HRCT of thorax:
   a. Ground-glass opacities and consolidation
   b. Peribronchovascular bundle thickening
   c. Interlobar septal thickening
   d. Reticular opacities
   e. Mediastinal and hilar lymphadenopathy

Follicular Bronchiolitis

Main findings are:
   a. Bronchiolocentric lymphocytic infiltration never extending to other interstitial compartments.
   b. Obstructive pattern with air trapping—it occurs due to:
      1. Extrinsic compression on the bronchus by the lymphoid tissue producing check-valve mechanism
      2. Bronchial ischemia due to vascular obstruction

HRCT findings:
   a. Centrilobular opacities with ground-glass opacities
   b. Lower lobe distribution along the peribroncho-vascular bundle

Light Chain Deposition Disease

It is characterized by deposition of light chain in different tissues in the body. It is seen electron microscopically as amorphous materials containing nodular deposits. Cysts are formed due to obstruction of bronchiole by this protein deposit.

Renal involvement is characterized by proteinuria and renal failure. It is followed by cardiac and hepatic involvement.

HRCT findings are:
   a. Lymphadenopathy
   b. Diffuse thin-walled cysts having 2 cm in diameter

Amyloidosis

It is characterized by extracellular deposition of soluble proteins in insoluble form that are stained by Congo red and has apple-green birefringence under polarized light. There are two amyloid proteins:

A. AL protein—it is derived from light chain of immunoglobulin, and it is associated with:
   - **a.** Primary amyloidosis
   - **b.** Amyloidosis associated with multiple myeloma
   - **c.** Isolated tracheobronchial amyloidosis
   - **d.** Pulmonary amyloidosis

B. Amyloid A (AA) protein—it is derived from the serum and is present in secondary amyloidosis.

Lung is formed in amyloid in three forms:

A. Pulmonary involvement in primary systemic amyloidosis
B. Pulmonary involvement in secondary amyloidosis
C. Isolated pulmonary amyloidosis

HRCT findings are:
   - **a.** Thin-walled cysts of varying sizes arranged in the periphery
   - **b.** Presence of nodules or masses
   - **c.** Thickening of interlobar septa
   - **d.** Presence of ground-glass opacities
   - **e.** Lymphadenopathy

Paracoccidioidomycosis

It is caused by *Paracoccidioides brasiliensis* and mostly occurs in male rural workers after inhalation of infectious particle into lung parenchyma in case of primary infection. There may be associated lymph node enlargement and mucocutaneous lesions as well as other glands such as kidney, CNS, liver, bones, adrenal glands and airways with deposition of epithelioid granuloma, abscesses, and necrosis.

Cysts are formed due to bronchial obstruction leading to dilatation of airway or central necrosis and loss of elastic recoil as a result of following factors:
   - **a.** Centrilobular fibrosis
   - **b.** Peribronchial granuloma formation

Following radiological patterns are described:
   - **a.** Reticular opacities
   - **b.** Consolidation
   - **c.** Reversed halo sign
   - **d.** Pulmonary cavitation
   - **e.** Paracicatricial emphysema

Desquamative Interstitial Pneumonia

It is characterized by extensive accumulation of macrophages in the alveoli. Male to female ratio is 2:1. Age of incidence is fifth decade of life. It occurs in smokers, more in case of connective tissue diseases such as rheumatoid arthritis and systemic sclerosis.

CT findings are:
   - **a.** Small round intervened by ground-glass opacities affecting mainly lower lobe
   - **b.** Mild distortion of lung architecture

Symptoms are cough and respiratory distress.

Hypersensitivity Pneumonitis

It is characterized by inflammation of lung parenchyma due to inhalation of fungal and avian antigen or chemical substances like isocyanates.

Pathology
   - **a.** Presence of bronchiolocentric and interstitial inflammation
   - **b.** Presence of granuloma
   - **c.** Fibrosis

Clinical Features
Respiratory distress and dry cough

HRCT Thorax
A. Randomly distributed cysts are sparse.
B. Centrilobular ground-glass appearances with micro-nodular opacities
C. Areas of mosaic attenuation
D. Nonspecific interstitial pattern

> **Q53. Management of HIV-positive patient with pulmonary tuberculosis.**
>
> **GMC/2016/MDIII (20)**
>
> **HIV associated tuberculosis.**
>
> **MGR UNI, TAMIL NADU, 2021 (10)**
>
> **NTR UNI OF HEALTH SC, VIJAYAWADA, JULY, 2021 (10)**

ANSWER

Following are the important links between HIV and tuberculosis:

A. Tuberculosis is the earliest opportunistic infection in HIV patients, when CD4 count is ≤300/cc.
B. It is the only transmissible opportunistic infection, and most common opportunistic infection; hence it is of immense importance.

C. HIV patients are more likely to have active tuberculosis by a factor of 100 as compared to non-HIV patients.
D. Most of the tuberculosis in HIV patients are either MDR-TB or XDR-TB; hence mortality is very high as compared to HIV-negative patients.
E. Early diagnosis and treatment can cure the patients.
F. Tuberculosis will accelerate the course of HIV as detected by HIV RNA level which can decline with successful treatment of tuberculosis.
G. Link between HIV and tuberculosis is bidirectional.
H. One-third of death of HIV patients is due to tuberculosis.

Risk from HIV Disease

A. HIV is the most important risk factor for converting latent tuberculosis to active phase.
B. Diabetes
C. Patients on hemodialysis
D. Patients receiving immunosuppressive treatment
E. Patients suffering from silicosis

Mechanism of Synergy between Tuberculosis and HIV Patients

CD4-positive T cells produce γ-interferon that activate macrophages to inhibit intracellular growth of *Mycobacterium tuberculosis*. But HIV inhibits these T cells selectively, thus inhibiting the production of γ-interferon and thereby increasing the risk of tuberculosis.

On the other hand, tuberculosis enhances the replication of HIV in the lung, thereby reducing the survival of these patients.

Clinical Features and Investigations

In HIV positive patients, it depends upon CD4+ cell count:

A. In patients with high CD4+ cell count, there are features of typical pulmonary reactivation such as:
   a. Fever with night sweats
   b. Cough
   c. Respiratory distress
   d. Loss of weight

   Chest X-ray demonstrates cavitary lesion in the upper lobe of the lung.
B. In patients with low CD4+ cell count, there will be the feature of disseminated tuberculosis. Chest X-ray demonstrates:
   a. Diffuse infiltrate or lower lobe reticulonodular infiltrate looking like miliary tuberculosis.
   b. Evidence of pleural effusion
   c. Hilar or mediastinal lymphadenopathy
   d. Spreading of tubercular lesion to other different organs such as bone, brain, cervical lymph nodes, and gastrointestinal tract.
C. In case of advanced HIV infection with active tuberculosis, there may be no symptom, so routine screening of tuberculosis is required for initial evaluation of HIV-positive patients.

Timing of tuberculosis in HIV patients:
Tuberculosis may occur at any time of HIV infection; it may occur prior to any other opportunistic infection.

Diagnosis

A. In HIV patients, CD4 cells go down producing energy; hence tuberculin test may be false negative. Centers for Disease Control and Prevention (CDC) recommends to perform tuberculin test with 5-TU purified protein derivative (PPD) with acceptable range of positivity of 5 mm reaction, and it should be routinely done in any HIV patient.

   In case of asymptomatic, HIV-negative patients having positive reaction with PPD and absence of any features of tuberculosis, risk of reactivation is 1% per year. On the other hand in case of untreated HIV infection with positive PPD test and no features of tuberculosis, risk of reactivation is 7–10% per year.
B. Interferon-γ release assay: It is very sensitive assay in HIV-positive patients. It may be difficult to interpret as a result if immune reactivation in the setting of fulminant HIV disease coinfected with tuberculosis where one cannot rely on negative PPD test.
C. Sputum microbiology is usually negative in HIV-positive patients; hence in case of clinical suspicion of tuberculosis empiric therapy should be started without delay.
D. Culture of the tubercular bacteria from the involved site is taken for definite diagnosis. Blood culture is positive in 15% patients.

Management of Coinfected HIV and Tuberculosis Patients

Patient should be kept in isolation ward with negative pressure. Treatment of tuberculosis is same as that in HIV-negative patients. Treatment is divided into two parts:

A. Tuberculosis treatment:
   a. Standard short course of chemotherapy with HREZ. But since incidence of MDR or extensively drug-resistant tuberculosis is very high in HIV patients, drug susceptibility testing has to be

performed which can guide the therapy. CDC guideline recommends 9 months treatment in patients who demonstrate clinical and bacteriological response.

b. Treatment should be direct observation therapy.

B. HIV treatment: Since HIV patient has high mortality, early introduction of antiretroviral therapy (ART) can improve the prognosis of these patients but monitoring both the therapies is very important to reduce drug-related toxicity, overlapping toxicity, drug interactions, paradoxical reactions, and immune reconstitution inflammatory syndrome (IRIS).

a. Increased incidence of drug toxicity:
   1. Incidence of hepatitis in patients receiving isoniazid
   2. Incidence of peripheral neuropathy in case of isoniazid
   3. Stevens–Johnson syndrome in patients receiving thiacetazone

b. Overlapping drug toxicity:
   1. Hepatitis may be due to isoniazid, rifampicin, pyrazinamide, and nevirapine (ART)
   2. Drug rashes may be due to antitubercular drugs or nevirapine, abacavir, and efavirenz.

c. Drug interactions:
   1. All PIs and some nonnucleoside reverse transcriptase inhibitors (NNRTs) will interact with rifampicin, because rifampicin is the potent inhibitor of cytochrome P450. So coadministration of rifampicin with the above drugs can increase the level of rifampicin leading to its toxicity and at the same time decrease the level of PI and NNRTs, thus reducing their efficacy. In this case, substitution of rifampicin with rifabutin, less potent inhibitor of this enzyme, takes place. Otherwise PIs can be replaced.

d. Paradoxical reactions: This can be defined as worsening of already present symptoms or appearance of new symptoms, signs, and changes in the radiographic appearances mainly in advanced HIV disease within 3 months of therapy or as early as 1 week of initiation of therapy. This is known as IRIS. There are two types of IRIS:
   1. Type 1 or paradoxical TB-IRIS: These patients are already diagnosed and on antitubercular treatment prior to starting of ART. So, there will be paradoxical worsening of tuberculosis with or without spreading of tuberculosis at different sites; it occurs usually within 3 months of therapy.
   2. Type 2 or unmasking TB-IRIS: It occurs in those patients who are not on antitubercular drugs prior to ART commencement. These patients will develop active tuberculosis within 3 months of commencement of ART. A large number of these patients already may have preexisting tuberculosis.

Mechanisms of IRIS

Main mechanism is restoration of immunity toward mycobacterial antigen. In the first month of ART, CD4+ count will rise leading to redistribution of memory cells from the area of immune reactivation which is followed by gradual recovery of native cells leading to:

A. Conversion of negative to positive tuberculin test
B. Improvement in CD4+ cell number and functions

Treatment

A. If CD4+ cell count is >50/c, ART can be delayed until 2–4 weeks following the initiation of antithyroid drug (ATD).
B. If CD4+ cell count is <50/cc, ART should be started as soon as possible in these patients.

Monitoring

A. Repeated CD4+ cell count should be done to see whether it is more or less than 200/cc.
B. Patient at risk of continued exposure should be tested yearly.
   a. PPD test is >5 mm in HIV patients.
   b. Patients with positive interferon-γ assay
   c. Those who are in close to household contact with active tuberculosis.

These patients should be treated with isoniazid along with pyridoxine for 9 months.

Atypical Mycobacterial Infection on HIV Patients

Epidemiology

There are 12 different mycobacteria involving lung in case of HIV-infected patients; most common atypical mycobacteria is *Mycobacterium avium* or intracellulare species—*Mycobacterium avium*-intracellulare complex or MAC. It is most common in US and rare in Africa.

Prior infection with *Mycobacterium tuberculosis* may decrease the risk of MAC infection.

MAC will arise from the organism that is ubiquitous in the environment like soil and water.

Transmission

Transmission occurs from person-to-person.

Portal of entry is respiratory tract or gastrointestinal tract. It is very late complication of HIV when CD4+ count is <50/cc.

Clinical Features

a. Fever with night sweat
b. Weight loss
c. Other clinical features are:
   1. Abdominal pain
   2. Diarrhea
   3. Lymphadenopathy

Investigations

a. Chest X-ray:
   1. Alveolar or nodular infiltrate
   2. Hilar or mediastinal lymphadenopathy
   3. Bilateral lower lobe infiltrate
b. Hematological:
   1. Anemia
   2. Raised alkaline phosphatase (ALP)
c. Culture of blood or involved tissue
d. Positive for MAC in two consecutive sputum samples—pulmonary infection

Treatment

A. Clarithromycin with ethambutol
B. In case of extensive disease, amikacin or ciprofloxacin or rifabutin has to be added.

Duration of Treatment

Indication of stoppage of treatment in the setting of ART therapy:

a. CD4+ count is >100/cc
b. Resolution of signs and symptoms
c. Negative culture

All should be present for 3–6 months.

Prevention of MAC in HIV-infected Patients along with Treatment

A. CD4+ cell <50/cc—azithromycin 1,200 mg weekly orally or 600 mg twice weekly or clarithromycin 500 mg twice daily orally.

   Alternative drug is rifabutin.

B. Prior documented disseminated disease

   Clarithromycin 500 mg twice daily orally plus ethambutol 15 mg/kg/day orally.

Duration of prophylactic treatment: Treatment should be continued till CD4+ cell count will reach >100/cc for >6 months.

Q54. Treatment of *Pneumocystis carinii* pneumonia.

MGR/APR2013/MDIII (7)

ANSWER

Treatment of Active *Pneumocystis Carinii* Infection of Lung in HIV-infected Patients

Treatment of choice is trimethoprim 160 mg plus 800 mg sulfamethoxazole—1 tablet thrice daily for 2–3 weeks.

Side effects are: skin rash and bone marrow suppression.

Alternative treatment is:

a. Dapsone 50 mg twice daily orally or 100 mg daily
   Or,
b. Dapsone 50 mg/day orally + pyrimethamine 50 mg/week orally + leucovorin 25 mg/week orally
   Or,
c. Clindamycin 300 mg orally thrice or four times daily + primaquine 15–30 mg orally once daily
   Or,
d. Atovaquone 1,500 mg/day orally

In case of severe infection, intravenous pentamidine should be given if patient is unable to tolerate trimethoprim-sulfamethoxazole.

Glucocorticoid should be given in following conditions:

a. If PaO_2 is <70 mm Hg.
b. Arterial-alveolar gradient is >35 mm Hg.

Steroids are effective, if they will be given within 72 hours of onset of this disease. They will act by blunting the inflammatory response.

Dose of the steroid is:

Prednisolone 40 mg twice daily for 5 days, then 40 mg daily for 5 days, then 20 mg daily for 11 days.

Total duration of treatment is 21 days.

Concurrent retroviral therapy will improve the survival of the patient.

Following are the possible causes of clinical deterioration of HIV patients with this infection in spite of continued treatment:

a. Drug-induced anemia
b. Methemoglobinemia
c. Pneumothorax
d. PE
e. Inappropriate dose

f. Severe PSP infection with persistent hypoxia in spite of ventilatory support
g. Associated CMV of *Mycobacterium avium-intracellulare* infection.

Prophylactic Treatment of PSP Infection in HIV-infected Patients

Prophylactic treatment should be given in following patients:

a. CD4 T cell count below 200/cc or CD4 percentage <15
b. Any patient with unexplained fever for >2 weeks
c. Patient with recent history of oropharyngeal candidiasis

Regimen of choice is trimethoprim-sulfamethoxazole (double strength)—1 tablet orally daily. This drug will protect against the following organisms:

a. *Toxoplasma gondii*
b. *Isospora belli*
c. *Listeria monocytogenes*
d. *Haemophilus influenza*
e. Staphylococci
f. Some gram-negative organisms

If the patient cannot tolerate this drug, following regime can be given:

a. Dapsone—100 mg/day + pyrimethamine 50 mg weekly + leucovorin 25 mg weekly
   Or,
b. Aerosolized pentamidine 300 mg via Respigard II nebulizer every month
c. Atovaquone 1,500 mg/day or 750 mg twice daily

Primary or secondary prophylaxis should be discontinued in patients on ART therapy in following patients:

a. Good suppression of HIV, i.e., <50 copies/mL
b. CD4+ cell count is >200/cc for at least 3 months.

Q55. Discuss the evaluation and management of pulmonary infections in retrovirus-infected patient.

MGR/APR2014/MDIII (15)

ANSWER

Organisms Involved in Case of HIV-related Pulmonary Infection

A. Bacterial infections:
   a. *Mycobacterium tuberculosis*
   b. Nontubercular mycobacteria
   c. Streptococcal pneumonia
   d. *Hemophilus influenzae*
   e. *Staphylococcus aureus*
   f. *Nocardia*
   g. *Listeria monocytogenis*
   h. *Klebsiella* species
   i. Gram-negative organisms
   j. *Rhodococcus*
B. Parasitic infections:
   a. *Toxoplasma gondii*
   b. *Strongyloides stercoralis*
   c. *Cryptosporidium* species
   d. *Microsporidium* species
   e. *Leishmania donovani*
C. Fungal infections:
   a. *Pneumocystis carinii*
   b. *Cryptococcus neoformans*
   c. *Histoplasma capsulatum*
   d. *Aspergillus* species
   e. *Coccidioides immitis*

Risk Factors

A. Geography: Certain geographical areas have influenced on the nature of infection like pulmonary tuberculosis which is most common infection in HIV—patients residing in India.
B. Severity of immunocompromise: Low CD4 count and high plasma viral load of HIV are associated with increased risk of pulmonary infection. If CD4 count is <200/cc, the patient may develop:
   a. Bacterial pneumonia
   b. Opportunistic organisms like *Pneumocystis carinii*
   c. Opportunistic fungi like *Penicillium marneffei* or *Aspergillus*
   d. Opportunistic bacteria like *Nocardia asteroides* and *Rhodococcus equi*
   e. Opportunistic viral infection, if the CD4 cell count is very low.
C. Addiction to drugs: Intravenous drug addicts are highly at risk for bacterial and mycobacterial pneumonia.
D. History of previous infections:
   a. There is high chance of recurrence if the patients suffered from bacterial pneumonia or episodes of *Pneumocystis jirovecii*.

b. Smokers with HIV are at high risk of pneumonia as compared to nonsmokers due to structural and functional damage of lungs.

E. Use of ART is associated with lowering of tempo of natural history of the disease as CD4 count will be gradually increased.

Evaluation of Infections in the Lung in HIV Patients

Pulmonary involvement is most common in HIV-infected patients. Three out of ten AIDs defining illness are bacterial pneumonia, mycobacterial infection, and *Pneumocystis jirovecii*, other causes being Kaposi sarcoma, nonspecific interstitial pneumonia, lymphoma, and fungal infection.

Bacterial Pneumonia

It is more common in case of HIV patients. Incidence is 0.8–2 cases/100 persons/year. Pneumonia usually occurs due to several bacterial or viral infections.

Risk Factors

a. Smoking
b. Intravenous drug users
c. Old age
d. Detectable load of HIV: 80% bacterial pneumonia occurs in case of CD4 count of <400/cc and recurrent bacterial pneumonia occurs if CD4 count is <300/cc.
e. Previous recurrent pneumonia

Pneumococcal infection is the earliest and serious infection to occur in HIV patients and can present as sinusitis, pneumonia, and bacteremia.

History of Present Illness

A. Acute symptoms of few days duration: Community-acquired bacterial pneumonia
B. Chronic and slowly progressive respiratory symptoms: Tuberculosis and *Pneumocystis jirovecii* (PSP), fungal pneumonia
C. Chronic cough of ≥2 weeks duration distinguishes bacterial from tubercular pneumonia
D. Chronic cough of months or years duration suggests COPD or malignancy
E. Productive cough—bacterial pneumonia
F. Dry or nonproductive cough—PSP
G. Dyspnea on exertion—PSP
H. High fever—bacterial pneumonia
I. Low-grade fever with night sweat and weight loss—tubercular or fungal infection, PSP

Medications

A. Adherence of ART and prophylaxis for opportunistic infection should be continued.
B. In patient on abacavir, respiratory symptoms such as cough and respiratory distress are seen in 30% of patients.

Social History

A. IV drug users are at high risk of infections with MRSA and pneumonia.
B. High incidence of smoking is associated with COPD and secondary pneumonia.
C. Direct contact with tuberculosis in high endemic area is associated with tubercular infection.
D. Recent travel to endemic area of fungi or resident of fungi is associated with fungal infection.

Physical Examinations

A. SaO_2 is normal at rest but decreases with exertion—PSP
B. Tachycardia with hypotension—bacterial pneumonia with sepsis
C. Diffuse crackles and occasional rhonchi in- PSP or viral pneumonia
D. Feature of focal consolidation—bacterial pneumonia
E. Normal chest auscultation and hypoxemia but significant symptoms—PSP
F. Features of pleural effusion—bacterial pneumonia or tuberculosis
G. Associated focal signs related to CNS—tuberculosis, fungal infection, or toxoplasmosis
H. Signs or right-sided heart failure as evidenced by pedal edema, enlarged tender liver, engorged pulsatile neck vein—due to pericarditis, due to tubercular infection, HIV-related cardiomyopathy
I. Hepatosplenomegaly, lymphadenopathy—disseminated tuberculosis and fungal infection
J. Patients with visual changes and slit-lamp examination and direct fundoscopy—CMV retinitis, tubercular uveitis, or fungal ophthalmitis

Laboratory Evaluation

A. CD4 count is the single important parameter as it can assess the immune status of the patient and can predict at what CD4 cell count with infection will be prevalent.

CD4 count	Lung infections
CD4 count is more than 200/cc	Bacterial pneumonia Tuberculosis COPD Influenza
100–200/cc	*Pneumocystis jirovecii* *Cryptococcus neoformans* pneumonia
<100/cc	*Toxoplasma gondii* pneumonia Kaposi sarcoma
<50/cc	*Pseudomonas aeruginosa* pneumonia *Mycobacterium avium* complex *Histoplasma capsulatum* *Aspergillus* species Cytomegalovirus infection *Coccidioides immitis*

B. Chest X-ray:

Chest X-ray findings	Lung disease
Normal	PSP
Unilateral focal infiltrate	Tubercular pneumonia Bacterial pneumonia Fungal pneumonia
Bilateral infiltrate	PSP Bacterial pneumonia Tuberculosis Fungal pneumonia Viral pneumonia *Toxoplasma gondii* pneumonia
Consolidation	Bacterial pneumonia Tuberculosis Fungal pneumonia
Interstitial infiltrate	PSP Fungal pneumonia Viral pneumonia Toxoplasma pneumonia *Haemophilus influenzae* pneumonia
Nodular infiltrate	Bacterial pneumonia Tuberculosis Fungal pneumonia
Miliary pattern	Tubercular pneumonia Fungal pneumonia
Masses	Fungal pneumonia
Cavitary lesion	Fungal lesion (*Aspergillus*, *Coccidioides*) Tubercular infection Bacterial pneumonia due to *Nocardia* or MRSA
Mediastinal and hilar lymphadenopathy	Tuberculosis Fungal pneumonia
Pneumothorax	Tubercular infection PSP
Pleural effusion	Bacterial pneumonia Tuberculosis Fungal pneumonia

Other Diagnostic Evaluation

A. Complete blood count with differential count

B. Liver function test

C. Renal function test

D. Bone marrow

E. CD4 count with last 3 months

F. Blood culture for bacteria, fungi, and acid-fast bacillus

G. Sputum culture for bacteria, fungus, and acid-fast bacillus

H. Induced sputum in case of nonproductive cough as in case of PSP, sometimes BAL fluid examination.

I. Serology in case of *Cryptococcus neoformans*, *Coccidioides immitis*, and *Histoplasma capsulatum*

J. Computerized tomography of chest if the chest X-ray is negative—it can diagnose PE, pulmonary hypertension, and pulmonary neoplasm.

K. Tuberculin skin test with PPD who was not prior positive for PPD. Induration of ≥5 mm in case of HIV-positive patient is considered as positive for active TB or latent TB infection.

L. Interferon-γ release assay: It can be done instead of PPD test and is more specific and sensitive.

M. Bronchoscopy with BAL: It should be done when chest X-ray and CT scan are inconclusive. It is highly sensitive for PSP.

N. Thoracentesis: It is considered where in spite of treatment there is worsening of pleural effusion. Fluid should be tested for cell type, cell count, protein, sugar, chloride, pH, LDH, cytology, bacterial, and fungal culture.

O. Pleural biopsy in case of suspected tubercular involvement of pleura

P. Bronchoscopy with transbronchial biopsies: It is done in case of suspected Cytomegalovirus, *Aspergillus*, and neoplasm and Kaposi sarcoma.

Q. Bronchoscopy with transbronchial aspiration: For evaluation of mediastinal and hilar lymphadenopathy where no diagnosis is possible with chest X-ray or CT scan of chest.

R. CT-guided percutaneous needle aspiration or biopsy: Tissue diagnosis is possible from perihilar lesion.

S. Open lung biopsy or video-assisted thoracic surgery: It is done, where the patient is not improving with current management.

Treatment

For treatment of tuberculosis and PSP, question numbers 54 is referenced. For bacterial pneumonia, see the treatment of community-acquired pneumonia in question number 7.

> **Q56. Enumerate the types of voice sounds in clinical examination of chest. Describe their characters and mechanisms.**
>
> **BF/JUN2016/MDIII (10)**

ANSWER

Sounds produced in the larynx are abnormally transmitted to the chest in certain diseases—it will provide a clue to the diagnosis.

It can be palpated on the chest wall by placing the ulnar side of the hand in the intercostal space.

Mechanism of Production of Vibration

During speech, vocal cord will set up a vibration in the air column in the bronchial cavity which will be conducted to the chest wall through the lung tissue that can be palpated on the chest wall.

A. Normal variation of vocal fremitus:
- **a.** In the parasternal region in the second right intercostal space close the bifurcation of bronchus—normal intense fremitus
- **b.** Interscapular region near the bronchi—increased fremitus
- **c.** High-pitched voice also produces intense unsatisfactory vibration

B. Diminished vocal fremitus:
- **a.** Blockage in the airways
- **b.** Presence of air or fluid in the pleural cavity
- **c.** Pleural fibrosis

C. Increased vocal fremitus:
- **a.** Pulmonary consolidation
- **b.** Lung fibrosis
- **c.** Collapse of the lung

During auscultation, voice can be heard by placing the stethoscope on the chest wall. These are called transmitted vocal sounds or vocal resonance. Four types of transmitted voice sounds:

A. Bronchophony: It is heard over the chest remote from bronchi or larynx, but this sound is as clear as over central bronchi or larynx.

B. Pectoriloquy: This type of sound is clear and intelligible words heard over the chest in the form of:
- **a.** Whispering (known as whispering pectoriloquy)
- **b.** Speaking (spoken pectoriloquy)

C. Egophony: It is characterized by goat-like bleating sound produced by patient's voice that is heard over the areas of consolidation or fibrosis or collapse.

D. E to A change: It is a variant of egophony.

Mechanism of Voice Sound Production and Transmission

Normally, voice sound is produced by vibration of vocal cords that will be transmitted upward toward mouth and downward toward the chest wall. Alveolar air acts as low pass filter and hence it will eliminate high frequency sounds of >3,000 Hz, and thus only low frequency sounds of 100–300 Hz are able to reach the chest wall. Since recognition of vowels is essential for comprehension of words, hence elimination of formants by the normal lung will make the voice sounds low pitched, mumbled, and unintelligible.

But in case of consolidation, collapse, and lung fibrosis, solidified lung will transmit sounds of high frequencies, so transmitted vowel sounds become louder, clear, and also intelligible.

Mechanism of Whispering Pectoriloquy

Whispering consists of high-frequency sounds—so they are not transmitted in the aerated lung but becomes audible when alveolar air will be lost and lungs become solidified.

Transformation of E to A in the Vocal Resonance in Consolidated Lung

E is a mixture of high- and low-frequency sounds—high-frequency sounds in the range of 2000—3,500 Hz and low-frequency sounds are in the range of 100–400 Hz.

A is the mixture of high- and low-frequency sounds—low-frequency sounds are higher than low-frequency sounds of E, i.e., 600 Hz.

When both E and A are heard over the chest none of their high frequencies will come across regardless of consolidation. Consolidated lung will transmit high-frequency sounds better that normal lung (close to 1,000 Hz instead of 400 Hz) but it cannot transmit high-frequency sounds of 2,000–3,500 Hz which is typical of E.

So consolidated lung can transmit low-frequency sound of 600 Hz better but cannot transmit high-frequency sounds of 2,000–3,500 Hz. So E becomes A.

Q57. Normal defense mechanism of lung.
BF/OCT2010/MDI (8)

ANSWER

During the process of exchanging, nearly 1,000 L of air during uptake of oxygen and elimination of carbon dioxide through the lungs, these will be exposed to a large number of injurious articulate matters and microorganisms. Again, during sleep, the patients are exposed to oropharyngeal contents regularly containing unwanted bacteria, particulate matters, and microorganisms. To protect the respiratory tract from the noxious materials, there are different components of protective mechanisms. These are as follows:

A. Anatomic or physical factors: Laminar flow of air while flowing through the airway, becomes turbulent at the different branching points and thus pariculate matter will be deposited on the bronchial mucosal surfaces in these locations but will never reach the distal airways and alveoli.

- **a.** Particulate matter of >10 µm in diameter will be deposited in the upper airways like nose.
- **b.** Particulate matter of 5–10 µm in diameter will be deposited in the trachea and upper airways but not reaching smaller airways and the alveoli.
- **c.** Particle size of <5 µm in diameter will reach the distal parenchyma; most of the bacteria are in this size. Particles of bronchodilators are <5 µm; hence they will reach the lung parenchyma easily.

When these particles will deposit in the trachea or bronchi, they will be cleared by the two following processes:

- **a.** Cough: This protective mechanism is triggered by stimulation of J-receptors present in the proximal airways by inhaled and aspirated foreign material, thus clearing the airways off foreign materials.
- **b.** Mucociliary clearance:
  1. Most superficial epithelial cells from trachea to respiratory bronchiol have cilia projecting into the lumen; the cross section of each cilia consists two central microtubules surrounded by nine pairs of microtubules around the periphery.
  2. Above the epithelial cells there is mucus layer—it has two sublayers:
     - Sol layer, which is directly adjacent to the epithelial cell. In this layer, cilia are present. In this layer, there are number of molecules which are part of innate system.
     - Gel layer produced by mucous glands and goblet cells and floats over the sol layer moves upward along with the particulate matters due to beating of cilia.

B. Antimicrobial peptides:

A number of substances consisting of small molecules, proteins, and cells present in the sol layer acts as fast-acting energy. An efficient and frontline defense system will protect the lungs in absence of prior sensitization and activation of immune system. This system does not require previous exposure to these particles but require pattern recognition receptors which are stimulated by conserved structures on the microbes. There are following components of innate immunity in the lung:

- **a.** Lysozyme: It is synthesized by respiratory epithelial cells, serous glandular cells and macrophages present throughout the airways but predominant proximally and is responsible for lysis of bacterial cells, mainly gram-positive organisms.
- **b.** Lactoferrin: It is produced by serous cells and neutrophils and through the recognition of carbohydrate moieties present on the bacterial surface responsible for:
  1. Agglutination and killing of bacteria
  2. Enhancement of neutrophilic adherence
  3. Production of neutrophil superoxide
  4. Blocking of iron from supporting metabolism
- **c.** Defensins: These small proteins having intrinsic microbial activity are present on the surface of the lung, gastrointestinal tract, and genitourinary tract. This protein is of two types: α-defensins produced by resident neutrophils and β-defensins produced by respiratory epithelial cells. Functions are:
  1. They will destroy the membrane potential of the bacteria by making the wall permeable and release of cellular contents.
  2. Being high sensitive to ionic concentration, they are inactivated in the abnormal milieu of the lungs in patients with cystic fibrosis.

3. SP-A and SP-B: These are the members of collectin family and are responsible for:
    - Binding and aggregating the microbes
    - Facilitating interaction with phagocytic cells
    - Regulating pulmonary macrophages activity
    - Regulating cytokine production
4. Respiratory IgA: It is constituted by respiratory epithelium and does not require prior exposure.

C. Phagocytic and inflammatory cells:

a. Pulmonary alveolar macrophages:

1. These cells are present in the alveoli escaping the deposition of upper airways. Its cytoplasm contains packed digestive enzymes which dispose the ingested foreign material and kill the microorganisms present in the lower respiratory tract.
2. They also secrete chemokines which help in recruiting the inflammatory cells.
    - Firstly, bacteria will be attached to the surface of the macrophages
    - Then these bacteria will be engulfed within the plasma membrane and ultimately produce phagosomes containing bacteria and enzymes. All these processes are sometimes enhanced by opsonins. The specific opsonins are IgG antibodies directed against foreign material, and nonspecific opsonins in the lungs are secretory IgA, complement, and fibronectin.
    - Phagosomes combine with lysozymes; lysosomal proteolytic enzymes digest, destroy, and detoxify the phagosomal contents.
    - Sometimes hydrogen peroxide product of oxidative metabolism, helps macrophages to kill the bacteria.
3. Activated macrophages release inflammatory mediators such as TNF-α, IL-1β, cytokines, and chemokines
4. Sometimes some foreign materials like inhaled silica being toxic to macrophages will kill these cells.
5. In some cases, the foreign material like *Mycobacterium tuberculosis* and HIV viruses being inert will reside in the macrophages as residue but cannot be cleared.
6. Small amount of inflammation of alveolar macrophages has negative effect on the gas exchange and thus it keeps the distal airways and alveoli free of infection.

b. Dendritic cells: It is present throughout the body, but bone marrow-derived cells are present in the airways, alveolar walls, and peribronchial connective tissue. Functions are:

1. Sampling the airway microenvironment
2. Ingesting and processing antigens.
3. Migrating to lymph nodes; here it will present antigens to T cells.

A special type of cell, Langerhans cells with abnormal proliferation, is responsible for Langerhans cell histiocytosis.

c. Polymorphonuclear leukocytes: These reside in the small airways and alveoli and are responsible for defense mechanisms against microorganisms in the lower respiratory tract by being attracted by products of complement activation and chemotactic factors from macrophages. These polymorphonuclear neutrophils (PMN) will be adherent to vascular endothelium aided by integrins present on the surface of PMNs and adhesion molecules present on the surface of vascular endothelial cells. PMN will engulf and kill the bacteria with the help of lysozymes, defensins, bacterial-permeability increasing protein, and lactoferrin.

d. Natural killer cells: Without prior sensitization, these cells kill viruses only by recognition. These cells have no surface markers that are present in either T or B lymphocytes.

D. Adaptive immune responses:

This process involves recognition and response to specific antigens. There are two components. These are:

a. Humoral immunity: It involves B lymphocytes and antibody production by plasma cells. Among the two main types, IgA are important in the nasopharynx and upper airways, also known as secretory IgA, that includes dimer of IgA plus extra secretory component glycoprotein. The functions of IgA are:

1. Binding to virus and bacteria
2. Prevent their attachment to epithelial cells
3. Agglutinate microorganisms

Another one is IgG, which is mostly locally produced in the lung but also originates from serum. Its functions are:

1. It agglutinate particles
2. It neutralize viruses
3. It serve as opsonins for phagocytosis of bacteria by macrophages
4. It activate complements
5. It is presence of complement causes lysis of the gram-negative bacteria

b. Cellular immunity: It involves T lymphocytes-based thymus differentiation, execution of function of certain lymphocytes, and cytokine production. It controls synthesis of antibody by humoral immune system. In the blood, T cells are abundant as compared to B cells but both are involved in the defense mechanisms against harmful microorganisms. Their functions are:

1. They produce varieties of soluble and biologically active cytokines. Among them interferon-γ attracts or activates macrophages.
2. They will interact with humoral immune system to modify production of antibodies.

On the basis of specific cell surface markers and functional characteristics, they are differentiated into two types of T lymphocytes:

- CD4+ or helper T cells: They will be differentiated into two types:
  T1 helper cells: These are responsible for cellular immune defense.
  T2 helper cells: These are responsible for allergic inflammation.
- CD8+ cells: There are two subtypes:
  Suppressor T cells
  Cytotoxic T cells

These two types of cells produce cytokines upon exposure to antigen. These cytokines interact with B lymphocytes and macrophages.

Q58. Fiberoptic bronchoscopy.

MGR/FEB2005/MDIII (5)

ANSWER

Introduction

It is an invasive procedure in the field of pulmonary medicine.

Indications of Bronchoscopy

A. Diagnostic indications:

a. Cough
b. Hoarseness of voice
c. Hemoptysis
d. Unexplained wheeze and stridor
e. Carcinoma of lung
f. Unresolved consolidation or collapse of lung
g. Suspected infections in the pulmonary parenchyma
h. Mediastinal masses
i. Assessment of endotracheal placement of the tube
j. Diagnostic BAL
k. Diagnosis of ILD

B. Therapeutic indications:

a. Hemoptysis
b. Removal of mucus plugs and clot
c. Tracheoesophageal fistula
d. Bronchogenic cyst
e. Endotracheal intubation
f. Debulking of the endobronchial tumor
g. In case of pulmonary alveolar proteinosis

C. Special procedures:

a. Laser therapy
b. Electrocautery
c. Cryotherapy
d. Brachytherapy
e. Photodynamic therapy
f. Bronchial thermoplasty
g. Argon plasma cauterization

Contraindications to Bronchoscopy

A. Refractory hypoxemia which will worsen during and after bronchoscopy.

B. Creatinine >3 mg/dL as it may produce platelet dysfunction during bronchoscopic biopsy.

C. Unstable status of cardiovascular system

D. Low platelet count is a contraindication of biopsies but not for collection of BAL through bronchoscope.

Procedure

Prior to procedure small dose of midazolam to be given intravenously and 4% lidocaine has to be sprayed on the back of the pharynx for suppressing cough during the procedure. Both oral and nasal approaches can be done.

Bronchoalveolar lavage is preferable from right middle lobe and lingual in absence of local lung pathology because these two areas are accessible. 20–60 mL of aliquots of sterile normal saline have to be given each time to a total of 100–200 mL. In case of normal patients, BAL can recover usually 50% of fluid. In normal individual, this recovered fluid is composed of mainly lymphocytes and alveolar macrophages.

Biopsies can be taken from diffuse and localized lung lesion.

Q59. Fungal pneumonia.

BF/OCT2010/MDIII (10)

ANSWER

Introduction

Pneumonia is the leading infectious cause of death in the developing countries. Fungi may be the true pathogen or colonize in the different sites in the body leading to production of broad variety of clinical syndromes. Fungal infection of the lung is the third most common infection following bacterial and viral infection in the lung; hence, it is very difficult to diagnose fungal infection of lung.

Risk Factors

A. Farmers having heavy exposure to droppings of bird, bat, and rodent—example is histoplasmosis due to heavy exposure to bat droppings.

B. Gardeners or farmers who are exposed to accidental cut or puncture while working in the soil—example is sporotrichosis.

With the use of broad-spectrum antibiotics, incidence of invasive fungal infection in the critical care unit is on rise in patients with following predisposing factors:

A. AIDS

B. Acute leukemia or lymphoma on myeloablative chemotherapy

C. Bone marrow transplantation

D. Peripheral blood stem cell transplantation

E. Postsplenectomy patients

F. Immunosuppressive therapy after solid organ transplantation

G. Prolonged neutropenia from various causes

H. Congenital immunodeficiency syndrome

I. Genetic predisposition

Following fungi are responsible for pneumonia:

Fungi	Diseases
Endemic fungal pneumonia	
Histoplasma capsulatum	Histoplasmosis
Coccidioides immitis	Coccidioidomycosis
Blastomyces dermatitidis	Blastomycosis
Paracoccidioides brasiliensis	Paracoccidioidomycosis
Opportunistic fungal pathogen producing pneumonia	
Candida species	Candidiasis
Aspergillus species	Aspergillosis
Mucor species	Mucormycosis
Cryptococcus neoformans	Cryptococcosis
Zygomycetes	

Basic pathologic process of fungal infection of lung has been divided into two types:

A. Allergic reaction to fungi

B. True infection

Following are the fungal infections of the lung:

Aspergillosis

According to invasion of lung or allergic reaction of the lung, *Aspergillus* can be divided into following types:

Simple colonization of the *Aspergillus*

Allergic alveolitis

Allergic bronchopulmonary aspergillosis

Criteria of ABPA:

International Society for Human and Animal Mycology (ISHAM) diagnostic criteria of ABPA:

Predisposing conditions (one must be present)
Asthma
Cystic fibrosis
Obligatory criteria (both must be present)
Aspergillosis skin test positivity or detectable IgE levels against *Aspergillus fumigatus*
Elevated total serum IgE concentration (typically >1,000 IU/mL) But if the patients meet all other criteria, IgE level of <1,000 IU/mL may be acceptable
Other criteria (at least must be present)
Precipitating serum antibodies to *Aspergillus fumigatus*
Radiographic pulmonary opacities consistent with ABPA
Total eosinophil count of >500/cc in glucocorticoid native patients (may be historical)

Stages of ABPA:

A. Acute stage

B. Stage of remission

C. Stage of exacerbation
D. Stage of steroid-dependent asthma
E. Stage of fibrosis

Radiographic pictures in ABPA:

A. Chest X-ray:
    a. Massive areas of consolidation
    b. Fungal debris blocking the bronchi (toothpaste shadow and gloved finger appearance)
    c. Inflammation of vascular and bronchial walls (tram shadow)
    d. Ring shadow in case of bronchiectasis
    e. Nodular shadow in the lung parenchyma
    f. Local areas of atelectasis
    g. Features of emphysema
B. CT bronchogram:
   It will demonstrate proximal bronchiectasis with distal sparing

Treatment of ABPA:

A. Steroid is used in acute phase and is slowly tapered as acute stage will be over.
B. Antifungal drugs such as amphotericin B or itraconazole.

Typical resolution can be defined as:

A. Control of attack of asthma
B. Disappearances of pulmonary opacities
C. Reduction of peripheral eosinophilia and reduction of IgE by >35%

Aspergilloma

It is a fungal ball containing *Aspergillus fumigatus* in the preexisting tubercular or in bronchiectatic cavities, in stage IV sarcoidosis, and healed lung abscess in the upper lobe in case ankylosing spondylitis.

Clinical features demonstrate hemoptysis and recurrent respiratory tract infection.

Diagnosis

A. Chest X-ray demonstrates mass in the cavity with air cresent level present on the top mainly in the upper lobe (Monods sign).
B. Immunological test: It demonstrates positive precipitin test to *Aspergillus* antigen.
C. Microscopic examination demonstrates fungal hyphae in the respiratory secretion or from the BAL.
D. Serology: Raised IgE level.

Treatment

A. Bronchial artery embolization
B. Surgical resection of lobe
C. Radiotherapy
D. Systemic antifungal therapy

In case of immunocompromised individual invasive aspergillosis:

It is clinically characterized by:

A. Bronchitis
B. Tracheitis
C. Pneumonia

Diagnosis is confirmed by:

A. Chest X-ray: Round pneumonia
B. Bronchoalveolar lavage

Treatment: Antifungal therapy.

Mixed Syndrome

It is a combination of any two or more of the above features.

Pulmonary Candidiasis

Risk factors are:

A. Oropharyngeal candidiasis
B. Malnourished diabetic patients
C. Patients on prolonged steroid therapy

Emerging species are:

A. *Candida tropicalis*
B. *Candida glabrata*
C. *Candida krusei*
D. *Candida parapsilosis*
E. *Candida lusitaniae*

Diagnosis

Demonstration of fungal hyphae in the BAL fluid

Treatment

Systemic antifungal drugs such as ketoconazole, amphotericin B, and fluconazole

Histoplasmosis

It is associated with construction projects due to contaminated soil. Inhaled spores are converted to yeasts after reaching the alveoli. These yeasts are ingested by macrophages where yeasts proliferate and disseminate to distant organs in the body.

In the lung these cells initiate cell-mediated immune response resulting in granuloma formation along with hilar and mediastinal lymphadenopathy.

Clinical Features

A. Nonspecific symptoms such as low-grade fever; later on lesion may heal or calcify.

B. If the disease progresses, caseous focus will cavitate producing cough with expectoration and occasionally hemoptysis.

Diagnosis

A. Associated features such as oral ulcers, adrenal enlargement, and tissue biopsy from these areas may demonstrate granuloma. Fungal and AFB stain have to be done.

B. Direct demonstration of BAL fluid, sputum of the fungus by PAS stain

C. Bone marrow may demonstrate *Histoplasma capsulatum*

D. Indirect diagnosis by:
   a. Complement fixation test
   b. Immunodiffusion test
   c. Radioimmunoassay

Treatment

A. Liposomal form of amphotericin B

B. Ketoconazole

C. Fluconazole

D. Itraconazole (200–400 mg/day)

Blastomycosis

Organism is B dermatitidis. Fungi grow in the soil and are inhaled to reach in the alveoli and produce yeasts. These will stimulate first PMNs and then cell-mediated immune response leading to formation of granulomas. This infection also involves skin, brain, bones, etc.

Clinical Features

A. Fever with chills

B. Cough with purulent sputum

C. Pleuritic pain

D. Hemoptysis and weight loss

Radiological Features

A. In milder form:
   a. Infiltrates
   b. Cavities
   c. Round opacities
   d. Miliary shadowing

B. In severe form: ARDS

Diagnosis

A. KOH preparation of the respiratory secretions and BAL fluid

B. Silver or PAS stain of the tissue demonstrates yeast form of fungus

Treatment

In milder case usually no treatment is required. But in severe cases:

A. Itraconazole

B. Ketoconazole

Coccidioidomycosis

It occurs mainly during hot and dry summer. Inhalation of spores will produce two types of lesions:

A. Cell-mediated immunity leading to formation of granulomatous disease.

B. Suppurative lesion

Clinical Features

A. Fever with chills

B. Cough

C. Arthralgia

D. Pleuritic chest pain

E. Respiratory distress

F. Hemoptysis in case of cavitary lesion

G. Signs of cavitation, consolidation, or pleural effusion

H. In case of dissemination, skin, bone, joints, or meninges may be involved.

Diagnosis

A. Chest X-ray:
   a. Consolidation
   b. Sometimes cavity
   c. Hilar lymphadenopathy

B. Microscopic examination in KOH preparation or silver staining of infected tissue demonstrates hyphae or yeasts respectively.

C. Skin test

D. Culture of sputum and BAL fluid

Treatment

A. In case of mild disease no specific therapy

B. In severe cases, fluconazole and itraconazole or ketoconazole

Cryptococcosis

It is usually uncommon infection and self-limiting and asymptomatic. But in case of immunocompromised individual, it may involve organs severely.

Clinical Features

A. Cough
B. Fever
C. Hemoptysis
D. Malaise

Diagnosis

India ink preparation of sputum demonstrates cryptococci.

Treatment

A. Ketoconazole
B. Fluconazole
C. Itraconazole

Pulmonary Mucormycosis

In case of immunocompromised and diabetic patients, granulomatous invasion of sinuses and upper respiratory tract.

> **Q60. Mechanism of dyspnea.**
>
> **BF/NOV2012/MDI (9)**

ANSWER

Definition

Dyspnea can be defined as awareness of own respiratory effort of varying intensity due to interactions of various factors such as psychological, social, environmental, and behavioral.

Mechanism of Dyspnea

Mechanism of dyspnea is complex producing various sensations like chest tightness, air-hunger, etc. It arises from various pathways:

A. Afferent signals:
- **a.** Afferent signal from following receptors due to hypoxemia, hypercapnia, and acidemia:
  - **1.** Various peripheral chemoreceptors such as carotid body and aortic body
  - **2.** Central chemoreceptors in the medulla
- **b.** Afferent signal from following mechanoreceptors activated in response to increased work load produced by the airway diseases such as bronchial asthma or COPD or decreased compliance of the lung and chest wall:
  - **1.** In the upper airways and lung, such as stretch receptors, irritant receptors, and J-receptors
  - **2.** Receptors from muscles like muscle spindle as stretch receptors and organ responsible for generation of force
- **c.** Afferent signals from pulmonary vessels also known as metaboreceptors in response to pulmonary artery pressure

All the above afferent signals are responsible for air hunger.

B. Efferent signals:
- **a.** Efferent output from brainstem to sensory cortex will contribute to sensation of effort
- **b.** Efferent signals like sensation of respiratory effort from motor cortex to sensory cortex
- **c.** Efferent signals from brainstem as well as from motor cortex will go to various respiratory muscle.

C. Various mismatches in between incoming afferent messages from chest wall and lung and various outgoing efferent messages to the various ventilatory muscles will produce dyspnea.

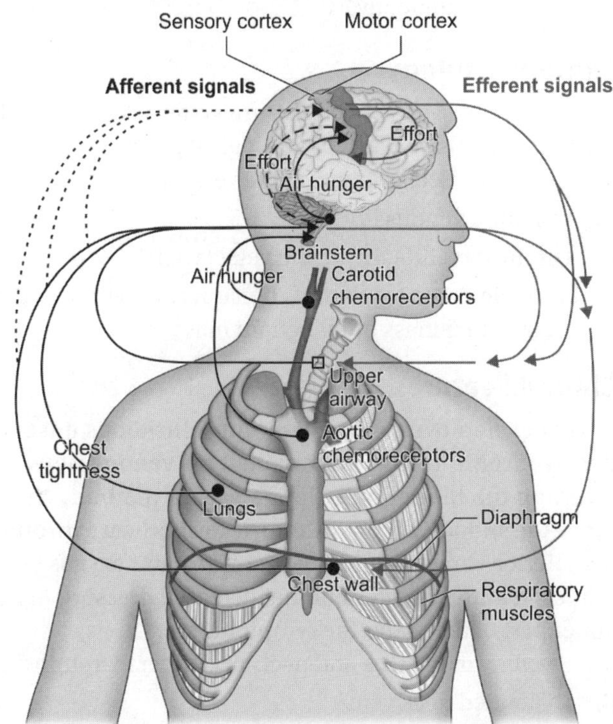

> **Q61. Enumerate the causes and discuss the diagnosis and treatment of superior vena caval syndrome.**
>
> **NNNDNB 2021 (10)**
>
> **Superior vena caval syndrome.**
>
> **TEERTHANKER MAHAVEER UNI, 2020 (10)**

ANSWER

Definition

Superior vena caval syndrome can be defined as a constellation of clinical features resulting from partial or complete obstruction of the superior vena cave leading to formation of thrombus or infiltration by the tumor.

Etiology

A. Bronchogenic carcinoma
B. Non-Hodgkin lymphoma
C. Metastatic tumor
D. Iatrogenic thrombus formation
E. Stenosis of superior vena cava due to:
   a. Pacemaker wires
   b. Semipermanent intravascular catheters used for:
      1. Chemotherapy
      2. Long term antibiotics
      3. Hemodialysis

Pathophysiology

Superior vena cava is low pressure system is susceptible to damage by three pathophysiological processes:

A. Compromised anatomy of the vessels
B. Impaired venous flow
C. Diminished integrity of the vessel wall.

Extrinsic compression of the superior vena cava by the mediastinal mass or malignant mass.

Clinical Features

It will develop over weeks to months. Insidious onset of this syndrome results from collateral venous network diverting the blood to the lower part of the body, from there the blood will again return to the heart through the inferior vena cava, intercostal veins and azygos vein. Clinical features result from the increased pressure in the upper part of the body. The symptoms are:

A. Swelling of the face and neck and upper extremity
B. Distended neck vein
C. Cough
D. Dyspnea
E. Orthopnea
F. Distended venous collaterals in the chest
G. Suffusion of the conjunctiva
H. Other less common symptoms are:
   a. Stridor
   b. Hoarseness of voice
   c. Dysphagia
   d. Pleural effusion
   e. Headache
   f. Plethora of head
   g. Nausea
   h. Lightheadedness
   i. Change in vision
   j. Papilledema
   k. Cyanosis
   l. Stupor and coma

Evaluation

A. CT scan/MRI of the chest with collaterals to detect the site and severity of the lesion or stenosis.
B. Ultrasound of the superior vena cava, jugular and subclavian vein to see the presence of thrombus.
C. Venography is the gold standard to diagnose and visualize the obstruction.

Treatment

A. Supportive treatment: Elevation of the head to decrease the venous pressure.
B. In case of thrombus related to indwelling catheter: Removal of the device along with anticoagulant therapy and catheter induced thrombolysis.
C. In case of tumor related obstruction by malignancy, treatment depends upon the type and extent of the tumor and whether it can be treated by surgery or radiotherapy.
D. Surgical therapy:
   a. Bypass grafting by saphenous vein, femoral vein polytetrafluoroethylene or Dacron graft.
   b. Endovascular therapy is the first line of treatment

Q62. Describe with a schematic diagram of alveolocapillary membrane. How will you assess functions of pulmonary interstitium?

WBUHS 2022 (10)

ANSWER

Assessment of the functions of pulmonary interstitium can be discussed in question number 25.

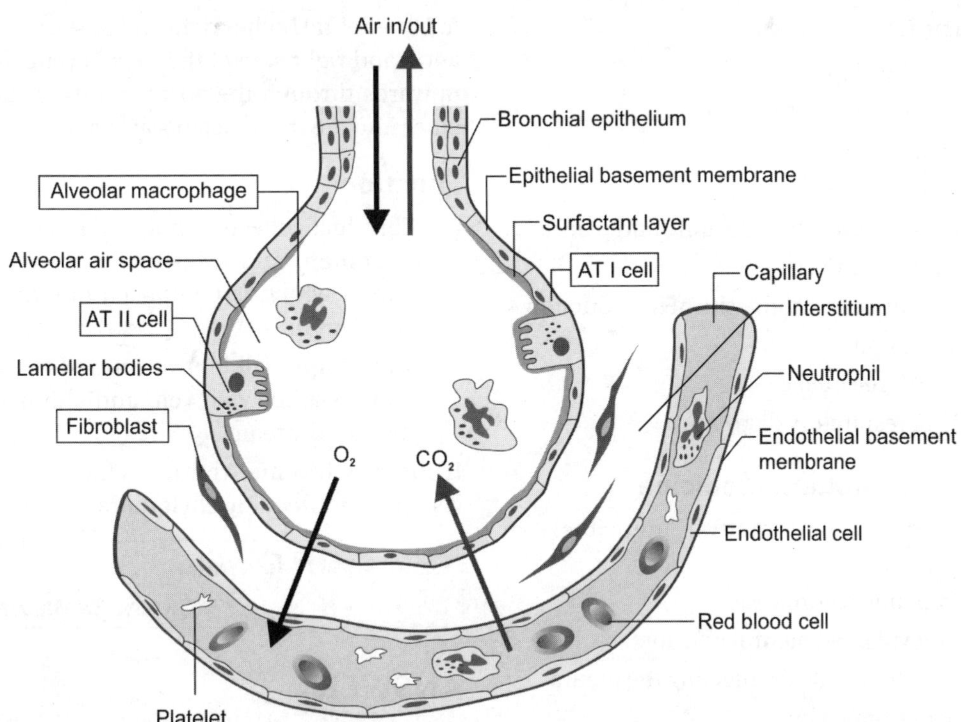

Q63. Discuss the medical thoracoscopy and its applications in modern medicine.

WBUHS 2022 (10)

ANSWER

Definition

Medical thoracoscopy is a specialized procedure by which the inside of the pleural cavity can be visualized by the introduction of cannula through the chest wall for diagnostic as well as therapeutic purpose.

Indications

A. *Diagnostic purpose*:

- **a.** To identify the causes of recurrent or undiagnosed pleural effusion.
- **b.** If the is suspicion of malignant pleural effusion.
- **c.** Presence of nodules inside the pleura.
- **d.** If there is localized thickening of the pleura
- **e.** To take the biopsy from the pleural surfaces.

B. *Therapeutic purposes*:

- **a.** To perform pleurodesis in case of recurrent pleural effusion as in case of malignancy, chronic renal disease, hepatopulmonary syndrome
- **b.** Drainage of the loculated pus from the cavity within the pleural cavity.
- **c.** Removal of septation from the pleural cavity in case of chronic pleural loculation.

Advantages

- **A.** It is a minimal invasive procedure as compared to surgical thoracoscopy.
- **B.** In case of high risk patient it can be performed through the local anesthesia.
- **C.** Direct visualization of the pleural cavity with high diagnostic yield.
- **D.** Simultaneous administration of administration of talc.
- **E.** Short recovery time.

Disadvantages

- **A.** All the mediastinal structures cannot be accessed.
- **B.** In case of extensive pleural effusion.
- **C.** Since this is operator dependent method, there may be complications.
- **D.** There is chance of:
  - **a.** Embolism
  - **b.** Infection
  - **c.** Pneumothorax

Contraindications

A. Absolute contraindications:
 a. Non-correctable coagulopathy
 b. Hemodynamic instability
 c. Reaction to anesthesia
 d. Suspected hydatid cyst in the lung and pleura
B. Relative contraindications:
 a. Presence of infection at the site of introduction
 b. Pleural adhesion
 c. Presence of large bullae
 d. Presence of respiratory distress

Its Applications in Modern Medicine

A. To diagnose a case of pleural metastasis or mesothelioma
B. Invasive therapeutic pleurodesis
C. To evaluate unexplained pleural effusion
D. Confirmation of tuberculosis infecting the pleura
E. Management of trapped lung.
F. For taking sampling for diagnosis cancer.

Q64. Cisterna chili.
MGR UNI, TAMIL NADU, 2022 (5)

ANSWER

Anatomy

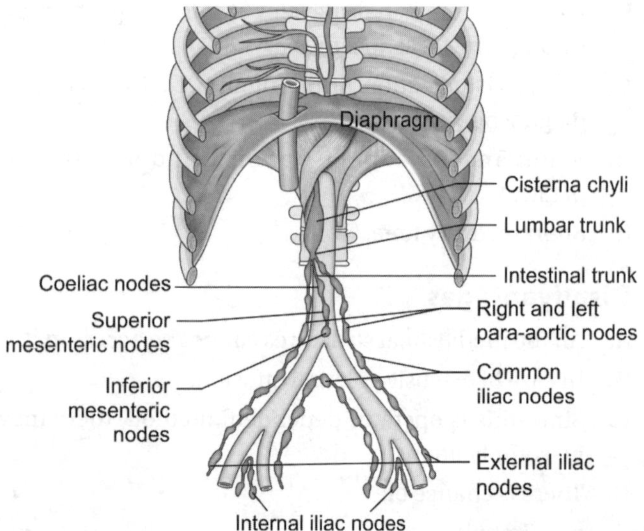

Cisterna chyli is a dilated sac composed of right and left lumbar lymphatic trunk and intestinal trunk, present at the lower end of thoracic duct acting as major collecting reservoir of lymph located retroperitoneally anterior to L1 to L2 vertebral bodies right and posterior to the abdominal aorta and right side of the azygos vein. This is continued upwards through the aortic hiatus of the diaphragm to enter into the thorax as thoracic duct.

Functions

A. This duct collects lymph from the lower limb, pelvis, abdomen, and intestinal tract act as reservoir of lymph which is composed of emulsified fat along with lymph.
B. This lymph will be transported to the thoracic duct then to subclavian vein and ultimately reaches into the blood stream.

If there is trauma, there is chance of damage of the cisterna chyli leading chylothorax or chylous ascites.

Q65. Cystic fibrosis.
MGR UNI, TAMIL NADU, 2022 (10)

ANSWER

Definition

Cystic fibrosis is a autosomal recessive disorder involving glandular and exocrine function of digestive, pulmonary and reproductive system affecting children and adult as evidenced by repeated pulmonary infection, pancreatic insufficiency, sinusitis, and infertility.

Etiology

This disease involves mutation of chromosome number 7 that codes for cystic fibrosis transmembrane conductance regulator protein. In case of clinically evident disease there are mutation of both the copies of the gene. There are more than 2000 types of mutations in this gene identified in cystic fibrosis.

These mutations have classified into five classes:

A. Class I: Defective synthesis of protein.
B. Class II: Defective processing of protein
C. Class III: Disorder in the regulation.
D. Class IV: Defective conductance of chloride
E. Class V: Accelerated turnover of the channels.

Pathophysiology

Most common mutation is ΔF508 in the axon 11, it is found in 70% of white patients in USA and two-third of all the cases Worldwide. It is class II mutation demonstrating abnormal folding of *CFTR* gene leading to premature destruction within the Golgi apparatus, it is mostly responsible for pancreatic exocrine insufficiency and increased incidence of meconium ileus.

Mutation of *CFTR* gene has been categorized into five dysfunctional variants:

A. Class I dysfunction results from the nonsense, splice-site or frameshift mutation leading to premature termination in the mRNA sequence resulting complete absence of CFTR expression.

B. Class II dysfunction result dysfunctional or abnormal post-translational processing of *CFTR* gene thereby prohibiting normal transit of intracellular protein.

C. Class III dysfunction results in diminished activity of protein in response to intracellular signaling.

D. Class IV dysfunction results decreased conduction of chloride ion and decreased duration of channel activation after stimulation.

E. Class V dysfunction results decreased concentration of CFTR channel in the cellular membrane due to rapid degradation by cellular processes. This class of dysfunction also alters the stability of mRNA.

Systemic Pathophysiologic Processes in the Cystic Fibrosis

There is decreased secretion of chloride along with increased resorption of sodium in the cellular spaces leading to increased resorption of water resulting thick mucus on the epithelial linings or thick secretion from the pancreas resulting plugging of the duct leading to obstruction affecting lung, hepatobiliary and pancreatic system, intestines and lastly sweat glands.

Disease of the Sinus

A. Obstruction of the ostia by thick viscid mucus.

B. Ciliary dysfunction

C. Increased inflammatory mediators

D. Increased colonization of the pathogenic bacteria mainly *Pseudomonas aeruginosa.*

All the above ultimately leads to secondary structural damage of sinus.

Pulmonary Disease

Lung of cystic fibrosis is normal in utero, after birth, but the disease is precipitated by infection and followed by inflammatory reaction. There is plugging of the bronchi by mucus that produces bronchial obstruction, it enhances the bacterial growth within the airways leading to development of bronchiectasis and in this bronchiectatic areas there is further production of purulent sputum.

During the inflammatory reaction epithelial cells produce neutrophil interleukin-8 that increases secretion of sputum thereby creating positive feedback loop between the mucus production and persistence of inflammation and structural changes in the bronchus—which ultimately leads to ventilatory failure if untreated.

Pancreatic Disease

As the gastric contents enter into the duodenal cavity, the pancreatic exocrine glands are stimulated to secrete enzymes into the duodenal cavity. But in cystic fibrosis thick viscid mucus obstructs the pancreatic duct, thereby the secretion of bicarbonates. As a result the gastric acidic pH cannot be neutralized and in acidic pH pancreatic enzyme will be degraded, as a result, intestinal chyme cannot be processed enzymatically leading to production of greasy stool.

Due to blockage of the pancreatic duct the enzyme accumulates in the duct leading to autodigestion of the pancreatic tissue. In severe cases there is autodigestion of the Islets of Langerhans leading development of diabetes mellitus.

Hepatic Disease

As a result of blockage of the biliary ductules by the thick mucus conjugated hyperbilirubinemia occurs leading to development of obstructive jaundice and cirrhosis hepatic failure.

Intestinal Disease

Meconium ileus at birth occurs due to increased absorption of fluid due to faulty CFTR channel. Intestinal obstruction in the later life is due to dehydration of the intestinal content leading to constipation and changes in the content in the lumen due to pancreatic insufficiency.

Sweat Gland Manifestation

Sweat gland moves chloride ion into intracellular spaces from the extracellular spaces. Thus, sodium along with water will be reabsorbed into the body from the tissues of the sweat gland. But in this disease failure of the chloride channel to reabsorb the chloride ion leads to loss of sodium ion onto the skin surface along with fluid loss resulting the salty skin—the pathognomonic in this disease.

Clinical Presentation

Adult with cystic fibrosis presents with exacerbation of one or more symptoms involving multiple organs:

A. Pulmonary system:

- **a.** Infections
- **b.** Bronchiectasis
- **c.** Chronic bronchitis

 d. Abnormal pulmonary function test
 e. Allergic bronchopulmonary aspergillosis
 f. Atypical asthma

B. Sinus involvement:
 a. Chronic postnasal drip
 b. Chronic rhinosinusitis
 c. Nasal polyp
 d. Panopacification of paranasal sinuses

C. Pancreatic involvement:
 a. Early onset diabetes
 b. Chronic pancreatitis
 c. Pancreatic insufficiency

D. Hepatobiliary manifestations:
 a. Cholelithiasis
 b. Focal biliary cirrhosis
 c. Hepatic cirrhosis
 d. Decompensating liver disease

E. Renal involvement:
 a. Nephrocalcinosis
 b. Nephrolithiasis
 c. Hyperoxaluria
 d. Hypercitraturia

F. Hematologic manifestations:
 a. Iron deficiency anemia
 b. Anemia of chronic disease

G. Dermatologic manifestations:
 a. Salty sweat
 b. Digital clubbing
 c. Cyanosis
 d. Acrodermatitis enteropathica due to zinc deficiency
 e. Wrinkling of the palm following brief immersion in the water test
 f. Scaly dermatitis following deficiency of fatty acids.

H. Infertility:
 a. Absence of vas deferens in male
 b. Thickened secretion in the cervix in female

I. Electrolyte abnormalities:
 a. Low chloride
 b. Low serum sodium
 c. Low potassium
 d. Metabolic alkalosis

J. Cardiovascular disease:
 a. Myocardial infarction
 b. Left sided heart failure
 c. Atrial fibrillation

Evaluation of Cystic Fibrosis

A. Clinical symptoms in cystic fibrosis criteria: Following symptoms along with positive screening are the clinical criteria:
 a. Siblings with cystic fibrosis
 b. Positive new born screening
 c. Clinical symptoms consistent with cystic fibrosis in one or more organ system:
  1. Chronic sinopulmonary disease
  2. Nutritional or gastrointestinal abnormalities
  3. Salt loss syndromes
  4. Obstructive azoospermia

B. Following are the laboratory criteria for CFTR dysfunction:
 a. Elevated chloride in sweat is more than 60 mEq/L
 b. Two diseases causing CFTR dysfunction
 c. Abnormal nasal potential difference

In symptomatic patient if first sweat chloride is normal, this should be repeated.

If initial sweat chloride content is high, in that case DNA test is indicated.

If CFTR mutation is found, in that case expanded DNA analysis should be done. But at least two cystic fibrosis related mutations are required for confirming the diagnosis.

Other Investigation Required for Diagnosis

A. Chest X-ray demonstrate fibrosis, bronchiectasis, hyperinflammation, atelectasis or abscess.

B. Sinus radiography demonstrates panopacification of the paranasal sinuses.

C. Abdominal straight X-ray demonstrates meconium ileus.

D. Bronchoalveolar lavage demonstrates different microorganisms.

E. Pulmonary function test demonstrates:
 a. Normal or high FEV_1 and low FVC—restrictive lung disease.
 b. Low FEV_1 and high FVC—obstructive lung disease and airway trapping.

Treatment

A. Pulmonary management:
 a. Control infection—where the main causative organism is *Pseudomonas aeruginosa* by broad spectrum antibiotics.

b. Improvement of oxygenation—inhaled bronchodilator like albuterol, ipratropium bromide help in bronchodilatation and oxygenation.
c. Inhalation of hypertonic saline should be administered to promote the clearance of the airway.
d. Provision of nasal cannula for administration of oxygen helps in:
    1. Enhances exercise endurance
    2. Improves quality of sleep
    3. Regular school attendance
e. Noninvasive ventilation helps in nighttime gas exchange more effectively.

B. Supportive therapies include supplementation of:
a. Pancreatic enzymes
b. Fat soluble vitamins
c. Bronchodilators
d. Mucolytic
e. Antibiotics
f. Anti-inflammatory agents

C. CFTR modulator therapies:
a. Ivacaftor: It will treat class III dysfunction where the primary aberration is mutation of G551D by binding the defective CFTR protein at the cells surface thereby opening the chloride channels and restoring the function of protein. Dosage are:
    1. 160 mg orally twice daily in patients having age more than 6 years.
    2. In case of younger patient having weight less than 14 14 kg—50 mg orally twice daily and more than 14 kg—75 mg orally twice daily.
b. Lumacaftor: Chaperone molecule acts by moving CFTR protein from the intracellular organelles onto the surface of the cells for processing. This drug is effective in case of mutation of *ΔF508* gene. Dose is Lumacaftor 200 mg along with Ivacaftor 125 mg should be administered orally twice daily.
c. Tezacaftor: It improves intracellular processing and trafficking.

D. Lung transplantation is the treatment of choice in case of end-stage lung disease. Following are the conditions according to International Society of Heart and Lung Transplantation:
a. Fall of FEV_1 to less than 30% of predicted value
b. Rapid fall of FEV_1 despite the optimal therapy
c. 6-minute walk distance is less than 400 meters
d. The development of pulmonary hypertension in absence of exacerbation of hypoxemia
e. Clinical declining of the conditions:
    1. Increased frequency of exacerbation like acute respiratory failure that requires noninvasive ventilation.
    2. Poor recovery from successive exacerbation
    3. Worsening of status of nutrition despite proper nutritional supplementation
    4. Pneumothorax
    5. Presence of life-threatening hemoptysis despite embolization of bronchial artery.

Q66. Various modes of oxygen delivery for hypoxia in COVID-19 patient.

MGR UNIVERSITY, 2021 (10)

ANSWER

The goal in COVID-19 patient with hypoxia is maintaining $SpO_2 \geq 90\%$ to prevent respiratory failure.

A. Low flow oxygen therapy:
a. By nasal cannula: In mild hypoxia flow rate should be 1 to 6 L/min and maintain FiO_2 near 24–40%.
b. By simple face mask when nasal cannula is not applicable, flow rate should be 6 to 10 L/min to maintain FiO_2 40–60%.

B. Moderate flow devices:
a. Venturi mask should be given to patient with chronic obstructive lung disease if controlled application of oxygen is required, FiO_2 of 24–40% should be maintained.
b. Non-rebreather mask: In case of patient with moderate to severe hypoxemia, it should be given at flow rate of 10 to 15 L/min to maintain FiO_2 up to 90%.

C. High flow nasal cannula: If the patient is suffering from moderate-to-severe hypoxemia and unresponsive to low flow oxygen, in that case flow rare should be maintained at 60 L/min with FiO_2 nearly 100%. Its advantages are
a. Work of breathing should be minimized.
b. It can avoid ventilation

D. Noninvasive ventilation: In patient with type 2 respiratory failure, or increased work of breathing, and patient refractory to high flow nasal cannula, BIPAP/CPAP should be of choice.

E. Invasive ventilation should be given to patients with ARDS, if the patient is hemodynamically unstable and altered mental status. Low tidal volume ventilation at a rate of 6 mL/kg of body weight should be preferred.

F. Prone position of the patient should be required in both intubated and non-intubated patient.

Q67. What is atypical pneumonia? When do you suspect it? Briefly outline the management strategies.

WBUHS, 2023 (10)

ANSWER

Definition

Atypical pneumonia is a community acquired pneumonia due to organisms not typically associated with classical bacterial pneumonia and is characterized by typical insidious onset of symptoms, evidences of extrapulmonary symptoms and atypical radiological features.

Etiology

A. Atypical bacteria:
- **a.** *Mycoplasma pneumoniae*
- **b.** *Chlamydophila pneumoniae*
- **c.** *Legionella pneumophila*
- **d.** *Coxiella burnetii*
- **e.** *Francisella tularensis*

B. Viral causes:
- **a.** Respiratory syncytial virus
- **b.** Influenza A and B
- **c.** Parainfluenza virus
- **d.** Adenovirus
- **e.** Coronaviruses

C. Fungi

Pathophysiology

A. Organ specific pathophysiology:
- **a.** *Mycoplasma pneumoniae* attaches to the respiratory epithelium producing dysfunction of the ciliary function leading to cellular injury.
- **b.** *Legionella pneumophila* invades the alveolar macrophages thereby prevents fusion of the phagolysosomal fusion, produces severe inflammation along with systemic symptoms.
- **c.** The intracellular pathogen *Chlamydophila* produces low grade inflammation.

Clinical Features

A. Low grade insidious onset features

B. Low grade to moderate fever without chill and rigor.

C. Dry or minimally productive cough

D. Respiratory distress: Minimal or absent.

E. Auscultation: Minimal feature in the form of minimal crackles.

F. Extrapulmonary features: Headache, myalgia, sore throat, diarrhea

Evaluation

A. Laboratory features:
- **a.** Complete blood count—mildly elevated leukocyte count
- **b.** Raised CRP
- **c.** Raised ESR

B. PCR for *Mycoplasma, Chlamydophila* and *Legionella*

C. Urinary antigen got serogroup 1 *Legionella pneumophila*

D. IgM antibodies for mycoplasma

E. Chest X-ray demonstrates diffuse bilateral infiltrate which may be disproportionate to clinical features.

Treatment

A. Empiric antibiotic as 1st line of therapy is macrolide group as
- **a.** 500 mg as 1st dose followed by 250 mg twice daily for 4 days.
- **b.** Doxycycline 100 mg twice daily for 7–10 days.

B. Alternative drugs are: Levofloxacin 500–700 mg daily for 7–10 days. In case of elderly or case of severe cases.

C. Supportive therapy—administration of oxygen, hydration

Q68. Describe newer modalities to diagnose tuberculosis and write about the National Tuberculosis Program in India.

SAURASHTRA UNI, RAJKOT, 2021 (20)

Discuss about recent changes in ENTCP and goal of National Tuberculosis Elimination Program.

WBUHS, 2020 (10)

ANSWER

Newer diagnostic modalities described in question number 14 in the chapter of Infectious Diseases.

In 2020 the name of the program has been changed from Revised National Tuberculosis Control Program to National Tuberculosis Elimination Program (NTEP) to eliminate tuberculosis by 2025, i.e., 5 years of the Global target at 2030.

The SDG target regarding to tuberculosis is:

A. 80% incidence reduction

B. 90% mortality reduction

C. Zero patients related to tuberculosis and their households face catastrophic cost as a result of tubercular disease.

Estimated Tuberculosis Burden in India as per Global Tuberculosis Report in 2023

A. Estimated incidence is 2.82 million new cases of tuberculosis in 2022—199 cases per 100,000 population.

B. Estimated mortality due to tuberculosis is 331,000 in 2022–2023 deaths per 100,000 population.

C. Approximately 2% tuberculosis patients are HIV positive.

D. Drug resistant tuberculosis: 2.5% new cases and 13% in previously treated cases.

Objectives of this program are:

A. Early diagnosis of the tuberculosis patients prompt treatment with quality assured drugs and treatment regimen.

B. Engaging with the patients seeking care in the private sector.

C. Prevention strategies include contact tracing in high risk/vulnerable population.

D. Control of air-borne infection

E. Multisectoral response for addressing social determinants.

Key Points in this Program

A. Early detection and diagnosis:

- **a.** Finding of active cases and detection of passive cases.
- **b.** Universal testing of drug susceptibility.
- **c.** Rapid molecular test like CBNAAT

B. Drug treatment and adhesion to the treatment:

- **a.** Administration of the fixed dose combination daily.
- **b.** Direct observed administration of drugs.
- **c.** Adherence to the new digital technologies

C. Engagement with the public sector:

- **a.** To notify and treat the patient Public–Private model
- **b.** Under Nikshay Poshan Yojana incentives to private providers.

D. Management of drug resistant tuberculosis:

- **a.** Surveillance for National Drug resistance
- **b.** Use of newer drugs like Bedaquiline, Delamanid

E. Supportive schemes:

- **a.** Under Nikshay Poshan Yojana Rs 500/- nutritional support to TB patients.
- **b.** Nikshay: To notify and monitor TB information technology-enabled surveillance system.

F. Preventive strategies:

- **a.** In case of high risk groups isoniazid preventive therapy.
- **b.** Tracing the contact and chemoprophylaxis.
- **c.** Just after birth BCG vaccination.

Achievement of this Program

A. In country model for estimation of burden of tuberculosis patient

B. Pradhan Mantri Tuberculosis Mukt Bharat Abhiyaan

C. Finding of cases of tuberculosis

D. Diagnostic services

E. Treatment services

F. Tuberculosis preventive services

G. Patient support systems

H. Active case findings

I. Medical college

Challenges in the Program

A. There is progressive increase in the burden of drug resistant tuberculosis

B. There is under-reporting of the incidence from the private sector

C. Village people becomes very afraid of social stigma

D. The patient being ignorant are poorly adherent to the anti-tubercular drugs

E. Due to search of the work the village people goes to urban areas hence there is chance of spreading of tuberculosis in the urban areas.

Q69. Non-resolving pneumonia.

NTR UNI OF HEALTH SC, VIJAYAWADA, ANDHRA, 2022 (10)

ANSWER

This can be defined as the failure of the clinical and radiological improvement of the pneumonia in spite of administration of antibiotics within 10 days or persisting beyond 2 weeks.

Etiology

A. Infectious causes:
- **a.** Organisms resistant to antibiotics: MRSA or multidrug resistant gram negative organism.
- **b.** Atypical bacteria like *Mycoplasma, Legionella* or *Chlamydophila*
- **c.** Fungal organism: *Histoplasma, Cryptococcus, Aspergillus*
- **d.** Mycobacterial infection
- **e.** Immunocompromised patients, *Strongyloides*

B. Noninfectious causes:
- **a.** Malignancy
- **b.** Pulmonary vasculitis
- **c.** Organizing pneumonia
- **d.** Eosinophilic pneumonia
- **e.** Pulmonary embolism leading to pulmonary infarction

Pathophysiology

A. Obstruction of the respiratory tract by foreign body or tumor leading to accumulation of the secretion as it cannot be cleared.

B. In case immunocompromised person, there is delayed clearance of the infection.

C. In some cases in spite of absence of infection, the inflammation may persists which mat invite further and new infection in future.

D. In spite of administration of broad spectrum antibiotics, there is failure to clear the pathogens.

Clinical Features

A. Cough with expectoration of sputum

B. Reappearance of fever of persistence of fever

C. Other constitutional symptoms are weight loss, weakness, lethargy, night sweat

D. No radiological improvement

E. There may be progression of symptoms and clinical signs like pleural effusion, consolidation

Evaluation

A. History of intake of drugs

B. History of provocating factors like smoking, obesity, hypertension

C. Use of recent administration of the antibiotics

D. Laboratory evaluation:
- **a.** Complete blood count, peripheral blood picture, ESR
- **b.** CRP
- **c.** Gram stain, culture of sputum
- **d.** Blood culture
- **e.** If possible bronchoscopy followed by examination of bronchoalveolar lavage fluid.
- **f.** Status of HIV which it common cause of unresolving pneumonia
- **g.** Serology for the different organisms

E. Chest X-ray demonstrating the persistence of infection or progression of infection.

F. CT scan of the thorax to detect the cause of nonresolution of pneumonias in the form of foreign body, tumor.

G. Bronchoscopy

H. PET-CT in case of suspicion of malignancy of lung is under suspicion.

Treatment

A. MRSA:
- **a.** Vancomycin—15–20 mg/kg intravenously thrice or twice daily.
- **b.** Linezolid—600 mg twice daily orally or intravenously depending upon the severity of the patient's condition.

B. Pseudomonas:
- **a.** Piperacillin-tazobactam—4.5 gram twice daily intravenously.
- **b.** Meropenem—1 gram intravenously twice daily.

C. Atypical bacteria:
- **a.** Voriconazole—6 mg/kg intravenously twice daily for 2 days.
- **b.** Liposomal amphotericin B 3–5 mg/kg/day intravenously

D. Tubercular bacteria:
- **a.** HRZE through the DOT therapy.

Q70. Brittle asthma.

NTR UNI OF HEALTH SC, VIJAYAWADA, ANDHRA, 2022 (10)

ANSWER

Definition

It is recurrent severe difficult to control asthma which can be life-threatening in spite of medical therapy.

Types:
There are two types of brittle asthma:

A. Type 1: Here there is variability in the wide peak expiratory flow rate in spite of intensive medical therapy.

B. Type 2: This is characterized by sudden and severe and intense attack of asthma on the background of well controlled bronchial asthma.

Following are the risk factor for developing brittle asthma:

A. Psychological factors like depression and anxiety

B. Poor perception bronchoconstriction

C. Repeated exposure to allergen

D. Irregular intake of medication

E. Hormonal changes

F. Exposure to environmental pollutants

G. Exposure to smoking

H. Triggering to allergen

I. History of anaphylaxis

J. Genetic predisposition

Pathophysiology

A. Hyperresponsive alveoli

B. Remodeling of the airways

C. Hypertrophy of the bronchial smooth muscle cells

D. Infiltration with increased number of eosinophils

E. In type 2 brittle asthma there is autonomic imbalance

F. Sudden bronchospasm in response to stress.

Clinical Features

A. In case of type 1 brittle asthma:

- **a.** More than 40% variable pulmonary expiratory flow
- **b.** Progressively worsening of symptoms in spite of administration of bronchodilator and corticosteroids requiring frequent hospitalization

B. In case of type 2 brittle asthma:

- **a.** In well controlled asthma, sudden deterioration of the respiratory distress.
- **b.** Female sex is more affected as compared to male.
- **c.** There is waxing and waning of the symptoms in the background well controlled asthma.
- **d.** There is sudden respiratory arrest

Laboratory Evaluation

A. Hematological features are:

- **a.** Increased eosinophil count

B. Increased level of IgE.

C. Spirometry demonstrated reversible airway obstruction

D. Peak expiratory flow rate demonstrated high variability in case of type 1.

E. Arterial blood gases demonstrates hypoxemia with or without hypercapnia

Treatment

A. Pharmacological treatment:

- **a.** Administration of intravenous corticosteroid or long acting beta agonists followed by oral corticosteroids
- **b.** Administration of leukotriene antagonist
- **c.** Theophylline

B. Non-pharmacological treatment:

- **a.** Triggering factors should be avoided.
- **b.** Arrangement of the portable oxygen
- **c.** Psychological support

Q71. Functional anatomy of lung.

MAHARASHTRA UNI OF HEALTH SC, VIJAYAWADA, 2020 (10)

ANSWER

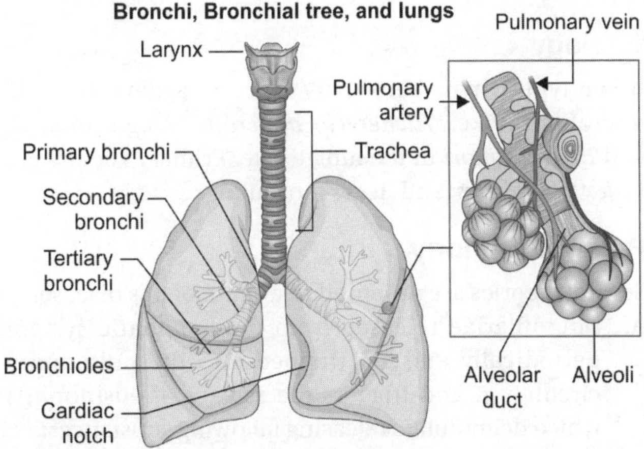

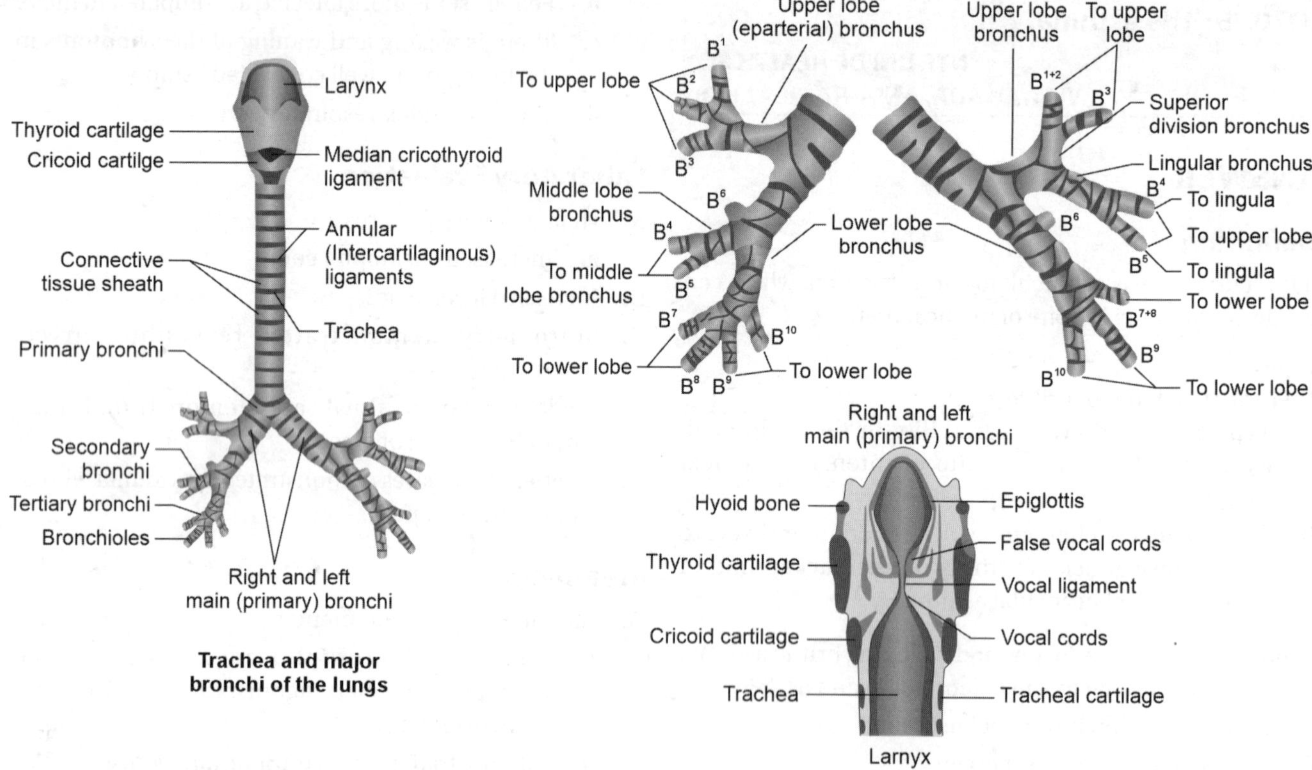

Q72. Tropical pulmonary eosinophilia.

NTR UNI OF HEALTH SC, VIJAYAWADA, ANDHRA, 2022 (10)

ANSWER

Definition

Tropical pulmonary eosinophilia is a hyperresponsive syndrome due to trapped microfilaria in the lung tissue developed in the endemic area and it is characterized by fever, nocturnal cough, and respiratory distress and wheezing.

Etiology

It is a type 1 hypersensitivity reaction against trapped microfilaria like *Wuchereria bancrofti*, *Brugia malayi*, and *Brugia timori* in the lung tissue. Primary vectors are *Culex*, *Anopheles*, and *Aedes* mosquito.

Pathophysiology

Several theories are proposed as a cause of this disease:

A. Microfilariae released from the lymphatic system periodically and get trapped into the pulmonary circulation and triggers the release of eosinophils which degranulate releasing following substances:
  - **a.** Eosinophilic cationic protein
  - **b.** Neurotoxins released from the eosinophils
  - **c.** Major basic proteins
  - **d.** Eosinophil peroxidase

  The above substances clear the microfilaria and also causes damage of the lung tissue.

B. Major basic protein-2 and interleukin-4 are associated with hyperactivity of the airways but interferon-gamma plays suppressive role.

C. In the pulmonary circulation, microfilaria generates systemic as well as pulmonary TH2 response leading to increased level of
  - **a.** Interleukin-4 activates eosinophils
  - **b.** Interleukin-5 promotes upregulation of eosinophil adhesion molecules on the endothelial cells
  - **c.** Interleukin-13
  - **d.** Filarial specific IgG, IgM and IgE specific antibodies
  - **e.** Significant pulmonary eosinophilia

D. Bm22-25, major antigen of the L3 stage larvae of *Brugia malayi* indices production of IgE in the patient with tropical pulmonary eosinophilia. Gamma glutamyl transpeptidase present on the pulmonary epithelium is similar to that which is found in Le stage of larvae—it showed that gamma glutamyl transpeptidase has a role in the pathogenesis of pulmonary eosinophilia.

E. Different types of oxidants like superoxide and hydrogen peroxide releasing from the respiratory tract epithelium plays an active role in the development of tropical pulmonary eosinophilia.

History and Physical Examination

Following are the clinical history:

A. Nocturnal and paroxysmal cough which is usually dry
B. Cough associated dyspnea
C. Systemic manifestations:
   a. Fever
   b. Malaise
   c. Anorexia
   d. Weight loss
D. Rarely extrapulmonary manifestations:
   a. Lymphadenopathy
   b. Hepatosplenomegaly
E. Peripheral blood eosinophilia of more than 3,000/cc.

Physical examination demonstrates:

A. Chest auscultation demonstrates crepitation, wheezing
B. Hepatosplenomegaly
C. Lymphadenopathy

Evaluation

Early diagnosis is very critical as delay in the diagnosis can lead to progressive interstitial fibrosis and respiratory impairment. Following findings guide the evaluation of tropical pulmonary eosinophilia:

A. Complete blood count demonstrates leukocytosis with eosinophil count of more than 3,000/cc.
B. Stool examination demonstrating other parasites producing pulmonary eosinophilia can exclude tropical pulmonary eosinophilia.
C. Increased level of immunoglobulin E can be seen.
D. Increased level of anti-filarial antibody.
E. Chest X-ray demonstrates:
   a. Reticulonodular opacities
   b. Miliary mottling in the middle or lower zone.
   c. Interlobular septal thickening
   d. May be completely normal in 20% patients
F. Chest CT scan demonstrates:
   a. Bronchiectasis
   b. Lymphadenopathy
   c. Pleural effusion
G. Pulmonary function test demonstrates predominant restrictive pattern with mild to moderate obstructive pattern.
H. Bronchoalveolar lavage contains intense presence of eosinophilia.

Diagnostic criteria of tropical pulmonary eosinophilia includes:

A. History of residence of travel to endemic area of filarial.
B. Paroxysmal and nocturnal cough with dyspnea
C. Leukocytosis with peripheral blood eosinophil count of more than 3,000/cc.
D. Increased level of IgE and filarial antibody titer.
E. Chest X-ray demonstrates pulmonary infiltrate.
F. Clinical improvement with diethylcarbamazine.

Treatment

A. Diethylcarbamazine citrate—6 mg/kg of body weight/day in 2 to 3 divided doses for 3 weeks as it will act against microfilaria and adults.
B. Concomitant therapy with corticosteroids will reduce the bronchial wall inflammation as it reduces release of superoxide and hydrogen peroxide.
C. Ivermectin acting on microfilariae and albendazole which acts on adult worm.
D. Alternate therapy is 200 mg doxycycline 200 orally daily coupled with corticosteroids for 4 to 6 weeks.

Q73. Diagnosis and management of bronchiectasis.

WBUHS, 2020 (10)

ANSWER

Definition

Bronchiectasis a chronic lung disease characterized by lifelong and persistent widening of the of the bronchial airways along with the weakening of the mucociliary function of the lining of the airways leading to recurrent invasion and mucus pooling of the airways by the different organisms.

Etiology:

A. Infections:
   a. Bacterial infection:
      1. *Mycobacterium*
      2. Tuberculosis
      3. *Haemophilus influenzae*
      4. *Staphylococcus aureus*
      5. *Pseudomonas*
      6. *Mycoplasma*
      7. HIV

b. Viral infection:
   1. Respiratory syncytial virus
   2. Measles virus
c. Fungal infection

B. Bronchial obstruction:
   a. Foreign body
   b. Mucus plug
   c. Tumors
   d. Hilar lymphadenopathy

C. Post-inflammatory:
   a. Chronic sinusitis
   b. Chronic infection
   c. Injury due to inhalation

D. Congenital:
   a. Cystic fibrosis
   b. Primary ciliary dyskinesia
   c. Young syndrome
   d. Hypogammaglobulinemia
   e. Alpha-1 antitrypsin deficiency

E. Inflammatory disease:
   a. Ulcerative colitis
   b. Rheumatoid arthritis
   c. Sjögren's syndrome

F. Lung diseases:
   a. Bronchial asthma
   b. COPD
   c. Bronchomalacia
   d. Idiopathic pulmonary fibrosis

G. Miscellaneous:
   a. Yellow nail syndrome

Pathophysiology

Three important causes of bronchiectasis:

A. Infection
B. Airway obstruction
C. Peribronchial fibrosis

At the site of bacterial accumulation I the bronchial tree due to poor mucociliary clearance, the chemoattractants like interleukin 8 and leukotriene B4 drive large number of neutrophils, but these neutrophils:

A. Fails to kill the bacteria by opsonophagocytosis.
B. Inability to clear apoptotic cells

TH17 cells play a significant role in the invasion of T cells.

Histology in the bronchiectasis includes:

A. Destruction of cartilage leading to fibrosis
B. Hyperplasia of mucosal and mucous gland
C. Infiltration of inflammatory cells
D. Increased amount of mucus and exudate

History and Physical Examinations

A. Progressive dyspnea
B. Hemoptysis—flecks of blood in the sputum, occasional life threatening.
C. Pleuritic chest pain
D. Intermittent wheezing
E. Fatigue
F. Weight loss
G. Chest pain secondary to coughing

Physical Examination

A. General survey includes:
   a. Clubbing
   b. Cyanosis
   c. Weight loss

B. Chest features include:
   a. On auscultation, crackles—75% at the basal areas and wheeze—22% due obstruction in the airflow due to secretion.

C. Clinical pictures associated with causative conditions:
   a. Allergic bronchopulmonary aspergillosis—widespread wheezing
   b. Connective tissue disease—arthritis sicca syndrome
   c. Localized bronchial obstruction—local wheezing
   d. Cystic fibrosis—recurrent sinusitis

Evaluation

A. Immunoglobulin test—IgA, IgE, IgG, and IgM
B. For ABPA, IgE and IgG to *Aspergillus* and absolute eosinophil count
C. Sputum culture for nontuberculous mycobacteria
D. Tests for cystic fibrosis:
   a. Sweat test and screening for cystic fibrosis mutation if the patient is younger than 40 years of age.
   b. Recurrent *Staphylococcus aureus, Pseudomonas aeruginosa*
   c. Upper lobe predominant disease

E. Imaging:

- **a.** Chest X-ray—findings includes:
  1. Parallel linear densities
  2. Tram-track appearances
  3. Ring shadows—indicating dilated thickened bronchial walls
  4. Patchy densities due to impaction of mucus.
  5. Consolidation volume loss secondary to mucoid bronchial obstruction
- **b.** Cardinal signs of bronchiectasis includes:
  1. Bronchoarterial ratio—greater than 1
  2. Lack of tapering of bronchus—normally airways taper gradually as the bronchi progress toward the periphery.
  3. Visibility of the airways within 1 cm of the pleural surface or abutting the mediastinal surface.
- **c.** Pattern of bronchial tree on CT scan:
  1. Cylindrical sign: Horizontally oriented dilated airways.
  2. Signet ring: Presence of dilated airways adjacent to pulmonary artery branch giving rise to appearance of ring—here the inner diameter of bronchus is greater than that of adjacent pulmonary artery.
  3. Varicose: It is non-uniform dilatation of bronchus.
  4. Cystic or saccular bronchus: It indicates cluster of thin walled cystic space.
  5. Mosaic lung attenuation: It is characterized by heterogenous density of the lung in the damaged lung segment due to trapping of air. On expiration this can be reproduced.
  6. Dilated bronchial arteries: The tortuous vessels extend toward the hila along the central airways.
  7. Lobar collapse
  8. Formation of mycetoma

F. Lung function test:

- **a.** Obstruction to airflow: Decreased FEV_1
- **b.** Trapping of air: Increased residual volume.

Treatment

Following are the treatment goals:

A. Identification of cause and treat the etiology

B. Improvement of the tracheobronchial clearance:

- **a.** Postural drainage—adoption of the position in which the upper lobe can be drained and it should be performed 5–10 minutes twice a day.
- **b.** Active cycle of breathing technique—deep breathing followed by forced expiratory maneuvers thereby allowing the mucus to gravitate down the bronchi toward trachea.
- **c.** Percussion of the chest wall with cupped hands will help dislodging the sputum
- **d.** With the help of mechanical device which helps the chest wall to oscillate.

C. Control of infection: Antibiotics should be administered based on the culture and sensitivity of the sputum. But if the patient is seriously ill and sputum culture is negative, in that case amoxicillin, macrolides or amoxiclav should be administered for at least 2 weeks.

D. If the sputum demonstrates *Haemophilus influenzae*, in the case 1 g amoxicillin 1 g orally twice daily for 2 weeks, or in case of *Pseudomonas* infection, 750 mg ciprofloxacin orally twice daily for 2 weeks should be of choice.

E. Treatment of *Pseudomonas* infection, intravenous antipseudomonal antibiotics along with nebulization with colistin for 3 months is of right choice.

Q74. Describe pathophysiology of breathlessness and causes of acute breathlessness. How can you approach?

KIMS, 2021 (10)

ANSWER

Introduction

Dyspnea can be defined as awareness of one's own respiratory effort. This symptom is responsible for nearly half of the admission in intensive care unit. The stimuli vary from individual to individual in developing cough in spite of their same pathology in lung or comorbid conditions. In different form patient may express, like, chest tightness, increased work of breathing or air hunger. It may be acute or chronic. It can be assessed according to its intensity, degree of distress during work of breathing, impact on instrumental activities of daily living. It is a cumulative results of different situations, like, physiological, social, psychological as well as environmental and behavioral factors.

Pathophysiology

There are three components for controlling the respiration: One is afferent pathway, central processing unit in the respiratory center in medulla and efferent pathways. Dyspnea occurs when there is mismatch between afferent (needs for ventilation) and efferent (physical breathing) signaling going to airways, lung, chest muscles and diaphragm.

A. Afferent signals are coming from following areas:
  a. Physiological pathways responsible for shortness of breath:
    1. Acid sensing ion channels
    2. Mechanoreceptors
    3. Receptors in the different zone of respiratory apparatus:
      - Juxtacapillary receptor sensitive to pulmonary interstitial edema
      - Stretch receptors in the bronchial smooth muscles.
      - Muscle spindles present in the respiratory muscles.

B. Efferent signal goes to respiratory muscles, most importantly diaphragm.

C. Central processing unit in the brain compares both signals. Afferent signal watches the efferent signals to ventilatory muscles are effective to satisfy the demands of airway pressure, air flow and movement of the lung. In case of mismatch degree of respiratory distress will increase

Causes of Dyspnea

A. Physiological:
  a. Normal aging
  b. Obesity
  c. Exercise
  d. Deconditioning

B. Pathological causes:
  a. Cardiological:
    1. Acquired causes:
      - Ischemic heart disease
      - Valvular diseases
      - Myocardial diseases
      - Pericardial diseases
    2. Congenital diseases:
      - Tetralogy of Fallot
      - Atrial septal defect
  b. Respiratory causes:
    1. Restrictive causes:
      - Interstitial lung disease
      - Obesity
      - Kyphoscoliosis
      - Sarcoidosis
    2. Pleural causes:
      - Pleural effusion
      - Pneumothorax
      - Hemothorax
      - Mesothelioma
    3. Obstructive causes:
      - Bronchial asthma
      - Chronic obstructive pulmonary disease
      - Obstructive sleep apnea
      - Bronchiolitis obliterans
      - Tracheomalacia
      - Intrabronchial tumor
    4. Lung alveoli:
      - Pneumonia
      - Tuberculosis
      - Bronchoalveolar carcinoma
      - Eosinophilic pneumonia
      - Aspiration pneumonitis
      - Hypersensitivity pneumonitis
    5. Interstitial involvement:
      - Drug-induced:
        - Methotrexate
        - Amiodarone
      - Radiation therapy
      - Pulmonary edema
      - Usual interstitial pneumonia
    6. Vascular involvement:
      - Pulmonary embolism
      - Pulmonary infarction
      - Idiopathic pulmonary hypertension
      - Pulmonary arteriovenous malformation
  c. Metabolic diseases:
    1. Thyroid disease
    2. Cushing's syndrome
  d. Hematological causes:
    1. Anemia
    2. Carbon monoxide poisoning
    3. Methemoglobinemia
    4. Sulfhemoglobinemia
    5. Thrombotic thrombocytopenic purpura
  e. Abdominal causes:
    1. Ascites
    2. Hepatic hydrothorax
    3. Gastroesophageal reflux disease
    4. Peptic ulcer disease

f. Neurological causes:
   1. Poliomyelitis
   2. Guillain-Barré syndrome
   3. Myasthenia gravis
   4. Amyotrophic lateral sclerosis
   5. Paraneoplastic myasthenia syndrome

g. Psychological causes:
   1. Anxiety
   2. Panic attack

h. Infective causes:
   1. Botulism
   2. Tetanus

Approach to a Case of Hypertension

When a patient comes with severe breathlessness, he or she should be admitted with immediate administration of oxygen through nasal cannula or endotracheal intubation with or without mechanical ventilation following assessment. Immediate assessment will establish degree of urgency, severity and duration of dyspnea and whether it is acute or acute on chronic. There are several "red-flag" signs requiring immediate attention. These are:

A. Tachypnea
B. Hypotension
C. Altered mental status
D. Retraction of chest wall
E. Unilateral deviation of trachea
F. Stridor
G. Cyanosis
H. Hypoxia
I. Absence of loss of breath sound unilaterally
J. Unstable arrhythmias

Presence of any one of the above requires immediate oxygenation. Usually two categories of patients are found. These are:

A. In an unknown patient with acute onset of breathlessness where the cause has to be ascertained. In this case main aim is to discover the underlying abnormality.

B. Already diagnosed case with onset of dyspnea. In this case the aim should be to search for the deterioration of the primary cause or search of the new cause over and above the primary event.

But psychogenic breathlessness requires special attention as it requires urgent intervention to motivate and guide the patient in a proper way.

Dyspnea is graded by the following methods:

A. Borg's scale
B. MMRC
C. American Thoracic society scale (ATS scale)
D. Fletcher's scale

Most commonly used scales are ATS and MMRC scale.

ATS scale:

Description	Scale	Degree
Patient is not troubled by shortness of breath when he is hurry in the same level or walking up a slight hill	0	None
He is troubled by shortness of breath when he is on the level or walking on straight hill	1	Mild
More slow walking than the people of same age on the level because of breathlessness or he has to stop breath when walking on the level at his own pace	2	Moderate
He has to stop for breath after walking about 100 yards or after a few minutes on the level	3	Severe
Patient is so severe breathless that he cannot leave the house or dress or cannot undress	4	Very severe

From history:

A. Acute episode of breathlessness, wheeze, sense of chest tightness, cough mainly in the morning with string like thick sputum—bronchial asthma.

B. Prolonged immobilized patient suddenly develop severe respiratory distress—suggest pulmonary embolism or pulmonary infarction.

C. History of acute respiratory distress during eating in case of semiconscious patient—suggest aspiration pneumonitis or aspiration of foreign body.

D. Sudden respiratory distress, cyanosis, gasping with loss of consciousness—foreign body aspiration producing complete respiratory obstruction.

E. Sudden respiratory distress with inspiratory stridor, localized wheezing—suggest partial respiratory tract obstruction.

F. History of severe respiratory distress, hyperventilation, tingling and numbness in the perioral region as well as extremities with history of anxiety—psychogenic hyperventilation.

G. History of severe respiratory distress with severe sweating, cough with pink frothy sputum in a diabetic patient—suggest acute pulmonary edema or acute myocardial infarction.

H. Chronic and recurrent respiratory distress exacerbated during exertion in previously suffered from respiratory disease—acute exacerbation of chronic obstructive respiratory disease, chronic cardiac failure, anemia, interstitial pulmonary disease.

I. History of chronic respiratory distress in one lateral position (trepopnea)—suggest pleural effusion of dependent side, disease of lung on non-dependent side.

J. History of breathlessness in upright position which can be relieved in lying down position (platypnea)—pulmonary arteriovenous malformation, intracardiac shunt,

K. History of sudden breathlessness at rest following cough—spontaneous pneumothorax.

L. History of severe breathlessness for more than 2 hours in hypertensive, hyperlipidemic diabetic patient—congestive cardiac failure.

M. History of paroxysmal nocturnal dyspnea, orthopnea—acute cardiac failure.

N. Morning headache with breathlessness—onset of respiratory failure, it occurs in case of musculoskeletal disease impairing respiratory function, e.g., Kyphoscoliosis, muscular dystrophy.

O. History of apprehension, sweating, with holding the site of pain firmly in a restless patient—suggests myocardial infarction, pulmonary infarction.

Associated symptoms:

A. History of chest pain with breathlessness—spontaneous pneumothorax, pulmonary embolism, acute myocardial infarction, pulmonary embolism

B. History of pricking chest pain, faintness occasionally unconsciousness—pulmonary embolism

C. Associated fever with chill and rigor—pneumonia

D. History of paroxysmal nocturnal dyspnea, swelling of leg bilaterally—heart failure

E. History of acute onset of anemia, dizziness, sweating, syncope—anemia

F. Associated lightheadedness, tingling and numbness of perioral areas, palpitation, and paresthesia—anxiety disorder.

G. History of primary lung disease, effort dyspnea, productive cough, rapid and shallow respiration with no relation with postural change, persistence of breathlessness for short time after cessation of exercise—dyspnea of pulmonary cause.

H. History of cardiac disease, breathlessness increased in lying down position, shallow but not rapid breath, relieve of distress after taking rest for longer time, increased volume of respiration at all level of exercise—dyspnea of cardiac cause.

Aggravating factors:

A. Smoking—chronic pulmonary disease

B. Exercise—aggravates breathlessness—bronchial asthma, chronic heart failure.

C. Exposure to pollen, cold, noxious—asthma

D. History of aggravating cough in lying down position—suggest gastroesophageal reflux.

E. History of aggravation of cough in specific decubitus position—suggest unilateral bronchiectasis, lung abscess

F. Beta blocker, calcium channel blocker—cardiac disease

G. Quinidine and penicillin—hemolytic anemia

H. Nitrates, nitrites—methemoglobinemia

I. Dapsone, amiodarone—chronic pulmonary fibrosis

Relieving factors:

A. Relief of breathlessness by sitting leaning forward or lying supine with head down—chronic obstructive pulmonary disease because in this position efficiency of accessary respiratory muscles and diaphragmatic muscles will be increased.

B. Heimlich maneuver (abdominal thrust) may dislodge the foreign body from respiratory tract.

Past history:

A. Cardiac disease:
   a. Paroxysmal nocturnal dyspnea
   b. Cough with pink frothy sputum
   c. Recurrent dyspnea
   d. Orthopnea
   e. History of taking increasing number of pillows during sleeping to relieve respiratory distress—heart failure

Social history:

History of:

A. Alcoholism

B. Illicit drug use

C. Smoking

Family history:

A. Cardiac disease:
   a. Coronary artery disease
   b. Cardiomyopathy
   c. Arrhythmias

Physical Examination

General survey:

A. Pallor—anemia, hemorrhagic shock,

B. Drowsy—metabolic acidosis, carbon monoxide poisoning, acute type 2 respiratory failure.

C. Cyanosis—acute respiratory failure, pulmonary edema, pulmonary embolism, COPD, asthma, congestive heart failure

D. Edema—congestive heart failure

E. Clubbing—interstitial pulmonary fibrosis, bronchogenic carcinoma, intracardiac shunt, mesothelioma, liver disease, lung abscess, bronchiectasis, biliary cirrhosis. Presence of associated hypertrophic osteoarthropathy suggest bronchogenic carcinoma.

F. Unilateral gynecomastia—bronchogenic carcinoma or pyopneumothorax of same side.

G. Pulse:

   a. Pulsus paradoxus—acute asthma, acute asthma
   b. Tachycardia—acute respiratory failure, asthma, cardiac failure, pulmonary edema.
   c. High volume pulse—anemia.
   d. Irregular beats—arrhythmias.

H. Tachypnea

I. Hypotension—pulmonary embolism, pulmonary infarction, hemorrhagic shock, myocardial infarction

J. Temperature—increased in case of aspiration pneumonia

K. Stridor—partial upper respiratory tract obstruction

L. Wheeze—severe bronchial asthma.

M. Extremities: Pedal edema—congestive cardiac failure, deep vein thrombosis, liver disease

N. Distended and pulsatile neck vein—congestive cardiac failure, severe chronic obstructive pulmonary disease, cardiac tamponade.

O. Dehydration, air hunger—metabolic acidosis

P. Evidence of carpopedal spasm—hyperventilation.

Q. Oral smell:

   a. Fetor hepaticus—hepatic encephalopathy
   b. Ammonia smell—uremic acidosis

Respiratory system examination:

A. Inspection:

   a. Accessary muscles of respiration—excessively active in all cases of respiratory failure.
   b. Excessively active respiratory muscles, tachypnea with unilateral loss of respiratory movement—suggest pneumothorax, pleural effusion or extensive lobar pneumonia of the same side.
   c. History of holding the chest with his or her palm—suggest pleurisy
   d. History of giving support with the other hand—pancoast tumor.
   e. Patient cannot lie down for a minute but can sit and take breath—suggest bilateral diaphragmatic paralysis.
   f. Tripod position, pursed lip breathing and negligible respiratory movements—suggest emphysema.
   g. Movement of chest is paradoxical in supine position during inspiration—suggest diaphragmatic weakness.
   h. Movement of abdomen is paradoxical during exhalation—suggest pulmonary edema.
   i. Unilateral flattening of chest with crowding of ribs—pulmonary fibrosis,
   j. Wheezing
      1. Unilateral—partial respiratory tract obstruction by foreign body, pulmonary embolism.
      2. Bilateral—bronchial asthma, pulmonary embolism, pulmonary edema

B. Palpation:

   a. Tracheal shifting:
      1. To the left:
         - Right sided pneumothorax
         - Right sided pleural effusion
         - Left sided collapse of lung
         - Left sided fibrosis of lung
      2. To the more right:
         - Left sided pneumothorax
         - Left sided pleural effusion
         - Right sided collapse of lung
         - Right sided fibrosis of lung
   b. Presence of intercostal tenderness suggests lung abscess, costochondritis, empyema, and pleurisy.
   c. Severe pain in a localized area in the chest suggests rib fracture by trauma or pathological, mesothelioma.
   d. Presence of crepitus on the chest suggests subcutaneous emphysema
   e. Presence of palpable rub—pleural rub

C. Percussion of chest:

   a. Hyperresonance—emphysema, COPD.
   b. Stony dull on one side—pleural effusion, emphysema
   c. Tympanic note unilaterally—unilateral pneumothorax, bullous emphysema.

   d. Woody dull in localized area—pulmonary consolidation, pulmonary fibrosis, collapse.

D. Auscultation of chest:

   a. Diminished vesicular breath sound with prolonged expiration—COPD, emphysema

   b. Absent breath sound in stony dull area—pleural effusion, empyema, pyopneumothorax

   c. Bronchial breath sound in the area of woody dullness—pulmonary consolidation, bronchogenic carcinoma, fibrosis, collapse.

   d. Rhonchi—bronchial asthma, pulmonary edema, pulmonary embolism (unilateral at a specific site).

   e. Crepitation—consolidation, pulmonary edema, interstitial pulmonary fibrosis.

   f. Basal crepitation—left ventricular failure

Cardiovascular examination:

A. Palpation:

   a. Apex beat—shifted toward midline or more toward left.

   b. S3 gallop—left ventricular failure with systolic dysfunction

   c. S4 gallop—left ventricular diastolic dysfunction in hypertension, ischemic heart disease.

   d. Palpable P2 suggests cor-pulmonale, pulmonary hypertension

B. Auscultation:

   a. Loud P2—pulmonary hypertension

   b. Murmurs—structural heart disease

   c. Pericardial rub—pericardial effusion

   d. Muffled and distant heart sound—pericardial effusion

Gastrointestinal system examination:

A. Palpation:

   a. Liver palpable—suggest COPD, alcoholic liver disease

   b. Spleen palpable—suggest portal hypertension, hepatic hydrothorax

   c. Presence of free fluid by shifting dullness and fluid thrill—ascites

   d. Hepatojugular reflux—positive in case of congestive cardiac failure

Investigations

A. Radiological investigation:

   a. Chest X-ray:

      1. Radiolucent area—pneumothorax

      2. Radiopaque area with Ellis S-shaped curve with highest point toward axilla—pleural effusion, empyema

      3. Radiopaque area bordered by pleural margin—consolidation

      4. Presence of radiolucent area above and radiopaque area below having a horizontal level—hydropneumothorax or pyopneumothorax.

      5. Triangular opaque area having apex toward center and base toward periphery—pulmonary embolism, pulmonary infarction.

      6. Prominent hilar markings with peripheral pruning of pulmonary vessels—pulmonary hypertension

      7. Bilateral basal patchy opacity—pulmonary edema.

      8. Tubular heart shadow—emphysema

      9. Boot shaped heart—Fallot's tetralogy

      10. Dilated heart—cardiomyopathy, valvular heart disease

      11. Water bottle configuration of heart—pericardial effusion

B. CT pulmonary angiography—pulmonary embolism, pulmonary infarction. If it is negative the diagnosis of pulmonary embolism is very unlikely and alternate diagnosis should be thought.

Wells criteria is used to detect pulmonary embolism:

   a. Clinical symptoms of deep venous thrombosis—3 points

   b. Other clinical diagnosis not more likely 3 points

   c. Heart rate greater than 100 beats/min—1.5 points

   d. Previous deep vein thrombosis or pulmonary embolism—1.5 points.

   e. Immobilization or surgery within past 4 weeks—1.5 points

   f. Hemoptysis—1 point

   g. Malignancy—1 point

If the score is >6: Highest risk for pulmonary embolism.

If the score is 2–6: Intermediate risk for pulmonary embolism

If the score is <2: Low risk for pulmonary embolism.

C. Electrocardiography:

   a. Tall peaked P in lead II and V1—cor pulmonale

   b. Ischemic heart disease, hypertension, myocardial infarction, arrhythmias

   c. Right bundle branch block, $S_1Q_3T_3$—pulmonary infarction

   d. Low voltage wave complexes (less than 5 small square QRS in limb lid and less than 10 small squares in V1–V6—suggestive of cardiomyopathy)
   e. Small waves throughout the all lead—pericardial effusion.

D. Echocardiography:
   a. Presence of valvular abnormality—valvular heart disease
   b. Presence of pericardial fluid—pericardial effusion

E. CT angiography: It is done in case of pulmonary embolism.

F. Doppler ultrasonography: It will measure the aortic blood flow during exercise and can distinguish the congestive heart failure from COPD because this blood flow will be lowered in case of heart failure but normal in COPD.

G. Hematological investigation:
   a. Hemoglobin low—anemia.
   b. Leukocytosis, raised ESR—infection, myocardial infarction
   c. Deranged liver function—liver disease
   d. D-dimer test: This will be increased in case of suspected pulmonary embolism. Its sensitivity is much greater than its specificity. Its positive predictive value is poor. But in following cases negative predictive value is poor:
      1. Patient of more than 60 years of age.
      2. Hospitalized patient after several days of hospitalization.
   e. Brain natriuretic peptide or NT-proBNP—if value is >100 pg/mL heart failure is likely but if <100 pg/mL heart failure is unlikely.
   f. Thyroid function test—TSH low and high T3 and or T4 in case of thyrotoxicosis

H. Bronchoscopy: It can diagnose foreign body, tumor

I. Pulmonary function test:
   a. In case of bronchitis, asthma, emphysema following results are found:
      1. Decreased air flow rates
      2. Decreased FEV_1
      3. Decreased peak expiratory flow rates
      4. Decreased mid-expiratory flow rate
      5. Decreased maximal voluntary ventilation
      6. Increased tidal volume
      7. Increased residual volume
   b. In case of lung fibrosis, kyphoscoliosis, pneumoconiosis, ascites, obesity, pulmonary edema following findings can be found:
      1. Decreased total lung capacity
      2. Increased respiratory minute volume
      3. Decreased compliance.
   c. FEV_1/FVC ratio:
      1. Decreased ratio (<0.7) FEV_1/FVC—COPD, bronchial asthma. These diagnoses can be differentiated by giving inhalation of bronchodilator—in bronchial asthma there is 12% reversibility, but in case of COPD it is not reversible.
      2. Normal ratio but there is suspicion of bronchial asthma, inhaled methacholine can provoke bronchoconstriction.
   d. In case of pulmonary vascular disease:
      1. Increased ventilation
      2. Increased dead space

J. Arterial blood gases:
   a. Acute severe asthma:
      1. Decreased PaO_2
      2. Decreased $PaCO_2$
   b. In case of acute COPD:
      1. PaO_2 decreased
      2. $PaCO_2$ increased
   c. In pulmonary edema:
      1. PaO_2 decreased
      2. $PaCO_2$ decreased.
   d. In psychogenic hyperventilation:
      1. PaO_2 is normal
      2. $PaCO_2$ decreased
      3. H^+ low

Section 8 Rheumatology

COLLAGEN VASCULAR DISEASE

Q1. Biological therapy in rheumatoid arthritis indications, contraindications, and monitoring.

DNBIV/JUN2010 (10)

Diagnostic criteria for rheumatoid arthritis.

DNBII/JUN2011 (10)

What are classification criteria for rheumatoid arthritis? Discuss role of biological management in management of rheumatoid arthritis.

DNBIIB/DEC2013 (10)

Extra-articular manifestations of rheumatoid arthritis.

DNBIIIA/DEC2014 (10)

Pathogenesis and diagnosis of rheumatoid arthritis.

DNBIIIA/DECJUN2015 (6)

Disease-modifying antirheumatic drugs (DMARDs) and biological therapy in rheumatoid arthritis.

DNBIIIB/JUN2015 (4)

Biologic DMARDs.

MGR/APR2014/MDII (7)
MGR/APR2014/MDIV (7)
KUHS/NOV2013(S)/MDIV (10)

Criteria for diagnosis of rheumatoid arthritis.

MGR/OCT2013/MDII (7)

Biological agents in rheumatoid arthritis.

MGR/OCT2012/MDII (7) GMC/2015/MDIV (25)

Discuss the pathogenesis, clinical features, evaluation, and management of rheumatoid arthritis.

MGR/SEP2007/MDI (15)

Disease-modifying drugs in the management of rheumatoid arthritis.

MGR/OCT2003/MDI (5)

Outline the pathogenesis of rheumatoid arthritis. Describe its clinical features and management. Add a note on its extra-articular manifestations.

RGUHS/SEP2002/MDII (25)

Hand in rheumatoid arthritis.

RGUHS/NOVE2001/MDII (10)

Biologicals in rheumatoid arthritis.

MJPRU/2015/MDIII (10) MJPRU/2015/MDIII (6)

Respiratory manifestations in rheumatoid arthritis.

MUHS/MAY2014/MDII (10)

Biologics in rheumatoid arthritis.

MUHS/MAY2014/MDIV (10)
MUHS/NOV2010/MDII (10)

Extra-articular manifestations of rheumatoid arthritis.

MUHS/MAY2012/MDII (10)

Discuss etiopathogenesis, clinical features, investigations, and management of rheumatoid arthritis.

MUHS/MAY2011/MDII (25)

Disease-modifying drugs in the treatment of rheumatoid arthritis.
MUHS/MAY2010/MDII (10)

Discuss recent advances in the management of rheumatoid arthritis.
BF/OCT2011/MDIV (20)

Management of refractory rheumatoid arthritis.
BF/OCT2010/MDIII (10)

Write down the management of rheumatoid arthritis.
MUZ/MAY2016/MDII (20)

ACR-EULAR classification of rheumatoid arthritis. Management of refractory rheumatoid arthritis. Microscopic polyangiitis.
DNB 2022 (10)

Significance of DAS in rheumatoid arthritis.
DNB 2021 (5)

Clinical features, diagnosis and treatment of rheumatoid arthritis.
DNB 2019 (10)

Enumerate and discuss role of biological agents in the management of rheumatoid arthritis. Enumerate their contraindications.
DNB 2018 (10)

Biologicals in rheumatoid arthritis.
MGR UNI, Tamil Nadu, 2022 (10)

Newer drug treatment in rheumatoid arthritis.
Maharashtra UNI of Health SC, Vijayawada, 2022 (10)

A 23-year-old female presents with bilateral swelling and pain of smaller joints. Discuss the differential diagnosis. Discuss the detail management of rheumatoid arthritis.
MGR UNI, Tamil Nadu, 2022 (15)

B cell targeted therapy in rheumatoid arthritis.
NTR UNI of Health SC, Vijayawada, AUG 2021 (10)

EULAR criteria for the diagnosis of rheumatoid arthritis.
NTR UNI of Health SC, Vijayawada, July 2021 (10)

Discuss etiopathogenesis, clinical features, diagnosis, and current guideline on management of rheumatoid arthritis.
Veer Narmad South Gujarat UNI, 2021 (20)

Biologics in treatment of rheumatoid arthritis.
Maharashtra UNI of Health SC, Vijayawada, 2020 (10)

Biologics in rheumatoid arthritis.
Kerala University, 2020 (8)

Biologicals in the treatment of rheumatoid arthritis.
NTR UNI of Health SC, Vijayawada, Septem, Andhra, 2020 (10)

Discuss sarcopenia in elderly. Describe late onset rheumatoid arthritis.
WBUHS, 2024 (10)

ANSWER

Microscopic polyangiitis has been described in question number 4.

Sarcopenia has been described in question of 117 in updated chapter.

Definition

Rheumatoid arthritis (RA) is chronic inflammatory disorder characterized by symmetrical polyarthritis with or without extra-articular manifestations.

Risk Factors for Rheumatoid Arthritis

A. Genetic risk factors:

- **a.** In 70% of patients with human leukocyte antigen (HLA)-DR4, there is three- to four-fold increased susceptibility to RA.

b. There is strong association of third hypervariable region DRβ1allele with RA—it is termed as susceptibility epitope.

c. Other genes associated with RA are:
   1. Protein tyrosine phosphate 22
   2. Peptidylarginine deiminase 4 (PADI-4)

B. Environmental factors:

a. Smoking: It acts as best-defined risk factors. It strongly stimulates citrullination to generate anti-citrullinated protein antibodies (ACPAs) which binds to HLA-susceptibility epitope and increases the risk to 40-fold.

b. Infections: Following are the infecting agents:
   1. Parvovirus 19
   2. Enteric bacteria
   3. Mycoplasma
   4. Epstein–Barr virus
   5. Chikungunya virus in India

   Following mechanisms are involved to produce RA:
   1. Molecular mimicry
   2. Toll-like receptor activation
   3. Direct invasion of synovium

c. Periodontitis: This chronic inflammation of gingiva is strongly associated with RA. Bacterium responsible for periodontitis is *Porphyromonas gingivalis* citrullinates through its own PADI enzyme leading to development of RA—it shows there is close relationship in between these chronic diseases.

d. Dietary factors:

   High-risk factors are:
   1. Red meat intake
   2. Vitamin D deficiency
   3. Excessive coffee consumption
   4. High-salt intake

   Protective factors:
   1. Omega-3 fatty acids
   2. Consumption of fish oils
   3. Antioxidants of fruits and vegetables:
      - Vitamin C
      - Vitamin E
      - Carotenoid
      - Lycopene

e. Hormonal factors: RA is three times more common in women as compared to men. Pregnancy reduces the risk of RA. Following factors increase the risk of RA:
   1. Estrogen-containing contraceptives
   2. Breastfeeding through the increased surge of proinflammatory cytokines
   3. Nulliparity
   4. Obesity increases the risk of RA in Western world, because:
      - It increases the level of circulatory cytokines
      - It stimulates the surge of proinflammatory cytokines such as interleukin-1 (IL-1) and tumor necrosis factor α (TNF-α)

Onset of rheumatoid arthritis is preceded by prerheumatoid arthritis, total period of established RA has been divided into the following phases:

A. Phase I: In this phase, there is interaction between genetic and environmental risk factors.

B. Phase II: In this phase, production autoantibodies such as like rheumatoid factor and anti-cyclic citrullinated peptide (CCP) antibodies.

C. Phase III: In this phase, there is evidence of arthralgia with or without joint stiffness without any evidence of arthritis.

D. Phase IV: There is arthritis involving 1 or 2 joints known as undifferentiated arthritis. If it intermittent, it is called palindromic rheumatism.

E. Phase V: Established rheumatoid arthritis

   In the early phase, there is synovial cell hyperplasia and activation of endothelial cells. In the later phase as the disease progresses, there is uncontrolled inflammation and consequent destruction of bones and cartilage.

   Following cells come into play in the pathophysiology of RA:
   a. CD4 T cells
   b. Mononuclear cells
   c. Phagocytes
   d. Fibroblasts
   e. Osteoclast
   f. Neutrophils

   B cells produce different autoantibodies.

   Following inflammatory mediators are involved in pathophysiology of RA:
   a. TNF-α
   b. IL-6, IL-1, IL-8
   c. Transforming growth factor beta (TGF-β)

d. Fibroblast growth factor (FGF)
e. Platelet-derived growth factor (PDGF)

Ultimately inflammation and exuberant proliferation of synovium with destroys various tissues such as bones, cartilage, tendon, ligaments, bursa, and blood vessels.

Classification of 2010 ACR-EULAR (American College of Rheumatology/European League Against Rheumatism) classification criteria for rheumatoid arthritis:

Target populations: Patents who have at least one joint with definite clinical synovitis. Patient with synovitis not better explained by another disease.		
Classification of rheumatoid arthritis: **A score of ≥6/10 is needed for classification of a patient as having definite rheumatoid arthritis.**		
	Criteria	**Score**
Joint involvement		
Large joint	1	0
Large joints	2–10	1
Small joints (with or without large joint involvement)	1–3	2
Small joints (with or without large joint involvement)	4–10	3
Joints with at least one small joint	>10	5
Serology (at least one test result is needed for classification)		
Rheumatoid factor and ACPA	Both negative	0
Rheumatoid factor and ACPA	Both are low positive	2
Rheumatoid factor and ACPA	Both are high positive	3
Acute phase reactant (at least one test result is needed for classification)		
C-reactive protein (CRP) and erythrocyte sedimentation rate (ESR)	Both are normal	0
CRP and ESR	Abnormal CRP Normal ESR	1
Duration of symptoms		
<6 weeks		0
>6 weeks		1

Articular manifestations:

A. General symptoms:
   a. Morning stiffness: To start with it will persist for >1 hour which ultimately extends to persist throughout the day.
   b. Stiffness following prolonged rest: Typical feature of inflammatory arthritis
   c. Limitation of joint movement: Stiffness is associated with swelling and movement limitation which ultimately terminates into complete immobility.
   d. Squeezing sign, i.e., tenderness following squeezing the hand—earliest indicator of RA.
   e. In late phase joint deformity with or without pain

B. Hands:
   a. In RA, metacarpophalangeal (MCP) joints and proximal interphalangeal (PIP) joints are involved but distal interphalangeal joints are not involved like psoriatic arthritis or osteoarthritis.
   b. In wrist involvement, there is flexion and extension movement at the wrist due to involvement of median nerve.
   c. There are several deformities of hand:
      1. Ulnar drifting of fingers at MCP joints characterized by drifting of fingers away from the thumb—it is unique and earliest deformity in RA.
      2. Boutonnière deformity characterized by flexion at PIP joints, hyperextension at distal phalangeal, and MCP joints
      3. Swan neck deformity characterized by hyperextension at PIP joint and flexion at distal interphalangeal joints
      4. Millet finger characterized by flexion at distal interphalangeal joints

C. Foot:
   a. Swelling of foot and stiffness at the ankles
   b. Lateral deviation of great toe that may override the second toe—it is most common deformity.
   c. Reduction in the ball of the toes
   d. Flattening and collapse of the arch of the foot and unstable ankles
   e. Hammer toe
   f. Flexion deformity at PIP joints

D. Larger joints:
   a. Knee, elbow, hip, and shoulder joint are involved.
   b. Deformities and dislocation of the articular surfaces leading to fibrous and bony ankyloses.
   c. Common dislocation of radioulnar joints at proximal annular point leading to early restriction of pronation and supination.

E. Back and spine:
   a. Atlantoaxial joint is involved, characterized by:
      1. Neck pain at the back of the neck
      2. Feeling of being pushed while walking
      3. Tingling sensation across the neck radiating down the neck
      4. Pain in the back
F. Other musculoskeletal involvement:
   a. Tendinitis: Vague pain at the insertion of tendon.
   b. Bursitis characterized by pain in the wrist and elbow.

Extra-articular manifestations:

A. Muscle: Degeneration of muscles occurs in the following five forms:
   a. Type II fiber atrophy
   b. Neuropathy and degeneration
   c. Steroid-induced myopathy
   d. Overlap myositis
   e. Chronic myopathy
B. Skin: Following types of skin manifestations are evidenced:
   a. Rheumatoid nodules in 30% of patients
   b. Skin atrophy
   c. Palmar erythema
   d. Raynaud's phenomenon
   e. Lesions related to vasculitis:
      1. Palpable purpura
      2. Digital infarct
      3. Nail-fold thrombi
      4. Livedo reticularis
      5. Pyoderma gangrenosum
C. Fistula connection: It will connect skin to joints and bursa.
D. Eye manifestation:
   a. Keratoconjunctivitis sicca—mainly associated with Sjögren's syndrome
   b. Scleritis—it may be localized, generalized, or necrotizing condition. It will produce severe pain and dark red discoloration.
   c. Episcleritis
   d. Secondary cataract
   e. Keratitis leading loss of vision
   f. Granulomatous resorption leading to formation of scleromalacia perforans
E. Hematological abnormalities:
   a. Normocytic normochromic anemia or anemia of chronic disease is found in 35% of patients.
   b. Eosinophilia
   c. Thrombocytosis
F. Vasculitis:
   a. Splinter hemorrhage
   b. Digital gangrene
   c. Cutaneous ulceration
   d. Peripheral neuropathy
   e. Palpable purpura
   f. Arteritis of viscera such as kidneys, lungs, heart, liver, spleen, pancreas, and testes
G. Neurovascular diseases:
   a. Severe distal sensory or motor neuropathy—common clinical presentation
   b. Rheumatoid pachymeningitis
   c. Autonomic nervous disturbances
   d. Compressive neuropathy
H. Renal involvement:
   a. Papillary necrosis due to salicylate and phenacetin ingestion
   b. Membranous nephropathy due to ingestion of gold and penicillamine
I. Pulmonary involvement:
   a. Pleural disease:
      1. Pleurisy
      2. Pleural effusion
      3. Pleural fibrosis
   b. Interstitial fibrosis of lung:
      1. Presence of diffuse dry rales without cough
      2. Breathlessness—but it may not be present due to limited mobility.
      3. X-ray demonstrates diffuse, reticulonodular shadow in both the lungs
      4. High-resolution computed tomography (HRCT) and pulmonary function tests confirm the diagnosis
   c. Nodular lung disease: It may be single or multiple and may cavitate.
   d. Bronchiolitis: In this disease, proteineous exudates in bronchioles produce respiratory insufficiency and death.
   e. Pulmonary hypertension
   f. Small airway diseases

J. Cardiac involvement:
   a. Pericardial involvement:
      1. Pericardial effusion
      2. Cardiac tamponade
      3. Constrictive pericarditis
   b. Granulomatous or interstitial myocarditis
   c. Endocardial involvement:
      1. Mitral regurgitation
      2. Aortic regurgitation.
   d. Conduction defect like atrioventricular block
   e. Amyloidosis producing heart block
   f. Myocardial infarction due to coronary arteritis

K. Psychiatric manifestations:
   a. Depression
   b. Anxiety
   c. Obsessive-compulsive disorders

Investigations

Laboratory parameters can be divided into three groups:

A. Markers of inflammation:
   a. C-reactive protein (CRP)—elevated
   b. Erythrocyte sedimentation rate (ESR)—elevated

B. Hematological parameters:
   a. Normochromic normocytic anemia
   b. If hypochromic—suggests blood loss from gastrointestinal tract due to nonsteroidal anti-inflammatory drugs (NSAIDs) use.
   c. Thrombocytosis—disease activity. If thrombocytopenia—suggests Felty's syndrome
   d. Leukocytosis—it may occur. If leukopenia—it suggests Felty's syndrome or as a consequence of therapy.

C. Immunological parameter:
   a. Rheumatoid factor: It can present in the following diseases:
      1. RA—it is not specific for this disease
      2. Other connective tissue diseases
      3. Infections
      4. Normal people
   b. Anti-CCP antibody: ACCP antibody positive RA is usually erosive. Its sensitivity and specificity is more than rheumatoid factor test.

Radiological features:

A. X-ray of involved bones and joints: Erosions, deformities of foot, hand bones, and joints.

B. Ultrasonography of joints to see any evidence of effusion

Instruments used for disease activity:

	Threshold for disease activity			
Instruments	**Remission**	**Low**	**Moderate**	**High**
Disease activity score in 28 joints (DAS28)	<2.6	≥2.6 to <3.2	≥3.2–5.1	>5.1
Simplified disease activity index (SDAI)	≥3.3	>3.3 to 11	>11 to ≤26	>26
Clinical disease activity index (CDAI)	≤2.8	>2.8–10	10–22	>22
Patient activity scale (PAS II)	<0.25	0.26–3.7	≥3.71–8	>8

Stages of Rheumatoid Arthritis According to ACR

A. *Stage 1*: No destructive changes in X-ray

B. *Stage 2*: Presence of X-ray evidence of periarticular osteoporosis, subchondral destruction of bone but no deformity of joint will be present.

C. *Stage 3*: X-ray evidence of destruction of bone and cartilage in addition to joint deformity and Periarticular osteoporosis.

D. *Stage 4*: Presence of fibrous or bony ankylosis plus stage 3 features.

Treatment

Pretherapy evaluation: It includes:

A. Staging of the disease—whether early, established, or long-standing disease

B. Assessing disease activity, functional capacity, physical capacity, quality of life, or radiological changes.

C. Target therapy determination.

Several developments in the treatment of RA have changed the therapeutic landscape in RA.

A. First choice of treatment in RA is methotrexate as initial drug of choice

B. New highly efficacious biologicals can be used alone or associated with methotrexate.

C. Proven superiority of DMARDs over methotrexate alone.

Pharmacotherapy:

The cornerstones of therapy are:

A. NSAIDs: Its anti-inflammatory activity is nonselective inhibition of cyclooxygenase-1 and 2 and analgesic activity. But it is not used as a core therapy of RA because of their side effects such as gastritis and nephrotoxicity.

B. Glucocorticoids: It can control the disease activity in several ways:

a. It can be administered in low-to-moderate doses to control the disease activity before the achievement of full effective dose.

b. It can be administered as 1–2 weeks pulse dose for the management of acute flare of the disease with dose and duration which can be guided by severity of exacerbation.

Chronic administration of low-dose steroid can control the disease activity according to several studies, but there is high risk of osteoporosis and other long-term complications. But high dose of steroid is necessary for the treatment of extra-articular manifestations of RA like interstitial lung disease.

If the patient complain of inflammation in one or two joints, intra-articular injection of intermediate-acting glucocorticoids like triamcinolone acetonide to control inflammation rapidly.

In case of osteoporosis:

a. Treatment with bisphosphonates should be the primary prevention of choice, which is based on the following factors:

1. Total dose of prednisolone
2. Length of treatment
3. Gender
4. Race
5. Bone density

b. Teriparatide

c. Denosumab

Indication of steroids:

a. Act as bridging therapy to tide over the time required, i.e., <6 months for the DMARDs to act.

b. High-dose pulse therapy to treat flares

c. Systemic complication of RA

d. Intra-articular injection of steroid in case of persistent synovitis

C. DMARDs: These drugs have their ability to slow and prevent structural progression of rheumatoid arthritis. It has been categorized into the following types:

a. Conventional synthetic DMARDs:

1. Methotrexate: It is the DMARD of choice. It stimulates release of adenosine from the cells which leads to its anti-inflammatory effect.
2. Leflunomide: It inhibits pyrimidine synthesis.
3. Sulfasalazine: It will reduce the progression of the disease.
4. Hydroxychloroquine: It delays the progression of the disease activity; hence, it is not considered as DMARDs. Hence, it can be given in very mild disease or as an adjunct to other DMARDs.
5. Gold salts
6. Minocycline
7. Penicillamine

b. Biological originator DMARDs: The drugs are the following:

1. TNF inhibitors:
   - Infliximab
   - Etanercept
   - Golimumab
   - Adalimumab
   - Certolizumab pegol
2. Anti-CD20 antibody: Rituximab
3. Anti-IL-6 receptor antibody: Tocilizumab
4. Anti-IL-1 antibody: Anakinra
5. Costimulation blocker: Abatacept

c. Targeted synthetic DMARDs:

1. Janus kinase inhibitors: Tofacitinib

d. Biosimilar DMARDs: It is therapeutic product which is similar in quality, safety, and efficacy.

1. Rituximab: Mabtas
2. Adalimumab: Adalirel
3. Etanercept: Intacept
4. Infliximab: Infimab

Advantages of biologics:

a. It acts on specific pathologic process

b. It acts faster to control the disease

c. It is effective when other DMARDs fail to act

d. It will prevent or retard the progression of the disease

Disadvantages of biologic:

a. It is costly

b. There is risk of infection

c. Parenteral route of administration

d. Unknown long-term adverse effect

Anti-TNF therapy

All anti-TNF-α therapy should be avoided in:

a. Infections

b. History of hypersensitivity reaction

Contraindications:

- **a.** Chronic hepatitis B
- **b.** Class III/IV congestive heart failure

Risk:

- **a.** Bacterial and fungal infections
- **b.** Reactivation of latent tuberculosis, hence, Mantoux test has to be done prior to start of therapy.

Infliximab:

- **a.** It is chimeric anti-TNF-α monoclonal antibody with predominant human amino acid sequences.
- **b.** It is used in giant cell arteritis, ankylosing spondylitis (AS) and polymyalgia rheumatic.
- **c.** Dose is 0.3 mg/kg at 0, 2, and 6 weeks followed by every 8 weekly.
- **d.** 100 mg intravenous methylprednisolone has to be given to prevent anaphylaxis.
- **e.** To rule out tuberculosis prior Mantoux test and chest radiograph has to be done to rule out tuberculosis.
- **f.** Before each dose disease activity score by DAS28 and functional activity score questionnaire has to be assessed and to compare with previous results.
- **g.** In patients being treated by this drug develop anti-infliximab antibody, but concomitant administration of methotrexate can reduce the formation

Etanercept:

- **a.** It is genetically engineered fusion protein—it has two identical chains of recombinant extracellular human TNF-receptor p75 monomer which is fused with Fc receptor domain of human IgG1.
- **b.** It will bind to TNF lymphotoxin-α and inhibits their activity.
- **c.** Dose is 25 mg subcutaneously twice weekly or 50 mg once weekly.
- **d.** It has minimal toxicity mainly in adult who does not respond to other DMARDs.
- **e.** It is effective in AS and psoriatic arthritis.

B cell Targeted Therapy

As B cells play a crucial role in the pathophysiology of rheumatoid arthritis through the following mechanisms:

- **A.** Autoantibody production
- **B.** Secretion of proinflammatory cytokines

Ectopic germinal center in the synovial tissue.

Adalimumab:

- **a.** It is recombinant fully humanized IgG1 monoclonal antibody.
- **b.** It binds typically to TNF-α.
- **c.** Dose is 40 mg subcutaneously weekly or 25 mg biweekly.

Golimumab:

- **a.** It is human G1 monoclonal antibody specific for TNF.
- **b.** It will bind to soluble and transmembrane forms of TNF thereby prevent TNF to bind to its receptors as a result inhibits the biological activity of TNF.
- **c.** Dose is 50 mg subcutaneously monthly.

Certolizumab:

- **a.** Its actions:
  1. It reduces signs and symptoms of the disease
  2. It reduces the radiological score in rheumatoid arthritis
- **b.** Dose is 400 mg subcutaneously at 0, 2, and 4 weeks then 200 mg every other week.

Other drugs are the following:

Drug	Dose	Toxicities	Initial evaluation	Monitoring
Abatacept	<60 kg: 500 mg 60–100 kg: 750 mg >100 kg: 1 g intravenously at 0, 2, and 4 weeks followed by every 4 weeks	• Increased risk of viral, bacterial infections • Headache • Nausea	Mantoux test	Reaction to infusion reaction
Anakinra	100 mg subcutaneously	• Increased risk of viral and bacterial infection • Reactivation of latent tuberculosis • Neutropenia • Headache • Reaction to injection sites	Mantoux test	Reaction to infusion reaction

Continued

Continued

Drug	Dose	Toxicities	Initial evaluation	Monitoring
Rituximab	1 g for 2 days at 0 and 14th, may be repeated at every 24 weeks IV infusion of methylprednisolone to prevent infusion reaction	• Increased risk of viral and bacterial infection • Reactivation of latent tuberculosis. • Neutropenia • Headache • Reaction to injection sites • Hepatitis B reactivation • Rash • Fever	Viral hepatitis panel Complete blood count	At regular interval complete blood count
Tocilizumab	4–8 mg/kg monthly	• Increased risk of infection • Reaction to infusion • Cytopenia • Deranged liver function test • Dyslipidemia	Mantoux test	At regular interval: • Liver function test • Complete blood count • Lipid profile
Tofacitinib	Orally 5 mg twice daily Or 11 mg orally daily	• Risk of infection • Dyslipidemia • Cytopenia • Elevation of liver function test • Headache • Diarrhea • Nasopharyngitis	Mantoux test	At regular interval: • Liver function test • Complete blood count • Lipid profile
Following targeted B cell directed therapies under research: • Ocrelizumab – humanized anti-CD20 monoclonal antibody • Obinutuzumab – glycoengineered anti-CD20 antibody • Belimumab – anti-B cell activating factor monoclonal antibody most commonly used in SLE • Atacicept – it targets both B cell activating factor as well as a proliferating inducing ligand				

According to ACR and EULAR Treatment Guidelines

A. According to ACR, patient with early rheumatoid arthritis not under disease modifying antirheumatic drug (DMARD) should start DMARD regardless the disease activity level.

B. In case of early with low disease activity, methotrexate is the preferred drug.

C. If the patient is intolerant to methotrexate or has contraindication to this drug, leflunomide or sulfasalazine should be started.

D. If the DMARD cannot control the disease activity (regardless the concomitant use of steroid), methotrexate should be discontinued or continued at this point. Additional therapy is either tumor necrosis factor inhibitor or nontumor necrosis factor inhibitor biologic agent should be given along with DMARD.

E. If the patient is having DMARD naïve established rheumatoid arthritis, in that case methotrexate should be the drug of initial choice regardless the disease activity level.

F. Patient having established rheumatoid arthritis uncontrolled by DMARD (regardless the concomitant steroid use), dual DMARD or TNF-α inhibitor = or non-TNF biologic agents or tofacitinib should be of choice.

G. If the disease activity is still high and the patient on TNF inhibitor monotherapy, in that case DMARD therapy should be started in addition to TNF-inhibitor.

H. If the disease activity is still high and the patient on TNF inhibitor monotherapy, treatment should be switched to non-TNF inhibitor biologic agents with or without methotrexate.

I. If the disease activity is still high and the patient on TNF inhibitor and non-TNF inhibitor, another non-TNF inhibitor should be tried before starting tofacitinib.

J. If the all trial fail, in that case tofacitinib should be started.

K. The high disease activity despite the above all treatment, short term low dose glucocorticoid should be given along with the previous treatment.

L. In case congestive cardiac failure, TNF inhibitor should be avoided.

Differential Diagnosis Bilateral Small Joint Arthritis

A. Osteoarthritis
B. Psoriatic arthritis
C. SLE
D. Sjögren's syndrome
E. Polymyalgia rheumatica
F. Chronic gouty arthritis
G. Calcium pyrophosphate deposition disease

Q2. Describe clinical features, diagnosis, and management of gouty arthritis.
DNBIIIB/DEC2013 (10)

Enumerate the causes of Hyperuricemia. Clinical features and management of gouty arthritis.
DNB 2018 (10)

ANSWER

Causes of Hyperuricemia

A. *Overproduction of uric acid*:
   a. *Purine rich diet*:
      1. Alcohol
      2. Beef
      3. Lamb
      4. Turkey
      5. Shellfish
   b. Fructose as this is metabolized in the liver through the aldolase reductase pathway to uric acid like full sugar containing soda, high fructose corn syrup
   c. Errors in purine metabolism like hypoxanthine-guanine phosphoribosyl transferase.
   d. High cell turn over in different malignancies

B. *Decreased uric acid secretion*:
   a. Acute or chronic kidney disease
   b. Metabolic acidosis
   c. Medications
   d. Toxins
   e. Hypovolemia
   f. Sarcoidosis
   g. Hyperparathyroidism

C. Diuretic induced:
   a. Thiazide
   b. Loop diuretics
   c. ACE inhibitor
   d. ARBs
   e. Allopurinol

Definition

Gouty arthritis is characterized by episodic acute arthritis or chronic arthritis as a result of deposition of monosodium urate crystals in the joints or connective tissue along with risk of deposition in the renal interstitium or presence of uric acid nephrolithiasis.

Clinical Pictures

A. Acute arthritis:
   a. It is the earliest clinical manifestation, joint affected is usually metatarsophalangeal joint of the great toe, but tarsal joints, knee or ankle joints may be involved.
   b. Usually, it is monoarticular to start with, but polyarticular manifestations may occur in the subsequent episode.
   c. In advanced disease or in elderly finger joints are involved.
   d. In some cases, inflammation of Heberden's node or Bouchard's node may be the first manifestation.
   e. First episode usually starts at night with severe pain in the joint, joints become swollen, warm, and tender. This attack will subside within 3–10 days spontaneously without any residual symptom until the next episode.
   f. Following factors will precipitate gouty arthritis:
      1. Dietary excess
      2. Trauma
      3. Surgery
      4. Ingestion of excess ethanol
      5. Hypouricemic therapy
      6. Any serious medical illness like myocardial infarction

B. Chronic arthritis:
   a. After repeated attack of acute monoarticular or polyarticular gout a significant proportion of

patients present with chronic gouty arthritis, it may be asymmetrical.

b. Sometimes chronic gouty arthritis may be the only manifestation.

c. Sometimes, this disease may present as tophaceous deposits without synovitis.

d. Affected women are usually:

1. Elderly
2. Menopause
3. Associated with osteoarthritis and arterial hypertension leading to mild renal insufficiency. But premenopausal women in presence of renal insufficiency or decreased urate clearance may develop gouty arthritis.

Risk Factors for Flares

A. More than 65 years of age having incidence of three or more flares.
B. Male gender
C. Use of diuretics
D. Presence of ≥3 comorbidities
E. Failure to attend serum uric acid goal
F. No change in the dose of initial urate-lowering therapy
G. Nonadherence to urate-lowering therapy

Complications of Gout

A. Severe degenerative arthritis
B. Severe infections
C. Uric acid nephropathy
D. Increased susceptibility to infection
E. Urate nephropathy
F. Renal stone
G. Impingement of spinal cord or nerves
H. Fractures of joint with tophaceous gout

Laboratory Diagnosis

A. Needle aspiration from the acutely or chronically involved joint mainly first metatarsophalangeal joint:

a. Physical color of the fluid appears cloudy due to increased number of leukocytes. But there is large number of crystals in the fluid; the fluid becomes thick, chalky.

b. Analysis of synovial fluid in acute gouty attack demonstrates needle-shaped monosodium urate crystals present both intracellularly and extracellularly.

c. With compensated polarized light crystals will present as brightly birefringent with negative elongation.

d. Synovial leukocyte count is 2,000–60,000/cc.

e. Culture of the synovial fluid to exclude septic arthritis

B. Serum uric acid: Usually there is hyperuricemia in 95% of patients with acute arthritis, but serum uric acid may be normal or low in acute attack due to:

a. Inflammatory cytokines may be uricosuric

b. Effective initiation of hypouricosuric therapy can precipitate the disease.

C. Hematology:

a. Raised ESR

b. Leukocytosis with leftward shift

D. Blood biochemistry:

a. Serum creatinine

b. Serum urea

c. Liver function test

d. Lipid profile

E. 24 hours urine collection for uric acid can assess:

a. Risk of stone formation

b. Overproduction or underproduction of uric acid

c. Whether to use uricosuric therapy or not

If the value is >800 mg/24 hours on regular diet—overproduction of purine is considered.

F. X-ray of the joint demonstrates:

a. Erosions with overhanging edges—pathognomonic of gout, it is distributed asymmetrically along the joints and strong predilection for distal joints.

b. Sclerotic border sometimes called punched out border

c. Absence of periarticular osteopenia

d. Maintenance of joint space

e. Location outside the joint capsule

G. Ultrasonographic findings are the following:

a. Double-contour sign—consists of hyperechoic irregular line of monosodium urate crystals present on the surface of the articular cartilage overlying hyperechoic bony contour

b. Wet clumps of sugar—suggesting presence of hyperechoic or hypoechoic tophaceous material surrounded by anechoic rim

c. Bony erosions just adjacent to tophaceous deposits

H. Dual-energy computed tomography demonstrates specific features suggestive of presence of crystals.

Treatment

Goals of the treatment are:

A. Treatment of acute attack

B. Provision of prophylaxis to prevent acute flare

C. Excess crystals should be lowered to prevent acute flare of arthritis.

D. Prevention of deposition of urate crystals

Asymptomatic hyperuricemia should not be treated in spite of ultrasonographic demonstration of deposition of urate crystals in the soft tissue.

Patients with uric acid level of >11 mg/dL with overexcretion of uric acids should be monitored regularly as there is high chance of developing renal stones.

Treatment targets are the following:

A. Serum uric acid level <6 or <5 mg/dL in patients with gouty arthritis or gouty tophi

B. Reduction in number and size of the tophi

C. Reduction of pain

D. Absence of attack

Monitoring should be done every 3–6 months whether the patient reaches the target or not.

Drugs used in acute gouty arthritis are:

A. NSAIDs are:

- **a.** Indomethacin 50 mg thrice daily
- **b.** Naproxen 500 mg twice daily
- **c.** Ibuprofen 800 mg thrice daily
- **d.** Diclofenac 50 mg thrice daily
- **e.** Celecoxib 800 mg stat followed by 400 mg 12 hours later followed by 400 mg twice daily

B. Colchicine: It should be started within 12–24 hours of start of symptoms, but incipient attack can be aborted by low dose of colchicine. Dose schedule for acute flare is:

- **a.** Initial dose of 1.2 mg followed by 0.6 mg 1 hour later—so total dose is 1.8 mg on the first day.
- **b.** 0.6 mg three times daily on the first day of treatment
- **c.** Once the significant response is achieved, treatment should be continued as 0.6 mg twice daily.

Adverse effect is abdominal cramping and loose motion. In that case drug should be stopped temporarily along with the symptomatic treatment for diarrhea.

C. Glucocorticoids: It can be given intramuscularly or orally or intra-articular injection.

- **a.** Initial dose is 30–50 mg/day for 2–3 days then gradually tapered over 2–3 weeks or with the resolution of the attack. If it is continued for >3 weeks, antiosteoporosis treatment should be initiated.
- **b.** Intra-articular injection of triamcinolone acetonide 20–40 mg or methylprednisolone 25–40 mg.

D. Anakinra: It is used to inhibit the of inflammasome and IL-1β receptor, it is safe and effective.

E. Urate-lowering therapy:

It is indicated where hyperuricemia cannot be corrected by simple means like low-purine diet, control of body weight, increased intake of liquid, limited use of alcohol, and decreased intake of fructose containing fruits. It should also be started in patients with chronic gouty arthritis and uric acid stones.

Decisions for starting hypouricemic therapy depend upon the following:

- **a.** Number of acute attacks
- **b.** Serum uric acid
- **c.** Patient's willingness to start the therapy
- **d.** Presence of uric acid stones

Drugs are the following:

- **a.** Probenecid:
  1. It is used in patients with good renal function and low uric acid excreter having <600 mg/day of uric acid in urine.
  2. Dose is 250 mg/day which can be gradually increased up to 3 g/day to achieve the target serum uric acid of <6 mg/mL.
  3. It is not effective when the creatinine level is >2 mg/dL.
- **b.** Allopurinol:
  1. It is xanthine oxidase inhibitor; hence, it will lower the uric acid production.
  2. Dose is to start with 100 mg daily to be taken in the morning which can be increased up to 800 mg/day.
  3. In case of chronic kidney disease with creatinine clearance of 10 mL/minute, dose should be 100 mg daily, but the target should be <6 mg/dL.
  4. Toxicity of this drug can be found in the following conditions:

- Concomitant use of thiazide diuretics
- Patient allergic to penicillin and ampicillin
- Asian population expressing HLA-B*58:01

5. Toxicities are:
   - Toxic epidermal necrolysis
   - Granulomatous hepatitis
   - Bone marrow suppression
   - Renal failure

c. Febuxostat:
   1. It is xanthine oxidase inhibitor.
   2. It can be started in patients allergic to allopurinol.
   3. Dose is 40–80 mg daily, this drug do not require dose adjustment in mild-to-moderate renal disease.

d. Pegloticase:
   1. It is pegylated uricase, can be given who cannot tolerate other drugs.
   2. Dose is 8 mg intravenously every 2 weeks—it can lower the uric acid level dramatically.

In resistant case of acute arthritis:

A. More prolonged course of NSAIDs therapy is required for some patients with persistent symptoms.

B. If there is no improvement with colchicine therapy after few days, in that case switching to NSAIDs. But if there is contraindication to the use of NSAIDs, glucocorticoid should be started.

Q3. Diagnosis and treatment of ankylosing spondylitis.

DNBIIIB/JUN2016 (10)

Clinical pictures and radiographic findings in a case of ankylosing spondylitis.

DNB 2018 (6)

Diagnosis and management of ankylosing spondylosis.

WBUHS, 2020 (10)

ANSWER

Diagnosis of ankylosing spondylitis includes clinical features and investigations specific for that disease.

Clinical Features

A. Age of onset is late adolescence or early childhood at an age of mid 20s. In 5% patient age of onset is after 40 years.

B. Initial symptoms are insidious onset dull aching pain in the lower lumbar or gluteal region with morning stiffness at low back which improves with activity and aggravates with period of inactivity. But within few months this pain becomes persistent and bilateral, but nocturnal low back pain will bound the patient to move around at night.

C. There is associated hip and shoulder joint (root joint) arthritis, which are considered as axial involvement, former may be present in 25–35% of patients and later occurs rarely.

D. Arthritis of the peripheral joints is asymmetric but occurs at any point of the disease. Neck pain with stiffness due to cervical spine involvement may be the late manifestation.

E. In juvenile spondyloarthritis, peripheral arthritis along with enthesitis predominates followed by features of axial involvement in late adolescence.

On physical examination:

A. Spinal mobility:
   a. Loss of spinal mobility
   b. Limitation of anterior and lateral flexion and extension of lumbar spine
   c. Limitation of chest expansion

   This limitation is out of proportion of the degree of bony ankyloses and it is due to muscle spasm as a result of pain and inflammation around the joints.

B. Common sites of bony tenderness are:
   a. Costochondral junctions
   b. Spinous processes
   c. Greater trochanters
   d. Iliac crests
   e. Ischial tuberosities
   f. Tibial tubercles

C. Limitation of mobility is measured modified Schober test as it can measure the forward flexion.
   a. Patient is asked to stand erect with heels together. Two marks are made in the following areas:
      1. At the lumbosacral junction on the spine which is marked by a horizontal line joining two posterosuperior iliac spines.
      2. Another mark at 10 cm above the first point.

b. Now patient is asked to bend forward maximally with knee fully extended.

c. If the distance will increase by ≥5 cm—it suggests normal mobility. If the distance is <4 cm—it suggests decreased mobility.

D. Chest expansion can be measured by the following methods:

a. Patient is asked to keep his hand resting on or behind his head.

b. Patient is asked to take maximal inspiration and hold his breath, measurement is taken.

c. Then patient is asked to take maximal deep expiration and hold his breath, measurement is taken.

d. In case male measurement is taken at the level of 4th intercostal space and in case of females just below the breast.

e. Normal expansion of chest is ≥5 cm. If it is below—it suggests restriction of mobility.

E. During maximal lateral bending, distance that the patient's middle finger travels down the leg normally >10 cm. Below this measurement suggests limitation of lateral bending.

F. In case of hip or shoulder involvement, there is limitation of movement of this joint. But in milder cases physical findings are subtle.

G. Tragus to wall distance

H. Occiput to wall distance

I. Intermalleolar distance:

a. In standing position, patient is asked to separate his leg as far as possible and distance in between the medial malleoli is measured.

b. In lying down position, patient is asked to separate the legs as far as possible with knee straight and toes pointing upward, then distance between the two medial malleoli is measured.

Extra-articular manifestations:

A. Eye:

a. Acute anterior uveitis—it is unilateral, causing photophobia, pain along with increased lacrimation, spreading to opposite eye.

b. Cataract

c. Secondary glaucoma

B. Gastrointestinal:

a. Inflammation of colon and ileum, in 5–10% case frank inflammatory bowel disease (IBD) may occur.

C. Cardiovascular:

a. Aortic insufficiency

b. Aortitis

c. Third-degree heart block may or may not occur with aortic insufficiency

d. Cardiomyopathy

e. Pericarditis

D. Respiratory system:

a. Upper lobe fibrosis

b. Bronchiolitis obliterans

E. Genitourinary tract: Urethritis

F. Renal involvement:

a. Immunoglobulin A (IgA) nephropathy

b. Mesangioproliferative glomerulonephritis

c. NSAIDs nephropathy

d. Secondary amyloidosis

G. Neurological:

a. Cauda equina syndrome

b. Spinal canal stenosis

H. Dermatological:

a. Psoriasis

b. SAPHO syndrome characterized by acne fulminans, hidradenitis suppurativa

Course of ankylosing spondylitis:

A. It has wide spectrum of distribution, at its one end, there is patient with mild stiffness with normal radiograph and its other end having totally disabled patient with fused spine, bilateral hip, and peripheral arthritis and extra-articular manifestations.

B. Pain usually persistent early in the disease, but as the disease progresses pain may be intermittent with alternating exacerbations.

C. In case of untreated patient, following types of progression will occur:

a. Spondylitis progresses to syndesmophyte formation.

b. Characteristic changes in the posture of the patient

c. Obliteration of lumbar lordosis

d. Atrophy of the buttock

e. Accentuation of thoracic kyphosis

f. Forward stoop of the neck

g. Flexure contracture at the hip with compensated knee flexion

D. Disease progression can be monitored by:
 a. Spinal flexion
 b. Chest expansion
 c. Occiput to wall distance

E. Factors most predictive of radiographic progression are the following:
 a. Presence of existing syndesmophytes
 b. High inflammatory markers
 c. Smoking

F. In adolescence, AS with early involvement of hip carries worse prognosis.

G. In case of women, AS progresses more slowly toward total ankyloses, but prevalence of isolated hip and peripheral arthritis is increased.

H. In case of pregnancy, AS may be improved or remains as it is or in one-third of pregnant patients.

Complications

A. Most serious complication is fracture to rigid osteoporotic spine with minor trauma affecting lower cervical spine mainly. Fractured spine may be displaced to produce spinal cord injury.

B. Fracture through discovertebral junction along with adjacent neural arch most commonly occurs in thoracolumbar spine—it is known as pseudoarthrosis—it may be responsible for localized persistent pain with neurological dysfunction.

C. Wedging of the thoracic vertebrae. Leading to accentuation of kyphosis.

Investigations

A. Laboratory findings:
 a. Hematological tests:
  1. Anemia—mild
  2. ESR—may be raised
  3. Alkaline phosphatase—increased in case of severe disease
 b. Serology:
  1. Rheumatoid factor, anti-CCP, antinuclear antibody (ANA) are with in normal limit unless specific disease is coexistent.
  2. Circulating CD8+ cells are low
  3. Serum matrix metalloproteinase will correlate with activity of the disease.
 c. HLA-B27 is positive in 75–90% of patients.
 d. Synovial fluid demonstrates the features of nonspecific inflammation
 e. Pulmonary function test: Decreased vital capacity, decreased ratio of forced expiratory volume in one second/forced vital capacity (FEV1/FVC)

B. Radiological features:
 a. Plain radiograph: It can demonstrate changes in the following areas of axial skeleton:
  1. Sacroiliac joints
  2. Discovertebral joints
  3. Costotransverse joints

 Findings are the following:
 a. Earliest change is sacroiliitis characterized by blurring of the cortical margins of the subchondral bone leading to bony erosions and sclerosis.
 b. Erosion progresses to "pseudowidening" of the joint space
 c. This is followed by fibrosis and ankyloses—thus joints become obliterated.
 d. In case of lumbar spine:
  1. Loss of lordosis
  2. Osteitis of the anterior corners of the vertebral bodies with subsequent erosion that lead to squatting or barreling of the vertebral bodies.
  3. Formation of syndesmophytes producing bony bridges anteriorly and laterally in the successive vertebral bodies.

 New York criteria for sacroiliitis (mean score of both sacroiliac joints) is as follows:
  1. Grade 0: Normal
  2. Grade 1: Suspicious
  3. Grade 2: Minimal abnormality—small localized areas of erosions with sclerosis and alteration of joint space width.
  4. Grade 3: Unequivocal abnormality—advanced sacroiliitis having the following features:
   - Erosions
   - Sclerosis
   - Widening
   - Narrowing or partial ankyloses
  5. Total ankyloses

 b. MRI features of acute sacroiliitis are:
  1. Edema of bone marrow
  2. Synovitis
  3. Enthesitis
  4. Capsulitis

c. MRI features of chronic sacroiliitis:
   1. Subchondral sclerosis
   2. Erosions
   3. Replacement of fatty marrow
   4. Bony ankyloses

Bath ankylosing spondylitis radiographic index for hips (BASRI-hips):

a. 0—normal
b. 1—suspicious (focal joint space narrowing)
c. 2—mild (circumferential joint space narrowing >2 mm)
d. 3—moderate (circumferential joint space narrowing 2 mm or bone-to-bone apposition of ≤2 cm)
e. 4—severe (bone-to-bone apposition of ≥2 cm)
f. Grade should be increased by 1 or 2 if following changes in the bone is present:
   1. Erosion
   2. Osteophytes
   3. Protrusion

BASRI-spine (for lumbar spine anteroposterior and lateral views are scored, views with highest score are taken, and for cervical spine lateral view is scored):

a. 0—normal
b. 1—suspicious (no definite change)
c. 2—mild (any number of erosions, squaring or sclerosis with or without syndesmophytes, on ≤2 vertebrae)
d. 3—moderate (syndesmophytes on more than or equal to vertebrae, with or without fusion involving two vertebrae)
e. 4—severe (fusion involving ≥3 vertebrae)

Treatment

A. First line in the pharmacologic therapy is NSAIDs. It will improve the following:
   a. Pain and tenderness of the joints
   b. The range of motion around the joints
   c. Radiological progression in patients with increased risk of progression
B. Sulfasalazine:
   a. Dose is 2–3 g/day, mainly in peripheral arthritis.
   b. It reduces pain and stiffness around the joints
   c. It is more effective in peripheral arthritis but not in spinal arthritis.
C. Methotrexate: It may provide some benefit in AS.
D. Leflunomide: It may provide some benefit in AS.
E. Thalidomide:
   a. It acts through inhibition of production of interleukin-12 and TNF-α by monocytes and macrophages thus acting as immunomodulatory and anti-inflammatory drug.
   b. It also inhibits chemotaxis of neutrophil at the site of inflammation.
   c. It will alter the density of TNF-α-induced adhesion molecules on the leukocytes.
   d. It will enhance the production of IL-4 and IL-5 by mononuclear cells.
   e. Dose is 100–300 mg/day for 6 months to 1 year.
F. Corticosteroids:
   a. Oral steroid is of little value as in this disease bone density will be lost already.
   b. Intra-articular steroid can provide relief of pain and stiffness.
   c. In the inflamed sacroiliac joint under CT scan guidance intra-articular triamcinolone can give substantial pain relief.
G. Bisphosphonates:
   a. Pamidronate is used in case of AS which is refractory to NSAIDs.
   b. Transient complication is arthralgia and myalgia.
H. Biologics:
   a. The drugs are:
      1. Infliximab:
         - It is chimeric human/mouse anti-TNF-α monoclonal antibody.
         - Dose is 5 mg/kg intravenously once followed by repeated injection 2 weeks and 6 weeks later followed by 6–8 weeks interval.
      2. Etanercept:
         - It is soluble p75 TNF-α receptor-Ig fusion protein.
         - Dose is 50 mg once weekly subcutaneous injection.
      3. Adalimumab:
         - It is human anti-TNF-α monoclonal antibody.
         - Dose is 40 mg biweekly subcutaneous injection.
      4. Golimumab:
         - It is human anti-TNF-α monoclonal antibody.
         - Dose is 50–100 mg subcutaneous injection every 4 weeks.

5. Certolizumab pegol:
   - It is humanized mouse anti-TNF-α monoclonal antibody.
   - Dose is 400 mg subcutaneous injection every 4 weeks.

b. Signs of good response: Improvement in both subjective and objective indicators of disease activity as well as function:
   1. Morning stiffness
   2. Joint pain
   3. Spinal mobility
   4. Peripheral swelling of the joints
   5. Decrease in CRP, ESR
   6. Increase in bone mineral density
   7. Improvement in the MRI features such as
      - Bone marrow edema
      - Joint effusion
      - Enthesitis

c. Best predictor of response:
   1. Younger age
   2. Disease duration
   3. Baseline inflammatory markers are higher
   4. Lower baseline functional disability

d. Adverse effects are the following:
   1. Increased risk of serious infection mainly disseminated tuberculosis. Hence prior to start, patient should be tested by tuberculin test and ≥5 mm will be suggested as positive tuberculin test. These patients should be treated with anti-tubercular drugs.
   2. Hypersensitivity reaction
   3. Reaction at the site of injection
   4. Anti-TNF-induced psoriasis
   5. Systemic lupus erythematosus (SLE)-related disease
   6. Demyelinating disease
   7. Pancytopenia
   8. Severe liver disease
   9. Congestive heart failure
   10. Hematologic malignancy

e. Contraindications are the following:
   1. Active infection
   2. Patient with high risk of infection
   3. Malignancy or premalignancy
   4. History of SLE
   5. History of multiple sclerosis

f. In case of pregnant lady:
   1. Pregnancy and breastfeeding are not contra-indication to therapy if proper measures are taken.
   2. If the fetus is exposed to anti-TNF-α therapy in utero, in that case the infants should not be immunized with live vaccines before 6 months of age.

g. Favorable response: The drug should be continued for > 12 weeks in the following conditions:
   1. If 50% reduction in bath AS disease activity index (BASDAI)
   2. If there is absolute reduction of ≥2 out of 10.

   If there is loss of response with the first TNF-α rather than primary failure, then second line of TNF-α should be introduced.

Q4. Churg–Strauss syndrome.

DNBI/JUN2011 (10)

NTR UNI of Health SC Vijayawada, Andhra, 2022 (10)

ANSWER

Definition

Eosinophilic granulomatosis with polyangiitis (EGPA) also known as Churg–Strauss syndrome is a necrotizing vasculitis involving small to medium size blood vessels characterized by the following six criteria according to American College of Rheumatology (ACR):

A. Asthma with the presence of expiratory rhonchi
B. More than 10% eosinophils in the peripheral blood
C. Paranasal sinusitis
D. Transient pulmonary infiltrate
E. Histologically proved vasculitis with extravascular eosinophils
F. Mononeuritis multiplex

Pathophysiology

A. The cause of this disease is not known but some features of autoimmunity are evident such as hypergammaglobulinemia, increased level of IgE in the blood, rheumatoid factor, and antineutrophil cytoplasmic antibody (ANCA). It may be an autoimmune or allergic reaction against drug or environmental agents.
B. It may be a rare complication of steroid-dependent asthma in whom dose of the steroid is reduced or

withdrawn after commencement of leukotriene receptor antagonist, because of the unmasking of underlying EGPA by steroid withdrawal.

C. Genetic factor HLA-DRB4 is a risk factor for the development of EBPA.

Clinical Manifestations

This disease will progress through the three different phases that may not be differentiated from each other.

A. First phase is prodromal phase—it is characterized by:
   a. Atopy
   b. New onset asthma: It occurs in 90% of patients and precedes the third phase by 8–10 years.
   c. Allergic rhinitis

B. Second phase is eosinophilic phase—it is characterized by:
   a. More than 10% of eosinophil in the peripheral blood
   b. Tissue eosinophilia as evidenced by presence of eosinophilia in the lung tissue as manifested by lung infiltrate

C. Third phase is vasculitic phase—it is characterized by:
   a. Involvement of small to medium size vessel involvement in different organs in the body.

Constitutional symptoms are: Fever, malaise, weight loss, flu-like symptoms, and myalgia.

Systematic features are the following:
Clinical features are:

A. Paranasal sinusitis which will respond to oral steroids.
B. Allergic rhinitis, it may be associated with nasal polyp.
C. Pulmonary symptoms such as
   a. Cough and hemoptysis
   b. Lung infiltrate
   c. Lung nodules
   d. Pleural effusion
   e. Alveolar hemorrhage
D. Dermatological manifestations:
   a. Palpable purpura
   b. Urticarial rash
   c. Digital ischemia
   d. Necrotic bulla
   e. Skin nodules
   f. Livedo reticularis
E. Cardiovascular features:
   a. Heart failure
   b. Pericarditis
   c. Constrictive pericarditis
   d. Myocardial infarction due to coronary artery vasculitis
   e. Deep vein thrombosis leading to pulmonary thromboembolism
   f. Hypertension
F. Gastrointestinal manifestations, the features are:
   a. Diarrhea
   b. Vomiting
   c. Abdominal pain
   d. Gastrointestinal bleeding
   e. Mesenteric vasculitis
   f. Bowel infarction with perforation of bowel
G. Peripheral neuropathy:
   a. Mononeuritis multiplex
   b. Peripheral neuropathy
H. Renal involvement:
   a. Proteinuria
   b. Microscopic hematuria
I. Central nervous system features:
   a. Stroke—ischemic or hemorrhagic type
   b. Cranial neuropathies

Investigations

A. Blood investigations:
   a. Peripheral blood:
      1. Eosinophilia
      2. Thrombocytosis
      3. Leukocytosis
   b. Raised ESR in active vasculitis
   c. CRP raised
   d. Hypoalbuminemia
   e. Specific IgE and IgG for *Aspergillus* species
   f. Sputum and bronchoalveolar lavage for *Aspergillus* species and eosinophilia.
   g. Tryptase and vitamin B12 levels
   h. Indirect immunofluorescence test for ANCA with detection of pattern of p-ANCA and c-ANCA
   i. Enzyme-linked immunosorbent assay (ELISA) test for proteinase-3 and myeloperoxidase can identify the antigen
   j. 50% patients are rheumatoid factor positive.
   k. Raised level of eosinophil cationic protein, soluble interleukin-2 receptor as well as soluble thrombomodulin.

B. Radiology:
   a. Chest X-ray demonstrates:
      1. Cavitation
      2. Pulmonary infiltrate
      3. Pleural effusion
   b. HRCT demonstrate: Cavitation, pleural effusion, and diffuse alveolar hemorrhage
   c. CT of paranasal sinuses demonstrates:
      1. Mucosal thickening
      2. Bony destruction
      3. Sinusitis
   d. Contrast-enhanced computed tomography (CECT) abdomen demonstrates:
      1. Mesenteric ischemia
      2. Dilated loop of bowel
      3. Target sign—bowel wall ischemia
      4. Comb sign—increased mesenteric vascularity
      5. Pneumatosis intestinalis
      6. Gangrene of the bowel leading to bowel wall perforation
   e. Neuroimaging includes:
      1. CECT of the head
      2. Contrast-enhanced magnetic resonance imaging (CEMRI)
   f. Fiberoptic bronchoscopy for diagnosis and taking tissue or bronchoalveolar fluid
   g. Nasal endoscopy for obtaining tissues
   h. Echocardiography
   i. Nerve conduction study
   j. Biopsy from the following areas:
      1. Lung
      2. Kidney
      3. Nerve
      4. Skin
      5. Muscles
   k. Histopathological examination demonstrates:
      1. Vessel wall infiltration with eosinophils
      2. Extravascular infiltration with eosinophils
      3. Extravascular necrotizing eosinophilic granuloma

Treatment

Treatment has been subdivided into two phases:

A. Induction of remission:
   a. Corticosteroid: To start with pulse intravenous methylprednisolone 1 g daily for 3 days followed by oral prednisolone 1 mg/kg/day to be continued till remission then it should be tapered to a dose of 5–7.5 mg/day by the end of sixth month.

      +

   b. Cyclosporine in pulse at a dose of 15 mg/kg every 2 weeks for three doses followed by every 3–6 months
   c. Rituximab, chimeric anti-CD20 monoclonal antibody—it is useful for steroid-resistant cases.
   d. Anti-IgE monoclonal antibody omalizumab can be given in patients refractory to steroids or relapse during steroid therapy.
   e. Plasma exchange: It is the procedure of choice in case of renal involvement with serum creatinine of >5.8 mg/dL or in presence of alveolar hemorrhage.
   f. In case of concomitant sepsis or infection intravenous immunoglobulin can be considered.
   g. In case of localized disease, combination of 15–25 mg/week with prednisolone in previously prescribed dose can be given.

B. Maintenance of remission: After achievement of remission to continue remission and to prevent relapse following drugs are of choice:
   a. Methotrexate
   b. Mycophenolate mofetil
   c. Azathioprine
   d. Rituximab

Q5. Clinical manifestations, laboratory and radiographic testing, and treatment of fibromyalgia.

DNBIIB/JUN2015 (10)

Diagnosis of fibromyalgia.

SNMC/MAY2013/MDII (10)

BF/MAY2011/MDIII (10)

Clinical features, diagnostic approach, and management of fibromyalgia.

DNB 2018 (10)

ANSWER

Clinical Manifestations of Fibromyalgia

A. Pain:
   a. It typically occurs on both sides of the body below and above the waist
   b. It also involves the axial skeleton such as neck, chest, and back

c. It is poorly localized, severe in intensity and difficult to ignore.
d. It should be present most of the day or may present most of the days in last 3 months.

Pain may be triggered by peripheral pain generators such as

a. Arthritis
b. Bursitis
c. Tendinitis
d. Neuropathies
e. Other degenerative arthropathies
f. Some subtle pain generators such as:
    1. Hypermobility of the joints
    2. Scoliosis
g. In case chronic fibromyalgia associated triggering factors are:
    1. Infectious conditions
    2. Metabolic conditions
    3. Psychiatric conditions

    It is necessary to distinguish the fibromyalgia occurred as a consequence of triggering factors from that occurring as a result of comorbid conditions as treatment strategies will vary.

According to the 1990 criteria of ACR, there are 18 tender points, out of which 11 positive tender points in the whole body are diagnostic of fibromyalgia. But newer criteria of ACR 2010 and modified in 2016 has replaced the old criteria, it focusses on clinical symptoms and neuropsychological symptoms. It shows increased prevalence of fibromyalgia and also changes in sex ratio.

B. Neuropsychological symptoms:
    a. Fatigue:
        1. It is present in most of the patients but not present all the times in a particular patient.
        2. It is aggravated along with pain and stiffness by unaccustomed activity or exercise.
    b. Sleep:
        1. Difficulty in falling asleep
        2. Early morning awakening
        3. After awakening patient feel unfreshed
        4. Sleep disordered breathing
        5. Frank sleep apnea
    c. Cognitive disorders:
        1. Difficulties in attention or concentration
        2. Problems with word retrieval
        3. Loss of short-term memory
    d. Anxiety and depression:
        1. Its lifetime prevalence is nearly 80%. Though it is not necessary for the diagnosis. Genetic factor analysis reveals that neurobiological pathways are shared by both fibromyalgia and mood disorders.

C. Overlap syndrome:
    a. Fibromyalgia overlaps with the following chronic pain conditions:
        1. Facial pain
        2. Headache
        3. Pain in jaw
        4. Regional myofascial pain involving neck and back
        5. Arthritis
    b. Fibromyalgia is associated with the following visceral pain:
        1. Bladder
        2. Gastrointestinal tract
        3. Pelvic region
        4. Perineal region

        These overlap syndromes occur due to shared pathways involved in both fibromyalgia and associated chronic regional or visceral pain, so effective treatment may cure both the conditions.

D. Comorbid conditions:

    Following comorbid conditions are associated with fibromyalgia:

    a. ≥20% of patients with fibromyalgia have comorbidity such as degenerative and inflammatory disorders.
    b. Chronic infectious conditions
    c. Metabolic conditions
    d. Psychiatric disorders

E. Psychosocial considerations:
    a. Fibromyalgia may start or be exacerbated during the period of perceived stress reflecting the interactions between central stress physiology, anxiety, vigilance, and central pain processing pathways. This understanding during management of fibromyalgia can be addressed by pharmacological interventions.
    b. In case of post-traumatic stress, this has to be addressed during providing treatment.

Diagnosis of Fibromyalgia

A. Routine investigations:
    a. ESR

   b. C-reactive protein
   c. Complete blood count
   d. Thyroid-stimulating hormone

B. Investigations according to history and clinical examinations:
   a. Complete metabolic panel:
      1. Liver function test
      2. Serum electrolytes
      3. Renal function test
      4. Thyroid function tests
   b. Serology:
      1. Antinuclear antibody
      2. Anti-SSA and anti-SSB antibodies
      3. Rheumatoid factor
      4. Anti-CCP antibody
      5. Creatine phosphokinase (CPK)
      6. Viral serology:
         - Hepatitis B surface antigen (HBsAg)
         - Hepatitis C virus (HCV) antibody
         - HIV I and II
         - Lyme serology
   c. X-ray of spine and joints

Treatment of Fibromyalgia

A. Nonpharmacological therapies:
   a. Low level aerobic exercise progressing toward consistent advancement
   b. In case of physically handicapped patients or who reports of post-exertional malaise, water-based exercise will be preferred.
   c. Strength training should be performed when the patient will reach their aerobic goals.
   d. Cognitive or behavioral therapies

B. Meditational therapies:
   a. Yoga therapy
   b. Tai chi
   c. Mindfulness
   d. Acupuncture
   e. Hydrotherapy

C. Pharmacological therapies:
   a. Anticonvulsants:
      1. Pregabalin
      2. Gabapentin
   b. Tricyclic antidepressant:
      1. Cyclobenzaprine
      2. Amitriptyline
   c. SNRIs:
      1. Duloxetine
      2. Milnacipran
   d. 5HT3 antagonists:
      1. Tropisetron

Q6. Crystal-induced arthritis.

MGR/OCT2013/MDII (7)

ANSWER

Definition

Crystal-induced arthritis is also known as type 1 autoinflammatory disease due to its clinical resemblance with monogenic autoinflammatory syndrome characterized by:

a. Its spontaneous onset with recurrence
b. Self-limitation
c. Its characteristic resolution
d. Inflammasome activation
e. Huge production of interleukin-1β
f. Prevention of involvement of innate immune system

Following are the crystal-induced arthritis:

a. Gouty arthritis due to deposition of monosodium urate crystals in the joints
b. Pseudogout due to deposition of calcium pyrophosphate crystals in the joint
c. Calcific periarthritis, osteoarthritis, and destructive arthropathies due to deposition of basic calcium phosphate crystals

Pathogenesis

Importance of interleukin-1β in case of crystal-induced arthritis is:

a. Uric acid crystal activates cytoplasmic NACHT-LRRPYD of pre-interleukin-1β to interleukin-1β
b. Interleukin-1β and MyD88 molecule in the nonmyeloid-derived cells leading to triggering and amplification inflammatory response through pathogenic crystals
c. Interleukin-1 induces its own gene expression, procession, and secretion. Hence triggering of IL-1 by interleukin-1β is considered as autoinflammatory process.

In case of gout: Purine is metabolized to inosine which in turn will be converted to hypoxanthine and lastly to uric acid through the enzyme xanthine oxidase, it is the major site to pharmacological intervention. Small amount of uric acid is excreted through the urine and intestinal tract. If the body is unable to excrete the uric acid, it will be precipitated in the soft tissues and synovial fluid. In the soft tissues, it will produce tissue damage leading to development of tophi. In the soft tissues and synovial fluid, it will activates monocytes and macrophages which in turn release proinflammatory cytokines and chemokines in the surrounding areas leading to acute influx of neutrophils into the joint cavity and soft tissues, as a result acute inflammatory reaction will be developed. But this inflammatory process is self-limiting within 1–2 weeks, which may be due to innate anti-inflammatory process mediated by anti-inflammatory cytokines.

Additional pathogenic mechanism involves action of inflammasome and IL-1 which is induced by monosodium urate crystals in case of gout and calcium pyrophosphate in case of pseudogout. One inflammasome cryopyrin detects both the crystals to activate IL-1 resulting inflammation cascade, which can be blocked by IL-1 inhibitors which can be used to treat gouty arthritis.

Clinical Features of Gout

In acute gouty arthritis can be presented as asymmetric monoarticular or oligoarticular arthritis involving upper and lower extremities lasing for 3–10 days and ultimately resolves spontaneously. But later on recurrent acute attack do not resolve spontaneously and ultimately leads to chronic gouty arthropathy in which there is erosion and destruction of the joints.

It starts as swelling and tenderness in the first metatarsophalangeal joints, called podagral. But ankle, knee, elbows, wrist, and hands are also involved. It may also involve prepatellar and olecranon bursae producing bursitis. This gouty attack trigger systemic inflammatory response such as fever, raised ESR, leukocytosis, and elevated CRP.

When urate is supersaturated, it will be deposited in the following areas:

- **a.** Helices in the ear
- **b.** Extensor areas of the limb
- **c.** Pressure areas like finger pad
- **d.** Tendo Achilles

Risk factors associated with gout:

A. Increased urate production:

- **a.** Obesity
- **b.** Excess consumption of alcohol
- **c.** Myeloproliferative and lymphoproliferative disorders
- **d.** Diet rich in purines—meat, seafood, and fructose-sweetened beverages

B. Reduced uric acid excretion:

- **a.** Chronic renal failure
- **b.** Diabetes
- **c.** Metabolic syndrome
- **d.** Medications responsible for increasing uric acid levels such as diuretics and cyclosporine

Synovial fluid analysis in gout and pseudogout:

Characteristics	Monosodium urate	Calcium pyrophosphate
Birefringence	Strong	Weak
Shape	Needle shaped	Rhomboid, rod like
Color parallel to polarizer	Yellow	Blue
Color perpendicular to polarizer	Blue	Yellow

Blood test:

A. In acute gout, serum uric acid is not helpful as it fluctuates from low to high level. But in chronic gout, it will be raised, and it can monitor the therapy.

B. Complete blood count, liver function test, and serum creatinine can evaluate the following:

- **a.** Other comorbid disease
- **b.** Monitor drug toxicity after starting the therapy
- **c.** Assess the contraindications to any specific drug

C. 24 hours urine for uric acid when uricosuric therapy is considered.

Treatment part has been written the answer of gouty arthritis.

Pseudogout

It is characterized by deposition of calcium pyrophosphate crystals in the fibrocartilage and hyaline cartilage leading to inflammation and calcification.

Following diseases are associated with pseudogout:

A. Strong association:

- **a.** Hypophosphatasia
- **b.** Hypomagnesemia
- **c.** Hemochromatosis

B. Possible associations:

- **a.** Wilson's disease
- **b.** Gout
- **c.** Hypothyroidism
- **d.** Ochronosis

e. Acromegaly
f. Familial hypocalciuric hypercalcemia (FHH)

Pathophysiology

A. Formation of CPP crystals: Increased level of local calcium or inorganic phosphate which is formed from adenosine triphosphate (ATP), this reaction is catalyzed by hormone known as nucleoside triphosphate pyrophosphohydrolase (NTPPH) present on the external surface of chondrocytes or in large quantities in the vesicles produced by collagen digestion of cartilage. This inorganic phosphate present in the extracellular fluid inhibits growth of basic calcium phosphate crystals. Following factors are responsible for inorganic phosphate:
   a. TGF-β
   b. Ascorbic acid
   c. Retinoic acid
   d. Thyroid hormone

B. Role of *ANK* gene: In familial form of pseudogout *ANK* gene is a transmembrane protein responsible for regulation and transportation of inorganic phosphate. Function of *ANK* gene:
   a. Its increased activity is responsible for calcium pyrophosphate crystal formation and deposition.
   b. Human analogue of *ANK* gene promotes the release of ATP by chondrocytes which provides substrate for NTPPH. Mutation of 5p locus of ANKH is identified in sporadic disease.
   c. Another variant of ANKH correlates with radiographic chondrocalcinosis independent of osteoporosis.

C. Role of calcium pyrophosphate crystals in pseudogout: Crystals activates induces assembly of NALP3 dependent inflammasome in the neutrophils and monocytes and activates NALP3 which in turn produces intereukin-1β from pro-interleukin-1β by activating latent caspase-1. This interleukin-1β will produce acute inflammation in joints and periarticular tissue.

D. Resolution of acute attack: These crystals will be phagocytosed and dissolved leading to resolution of the acute attack.

Etiology

A. Age: It occurs in old age, after 45 years the incidence is doubled in every decade.

B. Trauma: Surgery in joints increases the risk of this disease.

C. Familial chondrocalcinosis: It can be suspected if it occurs in earlier age and presentation is polyarticular. Two mutations like CCAL1 mutation related to 8q and CCLA2 mutation related to 5p are responsible for this disease.

D. Different metabolic and endocrine diseases

E. Intra-articular injection of hyaluronidase may be responsible for isolated calcium pyrophosphate deposition disease (CPPD) disease.

Clinical Pictures

According to EULAR criteria the classification of CPPD disease:

A. Asymptomatic/lanthanic chondrocalcinosis: These patients are usually old, clinically silent but X-ray will demonstrate chondrocalcinosis.

B. Osteoarthritis with CPPD

C. Acute CPP crystal arthritis

D. Chronic pyrophosphate arthropathy

Pseudogout: It is characterized by the following characteristics:
   a. Acute attack of synovitis involving knee, wrist, ankle, elbows, toes, shoulder, and hip in decreasing order
   b. It takes longer time to reach its peak and persists for >3 months in spite of treatment
   c. It is precipitated by trauma, surgery, or pamidronate therapy.
   d. It may coexist with gout in a single patient.

Pseudarthritis: It is characterized by the following characteristics:
   a. It is degenerative disorders involving multiple joints involving knee, wrists, MCP joints, hips, shoulders, spine, ankles, and elbows.
   b. Osteoarthritis involving typical multiple joints like wrists, ankles, elbows, and MCP joints will raise the suspicion of CPPD disease.

Pseudorheumatoid arthritis: It is characterized by the following characteristics:
   a. Chronic nonerosive, asynchronous, and inflammatory arthritis
   b. Associated features are early morning stiffness, symmetrical involvement, and flexion contracture along with raised CRP.
   c. In CPPD, typical crystals and typical radiographic features suggest CPPD disease. But positive anti-CCP antibody along with radiographic features of bony erosions suggests rheumatoid arthritis.

Pseudoneuropathic joints: It is characterized by the following:

a. Destructive arthropathy affecting knee joints
b. Presence of chondrocalcinosis
c. Absence of neurologic disorder

Atypical CPPD:

a. Deposition of CPPD crystals in tendons, bursae, ligaments, and joint recesses may lead to carpal tunnel syndrome, periarthritis, tenosynovitis, etc.
b. Involvement of spine will produce spinal stenosis and bony ankyloses.

Investigations

A. X-ray features:
  a. Chondrocalcinosis characterized by linear or wedge-shaped calcification due to deposition of CPPD crystals in the hyaline and fibrous cartilage of knees, pubis symphysis, wrist joints, glenoid, and acetabular labra.
  b. CPPD arthropathy: It is characterized by the following features:
    1. Chondrocalcinosis
    2. Normal bone mineralization
    3. Uniform loss of joint space
    4. Subchondral new bone formation
    5. Large subchondral cysts
    6. Bilateral distribution
    7. Occasional neuropathic changes
    8. Following joints are involved in decreasing order:
       - Elbow
       - Wrist
       - Hips
       - Hands
    9. Calcification of ligaments, bursa, and tendons.
    10. Multiple levels of degenerative disk disease involving cervical through lumbar spine.

B. Ultrasonography: Following findings are found in the cartilages:
  a. Presence of thin hyperechoic band parallels the bony cortex in the hyaline cartilage
  b. Small round hyperechoic amorphous regions with acoustic shadow in the triangular fibrocartilage in the wrist, tendons, and menisci of knee.
  c. Nodular hyperechoic deposits in the bursa and joint recesses
  d. Presence of linear calcifications along the tendo Achilles and plantar fascia

C. Synovial fluid: Presence of rhomboid long or short rod-shaped crystals having weak or weakly positive birefringence.

Treatment

Following are the aims of treatment of pseudogout:

A. Treatment of acute pseudogout attack:
  a. Nonpharmacological treatment:
    1. Application of ice-packs
    2. Rest to afforded joints
    3. Immobilization of the affected part
  b. Pharmacotherapy:
    1. Intra-articular injection of triamcinolone 40 mg with 2% lidocaine for large joints and small joints
    2. NSAIDs: Preferred short-acting drugs are the following:
       - Naproxen 500 mg twice daily
       - Sulindac 200 mg twice daily
       - Indomethacin 50 mg thrice daily

       These drugs are avoided in:
       - Chronic renal failure
       - Gastric ulcer
       - Duodenal ulcer
       - Heart failure
       - Poorly controlled hypertension

       After disappearances of symptoms it can be stopped after 1–2 days.
    3. Oral colchicine: 0.5 mg up to 3 times daily following loading dose of 1 mg is recommended.
    4. Oral prednisolone: 30–50 mg daily in 2–3 divided doses until the symptoms remission followed by slow tapering of dose. Equivalent dose of methylprednisolone can be given instead.

B. Prophylaxis against recurrent pseudogout:
   The aim to reduce the frequency of recurrent attacks:
  a. Colchicine 0.5 mg twice daily is preferred. But in presence of adverse effects such as abdominal pain and diarrhea once daily dose can be given.
  b. In absence of colchicine NSAIDs can be administered.

C. Correction of associated metabolic and endocrine diseases

D. Treatment of chronic inflammatory arthritis:

NSAIDs, oral colchicine or corticosteroids are given as initial treatment

Newer rugs which will block NLRP3 inflammasome:

a. IL-1 pathway

Other drugs are:

a. Polyphosphates
b. Probenecid
c. Transglutaminase 2
d. Phosphocitrate

Basic Calcium Phosphate Hydroxyapatite Deposition Disease

Clinical Features

In this, there is deposition of mixture of carbonate substituted hydroxyapatite and octacalcium phosphate in the shoulder and metatarsophalangeal joints followed by knees, elbows, wrists, and digits. Deposition leads to rotator cuff degeneration along with instability of glenohumeral region known as "Milwaukee shoulder syndrome."

There are also evidences of tendinitis, periarthritis, enthesitis, bursitis, and also calcification of soft tissues.

Investigations

A. Synovial fluid demonstrates nonbirefringent specific crystals which show bright red intracellular and extracellular crystals by the stain "alizarin red." It also can be demonstrated by electron microscopy, energy dispersive elemental analysis, infrared spectroscopy, X-ray diffraction, and Raman micro-spectroscopy.

B. Radiology:

a. Intra-articular and periarticular calcification

Treatment

A. Acute attack may be self-limiting and resolved within few weeks by nonpharmacological intervention.

B. Drugs used to decreasing intensity and duration of attack are:

a. Intra-articular aspiration of synovial fluid and intra-articular corticosteroid
b. NSAIDs
c. Oral colchicine

C. Local injection of following drugs can be given:

a. Intravenous immunoglobulin
b. Anakinra
c. Bisphosphonate

Calcium oxalate deposition disease:
It occurs in the following conditions:

a. Renal failure on maintenance hemodialysis
b. Chronic kidney disease (CKD) on peritoneal dialysis
c. Patients treated with vitamin C metabolized to oxalate

Patients present with chronic arthritis of the knee, ankle, feet or bursitis of tendon sheath, and bursa.

Crystals are bipyramidal or envelope like and strongly birefringent.

It looks like dense foamy deposits in electron microscopy.

Cholesterol deposition disease: It is seen in rheumatoid arthritis or in case of trauma or hemarthrosis. Synovial fluid is "glossy golden" appearance.

Synovial fluid demonstrates:

a. Cholesterol monohydrate crystal as broad plates with notched corners
b. Anhydrate cholesterol crystals as rod-shaped birefringent helical crystal

Lipid liquid crystals:
It is seen in:

a. Type II and IV hyperlipoproteinemia
b. Antecedent infection
c. Idiopathic

Synovial fluid demonstrates "maltese cross-like microspherules"

Rice bodies:
It is composed of fibrin, found in the joints, tendon in case of:

a. Rheumatoid arthritis
b. Tubercular arthritis
c. Tenosynovitis

Macroscopic features in the synovial fluid are policed grain of rice. Shape of the crystal is huge semicircular balloon having birefringent edges.

Protein crystals:
It includes:

a. IgG cryoprecipitable paraprotein
b. Charcot–Leyden crystals
c. Hemosiderin crystals

Q7. Reactive arthritis.

MGR/OCT2015/MDII (7) MJPRU/2015/MDII (10)
RGUHS/APR2001/MDII (10)

How will you differentiate reactive arthritis from seropositive arthritis? Write down the management of reactive arthritis.

MJPRU/2016/MDIV (10)

Reiter's disease.

RGUHS/NOV2001/MDII (10)

Reactive arthritis.

MGR UNI, Tamil Nadu 2022 (10)

What is reactive arthritis? When do you suspect that a patient is suffering from it? How do you treat such patients?

WBUHS, 2023 (10)

ANSWER

Definition

It is a type of inflammatory arthritis occurring within several days to weeks after gastrointestinal or genitourinary tract infection and characterized by the clinical triad of conjunctivitis, arthritis, and urethritis.

Epidemiology

It occurs in young adult between the ages of 20–40 years, both sexes are equally affected. But in case of chlamydia infection there is male predominance.

Etiopathogenesis

A. Gastrointestinal infection:
- **a.** *Shigella flexneri*
- **b.** *Campylobacter jejuni*
- **c.** *Campylobacter coli*
- **d.** *Yersinia enterocolitica*
- **e.** *Yersinia pseudotuberculosis*

B. Genitourinary tract infection:
- **a.** *Chlamydia trachomatis*

C. Respiratory tract infection:
- **a.** *Chlamydia pneumoniae*

D. Other organisms:
- **a.** *Clostridium difficile*
- **b.** *Salmonella typhimurium*
- **c.** *Ureaplasma urealyticum*
- **d.** Salmonella enteritidis

Genetic and infective agent interaction is responsible for reactive arthritis. As compared to different types of arthritis which is the result of overactive immune response, reactive arthritis occurs due to downregulation of cytokines, i.e., TNF-α and interferon-γ. Gram-negative and intracellular organisms like chlamydia containing lipopolysaccharide present in the cell membrane, present in the synovial cavity in dormant state in genetically predisposed individual.

In chlamydia infection, as a result of type 1 immune response interferon-γ will be increased which ultimately kills the bacteria leading to production of sterile arthritis. Again, if the type II response becomes dominant, patient will be susceptible to chronic infection.

Antigen presenting cells, macrophages are responsible for innate immune response. Depending upon the differentiation of T cell profile, macrophages are subdivided into two types:
- **a.** M1 macrophages—produce Th1 profile—these are responsible for control of infection.
- **b.** M2 macrophages—produce Th2 profile—these are responsible for spondyloarthropathies.

Ribosomal ribonucleic acid (RNA) transcripts of *Chlamydia trachomatis, Chlamydia pneumoniae*, enteric bacterial deoxyribonucleic acid (DNA), and bacterial degradation products in the synovial fluid. Following factors of chlamydia dictate the duration of infection:
- **a.** Ability to survive hypoxic environment
- **b.** Variation in the protein present in the outer membrane

Following factors are responsible for susceptibility to infection:
- **a.** Sensitization with heavy metal
- **b.** Repeated infection
- **c.** Host genetic variability—polymorphism in toll-like receptor 2 (TLR2).
- **d.** Deficiency in IL-12
- **e.** HLA-B27—it will present the bacterial antigen to T cells leading to development of reactive arthritis through the following mechanisms:
  1. Alteration of self-tolerance of host immune system
  2. Increased production of TNF-α
  3. Promotion of invasion of the gut by microbes
  4. Delayed clearance of responsible organisms

Following factors are responsible for resistance to infection:

f. Interferon-γ
g. Interleukin-10

Clinical Features

Clinical manifestation will start 1–4 weeks after infection in the gastrointestinal or genitourinary tract.

A. Articular manifestations:
  a. Most common is oligoarticular with lower limb predominance
  b. But polyarthritis involving upper and lower limb may occur.
  c. In 30% patient, there is inflammatory back pain.

B. Extra-articular manifestations:
  a. Ocular involvement: It is more common with chlamydia-induced reactive arthritis. Features are:
    1. Conjunctivitis: It typically occurs after urethritis, usually bilateral, in the early course of the disease. It is more common in sexually acquired males and after Shigella infections. Male-to-female ratio is 1.3: 1.
    2. Acute unilateral anterior uveitis presenting with ocular pain and photophobia
    3. Chronic infection leads to intraocular damage and ultimately visual loss
  b. Cutaneous manifestation: It occurs in 50% of patients.
    1. Keratoderma blenorrhagicum—it is characterized by clear vesicle around an erythematous base developing into nodules and eventually coalesce into crust present on the palms and soles.
    2. Circinate balanitis—it is characterized by painless shallow ulcers at the glans penis which varies according to presence or absence of circumcision.
      - In circumscribed male—the ulcer is dry, hyperkeratotic, and plaque like.
      - In uncircumscribed male—the ulcer is moist, shallow, and present around the meatus.
  c. Oral ulcer mainly presents in the hard palate or tongue but also found in cheek, gingiva, and soft palate.
  d. Cardiac involvement (10% of cases): Following features are:
    1. Aortic regurgitation
    2. Atrioventricular block
    3. Pericarditis

Evaluation of reactive arthritis according to ACR diagnostic guideline 1999:

A. Major criteria:
  a. Asymmetric oligoarticular or monoarthritis involving lower extremities
  b. Preceding enteric infection with one or two of the following findings:
    1. Enteritis-like diarrhea for at least 1 day, 3 days to 6 weeks before the onset of arthritis
    2. Urethritis like dysuria or discharge for 1 day, 3 days to 6 weeks before the onset of arthritis

B. Minor criteria:
  a. Evidence of triggering factors:
    1. Morning urine or urethral or cervical swab for nucleic acid amplification test positive for chlamydia.
    2. Stool culture positive for enteric pathogen-associated reactive arthritis
  b. Evidence of persistent synovial infection [positive test results on immunohistologic analysis or polymerase chain reaction (PCR) assay for chlamydia].

Investigations

A. Hematological test:
  a. ESR raised
  b. Raised CRP
  c. Leukocytosis
  d. Thrombocytosis

B. Isolation of organisms:
  a. Nucleic acid amplification test for chlamydia in the morning urine sample or urogenital swab
  b. ELISA test, complement fixation test, and micro-immunofluorescence test for upper genital tract infection by chlamydia infection
  c. Stool culture is negative in patients who have been already recovered from infection. But *Salmonella* and *Yersinia* may be present even after recovery from infection from stool sample provided; it will be preserved at 4–8°C.

C. HLA-B12 positivity associated with raised inflammatory biomarkers, involvement of metatarsophalangeal joint, and genitourinary tract can predict reactive arthritis with 70% specificity and 93% sensitivity.

D. Imaging: Ultrasonography, MRI or power Doppler studies can detect enthesitis, bursitis, or subclinical synovitis.

Differentiation of reactive arthritis and seropositive arthritis consult question number 1.

Treatment

A. Disease-modifying antirheumatic drugs (DMARDs): It is useful for:
   a. Chronic arthritis
   b. HLA-B27 positive severe arthritis
   c. Polyarthritis

B. Acute anterior uveitis—it can be treated with topical glucocorticoids and mydriatics.

C. Keratoderma blenorrhagicum can be treated with topical glucocorticoids, and in severe cases methotrexate.

D. Circinate balanitis can be treated with mild topical glucocorticoids.

E. Biologics like TNF-α inhibitors, i.e., infliximab, etanercept and adalimumab can provide good response in tender swollen joints and associated extra-articular manifestations.

Complications

A. Recurrent arthritis
B. Chronic arthritis
C. Sacroiliitis
D. Ankylosing spondylitis
E. Urethral stricture
F. Aortic root necrosis
G. Cystoid macular edema
H. Cataracts

Q8. Charcot's joint.

MGR/OCT2013/MDII (7)

ANSWER

Definition

Charcot joint can be defined as dislocations, pathological fractures, and debilitating deformities.

Classifications

Among the different classifications anatomical classification is most accepted as it has added benefit of predicting prognosis and outcome. According to Saunders and Mrdjenovich classification based on the location of arthropathy, charcot arthropathy has the following patterns:

A. Pattern 1—involves forefoot including interphalangeal joints, phalanges, and metatarsophalangeal joints
B. Patter 2—involves tarsometatarsal joints
C. Pattern 3—it involves cuneonavicular, talonavicular, and calcaneocuboid joints
D. Pattern 4—it involves talocrural or ankle joint, which is articulation of tibia, fibula, and talus.
E. Pattern 5—it involves posterior calcaneus

Another commonly used classification of Brodsky and Rouse:

A. Type 1—it involves mid foot
B. Type 2—it involves hind foot
C. Type 3a—it involves ankle
D. Type 3b—in involves pathological fracture of os calcis tubercle

Etiology

A. Diabetes
B. Syphilis
C. Chronic alcoholism
D. Leprosy
E. Spinal cord injury
F. Syringomyelia
G. Meningomyelocele
H. Renal dialysis
I. Congenital insensitivity to pain

Pathophysiology

There are two theories regarding the pathophysiology of Charcot joint:

A. Neurotraumatic theory: According to this theory, neuropathy and repeated microtrauma are responsible for joint destruction.

B. Neurovascular theory: According to this theory, increased peripheral blood flow is responsible for osteolysis and bone destruction.

Key inflammatory markers contributing to the development of Charcot joint. Calcium gene-related peptide antagonizes the synthesis of cytokine involved in the inflammatory process, nuclear factory kappa B ligand (RANKL) at the nerve terminal. But due to nonfunctioning of this peptide increasingly synthesized RANKL without any inhibition which leads to proliferation of osteoclastogenesis.

Again, normally, the osteoclastic activity of RANKL is moderated by osteoprotegerin which acts as decoy receptor of RANKL. This relation is also disrupted in Charcot joint leading to unregulated turnover of bones and accumulation in the Charcot limb.

Calcium gene-related peptide upholds the integrity of joint capsule in the Charcot joint thus leading to destruction and dislocation of joint—characteristic of Charcot joint.

Clinical Presentation

Presentation will vary from mild swelling without deformity to moderate deformity with significant swelling depending upon the stage of the disease.

Acute case presents with signs of inflammation, profound unilateral swelling, increased temperature, erythema, joint effusion, and resorption of bone along with presence of intact skin and loss of protective sensation. There is joint instability, loss of joint function, during passive movement there is feeling of "loose bag of bone."

Complications

A. In case of overlook, there is marked joint deformity and ulceration of skin over the bony prominence which may lead to severe infection and if required amputation of the affected limb.

B. Ossification of ligamentous structure

C. Formation of intra-articular exostoses

D. Club foot

E. Rocket-bottom foot—there is collapse and inversion of plantar arch.

F. Acute fracture and dislocation at Lisfranc joint complex.

G. Collapse of plantar arch

H. Development of osteomyelitis

Investigations

A. Normal or elevated WBC

B. Raised ESR

C. Elevated urea and creatinine

D. HbA1c increased in case of uncontrolled diabetes

E. Serum calcium, phosphorus, parathormone, and alkaline phosphatase can identify the bone disease like Paget's disease.

F. Vitamin B12 or folic acid deficiency—suggests peripheral neuropathy or chronic alcoholism

G. Abnormal liver function test—suggests chronic alcoholism

H. Radiology can help:

- **a.** To identify the stage of the disease
- **b.** To determine the activity of the disease
- **c.** To identify osteopenia like fragments of the bone, subluxation, dislocation, generalized destruction, and fractures

I. Doppler study should be done to identify deep vein thrombosis.

Diagnostic Procedures

A. Lumbar puncture should be done if rapid plasma reagin (RPR) is positive.

B. Bone probing with blunt sterile surgical probe—if the probe is passed down the bone or bone is exposed at the ulcer base—this establishes the diagnosis of osteomyelitis.

C. Portable infrared dermal thermometry to assess the skin temperature

D. In case of septic joint—joint aspiration

E. Synovial biopsy

Treatment

A. Medical therapy:

- **a.** Total contact casting helps the patient to become mobile and at the same time prevents the progression of the deformity. It should be reduced at every 1–2 weeks. In case of associated ulcer cast should be changed weekly along with ulcer debridement. In acute case, serial X-ray should be taken every month to evaluate progress. Cast should be discontinued on the basis of radiographic, clinical, and dermal thermometric signs. After removal, lifelong protection of the limb is advised.
- **b.** Metal braces
- **c.** Ankle orthoses
- **d.** Custom footwear after removal of cast is extra-depth shoes with rigid soles and plastic or metal shank.

B. Surgical therapies are the following:

- **a.** Osteotomy
- **b.** Arthrodesis
- **c.** Reconstructive surgery
- **d.** Amputation
- **e.** Autologous bone grafting
- **f.** Screw and plate fixation
- **g.** Exostectomy of bony prominence

Prognosis

Outcome depends upon:

- **a.** Outcome of treatment
- **b.** Prognosis: It is favorable when the joints are treated within 2 weeks of injury.

c. Healing time is increased in case of diabetes.
d. Extent of injury
e. Severity of injury: More severe is the more time is required.

Q9. Young onset osteoarthritis (OA).
MGR/OCT2011/MDII (7)

Pathological changes in osteoarthritis. Notes on young onset OA.
MGR/APR2012/MDIV (7)

Osteoarthritis.
NTR UNI of Health SC, Vijayawada, Aug 2022 (10)

ANSWER

Pathogenesis of Osteoarthritis

Chondrocytes in the hyaline cartilage in the joint is composed of water, type II collagen, and proteoglycan embedded in extracellular matrix. Cartilage maintains its stability through the process of degeneration and regeneration. When the process of degeneration exceeds the regeneration, osteoarthritis results.

Chondrocytes secrete following inactive matrix metalloproteinases such as stromelysin, collagenase, and gelatinase, these can destroy cartilage framework. These are activated by plasmin and activated stromelysin.

Tissue plasminogen activator released from chondrocytes converts blood and chondrocytes derived plasminogen to active plasmin.

Above cascade is modulated by inhibitor of matrix metalloproteinase as well as plasminogen activator inhibitor.

Interleukin-1 plays a pivotal role in the genesis of osteoarthritis in the following mechanisms:

a. It increases synthesis and secretion of inactive matrix metalloproteinase and tissue plasminogen activator
b. It will suppress the synthesis of proteoglycans and thus repair of cartilage.
c. It will decrease tissue inhibitor of matrix metalloproteinase and plasminogen activator inhibitor.
d. It will increase the osteoblast proliferation which leads to formation of osteophytes.

Osteoarthritis is an inflammatory disorder, inflammation worsens it.

a. Damage of chondrocytes will be started through stimulation of crystals and mechanical stress. As a result, nuclear factor kappa B (NF-κB) and mitogen-activated protein kinase (MAPK) pathways are stimulated which leads to activation of cytokine genes resulting in formation of pro-IL-1β.
b. Large size chondrocytes containing phagosomes and cathepsin B and other proteolytic enzymes are produced from damaged chondrocytes. These enzymes aid in degeneration of matrix and activate inflammasome, this activated inflammasome release caspase-1 which converts pro-IL-1β to IL-1β which is powerful mediator of inflammation leading to stimulation of chondrocytes and these activated chondrocytes take an active part in degeneration of cartilage by above methods.
c. On the other hand, matrix increases synthesis of insulin-like growth factor, TGF-β, and FGF
    1. In the early stage, there is degeneration of matrix and cartilage on one hand and replication of chondrocytes along with biosynthesis on the other hand leading to a state equilibrium of synthesis and degeneration—it is known as compensated osteoarthritis.
    2. But in the later life, there is exhaustion of repairing process leading to unopposed action of degeneration, as result there is progression of osteoarthritis.

Osteoarthritis in Young

Osteoarthritis though a devastating heterogenous clinical condition affecting mainly elderly, but it may occur in genetically predisposed young individuals where there are history of injury, occupational activities and obesity, it is associated with defective articular cartilage and associated changes in the bony morphology.

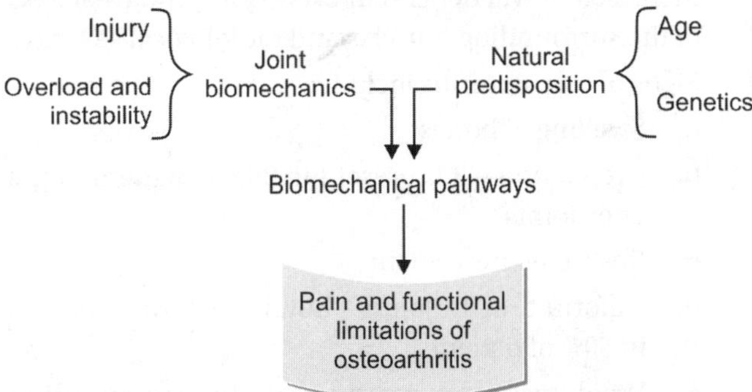

There is strong association of OA with obesity and occupational injury. As the athletes are engaged with the recreational activities hence they are predisposed to knee injury. Joint is made up of articular cartilage which is made up of macromolecular framework along with waters and cells, mainly chondrocytes. Any alteration in the structure of the articular cartilage will lead to articular injury followed by degeneration. In athlete, degeneration of knee and hip joints occurs due to damage in articular cartilage as a result of repetitive impact of loading, main game involved are football, hockey, basketball, rugby and lacrosse. Amount of joint injuries depends upon the amount of loading and frequency of impact which leads to degeneration and instability of the affected joints. These patients may develop osteoarthritis within next 20 years. Since there are no nerve endings in the articular cartilage, hence the patient becomes unaware of the repetitive exposure to high level of impact and loading. In the athlete there are other factors that make the patient more susceptible, these are high body mass index as in case of sumo wrestlers, strength and genetics.

Clinical Features

A. Main symptom is pain, which may vary according to tolerability of individual. There are different theories for pain. According to one theory, pain may occur due to stretching of the periosteum by the osteophytes; according to one, it may be due to inflammation of the joint involved. Pain waxes and wanes and ultimately resolute with the development and resolution of bone marrow lesion. The hallmark of osteoarthritis is bone marrow lesion. It will start as deep ache aggravated by use of joints and relieved by rest. In advanced cases night may arise which may be very disturbing. In some case, there may be locking and buckling of the joints.

B. Next common symptom is morning stiffness in the finger, knees, spine, and hips which will be healed within 30 minutes of activity but again recurs with inactivity. As the disease progresses, stiffness will be increased. It will depend upon wasting and weakness of the surrounding muscles and radiological severity.

C. Signs of osteoarthritis include:

- **a.** Swelling of bones
- **b.** Crepitation—it is present in 90% of patient in the knee joints.
- **c.** Restricted movement
- **d.** Deformity of the joints—bow leg deformity occurs in 50% of patients
- **e.** Weakness and wasting of the surrounding muscles

D. Common joints to be involved are:

- **a.** Knee
- **b.** Small joint of the hand:
  - **1.** Distal interphalangeal joints
  - **2.** First carpometacarpal joint
  - **3.** Proximal interphalangeal joints
- **c.** Spinal apophyseal joints

Investigations

A. Radiography of the knee joints: Classical radiological features include:

- **a.** Joint space narrowing
- **b.** Presence of osteophytes—it indicates advanced joint disease
- **c.** Subchondral bone sclerosis
- **d.** Subchondral bony cyst
- **e.** Presence of calcification:
  - **1.** Linear deposition of calcium pyrophosphate dehydrate crystals
  - **2.** Spotty due to hydroxyapatite deposition

B. MRI feature of joints:

- **a.** Fibrillation and defect in surface
- **b.** Cartilage quality
- **c.** Damage of meniscus or ligaments
- **d.** Edema of bone marrow
- **e.** Synovitis
- **f.** Synovial effusions

C. Synovial fluid analysis:

- **a.** Leukocytosis <2,000/cc
- **b.** Crystals depending on the used technique

D. Following levels are seen:

- **a.** Serum osteocalcin—noncollagenous marker of bone formation is increased.
- **b.** Urinary C peptide level of type I collagen—marker of bone formation is decreased.
- **c.** Serum cartilage oligomeric protein—noncollagenous marker of bone formation is increased.
- **d.** Urinary C peptide level of type II collagen—marker of cartilage turnover is increased.

Diagnostic criteria for the OA of knee joints

Presence of knee pain along with any three criteria of the following:

- **a.** Morning stiffness for <30 minutes
- **b.** Presence of crepitus on active knee motion
- **c.** Older than 50 years of age
- **d.** Bony enlargement
- **e.** No palpable warmth
- **f.** Bony tenderness

Diagnostic criteria for the hand

Presence of pain with or without stiffness along with any three of the following:

- **a.** Fewer than three swollen MCP joints.
- **b.** Hard enlargement of two or more DIP joints
- **c.** Deformity of at least one of the ten selected joints second and third distal interphalangeal joints, first carpometacarpal joints and second and third PIP joints.
- **d.** Hard tissue enlargement of two or more of the 10 selected joints.

Treatment

Main aim of treatment is to minimize pain and improve joint stability.

A. Nonpharmacological treatment:

- **a.** Aerobic exercise: Benefit of exercise are:
  1. Reduction of pain and stability
  2. Increases the strength, stability, and flexibility of the muscles
- **b.** Bracing:
  1. It will prevent changes in the alignment and biomechanical forces in the knee since malalignment is associated with radiographic changes of joint loss and functional deterioration.
  2. It will prevent instability secondary to torn ligaments and menisci.

B. Pharmacotherapy:

- **a.** NSAIDs: It reduces pain and inflammation around the joints.
- **b.** Intra-articular injection of steroids: It will relieve pain due to its anti-inflammatory properties. Adverse effect is cytotoxicity of steroids to chondrocytes.
- **c.** Intra-articular injection of hyaluronic acid. It has:
  1. Viscoelastic properties
  2. Anti-inflammatory properties—reduce pro-inflammatory cytokines and matrix metalloproteinases. It cannot modify the disease progression.
  3. Analgesic properties
- **d.** Duloxetine: It is selective serotonin and norepinephrine reuptake inhibitors. Dose is 120 mg/day. Effect can be seen within 2 weeks.

C. Surgical therapy:

- **a.** Minimal invasive joint surgery:
  1. In patient with varus or valgus deformities can be benefited from:
     - High tibial and distal femoral osteotomy
     - Unicompartmental arthroplasty because of:
       - ◆ Shorter recovery time
       - ◆ Better range of motion
     - Arthroscopic lavage and debridement—it is helpful in case of labral tear or femoroacetabular impingement.

Following methods are not recommended:

- **a.** Joint irrigation: It is associated with deep vein thrombosis, infection followed by death.
- **b.** Abrasion arthroplasty: It can worsen the symptoms and hasten the need for joint replacement.
- **c.** Arthroscopic synovectomy: It can be done in case of secondary osteoarthritis.

C. Total joint arthroplasty:

- **a.** Indication of joint replacement:
  1. Severe limitation of function
  2. Inequality of limb length
  3. Moderate to severe pain not responding to conservative drugs
- **b.** Contraindications of total hip replacement:
  1. Absolute contraindications:
     - Active infection
     - Medical illness increasing the risk of morbidity and mortality
  2. Relative contraindications:
     - Neuropathic arthropathy
     - Insufficiency of abductor musculature
     - Rapidly progressive neurologic diseases
- **c.** Contraindications of total knee replacement:
  1. Absolute contraindications:
     - Recent or current infection in the affected knee
     - Dysfunction of extensor mechanism
     - Recurvatum deformity secondary to weakness of muscles
     - Presence of painless arthrodesis which is well functioning
  2. Relative contraindications:
     - Morbid obesity
     - Neuropathic arthropathy
     - Features of peripheral vascular diseases
- **d.** Sequences of arthroplasty:
  1. Lower limb arthroplasty should be done before upper limb arthroplasty

2. Sequences in lower limb surgery:
   - Fore foot
   - Hip
   - Knee
   - Hind foot
   - Ankle

e. Functional limitation after hip or knee replacement: Following should be avoided:
   1. Contact sports and high-impact arthropathies
   2. Flexion of >90°
   3. Hip will always be at high level as compared to knee in sitting position.

Q10. Paget's disease.

MGR/MAR2010/MDII (6)

ANSWER

Definition

It is a type of bone disorder which is characterized by excessive bone resorption due to osteoclastic overactivity which is followed by increased formation of bones due to compensatory osteoblastic activity.

Bone Involvement

It has predilection of axial skeleton in descending order such as spine, pelvis, femur, sacrum, and skull. After onset, this disease does not spread from bone to bone. Sarcomatous degeneration may occur and it is deadly fatal.

Etiology

A. Clear genetic basis has been established with this disease.
   a. Homozygous deletion of *TNFRSF11B* gene encoding osteoprotegerin responsible for juvenile Paget's disease characterized by uncontrolled differentiation of osteoclast and resorption, it is autosomal dominant with variable penetrance.
   b. Mutation of *TNFRSF11A* encoding RANK, receptor activator of NF-κB is associated with early onset Paget's disease.
   c. Mutation of gene encoding valosin-containing protein is associated with inclusion body myopathy with Paget's disease and frontotemporal dementia, it is autosomal dominant with variable penetrance.
   d. Mutation of *SQSTM1* gene present in the C-terminal ubiquitin-binding domain is associated with sporadic cases of Paget's disease.
   e. Other genes are:
      1. CSF-1 encoding macrophage colony-stimulating factor, cytokine responsible for differentiation of osteoclast
      2. RIN3 encoding guanine exchange factor known as Rab and Ras interactor 3
      3. OPTN responsible for regulating NF-κB
      4. *TNFRSF11A* encoding receptor activator of NF-κB, which is essential for differentiation of osteoclast.

B. Viral factor: Following factors suggest the association between viral infection and Paget's disease:
   a. Presence of nuclear and cytoplasmic inclusions like that of measles virus and respiratory syncytial virus in patients of Paget's disease.
   b. Osteoclast precursors conversion to pagetic like osteoclasts by measles virus nucleocapsid or matrix genes.

   This can be supported by the decreased incidence of Paget's disease with the vaccination against measles.

Pathophysiology

Main abnormality in Paget's disease is increased number as well as activity of osteoclast. Osteoclast of Paget's disease is large having large number of nuclei and increased resorptive surfaces with erosion rate of 9 μg/day. Several causes of increased number and activity of osteoclasts are:

A. Precursors of osteoclasts are 1, 25-dihydroxy vitamin D3
B. Osteoclast is hyperresponsive to RANKL.
C. Stromal cells in the marrow from pagetic lesion have increased expression of RANKL.
D. IL-6 is increased in the peripheral blood with active Paget's disease recruit osteoclast precursors and it is overexpressed in pagetic osteoclasts.
E. Expression of Proto-oncogene c-fos with increased osteoclastic activity
F. Overexpression of Bcl-2 apoptotic oncogene in pagetic bone

Characteristic features are:

A. In the first phase or osteoclastic phase, prominent bone resorption along with marked hypervascularization. It can be evidenced radiologically as "Blade of Grass" lesion or advancing lytic wedge.

B. In the second phase or bone formation phase, resorption of lamellar bone will be replaced by woven or haphazard bone along with normal bone marrow will be replaced by fibrous connective tissue.

C. In the final sclerotic phase, there is progressive decline of bone resorption leading to formation of less vascular, hard, dense pagetic, or mosaic bone formation. This is the blunt-out phase of Paget's disease.

Clinical Features

A. Pain in the bone resulting from:
   a. Increased bony vascularity
   b. Expansion of lytic lesion
   c. Bowing of bones
   d. Fractures
   e. Deformities

B. Gait deformities from due to:
   a. Bowing of tibia and femur
   b. Abnormal mechanical stresses as a result of osteoarthritis of hip and knee joints

C. Extremity pain from:
   a. Bowing of the long bones
   b. Stretching of muscles attached to soft pagetic bones

D. Back pain results from:
   a. Enlarged pagetic vertebrae
   b. Spinal stenosis
   c. Compression of vertebrae
   d. Degenerative changes in the joints
   e. Alteration of body mechanics resulting from kyphosis and forward tilt of upper back

E. Feature of spinal cord syndrome resulting from:
   a. Enlargement of bones
   b. Vascular steal syndrome

F. Skull involvement:
   a. Headache
   b. Frontal bossing
   c. Increased size of the head
   d. Narrowing of the cranial foramen resulting neurologic complications:
      1. Hearing loss from damage of cochlear nerve due to temporal bone involvement as well as softening of the base of the skull. It may lead to brainstem compression.
   e. Facial deformity from involvement of facial bone involvement.
   f. Loss of teeth

Complications

A. Fracture of the shaft femur and subtrochanteric regions

B. Sarcoma—its incidence is now decreasing due to timely commencement of antiresorptive treatment. Major tumor is osteosarcoma.

C. Osteoclast-rich benign giant cell tumor arising from the areas adjacent to pagetic bones.

D. Cardiovascular complications develop in patients with increased disease activity and involvement of large portion of skeleton.
   a. High output state and cardiac enlargement due to:
      1. Increased blood flow through the vascular pagetic bone
      2. Extensive arteriovenous shunting
   b. High-output heart failure
   c. Calcific aortic stenosis
   d. Diffuse vascular calcifications

Diagnosis

A. Radiological features:
   a. In case of lone bones:
      1. Enlargement and expansion of entire bone area
      2. Cortical thickening
      3. Coarsening of trabecular markings
      4. Bowing deformity
   b. In case of skull:
      1. Cotton wool or osteoporosis circumscripta
      2. Thickening of diploic areas
      3. Enlargement and sclerosis
   c. In case of vertebra:
      1. Thickening of superior and inferior end plate producing "picture frame" vertebrae
      2. Diffuse radiodense enlargement producing "ivory vertebra"
   d. In case of pelvic bone:
      1. Fusion or disruption of sacroiliac joints
      2. Porotic and radiodense lesion in the ilium along with whorls and trabeculation
      3. Thickening and sclerotic iliopectineal line—Brim sign
      4. Softening with protrusion acetabuli
      5. Axial migration of hips with functional flexion contracture

e. Radionuclide ^{99m}Tc bone scan demonstrate can identify the bony lesion.
f. MRI: It can demonstrate:
 1. Sarcoma
 2. Giant cell tumor
 3. Metastatic disease

B. Biochemical evaluation: Parallel rise of bone markers for bone resorption and bone formation will confirm both bone formation and bone resorption.
 a. Measurement of serum alkaline phosphatase is required for diagnosis and assessing the response to therapy. Progression of bony lesion is associated with bone-specific alkaline phosphatase.
 b. Serum osteocalcin, marker of bone formation is not useful for the diagnosis and management of Paget's disease.
 c. Bone formation marker P1NP reflects the activity of the disease
 d. Serum or urine N-telopeptide or C-telopeptide are elevated in Paget's disease.
 e. Serum calcium and phosphate are normal in Paget's disease, but hypocalcemia with mild hyperparathyroidism may occur in case of active bone formation and insufficient intake of vitamin D particularly when patient is under bisphosphonate therapy suppressing bone resorption.

Treatment

It is initiated to control the metabolically active Paget's bone disease such as:

a. Bone fracture
b. Bone pain
c. Headache
d. Pain from pagetic radiculopathy
e. Pagetic arthropathy
f. Neurologic complications
g. To decrease local blood flow
h. To minimize operative blood loss in patients who need surgery
i. To reduce hypercalciuria occurring during immobilization
j. During the highly active disease to reduce complications

Drugs	Dose with mode of administration
Zoledronic acid	5 mg intravenously over 15 minutes
Pamidronate	30 mg/day intravenously on 3 days
Risedronate	30 mg/day orally for 2 months
Alendronate	40 mg/day orally for 6 months
Tiludronate	800 mg/day orally for 3 months
Etidronate	200–400 mg/day for 6 months
Calcitonin	100 unit/day subcutaneously for 6–18 months

Q11. Polymyositis.

MGR/SEP2009/MDIII (6)

ANSWER

Definitions

It is idiopathic inflammatory myopathy characterized by the following features:

a. Proximal symmetrical muscle weakness
b. Raised skeletal muscle enzyme levels
c. Characteristic electromyographic and muscle biopsy findings

Pathophysiology

Pathogenesis is mainly T cell-mediated cytotoxicity against unidentified muscle antigens. There is accumulation of CD8 T cells along with macrophages around the healthy nonnecrotic muscle fibers leading to eventual necrosis of them. Following factors are responsible for T cell-mediated reaction:

a. Virus—human retroviruses, human immuno-deficiency viruses and human T-lymphotropic virus type 1 (HTLV-1), simian retrovirus and Coxsackie virus B, influenza, echovirus, and adenovirus.
 These viruses invade muscle tissue, damage the vascular endothelium leading to release of cytokines which in turn induces abnormal expression of major histocompatibility complex (MHC) making the muscle fibers to destruction.
b. Autoantibodies to nuclear and cytoplasmic antigens are detected in 60–80% of patients. Some autoantibodies are shared by other autoimmune diseases. It is called myositis associated antibodies.

c. Some are unique to myositis—called myositis-specific antibodies. It includes three groups of proteins:
   1. Aminoacyl transfer RNA synthetase—anti-jo-1
   2. Nuclear Mi-2 protein
   3. Components of signal recognition particle (SRP)

Clinical Features

A. Insidious onset of symmetrical bilateral proximal muscle weakness
B. Pain is not a predominant symptoms
C. Associated arthralgia
D. In case of involvement of esophageal and pharyngeal muscles producing dysphagia and aspiration.
E. Difficulty in climbing, kneeling, and descending stairs
F. Difficulty in holding the head up due to weakness of head extensors
G. Involvement of pelvic girdle muscles
H. Cardiac muscle involvement producing pericarditis and cardiomyopathy
I. Ocular muscles are never involved, facial and bulbar muscle weaknesses are extremely rare.
J. Constitutional symptoms are fatigue, weakness, anorexia, morning stiffness, and weight loss.

Laboratory Investigations

A. Hematological findings:
   a. Complete blood count: Leukocytosis, thrombocytosis
   b. Raised ESR
   c. Raised muscle enzymes: CPK and aldolase, serum glutamate oxalate transaminase (SGOT), lactate dehydrogenase (LDH)
   d. Autoantibodies
   e. Rheumatoid factor—positive in 50% of patients
B. Urine for myoglobinuria
C. Radiological investigations:
   a. Chest X-ray
   b. CT scan
   c. MRI
   d. Pelvic ultrasonography
   e. Mammography
D. Other studies:
   a. Pulmonary function test
   b. Upper and lower gastrointestinal endoscopy
   c. ECG
   d. Echocardiography
   e. Swallowing study

Complications

a. Aspiration pneumonia
b. Interstitial lung disease
c. Pneumonia
d. Arrhythmias
e. Heart block
f. Pericarditis
g. Myocardial infarction
h. Congestive heart failure
i. Malabsorption
j. Infection
k. Breast and lung carcinoma
l. Steroid myopathy

Treatment

A. Corticosteroid is the drug of choice. The dose is 1 mg/kg/day for 4–8 weeks until the normalization of CPK level, then it should be tapered by 5–10 mg monthly until the lowest dose which can control the disease.
B. Immunosuppressants: These drugs should be used who is unable to get benefit with steroid with 4 weeks or there is steroid induced adverse effect. Patients with dysphagia and dysphonia should be started with these drugs. Methotrexate is the second line of choice. Azathioprine, cyclophosphamide or cyclosporine can be administered with varying success.

Drugs	Route	Dose	Adverse effect	Monitor
Azathioprine	Orally	2–3 mg/kg/day	• Hepatotoxicity • Pancreatitis • Infection • Neoplasia • Flu-like illness • Teratogenicity	LFT, CBC
Methotrexate	Orally	7.5–20 mg weekly	• Pulmonary fibrosis • Hepatotoxicity • Leukopenia • Gastric irritation • Infection • Infertility	CBC, LFT
Cyclophosphamide	Orally	1.5–2 mg/kg/day for 6–12 months	• Bone marrow suppression • Hemorrhagic cystitis • Teratogenicity • Infertility • Infection	Urine analysis CBC
Cyclosporine	Orally	4–6 mg/kg/day in divided doses	• Nephrotoxicity • Hypertension • Infection • Hepatotoxicity • Hirsutism • Gum hyperplasia	• LFT, blood pressure, Creatinine • Urea • Cyclosporine level
Tacrolimus	Orally	0.1–0.2 mg/kg/day in two divided doses	• Nephrotoxicity • Hypertension • Infection • Teratogenicity • Hepatotoxicity • Hirsutism • Gum hyperplasia	• LFT, blood pressure, Creatinine • Urea • Tacrolimus level
Mycophenolate mofetil	Orally	1–1.5 g twice daily	• Bone marrow depression, tremor, diarrhea, vomiting, confusion, amblyopia • Teratogenicity • Infection	CBC
Intravenous immunoglobulin	Intravenously	2 g/kg over 2–5 days followed by 1 g/kg every 4–8 weeks as required	• Arrhythmias • Hypotension • Nephrotoxicity • Anaphylaxis • Stroke • Aseptic meningitis	• Heart rate • Blood pressure • Serum creatinine • Urea
Rituximab	Intravenously	• 750 mg/m^2 up to 1 g repeated in 2 weeks • It can be repeated every 6–18 months	• Infusion reaction • Infection • Progressive multifocal leukoencephalopathy	Checking of B cell count prior to next dose

(CBC: complete blood count; LFT: liver function test)

Q12. Discuss the pathogenesis, clinical manifestations, pathology, and management of systemic lupus erythematosus (SLE).

MGR/SEP2009/MDII (20)

Systemic manifestations of SLE.

MGR/MAR2006/MDI (5)

Describe the pathogenesis, pathology, clinical features, and treatment of SLE.

MGR/MAR2002/MDII (25)

Complications of SLE.

GMC/2015/MDII (10)

Current status of biologicals in SLE.

KUHS/MAY2013/MDIV (10)

Describe diagnosis and management of SLE.

ERA/MAY2012/MDII (10)

What are the various autoantibodies that can be detected in systemic lupus erythematosus? Enumerate their target antigens and clinical significance. SLICC criteria for classification of SLE?

DNB 2020 (10)

Diagnosis, hematological, cutaneous, and renal manifestations of systemic lupus erythematosus.

DNB 2019 (10)

SLICC classification of systemic lupus erythematosus.

DNB 2018(4)

Management of systemic lupus erythematosus.

Kerala UNI, 2022 (10)

Describe etiopathogenesis, clinical pictures, diagnosis and management of SLE.

Veer Narmad South Gujarat UNI, 2021 (20)

Serological tests for systemic lupus erythematosus.

MGR University, Tamil Nadu, 2020 (5)

Describe the emergencies in SLE.

WBUHS, 2023 (10)

Mention the emergencies in SLE and management.

WBUHS, 2020 (10)

Discuss the autoantibodies present in SLE. What are its cutaneous manifestations?

WBUHS, 2024 (10)

ANSWER

Definition

Systemic lupus erythematosus is an autoimmune disease characterized by autoimmune antibody-mediated tissue destruction leading to dysfunction of organ system in the body.

Pathogenesis

Ribonucleic acid, DNA, and proteins of different cells bind to toll-like receptors leading to activation of autoimmunity production innate immunity, such as

a. Dendritic cells produce interferon-α
b. Macrophages produce inflammatory cytokine/ chemokines, i.e., TNF-α, interleukin-12
c. B-cell maturation/survival factor

Neutrophil releasing DNA/protein containing nets and natural killer cells are unable to:

a. Kill autoreactive T and B cells
b. Produce TGF-β to develop regulatory T cells

Interferons upregulate genes which become "genetic signature" in peripheral blood cells.

Innate immunity interacts with T and B cells of adaptive immunity to further drive the autoimmune response, as result T cell develops:

a. Altered metabolism
b. Increased utilization of glucose
c. Increased production of pyruvate
d. Activation of mammalian target of rapamycin (mTOR)
e. Increased autophagy

T and B cells being activated to produce auto-antibodies that bind to the antigen presenting cells leading to apoptosis of cells and abnormal signaling after engagement of the surface molecules leading lowered production of IL-2 which is required for survival of T cells. B cells on the other hand present antigen and secretes IL-6 and IL-10 which promote survival of B cells.

Lupus phagocytic cells are unable to clear immune complexes, DNA/RNA/Ro/La and apoptotic cells and phospholipid containing surface blebs resulting in:

- **a.** Production of large quantities of autoantigens leading to production of large quantities of autoantibodies
- **b.** Increased production of activated B cells, plasmablast/plasma cells
- **c.** Autoreactive T cells with shift toward increased number and function of Th1, T17, and Tfh cells all of which are able to produce autoantibodies leading to tissue damage.

Deposition of immune-complexes and/or autoantibodies in the tissues followed by activation of complement pathways leading release of large amount of proinflammatory cytokines/chemokines. At the same time, nonimmune tissue fixed-cells are also activated to more and more inflammation and damage the following cells:

- **a.** Basal cells in the dermis
- **b.** Mesangial cells, podocytes, and tubular epithelium in kidney
- **c.** Synovial fibroblasts in the joint cavity
- **d.** Endothelial cells throughout the body

Initial immune attack will attract following cells in the affected tissue:

- **a.** T and B cells
- **b.** Monocytes/macrophages
- **c.** Plasma cells
- **d.** Dendritic cells

Following mediators are also released to produce sclerosis and fibrosis with irreversible tissue damage in multiple organs:

- **a.** Fibroblastic growth factor
- **b.** Vasoactive peptides
- **c.** Oxidative damage growth factors

As a result, following tissues are damaged:

- **a.** Kidney
- **b.** Skin
- **c.** Joints
- **d.** Lung
- **e.** Blood vessels

All the above processes require following factor interaction:

- **a.** Genetic factors
- **b.** Environmental factors
- **c.** Epigenetics

Systemic lupus erythematosus is a multigenic disease, but rare monogenic deficiencies are responsible for SLE:

- **a.** Early complement components such as C1q, C1r, C1s, C2, and C4
- **b.** Mutation of TREX1 on the X chromosome

A. Genetic factors:

- **a.** Each of normal alleles of multiple genes contributes a small amount of inflammation and immune-mediated destruction of the tissue leading to expression of the full-blown disease. According to recent genomic analysis, nearly 60 genes with alleles are associated with increased risk of this disease.
- **b.** In multiple ethnic groups antigen presenting HLA molecules (DRB1*0301, DRB1 *1501, DR3, DQA2) are present along with multiple genes across the MHC 120-gene region.
- **c.** Enhancing innate immunity, including production of interferons—TNFAIP3, IRF5/TNPO3, IRF7/PHRF1
- **d.** Alteration of adaptive immunity, B and T cell abnormal signaling—BANK1, STAT4, MSHS
- **e.** Genes responsible for lupus nephritis: HLA-DR3, APOL1, STAT4, FCGR3A, ITGAM

B. Environmental factor:

- **a.** Exposure to ultraviolet rays increases the SLE flare by:
  1. Increasing apoptosis in the cells in the skin
  2. Altering the DNA or intracellular proteins to make them antigenic
- **b.** Lupus containing drugs—these will activate autoreactive T and B cells leading to increased production of autoantibody.
- **c.** Epstein–Barr virus infection triggers SLE in children and young adults. Amino acid sequence of this virus mimics RNA/protein antigen sequence on human spliceosomes and this leads to production of autoantibodies.
- **d.** Tobacco smoking
- **e.** Exposure to crystalline silica
- **f.** Drinking of glass glasses of wine
- **g.** African–European women

C. Epigenetics:

- **a.** Hypomethylation of DNA in CD+ 4 lymphocytes, B cells, and monocytes
- **b.** Modification of histones: Some increases expression in predisposing genes
- **c.** Expression of genes affected by microRNA

Pathology

A. In the skin:

a. In the affected skin:

1. Deposition of IgG in the dermoepidermal junction
2. Injury to basal keratinocytes
3. Inflammation is dominated by T lymphocytes in:
   - Dermoepidermal junction
   - Blood vessels
   - Dermal appendages

b. In clinically unaffected skin: There is deposition of Ig in the dermoepidermal junction.

These are not specific of SLE but suggestive of SLE.

B. Renal changes:

a. Class I: Minimal mesangial lupus nephritis:

1. Normal glomeruli in normal microscopy but by immunofluorescence mesangial immune deposits

b. Class II: Mesangial proliferative lupus nephritis:

1. Mesangial hypercellularity or expansion of mesangial matrix by light microscopy
2. By immunofluorescence isolated subepithelial or subendothelial deposits

c. Class III: Focal lupus nephritis:

1. Active or inactive focal or segmental or global or extracapillary or endocapillary glomerulonephritis, ≤50% glomeruli are involved.
   - Class III (A): Active lesion—focal proliferative lupus nephritis
   - Class III (A/C): Active and chronic lesions—focal proliferative and sclerosing lupus nephritis.
   - Class III (C): Chronic inactive lesions along with glomerular scar—focal sclerosing lupus nephritis.

d. Class IV: Diffuse lupus nephritis:

1. Active or inactive focal or segmental or global or extracapillary or endocapillary glomerulonephritis, ≥50% glomeruli are involved.
   - Class IV-S (A): Active lesions—diffuse segmental proliferative lupus nephritis
   - Class IV-G (A): Active—diffuse global proliferative lupus nephritis
   - Class IV-S (A/C): Both active and chronic lesions—diffuse segmental proliferative and sclerosing lupus nephritis
   - Class IV-G (A/C): Both active and chronic lesions—diffuse global proliferative and sclerosing lupus nephritis
   - Class IV-S (C): Chronic inactive lesions with scar—Diffuse segmental sclerosing lupus nephritis.
   - Class IV-G (C): Chronic scars with inactive lesions—diffuse global sclerosing lupus nephritis

e. Class V: Membranous lupus nephritis: Global or segmental subepithelial deposits of immune complexes in immunofluorescent microscopy. It shows advanced sclerosis.

f. Class VI: Advanced sclerotic lupus nephritis: Here ≥90% glomeruli are sclerosed without any residual activity.

C. Blood vessels: Evidence of inflammation in the vascular endothelium

Diagnostic criteria of SLE:

Clinical manifestations	Immunological manifestations
Skin: • Acute, subacute cutaneous LE (photosensitive, malar, maculopapular, bulbous) • Chronic cutaneous LE (discoid lupus, panniculitis, lichen planus-like, hypertrophic verrucous, chilblains)	ANA > reference negative value
Oral or nasal ulcers	Anti-dsDNA > reference, if by ELISA 2X reference
Nonscarring alopecia	Anti-smooth muscle cell antibody
Synovitis involving ≥2 joints	Antiphospholipid: • Any of lupus anticoagulant, false-positive RPR, • Anticardiolipin antibody • Anti-β glycoprotein I antibody • Low complement C3, C4, and CH50 • Positive direct Coombs test in absence of hemolytic anemia
Serositis (pleuritis, pericarditis)	
Renal: • Protein/creatinine ≥0.5 • RBC cast • Biopsy	

Continued

Continued

Clinical manifestations	Immunological manifestations
Neurologic: • Seizures • Psychosis • Mononeuritis • Myelitis • Peripheral or cranial neuropathies • Acute confusional state	
Hemolytic anemia	
Leukopenia <4,000/cc Or Lymphopenia <1,000/cc	
Thrombocytopenia	
Presence of any four criteria (must have at least 1 in each category—indicates SLE with 93% specificity and 92% sensitivity	

(ANA: antinuclear antibodies; dsDNA: anti-double stranded DNA; ELISA: enzyme-linked immunoassay; LE: lupus erythematosus; SLE: systemic lupus erythematosus)

Clinical Features

A. Musculoskeletal manifestations:

- **a.** Arthralgia—in 90% of patients
- **b.** Polyarticular symmetrical arthritis involving hands and feet
- **c.** Synovitis—mild to moderate with minimal effusion
- **d.** Rhupus—a few patients may present with erosive symmetrical arthritis similar to RA
- **e.** Avascular necrosis of hip and shoulder—may be due to:
  1. Antiphospholipid syndrome
  2. Prolonged steroid therapy
  3. Prolonged immobilization
- **f.** Osteoporosis—may occur due to:
  1. Disease activity
  2. Prolonged steroid therapy
- **g.** Tenosynovitis or tendon rupture
- **h.** Myalgia or proximal weakness of muscles—it may be due to:
  1. Steroid therapy
  2. Chloroquine therapy
  3. Myasthenia-like syndrome

B. Mucocutaneous manifestations:

- **a.** Specific skin lesion shows features of interface dermatitis.
  1. Butterfly photosensitive raised scaly erythematous rash involving cheeks, bridge of the nose
  2. Rash involving chin, V region in the neck, chest, upper back, and extensor surface of arms
- **b.** Discoid lupus: It is characterized by roughly circular, scaly hyperpigmented slightly raised erythematous rim with depigmented scaly center where dermal appendages are destroyed, it may be disfiguring. 5% of discoid lupus erythematosus (DLE) may develop SLE.
- **c.** In the scalp—scarring or nonscarring alopecia
- **d.** Subacute cutaneous lupus erythematosus—photosensitive nonindurated nonscarring papulosquamous or annular psoriasis like lesion
- **e.** Raynaud's phenomenon—uncommon
- **f.** Diffuse hyperpigmentation or diffuse maculopapular rash
- **g.** Other lesions are:
  1. Planus-like dermatitis
  2. Bullae
  3. Panniculitis—also known as lupus profundus

C. Neurological manifestations:

- **a.** Central nervous system manifestations:
  1. Cerebrovascular disease
  2. Cognitive dysfunction
  3. Demyelinating syndrome
  4. Septic meningitis
  5. Headache
  6. Myelopathy
  7. Seizure disorder
  8. Psychosis
  9. Acute confusional state
- **b.** Peripheral nervous system:
  1. Autonomic disorders
  2. Acute demyelinating polyradiculopathy
  3. Single mononeuropathy
  4. Mononeuropathy multiplex
  5. Myasthenia gravis
  6. Plexopathy
  7. Polyneuropathy
  8. Cranial neuropathy

D. Renal manifestations:

- **a.** Asymptomatic in most of the cases
- **b.** In class II and IV nephritis: Asymptomatic proteinuria >500 mg/24 hours

c. One half develops nephrotic syndrome
d. Mostly develop hypertension
e. Stage V and VI nephritis develop end-stage renal failure
f. Renal biopsy indicated in case of following:
   1. Increasing serum creatinine without compelling alternative causes
   2. Confirmed proteinuria ≥1 g/24 hours
   3. Proteinuria >0.5 g/day plus hematuria
   4. Proteinuria >0.5 g/day plus cellular casts

E. Pulmonary manifestations:
   a. Pleurisy with or without effusion
   b. Pulmonary infiltrate
   c. Interstitial pneumonia leading to fibrosis
   d. Intra-alveolar hemorrhage
   e. Pulmonary tuberculosis—infiltrative or cavitary type present in case of immunosuppression
   f. Shrinking lung syndrome presenting with dyspnea on exertion
   g. Pulmonary hypertension

F. Cardiac involvement:
   a. Pericarditis—most common
   b. Pericardial effusion may lead to pericardial tamponade
   c. Myocarditis
   d. Libman–Sacks endocarditis involving mitral and aortic valves
   e. Heart failure
   f. Cardiac arrhythmia
   g. Embolic manifestation
   h. Accelerated atherosclerosis

G. Gastrointestinal manifestations
   a. Diffuse abdominal pain
   b. Nausea, vomiting, and diarrhea
   c. Subclinical liver dysfunction
   d. Acute pancreatitis
   e. Mesenteric vasculitis leading to intestinal ischemia, bleeding, or perforation

H. Ocular manifestations:
   a. Nonspecific conjunctivitis
   b. Sicca syndrome
   c. Retinal vasculitis
   d. Optic neuritis—threatening vision
   e. Cataract
   f. Glaucoma

   Last two are complications of systemic and intraorbital glucocorticoid.

I. Antiphospholipid syndrome: 20% of case with SLE develops this syndrome.
   a. Systemic vascular thrombosis
   b. Recurrent abortion
   c. Livedo reticularis
   d. Thrombocytopenia
   e. Seizures
   f. Ischemic central nervous system disease

Diagnosis

A. Tests for autoantibodies:
   a. Antinuclear antibodies are present in 95% of patients.
   b. In case of ANA negative lupus, there may be presence of other autoantibodies—anti-Ro and anti-DNA antibodies.
   c. Antibodies to anti-Sm antibodies though assist in the diagnosis of SLE, but it does not correlate with disease activity.
   d. There are three different tests that measure three different antibodies:
      1. ELISA test for anticardiolipin antibody
      2. ELISA test for anti-β_2 glycoprotein antibody
      3. Russell venom test to identify lupus anti-coagulant

   Higher the titer of anticardiolipin antibody >40 IU along with the greater number of different antiphospholipid antibodies, there is greater risk of clotting.

   e. Other autoantibodies having higher predictive value:
      1. Anti-Ro/Anti-SS-A, it will increase the risk of:
         - Neonatal lupus
         - Sicca syndrome
         - SLCE

B. Hematological tests:
   a. Chronic anemia
   b. Leukopenia <4,000/cc
   c. Lymphopenia <1,500/cc
   d. Thrombocytopenia <100,000/cc

C. Following tests to detect the course of the disease:
   a. Following tests can detect the organ involvement:
      1. Urine for hematuria an proteinuria
      2. Platelet count
      3. Hemoglobin
      4. Serum albumin
      5. Serum creatinine

b. Following tests are done to detect the disease activity:

1. Anti-DNA antibody
2. Anti-C1q antibody
3. Several component of complement
4. Activated complement product—it can measure the binding to the C4d receptor on the RBC and B cells.
5. IFN-inducible gene expression in the peripheral blood cells
6. Serum level of BLyS (B lymphocyte stimulator)
7. Urinary level of TNF-like weak inducer of apoptosis (TWEAK)
8. Neutrophil gelatinase-associated lipocalin
9. Monocyte chemotactic protein-1

Treatment

Medicines	Dose	Adverse effects
Topical steroids	Mid-potency for the face	• Contact dermatitis • Skin atrophy • Folliculitis • Hyperpigmentation • Infection
Topical sunscreens Hydroxychloroquine	200–400 mg four times daily	• Renal damage • Aplastic anemia, thrombocytosis • Ataxia • Cardiomyopathy • Peripheral neuropathy • Pigmentation of skin
Dehydroepiandrosterone	200 mg four times daily	• Acne • Menstrual irregularities • High serum level of testosterone
Methotrexate	10–25 mg weekly with daily administration of folic acid daily except the day when methotrexate will be given. Dose should be reduced if creatinine clearance <60 mL/min	• Anemia • Bone marrow suppression • Hepatotoxicity • Nephrotoxicity • Pulmonary fibrosis • Pneumonia • Seizures
Oral steroids	For severe SLE: • 0.5–1 mg/kg/day For mild case: • 0.3 mg/kg/day	• Infection • Hyperglycemia • Hypokalemia • Hypertension • Aseptic necrosis of femur • Cushingoid changes • Congestive heart failure • Menstrual irregularities
Methylprednisolone	0.5–1 g intravenously four times daily for 3 days	As above
Cyclophosphamide	Low dose: • 500 mg every 2 weeks for 6 weeks followed by maintenance by mycophenolate mofetil or azathioprine High dose: • 7–25 mg/kg twice monthly for 6 dose Orally: 1.5–3 mg/kg/day If creatinine clearance is <25 mL/min, dose should be reduced	• Infection • Bone marrow suppression • Hemorrhagic cystitis • Carcinoma of bladder • Alopecia • Nausea, vomiting • Ovarian and testicular failure
Mycophenolate mofetil	Orally 2–3 g/day in two divided doses as induction followed by 1–2 g/day in two divided dose for maintenance therapy If creatinine clearance is <25 mL/min, 1 g/day in two divided doses	• Infection • Aplastic anemia • Lymphoproliferative disorder • Malignancy • Gastrointestinal symptoms • Headache • Hypertension • Hypercholesterolemia • Liver function dysfunction • Tremor • Rash

Continued

Continued

Medicines	Dose	Adverse effects
Azathioprine	2–3 mg/kg/day orally for induction followed by 1–2 mg/kg/day for maintenance therapy	• Infection • Aplastic anemia • Lymphoproliferative disorder • Malignancy • Gastrointestinal symptoms • Headache • Hypertension • Hypercholesterolemia • Liver function dysfunction • Tremor • Rash
Belimumab	10 mg/kg intravenously at 0, 2, and 4 weeks followed by monthly Or 200 mg subcutaneously weekly	• Allergy • Infection • Infusion reaction • Headache
Rituximab	• 375 mg/m^2 weekly × 4 weeks • 1 g every 2 weeks × 2	• Allergy • Infection • Infusion reaction • Headache • Arrhythmias
Tacrolimus	2 mg twice daily to maintain blood level of 5.5 ng/mL	• Nephrotoxicity • Infection • Neural toxicity

SLICC Classifications of SLE

At least four criteria should be met with one clinical and one immunologic criterion or, biopsy proven lupus nephritis or presence of ANA or anti-DsDNA antibody.

Clinical Criteria

A. Acute cutaneous lupus
B. Chronic cutaneous lupus
C. Oral/nasal ulcer
D. Nonscarring alopecia
E. Synovitis
F. Serositis
G. Renal manifestation
H. Neurologic manifestation
I. Hemolytic anemia
J. Leukopenia
K. Thrombocytopenia

Immunologic Criteria

A. ANA above the normal reference range.
B. Anti-Ds DNA—above the normal reference range.
C. Anti-Sm—any level
D. Anti-phospholipid antibodies—
  a. Lupus anticoagulant
  b. Anti-cardiolipin antibodies IgA, IgG and IgM
  c. Low complement C3, C4 and CH50
  d. Positive direct Coombs test

Q13. Enumerate the various vasculitis syndromes and discuss the clinical features and management of polyarteritis nodosa (PAN).

MGR/APR2013/MDIV (15)

Classify vasculitis syndrome. Discuss the pathogenesis, clinical features, diagnosis, and treatment of granulomatosis with polyangiitis.

DNB 2021 (10)

Enumerate the various vasculitis syndrome and add a note on polyarteritis nodosa.

Kerala University, 2021 (10)

Classify various vasculitis syndrome and discuss the clinical features and management of polyarteritis nodosa.

MGR University, Tamil Nadu, 2022 (15)

Outline the approach to a case of vasculitis.

WBUHS, 2020 (10)

Classify vasculitis. Outline the approach to a case of vasculitis.

WBUHS, 2024 (10)

ANSWER

Last part has been described in question number 35 in pulmonology section.

Systemic vasculitis can be divided into two categories:

A. Primary vasculitis: It is characterized by inflammation of different types of primary blood vessels.
B. Secondary vasculitis: This condition is due to:
  a. Connective tissue disease
  b. Infection

c. Tumor
d. Drug allergy

Vessels	Disease	Types of arteries involved
Large vessel vasculitis	Takayasu arteritis Giant cell arteritis	• Vasculitis affecting large vessels: These are aorta and its branches • Any size may be affected
Medium vessels vasculitis	Polyarteritis nodosa Kawasaki disease	• Medium size blood vessels are affected involving visceral arteries and their branches • Any size of the arteries may be affected. • Inflammatory aneurysm and stenosis are common
Small vessel vasculitis		• Vasculitis affecting intraparenchymal arteries, arterioles, capillaries, and venules • Medium size arteries are affected
ANA-associated vasculitis	Microscopic polyangiitis Granulomatosis with polyangiitis Eosinophilic granulomatosis with polyangiitis	Necrotizing vasculitis predominantly affecting small and medium size blood vessels, i.e., small arteries, arterioles, capillaries, and venules. It is associated with myeloperoxidase ANCA and proteinase-3 ANCA but not in all the patients. So they are called MPO-ANCA, pr3-ANCA, and ANCA negative
Immune complex vasculitis	• Antiglomerular basement disease • Cryoglobulinemic vasculitis • Henoch–Schönlein purpura • Hypocomplementemic urticarial vasculitis	Vasculitis is associated with deposits of immune complexes and/or complement affecting predominantly small blood vessels. Glomerulonephritis frequently occurs

Continued

Continued

Vessels	Disease	Types of arteries involved
Variable vessel vasculitis	Behçet's syndrome Cogan syndrome	Vasculitis can affect any size of vessels (small, medial, and large) and any type (arteries, arterioles, capillaries, and venules)
Single organ vasculitis	Cutaneous leukoclastic vasculitis Cutaneous arteritis Primary central nervous system vasculitis Isolated aortitis Testicular arteritis	• Any type and any size of vessels are involved in one organ. Involved organ and type of vessels will be included in the name • Distribution of vasculitis is unifocal or multifocal in one organ • Some patient firstly identified as single organ vasculitis may develop additional manifestation later which redefines the disease. Cutaneous vasculitis can be turned into polyarteritis nodosa.
Vasculitis associated with systemic diseases	Lupus vasculitis Rheumatoid vasculitis Relapsing polychondritis	Vasculitis may be secondary to systemic diseases
Vasculitis associated with probable etiology	HEV associated Cryoglobulinemic vasculitis HBV-associated vasculitis Syphilitic aortitis Drug-associated immune complex-mediated vasculitis Drug–associated, ANCA-associated vasculitis Cancer associated vasculitis	Vasculitis is associated with etiology of the disease. Etiology should be prefixed

(ANA: antinuclear antibody; ANCA: antineutrophil cytoplasmic antibody; HBV: hepatitis B virus; HEV: hepatitis E virus; MPO: myeloperoxidase)

Clinical Features of Polyarteritis Nodosa

A. Constitutional features:
- **a.** Fever
- **b.** Fatigue
- **c.** Weight loss

B. Musculoskeletal features:
- **a.** Arthralgia
- **b.** Arthritis

C. Eye manifestations:
- **a.** Episcleritis
- **b.** Choroiditis
- **c.** Iritis
- **d.** Retinal vasculitis

D. Dermatological manifestations:
- **a.** Palpable purpura
- **b.** Necrotic purpura
- **c.** Subcutaneous nodules
- **d.** Digital ulcerations
- **e.** Digital infarction
- **f.** Digital gangrene

E. Renal manifestations:
- **a.** Hypertension—it may be malignant
- **b.** Renal impairment due to ischemic nephropathy
- **c.** Perineal hemorrhage
- **d.** Rupture of microaneurysm
- **e.** Intraperitoneal hemorrhage

F. Cardiac manifestations:
- **a.** Coronary arteritis
- **b.** Dissection aneurysm of aorta and other large arteries

G. Gastrointestinal manifestations:
- **a.** Ischemic vasculitis leading to hemorrhage or small bowel perforation
- **b.** Acute necrotizing pancreatitis

H. Central nervous system manifestations:
- **a.** Encephalopathy
- **b.** Seizures
- **c.** Stroke
- **d.** Subarachnoid hemorrhage
- **e.** Cranial nerve palsies

According to criteria of ACR:

A. Weight loss of ≥4 g

B. Livedo reticularis

C. Testicular pain/tenderness

D. Myalgia or leg weakness/tenderness

E. Mononeuropathy or polyneuropathy

F. Diastolic blood pressure >90 mm Hg

G. Elevated blood urea nitrogen >40 mg/dL or creatinine >1.5 mg/dL

H. Presence of HBsAg or antibody in the serum

I. Arteriogram demonstrating aneurysms or occlusions of the visceral arteries

J. Biopsy of small or medium-sized artery showing granulocytes and mononuclear leukocytes in the arterial wall

Three of above 10 criteria should be present to classify as polyarteritis nodosa (PAN).

Prognosis

In case of untreated patients: 5-year survival rate is 13%, 50% patients will in the first year.

If the patient is on steroid 5 years survival rate is 50–60%.

Death occurs due to the following cases:
- **a.** Uncontrolled vasculitis
- **b.** Infections related to immunosuppression
- **c.** Vascular complications:
  1. Myocardial infarction
  2. Stroke

Treatment

Five factors score can be used to predict survival and to guide decision for treatment guidelines:

Five factors parameters	5 years mortality rate	Treatment guidance
Proteinuria >1 g/ 24 hours	FFS: 12%	FFS 0: Steroids alone
Serum creatinine is 58 mg/dL	FFS: 25.9%	FFS ≥1: Induction Steroids + cyclophosphamide Maintenance: Steroid + azathioprine/ methotrexate
Gastrointestinal involvement	FFS: ≥2 (45.9%)	
Cardiomyopathy		
Central nervous system (CNS) involvement		

A. Intravenous methylprednisolone can be used in life-threatening conditions or severe dysfunctions of organs.

B. Orally prednisolone 1 mg/kg/day in divided doses to start with and after remission, it should be tapered gradually to stop after 12–18 months.

C. Cyclophosphamide in intravenous pulses—6 pulses at 600 mg/m^2—3 pulses fortnightly followed by three infusions at 3 weeks interval.

D. Maintenance therapy with methotrexate and azathioprine is recommended for 18 months.

HBV-PAN can be treated with the following drugs:

A. Antiviral therapy with entecavir or tenofovir

B. Plasma exchange—it will remove circulating immune complexes. It can be useful until seroconversion occurs.

C. Lower dose of steroids

Q14. Secondary vasculitis syndrome.

MGR/SEP2008/MDIV (6)

ANSWER

Secondary causes of vasculitis syndrome:

A. Inflammatory diseases of unknown etiology:
- **a.** Rheumatoid vasculitis
- **b.** Systemic lupus erythematosus
- **c.** Sjögren's syndrome
- **d.** Sarcoidosis
- **e.** Inflammatory bowel disease

B. Infectious diseases:
- **a.** Hepatitis B
- **b.** Hepatitis C
- **c.** Human immunodeficiency disease
- **d.** Mycobacteria
- **e.** Syphilis
- **f.** Infective endocarditis

C. Neoplasm:
- **a.** Myeloproliferative syndrome
- **b.** Lymphoproliferative syndrome
- **c.** Solid tumor

D. Drugs: Hydralazine, propylthiouracil, and montelukast

Following diseases mimic vasculitis:

A. Antiphospholipid syndrome

B. Thrombotic thrombocytopenic purpura (TTP)

C. Sickle cell disease

D. Embolization from atrial myxoma

E. Cholesterol emboli from atheroma

F. Noninflammatory disorders such as
- **a.** Scurvy
- **b.** Amyloidosis
- **c.** Fibrovascular dysplasia

In case of secondary vasculitis, features of different organ involvement are due to involvement of different size of blood vessels. Clinical features are the following:

Size of vessels involved	Blood vessels involved	Features
Small vessel vasculitis involving capillaries and venules	Cutaneous postcapillary venules	Palpable purpura
	Glomerular capillaries	• Hematuria • Proteinuria • Red cell casts in urine • Decline in renal function
	Pulmonary capillaries	Lung hemorrhages manifested by: • Cough • Hemoptysis • Breathlessness
Medium vessel vasculitis involving small- and medium-sized vessels	Small cutaneous arteries	• Necrotic lesions • Ulcer • Digital infarct • Nail fold infarct
	Epinural arteries	Mononeuritis multiplex
	Mesenteric artery	• Pain abdomen • Gastrointestinal bleeding • Perforation of gut
	Branches of celiac artery	• Spleen infarction • Pancreas infarction • Liver infarction
	Renal artery	Infarction in the kidney
	Coronary arteries	• Angina • Myocardial infarction • Aneurysm • Ischemic cardiomyopathy
	Pulmonary arteries	Cavitary shadow in the lung in the chest radiograph due to necrotic lesion in the lung
	Small arteries in the ear, nose, and throat	• Nasal crusting • Epistaxis • Sinusitis • Stridor • Deafness
Large vessel vasculitis involving aorta and its branches	Extracranial branches of carotid artery	• Temporal artery—headache • Ophthalmic artery—blindness • Vessels supplying the muscles of mastication—jaw claudication
	Thoracic aorta and its branches	• Absent pulses • Unequal blood pressure • Claudication of limb • Thoracic artery aneurysm

Underlying infection can change the treatment protocol of management of vasculitis because the etiology should be taken care of first followed by treatment of vasculitis.

Q15. Systemic mastocytosis.

MGR/SEP2008/MDIII (6)

ANSWER

Mastocytosis: It can be defined as clonal expansion of mast cells in the skin, gut, spleen, and liver. Mastocytosis can be classified into main two types:

A. Cutaneous mastocytosis

B. Systemic mastocytosis:

- **a.** Indolent systemic mastocytosis: It is diagnosed when there is no evidence of associated hematologic disorders, it is characterized by >30% bone marrow infiltrated by mast cells and baseline serum tryptase >200 ng/mL.
- **b.** Smoldering systemic mastocytosis
- **c.** Aggressive systemic mastocytosis: It is associated with mast cell infiltration in multiple organs such as gut, bone, liver, spleen, and bone marrow.
- **d.** Systemic mastocytosis with an associated clonal hematologic no-mast cell lineage disease
- **e.** Mast cell leukemia

B findings: Two or more in absence of C findings are required for diagnosis of systemic smoldering mastocytosis:

A. Mast cell infiltration in bone marrow biopsy >30% and basal serum level of tryptase is >200 ng/mL.

B. Hypercellular bone marrow with signs of dysmyelopoiesis but without cytopenias meeting C criteria or who criteria of myelodysplastic syndrome or myeloproliferative disorders.

C. Palpable hepatomegaly and splenomegaly or lymphadenopathy (on CT scan or ultrasound: >2 cm)

C findings (one or more required for diagnosis of aggressive systemic mastocytosis): C findings reasonably are attributable to high tissue infiltration of mast cells.

A. Cytopenia(s): Absolute neutrophil count <1,000/cc or hemoglobin <10 g/dL or platelet count <100,000/cc

B. Hepatomegaly with ascites and impaired liver function

C. Palpable splenomegaly associated with hypersplenism

D. Malabsorption with hypoalbuminemia and weight loss

E. Skeletal lesions: Large areas of osteolysis with pathological fractures (large areas of osteoporosis alone without osteolytic lesion does not fit the criterion.

Clinical Features

A. Systemic manifestations is different from leukemic complications due to:

- **a.** Release of bioactive substance acting on both local and distant sites
- **b.** Tissue occupancy by the mast cell mass
- **c.** Tissue response to mast cell mass

B. Pharmacologically induced manifestations are:

- **a.** Intermittent flushing
- **b.** Tachycardia
- **c.** Vascular collapse
- **d.** Gastric distress
- **e.** Lower abdominal cramping pain
- **f.** Diarrhea

C. Due to increased local burden of mast cells:

- **a.** Urticaria pigmentosa

D. Internal organ biopsies from bone marrow and gastrointestinal tract

E. Mast cell-induced fibrosis is present in liver, bone marrow, and spleen but never in skin and gastrointestinal tract.

F. Immunofluorescent analysis of bone marrow and skin in case of indolent systemic mastocytosis and from spleen and lymph nodes and skin in case of aggressive systemic mastocytosis revealed one mast cells phenotype like scroll-poor cells that expresses carboxypeptidase A (CPA), tryptase, and chymase.

Diagnostic Criteria

A. Major criteria:

- **a.** Multiple dense infiltrates of mast cells (>15 mast cells per aggregate) in the bone marrow or exracutaneous tissues

B. Minor criteria:

- **a.** Abnormal mast cells morphology (spindle shape, bi- or multilobed or eccentric nucleus, hypogranulated cytoplasm)
- **b.** Aberrant mast cell surface phenotype with expression of CD25 (interleukin-2 receptor α chain) and/or CD2
- **c.** Detection of codon 816 mutation in peripheral blood cells, bone marrow cells, or an exracutaneous lesional tissue
- **d.** Total serum tryptase >20 ng/mL

Treatment

Stepwise approach is required to treat systemic mastocytosis:

A. H1 antihistaminic drugs to treat flushing and pruritus
B. H2 antihistaminic or proton pump inhibitor (PPI) to treat gastric acid hypersecretion
C. Oral cromolyn sodium to treat diarrhea and abdominal pain
D. Aspirin for severe flushing with or without vascular collapse
E. Systemic steroids to treat malabsorption
F. Mast cell cytoprotective therapy: It consists of:
  a. Midostaurin—it is multikinase inhibitor having activity against D816V mutated and wild type kit—it approved for treatment of severe systemic mastocytosis. Its efficacy is restricted because of its dose limitations to prevent side effects.
  b. Cladribine or INF-α
G. Stem cell transplantation can be effective in small subsets of patients.
H. Self-injectable epinephrine is effective in case of increased incidence of anaphylaxis.
I. In patients with history of systemic hypometria venom reaction:
  a. Test should be done for venom specific IgE.
  b. These patients should be treated with lifelong venom immunotherapy.
J. Tyrosine kinase inhibitor inhibits D816V KIT mutation is under investigation.

Q16. Clinical features, diagnosis, and treatment of mixed connective tissue disease.
MGR/SEP2006/MDI (15)

Mixed connective tissue disorders.
MJPRU/2015/MDIII (6)

MCTD.
NTR UNI of Health SC, Vijayawada, Aug 2022 (10)

ANSWER

Definition

Mixed connective tissue disease (MCTD) is characterized by overlapping features of:

  a. SLE
  b. Scleroderma
  c. Polymyositis/dermatomyositis
  d. High serum titer of anti-U1RNP antibodies

Classification Criteria

According to Alarcon-Segovia criteria:

A. Serologic criteria:
  a. Anti-RNP at hemagglutination titer of >1: 1,600
B. Clinical criteria:
  a. Swollen hands
  b. Myositis
  c. Synovitis
  d. Raynaud's phenomenon
  e. Acrosclerosis

If A along with three or more clinical criteria among which one must be synovitis or myositis—diagnostic of MCTD

Etiopathogenesis:

A. There is genetic association with major histocompatibility gene—HLA-DRB1*04/*15.
B. Innate immunity acts through TLR7 and TLR3.
C. Adaptive immunity: It involves B cells production leads to formation of anti-U1RNP. Small nuclear ribonucleoprotein (SnRNP) is made up of 5 small RNA (smRNA) molecules—U1, U2, U4, U6, and U7. They are all uridine rich. U1RNP resides on p70 protein, hence antibody to p70 is associated with anti-RNP specificity.

Clinical Features

A. Skin:
  a. Raynaud's phenomenon—it is characterized by initial pallor during exposure to cold (white color), followed by cyanosis (blue color) due to depletion of oxygen supply, this is followed by rubor (red color) of the skin during normalization of blood supply and the area becomes warm and lastly skin color becomes normal. It is accompanied by puffy fingers and edema of the hands.
  b. Sclerodactyly
  c. Digital infarction
  d. Digital ulceration
  e. Photosensitive skin rash
  f. Telangiectasia over the face
  g. Heliotrope rash
  h. Gottron's papule
B. Joint:
  a. In 90% cases, arthralgia or nonerosive symmetrical arthritis of hands and wrists. At the rate 5% patients are rheumatoid factor positive.
  b. Jaccouds arthropathy.

C. Muscles:

a. Myositis is infrequent at onset of MCTD, but during follow-up muscle discomfort with elevated CPK. It is less severe than in dermatomyositis.

b. Myalgia

D. Fever

E. Cardiac involvement:

a. Pericarditis is the most common presentation

b. Cardiac tamponade is rare.

F. Lung involvement:

a. Pulmonary hypertension:

1. Primary pulmonary hypertension

2. Secondary pulmonary hypertension due to interstitial lung disease. In 2D echocardiography, right ventricular pressure should be measured. By cardiac catheterization if the right ventricular systolic pressure is >25 mm Hg.

b. Interstitial lung disease: In HRCT, it can be diagnosed as septal thickening, ground glass opacities.

c. Pleuritis

d. Pulmonary hemorrhage

G. Gut:

a. Esophageal reflux presenting with dysphagia, odynophagia, and regurgitation of food

b. Bacterial overgrowth

c. Malabsorption syndrome

d. In patients with positive for anti-SSA antibody, there is evidence of sicca syndrome.

e. Enlargement of submandibular gland

H. Nervous system:

a. Trigeminal neuralgia

b. Sensorineural deafness

c. Psychosis

d. Meningitis

e. Stroke

f. Seizures

g. Transverse myelitis

h. Cauda equina syndrome

i. Cerebral hemorrhage

I. Kidney:

a. Patients present with anti-dsDNA antibodies may have membranoproliferative glomerulonephritis.

b. Membranous nephropathy

c. Interstitial nephritis in patient with Sjögren's syndrome

d. Scleroderma renal crisis

Management

Clinical features	Mild	Moderate to severe
Arthralgia/ arthritis	• NSAIDs • Hydroxychloro-quine	• Systemic corticosteroids • Rituximab
Raynaud's phenomenon	• Minimize the cold exposure • Protective gloves • Avoidance of trauma • Avoidance of β-blockers • Cessation of smoking	• Calcium channel blockers • Local nitrate • Analog of prostaglandin—iloprost • PDE5 inhibitors • Anticoagulation for digital gangrene
Rash	• Avoidance of exposure to sun • Hydroxychloro-quine • Topical steroids	• Systemic steroids • Azathioprine • Methotrexate
Esophageal reflux	• Elevation of head during sleeping • Avoid smoking and caffeine	• Administration of PPI • H2 receptor antagonists
Myositis	• Steroids • Hydroxychloro-quine	• Steroids • Azathioprine • Methotrexate • Intravenous immunoglobulin
Pulmonary hypertension	Prostaglandin E5 inhibitors	• Calcium channel blocker • PGDE5 inhibitors • Cyclophosphamide • Endothelin receptor antagonists—bosentan, ambrisentan
Pleuritis/ pericarditis	• Steroids • NSAIDs	• NSAIDs • Steroids • Azathioprine

(PDE5: phosphodiesterase-5; PPI: proton pump inhibitor)

Q17. Felty's syndrome.

MGR/MAR2002/MDI (10)

ANSWER

Definition

This is a rare complication in patients with seropositive rheumatoid arthritis and is characterized by associated features of splenomegaly and neutropenia.

Etiopathogenesis

- **A.** High titer of rheumatoid factor
- **B.** Long-standing rheumatoid disease
- **C.** Presence of HLA0DR4 in severe seropositive rheumatoid arthritis
- **D.** Aggressive and erosive synovitis
- **E.** Extra-articular manifestations of rheumatoid arthritis

Pathophysiology

In genetically predisposed individual, autoantibodies to histones and other components in the neutrophil bind to activated neutrophils, autoantibodies against granulocyte surface antigens which are sequestrated in the spleen and are destroyed.

Cytotoxic T lymphocytes also can destroy granulocytes.

Clinical Features

- **A.** It is most common in fifth through seventh decade of life with history of >10 years history of rheumatoid arthritis.
- **B.** Men are affected earlier than women in the course of rheumatoid arthritis and the ratio is 3 : 1 in women : men.
- **C.** More aggressive destructive arthritis
- **D.** History of extra-articular manifestations of rheumatoid arthritis such as:
  - **a.** Pericarditis
  - **b.** Rheumatoid nodules
  - **c.** Peripheral neuropathy
  - **d.** Eye involvement
  - **e.** Skin ulcer
- **E.** Presence of bacterial infections in the skin and respiratory tract
- **F.** Presence of left upper quadrant pain due to:
  - **a.** Splenic infarct
  - **b.** Stretching of the splenic capsule as a result of splenic enlargement
- **G.** Physical examinations:
  - **a.** Splenomegaly which may be nonpalpable
  - **b.** Mild hepatomegaly
  - **c.** Weight loss
  - **d.** Lymphadenopathy
  - **e.** Sjögren's syndrome
  - **f.** Articular findings in the involved joints:
    - **1.** Deformities of the joints
    - **2.** Joint swelling and tenderness.
  - **g.** Features of small vessel vasculitis:
    - **1.** Palpable purpura
    - **2.** Ulcers in the lower extremities
    - **3.** Brownish pigmentary changes in the lower extremities
    - **4.** Infarct in the periungual region
  - **h.** Features of systemic vasculitis:
    - **1.** Mononeuritis multiplex
    - **2.** Ischemia in the extremities
  - **i.** Other findings:
    - **1.** Peripheral neuropathy
    - **2.** Pleuritis
    - **3.** Episcleritis
    - **4.** Portal hypertension

Complications

- **A.** Splenic rupture
- **B.** Life-threatening infection
- **C.** Toxicities of immunosuppressive agents
- **D.** Upper gastrointestinal bleeding due to portal hypertension as a result of nodular regenerative hyperplasia

Laboratory Investigations

- **A.** Neutropenia, but there is chance of infection if the neutrophil count is <1,000/cc.
- **B.** Anemia—it may be due to chronic inflammatory disease.
- **C.** Thrombocytopenia
- **D.** ESR is invariably raised.
- **E.** Serum immunoglobulins are also raised.
- **F.** Mild elevation of transaminases and alkaline phosphatases
- **G.** Antinuclear antibodies and ANCAs are present in 65–80% of these patients.
- **H.** High titer of rheumatoid factor and anti-CCP antibodies are present in nearly 98% of patients.

I. Antihistone antibodies

J. Bone marrow demonstrates:

- **a.** Myeloid hyperplasia with relative immature form excess
- **b.** Adequate megakaryocytes
- **c.** Sometimes hypocellular marrow—suggestive of large granular lymphocyte (LGL) syndrome

Differential Diagnosis

A. SLE: Presence of the following differentiating features:

- **a.** Central nervous system disease
- **b.** Nephritis
- **c.** Photosensitive rash
- **d.** Laboratory features of:
  - **1.** Hemolytic anemia
  - **2.** Lymphopenia

B. Large granular lymphocyte syndrome: It has the following differentiating features:

- **a.** Increased proportion of LGL cells present in the peripheral smear, bone marrow, or biopsy.
- **b.** Immunophenotyping indicates presence of cytotoxic T cell lymphocyte population that expresses a set of surface markers.

Treatment

A. Methotrexate weekly along with folic acids daily to minimize the adverse effect of methotrexate is the drug of choice. Beneficial effect of methotrexate is not evident until 4–8 weeks of initiation of therapy. It has the following effects:

- **a.** It will improve both articular disease
- **b.** It improves neutropenia
- **c.** Frequency of infection will be decreased.

B. Alternatively leflunomide can be given.

C. Small proportion of patients may benefit from high-dose cyclophosphamide.

D. TNF-inhibitors: The drugs are etanercept, adalimumab, and infliximab. These drugs are very effective in rheumatoid arthritis but its effect in Felty's syndrome is limited.

E. Rituximab: It will improve in synovitis and neutropenia.

F. Glucocorticoids in moderate to high dose can be given as bridging therapy until the occurrence of full effect with DMARDs and biologicals.

G. In case of recurrent severe infection in presence of neutropenia of <1,000/cc: granulocyte colony-stimulating factor may be given as short-term use. As the neutropenia resolves this drug should be stopped but other treatment has to be continued.

H. Splenectomy: It is indicated in Felty's syndrome with recurrent or severe infection in spite of optimum medical treatment, but prophylactic splenectomy is not justified even in case of marked neutropenia because other causes of neutropenia has to be ruled out.

Result of splenectomy:

- **a.** Within minutes to hours neutrophil count will be increased in 80% cases of Felty's syndrome but in one-fourth cases it may recur but it will be above the presplenectomy level.
- **b.** Platelet count will be improved.
- **c.** Resolution of leg ulcer
- **d.** Improvement of esophageal varices

Q18. Juvenile rheumatoid arthritis.

MGR/MAR2006/MDIV (5)

SNMC/MAY2013/MDI (10)

ANSWER

Definition

Juvenile rheumatoid arthritis is characterized by arthritis before the 16th birthday and persisting for at least 6 weeks provided other conditions are excluded.

Classifications

According to International League of Association of Rheumatology:

Category	Definition
Oligoarthritis affecting ≤4 joints	1–4 joints are involved in first 6 months of the disease
Rheumatoid factor negative polyarthritis	≥5 joints are involved during 6 months of life
	Rheumatoid factor is negative.
Rheumatoid factor positive polyarthritis	≥5 joints are involved during 6 months of life
	≥2 positive rheumatoid factor tests at least 3 months apart during the 6 months of disease affection

Continued

Continued

Category	Definition
Psoriatic arthritis	Arthritis and psoriasis
	Arthritis and at least two of the following: • Dactylitis • Minimum two pits on one or more at a time • Onycholysis
	Psoriasis in first-degree relative
Enthesitis-related arthritis	Arthritis and enthesitis
	Arthritis or enthesitis and two of the following: • Positive HLA-B27 • Presence of/or history of sacroiliac joint tenderness and/or inflammatory lumbosacral pain • In male onset of arthritis >6 years of age • Acute symptomatic anterior uveitis • History of ankylosing spondylitis, enthesitis-related arthritis, sacroiliitis with inflammatory bowel disease, reactive arthritis, or acute anterior uveitis in first-degree relative
Systemic juvenile idiopathic arthritis	Arthritis involving one or more joints with/or preceded by daily documented fever for at least 2 weeks duration and quotidian (fever rises up to ≥39°C once in a day and returns to ≤37°C in-between the febrile episode) for at least 3 days which is accompanied by ≥1 of the following: • Nonfixed evanescent erythematous rash • Generalized enlargement of lymph nodes • Hepatomegaly and/or splenomegaly • Serositis
Undifferentiated arthritis	Arthritis fulfilling the criteria in no category or in ≤2 of the above categories

Pathogenesis

Two factors are responsible for juvenile rheumatoid arthritis:

A. Genetic factors: Monozygotic twins have 25–40% concordance rate in this disease and >100-fold risk as compared to general population. Genes involved in this juvenile idiopathic arthritis (JIA) has been subdivided into two categories:

a. HLA-related genes: *MHC* genes have strongest genetic association. There are two classes of *MHC* genes:

1. Class I *MHC* genes:
- There is strongest association of HLA-B27 with enthesitis-related arthritis.
- HLA-A2—A0261 is associated with oligoarticular JIA.
- HLAC*0202 is implicated in persistent JIA.

2. Class II *MHC* genes:
- DRB1*0801 and 11 are associated with oligoarticular JIA.
- Some alleles are associated with all form of arthritis.

b. Non-HLA-related genes: More than 100 genes are associated with JIA. Some of them are:

1. Chemokines

2. Cytokines—interleukin-2, interleukin-21, interleukin-2RA

3. Signaling molecules—PTPN22, STAT4, TNFAIP3, and TRAF1-C5

In India, most common are HLA-B27, of which two subtypes are HLAB*2705 and B*2704.

B. Environmental factor: In genetically predisposed individual following environmental factors are responsible for JIA through the modulation of immune system.

a. Breastfeeding: Here duration of breastfeeding is most important.

b. Infection: It is an important triggering factor. Early life infection will shape the immune system. Macrophage activation syndrome which is a complication of JIA may be precipitated by viral infections.

c. Gastrointestinal infection is linked to enthesitis-related arthritis.

d. Alteration of gut microbiota due to infection or administration of antibiotics may alter the immune system.

e. Streptococcal infection may be responsible for reactive arthritis.

Complex interactions between the genetic and environmental factors lead to development of persistent immune inflammation state by two mechanisms:

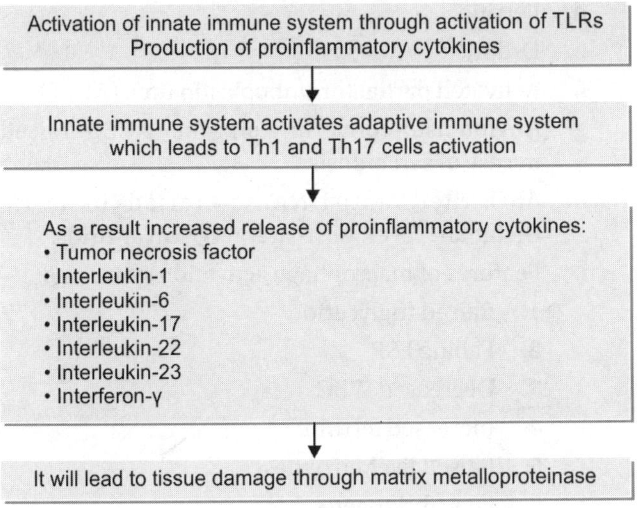

Activation of innate immune system through activation of TLRs
Production of proinflammatory cytokines

↓

Innate immune system activates adaptive immune system which leads to Th1 and Th17 cells activation

↓

As a result increased release of proinflammatory cytokines:
- Tumor necrosis factor
- Interleukin-1
- Interleukin-6
- Interleukin-17
- Interleukin-22
- Interleukin-23
- Interferon-γ

↓

It will lead to tissue damage through matrix metalloproteinase

Clinical Features

A. Articular manifestations:

a. Presence of cardinal signs of inflammation in the joints, these are:

1. Swelling: It occurs due to:
- Edema of the periarticular soft tissue
- Intra-articular effusion
- Hypertrophy of the synovial membrane
- Large joint cyst—called Baker cyst

2. Raised temperature

3. Pain in the joint

4. Redness of the joint

b. Morning stiffness: Though it is common but young children may not complain of this symptom.

c. Joint distribution: It is classified into two types:

1. Oligoarticular variety: Knee joints are most commonly affected followed by ankle joints, but hips and small joints of hands and feet are rarely affected. It is usually asymmetrical large joint arthritis mainly in female associated with positive ANA and asymptomatic anterior uveitis.

2. Polyarticular variety: It usually involves five or more joints in first 6 months of disease. It is symmetrical involving large and small joints of hands and feet, also involving axial skeleton and temporomandibular joints. These are of the following types:
- Rheumatoid factor positive arthritis
- Rheumatoid factor negative arthritis

These are more common in females than males.

- Enthesitis-related arthritis involving joints involving lower extremities and sacroiliac joints
- Psoriatic arthritis: It is asymmetrical involving both large and small joints mainly distal interphalangeal joints.
- In case of children, cervical, thoracic, and lumbar spines are involved along with impaction or subluxation of anterior atlantoaxial joints.

d. Enthesitis: It is inflammation of the site of bones where tendon, ligament, or joint capsules are attached. Most common affected sites are:

1. Inferior pole of patella where patellar ligament is attached.

2. Calcaneus at the site of insertion of plantar fascia

3. Calcaneus at the site of insertion of tendo Achilles

4. Greater trochanter at the site of insertion of hip extensors

e. Dactylitis: It can be defined as diffuse swelling of the digit—hallmark features of spondyloarthropathies in psoriatic arthritis. It involves involving fingers and toes.

f. Tenosynovitis: It is most common in children with JIA. Most common sites of affection:

1. Extensor tendon sheaths on the dorsum of the hand

2. On the dorsum of the foot extensor sheath

3. Posterior tibial tendon

4. Peroneus longus and bravis tendons around the ankle

g. Constitutional symptoms: Anorexia and weight loss, sleep disturbances, and night pain leading to fatigue.

B. Extra-articular manifestations:

a. Classical systemic arthritis: Fever rises to 39°C daily or twice daily basis followed by return to baseline or below the baseline. In case of children, it typically presents in the late afternoon to evening along with rash.

b. Classical rash: Evanescent, discrete, circumscribed, and salmon-pink macular rash surrounded by ring of pallor or with central clearing present in the trunk, lower extremities, inguinal and axillary areas but also on face, palms, and soles.

c. Pericarditis: It may precede or during the time of arthritis. It may be asymptomatic or present with dyspnea or precordial pain.
d. Pneumonitis
e. Pleural effusion
f. Rheumatic nodules
g. Lymphadenopathy or splenomegaly alone or in combination
h. Hepatomegaly is less common.
i. Macrophage activation syndrome: It is rare but life-threatening syndrome characterized by the presence of histiophagocytosis in the bone marrow. Clinical features are fever, lymphadenopathy, hepatosplenomegaly, cytopenias, disseminated intravascular coagulation (DIC), and liver disease.
j. Growth abnormalities. There is linear growth retardation.

C. Uveitis: Chronic anterior nongranulomatous uveitis

Investigations

A. Inflammatory markers:
a. Raised ESR
b. Raised CRP
c. Thrombocytosis
d. Leukocytosis
e. Low hemoglobin
f. Low albumin

B. Metabolic panel:
a. Liver function test to exclude autoimmune hepatitis
b. Assessment of renal function prior to starting NSAIDs, methotrexate, TNF-α inhibitors

C. Serological testing:
a. Antinuclear antibody
b. Rheumatoid factor
c. Anti-CCP antibody

D. Additional testing:
a. Uric acid
b. LDH
c. Fibrinogen
d. Ferritin
e. D-dimer
f. Activated partial thromboplastin time (APTT)
g. Angiotensin-converting enzyme (ACE)—raised in case of sarcoidosis
h. ASO titer, anti-DNAase—raised in acute rheumatic fever, post-streptococcal arthritis.
i. Features of macrophage activation syndrome:
1. Raised triglyceride
2. Falling ESR
3. Decreased WBC
4. Increased ferritin
5. Raised liver enzymes
6. Low fibrinogen
7. Hemorrhages

E. Radiological investigations:
a. Joint demonstrate:
1. Soft tissue swelling
2. Joint space narrowing
3. Bony erosion
4. Intra-articular bony ankyloses
5. Epiphyseal compression fracture
6. Joint subluxation
7. Synovial cyst
b. MRI with intravenous gadolinium or CT scan demonstrate active synovitis in the inflamed joints

Treatment

Previously NSAIDs were used for the treatment of juvenile rheumatoid arthritis (JRA). Aspirin is not commonly used because of:
a. Frequent dosing
b. Greater frequency of abnormality of liver enzyme
c. Association with liver enzymes

Now a days:
A. Naproxen 20 mg/kg/day in divided doses is given.
B. Ibuprofen 40 mg/kg/day is given.
C. Indomethacin 1–3 mg/kg/day 3–4 times daily.

Drugs	Dose	Considerations
	DMARDs	
Hydroxychloroquine	400 mg once or twice daily	• Eye examination recommended yearly as there is chance of retinal toxicity • Gray-tone change in skin color

Continued

Continued

Drugs	Dose	Considerations
Methotrexate	15 mg/week up to 25 mg/week. Patient will responds within 3 months	• Higher dose well tolerated • Avoid concomitant sulfa, tetracycline • No live vaccination, avoid alcohol • Regular monitoring of WBC, hemoglobin, LFT, platelets every 10–12 weeks
Sulfasalazine	600 mg once or twice daily up to 3 g/day in divided doses	Side effects are nausea, skin rash, raised LFT, and cytopenias. Monitoring of LFT and CBC every 8 weeks
Leflunomide	5–20 mg/day	• Avoid pregnancy as it is teratogenic, diarrhea • LFT and CBC to be checked every 10–12 weeks
TNF inhibitors		
Etanercept (fully humanized)	0.8 mg/kg/dose SC weekly	Risk of tuberculosis
Infliximab (mouse chimeric)	3–6 mg/kg/dose IV at 0, 2, and 6 weeks and then every 8th week	Risk of tuberculosis is high
Adalimumab (fully humanized)	24 mg every 2 weeks	Risk of tuberculosis is very high
Anakinra (IL-1 receptor antagonist, human recombinant form)	1–2 mg/kg/day SC	Very effective in systemic JRA
Tocilizumab (genetically engineered humanized monoclonal antibody against IL-6 receptor)	12 mg/kg in <30 kg and 8 mg/kg in >30 kg children	
Abatacept—it blocks costimulatory interaction between T and B cells	10 mg/kg IV at 0, 2, and 4 weeks followed by every 4th week up to maximum 1,000 mg/dose	Long-term study is required
Stem cell transplantation: Autologous stem cell transplantation can be done in case of severe autoimmune disease which refractory to conventional therapy.		

(CBC: complete blood count; JRA: juvenile rheumatoid arthritis; LFT: liver function test; TNF: tumor necrosis factor)

Q19. Discuss the pathogenic mechanisms of vessel damage in vasculitis syndrome. Outline the diagnosis and clinical features of small vessel vasculitis.

MGR/MAR2007/MDIV (20)

ANCA Small vessel vasculitis.

NTR UNI of Health SC Vijayawada, Andhra, 2022 (10)

ANSWER

All most all the subjects are exposed to a number of stimuli, but a subsets of patients develop vasculitis but other do not. A number of factors are responsible for vasculitic syndrome, these are:

- **a.** Genetic predisposition
- **b.** Environmental factor
- **c.** Regulatory mechanisms associated with immune response to a variety of antigens.

Following three hypothesized mechanism for vasculitis syndrome:

- **A.** Immune complex formation: It is the most widely accepted pathogenic mechanism for vasculitis syndrome, but the role of immune-complexes is not established in most of the syndrome. In this vasculitis, there is no need of deposition of immune-complexes in the wall of the blood vessels and there is no demonstrable immune-complexes in the circulation or in the wall of blood vessels. Actual antigen is rarely identified in the immune complexes:
  - **a.** In case of polyarteritis nodosa in the immune complexes hepatitis B antigen is identified.
  - **b.** In case of cryoglobulinemic vasculitis, HCV antigen or hepatitis C antigen-antibody complexes are identified.

  In case of serum sickness antigen-antibody complexes with antigen excess are deposited in the wall of the vessel and produces following reactions:
  - **a.** Release of vasoactive amines like bradykinin, histamine leukotrienes from platelets and mast

cells by IgE trigger that increase the vascular permeability.

b. Activation of C5a complements which is chemotactic to neutrophils that infiltrate wall of the vessels; they phagocytose the immune complexes and release intracytoplasmic enzymes that damage the wall of the vessels.

c. In case of subacute of chronic cases, there will be infiltration of the vessel wall with mononuclear cells.

But the resultant effect is damage of the vessels and ischemic changes of the tissues supplied by that vessels. Following factors can explain why certain types of immune complexes responsible for vasculitis and why certain types of vessels are involved:

a. The ability of the reticuloendothelial system to clear the circulating immune complexes from the blood
b. Physicochemical and size of the immune complexes
c. Relative degree of turbulence in the blood flow
d. Intravascular hydrostatic pressure in different blood vessels
e. Preexisting integrity of vascular endothelium

B. Antineutrophil cytoplasmic antibodies: These antibodies are directed toward certain proteins in the cytoplasmic granules in the neutrophils and monocytes.

a. In some disease, these are present in high percentages:
   1. Granulomatosis with polyangiitis
   2. Microscopic polyangiitis
b. In some disease, it is present in small percentages: Eosinophilic granulomatosis with polyangiitis.

Since all the above diseases share common antibodies such as ANCA and small vessel vasculitis, hence they are collectively called "ANCA-associated vasculitis."

There are two major types of antibodies based on different target antigens:

a. Cytoplasmic ANCA—here antibodies are directed against 29 kDa neutral serine protein proteinase-3 present in the azurophilic granules. About 90% of patients with granulomatosis with polyangiitis have these antibodies.

b. Perinuclear ANCA: Here the major target of these antibodies is myeloperoxidase, but other targets are elastase, lactoferrin, cathepsin G, lysozyme, and bactericidal/permeability increasing protein. But antibodies to myeloperoxidase are associated with vasculitis. This antibodies are associated with the following diseases:
   1. Microscopic polyangiitis
   2. Eosinophilic granulomatosis with polyangiitis
   3. Isolated crescentic glomerulonephritis
   4. Granulomatosis with polyangiitis

But pANCA pattern of staining which is not due to antimyeloperoxidase antibodies are associated with nonvasculitis entities like:

a. Rheumatic autoimmune diseases
b. Nonrheumatic autoimmune diseases
c. Inflammatory bowel disease
d. Infective endocarditis
e. Bacterial airway infections

It is unclear that why patients with vasculitis develop antibodies to proteinase-3 and myeloperoxidase. But a number of observations suggest the possible mechanisms by which these antibodies play a role in the pathogenesis of vasculitis. Normally, myeloperoxidase and proteinase-3 reside inside the azurophilic granules of neutrophil and monocytes. But as neutrophil and monocytes are primed by TNF-α or IL-1, myeloperoxidase and proteinase-3 will translocate toward cell membrane and react with extracellular ANCA.

a. As a result neutrophil degranulate to release reactive oxygen species leading to tissue damage
b. ANCA-activated neutrophil adheres and kills the endothelial cells
c. Activated neutrophils and monocytes release proinflammatory cytokines like IL-1 and IL-8.

But according to a number of laboratory tests, it is shown that in a certain number of patients with active granulomatosis with polyangiitis have no ANCA.

There is no correlation between the height of antibody titer and disease activity.

C. Pathogenic T lymphocyte responses and granuloma formation:

Histopathologic features in case of granulomatous vasculitis demonstrate the role of pathogenic T lymphocyte response leading to cell-mediated injury.

a. Interferon-γ activates expression of HLA class II molecules on the vascular endothelial cells which will participate in the immunological reactions like interactions with CD4+ T lymphocytes.
b. Endothelial cells also secrete IL-1 which activates T lymphocytes and propagates immunological process within the blood vessels.

c. IL-1 and TNF-α induce endothelial-leukocyte adhesion molecule 1 and vascular cell adhesion molecule 1. These two adhesion molecule enhance leukocytes to adhere to the endothelial cells of the blood vessels.

Granulomatosis with Polyangiitis

Clinical Features

There is wide spectrum of clinical features having constitutional symptoms such as fever, malaise, anorexia at one end and severe multisystem involvement, multiorgan failure, and death at other end.

Following systems are involved:

A. Respiratory tract:
- **a.** Nasal crusting leads to nasal obstruction.
- **b.** Persistent rhinorrhea
- **c.** Nasal discharge
- **d.** Nasal ulcer
- **e.** Septal perforation
- **f.** Collapse of nasal bridge

B. Ear:
- **a.** Ear ache
- **b.** Purulent or bloody ear discharge
- **c.** Conductive and sensorineural deafness

C. Gastrointestinal tract:
- **a.** Oral ulcer
- **b.** Strawberry gingivitis
- **c.** Upper gastrointestinal bleeding
- **d.** Mesenteric ischemia
- **e.** Perforation of bowel

D. Pulmonary involvement:
- **a.** Pulmonary nodules
- **b.** Pulmonary infiltrate
- **c.** Reticulonodular opacities
- **d.** Pulmonary consolidation
- **e.** Pleural effusion
- **f.** Diffuse alveolar hemorrhage

E. Renal involvement:
- **a.** Asymptomatic proteinuria to 500 mg/day to rapidly progressive glomerulonephritis
- **b.** Microscopic hematuria
- **c.** Urine analysis demonstrates RBC cast
- **d.** Elevated serum creatinine
- **e.** Kidney biopsy demonstrates Pauci-immune glomerulonephritis

F. Skin:
- **a.** Palpable purpura
- **b.** Livedo reticularis
- **c.** Urticaria
- **d.** Erythema nodosum
- **e.** Pyoderma gangrenosum
- **f.** Histopathology demonstrates leukoclastic vasculitis.

G. Eye involvement:
- **a.** Uveitis
- **b.** Scleritis
- **c.** Retinal vasculitis
- **d.** Episcleritis
- **e.** Conjunctivitis
- **f.** Corneal ulceration
- **g.** Retro-orbital mass
- **h.** Optic atrophy

H. Central nervous system:
- **a.** Pachymeningitis
- **b.** Cranial neuropathies

I. Cardiac involvement:
- **a.** Myocarditis
- **b.** Pericarditis
- **c.** Conduction abnormalities

For rest of the answer add question number 4.

Q20. Seronegative arthropathy.
MGR/FEB2005/MDIII (5)

Seronegative spondyloarthropathies.
BF/MAY2009/MDIII (10)

Seronegative arthritis.
NTR UNI of Health SC, Vijayawada, 2021 (10)

Seronegative spondyloarthropathies.
Kerala University, 2020 (8)

What are the seronegative arthropathies? Discuss the management of ankylosing spondylitis.
NWBUHS, 2025 (10)

ANSWER

Current Classification of Spondyloarthritis

A. Current classifications:
   a. Axial spondyloarthritis:
      1. With radiographic sacroiliitis
      2. Without radiographic sacroiliitis
         - Sacroiliitis on MRI
         - HLA-B27 positivity plus two clinical or laboratory criteria
   b. Peripheral spondyloarthritis:
      1. With psoriasis
      2. With inflammatory bowel disease
      3. With preceding infection
      4. Without psoriasis or inflammatory bowel disease or preceding infection

B. Classic classifications:
   a. Ankylosing spondylitis
   b. Reactive arthritis
   c. Psoriatic spondylitis
      1. Predominantly peripheral
      2. Predominantly axial
   d. Enteropathic spondyloarthritis:
      1. Predominantly peripheral
      2. Predominantly axial
   e. Juvenile onset spondyloarthritis
   f. Undifferentiated spondyloarthritis

Etiology

A. There is classical relationship between spondyloarthropathies and HLA-B27, strongest being with AS.

B. In case of psoriatic arthropathy, the associated HLA molecules being HLA-B27, HLA-DR7, and HLA-DQ3.

C. In case of IBD-associated arthritis, the relation will be weak.

D. In case reactive arthritis relationship with HLA is variable.

E. In case of juvenile spondyloarthropathy (SpA) relationship with HLA-B27 is 60%.

Pathophysiology

Inflammation at the site of attachment of tendon or ligament with the bone, enthesitis is the key manifestation in SpA and this will differentiate is from rheumatoid arthritis and other polyarthritides. Major gene involved in the pathogenesis is HLA-B27, but other non-HLA genes are also involved in the pathogenesis. Following factors are involved in the pathogenesis of SpA, these are:

   a. Environmental factor
   b. Microorganisms
   c. Several cytokines
   d. Tumor necrosis factor

Clinical Features

A. Inflammatory joint pain is associated with morning stiffness for >1 hour, improves with activity, worsening with rest.

B. In case of axial SpA:
   a. History of low back pain for >3 months having onset before the age of 45 years.
   b. Schober test for assessment of lumbar flexion is positive.
   c. Occiput to wall test to assess the mobility of thoracic and cervical spine will be positive.

C. In case of peripheral SpA:
   a. Acute onset involving ankle and knee joints, asymmetric involvement.
   b. Enthesitis occurs at the insertion of tendon at the calcaneus. Hence, there is difficulty in walking, tender on palpation.
   c. Dactylitis: This nonspecific finding is present in psoriatic and reactive arthritis.

Nonskeletal manifestations are:

A. Ocular involvement:
   a. Uveitis
   b. Iritis
   c. Conjunctivitis

B. Gastrointestinal infection

C. Genitourinary infection

Evaluation

A. In patients with inflammatory low back pain:
   a. Plain X-ray of lumbosacral spine: Sacroiliitis.
   b. Inflammatory markers should be elevated.

B. In case of ankylosing spondylitis, the following features are:
   a. Shiny corner—sclerosis at the attachment of annulus fibrosis up to the anterior corner of vertebral end plate.
   b. Calcification of fibrous ring of the intervertebral disk to form marginal syndesmophytes—bamboo spine.

C. MRI can be also done to detect signs of inflammation.

D. In presence of predisposing condition, psoriatic arthritis, IBD-associated arthritis or reactive arthritis should be suspected.

E. In absence of predisposing condition autoimmune and inflammatory markers, radiographic feature of joints should be done.

Assessment in Spondyloarthritis International Society classification criteria for peripheral arthritis

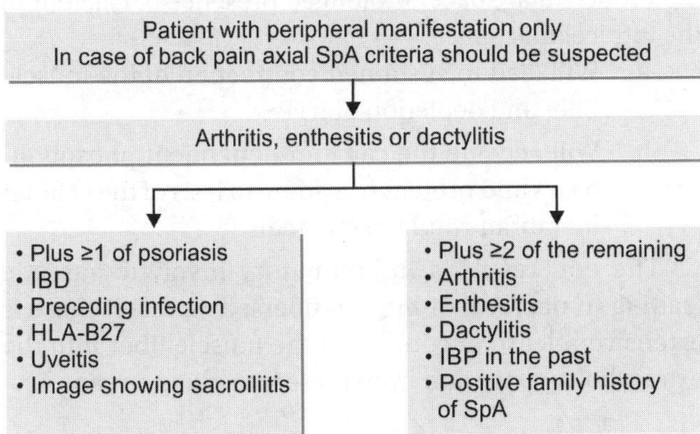

Q21. Rhabdomyolysis: Causes and consequences.

PGI/NOV2012/MDI (10)

ANSWER

Definition

It is a complex medical condition characterized by dissolution of damaged or injured skeletal muscles leading to release of intracellular components including creatine kinase, myoglobin, aldolase, and LDH along with electrolytes into the extracellular space and blood stream.

According to clinical advisory, rhabdomyolysis can be defined as muscle symptoms along with serum creatine kinase level of >11 time of the upper limit of normal, elevation of creatine is consistent with pigmentary nephropathy and brown urine with myoglobinuria.

Etiology

A. Physical causes:

- **a.** Trauma and compression:
  - **1.** Crush syndrome
  - **2.** Motor accident
  - **3.** Prolonged immobilization
- **b.** Exertion:
  - **1.** Seizures
  - **2.** Strenuous exercise
  - **3.** Delirium tremens
- **c.** Muscle hypoxia:
  - **1.** Major artery occlusion
  - **2.** Clamping of vessels during surgery
- **d.** Changes in body temperature:
  - **1.** Malignant hyperthermia
  - **2.** Neuroleptic malignant syndrome
  - **3.** Heat stroke
  - **4.** Hypothermia

B. Nonphysiological causes:

- **a.** Drugs and toxins
- **b.** Infections:
  - **1.** Influenza A and B
  - **2.** Epstein–Barr virus
  - **3.** *Legionella*
  - **4.** Herpes virus
- **c.** Electrolyte imbalance:
  - **1.** Hypokalemia
  - **2.** Hypophosphatemia
  - **3.** Hypocalcemia
  - **4.** Hyponatremia
  - **5.** Hypernatremia
  - **6.** Nonketotic hyperosmolar state
- **d.** Endocrine disorders:
  - **1.** Hyperaldosteronism
  - **2.** Hypothyroidism
  - **3.** Diabetic ketoacidosis (DKA)
- **e.** Autoimmune disorders:
  - **1.** Dermatomyositis
  - **2.** Polymyositis
- **f.** Genetic defect

Risk factors for rhabdomyolysis:

A. Endogenous factors:

- **a.** Age >80 years
- **b.** Increased frailty
- **c.** Multisystem diseases:
  - **1.** Hepatic dysfunction
  - **2.** Renal dysfunction
- **d.** Hypertriglyceridemia
- **e.** Hypothyroidism

f. Metabolic muscle disease:
   1. Carnitine palmitoyltransferase II deficiency
   2. McArdle's disease

B. Exogenous risks:
   a. Consumption of alcohol
   b. Heavy exercise
   c. Surgery with increased metabolic demand
   d. Agents affecting the P450 system:
      1. Fibrate
      2. Nicotinic acid
      3. Cyclosporine
      4. Verapamil
      5. Amlodipine

Pathophysiology

At rest, ion channels present on the sarcolemmal membrane to maintain high intracellular potassium and low intracellular sodium and calcium concentration. During depolarization of muscle fiber there is influx of calcium into the cytoplasm from the reserves stored in the sarcoplasmic reticulum leading to contraction of actin and myosin cross-linking producing muscle contraction. All these processes depend upon the availability of reserved energy in the form of ATP.

So, if any insult produces injury to the muscles or reduces the availability of ATP which leads to disruption of intracellular electrolyte concentration, so there will be excessive intracellular concentration of sodium and calcium. Increased intracellular sodium draws large amount of water intracellularly and disrupt the integrity of the intracellular space. Prolonged presence of calcium in the intracellular space.

a. Will lead to sustained contraction of the muscle fiber and depletion of ATP.
b. Will activate the calcium-dependent phospholipases and proteases leading to lysis of the cellular membrane and ion channels.

The end result is inflammatory myolytic cascade leading to necrosis of muscle fibers, as a result there is extensive release of content of the muscle fiber into the extracellular space and from there into blood stream.

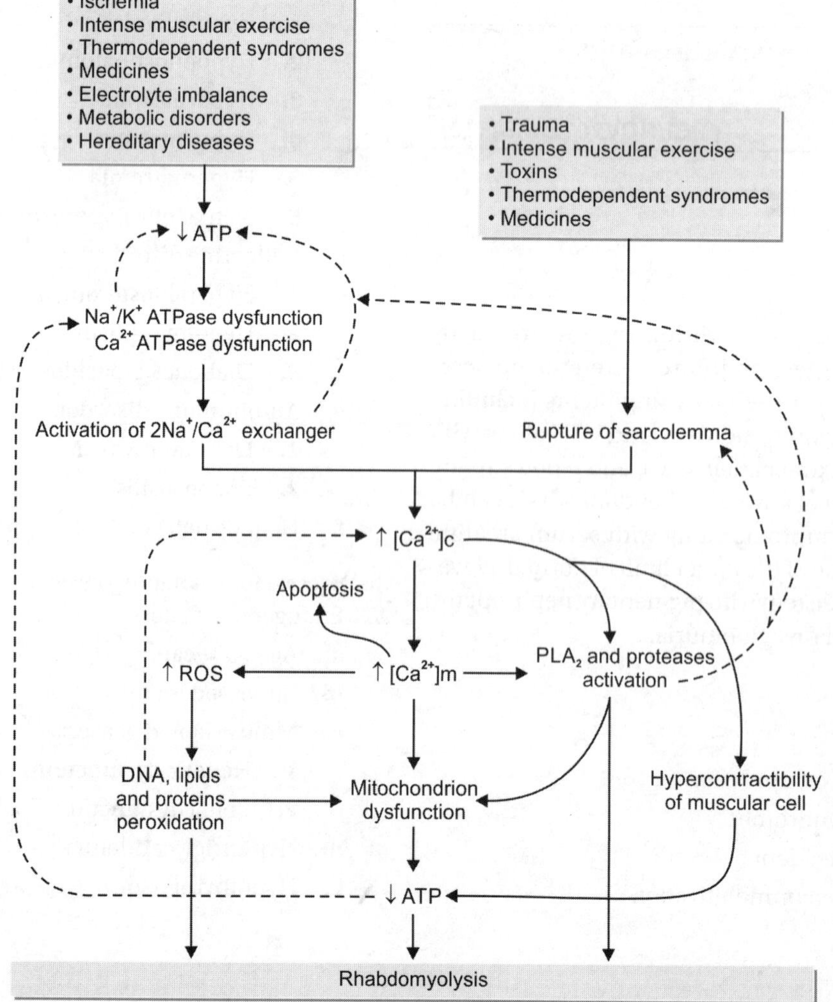

Clinical Features

Classical symptoms triad are:

A. Myalgia

B. Weakness

C. Tea-colored urine

This triad is present in <10% of patients.

Color of the urine is controlled by muscle mass, concentration of urine, and glomerular filtration.

On examination, the muscles will be tense and swollen.

D. Systemic manifestations include:

- **a.** Malaise
- **b.** Fever
- **c.** Nausea with or without vomiting
- **d.** Tachycardia

If not treated patient may develop:

- **a.** Acute kidney injury
- **b.** DIC
- **c.** Multiorgan failure

Diagnosis

A. The gold standard of the diagnosis is the measurement of creatine kinase which should be at least five times of upper limit of normal and it is closely related to kidney damage.

B. Serum myoglobin is not sensitive marker for the diagnosis of rhabdomyolysis.

C. Urine myoglobin demonstrates erythrocyte positivity on urine dip stick.

Complications

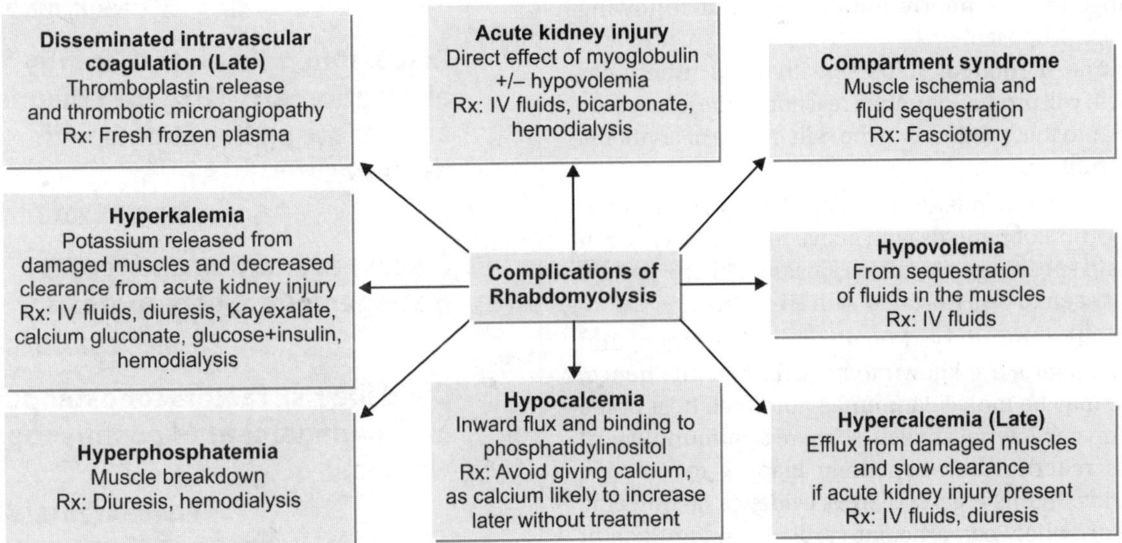

Management

A. Most important goal in rhabdomyolysis is to avoid acute kidney injury. Due to accumulation of fluid in the muscle compartment, there is associated hypovolemia leading to prerenal azotemia.

- **a.** This can be prevented by administration of intravenous fluid at a rate of 0.5 L/h.
- **b.** Another option is 500 mL/h normal saline alternated with 500 mL/h 5% dextrose with 50 mmol sodium bicarbonate for each subsequent 2–3 L solution. The goal is:
  1. Urine output 200 mL/h
  2. Urine pH >6.5
  3. Plasma pH <7.5

B. Correction of electrolyte and acid-base imbalance

C. Alkalinization of urine to protect the kidney from nephrotoxic injury of hyperuricosuria and myoglobinuria

D. Decompression of muscle compartments through the mobilization of edematous fluid

E. Restoration of arteriolar contractility in the injured muscles by reversion of arteriolar vasodilatation through correction of acidosis and hyperkalemia.

Q22. Poncet's syndrome.

PGI/NOV2012/MDI (10)

ANSWER

Definition

It is a type of reactive arthritis known as "polyarthritis associated with visceral tuberculosis" is characterized by visceral tuberculosis where there is no evidence of bacteriologic involvement of the joint itself. It was first described by Antonin Poncet in 1897. It is described as nondestructive postinfective polyarthritis in patients suffering from active tuberculosis which can be resolved by proper antitubercular therapy.

Age of incidence: Younger population age affected mainly. Female is mostly affected.

Pathogenesis

Its pathogenesis is poorly understood, but following theories are proposed:

A. Immune mediated: Hypersensitivity to tubercular protein will produce immune reaction in the joint cavity similar to that produced in the skin in case of erythema nodosum.

B. Genetic predisposition: Since it occurs in small proportion of patients with active tuberculosis, it can explain specific genetic predisposition, in one patient it was seen to be associated with HLA DR-4.

C. Molecular mimicry: Mycobacterial antigen and mycobacteria are known to be arthritogenic, hence, there may be molecular mimicry between host tissue and mycobacterial antigen, so there is immunological cross reaction between them leading to reactive arthritis. In this regard, there is evidence of antigenic similarity between articular cartilage and antigen of mycobacterium tuberculosis.

Clinical Features

A. Fever

B. Malaise

C. Symmetrical polyarthritis involving mainly large joints but small joints may be involved. But according to different literature, it is symmetrical and pauciarticular.

D. There may be presence of lymphadenopathy.

Diagnosis

A. This disease can be diagnosed by exclusion of other causes of arthritis.

B. Tuberculin test is frequently positive.

C. Biopsy of the enlarged lymph nodes

Treatment

A. Antitubercular therapy for active disease

B. NSAIDs for reactive arthritis

Q23. Diagnosis of osteoporosis.

SNMC/MAY2013/MDIV (10)

Management of osteoporosis.

SNMC/MAY2013/MDI (10)

Osteoporosis.

SNMC/MAY2005/MDIV (10)

KUHS/MAY2014/MDIII (10)

RGUHS/NOV2001/MDII (10)

MGR/SEP2007/MDI (5)

DNBIII/JUN2011 (10)

Discuss the role of dual-energy X-ray absorptiometry (DEXA) in diagnosis and follow-up in patients with osteoporosis.

BF/NOV2013/MDIV (10)

Discuss evaluation and recent management of osteoporosis.

BF/OCT2010/MDIV (20)

Describe risk factors for osteoporosis and management of postmenopausal women.

ERA/MAY2012/MDIII (10)

Newer drugs in osteoporosis.

MJPRU/2016/MDIV (10)

Discuss an approach to a case of osteoporosis. Outline its treatment.

MUHS/MAY2011/MDIII (25)

ANSWER

It has been discussed in parathyroid and metabolism chapter, question number 4.

Q24. Systemic sclerosis.

ERA/NOV2012(S)/MDII (15)

What is systemic sclerosis? Discuss its management.

ERA/MAY2011/MDII (10)

Write briefly about the pathogenesis of systemic sclerosis. How will you differentiate between limited and diffuse cutaneous systemic sclerosis? How will you manage a case of scleroderma renal crisis?

WBUHS 2022 (10)

Clinical features and diagnosis of systemic sclerosis.

NTR UNI of Health SC, Vijayawada, Andhra, 2022 (10)

ANSWER

Definition

It is chronic and progressive heterogeneous orphan disease characterized by protean clinical manifestations involving all the organ systems in the body leading to disfigurement and significant disability.

Risk Factors

A. Genetic contribution in the disease pathogenesis: Systemic sclerosis is polygenic disease, having each gene in very little contribution to the disease. In case of monozygotic twin, concordance rate is low. Incidence rate of Raynaud's phenomenon with SLE, RA, and autoimmune thyroiditis in first-degree relatives is high. Gene sequencing analysis and single nucleotide polymorphism analysis of candidate genes and analysis of entire genome demonstrate the following:

- **a.** Initial triggering mechanism for developing adaptive and innate immunity are robustly validate susceptibility loci for systemic sclerosis.
- **b.** Association with common variants of genes related to activated B and T lymphocytes and abnormal signaling like BLK, BANK1, CD247, CCR6, PTPN22, etc.
- **c.** Identification of strong association with HLA-class II haplotypes on chromosome 6 like DRB1*11:04, DQB1*03:01, and non-HLA molecule genes NOTCH4.
- **d.** Some genetic variants associated with systemic sclerosis are involved in innate immunity and interferon pathways like IRF5, IRF7, and STAT4, etc.
- **e.** Other associated genes are: apoptosis-related genes DNA-SEIL3 and SOX5, fibrosis-related genes.
- **f.** Some genes are associated with specific disease manifestation of diseases like interstitial lung disease like CTGF, CD226, and scleroderma renal crisis like HLA-DRB1, other autoimmune genetic disorders like SLE, RA, and psoriasis.

B. Environmental factors:

- **a.** Infecting agents:
  1. Epstein–Barr virus
  2. Parvovirus B19 infection
  3. Cytomegalovirus
  4. Rhodotorula glutinis
- **b.** Toxic oil syndrome: It is associated with contaminated rapeseed oil for cooking.
- **c.** Eosinophilia-myalgia syndrome associated with consumption of L-tryptophan-containing dietary supplements
- **d.** Nephrogenic systemic sclerosis is associated with use of gadolinium-containing contrast medium.
- **e.** Occupational exposure is associated with systemic sclerosis results epigamic changes like methylation of DNA and modification of histones.
  1. Particulate silica
  2. Polyvinyl chloride
  3. Epoxy resins
  4. Welding fumes
  5. Aromatic hydrocarbons—pan thinners, xylene, toluene, etc.
- **f.** Drugs:
  1. Bleomycin
  2. Cocaine
  3. Pentazocine
  4. Appetite suppressants

Pathogenesis

There are three cardinal features which lead to different clinical manifestations:

A. Diffuse microangiopathy: It involves small arteries, arterioles, capillary vascular beds involving lung, heart, kidney, and skins. Following are the triggering factors which are involved in vasculopathy:

- **a.** Viruses
- **b.** Cytotoxic factors

c. Chemokines, thrombogenic microparticles
d. Activation of alternate pathway of complement
e. Autoantibodies directing endothelial cells
f. Phospholipids
g. B2 glycoprotein 1

Following are the results of endothelial injury:

a. Production of vasodilatory substances such as prostacyclin and nitric oxide
b. Production of vasoconstrictor like endothelin-1
c. Upregulation of intercellular adhesion molecules

Microvasculature demonstrates:

a. Increased permeability
b. Transendothelial leukocyte diapedesis
c. Abnormal activation of coagulation cascade
d. Increased thrombin production
e. Impaired fibrinolysis
f. Spontaneous aggregation of platelets it releases:
   1. Serotonin
   2. Platelet-derived growth factor
   3. Platelet α granules like thromboxane
g. There is thickening of basement membrane
h. Proliferation of myointimal cells in the media

Above processes lead to proliferation of intima, hypertrophy of media along with fibrosis of adventitia, and perivascular area lead to progressive luminal obstruction, reduction of blood flow, tissue ischemia. So widespread loss of capillary, small- and medium-sized vessels vasculopathy along with impaired ability to repair and replace damaged vessels are the hallmark of this disease.

B. Inflammation and autoimmunity:

Cellular immunity:

Following features are suggestive of inflammatory and autoimmune nature of the diseases:

a. Universal presence of organ-specific antibodies in the circulation
b. Familial clustering of systemic sclerosis with other autoimmune diseases.
c. Detection of activated immune cells like activated immune cells—T cells with oligoclonal antigen receptors and T follicular helper-like cells
d. Elevated interferon signatures such as
   1. Elevated expression of interferon-regulate genes in different tissue
   2. Increased level of cytokines and chemokines secreted from mononuclear cells like IL-6, IL-4, IL-10, IL-17, IL-33, TNF-α, CCL-2, and CXCL4
e. There is association of systemic sclerosis with MHC molecules implicated in immune response.

In early phase, there is accumulation of activated T cells, macrophages, monocytes, dendritic cells in different organs such as skin, kidney, lungs prior to vasculopathy, and fibrosis.

Dendritic cells in the close proximity to activated fibroblasts and myofibroblasts expresses toll-like receptors that secrete IL-10 and interferon, thymic stromal lymphopoietin, and CXCL4 leading to loss of immunologic tolerance as well modifying adaptive immune response.

Circulating T cells bind with high affinity with endothelium and fibroblasts through the expression of chemokine receptors and α_1 integrin. Endothelial cells facilitate diapedesis of leukocytes through the expression of intercellular adhesion molecule-1 (ICAM-1) and other adhesion molecules.

T cells being activated by dendritic cells demonstrate Th2 immune response leading to release of IL-4, IL-13, IL-33, and TSP that activate fibroblast whereas, Th1 cytokine INF-γ will blocks the activation of fibroblast due to its antifibrotic properties.

Type-2 innate lymphoid cells is implicated in type-2 immunity and remodeling of tissues and TGF-β produced by M2 macrophages promoting angiogenesis and tissue remodeling are elevated in skin in scleroderma.

Although regulatory T cells responsible for enforcing immune tolerance are elevated in the circulation but this immunosuppressive functions are defective.

Following are the features of chronic B cell activation:

a. Elevation of CD19
b. Elevation costimulatory molecules CD80 and CD86

Following factors are elevated in the serum:

a. Proliferation inducing ligands (APRIL)
b. B cell activating factor
c. Members of TNF superfamily having potent activator of B cells

Humoral immunity:

Target antigen	Scleroderma antibody	Clinical presentation
DNA topoisomerase	dcSSc	• Digital ischemic ulcer • Scleroderma • Scleroderma renal crisis • Extensive skin involvement • Tendon friction
Centromere protein	lcSSc	• Digital ischemic ulcer • Isolated pulmonary hypertension • Calcinosis cutis
RNA polymerase III	dcSSc	• Tendon friction rub • Rapidly progressive skin • Joint contracture • Renal crisis • Contemporaneous ulcer
U3-RNP nuclear protein Nucleolar pattern	Dc/lcSSc	• Interstitial lung disease • Pulmonary hypertension • Renal crisis • Myositis • Involvement of gastrointestinal tract
Th/To (fibrillarin) Nucleolar pattern	lcSSc	• Interstitial lung disease • Isolated pulmonary hypertension
PM/Sci Nucleolar pattern	lcSSc	• Interstitial lung disease • Myositis overlap • Calcinosis cutis
Ku Speckled pattern	Overlap	• Myositis overlap • SLE
U1-RNP Speckled pattern	MCTD	• Inflammatory myositis • Pulmonary arterial hypertension • Myositis overlap
U11/U12 RNP Speckled pattern	Dc/lcSSc	Interstitial lung disease

(MCTD: mixed connective-tissue disease; SLE: systemic lupus erythematosus)

C. Fibrosis: Fibrosis is nothing but replacement of normal tissue by fibrotic tissue, in case of scleroderma it is result of inflammation, autoimmunity, and microvascular damage. Epithelial cells, endothelial cells, mesenchymal progenitor cells and preadipocytes and tissue fibroblasts are the source of myofibroblasts. Upon activation by T and B cell fibroblasts proliferate, secrete collagen and other molecules of matrix, chemokines, proinflammatory cytokines, growth factors, and ultimately transdifferentiate into contractile myofibroblasts, in normal physiological conditions repairing process is self-limiting. But if pathological conditions this fibrotic process will be amplified to maintain sustained fibrotic process, the factors responsible are:

a. Endogenous TGF-β
b. Paracrine fibrotic mediators like IL-6, IL-13
c. Connective tissue growth factor
d. Platelet-derived growth factor
e. Endothelin-1
f. Hypoxia
g. ROS
h. Thrombin
i. Mechanical forces responsible for continued activation of fibroblast

Bone marrow-derived mesenchyme progenitor cells will contribute to fibrosis.

Clinical Features

Characteristic clinical presentation: Within 4 years of onset there may be involvement of pulmonary and renal damage. But there is no organ failure, systemic process will be stabilized.

A. In localized cutaneous form:
- **a.** Interval between the Raynaud's phenomenon and organ involvement is more than years.
- **b.** Here distal limb is involved.
- **c.** There is dilatation of capillaries.
- **d.** Here the autoantigen is centromere.

Organ involvement:

A. Raynaud's phenomenon:
- **a.** It occurs in 95% of patients
- **b.** It is characterized by episodic vasoconstriction of small arteries and arterioles in the finger and toes, ear lobes or tip of the toes leading to pallor and/or cyanosis, coldness and numbness followed by vasodilatation on rewarming leading to rubor.
- **c.** Triggering factors are:
  - **1.** Cold exposure
  - **2.** Vibration
  - **3.** Emotional stress
- **d.** Pathogenic mechanism: There is gross imbalance between vasoconstrictor and vasodilator in response to triggering factors.

B. Localized scleroderma:

a. Morphea: It is characterized by plaques of fibrotic skin and subcutaneous tissue in absence of systemic disease.

b. Linear scleroderma: It is characterized by fibrotic bands occurring in extremities involving skin and deeper tissues.

C. Skin features:

a. Localized scleroderma:

1. Cutaneous changes affect face, neck, and extremities distal to knees, and elbows
2. In the edematous phase hands become edematous, puffy
3. But in fibrotic phase skin becomes thick, tight, fibrosis of tendon followed by contracture of the hands but thumb is spared.
4. In the face, there is perioral fibrosis leading to "puckered mouth" or "fish-mouth appearance"—microstomia.
5. Face is "mauskopf" appearance characterized by:
   - Taught and shine skin
   - Loss of wrinkle
   - Expressionless face due to reduced eyelids, cheeks, and mouth mobility
   - Lips are thin
   - Accentuation of central incisor teeth
   - Prominent perioral radial furrowing—Rhytides
6. Nose is inched-up, beak like.
7. In the late phase, skin is atrophic, strictly bound to underlying subcutaneous fat—tethering.
8. Dilated capillaries in the skin on the face—telangiectasia—demonstrated by wide angle microscopy

b. Diffuse scleroderma: In diffuse cutaneous form, interval between Raynaud's phenomenon and disease onset is weeks to months. There are two phases:

1. In edematous phase, intense pruritus with signs of inflammation involving limbs distal to knees and elbows advancing proximally, face and fingers first, this is associated with diffuse hyperpigmentation of skin with sparing around the hair follicles looking like "salt and paper" appearances, fatigue, muscle weakness, arthralgia, decreased mobility of joints.
2. In the indurated phase, skin becomes indurated with hair loss. Decreased sweating, reduced production of skin oils.
3. In the fibrotic phase, there is flexion contracture, stiff elbow hip, shoulder and knee, and ankle due to fibrosis of supporting structure.
4. Ulcer is present in the volar pads of fingertips which leads to pitting scars.
5. Skin changes usually peaks for 3–5 years followed by slow improvement.
6. There is dilatation and loss of capillaries—demonstrated by wide angle microscopy.
7. Here the autoantigen is topoisomerase 1.

D. Musculoskeletal features:

a. Swelling and stiffness of fingers and knees

b. Symmetrical polyarthritis resembling RA

c. Proximal myositis resembling polymyositis

d. In advanced cases leathery crepitation

E. Pulmonary manifestations:

a. Interstitial lung disease:

1. Present with progressive dyspnea on exertion, dry cough, and bibasilar Velcro crepitation on auscultation
2. Pulmonary function test demonstrates reduced vital capacity and low diffusing capacity
3. Chest X-ray shows reticular shadows in lung field
4. HRCT demonstrates ground-glass appearance due to alveolitis
5. Bronchoalveolar lavage shows increased number of alveolar macrophages and/or neutrophils
6. In case of diffuse scleroderma, there is chance of developing pulmonary fibrosis.
7. In case of limited scleroderma after many years, pulmonary hypertension may develop which is due to obliteration of arterioles due to medial hypertrophy and intimal fibrosis. Patients present with exertional dyspnea and features of right-sided heart failure. Prognosis is poor. Factors associated with poor prognosis are:
   - Male sex
   - Low DLCO
   - Early lung involvement
   - Severe Raynaud's phenomenon
   - Cigarette smoking

b. Pulmonary arterial hypertension:
   1. Features are:
      - Dyspnea on exertion
      - Chest pain
      - Fatigue
      - Systolic murmur of tricuspid regurgitation
      - Loud pulmonary component of S2
      - S3 gallop
      - Pedal edema
      - Engorged pulsatile neck vein
      - Enlarged liver
      - Right heart catheterization reveals mean pulmonary arterial pressure >25 mm Hg.
      - Increased level of N-terminal pro-brain natriuretic peptide (NT-proBNP)—indicates pulmonary arterial hypertension—it is poor prognostic marker.

F. Gastrointestinal tract:
   a. Upper gastrointestinal tract:
      1. Xerostomia
      2. Shortened frenulum
      3. Teeth may be loosened due to loss of attachment of the periodontal ligament with the alveolar bone
      4. Resorption of mandibular condyles
      5. Gastroesophageal reflux disease (GERD) due to:
         - Relaxed lower esophageal sphincter pressure
         - Impaired clearance of refluxed gastric contents due to deceased esophageal motility
         - Delayed gastric emptying
         - Use of calcium channel blockers and phosphodiesterase inhibitors to treat Raynaud's phenomenon

         Extraesophageal manifestations due to GERD:
         - Chronic cough
         - Microaspiration resulting aggravation of interstitial lung disease

         Intestinal complication of GERD:
         - Barrett's esophagus
         - Esophageal stricture

         Chest CT demonstrates dilated esophagus with intraluminal air

         Endoscopy should be done to exclude infection with candida, cytomegalovirus, and herpes virus.
      6. Gastroparesis resulting:
         - Abdominal distension
         - Early satiety
         - Aggravation of GERD
      7. Gastric antral vascular ectasia—resulting from small vessel vasculopathy which can be described as "watermelon" stomach.
   b. Lower gastrointestinal tract involvement:
      1. Weight and malnutrition from:
         - Intestinal motility impairment
         - Malabsorption of nutrients like fat and protein
         - Chronic diarrhea
      2. Pancreatic insufficiency resulting:
         - Vitamin B12 and vitamin D deficiency
         - Malabsorption of fat and protein
      3. Intestinal pseudo-obstruction results from disturbed motility of intestine and patients presents with:
         - Recurrent abdominal pain
         - Nausea
         - Vomiting
      4. Colonic features are:
         - Constipation
         - Sigmoid volvulus
         - Fecal incontinence
         - Rectal prolapse
      5. Gastrointestinal bleeding from intestinal ectatic vessels
      6. In late stage diverticula producing:
         - Perforation
         - Bleeding
      7. Rarely pneumatosis intestinalis from trapping of bowel air which may rupture leading to benign pneumoperitoneum.

G. Renal involvement:
   a. Scleroderma renal crisis occurs in 10–15% of scleroderma patients resulting:
      1. Accelerated hypertension (blood pressure >150/90 mm Hg. Patients may present with:
         - Headache
         - Blurred vision
         - Congestive heart failure
         - Pulmonary edema

2. Acute renal injury
3. Progressive oliguric renal failure

This occurs due to the following mechanisms:

1. Obliterative vasculopathy and narrowing of the lumen of renal arcuate and interlobar arteries
2. Intravascular hemolysis
3. Activation of compliment pathways
4. Glucocorticoid administration
5. Progressive reduction of renal blood flow aggravated by renal vasospasm leads to:
    - Renin secretion from juxtaglomerular apparatus
    - Activation of angiotensin II

    Risk factors are:
    - African-American race
    - Male sex
    - Diffuse or progressive skin involvement

    50% patients demonstrate anti-RNA polymerase III antibodies, but presence of anti-centromere antibodies protects the patients from renal involvement

    Creatinine >3 mg/dL is associated with poor outcome.

    Following features suggest impending renal crisis:
    - Palpable tendon friction rub
    - Pericardial effusion
    - Unexplained anemia
    - Thrombocytopenia

    Urine analysis demonstrates:
    - Granular cast
    - Microscopic hematuria

    Peripheral blood picture demonstrate:
    - Microangiopathic hemolysis
    - Moderate thrombocytopenia
    - Fragmented red blood cells

b. Crescentic glomerulonephritis—it is associated with myeloperoxidase specific ANCAs.

c. Membranous glomerulonephritis can occur in patients treated with d-penicillamine.

d. Asymptomatic impairment of renal function

H. Cardiac involvement: It is affected in case of diffuse scleroderma and may be due to secondary or primary pulmonary hypertension.

a. Pericardial involvement resulting:
1. Pericarditis
2. Pericardial effusion
3. Constrictive pericarditis
4. Cardiac tamponade

b. Myocardial involvement:
1. Secondary to vasospasm of cardiac microvessels and ischemic reperfusion injury—all may lead to patchy myocardial fibrosis resulting:
    - Asymptomatic systolic or diastolic myocardial dysfunction
    - Progressing to overt heart failure
2. Myocarditis leading to left ventricular dysfunction—diagnosed by MRI and endomyocardial biopsy. Doppler echocardiography and nuclear imaging like single photon beam emission CT demonstrate abnormal myocardial perfusion.

c. Endocardial involvement in the form of conduction system involvement leading to different types of arrhythmias.

I. Less common recognized manifestations:

a. Dry eyes and dry mouth—resulting from fibrosis of the gland rather than lymphocytic infiltration

b. Hypothyroidism resulting from Hashimoto disease

c. Erectile dysfunction resulting from:
    - Vascular insufficiency
    - Fibrosis of corporeal smooth muscle

d. Impaired sexual function in women

e. High risk of adverse outcome in pregnancy

f. Central nervous system is least commonly affected. But trigeminal neuropathy may occur.

According to 2013 American College of Rheumatology/European League classification:

Items	Subitems	Score
Skin thickening of fingers of both hands extending proximal to MCP joints (sufficient criteria)		9
Skin thickening of fingers	Puffy fingers	2
	Sclerodactyly of fingers (distal to MCP but proximal to PIP joints)	4
Fingertips lesions (only count the highest score)	Digital tip ulcer	2
	Pitting scar	3
Telangiectasia		2

Continued

Continued

Items	Subitems	Score
Abnormal nail fold capillaries		2
Pulmonary arterial hypertension and/or interstitial lung disease (maximum score 2)	Pulmonary arterial hypertension	2
	Interstitial lung disease	2
Raynaud's phenomenon		3
SSc-related autoantibodies [anticentromere, antitopoisomerase (anti-Scl-70), anti-RNA polymerase III]		3

(MCP: metacarpophalangeal; PIP: proximal interphalangeal; RNA: ribonucleic acid)

If total above score is ≥9—it is classified as systemic sclerosis.

Treatment of Systemic Sclerosis

A. Skin involvement:

a. Penicillamine:

1. Action:

- It reduces thickening of skin
- Prevent development of significant skin involvement through interfering inter- and intramolecular cross-linking of collagen and immunosuppressant action.

2. Dose: 125 mg/day with increase to 1.5 g/day within 1–3 months

3. Adverse effects:

- Glomerulonephritis
- Aplastic anemia
- Leukopenia
- Thrombocytopenia
- Myasthenia gravis
- Fever
- Rash
- Loss of taste

b. Other drugs used for rapidly progressive disease are:

1. Cyclophosphamide
2. Methotrexate
3. Chlorambucil
4. 5-fluorouracil

c. Intense pruritus can be treated by:

1. Antihistaminic
2. Skin lubricating creams
3. Low-dose oral steroids

d. Telangiectasia can be treated by laser therapy.

e. Calcinosis can be treated by calcium channel blockers, diltiazem. It can be removed surgically.

f. Treatment of skin thickening include:

1. Thalidomide
2. Humanized anti-transforming growth factor
3. Beta-1 monoclonal antibody
4. Relaxing hormone

B. Raynaud's phenomenon can be treated by:

a. Calcium channel blocker: Nifedipine—60–90 mg/day

b. Vasodilators: Methyldopa and prazosin

c. Prostacyclin analog: Epoprostenol, iloprost—0.5–3 mg/kg/minute intravenously for 3–5 days or orally 50–150 µg twice daily can be given.

1. Mechanism of action of iloprost:

- Potent vasodilator
- Inhibits adhesion and aggregation of platelets
- Alters function of neutrophils
- Repairs damaged endothelium
- Reduces the severity of Raynaud's phenomenon

d. Pentoxifylline:

1. Improves blood flow
2. Increases the deformability of RBC

e. Nitroglycerin patch

f. Ketanserin, losartan, bosentan

g. Antiplatelet drugs—dipyridamole and aspirin:

1. Improves blood flow
2. Reduces platelet adhesion

h. Surgical therapy:

1. Surgical sympathectomy
2. Digital sympathectomy

C. Treatment of digital ulcers:

a. Soak and warm water
b. Topical and oral antibiotics
c. Debridement
d. Amputation

D. Treatment of lung involvement:

a. Fibrosing alveolitis progressing to interstitial lung disease

1. Immunosuppressants:

- Prednisolone 30–40 mg/day orally plus 600–800 mg monthly intravenously or 2 mg/kg orally daily. Steroids should be tapered over 3 months. Condition of the lungs should be reassessed after 6 months and according this the dose of cyclophosphamide should be individualized. Otherwise, cyclophosphamide should be replaced by azathioprine.
- Mycophenolate mofetil is less toxic and safe alternative, dose is orally 1.5 g/day for 2 years.
- Rituximab: It is monoclonal antibody against B cells CD20.

2. Autologous hematopoietic stem cell transplantation: It can be administered in interstitial lung disease (ILD). But there are treatment-related infections and mortality.

3. Lung transplantation can be considered as life-prolonging procedure, but there is chance of recurrence of scleroderma-induced ILD.

b. Pulmonary hypertension:

1. Nifedipine: 60–90 mg/day

2. Anticoagulation—dose of it should be adjusted accordingly to maintain the INR of 2.5.

3. Endothelin receptor antagonist—bosentan: daily dose is 125–250 mg twice daily orally, it will improve:

- Exercise capacity
- Hemodynamic measures
- Functional class
- It will increase serum aminotransferase level.

Ambrisentan—due to its longer duration of action it is used as 5–10 mg daily.

4. Prostacyclin analog like iloprost should be given 5-day infusion (daily 6 hours) every 3 months. It will improve DLCO and improve the skin condition.

5. Phosphodiesterase 5 inhibitor:

- Sildenafil—thrice or four times daily
- Tadalafil—once daily dose is preferable.
- Vardenafil

Actions:

- Reduce pulmonary vascular resistance
- Improves ventilation-perfusion matching
- Improves oxygenation

6. Soluble guanylate cyclase stimulator, riociguat, can be used in pulmonary hypertension.

7. Heat-lung or single lung transplantation in medical therapy refractory cases.

E. Treatment of gastrointestinal involvement:

a. GERD can be treated by:

1. Small frequent meals

2. Antacids

3. Elevation of head

4. Proton pump inhibitors

5. Avoidance of tea, coffee, alcohol, and chocolates-containing foods

6. Motility agents such as metoclopramide and itopride

b. Malabsorption and bacterial overgrowth can be treated by:

1. Antibiotics such as ciprofloxacin, doxycycline, and metronidazole

2. Parenteral nutrition

c. Intestinal pseudo-obstruction can be treated by octreotide.

F. Treatment of renal involvement:

a. Hypertension is the mainstay of treatment in this patient and can be treated by:

1. ACE inhibitor

2. CCB

3. Beta blockers

4. Clonidine

b. Dialysis is of choice in case progressive renal failure.

c. Renal transplantation—it is not a choice because these patients suffer from other system involvement.

d. Endothelin-1 receptor blockers

e. Prostacyclin analog

In patients with progressive and extensive skin involvement, tendon friction rubs and presence of antiRNA polymerase antibody III blood pressure should be monitored daily.

f. Potentially nephrotoxic drugs should be avoided or can be given at very low dose.

G. Treatment of musculoskeletal involvement:

a. For arthritis:

1. Low-dose glucocorticoids
2. NSAIDs
3. Active and passive exercise
4. Surgery in case of contracture of ligaments

b. Myositis can be treated by:

1. Glucocorticoids
2. Methotrexate
3. Cyclophosphamide
4. Azathioprine

H. Treatment of cardiac involvement:

a. Pericarditis without cardiac tamponade can be treated by:

1. NSAIDs
2. Steroids

b. Pericardial tamponade can be treated by pericardiocentesis.

c. Myocarditis can respond to steroid and cyclosporine.

d. Heart failure can be treated by digoxin, diuretics, and antiarrhythmatics.

Differentiating point between the limited and diffuse systemic sclerosis:

Features	Limited scleroderma	Diffuse scleroderma
Onset	Slow	Rapid
Skin affected	Distal to elbow and knee, face	Proximal limb, face and trunk
Raynaud's phenomenon	It precedes skin changes	Simultaneously with involvement of skin
Involved organ	CREST syndrome Pulmonary hypertension	Renal crisis Cardiac fibrosis ILD
CREST syndrome	Common	Rare
Renal crisis	Rare	Common
Serology	Positive centromere antibody	Anti-topoisomerase antibody, Anti-RNA antibody
Prognosis	Better	Worse

Q25. Osteopenia.

BF/MAY2012/MDII (10)

ANSWER

Definition

According to WHO, osteopenia can be defined as t-score between –1 and –2.5, whereas, <–2.5 is diagnose as osteoporosis. It can be described as decreased bone mineral density below normal reference value, it can be measured by DEXA bone scan.

Etiology

Acquisition of bone mineral from the time of birth to adulthood varies according to age and sex. Bone mineral increases to a maximum level till the maximum height will be achieved by adolescence. Accretion rate of bone mineral will be greatest for about 4 years in both sexes after achieving peak accretion and it will be 17 years in female and 21 years in male. Failing to achieve this peak bone mass is known as osteopenia and the bone is liable to fragility fracture in adolescence and early adulthood. After the age of 30 years, bone mass gradually decreases over the ensuing decades till the late life. Causes of osteopenia:

A. Heritable factor in 80% of cases

B. Modifiable factors responsible for reduction in the bone mass in adulthood:

a. Weight bearing exercise

b. Nutrition status:

1. Inadequate calcium intake
2. Inadequate vitamin D intake
3. Body mass
4. Hormonal factors

C. Natural loss during adulthood

D. Secondary causes hastening the processes:

a. Alcohol use disorders

b. Smoking

c. Sedentary lifestyle

d. Thin body habitus (BMI < 18.5 kg/m^2)

E. Medical conditions:

a. Anorexia

b. Hyperparathyroidism

c. Hyperthyroidism

d. Malabsorption syndrome

e. Hypogonadism

f. Chronic renal failure

g. Amenorrhea

h. Oligomenorrhea

i. Early onset menopause

F. Medication:
  a. Chronic steroid use
  b. PPI
  c. Valproic acid
  d. Chemotherapeutic agents
  e. Antiepileptic drugs
G. White and Asian race

Pathophysiology

Osteopenia results from uncoupling of osteoblast and osteoclast activity resulting reduction in bone mass. Peak bone mass is achieved in the second decade and early third decade of life. After the age 30 years bone remodeling continues but it will be in favor of bone resorption and it will be continued till the later decade.

Histopathology

It will demonstrate:
  a. Thin trabeculae
  b. Decreased osteon size
  c. Enlarged-Haversian spaces
  d. Enlarged marrow spaces

Clinical Features

A. Proper history regarding to risk factors
B. Proper social history, alcohol and smoking
C. Family history of osteoporosis
D. History of prior fracture

Physical examination usually normal except under stressful condition. In absence of any risk factor, the male person at the age of 70 years and women advancing toward menopause are advised to do DEXA scan.

Patient with early fragility fracture proper attention should be paid to do DEXA scan. But women with normal DEXA score should not do further follow-up as they will not progress to osteoporosis.

Diagnosis

A. According to WHO, DEXA scan is the gold standard for assessing bone mineral density as it is most accurate with very little radiation exposure. Following areas are included in the DEXA scan:
  a. Lumbar region—L2 to L4
  b. Hip including femoral neck, trochanter, and intertrochanteric region
  c. Wrist
B. T-score: It is measured in standard deviations; it will reflect difference between BMD measured of that patient and the mean value of the BMD in young-matched control (women of 30 years of age). According to the definition, a normal BMD measurement is within 1 standard deviation of young adult mean. According to WHO, BMD is -1.20 to -2.5, suggests osteopenia, and >-2.5 suggests osteoporosis.
C. Z-score: It is measured in standard deviation, but it is compared to adult healthy age-matched control group. Z-score of <-1.5 suggests secondary osteoporosis.
D. Other laboratory tests include:
  a. LFT
  b. Calcium and phosphorus
  c. Thyroid function test
  d. Renal function test
  e. Vitamin D
E. Serum or urinary tests for the following:
  a. Cross-links of type I collagen
  b. N-telopeptide of type I collagen
  c. C-telopeptide of type I collagen
F. Fracture risk assessment score tool as suggested by WHO for prediction of 10 years risk of sustaining hip or other osteoporotic fracture, other sites include spine, wrist, humerus, and forearm. This tool consists of 12 questions related to future frailty fracture.

Treatment

A. Lifestyle modification:
  a. Avoidance of alcohol and smoking
  b. Cessation of weight-bearing physical activities
  c. Regular exercise programs
  d. Daily intake of vitamin D—800-1,000 IU/day over the age of 50 years
  e. Daily calcium—1,200-1,500 mg/day over the age of 50 years
B. Prevention of fall by:
  a. Removing loose carpet in the floor
  b. Reduction of dose of sleep medicine
  c. Correction of visual impairment
C. Risk stratification for probability of fracture in next 10 years and advice for taking medication who are prone to develop osteoporotic fracture.
D. Recommendation of pharmacotherapy:
  a. Treatment recommendation for history of nonvertebral fracture:
    1. Treatment should be started in all postmenopausal women with history of fragility fracture.

2. DEXA scan should be performed in patients sustaining nonvertebral fragility fracture and decision should be taken regarding the therapy in patients based on t-score and z-score.

E. Medicines to be given:
   a. Alendronate reduce the risk of fracture by 50% in hip, spine, and wrist.
   b. Risedronate reduces vertebral and nonvertebral fracture by 40%
   c. Intravenous zoledronic acid will reduce hip fracture by 40% over 3 years.
   d. Other medications are:
      1. Conjugated estrogen-progesterone hormone replacement
      2. Salmon calcium
      3. Only estrogen replacement
      4. Selective estrogen receptor modulator—raloxifene is estrogen receptor agonist
      5. Anabolic hormone—teriparatide—a recombinant form of parathyroid hormone stimulating osteoblast to produce more bones.
      6. RANKL inhibitors: Denosumab, a monoclonal Ig2 targeting RANKL and thus inhibiting its ability to bind with RANK, which in turn inhibits osteoclastic activity.

Q26. Inflammatory myositis.

PGI/NOV2012/MDIV (10)

Inflammatory myopathies

NTR UNI of Health SC Vijayawada, Andhra, 2022 (10)

ANSWER

Definition

It is a heterogeneous group of autoimmune myopathies where inflammation of the skeletal muscles leads to weakness along with involvement of other organ systems such as skin, cardiac, and gastrointestinal systems.

Classifications

Inflammatory myositis can be classified into five categories:

A. Idiopathic polymyositis
B. Idiopathic dermatomyositis
C. Idiopathic inflammatory myositis associated with malignancy
D. Childhood idiopathic inflammatory myositis often associated vasculitis
E. Idiopathic inflammatory myositis associated with collagen vascular disease

Exclusion criteria are the following:

A. Signs of central and peripheral neurological disease
B. Family history of muscle disease
C. Clinical features suggestive of muscular dystrophy
D. Granulomatous myositis
E. Infection of the muscles such as trichinosis, schistosomiasis, and trypanosomiasis

International myositis assessment and clinical studies has included the need of muscle biopsy to diagnose polymyositis and skin feature to diagnose dermatomyositis.

Recently, >30 specific autoantibodies have been identified for inflammatory myopathies.

Pathogenesis

There are multiple pathogenic pathways which are responsible for weakness and muscle damage and it is due to development of autoantibodies against muscle specific antigen. The result is:

a. Formation of autoantibodies
b. Formation of autoreactive lymphocytes
c. Unusual overexpression of MHC class I molecules to be present on the affected muscle fibers.

As a result, there is activation of innate and adaptive immunity and defect in the metabolic pathways in the skeletal muscles, innate immunity acting as bridge between adaptive immunity and metabolic defect. All the above factors interact with each other to produce muscle damage leading to development of myositis.

Clinical Presentation

A. Subtle symptoms of fatigue and tiredness
B. Weight loss—usually mild, but if it is persistent, it suggests myositis due to malignancy.
C. Fever—more common in childhood, in case of adult, antisynthetase antibody syndrome is associated with fever.
D. Gradual onset over several months, symmetrical painless, progressive proximal muscle weakness. But in children and young adult, painful weakness of muscles occurs acutely.
E. In a small subsets, slowly evolving weakness over many years, mainly occurring in older male of >60 years.
F. Other features are:
   a. Pitting edema in the extremities

b. Hoarseness of voice
c. Dysphagia due to bulbar palsy
d. Nasal regurgitation of fluid due to pharyngeal striated muscle involvement
e. Breathlessness due to ILD

G. Skeletal muscle involvement:
a. In case of polymyositis, there is gradual progressive symmetrical weakness of the proximal muscles leading to difficulty in climbing upstairs, getting up from squatting position. Patient develop waddling gait.
b. Gradually muscles of upper extremities are involved leading to difficulty in lifting the arm overhead, combing hair, etc.
c. Neck flexor muscles are involved leading to drooping of the head.
d. Muscle pain is rare. Oculofacial weakness never occurs.

H. Skin involvement:
a. Gottron's papule—scaly, erythematous violaceous plaques over the skin of MCP and PIP joints
b. Gottron's sign—macular erythema over the same bony prominences and over the knee and elbows
c. Heliotrope rash—present on the periorbital region with edema—specific sign of dermatomyositis
d. Other signs include:
1. Photosensitive scalp involvement
2. Shawl sign
3. V sign
4. Mechanic's hand—crackling and fissuring involving palmar and radial aspects of fingers
5. Panniculitis
6. Calcinosis
7. Acanthosis nigricans
8. Poikiloderma
9. In children multifocal lipoatrophy
10. Amyopathic dermatomyositis—presence of biopsy proven rash but without muscle weakness and normal muscle enzymes and normal electromyography

I. Articular involvement: It is usually polyarticular, rheumatoid like distribution.

J. Pulmonary involvement:
a. Interstitial lung disease
b. Bronchiolitis obliterans
c. Organizing pneumonia
d. Acute respiratory distress syndrome (ARDS)
e. Pulmonary hypertension
f. Pleural effusion
g. Alveolar hemorrhage
h. Pneumomediastinum

K. Cardiac involvement:
a. Rhythm disturbances
b. Pericardial effusion
c. Congestive cardiac failure
d. Myocarditis
e. Cardiomyopathy

L. Gastrointestinal involvement:
a. Dysphagia
b. Dysphonia
c. Nasal regurgitation of fluid
d. Esophageal stricture
e. Postprandial abdominal distension due involvement of small bowel

M. Peripheral vascular system:
a. Raynaud's phenomenon
b. Digital ulceration
c. Periungual infarct

N. Renal involvement:
a. Nonoliguric acute renal failure
b. Mesangioproliferative glomerulonephritis
c. Crescentic glomerulonephritis
d. Focal segmental glomerular sclerosis (FSGS)
e. Membranous nephropathy
f. Minimal change disease

O. Malignant myositis:
a. It occurs in following malignancies:
1. Lung
2. Pancreas
3. Stomach
4. Colorectal cancer
5. Non-Hodgkin's lymphoma
b. Following are the clinical features:
1. Epidermal necrosis
2. Cutaneous leukocytoclastic vasculitis
3. Amyopathic dermatomyositis

Investigations

A. Muscle biopsy: It will demonstrate:
a. Presence of chronic inflammatory infiltrate in the endomysial and perimysial regions around the blood vessel
b. Presence of necrosis and regeneration of myofibers
c. Intact muscle fibers are invaded by autoreactive T cells.

d. Connective tissue labeling with alkaline phosphatase by histochemical stain
e. Rimmed vacuoles, amyloid deposits
f. De novo expression of MHC-1 molecule, perifascicular atrophy

B. Electromyography:
  a. On needle insertion at rest:
    1. Fibrillation potential
    2. Positive sharp waves
    3. Complex repetitive discharge
    4. Short duration and low amplitude complex
  b. Single fiber electromyography
  c. Macro-electromyography
  d. Motor unit action potential analysis

C. MRI: It will demonstrate:
  a. Anatomy
  b. Morphology
  c. Potential functionality of muscles
  d. Muscle edema
  e. Areas of active involvement
  f. Potentially subclinical disease
  g. Provide guidelines for muscle biopsy

D. Ultrasound can demonstrate the following:
  a. Assess the dynamic function of the muscles on real-time
  b. Doppler evaluation of vascularity
  c. Image-guided biopsy

E. Capillaroscopy:
  a. Scleroderma spectrum diseases
  b. Microhemorrhages
  c. Giant capillaries
  d. Dilated capillaries

  All the above are consistent with microvasculopathy and involvement of capillaries that is observed in muscle biopsies.

  e. Capillary neoformation seen as tortuosity, bushy, clustering, or arboreal appearances.

Treatment

A. Corticosteroid:
  a. In case PM, DM and necrotizing autoimmune myositis can be treated by oral prednisolone at a dose of 1 mg/kg/day.
  b. In case of rapidly worsening of the disease or weakness of respiratory or bulbar muscles 1 g intravenous methylprednisolone for 3–5 days followed by oral prednisolone.

B. Immunosuppressive drugs:
  a. After 3–6 weeks continuous treatment with prednisolone, it should be tapered according to the response, then alternate day dose of steroid should be given. Muscle will regain its power after several months along with decease in serum CPK level.
  b. Those who are responsive to steroids, immunosuppressants such as methotrexate, cyclosporine A, and mycophenolate mofetil can be given as glucocorticoid sparing agents.
  c. In case of interstitial lung disease, cyclophosphamide or tacrolimus can be administered.
  d. In patients with myositis and interstitial lung disease along with steroids, immunosuppressant can be added.

C. Intravenous immunoglobulin:

  It is indicated in the following cases:
  a. Where glucocorticoid fails to induce remission
  b. In severe rapidly progressive cases
  c. Where high-dose pulse therapy of steroid is contraindicated due to concomitant infection.

  Dose of immunoglobulin is 2 g/kg in divided doses over 2–5 consecutive days. In severe cases, monthly infusion is required to maintain remission.

  In patients with dermatomyositis topical glucocorticoids and calcineurin inhibitors along with avoidance of sun exposure are advised.

D. Biologics:
  a. In patients with anti-Jo-1, anti-Mi-2, or anti-SRP antibodies: rituximab 2 g in divided into two infusions at 2 weeks apart is effective.
  b. Other biologics included are:
    1. Alemtuzumab
    2. Anti-complement C3—eculizumab
    3. Anti-interleukin-6 receptor—tocilizumab
    4. Anti-interleukin-1 receptor—anakinra

Treatment of Inclusion Body Myositis

The drugs are:

A. Intravenous immunoglobulin
B. Anakinra
C. Alemtuzumab—it may provide short-term stabilization.

Q27. Serum antibodies assay in different rheumatological disorders and its relevance in reactive arthritis.

MGR/APRIL2012/MDII(7)

ANSWER

Following are the antibodies in rheumatology:

A. Rheumatoid factor:

a. This antibody is directed against Fc portion of IgM.

b. It can be detected by nephelometry, latex agglutination, and ELISA test.

c. It is present in 80–85% of rheumatoid arthritis—seropositive arthritis, rest are seronegatives.

d. Its presence suggests—the disease is more aggressive and extra-articular manifestations are present and prognosis is poor.

e. It is also present in the following conditions:

1. Chronic inflammatory conditions:
   - Sjögren's syndrome
   - Autoimmune hepatitis
   - Primary biliary cirrhosis
   - SLE
   - Sarcoidosis
2. Chronic infections:
   - Malaria
   - Tuberculosis
   - Leprosy
   - Hepatitis C
3. Rarely malignancies

B. Antibodies to citrullinated peptides:

a. It is directed against citrullinated self-peptides.

b. It is highly specific for rheumatoid arthritis.

c. It is positive in one-third of patients with negative rheumatoid factor.

d. It is rarely seen in other connective tissue diseases and infections.

C. Antinuclear antibodies:

a. It is heterogeneous group of antibodies directed against different components of nucleus, centromere, and nucleolar protein.

b. Gold standard method of detection is immuno-fluorescence test.

c. Three pattern of positivity seen in immunofluorescence:

1. Rim or homozygous pattern:
   - Directed against DNA/DNA histone
   - Found in SLE and drug-induced lupus
2. Centromere pattern:
   - Directed against centromere protein A and B
   - Found in limited scleroderma
3. Speckled pattern:
   - Directed against smooth muscle, RNP, Ro/SSA, LA/SS, Scl-70, RNA, polymerase II and III
   - Found in SLE, systemic sclerosis, progressive systemic sclerosis, MCTD, and proximal myositis

D. Antibodies to dsDNA:

a. It is a hallmark of SLE.

b. They are detected by IIF using a protozoan parasite *Crithidia luciliae* of Leishmania family that has prominent kinetoplast made of DsDNA.

E. Antibodies to extractable nuclear antigens: The antigens are:

a. Anti-Sm: SLE

b. Anti-RNP: Mixed connective tissue disease

c. Anti-Scl-70: Scleroderma

d. Anti-La and anti-Ro: Sjögren's syndrome

e. Anti-Jo: Inflammatory myositis

This qualitative test should be done if ANA is positive. Quantitative estimation should be done by immunoblotting or line assay.

F. Antiphospholipid antibody:

a. Cardiolipin is the most commonly used substrate.

b. Antibodies detected are IgM and IgG. IgA may be present but is of less diagnostic value.

c. It can be measured as mild, moderate, and marked elevation.

G. Anti-beta 2 glycoprotein 1 antibodies:

a. Antibodies directed against cofactor which is required for binding of cardiolipin

b. It is more specific for diagnosis and can be detected by ELISA.

H. Antiprothrombin antibodies: It is used for assay of lupus anticoagulant.

I. Antibodies against phosphatidylserine and annexin-V

J. Antibodies to neutrophil cytoplasmic antigen:

a. It is positive for:

1. Granulomatosis with polyangiitis previously known as Wegener's granulomatosis
2. Eosinophilic granulomatosis with polyangiitis previously known as Churg-Strauss syndrome.
3. Microscopic polyangiitis—polyarteritis nodosa

b. There are two pattern of results:

1. Cytoplasmic pattern (cANCA): Antigenic target is proteinase 3—specific for diagnosis of GPA.
2. Perinuclear pattern (pANCA): Antigenic target is myeloperoxidase—specific for PAN. But it may be positive for ulcerative colitis, rheumatoid arthritis, and SLE.
3. These can be quantitatively measured by ELISA and is useful for monitoring the disease activity in vasculitis.

Reactive arthritis has been described in question number 7.

Q28. What are the various patterns of arthropathy seen in psoriatic arthritis?

DNB 2020 (5)

ANSWER

There are five types of joint involvements in psoriatic arthritis:

A. Asymmetric oligoarthritis involving five small or large joints.
B. Symmetric polyarticular arthritis involving distal interphalangeal joints and rheumatoid factor negative.
C. Distal arthritis involving distal small joints
D. Destructive joint disease with deformities known as arthritis mutilans involving hands and feet.
E. Spondyloarthritis involving sacroiliitis but not involving peripheral joints.

Q29. How will you differentiate articular pain from non-articular pain?

DNB 2020 (5)

ANSWER

Articular structures include:

A. Synovium
B. Synovial fluid
C. Articular cartilage
D. Joint capsule
E. Intraarticular ligaments
F. Juxta-articular bone

Periarticular structures include:

A. Extra-articular ligaments
B. Muscles
C. Fascia
D. Nerves
E. Bones
F. Tendons
G. Overlying skin

So, first thing is to differentiate articular pain from extra-articular pain, next to isolate the arthritis into acute and chronic, lastly, whether single joint or multiple joints are involved. Except articular pain other pains around the joints are:

A. Periarticular pain
B. Neurogenic pain
C. Referred pain

Following questions can differentiate the above conditions.

A. *Regarding motion*:
   a. Only selected movements are restricted due to pain - periarticular pain
   b. If all the movement of any particular joint are painful - articular pain
   c. If the pain around the joint is aggravated by compression on the nerve or spinal movement - neurogenic pain
   d. If the pain is not present in the joint but comes from distant organ and may be improved by rubbing - referred pain.
B. *Pain during different types of movement*:
   a. If pain mainly occurs during active movement than passive movement - periarticular pain
   b. If pain occurs during both active and passive movement - articular pain
   c. If there is no pain during any movement of that joint - referred pain
   d. If pain occurs during movement of the spine but normal if joint pain is due to root compression - neuropathic pain.
C. *In case of range of motion*:
   a. Restriction of active movement but passive movement is normal - periarticular pain
   b. Normal movement:
      1. Neuropathic pain
      2. Referred pain
   c. All the movement is restricted - articular pain
D. Resistance given during movement:
   a. Occurs during in specific movement: Periarticular pain
   b. No effect on resistance:
      1. Articular pain

2. Referred pain
3. Neurogenic pain

E. *Neurological examination*:
- **a.** Normal:
  1. Periarticular pain
  2. Referred pain
  3. Articular pain
- **b.** There may be root pain - neurogenic pain

F. On examination tenderness on local palpation:
- **a.** Absent:
  1. Neuropathic pain
  2. Referred pain
- **b.** Present of the periarticular structure - periarticular pain
- **c.** Present on the joint line - articular pain

Q30. Definition and enumerate causes of migratory arthritis.

DNB 2018 (4)

ANSWER

Definition

Migratory arthritis can be defined as inflammation of one joint followed by involvement of another joint when the previous joint will recover.

Causes of Migratory Arthritis

A. Infective causes:
- **a.** Rheumatic fever where large joints are involved.
- **b.** Lyme disease where in the early disseminated phase the joints are involved.
- **c.** Disseminated gonococcal arthritis where there is migratory polyarthritis along with rash.
- *d.* *Viral causes*:
  1. Parvovirus B19
  2. Hepatitis B infection
  3. Chikungunya virus

B. Post-infectious causes:
- **a.** Post-streptococcal
- **b.** Reactive arthritis like Reiter's syndrome

C. Rheumatologic causes:
- **a.** SLE where the feature is migratory but non-erosive and intermittent.
- **b.** Serum sickness - there is present of rash along with arthritis.
- **c.** Palindromic rheumatism - here this arthritis is short-lived and recurrent.

D. Miscellaneous causes: Here the arthritis may precede gastrointestinal symptom.

Q31. Temporal arteritis.

MGR UNI, Tamil Nadu, 2022 (10)

ANSWER

Definition

This temporal arteritis is a chronic inflammatory vasculitis involving large and medium sized arteries, mostly cranial arteries in patient of more than 50 years of age.

Etiology

A. *Genetic factors*: There is common association between this disease and specific polymorphisms in the major histocompatibility antigens like HLA DRB1*04:04, HLA DQA1*03:01, HLA-DQB1*03:02.

B. Other variants involving T helper cells 1, 17.

Epidemiology

A. Age incidence is between 70 and 79 years with mean age of 75 years.

B. *Race*: Highest incidence in the Scandinavian countries. And lowest in African-American, Asian and Japanese people.

C. *Sex*: Females are predominantly affected.

Pathophysiology

A. It is an immune-mediated disease where vascular dendritic cells are activated produce chemokines like granulocyte-macrophage colony stimulating factor which in turn attract more dendritic cells, macrophages and lymphocytes. These dendritic cells present and process the antigens, express the activation markers and major histocompatibility complex class II and costimulatory molecules that will lead to activation of T cells.

B. Activated vascular dendritic cells present in the tunica adventitia in the large vessels recruit T cells in the arterial wall which in turn differentiate into interferon-γ- producing T helper cells and interleukin-17 producing T-helper 17 cells. These cytokines after being produced activate macrophages leading to hyperplasia of vascular smooth muscle cells leading to formation of GIANT cells.

C. Macrophages release interleukin-1β and interleukin-6 leading to production systemic inflammatory response resulting disease specific constitutional symptoms.

Histopathology

A. In the early stage of the disease, collection of the lymphocytes in the internal and external elastic lamina or adventitia and intimal thickening.

B. With the progression of the disease, there is transmural inflammation and areas of necrosis and presence of granuloma consisting of multinucleated histiocytes as well as foreign body giant cells, histiocytes, T lymphocytes, plasma cells and fibroblasts.

C. There may be thrombotic changes during active inflammation.

D. There may be the evidence of skip lesions.

Clinical Features

A. Headache: Classically it is waxing and waning temporal headache associated with scalp tenderness, but in some cases, it may be unilateral frontal or occipital or generalized and may subside before commencement of treatment. Clinically there is presence of nodular tender temporal artery with absence of pulses unilaterally or bilaterally in the temporal artery.

B. In 50% of patients there may be claudication of jaw as evidenced by fatigue or pain in the mandible or may be in the tongue that may be triggered by chewing and subsided after cessation of chewing.

C. In 50% patients there are constitutional symptoms, these are:

- **a.** Low grade fever but may increase up to 102°F.
- **b.** Malaise
- **c.** Weight loss
- **d.** Anorexia

D. *Visual symptoms*:

- **a.** 20 to 30% patients may present with transient or permanent visual loss, presented with abrupt partial field defect or there may be feeling of presence of curtain in 1 eye.
- **b.** Permanent visual loss in the form of anterior ischemic optic neuropathy as evidenced by painless unilateral or bilateral partial or complete loss of vision. Diplopia is specific for this disease.
- **c.** Fundoscopy demonstrates:
  - **1.** Pallor or edema of optic disc.
  - **2.** Optic atrophy
  - **3.** Retinal ischemia
  - **4.** Choroid ischemia
- **d.** Rare finding is Charles Bonnet syndrome where there is visual hallucination and loss of vision due to loss of central or peripheral visual pathways.

E. *Musculoskeletal system*: There may be the features of polymyalgia rheumatica in 45 to 60% of patients as featured by pain, stiffness and limiting in the range of motion around the shoulder girdle, neck and also hips. There may be difficulty in the combing hair or standing from the sitting position.

F. *Large vessel involvement*: Involvement of aorta and its proximal branches leads to claudication of the upper extremities, chest or back pain – it may be due to aortitis or aortic dissection. Physical findings are:

- **a.** Auscultatory bruit present over abdominal aorta, axillary, brachial and femoral arteries.
- **b.** Lack of pulses, asymmetric pulses or blood pressure in the upper extremities.
- **c.** May be features of Raynaud's phenomenon without any evidence of ischemia
- **d.** Early diastolic murmur in the aortic area may signify ascending aortic aneurysm.

G. *Involvement of central nervous system*: There may be evidence of transient ischemic attack due to involvement of posterior circulation risk is higher within 4 weeks after diagnosis. Associated risk factors are hypertension and peripheral vascular disease.

H. *Additional features*:

- **a.** Symptoms of upper respiratory tract
- **b.** Dental pain
- **c.** Macroglossia
- **d.** Dysarthria
- **e.** Sensorineural hearing loss
- **f.** Breast mass
- **g.** Involvement of female genital tract
- **h.** Pericarditis

Evaluation

A. *Laboratory testing*:

- **a.** Complete blood count
- **b.** ESR: Raised, in some biopsy confirmed case it may be normal. In corticosteroid native cases it is more than 50 mm/1st hour.
- **c.** CRP: It is more significant marker in this disease
- **d.** Serum transaminases
- **e.** Blood glucose
- **f.** Serum creatinine kinase

- **g.** Serum aldolase
- **h.** Serum electrolytes
- **i.** Serum creatinine
- **j.** Serum protein electrophoresis
- **k.** Serum 25-hydroxyvitamin D
- **l.** Total proteins

B. Temporal artery biopsy at least 1 cm of artery is required to increase the positivity as sensitivity is decreased in the following conditions:

- **a.** Skip lesions
- **b.** Lack of involvement of temporal artery
- **c.** Inadequate specimens
- **d.** Glucocorticoid therapy

In case of symptomatic patient, biopsy should be taken from the symptomatic side.

C. *Carotid Doppler ultrasound*: It should be done in suspected case of temporal arteritis or within 1 week of commencing glucocorticoid therapy as this drug will lower the sensitivity. The hallmark is "Hallo Sign" that can be described as hypoechoic ring of inflamed edematous vessels surrounded by Doppler signal of internal carotid artery. Bilateral "Halo Sign" is specific for giant cell arteritis. It can visualize axillary, subclavian and carotid arteries.

Specificity of the biopsy is 100% as compared to 80% specificity of carotid Doppler ultrasound.

D. *Other imaging*:

- **a.** If carotid Doppler ultrasound and temporal artery biopsy are negative, high-resolution MRI of neck, chest, abdomen and pelvis with magnetic resonance angiography.
- **b.** Images for the large vessel disease include:
  - **1.** CT angiography
  - **2.** PET with FDG
  - **3.** PET with CT: PET can visualize the abdominal aorta.

Treatment

A. *Corticosteroids*: It is initial treatment of choice.

- **a.** It should be administered as 40–60 mg daily and to be continued for 2–4 weeks till the normalization of symptoms and acute phase reactant.
- **b.** After clinical remission, its dose should be decreased by 10 mg daily every 2 weeks to 20 mg daily after the patient is in remission for 4–8 weeks.
- **c.** Then the dose should be reduced by 2.5 mg every 2–4 weeks till dose comes down to 10 mg daily.
- **d.** Then the dose can be reduced by 1 mg every 12 to 18 months with supervision maintaining of clinical remission or normalization of clinical markers.

B. *Steroid sparing agents*: If there is risk of developing complications or there is 1st relapse, following agents should be given according to ACR:

- **a.** Tocilizumab weekly injection of 162 mg subcutaneously or monthly intravenous infusion of 8 mg/kg along with corticosteroids with maximum dose up to 800 mg. This drug can be continued up to 12–18 months. Tocilizumab completely inhibits interleukin-6.
- **b.** If the patient is unable to take Tocilizumab, in that case methotrexate can be started at a dose of 10–15 mg weekly orally with increase of 5 mg per week till the dose reaches maximum up to 25 mg weekly.

C. In case of threatened or established visual loss intravenous methylprednisolone 500–1000 mg for 3 consecutive days. In case of unavailability of methylprednisolone, 1 mg prednisolone orally can be administered. After pulse therapy of methylprednisolone, high dose of oral prednisolone should be recommended.

D. In case extracranial large vessels involvement, longer duration of steroids and steroid sparing immunosuppressive drugs are recommended.

Complications

- **A.** Visual loss
- **B.** Aortic aneurysm and aortic dissection
- **C.** Stroke
- **D.** Tongue necrosis
- **E.** Side effects of steroids
- **F.** Adverse effects of Tocilizumab

Q32. Sjögren's syndrome.

MGR UNI, Tamil Nadu, 2022 (10)

Clinical features and diagnosis of Sjögren's syndrome.

DR YSR UNI of Health SC, Vijayawada, Andhra, 2022 (10)

ANSWER

Definition

Primary Sjögren's syndrome is an autoimmune disorder defined as the dryness of the eyes and mouth due to inflammation of lacrimal and salivary glands.

Etiology

A. Primary Sjögren's syndrome - genetic predisposition involving major histocompatibility locus seen in the individual sharing haplotypes in HLA-DQA_DQB, these patients have increased risk.

B. Sjögren's syndrome may be associated with rheumatoid arthritis and SLE.

Pathophysiology

The characteristic lesion is focal lymphocytic sialadenitis involving exocrine glands consisting of foci of mononuclear cells including T lymphocytes, B lymphocytes and plasma cells seen adjacent to blood vessels and excretory duct. These infiltrate release cytokines and antibodies resulting dysfunction of exocrine glands leading to decreased production of tears and saliva from the lacrimal gland and salivary glands respectively. Other exocrine glands other than the head and neck are also involved leading to dryness of skin, vagina and tracheobronchial tree and also dysfunction of the kidney and lung.

In rare cases malignant transformation of the B lymphocytes results Hodgkin's lymphoma.

There is deposition of immune complexes in the skin and joints leading to systemic vasculitis.

History and Clinical Examination

A. Foreign body sensation in the eyes

B. Dry mouth

C. Eye examination demonstrates:

- **a.** Absence of tears in the inferior conjunctival sac.
- **b.** Injection of the eyes
- **c.** Examination of the eye in presence of vital dye staining can demonstrate keratoconjunctivitis sicca.
- **d.** Schirmer test can also demonstrate dryness of the conjunctiva.

D. In 50% cases there is enlargement of parotid and/or submandibular gland

E. Mouth looks parched,

F. Smooth tongue and thin mucosae.

G. Extraglandular involvement:

- **a.** Polyarthritis
- **b.** Features of peripheral neuropathy
- **c.** Purpura in the lower extremity

Evaluation

A. Eye examination:

- **a.** Schirmer test
- **b.** Vital dye staining
- **c.** Slit lamp examination
- **d.** Salivary flow rate

B. Assessment of autoantibodies like ANA, Rheumatoid factor, SS-A and SS-B, amongst which SS-A is most sensitive and specific for Sjögren's syndrome.

C. Most specific test is the biopsy of minor salivary gland—it can demonstrate focal lymphocytic sialadenitis.

Treatment

A. Dry eyes will respond to during daytime artificial tears and at night application of gel.

B. In severe cases punctual occlusion or cauterization but later should be done after trial of plugs to ensure the affected patient cannot be released with excessive tearing.

C. Instillation of cyclosporine in the eyes to reduce inflammation as well as increased production of tears.

D. Nowadays in most of the hospitals patient's whole blood is used to make serum tears.

E. To get recovery of dry mouth, drinking water and chewing gum can be used.

F. Administration of pilocarpine or cevimeline to increase the flow of saliva in the mouth.

G. Irrigation with nasal saline and humidifier can improve nasal dryness.

H. Proton pump inhibitors can be used to prevent the symptoms of acid reflux.

I. In case of yeast infection, anti-fungal therapy should be used.

J. Oral or parenteral corticosteroids can be used to treat Extraglandular involvement.

K. Methotrexate, azathioprine should be used as steroid sparing agents in this case.

L. Inflammatory arthritis can be treated by hydroxychloroquine.

Q33. Behçet's disease.

Maharashtra UNI of Health SC, Vijayawada, 2022 (10)

ANSWER

Behçet's disease has been described in 1937 by Hulusi Behçet.

Etiology

There is increased prevalence along the "Silk route" as well as familial aggregation indicating genetic element like association with HLA B51/B5 as compared to non-carriers. HLA-B51 is common Japanese, middle eastern and Turkish populations.

Several other genes identified are:

A. Tumor necrosis factor

B. Heat shock protein

C. Major histocompatibility complex class I chain related genes.

Following also act as potential culprits:

A. *Streptococcus sanguinis*

B. *Staphylococcus aureus*

C. Herpes simplex virus type 1.

D. *Prevotella* species

Epidemiology

A. It affects mostly young adult of 20–40 years of age and less frequently children.

B. Though both sexes are equally affected, but in Arabian population there is male preponderance.

C. Female preponderance is in Korea, China, and USA.

Pathophysiology

A. Though it is auto-inflammatory vasculitis involving veins and arteries of any size, but it is lack in giant cell formation and necrotizing vasculitis.

B. The unique of this disease is involvement of veins and pulmonary and arterial aneurysms.

C. There is lack of specific autoantibodies as compared to other autoimmune disorders.

D. There is significant role of cell mediated immunity in this disease as high level of circulating T lymphocytes resulting from T-1 helper cell activation.

E. Increased level of circulation proinflammatory cytokines like interleukin-1, 8, 12, 17 and 37 and tumor necrosis factor found in this disease.

F. Enhanced activation of macrophages, neutrophil chemotaxis followed by phagocytosis in these lesions like muco-cutaneous lesions, i.e., oral ulcers, skin pustules and erythema nodosum.

G. Circulating immune complexes, especially anti-endothelial antibodies are responsible for neutrophilic vascular reaction.

Clinical Features

A. *Aphthous ulcers like*:

- **a.** Oral ulcers present in nearly 95% patients. It can be described as painful, recurrent multiple superficial ulcers involving soft and hard palate, buccal mucosa, tongue, gingiva, lips and tonsils. Most of these ulcers heal without scarring.
- **b.** Genital ulcers in scrotum in males and vagina or valve in females occurs in 80% of patients, like oral ulcers. But these ulcers heal with scarring.

B. Cutaneous manifestations:

- **a.** Erythema nodosum in this disease is more vasculitic as compared to erythema nodosum from other causes.
- **b.** Superficial thrombophlebitis presents as nodular lesion which is usually associated with deep vein thrombosis.
- **c.** Acuneiform or pseudofolliculitis may be present which may not be possible to distinguish from acne.
- **d.** *Pyoderma gangrenosum* like lesion
- **e.** Pustular vasculitic lesions
- **f.** Cutaneous small vessel vasculitis
- **g.** Sweet syndrome like lesion
- **h.** Cutaneous pathergy reaction is very pathognomonic of this disease which is characterized by erythematous papules or pustules appearing 24 to 48 hours after insertion of needles mostly observed in patients from Turkey or Japan.

C. *Ocular involvement*: In 50% cases in patients with acneiform lesions.

- **a.** Uveitis – characterized by relapsing bilateral chronic involving both anterior and posterior uveal tracts.
    1. Involvement of anterior uveal tract leads to photophobia and erythema
    2. Involvement of posterior tract leads to loss of vision.
- **b.** Hypopyon related uveitis is less common but very severe and is associated with retinal disease.
- **c.** Retinal involvement leads to vision loss.
- **d.** Conjunctivitis and isolated anterior uveitis may occur but rare.

D. Musculoskeletal manifestations:

- **a.** Asymmetric but may be peripheral symmetric, oligoarticular or polyarticular joint involvement.
- **b.** Knee is commonly followed by ankles, wrist and elbow.
- **c.** Sacroiliitis is not usually seen, if present it is not erosive and HLA B-27 negative.

E. *Vascular manifestation*: Any size arterial and venular involvement are specific for this disease in 25% of patients.

a. Superficial and deep thrombophlebitis invo9lving lower extremities are most common features.
b. Involvement inferior vena caval obstruction may be seen.
c. Arterial vasculitis leading to aneurysm or occlusion may be the features.
d. Carotid, femoral and popliteal arteritis may be present.
e. The leading cause of death is involvement of pulmonary artery and aneurysm.

F. *Neurological manifestation*:
a. In 5% to 10% patient neurological manifestation, amongst 80% are brain parenchymal involvement leading to features of cerebellar, pyramidal and sensory features. Due to thrombi in the dural sinuses.
b. There may be papilledema, headache.

G. *Gastrointestinal involvement*:
a. Mucosal ulcerations involve ileum, cecum, colon and esophagus.
b. Extensive ulcerations involving ileum may be present. In this case inflammatory bowel disease should be ruled out.

H. *Cardiological features*:
a. Pericarditis
b. Myocarditis
c. Endocarditis
d. Coronary artery vasculitis
e. Coronary artery aneurysm

I. *Renal manifestations*:
a. AA-amyloidosis
b. Glomerulonephritis
c. Epididymitis

Evaluation

A. Complete blood count- anemia, leukocytosis, thrombocytopenia
B. Elevation of markers of inflammation
C. X-ray of joints and arthrocentesis to detect arthritis.
D. CT scan brain to detect cerebral edema, bleeding, thrombosis or cerebral aneurysm
E. Lumbar puncture to detect meningitis.

Revised International criteria of Behcet's disease are:

A. 1point each to oral aphthous ulcers and skin manifestations, vascular lesions, positive pathergy test.
B. 2 points each to genital aphthous ulcers and ocular lesions.

3 or more points suggest the diagnosis.

Treatment

A. Mucosa ulcers:
a. Isolated oral and genital aphthous ulcers:
1. Topical triamcinolone cream 3 to 4 times daily until the pain will be relieved.
2. Alternative to topical steroid is topical sucralfate 1 g/5 mL.
3. Topical anesthetic may provide temporary relief.

B. Prevention of recurrence of ulcers in mouth and genitalia:
a. Colchicine 1 to 2 mg/day in divided doses:
1. 1st line of drug
2. Narrow therapeutic index
3. More effective in genital ulcers
4. Significant side effects in neutropenia.
b. Apremilast should be titrated at a rate of 10 mg daily over 6 days lastly to attain maintenance dose of 30 mg twice daily.
1. It is more effective in oral ulcers.
2. Adverse effects are nausea, vomiting and diarrhea.

C. Oral, genital ulcers refractory to therapy:
a. Prednisolone 15 mg daily to start with and reduce the dose to 10 mg daily after 1 week and stop the dose completely after 2 to 3 weeks.

D. If all the treatment fails:
a. Azathioprine:
1. Initial dose is 50 mg daily and dose to be increased by 50 mg every month.
2. Dose should be 2.5 mg/kg/day.
3. CBC should be done every 15 days till the maximum dose should be reached then every 6 to 12 weeks.
4. Genetic counselling thiopurine methyl-transferase before commencement of therapy.
5. It can be combined TNF like infliximab, adalimumab and etanercept.
b. Interferon: Interferon-alfa and interferon-beta – 3 to 6 million units thrice weekly.

E. Cutaneous lesions:
a. Mild case – colchicine 1 to 2 mg in divided dose.

b. *If unresponsive to colchicine*: 40 mg prednisolone to start with followed by 5 to 10 mg as maintenance dose.

F. Erythema nodosum:

a. Prednisolone 40 to 60 mg daily plus:

1. Azathioprine initial dose is 50 mg daily, if tolerated dose should be increased by 50 mg weekly reaching to 2.5 mg/kg/day.

2. Complications are described above.

3. Dose of steroid should be reduced every 2 weeks to start after 1 month of therapy in full dose then the total treatment should be completed within 4 months.

G. Pyoderma gangrenosum:

a. No extensive debridement.

b. Mild localized case:

1. Topical steroid or topical Tacrolimus

c. More extensive and progressive case:

1. Systemic steroid:

- Oral prednisolone 0.5 to 1.5 mg/kg/day to be started initially with maximal dose of 60 mg/day for 4 to 10 weeks followed by tapering of the steroid.
- Intravenous methyl prednisolone 1 g intravenously for 5 days followed by oral prednisolone as above.

2. Systemic cyclosporine:

- It is an alternative solution to prednisolone or steroid refractory cases.
- Initial dose is 4 to 5 mg/kg followed by gradual tapering of the dose.
- In case of renal toxicity or hypertension the treatment should be limited to 1 year.

H. *Arthritis*:

a. Initial drug is colchicine at a dose of 1 to 2 mg/day in divided dose.

b. In case of refractory to colchicine, initial dose of prednisolone is 60 mg daily, in case of prolonged therapy requirement 5 mg daily should be given.

c. In refractory of persistent case azathioprine or TNF-α inhibitor.

d. If all the therapy is refractory, interferon-α or Apremilast

I. Gastrointestinal ulcerations: Prednisolone plus azathioprine

a. Prednisolone 1 mg/kg daily to start with for 1 month or till the resolution of the symptoms followed by decrease in the dose to 10 mg/day over 2 to 3 months.

b. Azathioprine to start with 50 mg daily and increasing the daily dose by 50 mg every 4 weeks to reach the target dose of 2.5 mg/kg daily with complete hematological monitoring every 2 weeks till the maximal dose then every 6 to 12 weeks.

c. *TNF-α inhibitor*: It should be used who will not respond to above drugs.

d. Infliximab and Adalimumab can also be used.

J. In case of renal manifestation, only in secondary amyloidosis, 1 to 1.2 mg colchicine can be administered orally.

K. Ocular involvement:

a. In anterior uveitis: topical corticosteroids like scopolamine 0.25% or cyclopentolate 1%. If unresponsive this therapy, oral steroid as 40 mg daily till the resolution of symptoms.

b. In case of posterior uveitis, Prednisolone and azathioprine as described above in gastrointestinal treatment.

c. Severe refractory cases, infliximab at a dose of 5/mg kg at 0, 4, 8, 16, 24 weeks or 0, 2, 6 and every 8 weeks; or Adalimumab at loading dose of 80 mg followed by 40 mg 4 weeks later and 40 mg every 2 weeks.

L. Vascular diseases:

a. Large artery disease:

1. High dose of steroids and cyclophosphamide should be given.

2. In case of inactive disease intervention surgeries can be performed.

b. Venous thrombosis:

1. In case of dural sinus thrombosis, anticoagulant should be recommended.

2. Glucocorticoids with immunosuppressive therapies

c. Neurological diseases: High dose of corticoids with immunosuppressive agents.

Q34. Antiphospholipid syndrome.

Maharashtra UNI of Health SC, Vijayawada, 2022 (10)

Define anti-phospholipid syndrome. Discuss the pathogenic mechanisms of organ involvement in the syndrome.

WBUHS, 2025(10)

ANSWER

Definition

It is an autoimmune multisystem disorder characterized by presence of Antiphospholipid antibodies i.e. anti-cardiolipin antibodies IgG or IgM, Lupus anticoagulant and Anti-beta 2 glycoprotein-I IgG and IgM in the setting of loss of pregnancy or arterial or venous thrombosis.

Etiology

A. Genetic factors:
  - **a.** Coagulation factor mutation,
  - **b.** HLA-DR7, DR4, DRw53, DQw7 and C4 null alleles

B. Infective etiology:
  - **a.** Borrelia Burgdorferi
  - **b.** *Coxiella burnetii*
  - **c.** Treponema
  - **d.** Hepatitis C
  - **e.** HIV
  - **f.** COVID-19
  - **g.** Leptospira
  - **h.** Epstein-Barr virus

C. *Drugs*:
  - **a.** Chlorpromazine
  - **b.** Procainamide
  - **c.** Quinidine
  - **d.** Phenytoin

Classification

APLA can be classified according to its clinical manifestation:

A. Thrombotic APLA: It is based on arterial or venous thrombosis, most common feature is DVT.

B. Obstetric APLA: It is based on pregnancy morbidity like Premature birth due to
  - **a.** Severe preeclampsia
  - **b.** Fetal death after 10 weeks of gestation.
  - **c.** Placental insufficiency
  - **d.** Multiple embryonic loss before 10 weeks of gestation
  - **e.** Persistent laboratory criteria for APLA

C. Catastrophic APLA: It is based on the life-threatening form involving thrombotic complications in micro and macro vessels in the multiple organs.

Epidemiology

In 10% individual anti-cardiolipin antibody may be seen. Positivity will increase with advancement of age. It is positive in 20% patients with rheumatoid arthritis.

Pathophysiology

If all the antibodies are positive the patient is at high risk of developing APLA.

Two hit thrombosis model is a proposed mechanism for formation of thrombus. 1st hit involves endothelial injury and 2nd hit is thrombus formation.

A. According to one hypothesis, the cause of injury is unidentified. The patient suffering from APS have low level of protective, reduced non-immunogenic beta-2 glycoprotein-I. Endothelial surface receptor, Annexin-2 will be unregulated in presence of oxidative stress.

B. Smoking can produce endothelial injury along with increase in pro-thrombotic susceptibilities in the patient is lupus anti-coagulant positive.

C. Reduced activity of endothelial nitric oxide synthetase leads to generation of peroxynitrite and superoxide. According to preclinical domain domain-1 of beta-2 glycoprotein-I antibodies will antagonize endothelial nitric oxide synthetase activity leading to adhesion of monocytes and inhibition of the nitric-oxide dependent relaxation of artery.

D. In this disease upregulation of expression of tissue factor through intracellular signaling pathways following binding of anti-beta-2 glycoprotein -I antibodies to the surface of monocytes as well as multiprotein complexes in the endothelial cells.

E. There is disruption of mitochondrial function of neutrophil and monocytes by the autoantibodies in this disease leads to increased production of reactive oxygen species resulting expression of tissue factors.

F. APS associated with pregnancy loss occurs due to:
  - **a.** Intraplacental thrombosis
  - **b.** Activation of complement pathway
  - **c.** Interference with trophoblastic growth factor as well as differentiation
  - **d.** Impaired trophoblastic invasion
  - **e.** Effects on production of hormone

Clinical Features

A. *Vascular thrombosis*:
  - **a.** Upper extremity thrombosis
  - **b.** Budd–Chiari syndrome

c. Sagittal sinus thrombosis
d. Deep vein thrombosis leading to pulmonary embolism results pulmonary hypertension
e. *Other sites of thrombosis are*:
   1. Pelvic vein
   2. Renal vein
   3. Mesenteric vein
   4. Hepatic vein
   5. Portal vein
   6. Axillary vein
   7. Ocular vein
   8. Sagittal vein
   9. Inferior vena cava

B. Arterial thrombosis:
a. Ischemic stroke
b. Retinal artery
c. Coronary artery
d. Brachial artery
e. Mesenteric artery
f. Peripheral arteries

C. Pregnancy morbidity:
a. Loss of pregnancy in less than 10 weeks of gestation
b. Loss of pregnancy after more than 20 weeks is associated with 10% positivity with APLA.
c. Other pregnancy related complications are:
   1. Fetal distress
   2. Preeclampsia
   3. Intrauterine growth retardation
   4. Premature birth
   5. Placental insufficiency
   6. Placental abruption
   7. HELLP syndrome:
      - Hemolysis
      - Elevated liver enzymes
      - Low platelet count

D. Cutaneous involvement:
a. Livedo reticularis
b. Small to large Skin ulceration involving extremities
c. Nail-ford thrombus
d. Digital gangrene
e. Superficial thrombophlebitis
f. Necrotizing purpura

E. Valvular involvement in the form of thickening, nodules and vegetations:
a. Mitral valve
b. Aortic valve

F. Hematological involvement:
a. Positive Coombs test
b. Thrombocytopenia

G. Cardiac involvement:
a. Non-ST elevated myocardial infarction
b. Cardiac emboli

H. Neurological involvement:
a. TIA
b. Ischemic stroke
c. Cognitive impairment
d. Seizures
e. Multi-infarct dementia
f. Blindness due to retinal artery involvement
g. Sensorineural hearing loss

I. Pulmonary involvement:
a. Pulmonary artery thromboembolism
b. Pulmonary artery hypertension

J. Renal involvement:
a. Hypertension
b. Proteinuria
c. Renal failure secondary to microangiopathy
d. Renal artery thrombosis leading to refractory hypertension as well as focal cortical atrophy.

K. Catastrophic Antiphospholipid syndrome: It is a life-threatening syndrome especially in patient with SLE or in patients with cardiac, renal or pulmonary and splenic involvement and characterized by thrombosis in the multiple organs over a short period. Following structures are involved:
a. DVT
b. Femoral or radial artery thrombosis
c. Pulmonary complications like:
   1. Acute respiratory distress syndrome
   2. Pulmonary embolism
   3. Pulmonary hemorrhage
d. Renal manifestations:
   1. Renal failure
   2. Thrombotic microangiopathy
e. Cutaneous manifestations:
   1. Digital ischemia
   2. Livedo reticularis

3. Digital gangrene
4. Skin ulcerations

f. Cerebral manifestations:
1. Encephalopathy
2. Ischemic stroke

g. Cardiac complications:
1. Valvular lesions
2. Myocardial infarction
3. Heart failure

h. Gastrointestinal features like bowel infarction

i. Hematological features like thrombocytopenia.

Evaluation

A. Lupus anticoagulant test: Positive test is the strongest predictor of catastrophic pregnancy related events.
  a. Positive lupus anticoagulant with positive for anticardiolipin antibodies - 20% patients.
  b. Positive anticardiolipin antibodies seen in positive for anticardiolipin antibodies - 80% patients.

B. Anticardiolipin antibodies and anti-beta-2c glycoprotein antibodies are of IgG and IgM types. IgG antibodies correlate with clinical manifestations better as compared to IgA and IgM antibodies. If the IgG titer is more than 40 units - it is associated with thrombotic events.

C. Other laboratory events:
  a. Thrombocytopenia
  b. Proteinuria
  c. In case of acute thrombotic events ESR will be high.
  d. ANA, Anti-Ds DNA positive in SLE
  e. Hypocomplementemia - its presence in APLA suggests renal involvement - lupus nephritis.
  f. In case of multiple thrombotic events and pregnancy loss:
    1. Hyperhomocysteinemia
    2. Mutation of factor V Leiden and Prothrombin
    3. Deficiency of protein C
    4. Deficiency of protein S
    5. Deficiency of anti-thrombin III.

Clinical criteria: On of the following findings should be confirmed to diagnose this disease.

A. Vascular thrombosis:
  a. One or more events involving arterial, venous small vessel thrombosis in any organ. Thrombosis should be confirmed objectively with appropriate histopathology or imaging. For histopathology, thrombosis is typically present without significant inflammation of vessel wall.
    1. A past thrombotic episode can be included as a criterion as long as long as it was appropriately confirmed by appropriate diagnostic means as there was no other cause of thrombosis.
    2. Superficial venous thrombosis is not included as a criterion.

B. *Pregnancy morbidity*:
  a. 1 or more unexplained fetal deaths of the morphologically normal fetuses, confirmed by ultrasound or direct examination at or beyond 10 weeks of gestation.
  b. 1 or more premature births of morphologically nor mal fetuses before 34th weeks of gestation. Prematurity must be secondary to Eclampsia or placental insufficiency.
  c. 3 or more consecutive spontaneous abortions before 10th weeks of gestation after ruling out any anatomical or hormonal abnormalities in the mother and parenteral chromosomal causes.

Laboratory criteria: 1 of the following laboratory findings should be confirmed to diagnose this disease.

A. Detection of lupus anticoagulant in plasma on 2 or more occasions, at least 12 weeks apart.

B. Detection of IgM or IgG anticardiolipin antibodies in serum or plasma at moderate or high titers [more than 40 IgG phospholipids (GPL) or IgM phospholipid (GPM) or GPL/GPM more than 99th percentile] measured by standard ELISA on 2 or more occasions at least 12 weeks apart.

C. Detection of IgG or IgM anti beta2GPI antibodies in serum or plasma at moderate to high titers (more than 99th percentiles) measured by standard ELISA on 2 or more occasions, 12 or more weeks apart.

According to the updated EULAR APS classification criteria at entry criterion of at least one positive Antiphospholipid antibody test within 3 years of an APS associated clinical criteria. These criteria are followed by additional weighted criteria having 1 to 7 points each which are clustered into 6 clinical domains, like macrovascular venous thromboembolism, macrovascular arterial thrombosis, microvascular, obstetric, cardiac valve and hematologic and 2 laboratory domains like lupus anticoagulant test and IgG/IgM anticardiolipin or IgG/IgM beta2GP1 b.

Patient having 3 points each from clinical and laboratory criteria are classified as a case of APS.

Treatment

Management of Thrombosis

A. Primary prevention: High risk patients with positive for lupus anticoagulant 2 or 3 positive for APLA or persistently high positive high APLA:

a. Patients with high risk Antiphospholipid profile bot without any history of thrombotic event should receive 75 to 10 mg aspirin.

b. Patient with SLE but no history of thrombosis or complications in pregnancy:

1. High risk of APLA: Low dose of aspirin
2. Low risk of APLA: Low dose aspirin
3. In case of non-pregnant woman having history of obstetric APLA only: Low dose aspirin after evaluation of adequate risk/ benefit

B. Secondary prevention:

a. Venous thrombosis:

1. Definite APS AND 1st venous thrombosis: Warfarin treatment with continuous monitoring of INR to 2 to 3.
2. Patient with unprovoked venous thrombosis: Anticoagulant should be continued lifelong.
3. Patient with unprovoked deep venous thrombosis and positive for lupus anticoagulant there is 40% risk of recurrent thrombosis if the anticoagulant is discontinued. But in presence of continuous anticoagulant therapy, 20% chance of recurrent thrombosis. Hence, lifelong anticoagulation should be continued.
4. In few selected patients with venous thrombosis and single or double antibody positivity direct anticoagulation therapy should be done.
5. In case of high risk for APLA in repeated test or with presence of other risk factor, longer anticoagulation should be considered.

b. Arterial thrombosis:

1. Warfarin is preferred over direct anti-coagulation therapy with continuous monitoring of INR between 2 to 3.
2. Low molecular weight heparin can be given if patient cannot tolerate warfarin.
3. In case of recurrent thrombosis in spite of aspirin should be given in addition to aspirin, LMWH with INR of more than 3.
4. DOAC should be considered in those patients on warfarin but there is complication of warfarin or contraindication to aspirin.
5. In DOAC dabigatran should be considered because of its anti-factor IIa mechanism.
6. Elderly patients with stroke and low titer of anticardiolipin antibodies, low dose aspirin should be considered.

c. Management of pregnancy: According to EULAR guideline:

1. Pregnant female and positive APLA and absence of any type of thrombosis:
    - 1st pregnancy: No treatment.
    - Single pregnancy loss at less than 10th week of gestation: No treatment.
    - High risk of APLA but absence history of thrombosis or pregnancy complication: Low dose aspirin.
2. History of loss of ≥3 pregnancy of less than 10 weeks of gestation: Low-dose aspirin along with prophylactic dose of unfractionated heparin of LMWH to be given throughout the pregnancy. Aspirin has to be started before conception and LMWH to be discontinued 6 to 12 weeks of postpartum. Anticoagulation can be started 6 to 12 hours after delivery or 4 to 6 hours after vaginal birth unless there is significant risk of bleeding.
3. If there is history of delivery before 34 weeks of gestation due to preeclampsia or Eclampsia, low dose aspirin with or without associated with prophylactic heparin can be given depending upon the patient's risk profile.

Q35. Arthritis associated with systemic diseases.

Kerala University, 2021 (10)

ANSWER

Disease	Key features
Rheumatoid arthritis	Symmetrical polyarthritis involving small joints with morning stiffness. Rheumatoid factor positive, anti-CCP positive
SLE	Non-erosive symmetrical polyarthritis with reversible deformities of the joints, Presence of Jaccoud's arthropathy, ANA positive

Continued

Continued

Disease	Key features
Systemic sclerosis	Mild arthritis along with features of Systemic sclerosis
Sjögren's syndrome	Non-erosive arthritis, Ro-SSA and anti-La SSB positive
Dermatomyositis Polymyositis	Arthralgia, positive CPK
Psoriatic arthritis	Asymmetric oligoarthritis involving distal interphalangeal joints, dactylitis and enthesitis
Mixed connective tissue disease	Overlap polyarthritis and anti U1 RNP antibodies
Vasculitis	Arthralgia along with systemic features of polyarteritis nodosa, granulomatosis polyangiitis
Reactive arthritis	Asymmetric oligoarthritis involving lower limb
Behcet's disease	Non-erosive arthritis, it is recurrent.
Hemochromatosis	Both large and small joints are involved, there may be deformity like rheumatoid arthritis
Inflammatory bowel diseases	Axial joints involvement, peripheral joint involvement

Q36. Write in detail about autoimmune polyglandular syndrome.

MGR UNI, Tamil Nadu, 2021 (15)

ANSWER

Type 1 Polyglandular Autoimmune Syndrome

Polyglandular autoimmune syndrome type 1 is also known as polyendocrinopathy-candidiasis-ectodermal dystrophy which is characterized by triad of hypoparathyroidism, Addison's disease and chronic mucocutaneous candidiasis.

Etiology

It is autosomal recessive disease due to mutation of autoimmune regulatory gene located in the short arm of chromosome number 21. There are 60 different types of mutations in the *AIRE* gene leading to variable presentation in the course of this disease. Any one of the following mutations may occur in 95% of cases:

- **a.** Substitution of Arginine at position 257
- **b.** Deletion of 13 base pairs in exon 8.

Pathophysiology

This disease occurs due to decreased central tolerance leading to autoimmunity. *AIRE* gene has been expressed in the thymic medullary cells encoding autoimmune regulator, DNA binding protein. This protein helps in regulating various thymic expression of tissue specific antigen thereby eliminating autoreactive T cells. So, in absence of this protein autoreactive cells will escape negative selection and will be released into the circulation.

Clinical Manifestations

- **A.** Mucocutaneous candidiasis presenting as ulcers at the angle of the mouth.
- **B.** Hypoparathyroidism - it is prevalent in females and clinically presenting as tingling and numbness in the fingertips and perioral areas, muscle cramps and seizures.
- **C.** Addison's disease - it appears in between 5 and 15 years.
- **D.** Alopecia - appears at 40 years of age presenting from patchy alopecia to alopecia totalis.
- **E.** Keratitis - appears around 20 years of age and characterized by decreased lacrimation, photophobia and blepharospasm.
- **F.** Gastritis and pernicious anemia - here anti-intrinsic factor antibodies are present in the serum.
- **G.** In 20% of cases there is asplenia.
- **H.** Primary hypogonadism
- **I.** Pituitary failure secondary to pituitary antibodies against Tudor domain protein.
- **J.** In 20% cases autoimmune hepatitis at the age of 20 years.
- **K.** Hashimoto thyroiditis
- **L.** In 75% of Finnish patient there is enamel dysplasia
- **M.** In 33% of cases there is vitiligo.

Diagnostic criteria

- **A.** Definite diagnosis:
  - **a.** Presence of 2 of the triad of mucocutaneous candidiasis, hypothyroidism and Addison's disease.
  - **b.** One of the above triad plus a sibling of with proven APS-1
  - **c.** Known disease causing mutation in the AIRE gene.

B. Probable diagnosis:
   a. Presence of 1 of the triad (before 30 years) and 1 of the following components:
      1. Chronic diarrhea
      2. Keratitis
      3. Periodic rash with fever
      4. Severe constipation
      5. Autoimmune hepatitis
      6. Vitiligo
      7. Alopecia
      8. Enamel hypoplasia
   b. Any 1 of the above triad plus anti-interferon antibodies
   c. Any 1 of the above plus antibodies against NALP5, aromatic amino acid decarboxylase, tryptophan hydroxylase or tyrosine hydroxylase.

Treatment

A. Mucocutaneous candidiasis can be treated by 2 topical polene antifungal drug for 4 to 6 weeks. Recurrent oral candidiasis can be treated by weekly plus prophylactic polyene antifungal drugs every three weeks.
B. Treatment of hypothyroidism.
C. Addison's disease can be treated by hydrocortisone, recommended dose being morning dose 10 mg and afternoon dose 5 mg at 3 to P.M.

Type 2 Autoimmune Polyglandular Syndrome

It is a cluster of two or more endocrine diseases in a single patient and is related to X-linked immune dysregulation polyendocrinopathy and enteropathy.

Etiology

A. PAS-1: It is autoimmune disease affecting multiple endocrine organs.
B. PAS-2: It is polygenic heterogenous disease due to multiple genetic loci along with environmental factors leading to damage of different organs. Affection of HLA-DR3 and DR4 haplotypes and class 2 HLADQ2 and DQ8 occurs in PAS-2 disease.
C. Non-HLA gene factors responsible for PAS-2 incudes:
   a. CD25 interleukin-2 receptor
   b. Cytokine T-lymphocyte protein 4
   c. Non-receptor type 22
   d. Protein tyrosine-protein phosphatase

Epidemiology

A. The age prevalence is between 20 and 40 years.
B. It is three times more common in women.

History and Physical Examination

A. Symptoms:
   a. Weight loss
   b. Fatigue
   c. Nausea
   d. Vomiting
   e. Anorexia
   f. Generalized weakness
   g. Abdominal pain
   h. Diarrhea
   i. Polyuria
   j. Polydipsia
B. Signs:
   a. If Addison's disease:
      1. Mucosal and cutaneous hyperpigmentation
      2. Hypoglycemia
      3. Orthostatic hypotension
      4. Tachycardia
      5. Altered mental status
   b. If T1DM:
      1. Polyuria, polydipsia
   c. If hypothyroidism:
      1. Bradycardia
      2. Delayed ankle jerk relaxation time
C. Other endocrine and non-endocrine manifestations:'
   a. Primary Hypogonadism
   b. Celiac disease
   c. Myasthenia gravis
   d. Alopecia
   e. Vitiligo
   f. Pernicious anemia
   g. Idiopathic heart block
   h. Parkinson's disease
   i. Stiff-man syndrome
   j. IgA deficiency
   k. Serositis
   l. Dermatitis herpetiformis
   m. Idiopathic thrombocytopenia
   n. Hypophysitis

Evaluation

A. It can be diagnosed if two out of following three are present:
   a. Addison's disease
   b. Graves' disease
   c. T1DM

Addison's disease can be diagnosed if:

A. Morning serum cortisol level is less than 6 μg/dL
B. Serum cortisol level is less than 18 μg/dL at 60 minutes by stimulation of ACTH after intramuscular or intravenous administration of bolus of cosyntropin
C. Presence of 21-hydroxylase or 17-hydroxylase antibodies - diagnose autoimmune adrenalitis. In that case morning serum for cortisol should be measured.

Evaluation of:

A. Serum TSH, T4 and T3 and TSH and T4 to diagnose Grave's' disease of Hashimoto thyroiditis respectively in case of euthyroid patients.
B. Anti-thyroglobulin antibodies or thyroid microsomal antibodies and thyroid receptor antibodies can detect risk of thyroid disease in fetus.

T1DM can be diagnosed if:

A. There is suggestive history
B. Fasting blood sugar more than 125 mg/dL
C. Random more than 200 mg/dL
D. HbA1C is more than 6.4%
E. Antiglutamic acid decarboxylase antibodies
F. Anti-Islet cell antigen-2 antibodies
G. Anti-Zn-transporter antibodies
H. Challenge with injection 1 mg glucagon plasma C peptide level is less than 0.6 ng/mL.

PAS-2 can be differentiated from PAS-1 due to late onset of clinical manifestation after the age of 20 years and different pattern of clinical presentation and no mucocutaneous candidiasis and types of inheritance.

Treatment

A. Replacement of hormones is the key treatment.
B. Patient should be followed up every 6 months.

Q37. Intrinsic muscles of the hand.

BBMGR University, Tamil Nadu, 2020 (5)

ANSWER

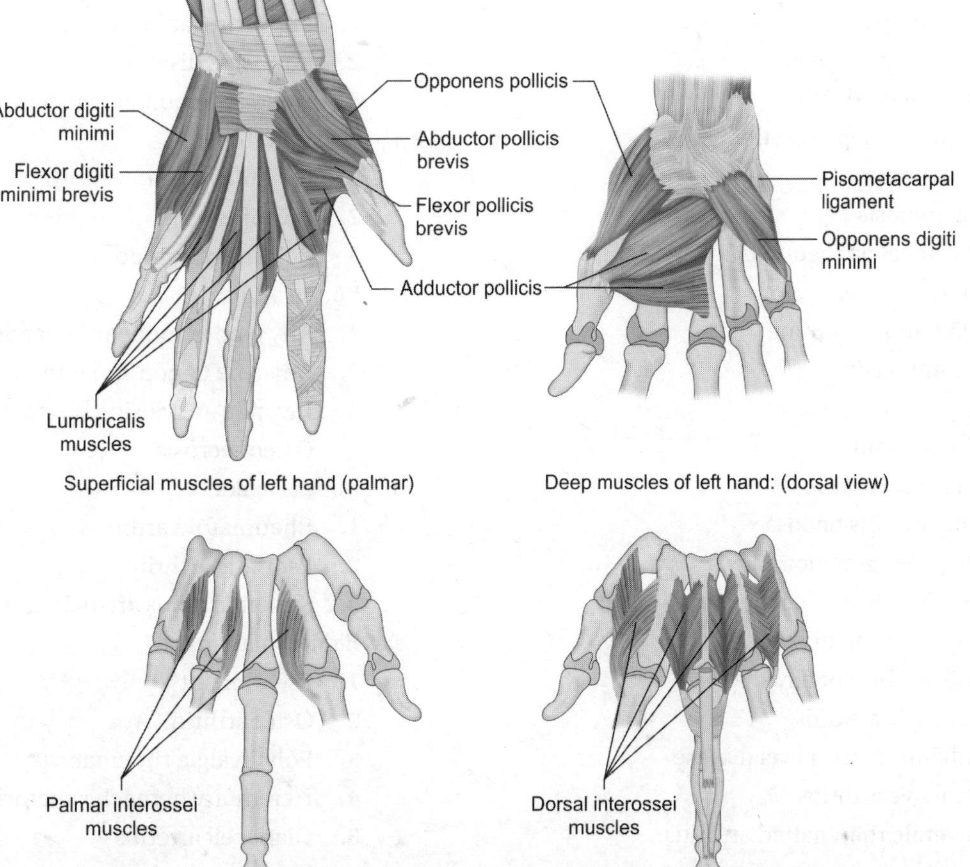

Q38. Describe approach to polyarthritis.

WBUHS, 2020 (10)

Describe the approach to a patient with polyarthritis. What are the common differential diagnoses?

WBUHS, 2024 (10)

ANSWER

A. Acute inflammatory polyarthritis (involvement of more than joints):
 a. Infectious causes:
  1. Bacterial:
   - Gonococcal arthritis
   - Lyme disease
   - Acute bacterial endocarditis
  2. Viral causes:
   - Rubella
   - HIV'
   - Hepatitis B
  3. *Postinfectious causes*:
   - Rheumatic fever
   - Enteric fever
   - Urogenital
 b. Rheumatologic causes:
  1. Rheumatoid arthritis
  2. Systemic Lupus Erythematosus
  3. Scleroderma
  4. Sarcoidosis
  5. Polymyalgia rheumatica
  6. Still's disease
  7. Sjögren's syndrome
 c. Crystal induced:
  1. Gout
  2. Pseudogout
 d. Systemic vasculitis:
  1. Polyarteritis nodosa
  2. Wegener granulomatosis
  3. Henoch-Schönlein purpura
 e. Spondyloarthropathies:
  1. Ankylosing spondylitis
  2. Psoriatic arthritis
  3. Inflammatory bowel disease
  4. Reactive arthritis
  5. Juvenile rheumatoid arthritis

B. Chronic polyarthritis:
 a. Osteoarthritis
 b. Fibromyalgia
 c. Amyloidosis
 d. Hyperparathyroidism

Approach to a Patient with a Patient with Polyarthritis

First step we have to diagnose it whether it is articular pain, neuropathic pain or referred pain. After excluding all the above pain following four patterns of articular involvement have to be defined:

A. The nature of the arthritis - whether it is inflammatory or non-inflammatory.

B. Temporal nature of involvement - whether it is acute (less than 6 weeks' duration) or chronically progressive (more than 6 weeks duration).

C. Observation of pattern of joint involvement - Primary monoarticular or polyarticular, progression from monoarticular to polyarticular involvement.

D. Whether extra articular involvement is present or not.

From History

A. Age:
 a. Early childhood:
  1. Polyarticular juvenile inflammatory arthritis
  2. Kawasaki disease
  3. Henoch-Schonlein purpura
 b. Mid childhood:
  1. Juvenile psoriatic arthritis
  2. Juvenile dermatomyositis
  3. Polyarteritis nodosa
 c. Young adult:
  1. Any type of monoarticular arthritis
  2. Any type of non-inflammatory arthritis
  3. Juvenile ankylosing spondylitis
  4. Osteonecrosis
 d. Middle aged:
  1. Rheumatoid arthritis
  2. Psoriatic arthritis
  3. Systemic lupus erythematosus
 e. Elderly patients:
  1. Pseudogout
  2. Osteoarthritis
  3. Polymyalgia rheumatica
  4. Hereditary hemochromatosis
  5. Giant cell arteritis

B. Sex:

a. Female:

1. Gonococcal arthritis – three times more common in females.
2. Rheumatoid arthritis (three to four times likely)
3. Collagen vascular disease
4. Undifferentiated polyarthritis
5. Systemic lupus erythematosus (nine times more likely)
6. Postmenopausal women—Gout

b. Male:

1. Gout
2. Kawasaki disease
3. Polyarteritis nodosa
4. Spondyloarthropathies

c. Male = female:

1. Polymyalgia rheumatica
2. Pseudogout
3. *After the age of 50 years*:
    - Systemic lupus erythematosus
    - Rheumatoid arthritis

C. Onset:

a. Acute onset:

1. Gonococcal arthritis
2. Septic arthritis
3. Hemarthrosis
4. Gout
5. Pseudogout

b. Chronic in nature:

1. Osteoarthritis
2. Rheumatoid arthritis
3. Spondyloarthropathies

D. Migratory in nature (it is characterized by rapid tender swelling of one or more joints with complete resolution within few days followed by similar tender swelling of other joints usually in asymmetric location.)

a. Gonococcal arthritis

b. Rheumatic fever

c. Lyme disease

d. Subacute bacterial endocarditis

e. Whipple's disease

f. Systemic lupus erythematosus

g. Sarcoidosis

E. Intermittent involvement (when the patient becomes asymptomatic in between the episodes):

a. Gout

b. Pseudogout

c. Reiter's syndrome

d. Behçet's syndrome

e. Intermittent hydrarthrosis

f. Palindromic rheumatism progressing to rheumatoid arthritis.

F. Additive involvement (Here addition of more and more joint in the disease)

a. Rheumatoid arthritis

b. Osteoarthritis

c. Psoriatic arthritis

d. Spondyloarthropathies

G. Ethnicity:

a. White race:

1. Polymyalgia rheumatica
2. Wegener granulomatosis

b. Black race:

1. Sarcoidosis
2. Systemic erythematosus

H. Pattern of joint involvement:

a. Involvement of distal interphalangeal and proximal interphalangeal joints but without involvement of metacarpophalangeal joints – osteoarthritis.

b. Involvement of metacarpophalangeal and proximal interphalangeal joints – rheumatoid arthritis.

c. Involvement of joints of lower extremities – spondyloarthropathies.

d. In acute phase polyarticular arthralgia followed by oligoarthritis involving mainly knee – Lyme disease

e. Involvement of metatarsophalangeal joint—gout

f. Involvement of knee:

1. Pseudogout.
2. Septic arthritis

g. Three general patterns of presentations in psoriatic arthritis:

1. Oligoarthritis – it involves large joints and hands.
2. PIP or MCP and DIP joints involvement.
3. Spinal joint involvement.

h. Involvement of elbow, wrist, hands, knee, ankle and feet in young patient – parvo viral disease.

1. Involving of knee, ankle, and spinal joints with tendinitis, enthesitis – reactive arthritis.

I. Mode of involvement:

a. Acute onset (less than 6 weeks):

1. Acute gout
2. Septic arthritis
3. Acute gonococcal arthritis
4. Reactive arthritis
5. Trauma

b. Chronic in onset (more than 6 weeks):

1. Rheumatoid arthritis
2. Spondyloarthritis
3. Osteoarthritis

J. Number of joints affected:

a. Single joint involvement:

1. Crystal arthropathy
2. Septic arthritis
3. Gonococcal arthritis

b. Oligoarticular involvement:

1. Psoriatic arthritis
2. Lyme disease
3. Juvenile idiopathic arthritis
4. Spondyloarthropathies

c. Polyarticular involvement:

1. Rheumatoid arthritis
2. Psoriatic arthropathy
3. Systemic lupus erythematosus
4. Reactive arthritis
5. Systemic sclerosis

K. Symmetry in joint involvement:

a. Symmetrical involvement (right 4th and 5th with left 2nd MCP defined as symmetry):

1. Rheumatoid arthritis
2. Systemic lupus erythematosus
3. Systemic sclerosis
4. Polymyalgia rheumatica
5. Viral arthritis

b. Asymmetrical involvement:

1. Psoriatic arthropathy
2. Reactive arthritis
3. Gout
4. Ankylosing spondylitis

L. Morning stiffness:

a. More than 30 minutes:

1. Rheumatoid arthritis
2. Systemic lupus erythematosus (SLE)
3. Spondyloarthropathies

b. Less than 30 minutes:

1. Osteoarthritis
2. Trauma

M. Type of joint involvement:

a. Small joints more than the large joint –

1. Rheumatoid arthritis
2. Psoriatic arthritis
3. Systemic lupus erythematosus (SLE)
4. Systemic sclerosis

b. Large joint more than the small joints – spondyloarthropathies.

N. Specific joint involvement:

a. Distal interphalangeal (DIP) joints –

1. Osteoarthritis
2. Psoriatic arthropathy
3. Scleroderma

b. Sparing of DIP with involvement of PIP and MCP joints – rheumatoid arthritis

O. Axial involvement:

a. Involvement of low back, neck or both areas along with involvement of peripheral joints – osteoarthritis.

b. Rare involvement of low back – rheumatoid arthritis

c. Chronic pain in low back with prolonged morning stiffness but improves on exercise –

1. Ankylosing spondylitis
2. Psoriatic arthritis
3. Reactive arthritis

P. Aggravation of pain:

a. Aggravation of pain on movement:

1. Osteoarthritis
2. Trauma

b. Aggravation of pain during rest:

1. Rheumatoid arthritis
2. Spondyloarthropathies
3. SLE

Q. Associated systemic symptoms:

a. Fever with chill, myalgia:

1. Septic arthritis (>39°C rare)

2. Acute gonococcal arthritis
3. Rheumatic fever

R. Other symptoms related to other organs:

a. Presence of burning eye with lacrimation and red eye:
    1. Reactive arthritis
    2. Ankylosing spondylitis

From past history:

a. Transient pain in heel and back pain or transient episode of red eye along with loss of vision indicating acute uveitis - Juvenile ankylosing spondylitis.

b. History of loose motion, acute conjunctivitis, urethritis - reactive arthritis

From family history:

a. Ankylosing spondylitis
b. Psoriatic arthritis
c. Inflammatory bowel disease

Drug history:

a. Prolonged course of steroid therapy:
    1. Infection
    2. Avascular necrosis
b. History of diuretic use, renal stones and intake of alcohol - Gout
c. History of intravenous drug use/immuno-suppression - Septic arthritis

Physical Examinations

Dermatologic Manifestations: Rash

1. Rash in malar area:
    - SLE
    - Lyme disease
    - Dermatomyositis
    - Parvo virus 19 infection
2. Heliotropic rash, Gottron's papule - dermatomyositis
3. Erythema nodosum:
    - Crohn's disease
    - Sarcoidosis
4. Silver plaques in navel, gluteal cleft, scalp - psoriasis
5. Erythema chronicum migrans - lyme disease
6. Palpable purpura:
    - Hypersensitivity vasculitis
    - Polyarteritis nodosa
7. Livedo reticularis - vasculitis
8. Erythema marginatum - rheumatic fever
9. Discoid skin lesion:
    - Discoid lupus erythematosus
    - SLE
    - Sarcoidosis
10. Vesiculopapular rash on erythematous base - gonococcal arthritis
11. Pyoderma gangrenosum:
    - Inflammatory bowel disease
    - SLE
    - Rheumatoid arthritis
    - Sarcoidosis
    - Ankylosing spondylitis
    - Wegener granulomatosis
12. Keratoderma blenorrhagicum:
    - Psoriatic arthritis
    - Reactive arthritis
13. Reticulated lacy rash, facial exanthema - human parvovirus 19 infection.
14. Jaundice:
    - Hemochromatosis
    - Hepatitis
15. Hyperpigmentation:
    - Whipple's disease
    - Hemochromatosis
16. Tightening of skin:
    - Scleroderma
    - Eosinophilic fasciitis
17. Telangiectasia - scleroderma

Eye Manifestation

1. Conjunctivitis:
    a. Spondyloarthropathies
    b. Wegener granulomatosis
    c. SLE
2. Uveitis with or without iritis:
    a. Spondyloarthropathies
    b. Wegener granulomatosis
    c. Sarcoidosis
3. Cytoid bodies - SLE
4. Scleritis - Rheumatoid arthritis
5. Ischemic optic neuritis:
    a. Wegener granulomatosis
    b. Giant cell arteritis

Nail Examination

1. Onycholysis, pitting - Psoriatic arthritis
2. Clubbing:
    a. Inflammatory bowel disease
    b. Whipple's disease

Nose, Throat

1. Ulcer in the mouth:
   - a. Behçet syndrome
   - b. Reactive arthritis
   - c. Wegener granulomatosis
2. Macroglossia – amyloidosis
3. Sinusitis with bloody discharge – Wegener granulomatosis
4. Parotid enlargement:
   - a. Sjögren syndrome
   - b. Amyloidosis
5. Inflammation of ear lobe – relapsing polychondritis

Nodules

1. Rheumatoid arthritis
2. Gout
3. Sarcoidosis
4. Osteoarthritis
5. Rheumatic fever

Musculoskeletal System

1. Different tender points in the muscles of the neck, trunk – fibromyalgia
2. Swan neck or/and boutonnière deformity in hand – rheumatoid arthritis
3. Heberden's node in distal interphalangeal joints and/or Bouchard's node in proximal interphalangeal joints–osteoarthritis.
4. Digital gangrene, Raynaud's phenomenon – scleroderma
5. Dactylitis (Sausage digits)–spondyloarthropathies
6. Tender bursa or tendon–spondyloarthropathies

Cardiovascular System

1. Different types of valvular damage, most common being mitral stenosis – rheumatic fever.
2. Cardiomyopathies –
   - a. Amyloidosis
   - b. Sarcoidosis
   - c. SLE
   - d. Polymyositis
   - e. Arteritis
3. Aortic regurgitation –
   - a. Ankylosing spondylitis
   - b. Rheumatic fever
   - c. Marfan syndrome
   - d. Relapsing polychondritis
   - e. Reactive arthritis
4. Variability in peripheral pulses –
   - a. Giant cell arteritis
   - b. Takayasu's arteritis
5. Appearances of new murmur –
   - a. Rheumatic fever
   - b. Bacterial endocarditis

Gastrointestinal System

1. Hepatomegaly –
   - a. Hemochromatosis
   - b. Whipple's disease
   - c. Inflammatory bowel disease
2. Splenomegaly –
   - a. Felty's syndrome
   - b. Still's disease
   - c. Subacute bacterial endocarditis

Genitourinary System

1. Urethritis/cervicitis –
   - a. Gonococcal urethritis
   - b. Reactive arthritis
2. Ulcer in the scrotum – Behçet's syndrome
3. Prostatitis –
   - a. Ankylosing spondylitis
   - b. Reactive arthritis
4. Balanitis circinata – Reactive arthritis

Neurological Manifestations

1. Facial palsy, lymphocytic meningitis, radiculopathy – Lyme disease
2. Chorea –
   - a. Rheumatic fever
   - b. SLE
3. Peripheral neuropathy –
   - a. Amyloidosis
   - b. SLE
4. Entrapment neuropathy – Rheumatoid arthritis

Lymphoglandular system:

1. Lymphadenopathy –
   - a. SLE
   - b. Tumor associated arthritis
   - c. Tubercular arthritis

Laboratory Investigations

A. *Hematological investigations*:

1. Anemia:
   - **a.** Rheumatoid arthritis
   - **b.** Inflammatory bowel disease
   - **c.** SLE
   - **d.** Parvovirus infection
   - **e.** Vasculitis
2. Leukopenia:
   - **a.** Rheumatoid arthritis
   - **b.** Felty's syndrome
   - **c.** Sjögren's syndrome
   - **d.** SLE
   - **e.** Parvo virus B19 infection
3. Leukocytosis:
   - **a.** Inflammatory bowel disease
   - **b.** Gonococcal arthritis
   - **c.** Septic arthritis (>10000/cc)
   - **d.** Tubercular arthritis
   - **e.** Rheumatoid arthritis
4. Thrombocytosis:
   - **a.** Vasculitis
   - **b.** Inflammation as acute phase reactant
   - **c.** Infection
5. Thrombocytopenia:
   - **a.** SLE
   - **b.** Human Parvo virus B19 infection
6. Eosinophilia:
   - **a.** Large and small vessel vasculitis
   - **b.** Inflammatory bowel disease
   - **c.** SLE
   - **d.** Sarcoidosis

B. Culture and sensitivity:

1. Positive – 50% positive in septic arthritis
2. Positive of gonococcus

C. Serological tests:

1. Antibody against *Borrelia burgdorferi* titer – 100% sensitive for Lyme disease.
2. Anti CCP antibody – Rheumatoid arthritis
3. Rheumatoid factor positive:
   - **a.** Rheumatoid arthritis
   - **b.** SLE
   - **c.** Sarcoidosis
   - **d.** Psoriatic arthritis
   - **e.** Reactive arthritis
4. Anti-DS DNA antibody anti smooth muscle cell antibody highly specific – SLE
5. Anti-Smith antibody, anti-ribosomal P highly specific for SLE.
6. Anti SS-A (anti-Ro) and anti-SS-B (anti-La) antibodies:
   - **a.** Sjögren syndrome
   - **b.** SLE
7. Anti-Scl antibody positive – Scleroderma
8. Anti-nuclear antibody positive:
   - **a.** SLE (most sensitive, negative ANA rules out SLE).
   - **b.** Rheumatoid arthritis
   - **c.** Sjögren syndrome
   - **d.** Scleroderma
   - **e.** Polymyositis

   Following are the staining patterns:

   Homogeneous pattern:
   - SLE
   - Rheumatoid arthritis
   - Drug induced lupus

   Peripheral staining:
   - SLE

   Speckled pattern:
   - Present in patient in absence of rheumatoid arthritis

   Nucleolar:
   - Scleroderma
   - Raynaud's phenomenon
9. Anti-histone antibody – drug-induced lupus
10. Cytoplasmic antineutrophil cytoplasmic antibody:
    - **a.** Wegener granulomatosis
    - **b.** Polyarteritis nodosa.
11. Anti-Jo-1 antibody positive – Polymyositis/ dermatomyositis.
12. Anti-ribosomal P antibody – Highly specific for SLE.
13. Anti-U1 RNP antibody – Mixed connective tissue disease
14. Complement C3, C4 and CH50 low – during lupus activity.
15. Raised or normal C3 and C4 in presence of positive ANA– rheumatoid arthritis.
16. Anti streptolysin O titer raised – Rheumatic fever

D. Blood biochemistry:

1. Raised uric acid:
   - **a.** Gout
   - **b.** Psoriatic arthritis
   - **c.** Paget's disease
2. Raised angiotensin converting enzyme – Sarcoidosis
3. VDRL false positive –
   - **a.** Anti-cardiolipin antibody syndrome
   - **b.** SLE
4. Creatine phosphokinase raised:
   - **a.** Polymyositis
   - **b.** Dermatomyositis
5. Raised calcium:
   - **a.** Cancer
   - **b.** Sarcoidosis
6. Serum aldolase will be increased in Polymyositis
7. Elevated liver enzyme:
   - **a.** SLE
   - **b.** Sarcoidosis
   - **c.** Polyarteritis nodosa
   - **d.** Hemochromatosis
   - **e.** Sjögren's syndrome

E. Synovial fluid tests:

Characteristics	Normal	Osteoarthritis	Rheumatoid arthritis	Septic arthritis
Color	Clear	Yellow	Yellow green	Cloudy
Volume (mL)	≤4	1–10	10–50	30–50
WBC/cc	<500	<2,000	2,500–50,000	10,000 to <1,00,000
Neutrophil (%)	<25	<50	>50	>75

1. Crystals:
   - **a.** Gout
   - **b.** Pseudogout
2. Gram stain demonstrates *Staphylococcus aureus* - Septic arthritis

F. Radiology:

1. Chest:

   Nodules:
   - **a.** Sarcoidosis
   - **b.** Rheumatoid arthritis
   - **c.** Wegener granulomatosis

   Reticular or reticulonodular pattern described as ground glass appearance which can progress to honey-comb appearance – RA

   Diffuse fibrosis:
   - **a.** Rheumatoid arthritis
   - **b.** Scleroderma
   - **c.** Polyserositis

   Upper lobe fibrosis – ankylosing spondylitis.
2. X-ray of knee:
   - **a.** Joint space narrowing, subchondral bone sclerosis, subchondral cyst, loose bodies, calcification (due to linear deposition of crystals of calcium pyrophosphate) and osteophytes – suggest osteoarthritis.
   - **b.** Presence of classical punctate and linear calcific densities commonly seen in the cartilages of knee, pelvis, wrist and hip – pseudogout.
   - **c.** In early phase of rheumatoid arthritis only tissue swelling is present. Later on, marginal erosion, uniform joint space narrowing, Juxta-articular osteopenia will be present.
   - **d.** Soft tissue swelling, periosteal reaction, exuberant Periarticular new bone formation, pencil-cup deformity, marginal erosion – suggest psoriatic arthritis.
   - **e.** Asymmetric soft tissue swelling, punch-out appearance and periarticular erosion – suggest tophaceous gout.
   - **f.** Evidence of soft tissue swelling, joint space narrowing, absence of erosions – suggest SLE.